Textbook of Small Animal Emergency Medicine

Textbook of Small Animal Emergency Medicine

VOLUME 2

Edited by

Kenneth J. Drobatz, DVM, MSCE, DACVIM (IM), DACVECC
Professor and Chief, Section of Critical Care
Department of Clinical Sciences and Advanced Medicine
University of Pennsylvania
Philadelphia, PA;

Senior Fellow of the Center for Public Health Initiatives
University of Pennsylvania
Philadelphia, PA
USA

Kate Hopper, BVSc, PhD, DACVECC
Associate Professor, Small Animal Emergency & Critical Care
Department of Veterinary Surgical and Radiological Sciences
School of Veterinary Medicine
University of California, Davis
Davis, CA
USA

Elizabeth Rozanski, DVM, DACVIM (SAIM), DACVECC
Associate Professor
Department of Clinical Sciences
Cummings School of Veterinary Medicine
Tufts University
North Grafton, MA
USA

Deborah C. Silverstein, DVM, DACVECC
Professor of Critical Care
Department of Clinical Sciences and Advanced Medicine
University of Pennsylvania
Philadelphia, PA;

Adjunct Professor
Temple University School of Pharmacy
Philadelphia, PA
USA

WILEY Blackwell

Registered Office
John Wiley & Sons, Inc., 111 River Street, Hoboken, NJ 07030, USA

Editorial Office
111 River Street, Hoboken, NJ 07030, USA

For details of our global editorial offices, customer services, and more information about Wiley products visit us at www.wiley.com.

Wiley also publishes its books in a variety of electronic formats and by print-on-demand. Some content that appears in standard print versions of this book may not be available in other formats.

Library of Congress Cataloging-in-Publication Data

Names: Drobatz, Kenneth J., editor. | Hopper, Kate, editor. | Rozanski, Elizabeth A., editor. |
   Silverstein, Deborah C., editor.
Title: Textbook of small animal emergency medicine / edited by Kenneth J. Drobatz, Kate Hopper,
   Elizabeth Rozanski, Deborah C. Silverstein.
Description: Hoboken, NJ : Wiley, 2019. | Includes bibliographical references and index.
Identifiers: LCCN 2018002995 (print) | LCCN 2018004342 (ebook) | ISBN
   9781119028949 (pdf) | ISBN 9781119028956 (epub) | ISBN 9781119028932
   (cloth)
Subjects: LCSH: Veterinary emergencies--Textbooks. | MESH:
   Emergencies--veterinary | Pets
Classification: LCC SF778 (ebook) | LCC SF778 .T49 2019 (print) | NLM SF 778
   | DDC 636.089/6025 – dc23
LC record available at https://lccn.loc.gov/2018002995

Cover Design: Wiley
Cover Images: (Top) © Jeffrey J Runge DVM, DACVS; (Bottom) © John Donges

Set in 10/12pt Warnock Pro by Aptara Inc., New Delhi, India

Printed and bound in Singapore by Markono Print Media Pte Ltd

V0B42E9D0-475D-4E4D-B258-C5763A871723_021221

Contents

Contributors

Amanda Abelson, *DVM, DACVAA, DACVECC*
Assistant Professor, Emergency and Critical
Care and Anesthesia
Department of Clinical Sciences
Cummings School of Veterinary Medicine
Tufts University
North Grafton, MA
USA

Elena S. Addison, *MA, VetMB, DECVS, MRCVS*
Clinician in Small Animal Surgery
University of Glasgow
Glasgow
UK

Ashley E. Allen-Durrance, *DVM, DACVECC*
Clinical Assistant Professor, Emergency Medicine and
Critical Care
Department of Small Animal Clinical Sciences
College of Veterinary Medicine
University of Florida
Gainesville, FL
USA

Alison Allukian, *DVM*
Staff Clinician
Angell Animal Medical Center
Jamaica Plain, MA
USA

Marisa K. Ames, *DVM, DACVIM (Cardiology)*
Assistant Professor
Colorado State University
College of Veterinary Medicine and Biomedical Sciences
Fort Collins, CO
USA

Jonathan Babyak, *MS, DVM, DACVECC*
Clinical Assistant Professor, Emergency and Critical Care
Cummings School of Veterinary Medicine
Tufts University
North Grafton, MA
USA

Anusha Balakrishnan, *BVSc, DACVECC*
Assistant Professor, Clinical
College of Veterinary Medicine
Ohio State University
Columbus, OH
USA

Ingrid M. Balsa, *MEd, DVM, DACVS-SA*
Assistant Professor of Clinical Soft Tissue Surgery
University of California, Davis
Davis, CA
USA

Dominic Barfield, *BSc, BVSc, MVetMed, DACVECC, DECVECC, FHEA, MRCVS*
Senior Lecturer in Emergency and Critical Care
Department of Clinical Science and Services
Royal Veterinary College
North Mymms
Hertfordshire
UK

James Barr, *DVM, DACVECC*
Group Medical Director
BluePearl Veterinary Partners
Tampa, FL
USA

Joseph Bartges, *DVM, PhD, DACVIM, DACVN*
Professor of Medicine and Nutrition
Department of Small Animal Medicine and Surgery
College of Veterinary Medicine
University of Georgia
Athens, GA
USA

Lisa J. Bazzle, *DVM, DACVECC*
Staff Criticalist
Animal Medical Center
New York, NY
USA

Matthew W. Beal, *DVM, DACVECC*
Professor HP, Emergency and Critical Care Medicine
College of Veterinary Medicine
Michigan State University
East Lansing, MI
USA

Kari Santoro Beer, *DVM, DACVECC*
Staff Criticalist
Oakland Veterinary Referral Services
Bloomsfield Hills, MI
USA

Kathryn Benavides, *DVM*
Resident, Emergency and Critical Care
Veterinary Specialists and Emergency
Service of Rochester
Rochester NY
USA

Leontine Benedicenti, *DVM, DACVIM (Neurology)*
Clinical Assistant Professor
University of Pennsylvania
School of Veterinary Medicine
Philadelphia, PA
USA

Marian E. Benitez, *DVM, MS, DACVS-SA*
Assistant Clinical Professor, Small Animal Surgery
Department of Small Animal Clinical Sciences
Virginia-Maryland College of Veterinary Medicine
Blacksburg, VA
USA

Allyson Berent, *DVM, DACVIM (SAIM)*
Director of Interventional Endoscopy
Staff Doctor Internal Medicine
Animal Medical Center
New York, NY
USA

Cara A. Blake, *DVM, DACVS-SA*
Certified Canine Rehabilitation Therapist
Department of Clinical Sciences and Advanced Medicine
School of Veterinary Medicine
University of Pennsylvania
Philadelphia, PA
USA

Amanda K. Boag, *MA VetMB, DACVIM, DACVECC, DECVECC, FHEA, MRCVS*
Clinical Director
Vets Now
Dunfermline
UK

Luiz Bolfer, *MV (Hons), DVM, DBCVECC*
Staff Criticalist
Affiliated Veterinary Specialists
Maitland, FL;
Small Animal Emergency and Critical Care Residency
PhD Candidate, Cardiology
Department of Small Animal Clinical Sciences
University of Florida
Gainesville, FL
USA

Elise Boller, *DVM, DACVECC*
Senior Lecturer, Emergency and Critical Care
Melbourne Veterinary School
Faculty of Veterinary and Agricultural Sciences
University of Melbourne
Melbourne
Australia

Manuel Boller, *DMV, MTR, DACVECC*
Senior Lecturer, Veterinary Emergency and Critical Care
Department of Veterinary Clinical Sciences
Melbourne Veterinary School
University of Melbourne
Werribee, Victoria
Australia

Angela Borchers, *DVM, DACVIM, DACVECC*
Associate Veterinarian in Small Animal Emergency
and Critical Care
William R. Pritchard Veterinary Medical
Teaching Hospital
University of California, Davis
Davis, CA
USA

Corrin Boyd, *BVMS (Hons), MVetClinStud, DACVECC*
Registrar
Section of Emergency and Critical Care
College of Veterinary Medicine
School of Veterinary and Life Sciences
Murdoch University
Murdoch, WA
Australia

Søren Boysen, *DVM, DACVECC*
Professor
Department of Veterinary Clinical and
Diagnostic Sciences
Faculty of Veterinary Medicine
University of Calgary
Calgary, AB
Canada

Benjamin M. Brainard, VMD, DACVAA, DACVECC
Edward H. Gunst Professor of Small Animal Critical Care
Director of Clinical Research
College of Veterinary Medicine
University of Georgia
Athens, GA
USA

Dorothy Cimino Brown, MS, DVM, DACVS
Senior Research Advisor
Translational & Comparative Medical Research
Elanco Animal Health
Greenfield, IN
USA

Yaron Bruchim, DVM, IVIMS, DACVECC, DECVECC
Senior Lecturer of Veterinary Medicine
The Hebrew University of Jerusalem
Jerusalem
Israel

Gareth Buckley, MA, VetMB, MRCVS, DACVECC, DECVECC
Medical Director, Small Animal Hospital
Associate Service Chief, Emergency and Critical Care
College of Veterinary Medicine
University of Florida
Gainesville, FL
USA

Melissa Bucknoff, DVM, DACVECC
Assistant Professor of Biomedical Sciences and
Clinical Pharmacology
School of Veterinary Medicine
Ross University
Basseterre, St Kitts
West Indies

Jesse Bullock, DVM
Resident in Emergency and Critical Care
Department of Small Animal Clinical Sciences
College of Veterinary Medicine
University of Florida
Gainesville, FL
USA

Yekaterina Buriko, DVM, DACVECC
Assistant Professor, Section of Critical Care
Department of Clinical Sciences and
Advanced Medicine
Matthew J. Ryan Veterinary Hospital
University of Pennsylvania
Philadelphia, PA
USA

Jamie M. Burkitt Creedon, DVM, DACVECC
Assistant Professor
Department of Veterinary Surgical and
Radiological Sciences
School of Veterinary Medicine
University of California, Davis
Davis, CA
USA

Andrew G. Burton, BVSc (Hons), DACVP
Clinical Pathologist
IDEXX Laboratories, Inc.
North Grafton, MA
USA

Laura Cagle, DVM
Small Animal Emergency and Critical Care
William R. Pritchard Veterinary Medical
Teaching Hospital
University of California, Davis
Davis, CA
USA

Samantha Campos, VMD
Emergency and Critical Care Resident
College of Veterinary Medicine
University of Florida
Gainesville, FL
USA

Jennifer Carr, DVM, MS, DACVS
Staff Surgeon
MedVet Medical and Cancer Center for Pets
Worthington, OH
USA

Sheila Carrera-Justiz, DVM, DACVIM (Neurology)
Service Chief & Clinical Assistant Professor, Neurology;
Medical Director, Small Animal Hospital
Small Animal Clinical Sciences
University of Florida
College of Veterinary Medicine
Gainesville, FL
USA

Margret L. Casal, DVM, MS, PhD
Professor of Medical Genetics, Reproduction
and Pediatrics
Section of Medical Genetics
Department of Clinical Sciences and Advanced Medicine
School of Veterinary Medicine
University of Pennsylvania
Philadelphia, PA
USA

Dava Cazzolli, *DVM, DACVECC*
Staff Criticalist
Animal Specialty Center
Yonkers, NY
USA

Daniel L. Chan, *DVM, DACVECC, DECVECC, DACVN, FHEA, MRCVS*
Professor of Emergency and Critical Care Medicine and Clinical Nutrition
Section of Emergency and Critical Care
Department of Clinical Science and Services
Royal Veterinary College
North Mymms
Hertfordshire
UK

Melissa Clark, *DVM, PhD, DACVCP*
Resident in Internal Medicine
Animal Medical Center
New York, NY
USA

Dana L. Clarke, *VMD, DACVECC*
Assistant Professor of Interventional Radiology & Critical Care
Department of Clinical Sciences and Advanced Medicine
University of Pennsylvania School of Veterinary Medicine
Philadelphia, PA
USA

Melissa A. Claus, *DVM, DACVECC*
Lecturer
Section of Emergency and Critical Care
College of Veterinary Medicine
School of Veterinary and Life Sciences
Murdoch University
Murdoch, WA
Australia

Craig A. Clifford, *DVM, MS, DACVIM (Oncology)*
Medical Oncologist
Director of Clinical Studies
Hope Veterinary Specialists
Malvern, PA
USA

Amanda E. Coleman, *DVM, DACVIM (Cardiology)*
Assistant Professor of Cardiology
College of Veterinary Medicine
University of Georgia
Athens, GA
USA

Edward Cooper, *VMD, MS, DACVECC*
Professor – Clinical
Small Animal Emergency and Critical Care
Veterinary Medical Center
Ohio State University
Columbus, OH
USA

William T.N. Culp, *VMD, DACVS*
ACVS Founding Fellow of Surgical Oncology
ACVS Founding Fellow of Minimally Invasive Surgery
Associate Professor, Small Animal Soft Tissue Surgery
University of California-Davis
School of Veterinary Medicine
Davis, CA
USA

Katherine A. Cummings, *DVM, DACVAA*
Staff Anesthesiologist
Angell Animal Medical Center
Boston, MA
USA

Suzanne M. Cunningham, *DVM, DACVIM (Cardiology)*
Assistant Professor of Cardiology
Department of Clinical Sciences
Cummings School of Veterinary Medicine
Tufts University
North Grafton, MA
USA

Gideon Daniel, *DVM, DACVIM*
Internist, Dialysis, Internal Medicine
Friendship Hospital for Animals
Washington, DC
USA

Autumn P. Davidson, *DVM, MS, DACVIM (SAIM)*
Staff Veterinarian
Department of Population Health and Reproduction
School of Veterinary Medicine
University of California, Davis
Davis, CA
USA

Rachel B. Davy-Moyle, *DVM, DACVECC*
Criticalist
Austin Veterinary Emergency and Specialty Center
Austin, TX
USA

Jonathan D. Dear, DVM, DACVIM
Assistant Professor of Clinical Internal Medicine
Department of Medicine and Epidemiology
School of Veterinary Medicine
University of California, Davis
Davis, CA
USA

Armelle de Laforcade, DVM, DACVECC
Associate Professor, Emergency Medicine and
Critical Care
Cummings School of Veterinary Medicine
Tufts University
North Grafton, MA
USA

Marlis L. de Rezende, DVM, PhD, DACVAA
Associate Professor, Veterinary Anesthesiology
Colorado State University
Fort Collins, CO
USA

Jillian DiFazio, DVM, DACVECC
Staff Criticalist
Veterinary Emergency and Referral Group
Brooklyn, NY
USA

Liam Donaldson, BVSc
Resident, Small Animal Emergency and Critical Care
University of Melbourne
Melbourne
Australia

Kenneth J. Drobatz, DVM, MSCE, DACVIM (IM), DACVECC
Professor and Chief, Section of Critical Care
Department of Clinical Sciences and Advanced Medicine
University of Pennsylvania
Philadelphia, PA;
Senior Fellow of the Center for Public Health Initiatives
University of Pennsylvania
Philadelphia, PA
USA

Steven Epstein, DVM, DACVECC
Associate Professor of Clinical Small Animal Emergency
and Critical Care
Department of Surgical and Radiological Sciences
School of Veterinary Medicine
University of California, Davis
Davis, CA
USA

Kate Farrell, DVM
Resident, Small Animal Emergency and Critical Care
William R. Pritchard Veterinary Medical Teaching
Hospital
University of California, Davis
Davis, CA
USA

Nuno Félix, DVM, MD, MSc, PhD
Resident in Pediatric Medicine
Centro Hospitalar Lisboa Central
Lisboa
Portugal

Daniel J. Fletcher, PhD, DVM, DACVECC
Associate Professor of Emergency and Critical Care
Cornell University College of Veterinary Medicine
Ithaca, NY
USA

Rebecca Flores, DVM
Resident, Small Animal Emergency and Critical Care
Department of Clinical Sciences and Advanced Medicine
Matthew J. Ryan Veterinary Hospital
University of Pennsylvania
Philadelphia, PA
USA

J.D. Foster, VMD, DACVIM
Internist, Dialysis, Internal Medicine
Friendship Hospital for Animals
Washington, DC
USA

Evelyn M. Galban, DVM, MS, DACVIM (Neurology)
Clinical Assistant Professor of Neurology and
Neurosurgery
Department of Clinical Sciences and Advanced Medicine
University of Pennsylvania
Philadelphia, PA
USA

Laura D. Garrett, DVM, DACVIM (Oncology)
Clinical Professor, Oncology
Coordinator of Communication Training
Department of Veterinary Clinical Medicine
College of Veterinary Medicine
University of Illinois Urbana-Champaign
Urbana, IL
USA

Anna R. Gelzer, DMV, PhD, DACVIM (Cardiology), DECVIM-CA (Cardiology)
Associate Professor of Cardiology
School of Veterinary Medicine
University of Pennsylvania
Philadelphia, PA
USA

Robert Goggs, BVSc, DACVECC, DECVECC, PhD, MRCVS
Assistant Professor, Emergency and Critical Care
Department of Clinical Sciences
College of Veterinary Medicine
Cornell University
Ithaca, NY
USA

Katherine J. Goldberg, DVM, LMSW
Founder/Owner
Whole Animal Veterinary Geriatrics & Hospice Services;
Courtesy Lecturer
Cornell University College of Veterinary Medicine
Cornell University
Ithaca, NY;
Core Instructor
University of Tennessee Veterinary Social Work Program
Knoxville, TN
USA

Anthony L. Gonzalez, DVM, DACVECC
Staff Criticalist
ACCESS Specialty Animal Hospitals
Los Angeles, CA
USA

Isabelle Goy-Thollot, MSc, PhD, DECVECC
Director SIAMU (SA-ICU)
Université de Lyon
VetAgro Sup Campus Vétérinaire Lyon
Agressions Pulmonaires et Circulatoires dans le Sepsis (APCSe)
Marcy L'Etoile
France

Reid Groman, DVM, DACVIM, DACVECC
Coordinator, Critical Care Service
Mount Laurel Animal Hospital
Mount Laurel, NJ
USA

Sophie A. Grundy, GVSc (Hons), MANZCVSc, DACVIM (Internal Medicine)
Internal Medicine Consultant
IDEXX Laboratories
Westbrook, ME
USA

Christine L. Guenther, DVM, DACVECC
Director, Critical Care Services
Pittsburgh Veterinary Specialty and Emergency Center
Pittsburgh, PA
USA

Julien Guillaumin, Doct. Vet., DACVECC, DECVECC
Associate Professor, Emergency and Critical Care Service
Department of Clinical Sciences
The Ohio State University
Columbus, OH
USA

Susan G. Hackner, BVSc, MRCVS, DACVIM, DACVECC
Chief Medical Officer
Cornell University Veterinary Specialists
Stamford, CT
USA

Kelly Hall, DVM, MS, DACVECC
Chair
ACVECC-Veterinary Committee on Trauma
Stillwater, MN
USA

Kayla Hanson, DVM
Practice Limited to Emergency and Critical Care
Lakeshore Veterinary Specialists
Oak Creek, WI
USA

Samantha Hart, BVMS (Hons), MS, DACVS, DACVECC
Criticalist, Emergency and Hospitalization
Hope Veterinary Specialists
Malvern, PA
USA

Laura Harvey, DVM, DACVIM (Neurology)
Associate Neurologist
Veterinary Neurology and Imaging of the Chesapeake
Annapolis, MD
USA

Geoff Heffner, DVM, DACVECC
Assistant Professor, Small Animal Emergency and Critical Care Medicine
Veterinary Teaching Hospital
Colorado State University
Fort Collins, CO
USA

Andrea Hesser, *DVM, DACT*
Associate Veterinarian
Advanced Care Veterinary Hospital
Sapulpa, OK
USA

Guillaume L. Hoareau, *DVM, PhD, DACVECC, DECVECC*
Trauma and Critical Illness Research Fellow
Clinical Investigation Facility
Travis Air Force Base
Fairfield, CA
USA

Sabrina N. Hoehne, *DMV, DACVECC*
Small Animal Emergency and Critical Care
William R. Pritchard Veterinary Medical
Teaching Hospital
University of California, Davis
Davis, CA
USA

Jayme E. Hoffberg, *DVM, DACVECC*
Department Head
Emergency and Critical Care Medicine
MedVet Medical and Cancer Centers for Pets
Chicago, IL
USA

Steven R. Hollingsworth, *DVM, DACVO*
Chief, Ophthalmology Service
Veterinary Medical Teaching Hospital
Professor of Clinical Ophthalmology
Department of Surgical and Radiological Sciences
School of Veterinary Medicine
University of California, Davis
Davis, CA
USA

Marie K. Holowaychuk, *DVM, DACVECC*
Speaker, Locum, and Consultant
Critical Care Vet Consulting
Calgary, AB
USA

David E. Holt, *BVSc*
Professor of Surgery
School of Veterinary Medicine
University of Pennsylvania
Philadelphia, PA
USA

Kate Hopper, *BVSc, PhD, DACVECC*
Associate Professor
Small Animal Emergency & Critical Care
Department of Veterinary Surgical and
Radiological Sciences
School of Veterinary Medicine
University of California, Davis
Davis, CA
USA

Karl E. Jandrey, *DVM, MAS, DACVECC*
Associate Professor, Clinical Small Animal Emergency
and Critical Care
School of Veterinary Medicine
University of California, Davis
Davis, CA
USA

Lynelle R. Johnson, *DVM, MS, PhD, DACVIM (SAIM)*
Professor, VM, Medicine and Epidemiology
School of Veterinary Medicine
University of California, Davis
Davis, CA
USA

Spencer A. Johnston, *VMD, DACVS*
James and Marjorie Waggoner Chair
Head, Department of Small Animal
Medicine and Surgery
College of Veterinary Medicine
University of Georgia
Athens, GA
USA

Alicia Z. Karas, *MS, DVM, DACVAA*
Assistant Professor, Clinical Sciences
Cummings School of Veterinary Medicine
Tufts University
North Grafton, MA
USA

Iain Keir, *BVMS, DACVECC, DECVECC*
Medical Director
Avets
Monroeville, PA
USA

Efrat Kelmer, *DVM, DACVECC, DECVECC*
Senior Clinical Lecturer
Department of Small Animal Emergency and
Critical Care
The Hebrew University Veterinary Teaching Hospital
Koret School of Veterinary Medicine
Israel

Patrick J. Kenny, *BVSc, DACVIM (Neurology), DECVN, FHEA, MRCVS*
Veterinary Neurologist & Neurosurgeon
Small Animal Specialist Hospital (SASH)
North Ryde, NSW
Australia

Lesley G. King, *MVB, DACVECC, DACVIM (Internal Medicine)*[†]
Professor, Section of Critical Care
Department of Clinical Sciences
School of Veterinary Medicine;
Director, Intensive Care Unit
Matthew J. Ryan Veterinary Hospital
University of Pennsylvania
Philadelphia, PA
USA

Amie Koenig, *DVM, DACVIM (SAIM), DACVECC*
Associate Professor, Emergency and Critical Care
Department of Small Animal Medicine and Surgery
College of Veterinary Medicine
University of Georgia
Athens, GA
USA

Amy Koenigshof, *DVM, MS, DACVECC*
Associate Professor, Emergency and Critical
Care Medicine
College of Veterinary Medicine
Michigan State University
East Lansing, MI
USA

Casey Kohen, *DVM, DACVECC*
Emergency Medical Director
MarQueen Veterinary Emergency and Specialty Group
Roseville, CA
USA

Jan P. Kovacic, *DVM, DACVECC*
President
Horizon Veterinary Services
Appleton, WI
USA

Marc S. Kraus, *DVM, DACVIM (Cardiology and Internal Medicine), DECVIM-CA (Cardiology)*
Professor of Clinical Cardiology
School of Veterinary Medicine
University of Pennsylvania
Philadelphia, PA
USA

Stephanie R. Krein, *DVM, DACVAA*
Anesthesiologist
Angell Animal Medical Center
Boston, MA
USA

Erika L. Krick, *VMD, DACVIM (Oncology)*
Staff Medical Oncologist
Mount Laurel Animal Hospital
Mount Laurel, NJ
USA

Michelle A. Kutzler, *DVM, PhD, DACT*
Associate Professor of Companion Animal Industries
Oregon State University
Corvallis, OR
USA

Mary A. Labato, *DVM, DACVIM*
Clinical Professor
Department of Clinical Sciences
Foster Hospital for Small Animals
Cummings School of Veterinary Medicine
Tufts University
North Grafton, MA
USA

Travis Lanaux, *DVM, DACVECC*
Clinical Assistant Professor, Emergency Medicine and Critical Care
Department of Small Animal Clinical Sciences
College of Veterinary Medicine
University of Florida
Gainesville, FL
USA

Selena L. Lane, *DVM, DACVECC*
Clinical Assistant Professor, Emergency and Critical Care
Department of Small Animal Medicine and Surgery
College of Veterinary Medicine
University of Georgia
Athens, GA
USA

James Lavely, *DVM, DACVIM (Neurology)*
Veterinary Neurologist
Neurology Department
VCA Animal Care Center
Rohnert Park, CA
USA

[†]Deceased

***Justine A. Lee**, DVM, DACVECC, DABT*
CEO
VETgirl LLC
Saint Paul;
Animal Emergency and Referral Center of Minnesota
St Paul, MN
USA

***Tekla Lee-Fowler**, DVM, MS, DACVIM*
Assistant Professor, Small Animal Internal Medicine
College of Veterinary Medicine
Auburn University
Auburn, AL
USA

***Jo-Annie Letendre**, DVM, DACVECC*
Criticalist
Centre Vétérinaire DMV
Montreal, QC
Canada

***Ronald Li**, DVM, MVetMed, PhD, DACVECC*
Assistant Professor of Small Animal Emergency and Critical Care
Department of Veterinary Surgical and Radiological Sciences
School of Veterinary Medicine
University of California, Davis
Davis, CA
USA

***Andrew Linklater**, DVM, DACVECC*
Clinical Instructor
Lakeshore Veterinary Specialists
Glendale, WI
USA

***Gregory R. Lisciandro**, DVM, DABVP, DACVECC*
CEO
FASTVet.com;
Owner
Hill Country Veterinary Specialists;
President
International Veterinary Point-of-Care Ultrasound Society (IVPOCUS)
Spicewood, TX
USA

***Meryl P. Littman**, VMD, DACVIM*
Professor Emerita of Medicine (CE)
School of Veterinary Medicine
University of Pennsylvania
Philadelphia, PA
USA

***Leo Londoño**, DVM, DACVECC*
Clinical Assistant Professor, Emergency and Critical Care
Hemodialysis Unit Director
Department of Small Animal Clinical Sciences
College of Veterinary Medicine
University of Florida
Gainesville, FL
USA

***Alycen P. Lundberg**, DVM*
Medical Oncology Clinical Instructor
PhD Candidate
College of Veterinary Medicine
University of Illinois Urbana-Champaign
Urbana, IL
USA

***Alex Lynch**, BVSc (Hons), DACVECC, MRCVS*
Assistant Professor in Emergency and Critical Care
Department of Small Animal Clinical Sciences
North Carolina State University
Raleigh, NC
USA

***John MacGregor**, DVM, DACVIM (Cardiology)*
Cardiologist
Portland Veterinary Specialists
Portland, ME
USA

***Sean B. Majoy**, DVM, DACVECC*
Clinical Assistant Professor
Department of Clinical Sciences
Tufts Cummings School of Veterinary Medicine
North Grafton, MA
USA

***Richard Malik**, DVSc, DipVetAn, MVetClinStud, PhD, FACVSc, FASM*
Valentine Charlton Veterinary Specialist
Veterinary Science Conference Centre
University of Sydney
Syndey;
Adjunct Professor
Charles Sturt University
Wagga Wagga, NSW
Australia

***Deborah C. Mandell**, VMD, DACVECC*
Professor, Small Animal Emergency Medicine
Department of Clinical Sciences and Advanced Medicine
Matthew J. Ryan Veterinary Hospital
University of Pennsylvania
Philadelphia, PA
USA

F.A. (Tony) Mann, DVM, MS, DACVS, DACVECC
Professor of Small Animal Surgery and Small Animal
Emergency and Critical Care
Veterinary Health Center
University of Missouri
Columbia, MO
USA

Carol A. Margolis, DVM, DACT
Lecturer, Medical Genetics
School of Veterinary Medicine
University of Pennsylvania
Philadelphia, PA
USA

Karol A. Mathews, DVM, DVSc, DACVECC
Professor Emerita
Ontario Veterinary College
University of Guelph
Guelph, ON
Canada

Brandi L. Mattison, DVM, DACVECC
Medical Director
Arizona Veterinary Emergency and Critical Care Center
Gilbert, AZ
USA

Katie D. Mauro, DVM
Resident, Emergency and Critical Care
Department of Clinical Sciences and Advanced Medicine
School of Veterinary Medicine
University of Pennsylvania
Philadelphia, PA
USA

Erin McGowan, VMD, DACVECC
Criticalist
BluePearl Veterinary Specialty and
Emergency Pet Hospital
Waltham, MA
USA

Maureen McMichael, DVM, DACVECC
Professor, Emergency and Critical Care
Veterinary Clinical Medicine
College of Veterinary Medicine;
Professor, Biomedical & Translational Sciences
Carle-Illinois College of Medicine
University of Illinois
Urbana, IL
USA

Margo Mehl, DVM, DACVS
Veterinary Specialist
VCA San Francisco Veterinary Specialists
San Francisco, CA
USA

Steve J. Mehler, DVM, DACVS
Staff Surgeon
Hope Veterinary Specialists
Philadelphia, PA
USA

Matthew Mellema, DVM, DACVECC
Professor of Small Animal Emergency and Critical Care
School of Veterinary Medicine
University of California, Davis
Davis, CA
USA

Kendra Mikoloski, DVM, DACVIM (Neurology)
Veterinary Specialist
Pittsburgh Veterinary Specialty and Emergency Center
Pittsburgh, PA
USA

Erin Mooney, BVSc, DACVECC
Staff Veterinarian
Unit Head, Emergency and Critical Care
University Veterinary Teaching Hospital
University of Sydney
Camperdown, NSW
Australia

Megan Morgan, VMD, DACVIM
Staff Internist
Cornell University Veterinary Specialists;
Adjunct Assistant Clinical Professor of Medicine
Cornell University College of Veterinary Medicine
Stamford, CT
USA

Lisa A. Murphy, MVB, DVM, DACVECC
Criticalist
Veterinary Specialty Center of Delaware
New Castle, DE
USA

Bob Murtaugh, DVM, MS, DACVECC, DACVIM
Medical Director
Pathway Vet Alliance
Austin, TX
USA

Reid K. Nakamura, DVM, DACVECC, DACVIM (Cardiology)
Staff Veterinarian
Veterinary Specialty and Emergency Center
Thousand Oaks, CA
USA

Lindsey Nielsen, DVM, DACVECC
Co-Medical Director and Criticalist
Veterinary Emergency and Specialty Centers of
New Mexico
Albuquerque, NM
USA

Christopher L. Norkus, DVM, DACVAA, CVPP
Emergency and Critical Care Fellow
Allegheny Veterinary Emergency Trauma and Speciality
Monroeville, PA
USA

Cassie Ostroski, DVM, DACVECC
Staff Criticalist
Mount Laurel Animal Hospital
Mount Laurel, NJ
USA

Therese E. O'Toole, DVM, DACVIM, DACVECC
Clinical Assistant Professor
Department of Clinical Sciences
Cummings School of Veterinary Medicine
Tufts University
North Grafton, MA
USA

Cynthia M. Otto, DVM, PhD, DACVECC, DACVSMR, CCRT
Director
Penn Vet Working Dog Center
School of Veterinary Medicine
University of Pennsylvania
Philadelphia, PA
USA

Mark A. Oyama, DVM, MSCE
Professor
Department of Clinical Sciences and
Advanced Medicine
School of Veterinary Medicine
University of Pennsylvania
Philadelphia, PA
USA

Carrie Palm, DVM, DACVIM
Associate Professor of Clinical Medicine
William R. Pritchard School of Veterinary Medicine
University of California, Davis
Davis, CA
USA

Lee Palmer, DVM, MS, DACVECC, NRP, EMT-T, WEMT, CCRP,
TP-C
Lieutenant Colonel
US Army Reserve
Veterinary Corps;
Chair
K9 Tactical Emergency Casualty Care
Working Group;
Veterinarian
Anti-terrorism Assistance Program
Canine Validation Center
Auburn, AL
USA

Medora Pashmakova, DVM, DACVECC
Staff Criticalist
BluePearl Veterinary Partners
Houston, TX
USA

April Paul, DVM, DACVECC
Specialist in Veterinary Emergency and Critical Care
Tufts VETS
Walpole, MA
USA

S. Anna Pesillo-Crosby, VMD, DACVECC
Owner/Chief Medical Officer
Moodus Veterinary Practice
Moodus, CT;
Director, Central Animal Blood Bank
Central Hospital for Veterinary Medicine
North Haven, CT
USA

Alexandra Pfaff, T, DACVECC
Emergency and Critical Care Specialist
Tufts VETS (Veterinary Emergency Treatment and
Specialties)
Walpole, MA
USA

Kursten V. Pierce, DVM, DACVIM (Cardiology)
Cardiology Specialist
Department of Clinical Sciences
Cummings School of Veterinary Medicine
Tufts University
North Grafton, MA
USA

Marko Pipan, *DVM, DACVECC*
Specialist in Emergency and Critical Care
Animal Hospital Postojna
Postojna
Slovenia

Lisa L. Powell, *DVM, DACVECC*
Associate Critical Care Clinician
BluePearl Veterinary Partners
Eden Prairie, MN;
Senior Consultant
Critical Consults, LLC
Dickson City, PA
USA

Chap Pratt, *DVM, DACVECC*
Emergency and Critical Care
Wheat Ridge Animal Hospital by Ethos
Veterinary Health
Wheat Ridge, CO
USA

Saya Press, *BVSc, MS, DACVECC*
Emergency and Critical Care Resident
College of Veterinary Medicine
Ohio State University
Columbus, OH
USA

Jennifer Prittie, *DVM, DACVIM (Internal Medicine), DACVECC*
Department Chair, Emergency and Critical Care (ECC)
Animal Medical Center
New York, NY
USA

Rebecca Quinn, *DVM, DACVIM (Internal Medicine, Cardiology)*
Staff Veterinarian
Angell Animal Medical Center
Boston, MA
USA

Rodrigo C. Rabelo, *DVM, EMT, MSc, PhD, DBVECC*
Medical and Quality Assurance Director
Emergency and Critical Care Department
Intensivet Veterinary Consulting
Brasília, DF
Brazil

Becca Reader, *DVM*
Resident, Anesthesia
Cummings School of Veterinary Medicine
Tufts University
North Grafton, MA
USA

Erica L. Reineke, *VMD, DACVECC*
Associate Professor of Emergency and
Critical Care Medicine
Department of Clinical Sciences and
Advanced Medicine
School of Veterinary Medicine
University of Pennsylvania
Philadelphia, PA
USA

Meghan Respess, *DVM, DACVECC*
Staff Clinician and Medical Director
BluePearl Veterinary Partners
Brooklyn, NY
USA

Leo Roa, *DVM*
Staff Veterinarian
Iowa Veterinary Referral Center
Des Moines, IA
USA

Brian K. Roberts, *DVM, DACVECC*
Medical Director
Mountain Emergency Animal Center
Blue Ridge, GA
USA

Mark P. Rondeau, *DVM, DACVIM (SAIM)*
Professor of Clinical Medicine
Department of Clinical Sciences and Advanced Medicine
School of Veterinary Medicine
University of Pennsylvania
Philadelphia, PA
USA

Melisa G. Rosenthal, *DVM*
Small Animal Internal Medicine Resident
Department of Clinical Sciences
Foster Hospital for Small Animals
Cummings School of Veterinary Medicine
Tufts University
North Grafton, MA
USA

Elizabeth Rozanski, *DVM, DACVIM (SAIM), DACVECC*
Associate Professor
Department of Clinical Sciences
Cummings School of Veterinary Medicine
Tufts University
North Grafton, MA
USA

Elke Rudloff, *DVM, DACVECC*
Critical Care Specialist
Lakeshore Veterinary Specialists
Glendale, WI
USA

John E. Rush, *DVM, MS, DACVIM (Cardiology), DACVECC*
Professor
Department of Clinical Sciences
Cummings School of Veterinary Medicine
Tufts University
North Grafton, MA
USA

Michael Schaer, *DVM, DACVIM (SAIM), DACVECC*
Emeritus Professor
Adjunct Professor, Emergency and Critical Care Medicine
Department of Small Animal Clinical Sciences
College of Veterinary Medicine
University of Florida
Gainesville, FL
USA

Dustin Schmid, *DVM*
Resident
VCA All Care Animal Referral Center
Fountain Valley, CA
USA

Claire R. Sharp, *BSc, BVMS (Hons), MS, DACVECC*
Senior Lecturer
Section of Emergency and Critical Care
College of Veterinary Medicine
School of Veterinary and Life Sciences
Murdoch University
Murdoch, WA
Australia

Nadja Sigrist, *DMV, FVH (Small Animals), DACVECC, DECVECC*
Senior Lecturer, Head of Critical Care Medicine
Vetsuisse Faculty of Zürich
Zürich
Switzerland

Deborah C. Silverstein, *DVM, DACVECC*
Professor of Critical Care
Department of Clinical Sciences and
Advanced Medicine
University of Pennsylvania
Philadelphia, PA;
Adjunct Professor
Temple University School of Pharmacy
Philadelphia, PA
USA

Meg M. Sleeper, *VMD, DACVIM (Cardiology)*
Clinical Professor of Cardiology
Department of Small Animal Clinical Sciences
College of Veterinary Medicine
University of Florida
Gainesville, FL
USA

Kim Slensky, *DVM, DACVECC*
Assistant Professor of Clinical Small Animal Critical
Care Medicine
Department of Clinical Sciences and Advanced Medicine
School of Veterinary Medicine
University of Pennsylvania
Philadelphia, PA
USA

Sean Smarick, *VMD, DACVECC*
Hospital Director
Avets
Monroeville, PA
USA

Lisa Smart, *BVSc (Hons), DACVECC*
Senior Lecturer
Section of Emergency and Critical Care
College of Veterinary Medicine
School of Veterinary and Life Sciences
Murdoch University
Murdoch, WA
Australia

Josh Smith, *DVM, DACVECC*
Criticalist
Veterinary Emergency Service
Middleton, WI
USA

Rachel E. Smith, *VMD*
Small Animal Internal Medicine Resident
Department of Veterinary Clinical Sciences
College of Veterinary Medicine
University of Minnesota
St Paul, MN
USA

Andrea M. Steele, *MSc, RVT, VTS(ECC)*
ICU Registered Veterinary Technical
Ontario Veterinary College
Health Sciences Centre
University of Guelph
Guelph, ON
Canada

Joshua A. Stern, *DVM, PhD, DACVIM (Cardiology)*
Associate Professor of Cardiology
Department of Medicine and Epidemiology
School of Veterinary Medicine
University of California, Davis
Davis, CA
USA

Elizabeth M. Streeter, *DVM, DACVECC*
Criticalist
Iowa Veterinary Referral Center
Des Moines, IA
USA

Lauren A. Sullivan, *DVM, MS, DACVECC*
Assistant Professor
College of Veterinary Medicine and Biomedical Sciences
Colorado State University
Fort Collins, CO
USA

Katrin Swindells, *BVSc, MANZCVS, DACVECC*
Criticalist, Department of Emergency and Critical Care
Western Australian Veterinary Emergency and Specialty
Perth, WA
Australia

Vincent Thawley, *VMD, DACVECC*
Staff Veterinarian, Emergency Services
Matthew J. Ryan Veterinary Hospital
University of Pennsylvania
Philadelphia, PA
USA

Philip Thomas, *BVSc, PhD, FANZCVS, DACT*
Specialist
Queensland Veterinary Specialists
Stafford Heights, QLD
Australia

Amanda Thomer, *VMD, DACVECC*
Staff Criticalist
ACCESS Specialty Animal Hospitals
Culver City, CA
USA

Erica Tinson, *BSc, BVSc (Hons), MVS, DACVECC*
Clinical Tutor, Emergency and Critical Care
Melbourne Veterinary School
Faculty of Veterinary and Agricultural Sciences
University of Melbourne
Melbourne
Australia

Yu Ueda, *DVM, DACVECC*
PhD Student/Morris Animal Foundation Fellow
Department of Medicine and Epidemiology
School of Veterinary Medicine
University of California, Davis
Davis, CA
USA

Meghan E. Vaught, *DVM*
Staff Criticalist
Port City Veterinary Referral Hospital
Portsmouth, NH
USA

Fabio Vigano', *DVM, SCMPA, GPCert E&S*
Clinical Director
Clinica Veterinaria San Giorgio
San Giorgio su Legnano (MI)
Italy

Lance C. Visser, *DVM, MS, DACVIM (Cardiology)*
Assistant Professor of Cardiology
Department of Medicine and Epidemiology
School of Veterinary Medicine
University of California, Davis
Davis, CA
USA

Lori Waddell, *DVM, DACVECC*
Professor, Clinical Critical Care
Department of Clinical Sciences & Advanced Medicine
School of Veterinary Medicine
University of Pennsylvania
Philadelphia, PA
USA

Jennifer E. Waldrop, *DVM , DACVECC*
Critical Care
BluePearl Veterinary Specialty and Emergency
Pet Hospital
Seattle, WA
USA

Julie M. Walker, *DVM, DACVECC*
Clinical Assistant Professor, Small Animal
Emergency and Critical Care
Department of Medical Sciences
School of Veterinary Medicine
University of Wisconsin-Madison
Madison, WI
USA

***Grayson B. Wallace**, DVM*
Associate Veterinarian
North Oatlands Veterinary Hospital
Leesburg, VA
USA

***Robert J. Washabau**, VMD, PhD, DACVIM*
Professor of Medicine
Department of Veterinary Clinical Sciences
College of Veterinary Medicine
University of Minnesota
St Paul, MN
USA

***Raegan J. Wells**, DVM, MS, DACVECC*
Medical Director
Emergency and Critical Care Specialist Veterinarian
Phoenix Veterinary Emergency and Referral
Phoenix, AZ
USA

***Lois A. Wetmore**, DVM, ScD, DACVAA*
Assistant Professor, Anesthesiology and
Pain Management
Foster Small Animal Hospital
Cummings School of Veterinary Medicine
Tufts University
North Grafton, MA
USA

***Ashley Wiese**, DVM, MS, DACVAA*
Veterinary Anesthesiologist
Regional Medical Director
MedVet Medical and Cancer Center for Pets
Cincinnati, OH
USA

***Tina A. Wismer**, DVM, DABVT, DABT, MS*
Medical Director
ASPCA Animal Poison Control Center
Urbana, IL
USA

***Jim Wohl**, DVM, MPA, DACVIM, ACVECC*
University Ombuds
University of Connecticut
Storrs, CT
USA

***Jonathan H. Wood**, VMD, DACVIM (Neurology)*
Veterinary Neurologist
School of Veterinary Medicine
University of Pennsylvania
Philadelphia, PA
USA

***Donald A. Yool**, BVMS, PhD, DECVS, CertSAS, MRCVS*
Professor of Soft Tissue Surgery
University of Glasgow
Glasgow
UK

Dedication

I would like to dedicate this book to my friend Dave. He was a true friend and was like a brother to me. His influence throughout my life has shaped the person that I am.

Kenneth J. Drobatz

To the animals, students and house officers who teach me something new on a daily basis and have made my career so worthwhile. I will be forever grateful.

Kate Hopper

This book is dedicated to my parents (Chester and Patricia Rozanski) and my sister (Catherine McNamara), for their support and love and to my colleagues in the ECC department at Tufts University who were vital in supporting me during the time and efforts that this book required.

Elizabeth Rozanski

As Franklin D. Roosevelt once said, "I'm not the smartest fellow in the world, but I can sure pick smart colleagues." I would like to dedicate this book to the phenomenal (and smart!) colleagues who co-edited this book, as well as the dedicated and talented contributors who made it possible. I am honored to contribute to such a rewarding profession that is filled with so many inspirational and caring colleagues. In addition, I would like to thank everyone at Wiley, especially Mirjana Misina, for their assistance as well as my family, Stefan, Maxwell and Henry, who put up with my hours at the computer to make this possible!

Deborah Silverstein

Preface

In the early to mid 1980's, the *Journal of Veterinary Emergency and Critical Care* was published once or twice per year with very few manuscripts included. There just simply was not much clinical evidence for veterinary emergency and critical care. There was no emergency specialty and ICU was run mostly by anesthesiologists. This struck me as strange, because when would you really want a specialist? When a life is on the line! Yet, here veterinary medicine was, similar to our MD colleagues years before that, where emergency was filled in mostly by people who were moonlighting and not really specialists in this area.

Now, let's fast-forward to today. *JVECCS* is a highly respected and frequently published clinical journal. The specialty has exploded with 639 diplomates, 69 approved residencies, and 176 residents in training along with numerous specialty internships. There are rigorous standards for veterinary emergency and critical centers. The ACVECC is a financially strong and still rapidly growing college. The IVECCS is one of the most highly attended and respected continuing education meetings in the world. Yet, despite all of this, there is no rigorous, evidence-based emergency medicine textbook. There are numerous excellent clinical emergency manuals but no real formal textbook. Deborah Silverstein's and Kate Hopper's *Small Animal Critical Care* textbook provided a rigorous format of excellent information for practicing in the ICU and has been the "go to" book for many experts practicing ICU medicine. Yet, there is no similarly formatted textbook for emergency medicine.

This frustrated Dr Rozanski and me as we both primarily focus our practice on emergency medicine. We decided to try to fill this gap with this book. Recognizing the great success of Drs. Silverstein and Hopper's textbook, we combined with them to bring this textbook together. I thought that the combination of editors who practice the "front-end" of emergency and critical care with two who practice the "back-end" of emergency and critical care would provide a well-rounded and integrated container of information and hence this book has come to fruition.

When putting this book together, we instructed the authors to provide cutting-edge, evidence-based emergency medicine information and combine that with their anecdotal expertise. We wanted the information to not only be cutting edge but provide physiology and pharmacological principles that are rigorous but clinically relevant. In reading this book cover to cover, I am impressed by what these chapter authors have done. It is truly remarkable and it reflects the rigor and high standards that this specialty has developed. I cannot thank them enough for their conscientious efforts, time, and energy. All of us editors are extremely grateful.

This book will provide you with a wealth of useful clinical information backed by clinical evidence and sound pathophysiological reasoning. Being my passion, I feel this area of veterinary medicine deserves nothing less.

Ken Drobatz
February 2018

About the Companion Website

This book is accompanied by a companion website:

www.wiley.com/go/drobatz/textbook

The website includes:

- PowerPoints of all figures from the book for downloading
- Video clips
- Additional figures that do not appear in the printed book

F. Urogenital Disorders

94

Acute Azotemia

Carrie Palm, DVM, DACVIM

William R. Pritchard School of Veterinary Medicine, University of California, Davis, CA, USA

Introduction

Azotemia is an increase in the concentration of nitrogen-containing substances in the blood, primarily BUN and creatinine. Since BUN and creatinine are both nitrogen-containing compounds, an increase in either compound by itself is therefore defined as azotemia. While azotemia is defined by any increase in BUN and/or creatinine, the term *uremia* is used to describe more severe azotemia, when adverse clinical manifestations are present. In current practice, BUN and creatinine are the most commonly measured "uremic toxins" or substances in the blood that are increased when the glomerular filtration rate (GFR) is compromised; however, these are relatively benign and non-toxic substances that act as surrogate markers for many other unmeasured uremic toxins.

Azotemia can be subcategorized into prerenal (or volume-responsive), intrinsic renal, and postrenal mechanisms. Azotemia, as traditionally defined by BUN and creatinine concentrations outside their defined reference ranges, does not occur until approximately 75% of kidney function has been impaired. Using this definition, many patients with significant kidney injury will not be diagnosed until late in their disease process once they have developed acute renal failure (ARF). As an example, a patient could have functional loss of an entire kidney and creatinine measurements could still be within the normal reference range. While it is critical for a clinician to recognize the presence of non-azotemic kidney injury, the focus of this chapter will be on azotemic kidney injury.

Acute renal failure is characterized by an abrupt and sustained decrease in GFR and is associated with high treatment costs and high morbidity and mortality. One of the speculated reasons for this high mortality is late recognition of disease and consequently the narrow window of opportunity for therapy. It is therefore critical for the attending clinician to look at changes outside established reference ranges, but also to evaluate for small changes in the serum concentration of these markers, which may indicate significant injury.

The term AKI has replaced the numerous definitions of ARF that had developed over the years, to allow for uniformity amongst clinicians when evaluating affected patients. AKI represents a spectrum of renal injury and disease severity, ranging from non-azotemic injury that is clinically non-detectable to severe damage resulting in fulminant ARF. ARF is the most severe stage of AKI and is associated with the highest morbidity and mortality. In the emergency setting, patients presenting with azotemia will likely be in the higher grades of kidney injury and this will therefore be the focus of this chapter. Nonetheless, it is crucial for any treating clinician to recognize that critical evaluation of creatinine is essential for identifying the development of kidney injury in patients presenting with other co-morbidities, such as pancreatitis.

An International Renal Interest Society (IRIS) grading system for AKI has been adopted from human medicine for use in veterinary medicine (Table 94.1) The term *grading* was used to confer the idea that grades of AKI are not static, but represent a time point during kidney injury and/or recovery. This grading system categorizes patients into five grades of AKI, ranging from non-azotemic AKI (where creatinine is still in the reference range) to severe AKI and ARF. These categorizations are based on absolute levels of creatinine, as well as changes in azotemia over a specified period of time. Patients can span through the various spectrums of AKI as they either progress or improve. An increase in creatinine by 0.3 mg/dL (even in the non-azotemic range) within a 48-hour period is consistent with an AKI. It is these small changes in creatinine that should be recognized as development of an AKI. Subgrading is also made based on urine output and on need for renal replacement therapy.

Textbook of Small Animal Emergency Medicine, First Edition. Edited by Kenneth J. Drobatz, Kate Hopper, Elizabeth Rozanski and Deborah C. Silverstein.
© 2019 John Wiley & Sons, Inc. Published 2019 by John Wiley & Sons, Inc.
Companion Website: www.wiley.com/go/drobatz/textbook

Table 94.1 The current International Renal Interest Society (IRIS) acute kidney injury (AKI) grading system. Note that grading is based on absolute creatinine values, and subgrading is based on urinary output, as well as a need for renal replacement therapy. For grade 1 AKI (non-azotemic AKI), grading is based on a ≥ 0.3 mg/dL increase in creatinine from baseline in a 48-hour period (http://iris-kidney.com/guidelines/grading.html)

AKI grade	Blood creatinine	Subgrade
Grade I	<1.6 mg/dL (<140 μmol/L)	Each grade of AKI is further subgraded as:
Grade II	1.7–2.5 mg/dL (141–220 μmol/L)	1. non-oliguric (NO) or oliguric (O)
Grade III	2.6–5.0 mg/dL (221–439 μmol/L)	2. requiring renal replacement therapy (RRT)
Grade IV	5.1–10.0 mg/dL (440–880 μmol/L)	
Grade V	>10.0 mg/dL (>880 μmol/L)	

Table 94.2 Common etiologies responsible for acute kidney injury (AKI) in dogs and cats. In many cases, the underlying etiology may not be definitively known, but each of these causes should be considered and ruled in or out with appropriate diagnostic testing, as indicated. Please note, this is not a comprehensive list of all causes of AKI.

Dog	Dog and cat	Cat
	Pyelonephritis	
	Hemodynamic instability (including hypertension)	
	Acute pancreatitis	
	Drugs, for example amphotericin B, aminoglycosides, non-steroidal anti-inflammatories	
Grape/raisin toxicity	Other nephrotoxins	Lily toxicity
	Ethylene glycol	
	Melamine/cyanuric acid	
Leptospirosis		Ureteral obstruction
Lyme nephritis		Renal lymphoma
		Feline infectious peritonitis

Prerenal Azotemia

Prerenal or volume-responsive azotemia is defined by a decreased GFR occurring secondary to hypoperfusion in a structurally normal kidney. Correction of hypoperfusion leads to rapid resolution of the azotemia, providing that intrinsic AKI has not developed. Hypovolemia, poor cardiac output secondary to cardiovascular dysfunction and pathological vasodilatory conditions (such as shock) are some of the common causes for prerenal azotemia in veterinary medicine. When prerenal azotemia occurs, the BUN to creatinine ratio is often increased (greater than approximately 20:1) due to the increased reabsorption of BUN in the nephron as physiological mechanisms function to re-establish a euvolemic state. In veterinary medicine, hypoadrenocorticism is commonly associated with prerenal azotemia and can be mistaken for intrinsic renal disease (see Chapter 115).

The assessment of azotemia should include determination of urine specific gravity. Suspicion for prerenal azotemia will increase when a corresponding urine sample is concentrated; however, in conditions where altered urinary concentrating ability is present, prerenal azotemia can occur without the presence of concentrated urine.

Intrinsic Renal Azotemia

Acute renal azotemia or AKI occurs due to intrinsic kidney dysfunction. Common causes for AKI in veterinary medicine include leptospirosis, pyelonephritis, and injury secondary to drugs, toxins, and ischemia (see Table 94.2 for a full list). With renal azotemia, crit-

ical evaluation of creatinine is crucial as misdiagnosis of renal disease can occur if the attending clinician simply uses established reference ranges. Significant renal dysfunction occurs before creatinine increases outside established reference ranges and earlier identification may lead to better outcomes. The search for novel biomarkers that are more sensitive than creatinine for early diagnosis of AKI is actively under way [1,2]. In addition, with application of the AKI grading system, patients can be appropriately categorized based on their severity of azotemia and early AKI will not be missed.

Postrenal Azotemia

Postrenal azotemia occurs secondary to obstruction of the urine drainage system (renal pelvis, ureter, bladder or urethra). When relief of obstruction is achieved, complete correction of azotemia often occurs rapidly if there is no concurrent prerenal and/or intrinsic renal disease. As discussed above, unilateral ureteral obstruction may lead to non-azotemic kidney disease, but astute clinicians may note the importance of small but significant increases (i.e. > 0.3 mg/dL increase) in creatinine that could lead to early detection. In the emergency setting, the most common causes for postrenal azotemia include ureteral obstruction(s) and urethral obstruction (see Chapters 97 and 98).

Diagnosis of Acute Azotemia

Physical Examination and History

Every patient with established AKI requires individualized treatment, but there are key aspects of evaluation and management that must be performed for each patient. A complete history should be obtained and can aid in prioritizing differential diagnoses (see Table 94.2) and in establishing the presence of more chronic kidney disease, which can be crucial for prognostication (Table 94.3).

A thorough physical examination should be performed, but the attending clinician should focus on the common abnormalities that can be found in a patient with acute azotemia.

Initial assessment should focus on fluid/hydration, cardiovascular and respiratory status, as well as evaluation for common consequences of uremia. AKI patients with oliguria or anuria readily develop overhydration when overzealous fluids are administered. Manifestations of fluid overload can include refractory hypertension, peripheral edema, pulmonary edema, and pleural effusion, the latter of which can lead to severe respiratory compromise. Life-threatening bradycardias and arrhythmias may be noted in patients with severe

hyperkalemia. Careful evaluation of the urinary bladder must be made so that urine production status can be assessed; this should be done in conjunction with evaluation of hydration status. A dehydrated patient with an empty urinary bladder may simply need restoration of vascular volume so that renal blood flow and urine output can be re-established. On the other hand, a severely overhydrated patient with an empty bladder is more likely to have intrinsic anuric or oliguric renal failure. Neurological status should also be evaluated as severe fluid overload can lead to cerebral edema, as can uremic and hypertensive encephalopathy. Abdominal palpation should be complete to detect possible underlying causes for AKI, but should focus on renal palpation. In cats, one small kidney and one large kidney may suggest an etiology of ureteral obstruction, while painful kidneys may suggest an underlying pyelonephritis or bilateral obstruction; it is important to note that any AKI can be painful due to renal capsular distension. In addition, renal swelling secondary to AKI can cause chronic, fibrotic kidneys to palpate within normal size limits. A careful oral examination should be performed, as severe oral ulceration can occur secondary to severe AKI (Figure 94.1).

Table 94.3 A comparison of some common findings in patients with acute kidney injury (AKI) versus chronic kidney disease (CKD). It is important to note that each individual patient has their own unique presentation and a single patient may have characteristics that fall within both the CKD and AKI categories.

Acute kidney injury	Chronic kidney disease
Shorter history of illness	Longer history of illness
Normal to increased body condition score (BCS)	Normal to decreased BCS
Normal hematocrit	Anemia
Normal to enlarged kidneys on palpation (often painful)	Normal to small, irregular kidneys on palpation
Normokalemia to hyperkalemia	Normokalemia to hypokalemia
Oliguria to anuria	Polyuria
More profound hyperphosphatemia	Moderate hyperphosphatemia
Normal sized to enlarged kidneys with hyperechoic cortices and perirenal fluid on ultrasound	Normal sized to small kidneys with irregular borders, cortical cysts, and previous infarcts on ultrasound

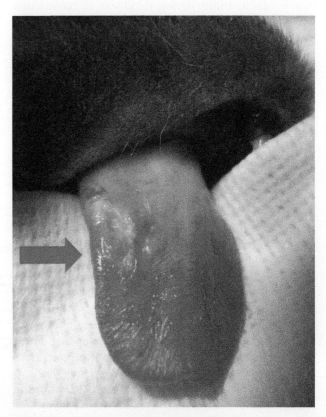

Figure 94.1 Image of a "uremic" oral ulcer (*red arrow*) in a feline patient with severe acute renal failure secondary to lily intoxication.

As discussed, a thorough examination should be performed to evaluate for underlying etiologies that may have caused AKI.

Initial Diagnostics

Initial diagnostics should be performed to fully assess patients with suspected AKI. Bloodwork, including a complete blood count and serum chemistry screen, is essential in the assessment of these patients. Complete blood counts may demonstrate a neutrophilia, which could suggest an underlying pyelonephritis or pancreatitis. Serum chemistry screens allow for evaluation of the severity of azotemia, and specific changes in the chemistry panel, such as a hepatopathy, can help to define underlying disease, such as leptospirosis or pancreatitis. As the kidney is largely responsible for potassium regulation, AKI can result in altered excretion of potassium and subsequent hyperkalemia that can lead to life-threatening cardiac arrhythmias (see Chapter 109). Other electrolytes that are often abnormal on the chemistry screen include phosphorus, sodium, and magnesium and these should be considered when devising a treatment plan (see Chapter 110). Metabolic acidosis is common in patients with AKI due to decreased bicarbonate production from damaged kidneys, in conjunction with increased concentrations of uremic and lactic acids (if dehydration is present) (see Chapter 107).

Evaluation of urine via urinalysis and urine culture is critical. The urine specific gravity (preferably obtained prior to fluid therapy) may assist in the determination of prerenal or volume-responsive azotemia and renal or postrenal azotemia, and should be monitored closely during AKI therapy. The degree of proteinuria should be evaluated in the context of urine specific gravity, as well as urine sediment. Tubular injury can lead to postglomerular proteinuria; however, in a patient with significant proteinuria (urine protein:creatinine ratio (UPC) > 10), especially in patients with exposure to ticks, testing for tick-borne infections should be submitted. A urine culture (obtained prior to antibiotic therapy) is an extremely important step in determining the pathogenesis of AKI and projected treatment regimen. In some cases of anuric renal failure, it is not possible to obtain a urine sample.

Imaging of patients with AKI may include thoracic and/or abdominal radiographs and abdominal ultrasound. Abdominal radiographs can identify urinary tract calculi and renal size, but are otherwise poorly sensitive in determining the underlying cause of AKI. Thoracic radiographs are important to assess AKI patients for other underlying disease processes, such as cardiac disease, aspiration pneumonia, and metastatic disease, and for secondary fluid overload. Abdominal ultrasound is the imaging diagnostic of choice for kidney assessment as an evaluation of corticomedullary distinction, kidney, renal pelvic and ureter size can be made. Additionally, ureteral obstructions may be noted, but it is important to recognize that acute obstructions are not always accompanied by significant hydronephrosis or hydroureter (especially if the patient is dehydrated at the time of initial evaluation).

Treatment

Initial therapy for an AKI patient in the emergency room should focus on life-threatening abnormalities. Serum potassium concentration should be evaluated immediately and hyperkalemia treated as appropriate (see Chapter 109).

Patients with AKI can present with a wide array of hydration and fluid volume statuses. Dehydrated or hypovolemic patients should be treated so that they become volume replete. Once euvolemia is achieved, more accurate assessments of urine output can be made. As many patients with AKI have ongoing losses via vomiting and diarrhea, it is crucial to maintain adequate hydration, so that the already damaged kidneys are not further compromised by decreased renal perfusion that can accompany hypovolemia. Careful and continual evaluation of hydration status is critical and this point cannot be overemphasized.

The presence of azotemia does not by definition require aggressive fluid therapy; instead, the goal of fluid therapy is to achieve and maintain hydration without creating overhydration, a condition that can be as life-threatening as the AKI itself. Successful monitoring can be achieved via serial assessments of skin turgor, body weight, respiratory rate and effort, PCV/TP, urinary output, and blood pressure. A urinary catheter is rarely necessary to monitor hydration status if careful attention is paid to the above factors.

In all cases of oliguria/anuria, it is essential to rule out the presence of a lower urinary tract obstruction. Initial treatment of oliguria/anuria is aimed at ensuring adequate hydration and ruling out a prerenal condition. Once this has been done, diuretics such as mannitol and furosemide should be considered. Furosemide may result in an increased urine output, but it is important to recognize that the increased urine output does not necessarily represent improved renal function. Other treatment options for oliguria/anuria include fenoldopam administration, hemodialysis (especially if fluid overload is present), and surgery (if ureteral obstruction is present). Fenoldopam has been shown to be relatively safe when used in dogs and cats, but there are no outcome data to show a definitive improvement with its use [3–5].

If oliguria/anuria is noted secondary to urinary tract obstruction (i.e. calculi, strictures, neoplasia), surgical intervention should be considered. Ureteral obstructions can typically be successfully managed with surgery, stenting or ureteral bypass. If no response is noted with the above therapies and surgery is not indicated, dialysis should be offered, especially in patients with severe hyperkalemia or fluid overload.

Consequences of metabolic acidosis include disrupted cellular metabolism, exacerbation of hyperkalemia, and increased protein and bone turnover (see Chapter 107). Treatment for metabolic acidosis is focused on correcting hypoperfusion to decrease lactic acidosis and the administration of sodium bicarbonate, once it is confirmed that a patient is volume replete. Dialysis can also correct acidemia.

Hypertension is a common sequela of AKI, and severe consequences such as retinal detachment, hypertensive encephalopathy with secondary seizures, progressive renal damage, and cerebral hemorrhage can all occur secondary to hypertension (see Chapter 63). Overhydration can significantly cause and/or exacerbate hypertension. The use of antihypertensive medications to maintain blood pressure within a safe range is imperative. Amlodipine, acepromazine, hydralazine, and nitroprusside can be considered. Angiotensin converting enzyme inhibitors can also be considered, but should be used cautiously in patients with significant azotemia, and are not administered as a first-line antihypertensive therapy to severely azotemic patients at this author's institution.

Pulmonary compromise occurs frequently in AKI patients. Underlying etiologies include iatrogenically induced fluid overload, aspiration pneumonia, and pulmonary hemorrhage secondary to leptospirosis infection. Therapy should be directed at preventing fluid overload, treatment of the underlying cause, if possible, as well as administration of supportive care to maintain patient stability. Given possible evidence for an immune-mediated component for the pulmonary manifestations of leptospirosis infections, plasmapheresis may be indicated in severely affected patients [6].

In any patient suspected to have pyelonephritis or an antibiotic-responsive infection, such as leptospirosis, antibiotic therapy should be instituted pending diagnostic testing (see Chapter 200). While judicious use of antibiotics is critical, so is the immediate treatment of conditions that are antibiotic responsive; this can improve outcome by allowing for more rapid renal recovery to occur. In addition, the primary underlying cause of disease should be evaluated for and treated accordingly.

Gastrointestinal issues, such as vomiting and GI ulceration, are seen regularly in patients with AKI (see Chapter 74). Vomiting can result from direct effects of uremic toxins on the chemoreceptor trigger zone (CRTZ), gastritis, gastrointestinal edema, and delayed gastric emptying/ileus. Gastrointestinal ulceration can occur secondary to decreased gastrin excretion or increased activity of urease-producing bacteria. Treatment for gastrointestinal-related disease is often focused on antiemetics (maropitant, ondansetron, phenothiazine derivatives, metoclopramide) and gastrointestinal protectants (H2 antagonists, proton pump inhibitors, sucralfate). Severe oral ulceration and stomatitis can also occur due to the conversion of urea by bacterial urease into ammonia, which is caustic to the oral mucosa (see Figure 94.1). Veterinary patients with stomatitis can be treated with oral chlorhexidine; as uremic stomatitis is often very painful, aggressive pain management is also indicated.

Hemodialysis should be considered in patients with severe azotemia with secondary adverse clinical signs, and in those with severe hyperkalemia (not correctable by medical intervention) or fluid overload. If a treatable condition, such as ureteral obstruction, is present, it is the author's recommendation to pursue definitive surgical treatment rather than hemodialysis, whenever possible. Hemodialysis can be a life-saving therapy that has the ability to improve patient well-being, quality of life, and ease of patient management while waiting for renal recovery to occur [7,8].

Acute kidney injury represents a spectrum of disease severity and clinicians should become astute at recognizing damage at an early stage, before it develops into a life-threatening problem. Established ARF is a severe disease process with life-threatening complications. Many affected patients can be managed successfully if careful and appropriate care is provided. The primary insult causing AKI, if identified, needs to be treated aggressively, as do the secondary complications of severe uremia. When medical management cannot maintain patient stability, hemodialysis should be offered, as it can be a life-saving treatment.

References

1 Segev G, Palm C, LeRoy B, et al. Evaluation of neutrophil gelatinase-associated lipocalin as a marker of kidney injury in dogs. *J Vet Intern Med* 2013;27:1362–1367.

2 Palm CA, Segev G, Cowgill LD, et al. Urinary neutrophil gelatinase-associated lipocalin as a marker for identification of acute kidney injury and recovery

in dogs with gentamicin-induced nephrotoxicity. *J Vet Intern Med* 2016;30:200–205.

3 Bloom CA, Labato MA, Hazarika S, et al. Preliminary pharmacokinetics and cardiovascular effects of fenoldopam continuous rate infusion in six healthy dogs. *J Vet Pharmacol Therapeut* 2012;35:224–230.

4 O'Neill KE, Labato MA, Court MH. The pharmacokinetics of intravenous fenoldopam in healthy, awake cats. *J Vet Pharmacol Therapeut* 2016;39:202–204.

5 Nielsen LK, Bracker K, Price LL. Administration of fenoldopam in critically ill small animal patients with acute kidney injury: 28 dogs and 34 cats (2008–2012). *J Vet Emerg Crit Care* 2015;25:396–404.

6 Schuller S, Callanan JJ, Worrall S, et al. Immunohistochemical detection of IgM and IgG in lung tissue of dogs with leptospiral pulmonary haemorrhage syndrome (LPHS). *Compar Immunol Microbiol Infect Dis* 2015;40:47–53.

7 Eatroff AE, Langston CE, Chalhoub S, et al. Long-term outcome of cats and dogs with acute kidney injury treated with intermittent hemodialysis: 135 cases (1997–2010). *J Am Vet Med Assoc* 2012;241:1471–1478.

8 Hoareau GL, Epstein SE, Palm C, et al. Resolution of anuric acute kidney injury in a dog with multiple organ dysfunction syndrome. *J Vet Emerg Crit Care* 2014;24:724–730.

95

Oliguria

J.D. Foster, VMD, DACVIM

Friendship Hospital for Animals, Washington, DC, USA

Pathogenesis of Oligoanuria

Urine output (UOP) is an important aspect of monitoring the hospitalized patient, as it can provide valuable information regarding kidney function and patency of the urinary tract, as well as helping to guide fluid therapy. This is particularly true for the patient with renal disease. Normal urine production has been reported to be 1–2 mL/kg/h in dogs and cats [1–3]. Renal dysfunction, such as acute kidney injury and chronic kidney disease, typically includes impaired tubular solute reabsorption. This results in a solute diuresis and subsequent polyuria (>2 mL/kg/h UOP). Numerous definitions have been used for anuria and oliguria in veterinary patients. Because most patients with renal disease will be polyuric, UOP < 2 mL/kg/h indicates relative oliguria. UOP < 1 mL/kg/h is considered absolute oliguria and anuria is defined as 0–0.5 mL/kg/h UOP.

While urine production is an important observance in monitoring renal function, UOP cannot be used as a surrogate for glomerular filtration rate (GFR). Rather, UOP is a function of GFR, tubular solute reabsorption, and tubular solute secretion. Patients with complete anuria will have a GFR of 0 mL/kg/min, but the restoration of UOP in these patients does not necessarily indicate improvement in GFR.

Oligoanuric acute kidney injury can occur due to several processes (Table 95.1) [4,5]. Dogs and cats with oligoanuric acute kidney injury (AKI) have higher mortality rates and as much as a 20-fold increased risk of death compared to polyuric animals [6,7].

Patient Assessment and Initial Diagnostics

Oligoanuric patients should be evaluated with a thorough physical examination with particular emphasis on detection of subcutaneous edema, cardiopulmonary auscultation, respiratory rate and effort, presence of

Table 95.1 Causes of oligoanuria.

Pathogenesis	Potential causes
Decreased renal blood flow	Hypovolemia or hypotension
	Decreased cardiac output
	Renal artery stenosis or thrombosis
	Sepsis
	Vasodilatory drugs
Tubular obstruction from casts or cellular debris	Pyelonephritis
	Acute interstitial nephritis
	Leptospirosis
	Acute tubular necrosis
	Nephrotoxicity
Backflow of glomerular filtrate into renal interstitium	Ureteral, renal pelvis, or urethral obstruction
	Tubular obstruction from casts and cellular debris
Intrarenal renin-angiotensin system activation	Failure of NaCl reabsorption within proximal tubule
	High chloride-containing intravenous fluid therapy
Altered permeability of glomerular filtration barrier	Glomerulonephritis
	Vasculitis

abdominal distension or pain, as well as urinary bladder size. Assessment of patient hydration status and intravascular volume should be made and noted within the patient's medical record. Blood pressure measurement and body weight are also very important to record.

Initial diagnostics should include imaging to document the size or volume of the urinary bladder (often achievable with bedside ultrasound machines), PCV/TS, serum chemistry with electrolytes, and acid–base analysis. Urine should be collected for analysis prior to the initiation of fluid therapy; cystocentesis is preferred to also

Textbook of Small Animal Emergency Medicine, First Edition. Edited by Kenneth J. Drobatz, Kate Hopper, Elizabeth Rozanski and Deborah C. Silverstein.
© 2019 John Wiley & Sons, Inc. Published 2019 by John Wiley & Sons, Inc.
Companion Website: www.wiley.com/go/drobatz/textbook

provide a sample for urine culture. The urine specific gravity can be helpful to determine if a prerenal cause of oligoanuria is present. Urine may be difficult to obtain in anuric patients. Thoracic radiographs and/or ultrasound should be performed in patients with any concern for pulmonary edema or pleural effusion.

Managing the Oligoanuric Patient

The therapeutic approach to the oligoanuric patient is dependent on their current volume and hydration status (Figure 95.1). Hypovolemic patients should be treated with boluses of isotonic replacement solutions, given rapidly through an intravenous route (see Chapter 167).

Patients with decreased renal perfusion will have an appropriate reduction in UOP secondary to activation of the renin-angiotensin-aldosterone system. Therefore, patients should be adequately hydrated with normal intravascular volume prior to definitively declaring an oliguric or anuric state. Patients that are cardiovascularly stable but dehydrated should have their degree of dehydration estimated from physical examination findings, and this volume calculated and replaced over 6–8 hours (unless cardiopulmonary disease is present that could create an intolerance of such fluid rates) [5]. Once the patient has been rehydrated, an appropriate UOP is 2–5 mL/kg/h depending on the rate of intravenous fluid administration. A UOP less than 2 mL/kg/h would be considered oliguria in a hydrated patient receiving intravenous fluids.

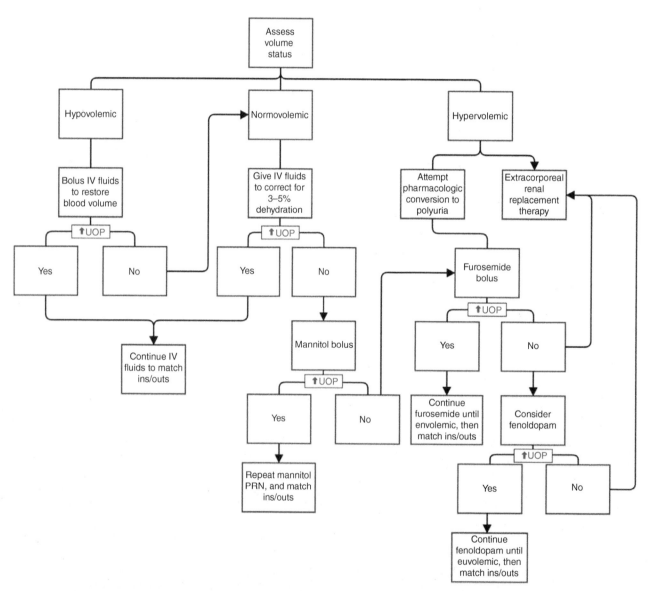

Figure 95.1 Therapeutic intervention for oligoanuria.

For euhydrated patients, an isotonic crystalloid of a volume of fluid equal to 3–5% of body weight should be administered because dehydration of less than 5% cannot be detected clinically. If UOP fails to reach an appropriate magnitude (2–5 mL/kg/h), pharmacological conversion to polyuria may be attempted (see below).

Oligoanuric patients who are hypervolemic often show evidence of serous ocular and nasal discharge, subcutaneous edema, pleural and abdominal effusion, pulmonary edema, and arterial hypertension. Although less commonly seen in veterinary oligoanuric patients, conditions such as systemic inflammatory response syndrome, vasculitis, sepsis, burns, trauma, or pancreatitis can result in intravascular volume depletion with interstitial overhydration in humans (see Chapter 159) [8]. Most patients have normal to increased intravascular and interstitial fluid volumes. Hypervolemic patients with systemic hypotension should be treated with pressors, and intravascular volume expansion should be performed in any patient with a decreased effective circulating volume.

Monitoring UOP in comparison to volume of fluids administered (sum of all IV and PO fluids, often referred to as "ins/outs") is very helpful in the assessment of oligoanuric patients. Aseptic placement of a urinary catheter and a closed collection system should be considered, as it is more accurate, allows for more frequent assessment of urine output, and protects hospital staff from potential zoonotic agents compared to weighing urine collected in pans and bedding. Hypervolemic patients should be managed so their "outs" exceed their "ins." GI fluid losses through diarrhea or vomitus should be estimated and included in this assessment. Euvolemic patients should be managed with a neutral or minimally negative total daily fluid balance. It has been documented in people that a positive fluid balance is associated with a worse prognosis in patients with AKI, greater risk of developing AKI, and a poorer chance of return of renal function following AKI [9,10].

The goal of fluid therapy is to maintain renal perfusion. Several studies have shown that supraphysiological rates of intravenous fluids fail to increase GFR in dogs and cats [11,12]. Therefore, patients should have frequent assessments and the fluid plan be adjusted to prevent fluid accumulation.

Converting Oligoanuria to Polyuria

It is now accepted that pharmacological conversion from an oligoanuric to a polyuric state is the mainstay of management in veterinary medicine. Studies in dogs and cats are lacking, but it should be noted that numerous studies in people have demonstrated that successful pharma-

cological induction of polyuria has no effect on patient mortality [13]. Hypervolemia in an oligoanuric patient is an indication for extracorporeal renal replacement therapy, and referral for this treatment should be considered early in the course of patient evaluation. In people, an increase in urine output with diuretic use often delays referral for dialysis, potentially at the expense of worse clinical outcomes [14]. Currently, there is scant evidence to show that pharmacological attempts at inducing polyuria are effective, or when it occurs that this carries an improved survival and return of renal function in veterinary patients with AKI.

Mannitol is an osmotic diuretic that decreases cellular swelling and may help to wash out obstructive casts and debris from the tubules. It may also serve as a free radical scavenger. Mannitol is administered as a intravenous bolus of 0.25–1.0 g/kg, administered over 15–20 minutes. If an increase in UOP is achieved, mannitol can be dosed intermittently q4–6h or administered as a CRI (60–120 mg/kg/h). Mannitol should not be given to patients that are dehydrated because it can further exacerbate intracellular dehydration. Importantly, it is contraindicated if overhydration is present, and may worsen pulmonary edema. Due to lack of evidence showing that mannitol can help prevent AKI and potential risks of hypervolemia secondary to administration, consensus guidelines in people suggest that mannitol not be used in patients with AKI [15]. It is still used in euvolemic veterinary patients, but no publications have reported its efficacy.

Furosemide is a loop diuretic, which inhibits the Na-K-2Cl transporter in the thick ascending loop of Henle. Experimental models have shown potential benefits, including decreased renal oxygen consumption and less ischemic damage. It should be noted that it is the concentration of furosemide within the tubular filtrate and not the blood that determines the observed effect [16]. Furosemide enters the tubular filtrate via active secretion within the proximal tubule as well as filtration of non-protein-bound furosemide across the glomerular filtration barrier. Anuric patients with minimal to no tubular flow are unlikely to have furosemide reach the site of activity, and therefore this drug is often ineffective in increasing UOP in these patients. Human patients who fail to respond to furosemide are more likely to have progression and greater severity of AKI [17]. Furosemide is typically administered as an intravenous bolus or intramuscular dose of 1–4 mg/kg. If an increased UOP is observed, the dose may be repeated every 6–12 hours as needed, or a constant-rate infusion may be administered. The function of the CRI is to maintain serum concentrations sufficient to allow continuous accumulation within the tubular filtrate. Patients who fail to respond to a bolus of furosemide are unlikely to respond to a CRI, as they likely have adequate serum concentrations for several hours following bolus administration. It should be noted that in people, consensus guidelines suggest that furosemide only be used in early or established AKI for management of fluid balance, hyperkalemia, and hypercalcemia, but any putative role in amelioration of the AKI course is unproven [18].

Renal dose dopamine has been advocated for the management of oliguric AKI for its effects on renal vasodilation. Human studies have shown limited to no improvement in morbidity, mortality, or need for dialysis in established AKI. Additionally, even at low doses, dopamine is potentially toxic in critically ill patients and can induce tachyarrhythmias and myocardial ischemia [19]. Based on these data, dopamine is not currently recommended for treating AKI in humans or animals [20].

Fenoldopam is a selective postsynaptic dopamine receptor (DA-1) agonist that causes more potent renal vasodilation and natriuresis than dopamine. However, it can also promote hypotension by decreasing systemic vascular resistance. Fenoldopam has been shown to increase UOP in healthy cats [21]. Compared to placebo, fenoldopam administration resulted in an increase in GFR and fractional exertion of sodium in healthy dogs [22]. Pharmacokinetic data exist for healthy dogs [23]. A retrospective study of fenoldopam use for both dogs and cats with AKI demonstrated no improvement in survival or length of hospitalization in patients who were administered fenoldopam compared to those who were not [24].

Diltiazem is a calcium channel blocker that may improve renal blood flow through afferent arteriolar vasodilation, which may increase GFR and UOP [25]. It may also be renoprotective by preventing the intracellular accumulation of calcium, which can trigger cellular necrosis. A retrospective study evaluating the effect of diltiazem in dogs with AKI secondary to leptospirosis did not identify significant improvements in rate of reduction of serum creatinine, recovery of renal function, or survival [26].

Extracorporeal Renal Replacement Therapy

The most significant complications of oligoanuria are hyperkalemia, hypervolemia, and uremia. Extracorporeal renal replacement therapy (ERRT) is extremely effective in correcting all three of these, as well as acid–base and other electrolyte disturbances. Both intermittent hemodialysis and continuous renal replacement therapy can perform ultrafiltration of blood, which removes plasma water to help correct hypervolemia. Referral to a hospital with ERRT capabilities should be discussed with the clients and offered early in the management of the oligoanuric patient, particularly those who are hypervolemic. By helping to normalize the patient's volume status, electrolytes, and uremia, ERRT affords greater opportunity and time to manage the oligoanuric patient. Volume can be controlled so that intravenous medications and nutrition can be administered without causing hypervolemia. Uremia may be improved to allow for initiation of enteral nutrition and fewer antinausea medications.

For clients for whom ERRT is not an option, due to financial restraints or geographic distance to the nearest hospital with ERRT capabilities, pharmacological conversion to polyuria should be attempted. Peritoneal dialysis should also be considered, as ultrafiltration can be achieved by use of hypertonic dialysate [27,28].

References

1 Worden AN, Waterhouse CE, Sellwood EHB. Studies on the composition of normal cat urine. *J Small Anim Pract* 1960;1(1–4):11–23.

2 Osborne CA, Stevens JB, Lulich JP, et al. A clinician's analysis of urinalysis. In: *Canine and Feline Nephrology and Urology* (eds Osborne CA, Finco DR). Williams and Wilkins, Baltimore, 1995. pp. 137–205.

3 Pelligand L, Lees P, Elliott J. Development and validation of a timed urinary collection system for use in the cat. *Lab Anim* 2011;45(3):196–203.

4 Klahr S, Miller SB. Acute oliguria. *N Engl J Med* 1998;338(10):671–675.

5 Ross LA. Fluid therapy for acute and chronic renal failure. *Vet Clin North Am Small Anim Pract* 1989;19(2):343–359.

6 Behrend EN, Grauer GF, Mani I, Groman RP, Salman MD, Greco DS. Hospital-acquired acute renal failure in dogs: 29 cases (1983–1992). *J Am Vet Med Assoc* 1996;208(4):537–541.

7 Brown N, Segev G, Francey T, Kass P, Cowgill LD. Glomerular filtration rate, urine production, and fractional clearance of electrolytes in acute kidney injury in dogs and their association with survival. *J Vet Intern Med* 2015;29(1):28–34.

8 DePriest J. Reversing oliguria in critically ill patients. *Postgrad Med* 1997;102(3):245–6, 251–2, 258 passim.

9 Bouchard J, Soroko SB, Chertow GM, et al. Fluid accumulation, survival and recovery of kidney function in critically ill patients with acute kidney injury. *Kidney Int* 2009;76(4):422–427.

10 Payen D, de Pont AC, Sakr Y, et al. A positive fluid balance is associated with a worse outcome in patients with acute renal failure. *Crit Care* 2008;12(3):R74.

11 McClellan JM, Goldstein RE, Erb HN, Dykes NL, Cowgill LD. Effects of administration of fluids and diuretics on glomerular filtration rate, renal blood flow, and urine output in healthy awake cats. *Am J Vet Res* 2006;67(4):715–722.

12 Boscan P, Pypendop BH, Siao KT, et al. Fluid balance, glomerular filtration rate, and urine output in dogs anesthetized for an orthopedic surgical procedure. *Am J Vet Res* 2010;71(5):501–507.

13 Shilliday IR, Quinn KJ, Allison ME. Loop diuretics in the management of acute renal failure: a prospective, double-blind, placebo-controlled, randomized study. *Nephrol Dial Transplant* 1997;12(12):2592–2596.

14 Mehta RL, Pascual MT, Soroko S, Chertow GM, PICARD Study Group. Diuretics, mortality, and nonrecovery of renal function in acute renal failure. *JAMA* 2002;288(20):2547–2553.

15 Kellum JA, Cerda J, Kaplan LJ, Nadim MK, Palevsky PM. Fluids for prevention and management of acute kidney injury. *Int J Artif Organs* 2008;31:96–110.

16 Abbott LM, Kovacic J. The pharmacologic spectrum of furosemide. *J Vet Emerg Crit Care* 2008;18(1):26–39.

17 Koyner JL, Davison DL, Brasha-Mitchell E, et al. Furosemide stress test and biomarkers for the prediction of AKI severity. *J Am Soc Nephrol* 2015;26(8):2023–2031.

18 Mehta RL, Cantarovich F, Shaw A, Hoste E, Murray P. Pharmacologic approaches for volume excess in acute kidney injury (AKI). *Int J Artif Organs* 2008;31:127–144.

19 Clarkson M, Friedewald J, Eustace J, Rabb H. Acute kidney injury. In: *The Kidney*, 8th edn (eds Brenner EBBM, Brenner BM, Levine S). Saunders Elsevier, Philadelphia, 2008, pp. 943–986.

20 Sigrist NE. Use of dopamine in acute renal failure. *J Vet Emerg Crit Care* 2007;17(2):117–126.

21 Simmons JP, Wohl JS, Schwartz DD, Edwards HG, Wright JC. Diuretic effects of fenoldopam in healthy cats. *J Vet Emerg Crit Care* 2006;16(2):96–103.

22 Kelly KL, Drobatz KJ, Foster JD. Effect of fenoldopam continuous infusion on glomerular filtration rate and fractional excretion of sodium in healthy dogs. *J Vet Intern Med* 2016;30(5):1655–1660.

23 Bloom CA, Labato MA, Hazarika S, Court MH. Preliminary pharmacokinetics and cardiovascular effects of fenoldopam continuous rate infusion in six healthy dogs. *J Vet Pharmacol Ther* 2012;35(3):224–230.

24 Nielsen LK, Bracker K, Price LL. Administration of fenoldopam in critically ill small animal patients with acute kidney injury: 28 dogs and 34 cats (2008–2012). *J Vet Emerg Crit Care* 2015;25(3):396–404.

25 Rodicio JL, Campo C, Ruilope LM. Renal effects of calcium antagonists. *Nephrol Dial Transplant* 1995;10 Suppl 9:17–22.

26 Mathews K, Montheith G. Evaluation of adding diltiazem therapy to standard treatment of acute renal failure caused by leptospirosis: 18 dogs (1998–2001). *J Vet Emerg Crit Care* 2007;12(2):149–158.

27 Cooper RL, Labato MA. Peritoneal dialysis in veterinary medicine. *Vet Clin North Am Small Anim Pract* 2011;41(1):91–113.

28 Bersenas AME. A clinical review of peritoneal dialysis. *J Vet Emerg Crit Care* 2011;21(6):605–617.

96

Urinary Tract Infections

Reid Groman, DVM, DACVIM, DACVECC

Mount Laurel Animal Hospital, Mount Laurel, NJ, USA

The therapy of uncomplicated urinary tract infections (UTIs) is exclusively antimicrobial, whereas successful treatment of complicated UTIs also includes identification and correction of predisposing conditions. Microscopic examination of appropriately stained urine sediment can be a valuable screening tool to support UTI in symptomatic patients. Fluoroquinolones and third-generation cephalosporins should not be routinely used for initial therapy of UTIs in small animals. Repeated treatment of animals without culture and susceptibility testing may lead to incorrect antimicrobial choices, unnecessary adverse effects of treatment, and possible selection of resistant bacterial populations.

Definition

A urinary tract infection (UTI) occurs when microbes, most commonly bacteria, adhere to, multiply and persist in the urinary tract [1–3]. UTIs are subdivided by anatomic site of involvement into lower UTI (cystitis) and upper UTI (pyelonephritis) [4,5]. Infections at these sites may occur together or independently, and may be subclinical or associated with a wide range of symptoms and clinicopathological findings in dogs and cats. Lower UTIs are generally superficial (or mucosal) infections whereas pyelonephritis and prostatitis signify tissue invasion.

Urinary tract infections can be further classified as simple or complicated infections in order to determine the extent of diagnostic testing, risk of recurrence, duration of treatment, prognosis, and requirements for follow-up evaluations in a given patient [1,3,4,6]. Simple UTIs involve the bladder and are typically initial or sporadic infections of the bladder with no concurrent disease or underlying structural or functional abnormalities (i.e. no compromise of host defense mechanisms). Complicated UTIs are associated with pyelonephritis,

prostatitis, concurrent systemic diseases and either systemic or local alterations in immunity that increase the risk of acquiring infection, or predispose to recurrent infection or treatment failure [3,4]. The majority of UTIs in dogs are simple (uncomplicated) and occur as a single episode [7].

While the stratification into "simple" and "complicated" has proven useful in human medicine, the applicability of this algorithm-based binary classification to UTIs to veterinary patients is less clear. Specifically, this classification scheme does not account for the diversity of "complicated" syndromes in veterinary patients. In companion animals, uncomplicated UTIs are by definition confined to the bladder, and uncomplicated or simple cystitis is a more relevant term. UTIs in intact male dogs are classified as complicated infections, since most have concurrent prostatic involvement. Recurrent UTIs (defined as three or more UTIs during a 12-month period) are classified as complicated infections, and any patient with an identifiable risk factor for UTI is considered to have a complicated infection [8]. Risk factors that predispose to UTI generally do so by compromising immune function, causing obstruction to urine flow, or by providing a nidus of infection that is not readily treated by antimicrobials (Table 96.1) [1,3].

The differentiation between UTI and non-pathogenic bacteriuria is becoming increasingly important because of the emergence of antimicrobial resistance among common uropathogens. Traditionally, the presence of bacteria in urine constituted evidence of infection, and the terms occult or silent UTI were used in veterinary medicine to indicate bacterial infection in the absence of clinical signs. However, bacteriuria does not indicate the presence of disease or potential for future disease. The term UTI implies not only that an organism multiplies in the urinary tract, but that it causes clinical disease [3].

Asymptomatic, or subclinical bacteriuria (SB) is a microbiological diagnosis, defined in the human literature

Textbook of Small Animal Emergency Medicine, First Edition. Edited by Kenneth J. Drobatz, Kate Hopper, Elizabeth Rozanski and Deborah C. Silverstein.
© 2019 John Wiley & Sons, Inc. Published 2019 by John Wiley & Sons, Inc.
Companion Website: www.wiley.com/go/drobatz/textbook

Table 96.1 Co-morbidities and risk factors that predispose patients to urinary tract infections.

Co-morbidity or risk factor	Examples
Anatomical abnormalities	Abnormal vulvar conformation (dogs)
	Ectopic ureters
	Uroepithelial neoplasia
	Cystic diverticulum
Systemic disorders	Diabetes mellitus
	Hyperadrenocorticism (dogs)
	Hyperthyroidism (cats)
Medication causing immunosuppression	Chemotherapeutic agents
	Corticosteroids, cyclosporine
Urinary tract disorders	Chronic kidney disease
	Urolithiasis
	Obstruction (structural, e.g. mass/stones, or functional, e.g. neurogenic urinary retention)
Urinary incontinence	Neurogenic bladder (thoracolumbar myelopathy)
	Urethral sphincter mechanism incompetency
Miscellaneous	Previous urethrostomy (especially cats)
	Cystostomy or nephrostomy urinary diversion
	Urinary instrumentation
	Urinary catheterization

as the isolation of bacteria in urine from an appropriately collected urine specimen obtained from a person without symptoms or signs referable to the urinary tract. In human medicine, SB is usually transient and does not require antibiotic therapy. SB is increasingly recognized in diverse populations of dogs and cats, although the significance of a positive urine culture in dogs and cats without overt clinical signs of infection remains unclear. Diseases or conditions commonly associated with SB include glucocorticoid excess, diabetes mellitus, obesity (dogs), hyperthyroidism (cats), chronic kidney disease, and presence of indwelling urinary catheters [1,2,6].

Incidence and Pathogenesis

Urinary tract infections are reported to occur commonly in dogs [1]. The true incidence is difficult to determine, largely because criteria for defining UTI differ among sources [9]. Spayed female dogs are more susceptible to UTIs than castrated male dogs and intact female dogs. UTIs are least commonly found in intact males. UTIs can occur in dogs at any age, but are more common in older dogs [1,10].

In contrast to dogs, bacterial UTIs are relatively rare in cats [1,9]. Young healthy cats have an innate resistance and rarely develop UTIs. Most young cats with lower urinary tract signs have disorders such as idiopathic cystitis or bladder stones, which are generally not associated with bacterial infection [1,11]. UTIs most often occur in older cats (>10 years) and the incidence increases with age [1,2,10,12]. Common metabolic diseases in cats, such as diabetes mellitus, hyperthyroidism and chronic kidney disease (CKD), or other co-morbidities, are often present at the time of diagnosis [2,11–13]. It is likely that cats with DM and CKD have impaired host defense mechanisms that allow colonization of bacteria in the urinary tract, although the exact reasons why cats with these disorders appear predisposed are unclear. As in dogs, the exact prevalence of UTI in cats is difficult to determine, because the inclusion criteria for establishing diagnosis of UTI vary between investigators [11].

The bacteria that most commonly cause UTIs are similar in dogs and cats [5,11]. Although UTIs can comprise mixed bacterial infections, most involve a single bacterial species [1,2,5,7]. *E. coli* infections are most common, accounting for one-third to one-half of all positive urine cultures [1,7]. Other relatively common genera are *Staphylococcus* spp, *Enterococcus* spp, *Proteus* spp, *Streptococcus* spp, and *Klebsiella* spp [1,2]. Cats appear to be infected with a unique staphylococcal strain, *Staphylococcus felis* [1,5]. *S. felis* is a normal commensal organism, but the high prevalence of *S. felis*-positive UTIs suggests that it is a common feline urinary tract pathogen [11].

Commercial phenotypic identification systems may not differentiate *S. felis* from other coagulase-negative *Staphylococcus* spp [5]. Gram-negative rods, including *Enterobacter* spp and *Pseudomonas* spp, assume increasing importance in recurrent and nosocomial UTIs [3,7,8]. Canine infections with *Staphylococcus*, *Proteus*, and *Corynebacterium* spp are often associated with formation of struvite calculi due to alkalinization of urine by urea metabolism by these organisms [1].

Primary fungal infections occur uncommonly in dogs and cats. Periodic infection with *Candida* spp is reported in animals that receive chronic antibiotics or are immunocompromised. The causative role of several more unusual pathogens, including *Mycoplasma* spp and *Ureaplasma* spp, remains poorly defined [1,5].

The urinary tract may be viewed as a single anatomic unit that is united by a continuous column of urine extending from the urethra to the kidney. In the vast majority of UTIs, enteric organisms residing in the bowel gain access to the urethra after colonizing the perineum and external genitalia [1,2,14]. The female urethra is particularly prone to colonization owing to its short length and proximity to the anus, and female dogs and cats are at increased risk for UTI. Ascent of bacteria from the bladder may follow and is the most common pathway for most renal infections in both dogs and cats [1,5]. Hematogenous spread is uncommon. Whether bladder infection ensues depends on the interacting effects of the pathogenicity of the strain, the inoculum size, and local and systemic host defenses [2]. Under normal circumstances, bacteria that gain access to the bladder are rapidly cleared, partly due to micturition and dilutional effects of voiding, but also as a result of antibacterial properties of urine and the bladder mucosa [1,2]. Owing mostly to high osmolality and and high urea concentration, the urine of dogs and cats inhibits bacterial growth [11]. Mucosal secretions such as immunoglobulin and glycosaminoglycan prevent the adherence of uropathogens to epithelium [1]. In male dogs, prostatic secretions possess antibacterial properties as well.

Escherichia coli is the most common pathogen associated with simple and complicated UTIs in dogs and cats [1]. Not all *E. coli* strains are equally capable of infecting the healthy urinary tract, and many strains that cause uncomplicated UTIs belong to a small number of uropathogenic subgroups that have a selective advantage for colonization and infection [11]. Uropathogenic *E. coli* (UPEC) is a specific subset of pathogenic extraintestinal *E. coli* that has the potential for enhanced virulence. Genes encoding virulence factors, including fimbriae, flagella, adhesins, siderophores, toxins and polysaccharide coatings, have been identified in canine and feline UPEC strains. Bacterial virulence factors enable bacteria to subvert host defenses, facilitate microbial entry into host tissue, and can markedly influence whether a given strain, once introduced into the bladder, will cause UTI. UPEC virulence determinants are thought to be less significant in the pathogenesis of complicated UTIs [15]. However, complicated UTIs often have a wider range of associated pathogens.

Less is known about the pathogenicity of other bacteria. Several uropathogens, including *Staphylococcus* spp, *Proteus* spp and *Corynebacterium* spp, possess high urease activity. The resultant cleavage of urea to ammonia is not only irritating to the bladder mucosa but increases urine pH and promotes crystalluria (dogs and cats) and struvite stone formation (dogs) [1].

Fungal UTIs are rare in dogs and cats, and generally occur in patients with altered host defense mechanisms [2,16]. Concurrent bacterial infection is common in animals with fungal UTIs and clinical signs are indistinguishable from bacterial UTIs [1]. If fungal elements are identified on urine sediment, fungal culture should be performed to identify the infecting species. Primary fungal UTIs are most commonly caused by *Candida* spp. Other ubiquitous fungi, including *Aspergillus* spp and *Cryptococcus* spp, occasionally cause UTIs in dogs and cats, respectively [2,16].

The organisms and predisposing causes of pyelonephritis are similar to those of lower UTIs [5]. Any impediment to normal flow of urine from the renal pelvis to the bladder, such as obstruction, ureteroliths, or any condition that may promote reflux of urine from the bladder into the ureters may contribute to the development of pyelonephritis [5]. In many instances, however, an underlying cause is not identified. Acute prostatitis is typically due to the same array of pathogens causing other UTIs, with *E. coli* being most common. *Brucella canis* should be considered as a cause of both acute and chronic prostatitis [5].

History and Physical Examination

Patient history and clinical signs of simple cystitis/lower UTI are those of lower urinary tract inflammation or irritative voiding. Clinical history may include varying degrees of pollakiuria, dysuria, and inappropriate urination [5]. Stranguria may persist after the bladder is empty, presumably from inflammation-induced detrusor hyperactivity or urethritis [2]. The bladder and proximal urethra are in close proximity so that inflammation in one is thought to affect the other and passage of urine may elicit discomfort. Primary infectious urethral disorders are rare in both dogs and cats, but when inflammation is confined to the urethra, the pain associated with voiding may cause some animals to retain urine and not fully empty their bladder. Hematuria, "cloudy" urine, or an offensive ammonia-like odor often prompt owners to seek veterinary attention. If a UTI is associated with an underlying or concurrent disorder (e.g. diabetes mellitus, hyperadrenocorticism), history and clinical signs of that condition may predominate [2].

Patients with lower UTI may exhibit mild sensitivity to bladder palpation but physical examination findings are otherwise unremarkable [2]. When lower UTIs are recurrent or long standing, bladder wall thickening and tenderness may be appreciated. Fever is an uncommon finding in patients with simple UTIs. Rectal examination should be performed in all dogs with signs of lower urinary tract disease to evaluate for urethral stones and irregularities. The urethra may be prominent with severe urethritis, or thickened in cases of urethral neoplasia. Rectal examination in male dogs may disclose pain and prostatomegaly. Inspection of external genitalia should be performed in all patients with suspected or confirmed UTI. Female dogs should be examined for vulvar recession/hypoplasia and regional pyoderma [2]. When possible, digital vaginal examination should be performed to identify vestibulovaginal abnormalities in dogs that may predispose to infection. In male dogs, the prepuce, ostium, glans, and meatus should be examined for discharge, foreign material, or mass lesions. Similar detailed evaluations are seldom possible in cats.

Acute or acute-on-chronic pyelonephritis is commonly associated with non-specific signs of severe systemic illness such as lethargy, anorexia, and vomiting [5]. Polyuria and polydipsia may occur despite minimal nephron damage owing to inhibition of antidiuretic hormone activity in the renal tubules [5]. Hematuria and signs of cystitis may or may not be present. With acute infection, physical examination often reveals dehydration, fever, renomegaly, and dorsal abdominal or lumbar tenderness.

Prostatitis should be suspected in any intact male dog with UTI. Dogs with acute prostatitis often have lower urinary tract signs as well as hemorrhagic or purulent urethral discharge, stiff gait and abdominal pain [5]. Tenesmus may occur if the enlarged prostate compresses the distal colon. Depression, diarrhea, and dehydration occur commonly. Rectal examination may reveal an enlarged, asymmetric painful prostate. Most dogs with prostatitis also have bacterial cystitis. Bacterial prostatitis is rarely identified in domestic cats.

Diagnosis

The diagnostic evaluation of a patient with suspected simple cystitis is the approach for any patient with lower urinary tract signs. The extent of diagnostic work-up varies depending on severity of illness, history of prior infection, and presence of co-morbidities. Although clinical signs are non-specific, a provisional diagnosis of simple cystitis is often made based on historical information and physical examination findings. Survey abdominal radiographs may reveal concurrent abnormalities that alter urinary tract immunity, including stones, masses or changes in renal size [10]. Simple cystitis does not generally result in changes to routine laboratory studies, and routine bloodwork is seldom helpful [10].

Challenges to evaluating and managing UTIs in the acute care setting often include limited history, lack of longitudinal follow-up, and lack of microbiological information. Urine culture is the gold standard for confirming bacterial infection in patients with clinical signs [3]. Final results are often not available for several days. In-house screening techniques provide timely results and are critical when investigating for the presence of infection [17]. Complete urinalysis is performed in all patients with suspected UTI, and includes measurement of urine specific gravity and microscopic examination of sediment, in addition to routine biochemical evaluation of urine supernatant with a commercially available reagent strip (dipstick) [1,3,10,12]. In human healthcare, the reagent strip (dipstick) is a useful screening test for UTI, where it is routinely used to detect pyuria and bacteriuria. In veterinary patients, the predictive ability of reagent pads is generally poor, and the urine dipstick does not have a prominent role in the diagnosis of UTI in dogs and cats. Leukocyte (WBC) and nitrite (bacteria) test pads are not reliable in dogs and cats [10]. Many dogs and cats with UTIs will have non-specific changes to urine test pads, including qualitative proteinuria and microscopic hematuria [3,10]. Positive results for glucose or bilirubin may indicate the presence of diseases outside the urinary tract.

Alkaline urine in association with UTI suggests infection with a urease-producing agent such as *Proteus* and *Staphylococcus* spp. *E. coli* is the most common agent causing UTIs and urine pH is often acidic with *E. coli* infections. Most healthy dogs and cats have relatively acidic urine, and pH is not always predictive of infection or the causative pathogen, particularly when pH is determined on a reagent strip and not a pH meter. Urine specific gravity is variable in dogs and cats with UTIs. Dilute or minimally concentrated urine may be identified in patients with concurrent diseases predisposing to UTI (e.g. diabetes mellitus, hyperadrenocorticism) or in patients with impaired renal concentrating ability (e.g. CKD).

Microscopic examination of urine from symptomatic patients is often useful as a rapid albeit imperfect screening tool to support a diagnosis of UTI [3,17,18]. Urine for routine sediment examination is prepared by placing a coverslip over a small drop of resuspended sediment on a glass slide, followed by prompt examination. Sediment findings that suggest UTI are white blood cells (WBCs) (pyuria), red blood cells (RBCs) (hematuria), and bacteriuria [10,16]. Although increased numbers of RBCs are often observed with UTI, hematuria (>5 RBC/high-power field) may also result from non-infectious causes such as interstitial cystitis, neoplasia or urinary calculi. Pyuria (>5 neutrophils/high-power field) is documented in some but not all patients with UTI [1,3,17].

Several non-infectious disorders, including obstruction, calculi and epithelial neoplasia, can cause inflammation and clinical signs of lower urinary tract inflammation [2]. The inflammatory response is often dampened in disorders that impair host defenses, such as diabetes mellitus, hyperadrenocorticism, and feline leukemia virus [1,2,10,16,17]. Thus, the presence of white blood cells in any number should not be used as a criterion for the presence or absence of infection.

In addition to cells, infectious elements are often identified [17,18]. Results of sediment findings have limitations and can yield discordant results [1,17–19]. False-positive results (i.e. bacteria observed in a sample with a negative urine culture) occur as a result of misidentification of amorphous debris as pathogens, or the presence of non-viable organisms. False negatives (i.e. no bacteria observed but positive urine culture) are common, particularly when bacteria are present in low numbers [17]. Examination of air-dried urine sediment stained with modified Wright stain (e.g. Diff Quik) is more sensitive and specific for detection of bacteria compared to routine wet-mount sediment evaluation [1,16]. The procedure is simple, and should be a component of routine microscopic evaluations. Gram staining of air-dried sediment further improves accuracy for identifying bacteria [1,2,10,18]. An additional advantage of gram staining is its ability to identify bacteria as gram negative or gram positive, since gram-staining characteristics may help narrow differentials and allow for improved empirical antibiotic selection [18]. The observation of bacteria and pyuria in patients with clinical signs of lower urinary tract disease is indicative of active inflammation associated with infection.

Not all bacteria are pathogenic, and the significance of bacteriuria in dogs and cats without clinical history and signs of infection remains unclear [3,10,20]. Identification of fungal elements in sediment is diagnostic for fungal UTI [10]. *Candida* spp are responsible for most fungal UTIs [2]. Most pathogenic yeasts grow on blood agar plates that support bacterial growth. Thus, separate submission of urine for fungal culture is not always indicated. Selective fungal media is more useful for rare instances in which there is a high probability that a UTI is caused by a more fastidious yeast or mold.

Urine is most often collected from dogs and cats by cystocentesis, since any observed cytological abnormalities or infectious agents likely originate in the bladder (or kidneys), and not the urethra or periurethral tissues [3]. Catheterized samples using aseptic technique are acceptable for interpretation of urinalysis and urine microscopy. However, infectious elements from the urethra may be introduced as the catheter advances. The examination of voided samples is generally discouraged, but it is not a pointless endeavor. While not ideal, midstream voided urine is often satisfactory for the initial evaluation of urinary disorders, and for screening purposes. Bacterial contamination from the urethra in voided samples usually does not result in enough organisms to be visualized microscopically. Nothing is gained by collecting urine by a more invasive method if microscopic findings of a voided sample are normal. Manual bladder expression should be avoided, as it can cause unnecessary bladder trauma, and increased hydrostatic pressure in the bladder may propel infectious elements into the ureters and kidneys.

A quantitative bacterial urine culture, from urine obtained by cystocentesis, confirms the presence of infection in dogs and cats with signs of lower urinary tract disease, and to identify resistant bacteria that may not respond to initial therapy [3,7]. Cystocentesis is considered the gold standard against which results using either voided or catheterized samples are compared. A quantitative urine culture includes identification of the organism and determination of the number of organisms.

The concept of relevant or significant bacteriuria was introduced to differentiate between bacterial contamination and infection, and quantitation of the number of bacteria in colony forming units/volume (cfu/mL) is standard when reporting urine culture results. It is recognized that low but variable numbers of commensal flora are occasionally identified by culture, and significant bacteriuria is the number inferred to define clinically relevant infection [2,6,21]. General guidelines based on quantitative bacterial counts and method of collection (cystocentesis, voided, catheter) are published for small animals, but there is limited evidence to support proposed veterinary "cut-off" values [3,22]. Whether colony counts are relevant in animals is unclear, and accurate interpretation of culture results must also rely on clinical information [3]. While the recovery of a single organism at $>10^4$ cfu/mL is proposed as a cut-off for significant bacteriuria, it is possible that lower counts may represent "significant" infection in patients with appropriate clinical signs. Conversely, the presence of $>10^4$ cfu/mL bacteria in a urine sample obtained by cystocentesis from an asymptomatic patient may signify transient colonization or subclinical bacteriuria, and skepticism is warranted before concluding that UTI is present [10]. Any amount of bacterial growth is significant in urine obtained by cystocentesis, particularly when signs of lower urinary tract disease are present. Midstream voided urine is least desirable for purposes of sampling urine for culture in dogs and cats [3,10,21].

Urine should be submitted in sterile tubes that do not contain additives [10]. To avoid false-positive and false-negative results, immediate culture after collection of a urine specimen is recommended [10]. Longer delays are often unavoidable, and samples should be refrigerated within 1 hour of collection and processed as soon as possible. Commercially available urine culture collection tubes containing preservative may be used to preserve refrigerated specimens for up to 72 hours. Culture swabs allow drying of liquid specimens and loss of viability and are not intended for submitting urine cultures. Further, culture swabs do not permit bacterial enumeration and are thus not suitable for submission of urine for quantitative culture.

Most veterinary diagnostic laboratories classify an organism as susceptible, intermediate, or resistant according to Clinical and Laboratory Standards Institutes (CLSI) recommendations for serum breakpoints. Most antimicrobials are eliminated through the kidneys, and attain higher concentrations in the urine than serum as long as renal function is normal. Therefore, a higher rate of susceptibility among isolates could be predicted if traditional (urinary) breakpoints are applied. Some investigators propose using urinary breakpoints for simple UTIs, whereas serum breakpoints are preferred for complicated UTIs and pyelonephritis [8]. Using urinary breakpoints for simple UTIs may be problematic if a pathogen invades the bladder wall, in which case tissue (i.e. serum) and not urine drug concentration is relevant Microbiology results could lead to ineffective or inappropriate therapy, and possible recurrent infection, in this example. Veterinary-specific urinary breakpoints have been developed for only a small number of currently available drugs, and the Antimicrobial Guidelines Working Group of the International Society of Companion Animal Infectious Diseases (ISCAID) recommends using serum interpretive criteria for UTIs [3].

In-clinic urine cultures allow immediate processing of urine and may decrease cost to owners by allowing veterinarians to select only positive samples for species identification by external laboratories. However, bacterial isolation should only be attempted in clinics with appropriate facilities, proper biosafety containment and waste management, and trained staff [3].

Point-of-care testing can reduce both turnround time and costs, and may serve as a bridge between urinalysis and urine culture. The Uricult Veterinary System™ is an in-house diagnostic test that identifies clinically relevant bacterial growth in canine and feline urine samples [13]. Although suitable as a screening test for UTIs, this test is not widely utilized in private practices. More recently, a point-of-care test that allows for the semi-quantitative

enumeration of bacteria in urine, presumptive identification of pathogens, and prediction of antimicrobial susceptibility after overnight incubation has been optimized for use in veterinary patients. The Flexicult Vet™ was found to be sensitive and specific for detection of bacteriuria in dogs and cats, and may have a role as a timely and cost-effective point-of-care test to guide antimicrobial therapy [9].

The role of in-house methods for the timely detection of bacteriuria and antimicrobial susceptibilities remains to be defined in veterinary medicine. If cost-effectiveness and diagnostic utility are corroborated by further studies, such tests could also represent a valuable approach to overcoming problems related to storage and transport of urine samples for culture.

While limited diagnostics are generally performed in patients with simple cystitis, patients with complicated infections and those with suspected prostatitis or pyelonephritis require more extensive evaluations, including urinalysis, urine culture, complete blood count, serum biochemical profile, and diagnostic imaging to evaluate for the presence of systemic inflammation, azotemia, concurrent illness and predisposing structural or systemic conditions that impair host immune defenses. Leukocytosis is a common finding with pyelonephritis. Azotemia may be present if both kidneys are affected, or if unilateral pyelonephritis occurs in a patient with pre-existing renal disease. If survey radiographs are unremarkable and a predisposing cause for infection is suspected, abdominal sonography is indicated. Contrast studies may be indicated to investigate for anatomic defects. Evaluation of endocrine function is indicated if suggested by presentation, such as measurement of serum thyroid hormone in an older cat with weight loss and polyphagia. There are no reliable methods to clinically distinguish renal pareynchymal infections from lower UTIs.

The diagnosis of pyelonephritis is generally based on clinical signs, laboratory studies (e.g. leukocytosis, azotemia), radiographic (e.g. renomegaly) and/or sonographic (e.g. pyelectasia) abnormalities. A positive culture of urine sampled from the renal pelvis confirms renal involvement, but pyelocentesis is seldom indicated. Similarly, sampling of prostatic fluid for culture is not usually warranted, or performed for acute infections. It is generally assumed that the causative pathogen will be identified in urine appropriately sampled from the urinary bladder [16].

Therapy

Successful antimicrobial therapy consists of avoidance of antimicrobials when appropriate, and when antimicrobials are indicated for UTI, optimizing the selection, dosing, route of administration, and duration of therapy [3,23]. Antibiotics are indicated to limit the spread of infection and alleviate pain. While selecting an antibiotic based on susceptibility information is ideal, therapy is often initiated on the basis of history, clinical signs, and urine sediment findings, and not withheld until culture results are available, particularly for patients in obvious discomfort. Important considerations for treating all UTIs include location of infection, history of antibiotic use, presence of complicating factors or concurrent illness, risk of adverse effects, and cost [10]. Most first-time UTIs are due to one of a limited number of common uropathogens with predictable antimicrobial susceptibilities. While susceptibility patterns can vary over time and regionally, local prevalence data are rarely available to most clinicians.

In addition to other patient variables, the decision to initiate therapy and select initial empirical antimicrobial(s) can often be guided by microscopic examination of urine sediment. When present in sufficient numbers, recognition of bacteria is often possible on standard wet-mount preparations of urine sediment, and modified Wright staining of dried sediment increases the likelihood of identifying bacteria. Recognition of bacterial morphology, particularly if gram staining is performed, affords clinicians an opportunity to make an educated guess about the type of organism present and a reasonable first-choice antibiotic [2]. Microscopic observations are often most useful when interpreted along with urinalysis and in tje context of history and clinical findings. For instance, *E. coli*, the most prevalent uropathogen in dogs and cats, is a gram-negative rod often associated with aciduria [2]. The identification of gram-positive cocci forming doublets or clusters suggests infection with enterococci or staphylococci. Occasionally, streptococci are observed lining up and forming long chains. Alkaline urine suggests possible infection with a urease-producing organism, with staphylococci (cocci) and *Proteus* spp (rods) being the most prevalent urease-producing bacteria causing UTIs in dogs and cats [2].

The most comprehensive source of information for management of UTIs in dogs and cats was developed by the Antimicrobial Guidelines Working Group of the International Society for Companion Animal Infections Diseases (ISCAID) and published in 2011 [3]. These guidelines, based on literature reviews, microbiological data and expert opinion, provide a detailed series of recommendations for the diagnosis and management of UTIs in dogs and cats, and most suggestions for therapy in this chapter are in line with them.

While the spectrum of micro-organisms causing UTIs is largely unchanged, patterns of resistance can change over time, and relevant companion animal-specific clinical reports and research studies have been published

since 2011. Further, it was recognized that present algorithms for subdividing UTIs in veterinary medicine, based on classification of UTIs in humans, could not easily be applied to define naturally occurring syndromes in both dogs and cats, and the process of revising the 2011 guidelines was initiated in 2015. Revised guidelines are not yet published, but will expand on information in current guidelines in both scope and depth. Treatment recommendations and definitions will likely supplant those in the 2011 version. Importantly, guidelines are intended to educate veterinarians about appropriate management of UTIs in dogs and cats, and recommendations for therapy should not be inferred to represent a standard of care, or to replace clinical judgment.

The microbiology of simple cystitis is generally limited to a relatively small number of bacteria, and guidelines for empiric therapy are based on the limited predictable spectrum of the most common etiological organisms [2,3]. Susceptibility patterns may exhibit regional differences, and can change over time. Updated regional antimicrobial surveillance data in dogs and cats would be useful to supplement therapeutic guidelines, but this information is generally not available [1,3,8]. Although urine culture is the reference standard for confirming the diagnosis of UTI, it provides no immediate diagnostic utility in the acute care setting. Urine microscopy is often sufficient, and many patients with simple cystitis are successfully managed without the benefit of pretreatment culture results. For example, if an otherwise healthy adult female dog develops acute clinical signs, and there is microscopic evidence to support infection, urine culture may be omitted and treatment initiated with an empirically selected antimicrobial. If there is no improvement after 48 hours of therapy, additional investigations, including urine culture, are required to determine the etiological agent and to exclude non-infectious causes [1,3]. Urine culture should always be performed in patients with recurrent clinical signs, history of recent antimicrobial use, and known or suspected risk factors for infection [2,3,8,24].

Clinical practice guidelines support the use of targeted, narrow-spectrum "first-line" antimicrobials for initial empiric therapy of simple cystitis [3]. However, practitioners commonly prescribe more familiar, typically broad-spectrum "second-line" drugs for simple infections even though narrower-spectrum and more cost-effective options are available. While many of these drugs (fluoroquinolones, third-generation cephalosporins) have a proven track record in treating infections, their spectrum and potency are not required for initial therapy of most first-time or sporadic UTIs [14,16].

Appropriate antimicrobial therapy optimizes clinical and microbiological cure and limits the possibility of acquiring infection with a resistant pathogen. ISCAID guidelines emphasize the importance of considering ecological adverse effects of antimicrobial agents (i.e. development of resistance to other antibiotics – so-called "collateral damage") along with drug effectiveness when selecting therapy. Initial use of a first-line agent minimizes the selection for antimicrobial-resistant organisms colonizing or infecting the urinary tract of the individual patient, whereas overuse of broader spectrum antimicrobials promotes antimicrobial resistance in the general population [8]. Particularly concerning in veterinary medicine is the increasing resistance to amoxicillin-clavulanic acid, fluoroquinolones, and third-generation cephalosporins, and the parallel development of co-resistance to other antibiotics [8,23,24].

Suggested first-line agents for simple cystitis in dogs include amoxicillin, cephalexin, and TMP/S (trimethoprim-sulfamethoxazole or trimethoprim-sulfadiazine) (Table 96.2) [2,3,7,16]. Amoxicillin is bactericidal and relatively non-toxic, with a spectrum of antibacterial activity greater than that of natural penicillins. Amoxicillin retains activity against streptococci, enterococci, and *Proteus*, and often achieves urinary concentrations high enough to be effective against staphylococci, and wild-type strains of *E. coli* and *Klebsiella*. Amoxicillin is a weak acid with a low volume of distribution, so therapeutic concentrations in renal and prostatic tissues are not often achieved. Amoxicillin, like most antimicrobials,

Table 96.2 Recommended antimicrobials for treating urinary tract infections.

Drug	Dose	Comments
Amoxicillin	11–15 mg/kg PO q12h	Suggested first-line therapy in dogs and cats
Amoxicillin-clavulanic acid	Dogs: 12.5–20 mg/kg PO q12h Cats: 62.5 mg/cat PO q12h	
Cephalexin	15–30 mg/kg PO q8–12h	Enterococci are resistant
Cefovecin	Dogs: 8 mg/kg SC q14 days	Appropriate for resistant infections and/or when oral treatment is problematic. Pharmacokinetic data support use in cats q21 days
Cefpodoxime	Dogs: 5–10 mg/kg PO q24h Cats: No dose established	Enterococci are resistant
Ceftiofur	Dogs: 2.2–4.4 mg/kg SC injection q24h Cats: No dose established	Enterococci are resistant
Ciprofloxacin	Dogs: 30 mg/kg PO q24h	Lower and more variable oral bioavailability than veterinary-approved fluoroquinolones. Difficult to justify use over approved fluoroquinolones. Dosing recommendations are empirical
Enrofloxacin	Dogs: 5–20 mg/kg PO/IM/IV q24h Cats: 5 mg/kg PO/IM/IV q24h	Reserved for documented resistant UTIs. Associated with retinopathy in cats at higher doses
Marbofloxacin	2.7–5.5 mg/kg PO q24h	Reserved for infections resistant to first-line antimicrobials. Not recommended for enterococci
Orbifloxacin	Tablets: 2.5–7.5 mg/kg PO q24h Oral suspension (cats): 7.5 mg/kg PO q24h	Reserved for documented resistant infections
Trimethoprim/sulfadiazine Trimethroprim/sulfamethoxazole	15 mg/kg PO/IV/SC q12h	Idiosyncratic and immune-mediated reactions reported in dogs. Initial and periodic monitoring of tear production recommended. Avoid in dogs of Doberman pinscher lineage. Hypersalivation and nausea common in cats. Not effective for enterococci
Pradofloxacin	Dogs: 3–5 mg/kg PO q24h Cats: 3–5 mg/kg PO q24h (tablets) Cats: 5–7.5 mg/kg PO q24h (suspension)	Reserved for documented resistant infections. Greater activity against some pathogens than other fluoroquinolones
Chloramphenicol	Dogs: 30–40 mg/kg PO/IV q8h Cats: 10–15 mg/kg PO/IV q12h (50 mg/cat q12h)	Reserved for multidrug-resistant infections. Avoid contact by humans (idiosyncratic bone marrow aplasia)

IM, intramuscular; IV, intravenous; PO, by mouth (*per os*); SC, subcutaneous.

achieves very high urine concentrations, such that urinary tract sterility is often possible when it appears that the drug would fail to do so based on concentrations achieved in plasma. For example, the majority of urinary *Staphylococcus pseudintermedius* produce beta-lactamase, and isolates are often reported to be resistant to amoxicillin yet lower UTIs due to these organisms are often successfully treated with amoxicillin, as a result of high concentration of active drug in urine. This is not inferred to mean that amoxicillin is appropriate therapy for such infections. Urinary staphylococci are becoming increasingly resistant to aminopenicillins, and initial therapy with a beta-lactamase stable antimicrobial (e.g. cephalexin, amoxicillin-clavulanic acid) should be chosen when staphylococci are suspected or preliminarily identified [7].

Amoxicillin-clavulanic acid is familiar to most veterinarians and approved for the treatment of UTIs. It has a spectrum of activity against gram-negative bacteria, often including *Proteus* and *Klebsiella* spp that are generally resistant to amoxicillin, and it is usually effective against beta-lactamase-producing staphylococci. It is a reasonable choice for initial therapy of simple cystitis, particularly when staphylococci are suspected. However, current ISCAID guidelines suggest that amoxicillin-clavulanic acid should not be included among first-line agents, because the need for clavulanic acid has not been demonstrated, and to encourage use of more narrow-spectrum agents when possible [3]. Clavulanic acid undergoes some hepatic metabolism and excretion, and the antimicrobial activity of amoxicillin-clavulanic acid against bladder pathogens is due in part to the high concentrations of amoxicillin achieved in urine.

Potentiated sulfonamides (TMP/S) are active against most urinary *E. coli* isolates in dogs and cats, and their spectrum often encompasses other gram-negative enteric pathogens and many veterinary staphylococci. All enterococci are resistant to TMP/S, despite information indicating otherwise in culture reports. While initial therapy with TMP/S is "microbiologically sound," the potential for infrequent but well-described adverse drug reactions has reduced the attractiveness of TMP/S for routine empirical use [23]. The routine clinical use of potentiated sulfonamides is limited by the potential for hypersensitivity reactions that include blood dyscrasias, hepatotoxicity, polyarthropathy and skin eruptions, as well as idiosyncratic events, such as keratoconjunctivitis sicca (KCS). TMP/S is most often prescribed to dogs without incident [1] but clients should be appropriately educated about potential toxicities. Normal hepatic function as assessed by routine liver chemistries and adequate tear production should be documented prior to initiating therapy in all dogs. Tear production should be monitored during therapy with TMP/S, especially in

small dog breeds [1]. TMP/S should not be used in dogs of Doberman pinscher lineage, due to increased incidence of adverse reactions in these breeds. Sulfonamide hypersensitivity reactions occur > 5 days after beginning therapy, and short courses of TMP/S may be effective and safe in some dogs with simple cystitis [23].

TMP/S is also suggested for initial therapy of UTIs in cats. However, hypersalivation and anorexia are frequently observed following oral administration, making it difficult to support recommendations for routine use in cats. If TMP/S therapy is indicated based on culture information or clinical judgment, oral administration in capsule (but not liquid) formulation or by subcutaneous injection may obviate objectionable acute events. Injectable trimethoprim/sulfadiazine (Tribrissen 24%™) is available outside the USA and approved for use in companion animals.

Cephalexin, a first-generation cephalosporin, is generally active against gram-positive and some gram-negative bacteria in the urinary tract. Some but not all sources support the use of cephalexin for initial empiric therapy of UTIs (see Table 96.2) [1]. Cephalexin is often effective for simple cystitis due to streptococci and beta-lactamase-producing staphylococci. Activity against Enterobacteriaceae, including *E. coli*, is less predictable compared with other first-line antimicrobials, and (as with all cephalosporins) enterococci are resistant to cephalexin [1]. Cephalexin is not effective for renal or prostatic infections.

The use of potentiated beta-lactams (amoxicillin-clavulanic acid), oral (cefpodoxime) and extended-release injectable (cefovicin) third-generation cephalosporins for initial therapy is generally discouraged. While these drugs exhibit activity against most aerobic pathogens associated with UTIs in dogs and cats, their use should be reserved for complicated and/or recurrent infections, and optimally, as indicated by culture and susceptibility data [2]. Fluoroquinolones also cover most expected pathogens and achieve high levels in urine. Resistance is increasing in dogs and cats at a rapid pace and has limited the usefulness of this class of drugs in veterinary medicine [2,16]. The use of fluoroquinolones for empiric therapy of simple cystitis is discouraged. Their use should be reserved for complicated UTIs and systemic infections.

While simple cystitis is by far the most common UTI in dogs, simple or "primary" UTIs are uncommon in cats [9,12]. Most young cats with lower urinary tract disease have idiopathic cystitis, which is generally not infectious, and the reflex action to associate irritative voiding and hematuria with a treatable infection and prescribe antimicrobial therapy without further evaluation in young cats is thus inappropriate. In older cats, UTIs (based on positive urine culture alone) are frequently documented in cats with one or more common endocrine diseases, yet only a small percentage of bacteriuric cats have histories or clinical signs supportive of lower urinary tract disease. For cats especially, the need for antibiotic therapy must be assessed before selecting or prescribing any agent.

While ISCAID guidelines recommend the same antimicrobials for initial empiric therapy of UTIs in dogs and cats (including amoxicillin and TMP/S), there is comparatively less information available to guide empiric therapy of UTI in cats. Amoxicillin is appropriate initial therapy for feline cystitis, especially when caused by gram-positive organisms [3,12]. Because the susceptibility of *E. coli* to aminopenicillins in cats is increasingly unpredictable, amoxicillin-clavulanic acid has been suggested for initial therapy of gram-negative infections, such as when rods are observed in urine sediment [9,10]. Currently, amoxicillin retains activity against many wild-type strains of common gram-negative uropathogens. It is still a suitable first-line agent in cats, considering its lower cost, narrow (targeted) spectrum, and reduced tendency to cause adverse gastrointestinal effects when compared to amoxicillin-clavulanic acid [11,19].

Simple cystitis in dogs is typically treated for 7–14 days, although the optimal duration of antimicrobial therapy has not been systematically studied [3]. Short-duration antimicrobial therapy is standard treatment for cystitis in women, and it is likely that both microbiological and clinical cures can be achieved with shorter courses of therapy in some dogs [5]. A multicenter clinical trial showed that a 3-day course of oral enrofloxacin dosed at 20 mg/kg/day showed comparable efficacy to conventional therapy with 2 weeks of amoxicillin-clavulanic acid in dogs with simple cystitis [25]. A more recent study compared 3 days of therapy with TMP/S to 10 days of cephalexin for treating simple cystitis in female dogs [23]. Both regimens were effective, with similar eradication rates following therapy. Advantages of short-term therapy include fewer adverse events, lower cost, decreased antimicrobial resistance, and better owner compliance. Appropriate duration of therapy for first-time UTIs is not well studied in cats, and recommendations vary. Since many cats with lower UTIs have concurrent systemic disease or other predisposing factors for "complicated" infection, it is recommended that all UTIs in cats, including initial occurrence of cystitis, be treated for at least 21 days. Further research is required to determine the optimal duration of antimicrobial therapy for initial UTIs in both dogs and cats.

Resolution of clinical signs is usually used as a marker for successful treatment of simple cystitis, particularly in female dogs. Clinical signs usually resolve within 48 hours after initiating therapy. Urinalysis results generally improve over a similar time frame, although posttreatment urinalysis and culture are generally not performed in the absence of clinical signs [3]. When patients with simple cystitis do not improve after 48 hours with an initially chosen antimicrobial, additional investigations are needed to determine the etiological agent or exclude non-infectious causes. Other diverse disease processes, including neoplasia and urolithiasis, result in inflammatory lesions of the urinary tract characterized by proteinuria, hematuria, and pyuria. In addition to initiating therapy with a broader spectrum agent, urinalysis, urine culture, survey abdominal radiographs and routine bloodwork should be performed to evaluate for important potential causes of apparent treatment failure.

In contrast to simple cystitis, complicated UTIs encompass an extraordinarily broad range of infections that often warrant a more extensive diagnostic evaluation. The variety of underlying conditions, and diverse bacterial agents with unpredictable susceptibilities make generalizations about antimicrobial therapy difficult. It is imperative that aerobic culture is performed for all complicated UTIs [7].

In antibiotic-naive patients, initial antibiotic recommendations for complicated cystitis are no different from first-line agents for managing simple cystitis. However, patients with complicated cystitis more often have UTIs that are recurrent or fail to respond to appropriate initial treatment. Ideally, antibiotic selection would be postponed until susceptibility information is available. However, when signs of lower urinary tract disease are present, a drug belonging to an antibiotic class different from that used to treat the most recent infection should be prescribed while awaiting culture results. Although the presence of a resistant strain on its own does not define a UTI as complicated, the prevalence of resistance among bacteria causing complicated UTIs is increasing and antibacterial susceptibilities are less predictable [8,15]. While isolates may remain susceptible to one commonly prescribed oral antimicrobial drug, it becomes increasingly less likely that first-line antimicrobials will be effective for complicated UTIs, highlighting the importance of urine culture in all cases [1,8].

Second-line antimicrobials include amoxicillin-clavulanic acid, third-generation cephalosporins, and fluoroquinolones (see Table 96.2) [16,23]. While empiric use is often indicated, none of these antimicrobials should be prescribed without culture and susceptibility information. Amoxicillin-clavulanic acid (or similar beta-lactam/beta-lactamase inhibitor) may be prescribed for complicated cystitis [16]. Amoxicillin-clavulanic acid often retains effectiveness against beta-lactamase-producing staphylococci and gram-negative pathogens resistant to amoxicillin, cephalexin, and TMP/S. Amoxicillin-clavulanic acid is an appropriate selection for dogs and cats with lower UTIs that have not been on repeated courses of antimicrobials.

Third-generation cephalosporins are also suitable second-line agents for managing complicated UTIs. Both oral (cefpodoxime) and extended-release injectable (cefovicin) products are effective against most major bacterial pathogens associated with UTIs in dogs and cats, although enterococci are universally resistant to all cephalosporins. Neither drug is approved for the treatment of UTIs in the United States. However, off-label use is reported, and treatment is often successful, particularly when culture information is used to guide therapy. Cefpodoxime is more active than cephalexin against Enterobacteriaceae. It is not registered for use in cats, but safe use in felines is reported. Cefovicin is given by subcutaneous injection every 14 days, eliminating problems with client compliance and ensuring that drug levels are consistently maintained above the MIC of common uropathogens. Cefovicin appears to be particularly effective against urinary isolates of *Staphylococcus pseudintermedius* and *Proteus* spp.

Ceftiofur, a third-generation cephalosporin used extensively in cattle, is approved for treatment of UTI in dogs due to susceptible strains of *E. coli* or *Proteus* spp. It is given by daily subcutaneous injection. It is economical, relative to the cost of therapy with other veterinary-approved third-generation antimicrobials. Beyond cost, specific indications for use are unclear. Indications may include treatment of UTI caused by a pathogen uniquely susceptible to ceftiofur, or when subcutaneous injection is preferable to oral treatment of UTI (i.e. dogs that experience unacceptable gastrointestinal side-effects with oral medication, or when a pet's disposition makes oral administration difficult). At the manufacturer's recommended dose, ceftiofur is not effective for infections outside the bladder. While a dose has not been established for cats, dose recommendations for dogs have been extrapolated for feline use.

Fluoroquinolones have a broad spectrum of activity against many uropathogens and are appropriate second-line agents as directed by susceptibility information. Fluoroquinolones are rapidly bactericidal, well tolerated and can be administered by a variety of routes. They are frequently useful against a broad range of gram-positive and gram-negative organisms, including *Staphylococcus pseudintermedius*, *E. coli*, *Klebsiella* and *Proteus* spp. Fluoroquinolones are often, though not uniformly, effective for infections caused by *Pseudomonas aeruginosa* and *Enterobacter* spp. They are generally ineffective for streptococcal and enterococcal infections, despite *in vitro* reporting of susceptibility.

Among fluoroquinolones, enrofloxacin is the most extensively studied. It is available in oral and injectable formulations. Enrofloxacin is registered for intramuscular injection only, but slow dilute intravenous injection has been used by veterinarians for many years. Fluo-roquinolones penetrate tissues well and enrofloxacin is considered the drug of choice for pyelonephritis and prostatitis in dogs. Enrofloxacin is not recommended for use in cats because of the risk of treatment failure with low doses and retinopathy at high doses.

Enrofloxacin is converted *in vivo* to ciprofloxacin. Ciprofloxacin is effective for susceptible pathogens in urine, including some isolates of *Pseudomonas aeruginosa*, but penetration into prostate and renal tissue is relatively poor. It is relatively inexpensive compared with fluoroquinolones approved for veterinary use. Beyond cost containment, it is difficult to support the use of ciprofloxacin over approved veterinary fluoroquinolones. There are no interpretive criteria for testing isolates from animals, and human breakpoints do not apply to veterinary patients.

Enrofloxacin (dogs) and marbofloxacin (dogs and cats) are generally most effective for *E. coli* UTIs. Difloxacin undergoes less renal excretion than other fluoroquinolones and is less likely to be effective against urinary pathogens. Studies have documented cross-resistance among fluoroquinolones [16]. More specifically, if an organism is reported as resistant to one fluoroquinolone, resistance to all other available fluoroquinolones (except pradofloxacin) should be assumed, regardless of susceptibility results [1]. Pradofloxacin is a third-generation fluoroquinolone developed to treat infections in dogs and cats. It is highly active against a wide range of canine and feline urinary pathogens, including strains of *E. coli* and *Staphylococcus* spp, and generally outperforms other fluoroquinolones in regard to both potency and efficacy. In the USA, pradofloxacin is only approved for treating skin infections in cats, but it is licensed in Europe for a wide variety of infections, including UTIs in dogs and cats. It may be a particularly attractive choice for pathogens with reduced susceptibility to other fluoroquinolones.

Fluoroquinolones have the potential to cause retinal degeneration and irreversible blindness in cats. Retinal damage is reported when enrofloxacin is administered to cats at higher doses (>5 mg/kg/day). Retinal damage is not reported with either pradofloxacin or marbofloxacin. Fluoroquinolones can cause damage to cartilage in weight-bearing joints of young growing dogs. Neurological signs including seizures are infrequently reported, particularly with intravenous or high-dose administration.

Fluconazole is recommended for initial treatment of fungal UTIs, given its favorable safety profile and efficacy against *Candida* spp. Some isolates may respond to intravesicular administration of 1% clotrimazole [2]. Secondary fungal UTIs occur when organisms are shed into the urine in patients with systemic fungal infections.

A uniform recommendation for treatment duration for complicated UTIs is likely not appropriate because of variation of types and severity of infections. Most veterinarians suggest treating complicated UTIs for 4–6 weeks. There is no supporting evidence for this recommendation and it is suspected that shorter courses of therapy might be effective in some patients. As with simple cystitis, clinical improvement should occur within 48 hours. However, resolution of clinical signs, hematuria and bacteriuria may be misleading, as these may resolve transiently because of reduced activity of infection, without eradication of the pathogen.

If the patient has not responded, the choice of antibiotic should be reviewed in light of culture and susceptibility results. Successful treatment is defined as sterile urine during and after antimicrobial administration. A urine culture should be obtained 7 days after antimicrobial therapy is initiated, and approximately 7 days after completing the full course of therapy [3]. Bacterial growth at either time point indicates treatment failure. With recurrent infections, urine culture should be performed 1 week before cessation of antimicrobial therapy, and repeated at 8, 12, and 24 weeks after therapy is discontinued.

Although appropriate antimicrobial therapy is critically important, it is often impossible to cure or prevent recurrence of complicated cystitis without identifying and correcting underlying functional, anatomic or metabolic defects [1,2]. When underlying conditions and predisposing factors cannot be determined, repeat courses of antibiotics typically prove ineffective at achieving bladder sterility. Instillation of antimicrobials into the urinary bladder is ineffective for treatment of bacterial UTIs.

Cystitis is not associated with signs of illness, and is generally managed on an outpatient basis with oral antibiotics. Dehydration, fever, nausea, unremitting discomfort or other signs of severe systemic disease are not present with lower urinary tract infections. Intravenous fluid support and parenteral antimicrobial therapy are indicated while further diagnostics, including bloodwork (CBC, serum chemistries/electrolytes), and imaging studies are performed to evaluate for prostatitis, pyelonephritis, and extraurinary sources of infection.

Management of Particular Conditions

Subclinical Bacteriuria

Circumstances in which bacterial growth should be classified as asymptomatic colonization, or SB, are currently undefined in the veterinary literature [3]. However, infection implies the presence of clinical and not just clinicopathological abnormalities. UTIs in small animals with underlying disease are frequently asymptomatic, or clinically silent, and there is no apparent correlation between occurrence of signs of lower urinary tract disease and the presence of a positive urine culture [11,14]. Since bacteria are not always harmful or pathological and therapy not always warranted, using the terms "silent" or "occult" UTI to characterize a non-pathological condition not requiring antimicrobials or other intervention may be misleading [3].

Veterinarians have justified therapy given reports that failure to do so is a risk factor for pyelonephritis, prostatitis, or urosepsis. Results of studies to prospectively determine the impact of treating SB on clinical outcome or on the frequency of antimicrobial resistance in companion animals have not been published. In general, antimicrobials are not routinely prescribed for animals with indwelling urinary catheters, or otherwise healthy dogs and cats with a positive urine culture and no clinical signs of infection. The risk of SB leading to cystitis or ascending infection or other possible complications in dogs and cats with underlying chronic disease, including hyperthyroidism, hyperadrenocorticism and diabetes mellitus, as well as dogs receiving chemotherapy and immunosuppressive drugs remains to be studied. The decision to screen for and treat SB in dogs and cats should be made on an individual basis. However, similar to recommendations in humans, treatment of SB is not recommended for most dogs and cats.

Some veterinary patients at high risk of complications may warrant a more aggressive approach to treatment, including those with anatomic abnormalities and patients undergoing urological surgery. It is likely that by treating SB with antimicrobials, patients stand little chance of benefit and are exposed to greater risk for antimicrobial resistance, and evidence-based guidelines are needed [1].

Urinary Tract Infections Associated with Urinary Catheters

Urinary catheters are a risk for UTI in dogs and cats [5,26]. However, judicious patient selection and vigilant management can decrease the morbidity associated with their use.

Subclinical bacterial colonization is common in catheterized patients and bacteriuria should not raise concern. If, however, there is an abrupt change in the gross appearance of urine (hematuria or turbidity) or urine changes supporting infection (pyuria) or clinical signs of illness (fever), urine culture and treatment are likely warranted. For patients that develop a catheter-associated UTI, treatment is more likely to be successful if the catheter can be removed. Urine for culture should be obtained by cystocentesis, and never sampled from the collection bag or catheter [3]. Concurrent use of antimicrobials in a patient with an indwelling urinary catheter is discouraged, and promotes infection or colonization with multidrug-resistant organisms.

To reduce catheter-associated infections:

- place a urinary catheter only when needed [5]
- educate personnel regarding aseptic placement, hand-washing, and wearing gloves when manipulating the catheter
- use collection bags with a distal drainage port, and periodically clean the port with a dilute chlorhexidine solution
- consider replacing the catheter every 48 hours, or sooner if gross contamination is evident
- avoid antibiotics while patient has a catheter in place [5]
- clean the outside of the penis/vulva and external catheter line several times daily with dilute chlorhexidine solution
- do NOT culture the urinary catheter tip, as this is not predictive of UTI or UTI risk [3].

Placement of urinary catheters is common in cats but few studies have examined the incidence of infection that may develop as a result. One study showed that 33% of catheterized cats developed significant bacteriuria during catheterization [26]. In another study, 26.9% of cats with multidrug-resistant *E. coli* infection had a history of urinary obstruction managed with catheterization [24].

Acute Prostatitis

Dogs with acute prostatitis are often severely ill, frequently requiring hospitalization, intravenous fluids, and analgesics, in addition to antimicrobial therapy. Initial outpatient management is often unsuccessful. Physical exam findings and associated clinical signs in conjunction with results of CBC, radiography, urinalysis, and urine culture are generally sufficient to establish a presumptive diagnosis. *E. coli* is the most common causative organism. Culture of prostatic fluid is generally not necessary for acute infections, and antimicrobial therapy can be guided based on urine culture results.

Parenteral therapy with a fluoroquinolone is initially selected while susceptibility data are pending. With the availability, predictable efficacy, and safety profile of fluoroquinolones, therapy with other drug classes is only pursued if clinical signs do not resolve and susceptibility to another drug is documented. Other lipid-soluble drugs, such as TMP/S and chloramphenicol, are also described for treating prostatic infections. Both achieve high concentrations in the prostate, and are available in intravenous and oral formulations. Chloramphenicol is not used for initial therapy but is occasionally prescribed for prostatic infections caused by methicillin-resistant staphylococci. Gastrointestinal upset, reversible bone marrow suppression, and peripheral neuropathy affecting predominantly pelvic limbs are the most commonly reported adverse events reported with chloramphenicol in dogs. Antibiotics are continued for no less than 4 weeks. Urine culture should be performed 5–7 days after treatment is concluded to document microbiological cure.

Acute prostatitis generally responds favorably to treatment. Abscess formation occurs, and should be suspected if signs do not improve, caudal abdominal pain worsens, or signs of sepsis develop. Culture of prostatic fluid is recommended for dogs with chronic prostatitis, and non-ionic lipid-soluble drugs such as chloramphenicol, fluoroquinolones, and TMP/S are sporadically required for therapy of chronic infection. However, the challenges of treating chronic prostatitis (selecting lipid-soluble drugs such as CHPC and TMP/S that cross the blood–prostate barrier) are less of a concern for acute infections in which the blood–prostate barrier is typically disrupted by inflammation. For some dogs, long-term microbiological cure and durable control of clinical signs may not be possible without castration.

Acute Pyelonephritis

Empirical antibiotic therapy should be initiated immediately in all patients with suspected pyelonephritis. Initial treatment should include an antibiotic with proven efficacy against gram-negative enteric organisms, due to the frequency of their involvement in pyelonephritis. Antibiotics diffuse into renal parenchyma from plasma so achieving high drug levels in plasma may be more important than urine. Urine culture and susceptibility testing should be performed, and initial therapy can be tailored to the individual pathogen, if appropriate, when results become available. Fluoroquinolones penetrate renal parenchyma and are recommended for initial therapy. Dogs with acute pyelonephritis are usually systemically ill and require monitoring and intravenous fluid support. Indications to hospitalize patients with acute pyelonephritis include pain, hemodynamic instability, azotemia, nausea or inability to tolerate oral medications. Opioids given by intermittent intravenous injection, or as a constant rate infusion, are often effective for pain management. Parenteral therapy is continued until patients eat and drink voluntarily.

There are no published systematic reviews of pyelonephritis in dogs or cats. Scientific evidence for appropriate duration of antimicrobial therapy is lacking. Treatment is generally continued for 6–8 weeks, with regular monitoring for recurrence of infection. Urine culture should be performed 5–7 days after antimicrobial therapy is discontinued. Progressive, sometimes irreversible renal damage is a possible consequence of infection, but uremic symptomatology and long-term renal functional impairment are not commonly reported when acute pyelonephritis is recognized and treatment initiated promptly [1].

References

1 Barsanti J. Genitourinary infections. In: *Infectious Diseases of the Dog and Cat*, 4th edn (ed. Greene CE). Elsevier-Saunders, Philadelphia, 2012, pp. 1013–1043.

2 Pressler B, Bartges JW. Urinary tract infections. In: *Textbook of Veterinary Internal Medicine*, 7th edn (eds Ettinger SJ, Feldman EC). Elsevier, St Louis, 2010, pp. 2037–2047.

3 Weese JS, Blondeau JM, Boothe D, et al. Antimicrobial Use Guidelines for Treatment of Urinary Tract Disease in Dogs and Cats: Antimicrobial Guidelines Working Group of the International Society for Companion Animal Infectious Diseases. *Vet Med Int* 2011;263768.

4 Wang A, Nizran P, Malone MA, Riley T. Urinary tract infections. *Prim Care* 2013;40(3):687–706.

5 Olin SJ, Bartges JW. Urinary tract infections: treatment/comparative therapeutics. *Vet Clin North Am Small Anim Pract* 2015;45(4):721–746.

6 Smee N, Loyd K, Grauer GF. UTIs in small animal patients: Part 2: diagnosis, treatment, and complications. *J Am Anim Hosp Assoc* 2013;49(2):83–94.

7 Windahl U, Holst BS, Nyman A, Grönlund U, Bengtsson B. Characterisation of bacterial growth and antimicrobial susceptibility patterns in canine urinary tract infections. *BMC Vet Res* 2014;10:217.

8 Wong C, Epstein SE, Westropp JL. Antimicrobial susceptibility patterns in urinary tract infections in dogs (2010–2013). *J Vet Intern Med* 2015;29(4):1045–1052.

9 Guardabassi L, Hedberg S, Jessen LR, Damborg P. Optimization and evaluation of Flexicult® Vet for detection, identification and antimicrobial susceptibility testing of bacterial uropathogens in small animal veterinary practice. *Acta Vet Scand* 2015;57:72.

10 Bartges JW. Diagnosis of urinary tract infections. *Vet Clin North Am Small Anim Pract* 2004;34(4): 923–933, vi.

11 Litster A, Thompson M, Moss S, Trott D. Feline bacterial urinary tract infections: an update on an evolving clinical problem. *Vet J* 2011; 187(1):18–22.

12 Bailiff NL, Westropp JL, Nelson RW, et al. Evaluation of urine specific gravity and urine sediment as risk factors for urinary tract infections in cats. *Vet Clin Pathol* 2008;37(3):317–322.

13 Ybarra WL, Sykes JE, Wang Y, Byrne BA, Westropp JL. Performance of a veterinary urine dipstick paddle system for diagnosis and identification of urinary tract infections in dogs and cats. *J Am Vet Med Assoc* 2014;244(7):814–819.

14 Thompson MF, Litster AL, Platell JL, Trott DJ. Canine bacterial urinary tract infections: new developments in old pathogens. *Vet J* 2011;190(1):22–27.

15 Wagner S, Gally DL, Argyle SA. Multidrug-resistant Escherichia coli from canine urinary tract infections tend to have commensal phylotypes, lower prevalence of virulence determinants and ampC-replicons. *Vet Microbiol* 2014;169(3–4):171–178.

16 Olin SJ, Bartges JW, Jones RD, Bemis DA. Diagnostic accuracy of a point-of-care urine bacteriologic culture test in dogs. *J Am Vet Med Assoc* 2013;243(12):1719–1725.

17 O'Neil E, Horney B, Burton S, Lewis PJ, MacKenzie A, Stryhn H. Comparison of wet-mount, Wright-Giemsa and Gram-stained urine sediment for predicting bacteriuria in dogs and cats. *Can Vet J* 2013;54(11):1061–1066.

18 Way LI, Sullivan LA, Johnson V, Morley PS. Comparison of routine urinalysis and urine Gram stain for detection of bacteriuria in dogs: Utilization of Gram stain to detect bacteriuria. *J Vet Emerg Crit Care* 2013;23(1):23–28.

19 Lund HS, Skogtun G, Sørum H, Eggertsdóttir AV. Antimicrobial susceptibility in bacterial isolates from Norwegian cats with lower urinary tract disease. *J Feline Med Surg* 2015;17(6):507–515.

20 Wan SY, Hartmann FA, Jooss MK, Viviano KR. Prevalence and clinical outcome of subclinical bacteriuria in female dogs. *J Am Vet Med Assoc* 2014;245(1):106–112.

21 Sorensen TM, Jensen AB, Damborg PP. Evaluation of different sampling methods and criteria for diagnnosing canine urinary tract infections by quantitative bacterial culture. *J Vet Intern Med* 2016;30(1):358.

22 Kvitko-White HL, Cook AK, Nabity MB, Zhang S, Lawhon SD. Evaluation of a catalase-based urine test for the detection of urinary tract infection in dogs and cats. *J Vet Intern Med* 2013;27(6):1379–1384.

23 Clare S, Hartmann FA, Jooss M, et al. Short- and long-term cure rates of short-duration trimethoprim-sulfamethoxazole treatment in female dogs with uncomplicated bacterial cystitis. *J Vet Intern Med* 2014;28(3):818–826.

24 Hernandez J, Bota D, Farbos M, Bernardin F, Ragetly G, Médaille C. Risk factors for urinary tract infection with multiple drug-resistant Escherichia coli in cats. *J Feline Med Surg* 2014;16(2):75–81.

25 Westropp JL, Sykes JE, Irom S, et al. Evaluation of the efficacy and safety of high dose short duration enrofloxacin treatment regimen for uncomplicated urinary tract infections in dogs. *J Vet Intern Med* 2012;26(3):506–512.

26 Hugonnard M, Chalvet-Monfray K, Dernis J, et al. Occurrence of bacteriuria in 18 catheterised cats with obstructive lower urinary tract disease: a pilot study. *J Feline Med Surg* 2013;15(10):843–848.

97

Urolithiasis

Joseph Bartges, DVM, PhD, DACVIM, DACVN

College of Veterinary Medicine, University of Georgia, Athens, GA, USA

Introduction

Formation of uroliths is not a disease, but rather a complication of several disorders. A common denominator of these disorders is that they can occasionally create oversaturation of urine with one or more crystal precursors, resulting in formation of crystals. If these crystals are retained and the urine remains oversaturated with the crystal precursors, the microscopic crystals may aggregate to form macroscopic uroliths.

Patients with uroliths may present with urinary tract obstruction (urethroliths or ureteroliths), lower urinary tract signs without urinary obstruction, or with no clinical signs and an inadvertent diagnosis of urolithiasis. In an emergency situation, patients will present usually with clinical signs associated or unassociated with urinary obstruction. Clinical signs may include vomiting, anorexia, and abdominal pain. If urethral obstruction is present, a large urinary bladder or uroabdomen may be present. With ureteral obstruction, renal pain may be found. Initial management is aimed at relieving the obstruction, correcting any metabolic abnormalities that result from obstruction, if present, and/or minimizing clinical signs until more definitive treatment is undertaken.

A detailed discussion of urolith formation and medical preventive therapy is beyond the scope of this chapter and the reader is referred to other sources for this information [1–3]. This chapter will focus on management of the emergent patient.

Diagnosis of Uroliths

Imaging is the most definitive diagnostic tool for detection of uroliths. Abdominal radiography is generally the first diagnostic imaging modality (Figure 97.1). Ultrasonography or contrast radiography (e.g. contrast and

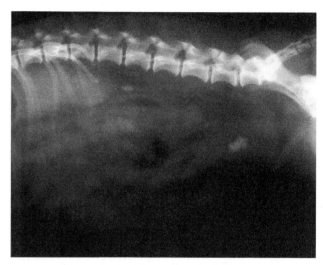

Figure 97.1 Lateral abdominal radiograph of an 8-year-old miniature schnauzer showing a ureterolith and two urocystoliths composed of calcium oxalate.

double contrast urocystography or excretory urography) can be used to detect uroliths, including those that are radiolucent [4]. These abdominal imaging techniques are used to verify the presence, location, number, size, shape, and density of the uroliths.

Urinalysis is an important part of the diagnostic evaluation. Crystalluria does not confirm the presence of uroliths but it does suggest risk, and some patients may have active urocystoliths but not have crystalluria [6]. Urine specific gravity and urine pH can help assess the chemical environment of urine. A high urine specific gravity suggests an increase in concentration of urolithic precursors [6]. Calcium oxalate, purines, and cystine uroliths form typically in urine with a pH less than 7.0, whereas struvite calculi form typically in urine with a pH greater than 7.0 [7]. Urine culture and susceptibility testing are indicated because urinary tract infections may occur secondary to uroliths or may induce urolith formation in the case of infection-induced struvite uroliths [2,8,9]. Factors contributing to this condition include mucosal damage induced by the stones, incomplete urine voiding, or micro-organism entrapment in the stone.

When uroliths are found, particularly when associated with urinary tract obstruction, it is important to obtain a blood biochemical profile; this may suggest presence of underlying diseases, such as hypercalcemia, that can predispose patients to urolith formation [10–13]. Because uroliths occasionally cause urinary tract obstruction, electrolyte, calcium, phosphorus, creatinine, and blood urea nitrogen concentrations should be closely monitored. Urate calculi may be caused by underlying liver disease, particularly congenital vascular anomalies, so hepatic function should be determined in patients with suspected or confirmed urate uroliths [14,15].

Management of Uroliths Associated with Urinary Obstruction

Urinary obstruction may be associated with azotemia, hyperkalemia, metabolic acidosis, and dehydration if there is urethral obstruction, uroabdomen, or bilateral ureteral obstruction, or if unilateral ureteral obstruction occurs in a patient with chronic kidney disease [16,17]. Treatment for urethral obstruction involves relieving the obstruction and correcting the metabolic imbalances. Performing perineal urethrostomy in cats, or urethrotomy or scrotal urethrostomy in dogs, on an emergency basis is unnecessary and not recommended. Relief of urethral obstruction by retrograde hydropropulsion allows time for additional diagnostic testing and stabilization of the patient. If urethroliths cannot be retropulsed into the urinary bladder, then passage of a small-diameter urethral catheter around the urethroliths or repeated cystocenteses may be done (see Chapter 106).

When ureteral obstruction is present, medical expulsion therapy utilizing intravenous fluids, amitriptyline, and prazosin may attempted; however, often a urinary diversion technique, such as a nephrostomy tube, ureteral stent, or subcutaneous bypass device, must be employed to preserve remaining renal function in the obstructed kidney.

Management of Uroliths Unassociated with Urinary Obstruction

Medical Treatment

Certain types of uroliths are amenable to medical dissolution therapy.

Struvite

Struvite is another name for magnesium ammonium phosphate hexahydrate. Struvite uroliths may occur as a consequence of a urinary tract infection with a urease-producing microbe (infection-induced struvite) or without the presence of a urinary tract infection (sterile struvite) [18]. Infection-induced struvite uroliths occur most commonly in dogs [19] and pediatric dogs and cats; sterile struvite uroliths occur most commonly in cats. Any animal that develops a bacterial urinary tract infection with a urease-producing micro-organism can develop infection-induced struvite uroliths (see Chapter 96). Sterile struvite uroliths have been documented to occur in dogs [20] but they are very rare.

Infection-induced struvite uroliths can be dissolved by feeding a "struvite dissolution" diet and administering an appropriate antimicrobial agent based on bacteriological culture and susceptibility testing, although there is a case report of dissolution with administration of an antimicrobial agent only [21] (see Chapter 200). Average dissolution time for infection-induced struvite uroliths is approximately 8–12 weeks [18]. An alternative dissolution protocol utilizing a urinary acidifier, d,l-methionine, administered at a dosage of 75–100 mg/kg PO q12h in combination with an appropriate antibiotic, induced medical dissolution in 1–4 months [22]. It is important that the patient receive an appropriate antimicrobial agent during the entire time of medical dissolution.

Sterile struvite uroliths can be dissolved by feeding a diet that is magnesium, phosphorus, and protein restricted, and that induces aciduria [18,23]. Average dissolution time of feline sterile struvite uroliths was 36.2 ± 26.6 days (range 14–141 days) [18,24]. In a more recent study of 32 cats with presumed struvite urocystoliths comparing two low-magnesium acidifying diets, one a "struvite dissolution" diet and the other a "struvite prevention" diet, the mean ($\pm$ SD) times for a 50% reduction in urolith size (0.69 ± 0.1 weeks) and complete urolith dissolution (13.0 ± 2.6 days) were significantly shorter for cats fed the struvite dissolution diet compared with those (1.75 ± 0.27 weeks and 27.0 ± 2.6 days, respectively) for cats fed the struvite prevention diet [25]. Therefore, sterile struvite urocystoliths often dissolve in 2–4 weeks.

Calcium Oxalate

Currently, it is impossible to dissolve calcium oxalate uroliths in dogs and cats so the only management strategy is removal by minimally invasive methods or surgery.

Purines
Urates

Most information concerning urate uroliths is derived from dogs, with very little information available for cats. Uric acid is one of several biodegradation products of purine nucleotide metabolism [26]. In most dogs and cats, allantoin is the major metabolic endproduct; it is the most soluble of the purine metabolic products excreted in urine. Ammonium urate (also known as ammonium acid urate and ammonium biurate) is the most common form of naturally occurring purine uroliths observed in dogs and cats. Urate is the third most common mineral found in uroliths in dogs and cats, accounting for 5–8% of uroliths, and the second most common urolith occurring in dogs and cats < 1 year of age (infection-induced struvite is the most common urolith in these patients). Urate uroliths form because of liver disease (usually a portosystemic vascular shunt) [14,15] or because of an inborn error of metabolism resulting in hyperuricosuria (e.g. Dalmatians and English bulldogs) [27,28]. They are more common in dogs and cats less than 7 years of age [27–29].

Dissolution is not possible in dogs and cats with uncorrected liver disease (e.g. non-surgical portovascular anomalies or microvascular dysplasia). Surgical removal, voiding urohydropropulsion, or cystoscopy ± laser lithotripsy remain the treatments of choice for animals with symptomatic urate stones that cannot be dissolved.

In dogs without underlying liver disease, dissolution may be attempted. Dissolution of urate uroliths in dogs is accomplished by feeding a purine-restricted, alkalinizing diet that induces a diuresis and administering the xanthine oxidase inhibitor allopurinol (15 mg/kg PO q12h) [26,30–34]; allopurinol has not been evaluated in cats and should not be used in this species. While "renal failure" diets are protein restricted and thus lower in purines, there are two commercially available diets formulated to be low in purines: Prescription Diet u/d (Hill's Pet Products) and UC Low Purine (Royal Canin). Canned diets may be better than dry diets. In one study, medical dissolution was effective in approximately 40% of Dalmatians, partial dissolution occurred in approximately 30%, and no dissolution or growth of uroliths due to xanthine formation occurred in approximately 30% [26].

Until further studies are performed to confirm the safety and efficacy of medical dissolution, surgical removal or minimally invasive procedures remain the treatment of choice for urate uroliths in cats.

Xanthine

Xanthine urolithiasis may occur with allopurinol administration to dogs, especially when dietary purines are not restricted. Management involves adjusting dosage of allopurinol and changing diet. Spontaneously occurring xanthine uroliths have been reported rarely in cats (0.14% of uroliths analyzed at the Minnesota Urolith Center). They are composed typically of pure xanthine and have been reported in cats less than 5 years of age with an average age of approximately 3 years; they occur with approximately even distribution between males and females.

Xanthine uroliths have also been found in a few Cavalier King Charles spaniels [35–37]. No medical dissolution protocol for naturally occurring xanthine uroliths exists.

Cystine

Cystinuria occurs when there is a proximal renal tubular defect in reabsorption and is often present with other amino acids (notably ornithine, lysine, and arginine) [38–43]. Affected animals also demonstrate altered intestinal transport of cystine [44–46]. Several genetic mutations that are associated with cystinuria have been identified in dogs and cats [47–50]. Cystinuria is only associated with urolith formation and is not associated with protein malnutrition or amino acid deficiency, although it can be associated with hypercarnitinuria and/or hypertaurinuria and associated dilated cardiomyopathy [51]. Cystinuria by itself does not result in urolithiasis, however, and many cystinuric dogs and human beings do not form uroliths [52].

Canine cystine uroliths can be dissolved medically by feeding a diet that is low in protein, alkalinizing, and induces a diuresis. While "renal failure" diets are protein restricted and thus lower in amino acids, there are two commercially available diets formulated to be low in sulfur-containing amino acids: Prescription Diet u/d (Hill's Pet Products) and UC Low Purine (Royal Canin). Canned diets may be better than dry diets.

Administration of 2-mercaptopropionylglycine (2-MPG, Tiopronin, Thiola) is recommended [38,39,53]. This drug is similar to D-penicillamine in that it binds to the individual cysteine molecules, preventing formation of the disulfide bond of cystine; however, it is associated with fewer side-effects and complications. Dosage is 15 mg/kg PO q12h for dissolution. There are studies showing that administration of 2-MPG without modifying diet may result in dissolution of cystine uroliths. Cats do not tolerate 2-MPG well and it is associated with GI signs, liver disease, and anemia; therefore, it should not be used in cats and dissolution of cystine uroliths has not been successful.

Compound and Mixed Uroliths

Between 5% and 15% of uroliths may be mixed or compound stones. This refers to a situation where more than one mineral is present within the stone, either mixed within layers or different parts of the stone are composed of various minerals (nidus versus major volume of the stone versus the outer layer or shell).

As mentioned previously, ammonium urate and calcium carbonate (or calcium apatite) may be mixed with struvite as part of infection-induced struvite stone formation. In this situation, the struvite caused by the infection is the primary focus for prevention. Some stones may be composed of both struvite and calcium oxalate. In this situation, usually calcium oxalate is the nidus (inner part of the stone) and struvite is layered around it.

This compound stone forms because the patient first formed a calcium oxalate stone and then developed a urinary tract infection and layered infection-induced struvite around the calcium oxalate nidus. Ammonium urate uroliths may contain xanthine in patients that receive allopurinol for dissolution or prevention. This may be due to (a) too high a dose of allopurinol, (b) lack of restriction of dietary protein/purine, or (c) individual patient metabolism of allopurinol despite appropriate allopurinol dosage and dietary management. Prevention is directed to (a) decreasing or discontinuing allopurinol, (b) changing the diet to a more protein/purine-restricted diet, or (c) both.

Minimally Invasive Techniques

There are several minimally invasive treatment options for retrieval of bladder and urethral stones. These include voiding urohydropropulsion, transurethral cystoscopic stone removal (with or without use of laser lithotripsy), and mini-laparotomy-assisted cystoscopic stone removal, also called percutaneous cystolithotomy (PCCL).

In catheter-assisted retrieval or voiding urohydropropulsion of calculi, the patient is sedated or anesthetized, a catheter is passed into the urinary bladder transurethrally, and the bladder is filled with sterile crystalloid solution [54]. In cats, a 3.5 Fr or 5 Fr catheter is used and in dogs a 5, 8, or 10 Fr catheter is used, depending on patient size. During catheter retrieval, the contents of the bladder are aspirated while the bladder is agitated by palpating and manipulating it or rotating the patient's body. This is difficult in most male cats and in small male dogs due to the limiting size of the urethra and the small size of the catheter.

With voiding urohydropropulsion, the patient is anesthetized and held vertically while the distended bladder is manually expressed [54]. Sizes of uroliths that may be retrieved with this technique are approximately 1 mm in male cats, up to 5 mm in female cats, 1–3 mm in male dogs, and up to 10 mm in female dogs.

These methods are used to eliminate small calculi and collect them for analysis to plan further treatment. These techniques will not be successful, however, if a patient presents with urethral obstruction as this situation indicates that there is at least one urolith that is too large to pass through the urethra.

Percutaneous cystolithotomy is a procedure where the bladder is approached through a small abdominal wall incision and is temporarily fastened to the incised linea, thus allowing for cystoscopic stone removal through a stab incision or a laparoscopic port placed in the urinary bladder [55,56]. This method is an effective, safe, and efficient means for managing urocystoliths.

Cystoscopy produces magnified images of the fluid-distended urinary bladder, allowing identification of abnormalities such as strictures, masses, and calculi [57,58]. This is the minimally invasive procedure of choice for male dogs and cats because the diameter of the male urethra limits insertion of a cystoscope with operating channel. Cystoscopic techniques are more efficient than surgical procedures, decreasing the risk of trauma and abdominal contamination [57,58]. When performing transurethral cystoscopy, a cystoscope is inserted into the urethra and passed into the urinary bladder. This procedure is preferred for use in females but has been described in male dogs because it is less invasive than other diagnostic and treatment methods. If calculi are small enough, they can be removed using stone retrieval devices such as stone baskets and graspers.

For larger calculi, lithotripsy may be used, if available [58]. Lithotripsy uses a laser fiber that is passed through the operating channel on the cystoscope. The fiber emits light at an infrared wavelength to fragment calculi [59–64], and the resulting fragments are removed transurethrally. This procedure is possible in female dogs and cats and male dogs, but not male cats due to the limiting size of the male cat urethra and inability to insert a large enough scope with an operating channel.

In patients with ureteral obstruction, minimally invasive techniques are primarily used to either bypass the obstruction or divert urine flow from the obstructed kidney to the urinary bladder. These techniques include placement of a nephrostomy tube, ureteral stent, or subcutaneous urinary bypass device. Nephrostomy tubes provide temporary relief of pressure within the obstructed kidney until more definitive therapy can be undertaken [65]. A ureteral stent may be placed fluoroscopically with or without cystoscopic guidance, depending on the patient, or using a surgical approach (Figure 97.2) [65]. Subcutaneous ureteral bypass devices are placed surgically, diverting urine flow down the path of least resistance, which is through the renal catheter, subcutaneous port, and urinary bladder catheter into the urinary bladder (Figure 97.3) [65].

Surgical Treatment

Detection of uroliths does not necessarily warrant surgical intervention; however, obstruction of urine outflow, an increase in size and/or number of calculi, persistent clinical signs, and a lack of response to therapy are indications for calculi removal [2]. Surgery is required in patients with non-dissolvable calculi and clinical signs. Traditional open surgical options are available for treatment of urolithiasis, including cystotomy, urethrotomy, and urethrostomy, and for ureteroliths, ureteral resection with neoureterocystostomy.

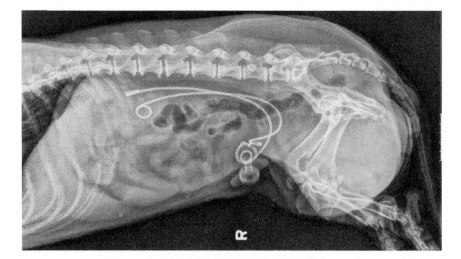

Figure 97.2 Lateral abdominal radiograph of a 10-year-old spayed female mixed breed dog with bilateral ureteral stents and a cystostomy tube due to urethral and ureteral obstruction by transitional cell carcinoma.

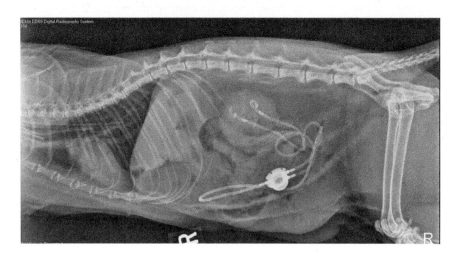

Figure 97.3 Lateral abdominal radiograph of a 14-year-old castrated male, domestic short-haired cat with bilateral subcutaneous ureteral bypass devices due to bilateral ureteral obstruction from uroliths.

References

1 Bartges JW, Callens AJ. Urolithiasis. *Vet Clin North Am Small Anim Pract* 2015;45:747–768.

2 Lulich JP, Osborne CA, Albasan H. Canine and feline urolithiasis: diagnosis, treatment, and prevention. In: *Nephrology and Urology of Small Animals* (eds Bartges J, Polzin DJ). Wiley-Blackwell, Chichester, 2011, pp. 687–706.

3 Osborne CA, Bartges JW, Lulich JP, et al. Canine urolithiasis. In: *Small Animal Clinical Nutrition*, 4th edn (eds Hand MS, Thatcher CD, Remillard RL, et al.). Wadsworth, Marceline, 2000, pp. 605–688.

4 Feeney DA, Anderson KL. Radiographic imaging in urinary tract disease. In: *Nephrology and Urology of Small Animals* (eds Bartges J, Polzin DJ). Wiley-Blackwell, Chichester, 2011, pp. 97–127.

5 Osborne CA, Lulich JP, Kruger JM, et al. Analysis of 451,891 canine uroliths, feline uroliths, and feline urethral plugs from 1981 to 2007: perspectives from the Minnesota Urolith Center. *Vet Clin North Am Small Anim Pract* 2009;39:183–197.

6 Bartges JW. Urinary saturation testing. In: *Nephrology and Urology of Small Animals* (eds Bartges J, Polzin DJ). Wiley-Blackwell, Chichester, 2011, pp. 75–85.

7 Langston C, Gisselman K, Palma D, et al. Diagnosis of urolithiasis. *Compend Contin Educ Vet* 2008;30:447–450, 452–444; quiz 455.

8 Seaman R, Bartges JW. Canine struvite urolithiasis. *Compen Contin Educ Pract Vet* 2001;23:407–429.

9 Palma D, Langston C, Gisselman K, et al. Canine struvite urolithiasis. *Compend Contin Educ Vet* 2013;35:E1; quiz E1.

10 Gisselman K, Langston CE, Douglas P, et al. Calcium oxalate urolithiasis. *Compend Contin Educ Vet* 2009;31:496–502.

11 McClain HM, Barsanti JA, Bartges JW. Hypercalcemia and calcium oxalate urolithiasis in cats: a report of five cases. *J Am Anim Hosp Assoc* 1999;35:297–301.

12 Midkiff AM, Chew DJ, Randolph JF, et al. Idiopathic hypercalcemia in cats. *J Vet Intern Med* 2000;14:619–626.

13 Savary KC, Price GS, Vaden SL. Hypercalcemia in cats: a retrospective study of 71 cases (1991–1997). *J Vet Intern Med* 2000;14:184–189.

14 Caporali EH, Phillips H, Underwood L, et al. Risk factors for urolithiasis in dogs with congenital extrahepatic portosystemic shunts: 95 cases (1999–2013). *J Am Vet Med Assoc* 2015;246:530–536.

15 Bartges JW, Cornelius LM, Osborne CA. Ammonium urate uroliths in dogs with portosystemic shunts. In: *Current Veterinary Therapy XIII* (ed. Bonagura JD). WB Saunders, Philadelphia, 1999, pp. 872–874.

16 Bartges JW, Finco DR, Polzin DJ, et al. Pathophysiology of urethral obstruction. *Vet Clin North Am Small Anim Pract* 1996;26:255–264.

17 Kyles AE, Hardie EM, Wooden BG, et al. Management and outcome of cats with ureteral calculi: 153 cases (1984–2002). *J Am Vet Med Assoc* 2005;226:937–944.

18 Osborne CA, Lulich JP, Kruger JM, et al. Medical dissolution of feline struvite urocystoliths. *J Am Vet Med Assoc* 1990;196:1053–1063.

19 Okafor CC, Pearl DL, Lefebvre SL, et al. Risk factors associated with struvite urolithiasis in dogs evaluated at general care veterinary hospitals in the United States. *J Am Vet Med Assoc* 2013;243:1737–1745.

20 Bartges JW, Osborne CA, Pozin DJ. Recurrent sterile struvite urocystolithiasis in three related Cocker Spaniels. *J Am Anim Hosp Assoc* 1992;28:459–469.

21 Rinkardt NE, Houston DM. Dissolution of infection-induced struvite bladder stones by using a noncalculolytic diet and antibiotic therapy. *Can Vet J* 2004;45:838–840.

22 Bartges J, Moyers T. Evaluation of d,l-methionine and antimicrobial agents for dissolution of spontaneously-occurring infection-induced struvite urocystoliths in dogs. Proceedings of the American College of Veterinary Internal Medicine, *Anaheim*, 2010.

23 Roudebush P, Forrester SD, Padgelek T. What is the evidence? Therapeutic foods to treat struvite uroliths in cats instead of surgery. *J Am Vet Med Assoc* 2010;236:965–966.

24 Houston DM, Rinkardt NE, Hilton J. Evaluation of the efficacy of a commercial diet in the dissolution of feline struvite bladder uroliths. *Vet Ther* 2004;5:187–201.

25 Lulich JP, Kruger JM, Macleay JM, et al. Efficacy of two commercially available, low-magnesium, urine-acidifying dry foods for the dissolution of struvite uroliths in cats. *J Am Vet Med Assoc* 2013;243:1147–1153.

26 Bartges JW, Osborne CA, Lulich JP, et al. Canine urate urolithiasis. Etiopathogenesis, diagnosis, and management. *Vet Clin North Am Small Anim Pract* 1999;29:161–191, xii–xiii.

27 Bartges JW, Osborne CA, Lulich JP, et al. Prevalence of cystine and urate uroliths in bulldogs and urate uroliths in dalmatians. *J Am Vet Med Assoc* 1994;204:1914–1918.

28 Case LC, Ling GV, Ruby AL, et al. Urolithiasis in Dalmations: 275 cases (1981–1990). *J Am Vet Med Assoc* 1993;203:96–100.

29 Albasan H, Osborne CA, Lulich JP, et al. Risk factors for urate uroliths in cats. *J Am Vet Med Assoc* 2012;240:842–847.

30 Bartges JW, Osborne CA, Felice LJ, et al. Influence of four diets containing approximately 11% protein (dry weight) on uric acid, sodium urate, and ammonium urate urine activity product ratios of healthy beagles. *Am J Vet Res* 1995;56:60–65.

31 Bartges JW, Osborne CA, Felice LJ, et al. Diet effect on activity product ratios of uric acid, sodium urate, and ammonium urate in urine formed by healthy beagles. *Am J Vet Res* 1995;56:329–333.

32 Bartges JW, Osborne CA, Felice LJ, et al. Influence of chronic allopurinol administration on urine acivty product ratios of uric acid, sodium urate, ammonium urate, and xanthine. *J Vet Intern Med* 1994;8:168A.

33 Bartges JW, Osborne CA, Felice LJ, et al. Influence of allopurinol and two diets on 24-hour urinary excretions of uric acid, xanthine, and ammonia by healthy dogs. *Am J Vet Res* 1995;56:595–599.

34 Bartges JW, Osborne CA, Koehler LA, et al. An algorithmic approach to canine urate uroliths. 12th Annual Veterinary Medical Forum of the American College of Veterinary Internal Medicine, 1994, pp. 476–477.

35 Jacinto AM, Mellanby RJ, Chandler M, et al. Urine concentrations of xanthine, hypoxanthine and uric acid in UK Cavalier King Charles spaniels. *J Small Anim Pract* 2013;54:395–398.

36 van Zuilen CD, Nickel RF, van Dijk TH, et al. Xanthinuria in a family of Cavalier King Charles spaniels. *Vet Q* 1997;19:172–174.

37 Gow AG, Fairbanks LD, Simpson JW, et al. Xanthine urolithiasis in a Cavalier King Charles spaniel. *Vet Rec* 2011;169:209.

38 Hoppe A, Denneberg T. Cystinuria in the dog: clinical studies during 14 years of medical treatment. *J Vet Intern Med* 2001;15:361–367.

39 Osborne CA, Sanderson SL, Lulich JP, et al. Canine cystine urolithiasis. Cause, detection, treatment, and prevention. *Vet Clin North Am Small Anim Pract* 1999;29:193–211, xiii.

40 Hoppe A, Denneberg T, Jeppsson JO, et al. Urinary excretion of amino acids in normal and cystinuric dogs. *Br Vet J* 1993;149:253–268.

41 Osborne CA, Lulich JP, Bartges JW, et al. Metabolic uroliths in cats. In: *Current Veterinary Therapy XI* (eds Kirk RW, Bonagura JD). WB Saunders Philadelphia, 1992, pp. 909–910.

42 DiBartola SP, Chew DJ, Horton ML. Cystinuria in a cat. *J Am Vet Med Assoc* 1991;198:102–104.

43 Bovee KC, Thier SO, Rea C, et al. Renal clearance of amino acids in canine cystinuria. *Metabolism* 1974;23:51–58.

44 Tsan MF, Jones TC, Wilson TH. Canine cystinuria: intestinal and renal amino acid transport. *Am J Vet Res* 1972;33:2463–2468.

45 Holtzapple PG, Rea C, Bovee K, et al. Characteristics of cystine and lysine transport in renal jejunal tissue from cystinuric dogs. *Metabolism* 1971;20:1016–1022.

46 Treacher RJ. Intestinal absorption of lysine in cystinuric dogs. *J Comp Pathol* 1965;75:309–322.

47 Mizukami K, Raj K, Giger U. Feline cystinuria caused by a missense mutation in the SLC3A1 gene. *J Vet Intern Med* 2015;29:120–125.

48 Brons AK, Henthorn PS, Raj K, et al. SLC3A1 and SLC7A9 mutations in autosomal recessive or dominant canine cystinuria: a new classification system. *J Vet Intern Med* 2013;27:1400–1408.

49 Harnevik L, Hoppe A, Soderkvist P. SLC7A9 cDNA cloning and mutational analysis of SLC3A1 and SLC7A9 in canine cystinuria. *Mamm Genome* 2006;17:769–776.

50 Henthorn PS, Liu J, Gidalevich T, et al. Canine cystinuria: polymorphism in the canine SLC3A1 gene and identification of a nonsense mutation in cystinuric Newfoundland dogs. *Hum Genet* 2000;107:295–303.

51 Sanderson SL, Osborne CA, Lulich JP, et al. Evaluation of urinary carnitine and taurine excretion in 5 cystinuric dogs with carnitine and taurine deficiency. *J Vet Intern Med* 2001;15:94–100.

52 Brand E, Cahill GF, Kassell B. Canine cystinuria V. Family history of cystinuric Irish terriers and cystine determinations in urine. *J Biol Chem* 1940;133:430.

53 Hoppe A, Denneberg T, Kågedal B. Treatment of clinically normal and cystinuric dogs with 2-mercaptopropionylglycine. *Am J Vet Res* 1988;49:923–928.

54 Lulich JP, Osborne CA. Voiding urohydropropulsion. In: *Nephrology and Urology of Small Animals* (eds Bartges J, Polzin DJ). Wiley-Blackwell, Chichester, 2011, pp. 375–378.

55 Bartges J, Sura P, Callens A. Minilaparotomy-assisted cystoscopy for urocystoliths. In: *Kirk's Current Veterinary Therapy* (eds Bonagura JD, Twedt DC). Elsevier, St Louis, 2014.

56 Runge JJ, Berent AC, Mayhew PD, et al. Transvesicular percutaneous cystolithotomy for the retrieval of cystic and urethral calculi in dogs and cats: 27 cases (2006–2008). *J Am Vet Med Assoc* 2011;239:344–349.

57 Rawlings C. Diagnostic rigid endoscopy: otoscopy, rhinoscopy, and cystoscopy. *Vet Clin North Am Small Anim Pract* 2009;39:849–868.

58 Rawlings C. Surgical views: endoscopic removal of urinary calculi. *Compend Contin Educ Vet* 2009;31:476–484.

59 Lulich JP, Osborne CA, Albasan H, et al. Efficacy and safety of laser lithotripsy in fragmentation of urocystoliths and urethroliths for removal in dogs. *J Am Vet Med Assoc* 2009;234:1279–1285.

60 Lulich JP, Adams LG, Grant D, et al. Changing paradigms in the treatment of uroliths by lithotripsy. *Vet Clin North Am Small Anim Pract* 2009;39:143–160.

61 Bevan JM, Lulich JP, Albasan H, et al. Comparison of laser lithotripsy and cystotomy for the management of dogs with urolithiasis. *J Am Vet Med Assoc* 2009;234:1286–1294.

62 Grant DC, Werre SR, Gevedon ML. Holmium:YAG laser lithotripsy for urolithiasis in dogs. *J Vet Intern Med* 2008;22:534–539.

63 Adams LG, Berent AC, Moore GE, et al. Use of laser lithotripsy for fragmentation of uroliths in dogs: 73 cases (2005–2006). *J Am Vet Med Assoc* 2008;232:1680–1687.

64 Davidson EB, Ritchey JW, Higbee RD, et al. Laser lithotripsy for treatment of canine uroliths. *Vet Surg* 2004;33:56–61.

65 Berent AC. Ureteral obstructions in dogs and cats: a review of traditional and new interventional diagnostic and therapeutic options. *J Vet Emerg Crit Care* 2011;21:86–103.

98

Feline Ureteral Obstruction: Diagnosis and Management

Allyson Berent, DVM, DACVIM (SAIM)

Animal Medical Center, New York, NY, USA

Introduction

An increasing incidence of problematic ureteroliths, ureteral strictures, obstructive pyonephrosis, and obstructive neoplasia has been seen in veterinary practice over the past decade, particularly for feline patients. The traditional invasiveness and morbidity associated with traditional surgical techniques [1–3], which are often even more complicated for non-stone-related obstructions, make the investigation of minimally invasive alternatives appealing. Interventional radiological (IR) and interventional endoscopic (IE) techniques, like ureteral stenting and the use of a subcutaneous ureteral bypass (SUB) device, have aided tremendously in the ability to treat difficult ureteral obstructions in a more minimally invasive manner, with long-term ureteral protection from future obstruction, while concurrently lowering the perioperative morbidity and mortality when compared to traditional surgical techniques (ureterotomy, neoureterocystostomy, ureteronephrectomy or renal transplantation) [4–12]. The treatment of ureteral obstructions in human medicine is routinely done using more minimally invasive endourological techniques, and this has recently been a similar trend in veterinary medicine.

This chapter will focus on the diagnosis, management, and treatment of cats with ureteral obstructions from various causes and will review data from what has been reported in the past, and some of the more recent data pertaining to more novel approaches and not to their management. Data from over 325 interventionally treated consecutive cases in the author's practice will be expanded upon.

Etiology

Greater than 90% of feline upper tract stones are reported to have a composition of calcium oxalate, meaning that they will not dissolve medically. They either need to pass spontaneously or be removed, or the urine needs to be diverted when an obstruction is present. Additionally, obstructions can occur for other reasons beyond stone disease, such as dried solidified blood clots (~8% cats) [6], strictures (25–30% or more of cats) [6,9,12], tumors (<5% of cats), accidental ureteral ligation during surgery, ureteral trauma, ureteral edema following ureteral surgery, and secondary to purulent material associated with pyelonephritis/pyonephrosis [6]. Obstruction can result in life-threatening azotemia, particularly when presenting bilaterally (~15–20%) in cats with concurrent pre-existing renal insufficiency/failure (>75–90%) [1,6]. For each of these conditions, different options exist and should be considered.

Regardless of the cause of the obstruction, treatment needs to be considered in an expedited manner and should not be delayed. The physiological response to a ureteral obstruction is very complex [13–17]. In dog models, it is shown that after a complete ureteral obstruction, an immediate increase in renal pelvic pressure occurs and the renal blood flow diminishes by 60% over the first 24 hours, and 80% within 2 weeks. This excessive pressure decreases the glomerular filtration rate (GFR). The contralateral kidney will increase its GFR in response, as long as that kidney is normal and has the potential for hypertrophic compensation [13–17]. It has been shown that the longer the ureter remains obstructed, the more progressive the damage (after 7 days the GFR is permanently diminished by 35%, and after 2 weeks by 54%).

Since this research model was performed in normal dogs with a complete ureteral obstruction, without pre-existing azotemia, chronic interstitial nephritis, fibrosis, or chronic obstruction, an extrapolation of a worse outcome might be expected in a clinical patient once the hypertrophy mechanisms are exhausted. Additionally, since over 30% of cats will develop renal azotemia as an adult, leaving less than 25% of renal function, and over 95% of cats diagnosed with a unilateral ureteral

Textbook of Small Animal Emergency Medicine, First Edition. Edited by Kenneth J. Drobatz, Kate Hopper, Elizabeth Rozanski and Deborah C. Silverstein.
© 2019 John Wiley & Sons, Inc. Published 2019 by John Wiley & Sons, Inc.
Companion Website: www.wiley.com/go/drobatz/textbook

obstruction are azotemic at the time of diagnosis, suggesting compromised renal function of the contralateral kidney [6], any preventable loss in GFR should be avoided. This encourages aggressive and timely intervention whenever possible.

Interestingly, in contrast to the irreversibility of a complete obstruction, partial obstructions have been shown to result in less severe and slower nephron destruction, giving more time for intervention when needed [18]. It is estimated in the author's practice that over 85% of feline ureteral obstructions are considered partial, based on ureteropyelography. In a dog model, it was found that after decompression, the GFR returned to normal after 4 weeks from a partial obstruction. Knowing that many patients are partially obstructed, with concurrent renal compromise, aggressive diagnosis, management, and obstruction relief are recommended whenever possible, regardless of the chronicity.

It is now clear that partial obstructions do result in permanent renal damage, just at a slower pace than a complete obstruction, so they should always be treated whenever possible, regardless of the degree of pelvic dilation noted on ultrasound or the suspected chronicity of the condition [6,8]. Knowing the cause of the obstruction is very important when deciding on traditional surgical fixation methods, as different therapeutic methods will be considered for a tumor, stricture, or stone-induced obstruction. For the newer interventional treatment options (double pigtail ureteral stents or a subcutaneous ureteral bypass device), these details are slightly less important, as all can safely be used to treat most causes of a ureteral obstruction effectively, regardless of obstruction cause, location, stone number, or presence of concurrent nephrolithiasis.

Treatment of Feline Ureteral Obstructions

Medical management should always be considered to stabilize a patient prior to any potential anesthetic event. Successful stone passage after medical management has been reported in approximately 8–13% of cases [2], with stones often moving into different positions to allow urine to pass, but the stone itself not actually moving out of the ureter. When this occurs, there is a high risk of reobstruction. The author's recommended approach is to consider fluid diuresis, a ureteral muscle relaxer (alpha-adrenergic blockade), and mannitol (0.25 g/kg bolus IV then 1 mg/kg/min CRI for 24 hours), as long as the patient is not overhydrated, hyperkalemic, oliguric, or showing evidence of progressive renal pelvic dilation on daily imaging. If no stone is seen and there is clear pyuria/bacteriuria (~10–30% of cats with a ureteral obstruction have a positive urine culture) [6,10] then

antibiotics should be started. Purulent plugs can cause a ureteral obstruction in the proximal ureter and medical management can be successful in decompression (Berent, unpublished data). If medical management fails to encourage stone passage after 24–48 hours, then immediate resolution of the obstruction should be considered.

The main interventional options considered in veterinary medicine include nephrostomy tube placement, ureteral stenting, and the placement of a subcutaneous ureteral bypass (SUB) device [4]. Decompression of the renal pelvis will decrease the hydrostatic pressure and stop the permanent damage that is occurring to the renal parenchyma, allowing for immediate renal recovery. When a patient is not stable then intermittent hemodialysis should be considered.

Traditional Surgery

Traditional intervention for *ureterolithiasis* has been accomplished surgically via ureterotomy, neoureterocystostomy, ureteronephrectomy, and renal transplantation [1–3]. In 2005, Kyles et al. reported two retrospective studies in a large number of cats [1,2]. There were high procedure-associated complications (over 30%) and perioperative mortality rates (21%). This study was from two universities that have extensive expertise with ureteral surgery. The morbidity and mortality may be higher in environments where operating microscopes and microsurgical experience are not as readily available. Nearly 10 years later, another study from a different university found the same perioperative mortality rate of 21% [3].

Many of the complications associated with surgery are due to site edema, recurrence of obstruction from stones that pass from the renal pelvis to the surgery site, stricture formation, and ureterotomy-associated or nephrostomy tube-associated urine leakage. In one study [2], over 10% of cats that survived their complications required a second surgical procedure during the same visit and 30% of those cats were then subsequently euthanized or died from serial complications associated with their ureteral stones/surgeries. Of the cats that had long-term imaging follow-up, 40% had evidence of ureteral stone recurrence, 85% percent of which had evidence of ipsilateral nephrolithiasis at the time of the first ureteral surgery [2]. The number of animals that did not have stone recurrence with prior nephrolithiasis was not evident in that study. Chronic kidney disease was found to be common at the time of diagnosis (>75% were azotemic with a unilateral obstruction), and persistent azotemia was commonly seen after a successful surgery (over 50–80% of cats). Even with all of the surgical concerns, survival rates were dramatically higher for cats that had surgical intervention compared to those treated with medical management alone (33% mortality prior to discharge; 87% failure to see any renal functional improvement).

Additionally, over the past 8 years, the number of stones found in the ureter and kidney have been much greater (median of four stones per ureter in our recent study of 79 ureters) [6], with over 60% of patients in that study not being considered good traditional surgical candidates due to the number of stones, location of stones, presence of a proximal stricture, etc. In this same study, over 86% of cats had evidence of ipsilateral nephrolithiasis, making the risk of ureteral reobstruction higher than that reported in previous studies.

Feline *ureteral strictures* were reported in 10 cats in 2011 by Zaid et al. [12], and have since been reported in a larger series of 79 feline ureteral obstruction [6] and a series of 22 cats with circumcaval ureters [9]. Ureteral strictures can occur for various reasons, and are most commonly seen secondary to a previous surgery of the ureter for stone disease, from a stone becoming embedded in the ureteral mucosa, as a congenital abnormality, associated with idiopathic renal hematuria, as an idiopathic process, and possibly associated with a circumcaval (retrocaval) ureter. Most ureteral strictures were found to occur in the very proximal ureter (<2.5 cm from the renal pelvis), in which traditional surgical approaches were difficult, requiring reimplantation with renal descensus and psoas cystopexy or a ureteral resection and anastomosis. With a cat ureter being < 0.4 mm in luminal diameter, this can be a very challenging situation, particularly in a potentially unstable patient.

The ideal procedure would result in immediate decompression and stabilization of the kidney, while concurrently allowing patency to be established quickly and effectively, for any cause of ureteral obstruction (stone, numerous stones, stricture, debris, blood clots, purulent debris, blood stones, tumors, etc.), while decreasing postoperative complications, mortality and long-term reobstruction.

The use of interventional radiological (IR) techniques has aided in circumventing the complications of tradi-

tional ureteral surgery (perioperative leakage, stricture, reobstruction, long anesthesia times, worsening renal function, etc.), particularly in cases that are not considered good surgical candidates. IR techniques have allowed successful and efficient stabilization of the patient regardless of the cause of ureteral obstruction, while decreasing renal pelvic pressure and stopping the cycle of pressure-induced nephron damage and loss [6–10]. It is important to realize when interpreting the current literature that most of what is reported is by groups that have expertise in a certain type of fixation approach. In the hands of an average operator who is not an expert in that particular modality, the outcomes would be expected to be worse, which is the case for traditional surgery and interventional treatment. Additionally, it is important to realize that making a decision between traditional surgery or interventional treatment is not always clear cut. Many, if not most, of the cases reported in the early stages of IR development were those that were considered poor surgical candidates and had failed a previous surgery or were not amenable to traditional surgery. This encouraged an interventional approach to be undertaken. Additionally, most of these early reported cases were in the learning stages of each interventional procedures. It would be unrealistic to try and compare the literature on traditional surgery versus IR techniques due to these reasons. The IR cases were commonly far more complicated, and not amenable to traditional surgery. Instead, the ideal procedure for each patient should be that which would provide the best ultimate outcome in the hands of a particular operator for a particular situation.

Interventional Options

Percutaneous Nephrostomy Tube Placement (Figure 98.1) Fixation procedures can be relatively prolonged and complicated in highly debilitated patients, especially in facilities where expertise in treating feline ureteral obstruction is not extensive. One possibility is to place

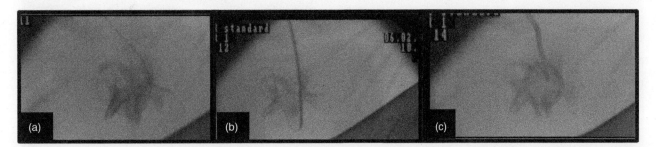

Figure 98.1 Nephrostomy tube placement in a cat with a ureteral obstruction using the modified Seldinger technique. (a) Renal puncture into the kidney of a cat for pyelocentesis and antegrade pyelogram. A guidewire is passed through the catheter and coiled inside the dilated renal pelvis. (b) The catheter is removed over the guidewire and the locking loop pigtail catheter is advanced over the guidewire and coiled inside the renal pelvis. (c) The guidewire is removed and the renal pelvis is drained.

a nephrostomy tube to quickly relieve the obstruction and determine whether adequate renal function remains before prolonged anesthesia for ureteral surgery, ureteral stent or SUB device placement can be performed. A locking loop pigtail catheter is recommended (5 or 6 Fr) to decrease the risk of inadvertent tube removal or urine leakage.

Historically, nephrostomy tubes have met with much resistance due to the high risk of postplacement complications (over 50%). These complications were usually due to premature removal or dislodgment, urine leakage, or poor drainage. With the advent of sturdy, multifenestrated tubes, that form a loop that will lock the catheter in the renal pelvis, these complications seem to have declined dramatically. We reported on the use of the locking loop pigtail catheter in 20 patients [19]. One patient developed leakage into the subcutaneous space and the remaining catheters worked without complication. These locking loop pigtail catheters were deemed to be safe, effective, and well tolerated in both dogs and cats. Placement is typically undertaken percutaneously in dogs using ultrasound and fluoroscopic guidance, and surgically assisted with fluoroscopy and a nephropexy in cats.

Subcutaneous Ureteral Bypass Device

The subcutaneous ureteral bypass device (Norfolk Vet Products) was initially created for feline patients as an alternative to ureteral stents when either a stricture was present (higher rate of stent occlusion, > 50%) or a stent could not be successfully placed due to excessive stones, very narrow lumen, or patient stability. The long-term outcomes documented with the SUB device, the long-term complications, and patient comfort were all found to be superior to those of stents and traditional surgery [8–11]. Due to these findings, the trend in the author's practice has moved toward using the SUB device as a primary treatment option for all-cause ureteral obstruction in cats. It is very important to understand the risks and benefits of traditional surgery, ureteral stenting, and SUB device placement prior to deciding the best treatment option for your patient, all of which should be carefully discussed with the pet owner.

The placement of nephrostomy catheters in veterinary medicine has demonstrated excellent success when the appropriate device is used [19], but the limitation is the externalized drainage, which is not a long-term fixation, requiring an additional surgery to create something more definitive. The development of an indwelling SUB device using a combination locking loop nephrostomy catheter and cystostomy catheter connected to a subcutaneous shunting port has been highly successful for the treatment of all causes of ureteral obstructions (stones, stricture, tumors, and obstructive pyelonephritis) (Figure 98.2). This device reduces the complications associated with externalized nephrostomy tubes and ureteral stents (see below), and has been shown to be associated with lower mortality and long-term complications than both traditional surgery and ureteral stents in cats [2,3,6,9].

We recently evaluated 174 SUBs in 137 cats, of which 33% were bilaterally obstructed. Twenty percent had bilateral SUBs placed, and 13% had the contralateral side treated with alternative options (a ureteral stent, traditional ureteral surgery, or successful medical management prior to SUB placement). The cause of the ureteral obstruction was stone related in 67%, a stricture in 13%, and a stricture with stones in 20%, documenting the high rate of concurrent strictures (33%) associated with ureteral obstructions in cats. The median preoperative creatinine was 6.6 mg/dL (mean 8) and the creatinine at discharge, 3 months, 6 months, 1 year, 2 year, 3 year,

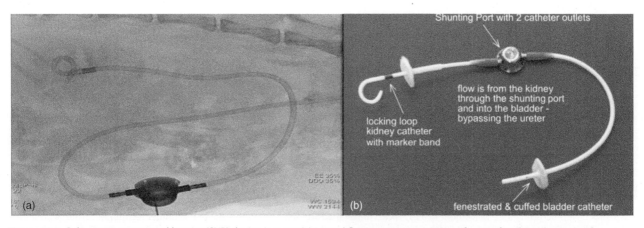

Figure 98.2 Subcutaneous ureteral bypass (SUB) device in a cat. (a) Lateral fluoroscopic projection of a cat after SUB placement for a unilateral ureteral obstruction. Note the nephrostomy tube in the renal pelvis, the cystostomy tube in the urinary bladder and the connection to the subcutaneous metallic shunting port. (b) Catheter hooked up outside the patient.

4 year, and 5 years postoperatively was 2.7, 2.6, 3.1, 2.5, 2.6, 2.2, 2.6 and 4.2 mg/dL, respectively. The perioperative mortality after surgery was 6.6%, with one death associated with an anesthetic-related complication, and none associated with the procedure. The remaining causes of death prior to discharge included failure of improvement of the CKD (2%), pancreatitis (0.7%), neurological signs (0.7%), cardiac causes (0.7%), and other unrelated causes (1.4%). This compares well to traditional surgery (21% perioperative mortality) and ureteral stenting (7.5%). The median survival time was 827 days (range 1 day to 6.6 years), with 51% of patients still alive at the time of data collection. At the time of death, 65% of cases that died were determined to have a renal cause of death as the primary diagnosis. Postoperative complications include leakage of urine (3.4%), kinking of the catheter (5%), and blockage of the system with blood clots or purulent debris (7.5%), or with stone deposition (25%). The need for device exchange from stone deposition in the long term, even in the face of device occlusion, was only apparent in 13% of cases due to the development of ureteral patency at some point after device placement. SUB occlusion was documented in four of 23 of cases with a primary stricture and 35 of 150 (23%) of cases with stones +/− a stricture, compared to 54% of stents in cases with primary strictures.

Dysuria was seen in 23% of cats pre-SUB placement and was uncommonly seen in cats post-SUB placement (8.2%), compared to those with ureteral stents (38%). Of the 8% that had evidence of postprocedural dysuria, 55% had reported dysuria prior to SUB placement, suggesting the possible presence of feline lower urinary tract disease rather than SUB-associated dysuria.

Urinary tract infections were carefully evaluated in this large series of cats after SUB placement, as device implantation and chronic infections had been of concern. Interestingly, chronic urinary tract infections were uncommonly seen after SUB placement in this study (12%) compared to cats after ureteral stenting (30%), with 60% being associated with *Enterococcus* infections, and those cases were nearly always asymptomatic and did not require therapy. Twenty-five percent of cats had a positive culture prior to SUB placement, 10.5% had one infection at any time after SUB placement, and 12% had more than one infection after SUB placement. Only 2.4% of cats had evidence of more than one UTI that did not have a UTI prior to SUB placement, suggesting the SUB device was likely not solely responsible for inducing new infections. Only 8.9% of cats with more than one UTI after SUB placement were considered symptomatic, only one of which (0.8%) was associated with a positive *Enterococcus* infection. Those cats that had urinary tract infections were commonly associated with cats that had externalized urinary catheters (32% of cats with one or more UTIs and 40% of cats with > 1 UTI) during or after SUB placement.

The SUB device is considered a functional option and is the author's treatment of choice in cats with ureteral obstructions. As with all interventional procedures, the learning curve is steep and the procedure should not be performed until the operator is properly trained and is comfortable with the associated risks.

Ureteral Stenting (Figure 98.3)
Ureteral stenting has been performed for a variety of disorders in both dogs and cats (over 400 cases to date). The goal of using a feline double pigtail ureteral stent (Infiniti Medical, LLC) is to divert urine from the renal pelvis into the urinary bladder during a ureteral obstruction (ureterolithiasis, obstructive neoplasia, ureteral stricture/stenosis, dried solidified blood clots or severe obstructive pyelonephritis or pyonephrosis). Stents also encourage passive ureteral dilation (for ureteral stenosis/strictures or future ureteroscopy, extracorporeal shockwave lithotripsy, etc.), which has recently been documented in normal dogs [20]. The double pigtail stent, which is recommended in cats, is completely intracorporeal, and can remain in place long term, maintaining ureteral patency and passive ureteral dilation (a 0.4 mm ureter was documented to dilate to 1.5–2.0 mm within 3–7 days in over 90% of cats in the author's experience). Each loop of the pigtail is curled (one in the bladder and one in the renal pelvis), allowing for direct urinary diversion from the kidney to the urinary bladder, around the stones, or through the stricture.

In most cats (male and female), the procedure is done using fluoroscopy and surgical assistance using nephrostomy needle access in an antegrade manner, although it can be attempted endoscopically in female cats with a reported 20% success rate (compared to over 95% success with antegrade surgical assistance). Endoscopic

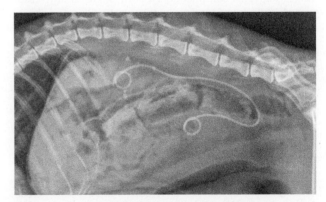

Figure 98.3 Lateral radiograph in a cat after ureteral stent placement for nephroureterolithiasis. Note one pigtail is in the renal pelvis and the other is in the urinary bladder. The shaft of the stent is within the lumen of the ureter.

approaches are not typically performed due to the technical complexity in most practices. This procedure requires special training and experience using wires, catheters and stents, and is not recommended in all patients with a ureteral obstruction. If the operator is not comfortable placing a locking loop pigtail catheter for a nephrostomy tube then this procedure should not be attempted because if stent placement is not successful, the ureter will experience severe edema and spasm and will be acutely obstructed, requiring another mechanism of drainage. Those that are using ureteral stents should be well trained in SUB device placement, nephrostomy tube placement and traditional ureteral surgery so that all options are available for each patient.

A recent study evaluating 69 feline patients (79 ureters) with ureteral obstructions treated with a ureteral stent had a 96% placement success, 14% were bilaterally obstructed, 28% were associated with strictures (+/− concurrent ureteroliths), and 85% of cases had concurrent nephroliths [6]. The median number of stones in the obstructed ureter was four. Approximately one-third of cats had documentation of a urinary tract infection prior to stent placement, and 30% of cats had at least one positive culture in their lifetime after stent placement. The median preoperative creatinine was 5.3 mg/dL and 2.1 mg/dL after stent placement. The perioperative mortality after surgery was 7.5%, with no death associated with a ureteral obstruction or the procedure. This compares to 6.6% mortality with the SUB device [6,9] and 21% with traditional surgery [2,3]. The most common long-term (>1 month) complications after ureteral stent placement were dysuria (38%, but only persistent in 2% after medical management), chronic hematuria (18%), stent occlusion (19%), stent migration (6%), and ureteritis/mucosal proliferation (4%). The dysuria typically resolved with short-term steroid therapy. A ureteral stent exchange with either a bigger stent or a SUB device was needed in 27% of cats for either occlusion or migration. This complication was most commonly associated with ureteral strictures (over 50% of strictured ureters experienced reocclusion) or an occlusion at a previous ureterotomy site. Ureters remained patent long term in most cats, with the longest stent in place and functional for over 5 years. The median survival time was 498 days in this study. The median survival time with a renal cause of death was over 1250 days, with only 21% of cats dying of suspected CKD. With evaluation of cases being treated with all the different options, the author finds that the SUB device is the safest and most expeditious procedure for most causes feline ureteral obstruction, especially in when performed by trained operators.

Another study evaluating preoperative prognostic factors for short- and long-term survivals and renal recovery did not identify any clinical, biochemical or imaging findings to suggest overall survival in patients. It is important to note that in this study, as well as the SUB device study, there was no association or prediction of renal pelvis size, or kidney size, on preoperative ultrasound and long-term survival. Making an assumption of chronicity and treatment success based on any preoperative information was not shown to be predictive of survival and the ultimate prognosis for renal recovery was considered good to great.

Extracorporeal Shockwave Lithotripsy for Ureterolithiasis

Extracorporeal shockwave lithotripsy (ESWL) is another minimally invasive alternative for the removal of ureteral calculi. ESWL delivers external shockwaves through a water medium directed under fluoroscopic guidance in two planes. The stone is shocked at different energy levels to allow for implosion and powdering. This procedure has been effective in only a small number of feline cases and is possible for very distal ureteroliths or small stones < 3 mm in diameter, but is not commonly done in cats. It is important to remember that the feline ureter is normally only 0.3–0.4 mm in diameter and the ESWL unit will break stones to approximately 1 mm in diameter. Without ureteral dilation (concurrent ureteral stent), most of these stones will therefore not pass, and if they do pass, it can take weeks to see that benefit, which promotes renal function deterioration. In addition, feline stones are typically embedded into the ureteral mucosa, so even if the stones fragment well with ESWL, they may not pass as effectively as seen in dogs.

Postoperative Management

Feline patients can have a substantial postobstructive diuresis after relieving a ureteral obstruction, necessitating a large quantity of fluids to maintain hydration. This should be carefully monitored and managed. The leading postoperative complication found in the ureteral stent series was the development of congestive heart failure associated with fluid overload [6]. Most of these patients had a normal echocardiogram prior to their procedure, but the volume of fluids required to maintain their hydration was overloading to their heart. Because of this finding, the author has advocated using a combination of a maintenance rate of enteral hydration (unflavored electrolyte solution – Pedialyte) through the use of an esophagostomy tube (placed at the time of ureteral decompression); a maintenance rate of a low sodium maintenance fluid (0.45% NaCl + 2.5% dextrose); and the remainder of fluids necessary as a replacement fluid. This has been found to lower the sodium load and decrease the risk of fluid overload in the author's experience. Body weights are monitored extremely carefully with fluid rate adjustments occurring throughout each weight assessment.

In the SUB patients, there was no one cause of death due to fluid overload, and all patients were managed similarly with the above protocol. Due to this improved fluid balance in these critically ill patients, the author advocates this approach. Once the creatinine level reaches a plateau, the patient can be weaned off IV fluids, discharged and monitored at 1 and 4 weeks postoperatively (with bloodwork and a urinary tract ultrasound), and a 4-week SUB flush. After this evaluation, they are evaluated every 3 months with bloodwork, a focal urinary tract ultrasound with a SUB flush, and a urinalysis and urine culture is obtained during this flush. Currently the SUB device is being regularly flushed with an antiseptic and anti-mineralization material called tetra-EDTA. Since starting this protocol less than 2% of patients have had any signs of SUB device mineralization or chronic infections.

Conclusion

The feline ureter is a frustrating area to gain access to for both diagnosis and treatment of disease. With recent advances in veterinary interventional endourological techniques, diagnosis and treatment have become less invasive, more effective, and safer. Proper training and the availability of specialized equipment are needed to help these procedures become more available in the future. With these new devices in veterinary medicine, we are hoping to find better alternatives for these problematic conditions, as we have seen in our human counterparts. These techniques offer an alternative option to traditional surgery, and as the data are published, the veterinary community can decide if, and when, interventional techniques will replace traditional surgery, as is the case in human medicine.

References

1 Kyles A, Hardie E, Wooden B, et al. Clinical, clinicopathologic, radiographic, and ultrasonographic abnormalties in cats with ureteral calculi: 163 cases (1984–2002). *J Am Vet Med Assoc* 2005;226(6):932–936.

2 Kyles A, Hardie E, Wooden B, et al. Management and outcome of cats with ureteral calculi: 153 cases (1984–2002). *J Am Vet Med Assoc* 2005;226(6):937–944.

3 Roberts S, Aronson L, Brown D. Postoperative mortality in cats after ureterolithotomy. *Vet Surg* 2011;40:438–443.

4 Berent A. New techniques on the horizon: interventional radiology and interventional endoscopy of the urinary tract ('endourology'). *J Feline Med Surg* 2014;16(1):51–65.

5 Berent A. Interventional urology: endourology in small animal veterinary medicine. *Vet Clin North Am Small Anim Pract* 2015;45(4):825–855.

6 Berent A, Weisse C, Bagley D. Ureteral stenting for benign feline ureteral obstructions: technical and clinical outcomes in 79 ureters (2006–2010). *J Am Vet Med Assoc* 2014;244:559–576.

7 Nicoli S, Morello E, Martano M, et al. Double-J ureteral stenting in nine cats with ureteral obstruction. *Vet J* 2012;194(1):60–65.

8 Horowitz C, Berent A, Weisse C, et al. Prognostic indicators of short and long-term outcome in cats with interventional management of ureteral obstructions. *J Feline Med Surg* 2013;15(12):1052–1062.

9 Steinhaus J, Berent A, Weisse C, et al. Presence of circumcaval ureters and ureteral obstructions in cats. *J Vet Intern Med* 2015;29(1):63–70.

10 Berent A, Weisse C, Bagley D, et al. The use of a subcutaneous ureteral bypass device for the treatment of feline ureteral obstructions. ECVIM, Seville, Spain, 2011.

11 Berent A. Ureteral obstructions in dogs and cats: a review of traditional and new interventinal diagnostic and therapeutic options. *J Vet Emerg Crit Care* 2011;21(2):86–103.

12 Zaid M, Berent A, Weisse C, et al. Feline ureteral strictures: 10 cases (2007–2009). *J Vet Intern Med* 2011;25(2):222–229.

13 Coroneos E, Assouad M, Krishnan B, et al. Urinary obstruction causes irreversible renal failure by inducing chronic tubuointerstitial nephritis. *Clin Nephrol* 1997;48:125–128.

14 Wilson DR. Renal function during and following obstruction. *Ann Rev Med* 1977;28:329–339.

15 Fink RW, Caradis DT, Chmiel R, et al. Renal impairment and its reversibility following variable periods of complete ureteric obstruction. *Aust NZ J Surg* 1980;50:77–83.

16 Kerr WS. Effect of complete ureteral obstruction for one week on kidney function. *J Appl Physiol* 1954;6:762–772.

17 Vaughan DE, Sweet RE, Gillenwater JY. Unilateral ureteral occlusion: pattern of nephron repair and compensatory response. *J Urol* 1973;109:979–982.

18 Shokeir A, Nijman R, El-Azab M, et al. Partial ureteral obstruction: role of renal resistive index in stages of obstruction and release. *Urology* 1997;49(4):528–535.

19 Berent A, Weisse C, Todd K, et al. Use of locking-loop pigtail nephrostomy catheters in dogs and cats: 20 cases (2004–2009). *J Am Vet Med Assoc* 2012;241:348–357.

20 Vachon C, Defrages A, Berent A, et al. Passive ureteral dilation and ureteroscopy following ureteral stent placement in normal dogs. *J Vet Intern Med* 2014;28:1073.

99

Feline Lower Urinary Tract Obstruction

Edward Cooper, VMD, MS, DACVECC

Veterinary Medical Center, Ohio State University, Columbus, OH, USA

Pathogenesis of Obstruction

Urethral obstruction (UO) is a potentially life-threatening manifestation of feline lower urinary tract disease. It has long been held that a physical obstruction, such as a calculus or urethral plug (or, much less commonly, stricture or neoplasia), is responsible for occluding the lumen of the urethra in these cases. However, there is evidence to suggest that functional (or "idiopathic") obstruction secondary to urethral spasm and edema may play an equally important role in up to 50% [1,2].

These conditions in the urethra are thought to be brought about by underlying feline idiopathic cystitis (FIC). The pathogenesis of FIC is still unclear but it appears to be a sterile inflammatory process as attempts to isolate a bacterial or viral cause have been unsuccessful [3,4]. Instead, documented neurohumoral alterations in cats with FIC suggest the disease may be related to a sympathetic and hypothalamic-pituitary-adrenal imbalance brought about by stressful situations [5]. This imbalance is thought to result in impaired blood flow and release of inflammatory mediators which cause edema, smooth muscle spasm, and pain within the lower urinary tract. These conditions, either independently or in conjunction with a physical obstruction such as a plug or stone, are ultimately what lead to urethral obstruction in cats.

Predisposing Factors

Given their long and narrow urethra (compared to females), it is generally thought that male cats are much more likely to develop obstruction. Further, the likely association with FIC suggests there is also potential cross-over with regard to predisposing factors for UO. In one study examining patients with FIC, it was determined that male, pedigreed and long-hair cats were at increased risk, as well as multi-cat households and known with a housemate [6]. No association was found with age, diet, and indoor–outdoor status. Another FIC study similarly found weight and number of household cats to be risk factors, but did not find an association with breed, long hair, or neuter status [7]. This study also found use of a litter pan, decreased water intake and predominant indoor status were risk factors, but number of litter boxes, conflict with a housemate, and feeding wet versus dry food were not.

In the only available study specifically investigating predisposing factors in cats with UO, it was determined that indoor–outdoor cats in the control population had a decreased likelihood of obstruction [8]. Obstructed cats were older, weighed more and were more likely to be fed dry food only [8]. This study did not reveal any association with breed, neuter or vaccination status, or number of pets in the household.

Pathophysiology of Obstruction

Regardless of underlying cause, complete obstruction of the urethra leads to the accumulation of urine and pressure within the urethra and urinary bladder. Once the tissue can no longer distend, pressure necrosis and mucosal injury will occur. Pressure within the urinary bladder is then transmitted up the ureters to the kidney, with subsequent reduction of glomerular filtration. Within 24–48 hours of obstruction, the kidney's excretory ability ceases, resulting in an accumulation of blood urea nitrogen, creatinine, phosphorus, potassium, and hydrogen ion in the blood which largely contributes to the clinical signs associated with UO.

Uremia can cause depression, nausea, vomiting, and anorexia. The combination of decreased intake of food and water, along with potential gastrointestinal losses (vomiting and diarrhea), can result in dehydration and potential for hypovolemia. Development of profound

Textbook of Small Animal Emergency Medicine, First Edition. Edited by Kenneth J. Drobatz, Kate Hopper, Elizabeth Rozanski and Deborah C. Silverstein.
© 2019 John Wiley & Sons, Inc. Published 2019 by John Wiley & Sons, Inc.
Companion Website: www.wiley.com/go/drobatz/textbook

metabolic acidosis can lead to denaturing of proteins, enzymatic dysfunction, and catecholamine hyposensitivity. Severe hyperkalemia is considered to be the most life-threatening aspect of UO because of its effects on the cardiovascular system. Elevations in serum potassium affect electrical conduction by raising resting membrane potential and causing diminished sodium conductance. As a result, the rate of depolarization is significantly diminished, resulting in bradycardia. If the serum potassium level gets high enough (typically greater than 10–12 mEq/L), electrical activity in the heart can cease altogether. Without intervention, these changes will ultimately progress to cardiovascular collapse and death, typically within 3–5 days.

History and Clinical Signs

The classic history associated with UO involves a male cat which has been vocalizing and straining unproductively in the litter box. However, these signs might be difficult to distinguish from a cat with FIC. In addition, FIC cats will often urinate very small amounts frequently, and sometimes outside the litter box, making it difficult to know for sure if urine is produced. Multicat households can also present challenges for owners to keep track of whether or not the cat has been urinating. One distinguishing feature of UO (versus FIC) is the development of systemic signs as the obstruction progresses. This could include vomiting, lethargy, anorexia, and abdominal pain which can eventually progress to changes in mentation and lateral recumbency. These signs are fairly non-specific if UO is not suspected, so obstruction should be considered as a differential for any sick male cat.

Clinical signs can vary considerably, depending on severity at the time of presentation. Patients that present early may not have any striking physical exam findings aside from a firm, moderate to large urinary bladder. In the "healthy" blocked cat, this is the most definitive way to help distinguish between obstruction and cystitis (as cystitis cats should have a small, barely palpable bladder). If the obstruction has been present for greater than 24 hours, the patient may be showing signs of systemic illness such as dehydration, bradycardia, and/or hypothermia. The presence of bradycardia in male cats should always raise concern for hyperkalemia as the normal stress response to hospital presentation should result in tachycardia (though cats in septic or cardiogenic shock can also demonstrate bradycardia). In fact, the combination of bradycardia (HR < 140) and hypothermia (T < 96.6 °F) has been found to be strongly predictive of severe hyperkalemia (serum level greater than 8 mEq/L) in cats with urethral obstruction [9].

Initial Stabilization

Presentation of the "sick" blocked cat warrants immediate medical attention. An IV catheter should be placed and initial blood samples obtained (PCV/TP, stat electrolyte/acid–base/renal values). Fluid therapy should be started immediately to support vascular volume and help dilute serum potassium concentration, even if bladder decompression cannot be performed immediately. While there are theoretical arguments for use of 0.9% NaCl versus a balanced electrolyte solution (potassium content and acid–base effects), two studies have shown no difference in outcome (survival, length of stay) or in reduction of serum potassium levels [10,11]. And while the acid–base abnormalities corrected more rapidly with a balanced electrolyte solution, overall it does not appear that fluid type has a significant clinical impact. Volume and rate of fluid administration should be dictated by cardiovascular stability, as well as hydration status and/or any concern for underlying cardiac disease.

An ECG is beneficial, even if the patient is not bradycardic, to determine any effects hyperkalemia might be having on cardiac electrical conduction. Classic ECG changes associated with hyperkalemia include prolonged P-R interval, diminished to absent P-waves, widened QRS and tall tented T-waves. As hyperkalemia worsens, ECG changes can progress to atrial standstill, ventricular fibrillation or asystole. While deobstruction and IV fluids will ultimately be the primary means of eliminating potassium and reversing the adverse affects of hyperkalemia, this process takes time. If the patient has significant bradycardia (HR < 140) then immediate intervention to protect the heart (calcium gluconate) and promote intracellular shift of potassium (regular insulin, dextrose, terbutaline, and/or sodium bicarbonate) should be employed (see Table 99.1 for dosing recommendations). Given that calcium gluconate does not serve to decrease potassium levels, if administration is needed to stabilize electrical conduction, the patient should also receive dextrose, or insulin and dextrose (note: dextrose should always be given with insulin to prevent the development of hypoglycemia).

Although controversial, cystocentesis can also be a part of initial stabilization by allowing immediate relief of pressure within the urinary tract and more rapid resumption of glomerular filtration. This could be especially important when busy emergency receiving does not afford the time which might be necessary to relieve the obstruction by passing a urinary catheter (particularly for a novice clinician). In addition, only moderate sedation is usually necessary to perform cystocentesis and a "pure" urine sample can be obtained for urinalysis or urine culture. Finally, relieving the backpressure against the obstruction (whether stone, plug or spasm) may make for easier passage of a urinary catheter, although this has not been substantiated.

Table 99.1 Emergency dosing for severe hyperkalemia. All medications given intravenously.

Medication	Dose	Rate of administration	When to administer
Calcium gluconate	50–150 mg/kg	3–5 minutes	Bradycardia, major ECG changes
Regular insulin	1 unit	IV bolus	If Ca gluconate given
			Potassium > 8 mEq/L
Dextrose	0.5 g/kg	3–5 minutes	If Ca gluconate given
			Potassium > 8 mEq/L
Terbutaline	0.01 mg/kg	IV bolus	If Ca gluconate given
			Potassium > 8 mEq/L
Sodium bicarbonate	1 mEq/kg	5 minutes	Potassium > 10 mEq/L
			pH < 7.0

The major concern raised against performing cystocentesis in UO cats is the potential for tearing or rupture of a distended and friable bladder with resultant uroabdomen. However, a recent retrospective study of 47 UO cats undergoing decompressive cystocentesis did not reveal any significant complications [12]. A prospective study of 45 blocked cats has also demonstrated that development of clinically significant abdominal effusion, as evidenced by abdominal ultrasound performed before and after cystocentesis, occurs very uncommonly and further suggests that this procedure can be safely performed [13].

To help limit the risk of complications, it is important to ensure adequate patient compliance and/or provide sedation so there is minimal patient movement during the procedure. A flexible collection system (syringe, three-way stopcock, extension tubing and 22–20 G needle) may also be beneficial (Figure 99.1).

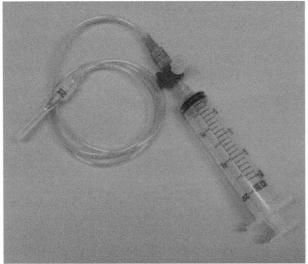

Figure 99.1 Set-up for performing cystocentesis including syringe, three-way stopcock, extension tubing, and 22 G needle.

Urethral Catheterization

Passage of a urinary catheter to relieve a physical obstruction is generally considered to be essential in the management of UO (see Chapter 187). In addition to successful catheter placement, every effort should be made to minimize urethral trauma as tearing or stricture formation can add significantly to morbidity, cost, and even mortality (from euthanasia) [14].

In order to optimize the likelihood of successful catheterization and minimize damage to the urethra, heavy sedation/analgesia or anesthesia is recommended (Box 99.1). Vocalizing or movement during catheterization attempts, reflecting insufficient sedation, is likely to be associated with significant urethral spasm and an increased risk of urethral trauma. In addition, creating a mixture of saline and sterile lubricant (10:1) as the flush solution can serve to deposit lubricant along the

---

Box 99.1 Suggested anesthesia protocols for urethral deobstruction.

Stable patient
  Premedication/sedation
    Ketamine (5–10 mg/kg) + diazepam/midazolam (0.25–0.5 mg/kg)
    Buprenorphine (0.01–0.02 mg/kg) and
    Acepromazine (0.01–0.05 mg/kg) or diazepam/ Midazolam (0.25–0.5 mg/kg)
  Induction
    Propofol (1–4 mg/kg, to effect)
  Maintenance
    Inhalant anesthesia (isoflurane, sevoflurane)
Unstable patient
    Buprenorphine (0.01–0.02 mg/kg) + diazepam/ Midazolam (0.25–0.5 mg/kg)
    Methadone (0.2–0.25 mg/kg) + diazepam/ Midazolam (0.25–0.5 mg/kg)

Figure 99.2 Catheter flushing apparatus including two syringes, three-way stopcock, extension tubing, sterile saline, and sterile lubricant.

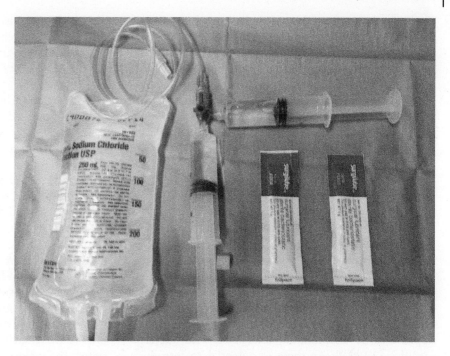

entire length of the urethra and potentially decrease urethral damage (Figure 99.2). Another helpful technique is to pull the prepuce caudally once the catheter is seeded in the penile urethra. This will straighten out the urethra, thus making passage of the catheter easier and less traumatic.

An open-ended catheter (polypropylene, polytetrafluoroethylene or polyurethane) is typically used to

initially relieve the obstruction (Figure 99.3). Given that a polypropylene catheter is rigid and can cause significant urethral irritation [15], it should be withdrawn and replaced by a softer indwelling catheter. Both polytetrafluoroethylene and polyurethane catheters carry the benefit of being firmer at room temperature to facilitate initial unblocking efforts, but then soften when warmed to body temperature (meaning they can be left in place).

Figure 99.3 Common types of catheter used for urethral deobstruction and/or indwelling management – polypropylene (a), polyvinyl (b), polytetrafluoroethylene (c), polyurethane (d).

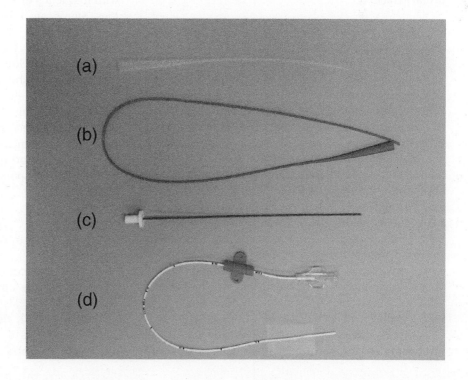

Findings of a recent study suggest that use of a 3.5 Fr urinary catheter may be associated with less risk of immediate reobstruction when compared to 5 Fr [16]. Given the retrospective nature of this study, care should be taken in interpreting the result, especially given that another similar study failed to find this association [17]. With the catheter securely in place, the urinary bladder can be emptied and flushed, and a closed sterile collection system placed to help decrease the risk of ascending infection.

Diagnostic Evaluation

Careful selection of additional diagnostics to be performed can be very important in UO, especially in cases with limited financial resources. A complete blood count will not often yield significant information beyond that provided by PCV/TP. Urinalysis may reveal crystalluria, along with hematuria and pyuria. Urinary culture at the time of presentation is unlikely to be useful as UO appears to be uncommonly associated with bacterial cystitis [12,18,19]. As there is potential to introduce a UTI, it is recommended that urine culture and sensitivity be performed at the time of catheter removal, although the overall incidence of catheter-associated UTI in UO is currently unknown (see Chapter 96). Given the significant potential for contamination during catheter removal, the practice of submitting the catheter tip for culture should be avoided. It is also prudent to perform abdominal radiographs to assess for cystic/urethral calculi, being certain to include the entire lower urinary tract.

Postobstructive Care

Fluid therapy and monitoring urine output are important aspects of postobstructive care. Patients which have had prolonged obstruction are at risk of a postobstructive diuresis (POD), resulting in massive urine production. This diuresis is thought to occur secondary to the accumulation of osmotically active substances in the blood, pressure necrosis, medullary washout and/or antidiuretic hormone resistance brought about during the obstructive process. It has been demonstrated that POD (defined as urine output > 2 mL/kg/h) may occur in 46% and 88% of postobstructive cats [20,21]. However, in the latter study, the proposed incidence decreased to 37% when corrected for rate of fluid administration. Regardless, it is very important to keep up with urinary losses in these patients as they can quickly become severely dehydrated and hypovolemic.

Another potential concern is for inadequate urine production (<1 mL/kg/h) after obstruction is relieved.

This could occur as a result of obstruction in the collection system or dehydration. True oliguria could occur as a result of progression to acute renal failure but this appears to be very uncommon in urethral obstruction (see Chapter 95).

Another important aspect of postobstructive care is analgesia and sedation (see Section 7; Chapters 190–193). Cystitis and obstruction, in addition to urethral catheterization, are painful and could be associated with risk of reobstruction. An opioid (such as buprenorphine or methadone) generally provides sufficient pain control. In addition to analgesia, acepromazine can provide adequate sedation to decrease stress and agitation (provided the patient is cardiovascularly stable). The alpha-antagonist effects of acepromazine might promote urethral relaxation [22]. Prazosin, an alpha-1-antagonist, could also be used for this purpose.

A frequent consideration in the postobstructive period is whether the patient should be placed on antibiotics, either to address existing UTI or prevent development of UTI from having a catheter in place. As previously stated, the incidence of UTI at presentation appears to be very low [12,18,19]. Further, it has been well documented that antibiotics do not prevent development of catheter-associated UTI [23,24] and in two studies investigating incidence of acquired UTI, rates of 13–33% were reported [18,19]. Given the low incidence, performing a urine culture and sensitivity after catheter removal is recommended to determine if a UTI has been introduced (see Chapter 96).

Electrolytes and renal values are serially monitored, with frequency dictated by initial severity of abnormalities. Significant reduction in renal values is expected within 24 hours, otherwise complications may have occurred (renal failure, uroabdomen, etc.). Hypokalemia can develop (especially in patients with POD) and potassium should be supplemented accordingly. The urinary catheter is typically left in place until the cat is clinically improved, bloodwork has normalized, POD has resolved, and urine is free of major debris, clots or plugs. Once the catheter has been removed, a 12–24-hour period of observation is recommended to ensure effective spontaneous urination is possible prior to discharge.

Alternative Management Protocols

Owner financial constraints may significantly affect the ability to provide optimal care for cats with UO. For severely affected cats (hypothermia, bradycardia, lateral recumbency, etc.), euthanasia may be the only option. As an alternative to euthanasia in stable UO cats, it has been demonstrated that an in-hospital protocol of pharmacological manipulation (analgesia and sedation), a low-stress environment, and intermittent cystocentesis can result in spontaneous urination without the need for catheterization [25]. Alternatively, patients that must be seen on an outpatient basis may be managed with bladder decompression through one-time passage of a urinary catheter to clear any physical obstruction. The patient is then discharged with recommendations as outlined below in the hope that continued analgesia and sedation will allow for spontaneous urination to occur.

At-Home Care

Given the potential for recurrence, at-home care may be extremely important to help decrease the likelihood of reobstruction either immediately or in the future. Continued analgesia and sedation after discharge may be helpful, with administration of acepromazine and buprenorphine or gabapentin for 5–7 days. For patients demonstrating significant straining/urethral spasm after catheter removal, it may be of benefit to also administer prazosin as an alpha-1 antagonist and urethral relaxant. Antibiotics should only be dispensed based on results of urine culture taken at the time of catheter removal (see

Chapter 96). Other recommendations which have been made to help decrease the risk of reobstruction include increasing water intake by switching to wet food, flavoring the water, or using a running-water bowl. Given the questionable role that urinary crystals play in the pathogenesis of obstruction, it is unclear whether dietary manipulation of urinary pH to address crystalluria is beneficial. Given the potential role that stress may play in the pathogenesis of this disease, environmental enrichment may also help [26].

Prognosis

The potential recurrence of UO has been reported as anywhere from 15% to 40% [2,16,17,27]. With a second obstructive episode, it becomes more likely that there will be subsequent occurrences, at which point it may be necessary to consider perineal urethrostomy (PU). This surgical procedure can significantly decrease the likelihood of UO, although it does not serve to resolve signs of underlying FIC. In addition, these patients may be at an increased risk for UTI. However, a study of 86 cats undergoing PU showed good long-term quality of life with minimal risk of recurrence [28].

References

1 Bartges JW, Finco DR, Polzin DJ, et al. Pathophysiology of urethral obstruction. *Vet Clin North Am Small Anim Pract* 1996;26(2):255–264.
2 Gerber B, Eichenberger S, Reusch CE. Guarded long-term prognosis in male cats with urethral obstruction. *J Feline Med Surg* 2008;10:16–23.
3 Kruger JM, Osborne CA, Lulich JP. Changing paradigms of feline idiopathic cystitis. *Vet Clin North Am Small Anim Pract* 2009;39(1):15–40.
4 Larson J, Kruger JM, Wise AG, et al. Nested case-control study of feline calicivirus viruria, oral carriage, and serum neutralizing antibodies in cats with idiopathic cystitis. *J Vet Intern Med* 2011; 5(2):199–205.
5 Buffington CA, Teng B, Somogyi GT. Norepinephrine content and adrenoceptor function in the bladder of cats with feline idiopathic cystitis. *J Urol* 2002;167(4):1876–1880.
6 Cameron ME, Casey RA, Bradshaw JWS, et al. A study of environmental and behavioural factors that may be associated with feline idiopathic cystitis. *J Small Anim Pract* 2004;45(3):144–147.
7 Defauw PA, van de Maele I, Duchateau L, et al. Risk factors and clinical presentation of cats with feline idiopathic cystitis. *J Feline Med Surg* 2011;13(12):967–975.
8 Segev G, Livne H, Ranen E, et al. Urethral obstruction in cats: predisposing factors, clinical, clinicopathological characteristics and prognosis. *J Feline Med Surg* 2011;13:101–108.
9 Lee JA, Drobatz KJ. Historical and physical parameters as predictors of severe hyperkalemia. *J Vet Emerg Crit Care* 2006;16(2):104–111.
10 Drobatz KJ, Cole SG. The influence of crystalloid type on acid-base and electrolyte status of cats with urethral obstruction. *J Vet Emerg Crit Care* 2008;18(4):355–361.
11 Cunha MG, Freitas GC, Carregaro AB, et al. Renal and cardiorespiratory effects of treatment with lactated Ringer's solution or physiologic saline (0.9% NaCl) solution in cats with experimentally induced urethral obstruction. *Am J Vet Res* 2010;71(7):840–846.
12 Hall J, Hall K, Powell LL, et al. Outcome of male cats managed for urethral obstruction with decompressive cystocentesis and urinary catheterization: 47 cats (2009–2012). *J Vet Emerg Crit Care* 2015;25(2):256–262.
13 Cooper ES, Weder C, Butler A, et al. Incidence of abdominal effusion associated with decompressive cystocentesis in male cats with urethral obstruction. Proceedings of the 19th Annual Veterinary Emergency and Critical Care Symposium, 2013, p. 801.
14 Addison ES, Halfacree Z, Moore AH, et al. A retrospective analysis of urethral rupture in 63 cats. *J Feline Med Surg* 2014;16(4):300–307.

15 Lees GE, Osborne CA, Stevens JB, et al. Adverse effects caused by polypropylene and polyvinyl feline urinary catheters. *Am J Vet Res* 1980;41(11):1836–1840.

16 Hetrick PF, Davidow EB. Initial treatment factors associated with feline urethral obstruction recurrence rate: 192 cases (2004–2010). *J Am Vet Med Assoc* 2013;243:512–519.

17 Eisenberg BW, Waldrop JE, Allen SE, et al. Evaluation of risk factors associated with recurrent obstruction in cats treated medically for urethral obstruction. *J Am Vet Med Assoc* 2013;243(8):1140–1146.

18 Hugonnard M, Chalvet-Monfray K, Dernis J, et al. Occurrence of bacteriuria in 18 catheterised cats with obstructive lower urinary tract disease: a pilot study. *J Feline Med Surg* 2013;15:843–848.

19 Cooper ES, Lasley E, Daniels J, et al. Incidence of urinary tract infection at presentation and after urinary catheterization in feline urethral obstruction. Proceedings of the 19th Annual Veterinary Emergency and Critical Care Symposium, 2013, p. 815.

20 Francis BJ, Wells RJ, Rao S, et al. Retrospective study to characterize post-obstructive diuresis in cats with urethral obstruction. *J Feline Med Surg* 2010;12:606–608.

21 Frohlich L, Hartmann K, Sautter-Loius C, et al. Postobstructive diuresis in cats with naturally occurring lower urinary tract obstruction: incidence, severity and association with laboratory parameters on admission. *J Feline Med Surg* 2016;18:809–817.

22 Marks SL, Straeter-Knowlen IM, Moore M, et al. Effects of acepromazine maleate and phenoxybenzamine on urethral pressure profiles of anesthetized, healthy, sexually intact male cats. *Am J Vet Res* 1996;57:1497–1500.

23 Barsanti JA, Shotts EB, Crowell WA, et al. Effect of therapy on susceptibility to urinary tract infection in male cats with indwelling urethral catheters. *J Vet Intern Med* 1992;6(2):64–70.

24 Lees GE, Osborne CA, Stevens JB, Ward GE. Adverse effects of open indwelling urethral catheterization in clinically normal male cats. *Am J Vet Res* 1981;42(5):825–833.

25 Cooper ES, Owens TJ, Chew DJ, et al. Managing urethral obstruction in male cats without urethral catheterization. *J Am Vet Med Assoc* 2010;237(11):1261–1266.

26 Buffington CAT, Westropp JL, Chew DJ, et al. Clinical evaluation of multimodal environmental modification (MEMO) in the management of cats with idiopathic cystitis. *J Feline Med Surg* 2006;8(4):261–268.

27 Segev G, Livne H, Ranen E, et al. Urethral obstruction in cats: predisposing factors, clinical, clinicopathological characteristics and prognosis. *J Feline Med Surg* 2011;13:101–108.

28 Ruda L, Heiene R. Short- and long-term outcome after perineal urethrostomy in 86 cats with feline lower urinary tract disease. *J Small Anim Pract* 2012;53(12):693–698.

100

Urethral Trauma

Elena S. Addison, MA, VetMB, DECVS, MRCVS and Donald A. Yool, BVMS, PhD, DECVS, CertSAS, MRCVS

University of Glasgow, Glasgow, UK

Incidence

The reported incidence of traumatic urethral rupture ranges from 0.003% to 5% [1,2] in dogs; however, the incidences in cats and of iatrogenic urethral injury are unknown. Males are more frequently affected in both dogs (85%) [3] and cats (88.9%) [4]. The ischiocavernosus and ischiourethralis muscles anchor the urethra to the ischium in the male [5,6], which may make it less tolerant to traumatic traction and shearing forces [7]. The male urethra also has a smaller diameter, predisposing it to obstruction [7]. This may increase the risk of iatrogenic injury through increased likelihood of urethral catheterization being performed. Differences in temperament with increasing roaming in males may also lead to a greater risk of vehicular trauma [8].

The most common cause of urethral injury in both dogs and cats is trauma, accounting for 70% of cases in dogs [4] and 55.6% of cases in cats [7]. In dogs, urethral injury is associated with pelvic fractures in 85.7% of cases [4]. However, in cats, pelvic fractures account for only 37.1% of cases [7], indicating that blunt trauma without pelvic fracture can lead to significant urethral injury in cats.

Patient Evaluation

Clinical signs are variable and include dysuria, stranguria, anuria, hematuria, abdominal distension and discomfort, anorexia, depression and hind imb, inguinal, and perineal swelling or bruising [4–9]. It is important to ascertain whether the animal has suffered any trauma or has a history of urolithiasis, urethral catheterization or previous surgery in the vicinity of the urethra.

During physical examination, particular attention should be paid to abdominal palpation for bladder assessment and for signs of pain. The hindlimbs, inguinal, and perineal area must be evaluated for swelling or discomfort, which may indicate subcutaneous urine extravasation. Assessment of hemodynamic status and correction of any metabolic abnormalities is important. Affected animals may be azotemic, hyperkalemic or develop metabolic acidosis. Further information regarding the pathophysiology and correction of electrolyte and acid–base disorders is given elsewhere in this text (see Chapters 107–110).

An emergency minimum database should be collected and ideally includes blood pressure measurement, biochemistry (urea, creatinine, lactate, electrolytes, total solids), packed cell volume, acid–base status, electrocardiogram and abdominal ultrasound to assess for free abdominal fluid (see Chapter 182). If an effusion is identified, fluid should be collected for analysis (see Chapter 186). If the creatinine and potassium levels of the peritoneal fluid exceed those of the serum by $>2:1$ and $>1.4:1$ respectively, then a diagnosis of uroabdomen is confirmed [10]. If an initial minimum database is not suggestive of urine leakage and the patient's status does not improve, the authors recommend re-evaluating the minimum database every 6–12 hours as low-volume urine leakage may take 24–48 hours to become apparent. Please see Chapter 103 for further information on uroabdomen

Diagnosis

Contrast radiography, such as retrograde urethrography, is the diagnostic test of choice for urethral rupture. The presence of urethral disruption is confirmed by extravasation of contrast along the course of the urethra (Figure 100.1). With complete disruption of the urethra, no contrast should flow beyond the urethral defect. However, with partial rupture contrast may reach the bladder.

Textbook of Small Animal Emergency Medicine, First Edition. Edited by Kenneth J. Drobatz, Kate Hopper, Elizabeth Rozanski and Deborah C. Silverstein.
© 2019 John Wiley & Sons, Inc. Published 2019 by John Wiley & Sons, Inc.
Companion Website: www.wiley.com/go/drobatz/textbook

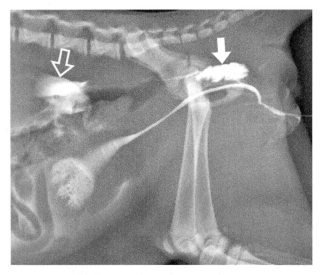

Figure 100.1 Retrograde urethrogram performed in an 8-week-old kitten with a history of urethral obstruction and catheterization. Notice the extravasation of contrast medium dorsally in the intrapelvic portion of the urethra (*closed arrow*), with contrast medium extending into the retroperitoneal space (*open arrow*). The cranial extension of contrast medium past the urethral disruption and into the bladder is consistent with a partial rupture.

It is not always possible to assess the severity of rupture from contrast radiography. Diagnostic urethral catheterization is an alternative but is controversial as it may cause further tearing. With partial rupture, it should be possible to pass the catheter into the bladder. However, with complete urethral rupture, displacement of the urethral ends prevents catheterization of the bladder [9]. Cystourethroscopy can also be considered but is rarely recommended. It can be difficult to perform in patients with urethral injury as leakage prevents fluid distension of the urethra that normally aids visualization [11]. There is also a risk of introducing bacteria into the abdominal cavity or perineal soft tissues [11].

Treatment

Urethral trauma can be managed conservatively through second intention healing, by surgical repair or by permanent urinary diversion (e.g. urethrostomy). Treatment planning should take into account the nature and extent of injury, and consider the requirement for temporary urinary diversion.

The two most important factors in promoting urethral healing are good mucosal continuity and prevention of urine extravasation. The urethral mucosa heals rapidly in as little as 7 days but regeneration of the corpus spongiosum can take 3–5 weeks [12]. The degree of urethral injury influences healing. Experimental resection of up

to two-thirds of the canine urethral circumference for a length of 1–5 cm still leads to good regeneration of the mucosa when a urethral catheter is placed during the healing phase, as long as a strip of urothelium connects the proximal and distal urethral ends [12]. However, with complete transection of the urethra, the urothelium contracts intraluminally due to spastic contraction of the muscle layer and this prevents healing. Periurethral tissue then covers the urethral ends and results in fibrous tissue proliferation [13]. In cases with partial rupture, conservative management with second intention healing can be attempted. However, in cases with complete rupture, surgery is indicated. Traumatic injury is more likely to lead to complete rupture [7] and so appropriate patient selection is important.

Urine is toxic to local tissues and leads to necrosis [7]. It also increases periurethral fibrosis, which in turn can increase stricture formation [13]. Temporary urinary diversion away from the site of injury to prevent extravasation should be utilized in all cases to promote healing.

Conservative Management

This is achieved by temporary urinary diversion whilst the urethral mucosa heals by second intention healing. Urinary diversion may be provided using a cystostomy tube, urethral catheter, or both. The authors' preference is to place a urethral catheter because it will act as a stent to aid alignment and healing [9]. Reported disadvantages of catheterization include mechanical irritation and the risk of ascending infection, both of which may promote stricture formation [13]. It is very important that the catheter is appropriately sized to prevent damage to the urethra during catheterization [13]. Most cases can be catheterized in a retrograde manner but some require normograde catheterization via a cystotomy incision [9]. See Chapters 97 and 189 for further information on how to perform urethral catheterization. In cases that have had urethral anastomosis, both methods of urinary diversion are as effective in promoting urethral healing [14] but the effect of cystostomy versus catheterization on healing in cases managed conservatively has not been established. In some patients, the use of both types of diversion simultaneously may be advantageous, particularly if the patient is fractious or difficult to manage.

The optimal duration of urinary diversion is unknown and has ranged from 3 to 37 days [7,15]. However, as the urethral mucosa takes 7 days to regenerate [12], a minimum period of 7 days urinary diversion is recommended in patients with significant trauma. Shorter periods are likely to only be suitable for cases with minor lacerations to the urethra.

Prior to cessation of urinary diversion, a retrograde urethrogram should be performed to assess for ongoing leakage. If further leakage is identified, the authors advise to continue urinary diversion for another 3–5 days prior to repeating the contrast study. If persistent leakage is still identified, surgical treatment is indicated. Once urinary diversion is stopped, urination should be monitored for a further 24–48 hours. Urethritis caused by catheterization [13] may lead to transient hematuria or incontinence.

Urinary tract infection occurs in up to 80% of cases even when closed urine collection systems are used [9]. The risk of infection increases with the duration of catheterization [16]. Antibiotics administered while indwelling urinary catheters are in place will not prevent the development of infection [9] (see Chapter 96) but may increase the risk of antibiotic-resistant bacteria. Antibiotics should not be prescribed prophylactically to cases with indwelling urinary catheters unless they are at risk of sepsis or there is a separate infectious process elsewhere. Regular urinalysis to screen for infection is recommended and urine culture should be performed if infection is suspected. Broad-spectrum antimicrobials should be initiated if infection is confirmed and altered dependent on culture results (see Chapter 96). Submission of the catheter tip for culture at the end of catheterization is not recommended. It is unreliable for identifying urinary tract infection in people because presence of bacteria on the catheter does not correlate with urinary tract infection [17]. In addition, some bacteria may be cleared after catheter removal [17]. The authors recommend urinalysis 24 hours after catheter removal even if normal urination is documented.

Success rates of up to 80% have been reported in patients managed conservatively with urethral catheterization [9]. Cats with iatrogenic injury following catheterization for lower urinary tract disease may require long-term ongoing medical management of their underlying disease. See Chapter 99 for further information on feline lower urinary tract obstruction and Chapter 97 on urolithiasis.

Surgical Management

Surgery is indicated for complete transections of the urethra or if conservative management with temporary urinary diversion fails.

Urethral Anastomosis

The surgical approach depends on the location of the defect but involves a caudal celiotomy and/or a pubic placed to identify and orientate the urethral ends. This is usually performed retrograde but a second catheter may need to be placed normograde if identification of the proximal end is difficult. The blood supply to the torn edges of the urethra is often compromised and the edges must be sharply debrided to promote healing.

After apposition of the urethral ends, the urethra is sutured using 4-0 or 5-0 absorbable monofilament suture in an interrupted pattern including mucosa and submucosa in each bite. The mucosa typically retracts into the lumen and must be identified for suturing to ensure correct apposition. Previous experimental work has found that the degree of stricture formation is reduced when suturing of the urethra occurs over a urethral catheter [18]. It is critical that there is no tension at the anastomosis site or dehiscence is likely [18,19]. Ischial ostectomy, ischial osteotomy, and crural release are reported to help decrease tension [19,20]. Once the anastomosis is completed, the authors' preference is to omentalize the surgical site.

Permanent Urethrostomy

Urethrostomy provides permanent urinary diversion by creating a stoma to bypass the area of injury. The location of the stoma depends on the position of the defect. There are higher complication rates associated with urethrostomies performed at more proximal locations so the most distal urethrostomy possible should be performed [7,21].

In male dogs, scrotal urethrostomy is preferred as the urethra in this region is superficial and relatively wide. The urethra is surrounded by less cavernous tissue at this site, which leads to a reduction in the amount of hemorrhage [22]. One of the main complications of this technique is postoperative hemorrhage but this is reduced when a simple continuous pattern and three-needle bite sequence (urethral mucosa first, then tunica albuginea, then skin) is used [23]. This is suggested to improve tissue apposition and uses fewer suture knots to reduce tissue irritation. However, a retrospective study reported postoperative hemorrhage in all cases, regardless of whether a continuous or interrupted suture pattern was used [22].

In male cats, perineal urethrostomy is most frequently performed by amputating the penis and prepuce and generating a urethrostomy at the level of the ischium using the pelvic urethra (Wilson and Harrison technique) [24]. The authors prefer a modified technique that retains the prepuce and anastomoses preputial and urethral mucosa to provide preputial cover to the site [25,26]. This reduces the opportunity for self-trauma and may decrease the incidence of postoperative stricture and urinary tract infection. Adequate dissection of the intrapelvic portion of the urethra from fibrous attachments to the pelvis and release of the ischiocavernosus muscle attachments are very important with both techniques to reduce tension at the stoma site and give access to the wide pelvic urethra.

For more proximal urethral defects, transpelvic urethrostomy and prepubic urethrostomy can be considered, of which the transpelvic urethrsotomy may have a lower complication rate [27].

Complications

Complications affect up to 57.1% of cases in the first 10 weeks following treatment and 27% in the long term [7]. They include urinary tract infections, strictures, stenosis of urethrostomy stoma, dehiscence, incontinence, urine scalding, urine extravasation with either peristomal skin necrosis or uroabdomen, and the development of lower urinary tract disease. The most common complication is urinary tract infection, which involves multidrug-resistant organisms in up to 28.6% of cases [7]. Patients requiring permanent urethrostomies have higher complication rates when the urethrostomy is performed at more proximal sites [7,21].

Stricture Management

Stricture development is a severe complication, which can lead to dysuria or complete urethral obstruction, typically seen when reduction of luminal diameter exceeds 60% [18]. Historically, these have been managed with urethral resection and anastomosis, permanent urinary diversion with cystostomy tube placement or, in mild cases, medical management to promote urethral relaxation [7,27,28]. Long-term management of permanent cystostomy tubes in animals can be problematic and bacterial cystitis is reported [29]. Dependent on the length and location of the stricture, repeat surgery with resection and anastomosis or permanent urethrostomy may not be possible.

Minimally invasive alternatives include repeated balloon dilation or urethral stent placement (Figure 100.2), with and without antifibrotic treatment. Disadvantages of balloon dilation include the requirement for multiple dilations in some cases [28]. Advantages of urethral stent placement include immediate relief of obstruction in a single procedure, which may decrease morbidity and save costs [28]. Complications of stent placement in dogs include incontinence (seen in 12.5% of cases with benign obstructions), inadvertent compression of the stent, tissue ingrowth through the stent or incomplete patency

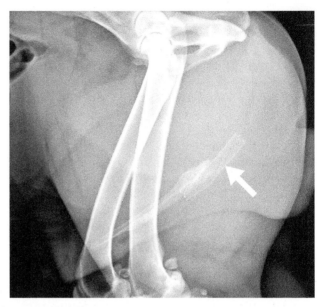

Figure 100.2 Urethral self-expanding metallic stent (*arrow*) placed in a 3-year-old male entire rottweiler with a urethral stricture secondary to chronic urethrolithiasis and a urethral tear.

after the first procedure [28]. For the latter three complications, a second stent can be placed to improve the outcome. Urethral stents have also been successfully placed in cats for management of urethral strictures [29,30] and incontinence rates appear to be similar to dogs. The proximity of the ureterovesicular junction to the proximal urethra in the cat means that ureteral obstruction is a concern when attempting to address strictures in this area [30].

Outcome

Outcome for patients that have iatrogenic injury is generally better than for those which have had traumatic rupture. A good outcome (survival to discharge and without long-term complications) is seen in 83.3–91.3% of cases after iatrogenic injury and 50–57.1% after trauma [4,7].

References

1 Kleine LJ, Thornton GW. Radiographic diagnosis of urinary tract trauma. *J am Anim Hosp Assoc* 1971;7:318–327.

2 Kolata RJ, Johnston DE. Motor vehicle accidents in urban dogs: a study of 600 cases. *J Am Vet Med Assoc* 1975;167:938–941.

3 Selcer BA. Urinary tract trauma associated with pelvic trauma. *J Am Anim Hosp Assoc* 1982;18: 785–793.

4 Anderson RB, Aronson LR, Drobatz KJ, et al. Prognostic factors for successful outcome following urethral rupture in dogs and cats. *J Am Anim Hosp Assoc* 2006;42:136–146.

5 Addison ES, Halfacree Z, Hotson Moore A, et al. A retrospective analysis of urethral rupture in 63 cats. *J Feline Med Surg* 2014;16:300–307.

6 Meige F, Sarrau S, Autefage A. Management of traumatic urethral rupture in 11 cats using primary

alignment with a urethral catheter. *Vet Comp Orthop Traumatol* 2008;21:76–84.

7 Holt PE. Hind limb skin loss associated with urethral rupture in two cats. *J Small Anim Pract* 1989;30:406–409.

8 Smith CW. Perineal urethrostomy. *Vet Clin North Am Small Anim Pract* 2002;32:917–925.

9 Tobias KM. Perineal urethrostomy in cats. In: *Manual of Small Animal Soft Tissue Surgery*. Wiley-Blackwell, Ames, 2010, pp. 313–321.

10 Schmiedt C, Tobias KM, Otto CM. Evaluation of abdominal fluid: peripheral blood creatinine and potassium ratios for diagnosis of uroperitoneum in dogs. *J Vet Emerg Crit Care* 2001;4:275–280.

11 Morgan M, Forman M. Cystoscopy in dogs and cats. *Vet Clin North Am Small Anim Pract* 2015;45:665–701.

12 Weaver RG, Schulte JW. Experimental and clinical studies of urethral regeneration. *Surg Gynecol Obstet* 1962;115:729–736.

13 Degner DA, Walshaw RW. Healing responses of the lower urinary tract. *Vet Clin North Am Small Anim Pract* 1996;26:197–206.

14 Cooley AJ, Waldron DR, Smith MM, et al. The effects of indwelling transurethral catheterisation and tube cystostomy on urethral anastomoses in dogs. *J Am Anim Hosp Assoc* 1999;35:341–347.

15 Bellah JR. Problems of the urethra. *Prob Vet Med* 1989;1:17–35.

16 Barsanti JA, Blue J, Edmunds J. Urinary tract infections due to indwelling bladder catheters in dogs and cats. *J Am Vet Med Assoc* 1985;187:384–388.

17 Smarick SD, Haskins SC, Aldrich J, et al. Incidence of catheter-associated urinary tract infection among dogs in a small animal intensive care unit. *J Am Vet Med Assoc* 2004;224:1936–1940.

18 Layton CE, Ferguson HR, Cook JE, et al. Intrapelvic urethral anastomosis: a comparison of three techniques. *Vet Surg* 1987;16:175–182.

19 Srithunyarat T, Pankhum S, Chuthatep S, et al. Ischial ostectomy in direct end-to-end anastomosis of the pelvic urethra in male dogs. *Res Vet Sci* 2012;93:473–477.

20 Zemer O, Benzioni H, Kaplan R, et al. Evaluation of crural release and ischial osteotomy for relief of tension in the repair of large segmental urethral defects in male cats. *Vet Surg* 2013;42:971–978.

21 Baines SJ, Rennie S, White RS. Prepubic urethrostomy: a long term study in 16 cats. *Vet Surg* 2001;30:107–113.

22 Burrow RD, Gregory SP, Giejda AA, et al. Penile amputation and scrotal urethrostomy in 18 dogs. *Vet Rec* 2011;169:657–664.

23 Smeak DD. Urethrotomy and urethrostomy in the dog. *Clin Tech Small Anim Pract* 2000;15:25–34.

24 Wilson GP 3rd, Harrison JW. Perineal urethrostomy in cats. *J Am Vet Med Assoc* 1971;159;1789–1793.

25 Yeh LS, Chin SC. Modified perineal urethrostomyusing preputial mucosa in cats. *J Am Vet Med Assoc* 2000;216:1092–1095.

26 Bernarde A, Viquier E. Transpelvic urethrostomy in 11 cats using an ischial ostectomy. *Vet Surg* 2004;33:246–252.

27 Salinardi BJ, Marks SL, Davidson JR, et al. The use of a low-profile cystostomy tube to relieve urethral obstruction in a dog. *J Am Anim Hosp Assoc* 2003;39:403–405.

28 Hill TL, Berent AC, Weisse CW. Evaluation of urethral stent placement for benign urethral obstructions in dogs. *J Vet Intern Med* 2014;28:1384–1390.

29 Hadar EN, Morgan MJ, Morgan OD. Use of a self-expanding metallic stent for the treatment of a urethral stricture in a young cat. *J Feline Med Surg* 2001;13:597–601.

30 Brace MA, Weisse C, Berent A. Preliminary experience with stenting for management of non-urolith urethral obstruction in eight cats. *Vet Surg* 2014;43:199–208.

101

Lyme Nephritis

Meryl P. Littman, VMD, DACVIM

School of Veterinary Medicine, University of Pennsylvania, Philadelphia, PA, USA

Introduction

When dogs present emergently with serious and sudden complications of protein-losing nephropathy (PLN) (e.g. thromboembolism (TE), hypertension, effusions/edema, and/or renal failure), criticalists are called upon to stabilize and support them, submit or save appropriate samples before starting antimicrobial therapy, and discuss estimates for diagnostic tests (to stage disease and rule out differentials), treatments, future monitoring, and overall prognosis, so that owners can make educated decisions concerning their options.

Lyme nephritis [1–4] is suspected in Lyme-seropositive PLN cases (Lyme+ PLN), but in endemic regions, being seropositive for antibodies against the agent ("Lyme+" status) is common in many healthy dogs and possibly coincidental in sick dogs, so other causes of illness need to be considered. Lyme+ status is a marker for tick and wildlife exposure; an important differential diagnosis that may mimic Lyme nephritis is leptospirosis and precautions (isolation) may be necessary due to its infectious and zoonotic potential [5].

Transmission, Prevalence, and an Experimental Model of Canine Lyme Disease

Exposure to the spirochete *Borrelia burgdorferi* is very common in Lyme-endemic areas (New England, Mid-Atlantic, Upper Midwest states, and adjacent Canada). In people, 95% of Lyme disease cases were reported in just 14 states (CT, DE, ME, MD, MA, MN, NH, NJ, NY, PA, RI, VT, VA, WI) [6]. Data concerning exposure rates among dogs are similar [7]. In some areas 70–90% of healthy dogs are Lyme+, but less than 5% showed Lyme arthritis (similar to seronegative dogs) over 20 months of observation [2]. Lyme arthritis is often overdiagnosed; 40% of dogs so diagnosed were later found to have another cause for their signs [8]. Roughly less than 1–2% of Lyme+ dogs show PLN, often attributed to Lyme nephritis but possibly due to other causes [1–4,9,10]. Proteinuria is rarely associated with Lyme+ status, even among Lyme+ retrievers, which are the predisposed breeds [11].

Transmission of the agent occurs via the bite of the three-host field deer tick or black-legged tick (*Ixodes scapularis* in the East/MidWest, *I. pacificus* in the West, and *I. ricinus* in Europe). Transstadial but not transovarial transmission occurs within the tick. The 2-year life cycle of an *I. scapularis* tick begins with six-legged larvae acquiring the agent during summer feeding on the first hosts, usually mice, small rodents, or migratory birds; after feeding for several days, the ticks fall off, molt to eight-legged nymphs, emerge and feed the following spring on small mammals, birds, and also larger species such as dogs, deer, and people, and transmit the agent to them after roughly 2 days of feeding. After feeding for several days, nymphs molt and emerge as adult ticks in the autumn, again able to transmit the agent to larger animals as the adult ticks quest on higher vegetation. Migratory birds spread infected ticks to new areas. Deer ticks in Lyme endemic areas may also carry *Anaplasma phagocytophilum*, *Babesia microti*, *Borrelia miyamotoi*, *Ehrlichia muris*-like agent, tick-borne encephalitis (Powassan) virus, and possibly *Bartonella* and *Mycoplasma* spp.

A natural tick exposure experimental model of Lyme disease in dogs demonstrated that adult beagles remained seropositive carriers, but showed no illness when observed for more than a year after tick exposure [12]. Exposed beagle puppies (6–12 weeks old) showed no acute signs; 2–5 months after tick exposure and well after seroconversion, they showed only 4 days of self-limiting anorexia, fever, and lameness in the leg closest to the tick bites, sometimes with several similar episodes every few weeks, associated with the agent's ability to hide from the immune system near collagen and fibroblasts, with antigenic variation during carrier status. Exposed

Textbook of Small Animal Emergency Medicine, First Edition. Edited by Kenneth J. Drobatz, Kate Hopper, Elizabeth Rozanski and Deborah C. Silverstein.
© 2019 John Wiley & Sons, Inc. Published 2019 by John Wiley & Sons, Inc.
Companion Website: www.wiley.com/go/drobatz/textbook

puppies aged 13–26 weeks showed milder signs (1–2 days) and fewer episodes [1].

Some experimental dogs were inadvertently co-infected with *A. phagocytophilum* and *B. microti*. Carrier dogs maintained high Lyme antibody titers; cultures of skin biopsies of the tick bite sites showed viable spirochetes even a year later while the dogs showed no further illness. When treated with antibiotics for 1 month, about 10–15% of dogs were not cleared of spirochetes in the skin [13]. There is no experimental model for Lyme nephritis; perhaps multiple exposures, different strains of the agent, co-infections, or predisposed breeds are necessary to induce the disease. Since retrievers appear to be at highest risk, a genetic predisposition may involve immunodysregulation or innately abnormal glomeruli that are unable to clear immune complexes normally (e.g. a podocytopathy) [14].

Presentation of Field Cases with Presumptive Lyme Nephritis [1–4,15]

A typical case of Lyme nephritis is a middle-aged Labrador or golden retriever (although any breed may be affected) living in a Lyme-endemic region, presenting with several days' to weeks' history of lethargy, anorexia, acute vomiting and/or diarrhea, mild-to-moderate systemic hypertension, Lyme+ status, hypoalbuminemia, hypercholesterolemia, mild-to-moderate azotemia, possible hyperphosphatemia and/or hyperkalemia, consumptive thrombocytopenia, urine specific gravity 1.020–1.030 (isosthenuria is a late sign), proteinuria/cylindruria, possibly glucosuria, mildly active sediment, and negative urine culture. Polyuria/polydipsia are relatively late signs due to tubular involvement. Oliguria/anuria may be due to acute kidney injury (AKI), therefore other causes should also be considered (e.g. leptospirosis, Rocky Mountain spotted fever) (see Chapter 94). Fever, pallor/anemia, icterus, liver enzyme elevation, petechiation/ecchymoses, lymphadenopathy, or hepatosplenomegaly are not commonly seen with Lyme disease and if present, may be due to co-infection or co-morbidity.

Other presentations may involve thromboembolic events due to vasculitis, hypertension, and hypercoagulability from the PLN and subsequent loss of antithrombin (e.g. dyspnea due to pulmonary TE; weakness/lameness due to a saddle or limb TE; collapse, seizure, or sudden death due to cardiac or neurovascular TE) (see Chapter 62), effusions/edema due to hypoalbuminemia (e.g. dyspnea due to pleural effusion, ascites, incipient edema with crystalloid therapy), hypertensive damage (e.g. blindness due to retinal hemorrhage/detachment, epistaxis, neurological signs) (see Chapter 63), and/or lameness (due to Lyme or other tick-borne arthritis or neurovascular

events). One study reported previous or concurrent lameness in less than 30% of cases and past Lyme vaccination in almost 30% [15]. Still other presentations may be occult (early/mild), so any Lyme+ dog, whether healthy or sick, should be screened for proteinuria. Early/mild cases may have hypoalbuminemia but with only mild (or no) azotemia, and these dogs have the best prognosis.

Recent tick exposure is not a prerequisite. In the experimental model of Lyme disease in young puppies, classic signs of illness (anorexia/fever/lameness) were not seen until 2–5 months after tick exposure, well after seroconversion [12]. The initiation and progression of Lyme nephritis is unknown (the experimental model did not develop PLN), but is assumed to be a later occurrence due to chronic immune stimulation by this stealth pathogen which manifests antigenic variation during the carrier state. A history of previous treatment for Lyme disease for 1 month does not ensure clearance, as 10–15% of experimental dogs so treated still showed cultivable organisms in biopsies taken from tick bite sites [13].

Physical examination is often unrewarding. Dogs with gastrointestinal signs secondary to azotemia may be dehydrated. Cavitary effusions or dependent edema may be evident in dogs with nephrotic syndrome. Dyspnea may be due to pleural effusion, aspiration pneumonia or pulmonary TE. Retinal changes (hemorrhage/detachment/intraocular exudation) and a soft cardiac murmur may be target organ damage from hypertension. Lameness may be due to oligo/polyarthropathy from Lyme or co-morbid tick-borne arthritis, saddle or limb TE (evaluate pulses carefully) or neurological events.

Diagnostic Work-Up to Stage Disease and Rule Out Other Differentials [1–4,9,10]

The diagnosis of Lyme nephritis is often presumed in Lyme+ dogs with PLN until proven otherwise. Diagnostic tests (Table 101.1) are helpful to localize proteinuria, rule out other causes of PLN, stage renal disease, and identify complications requiring special tests or management. Other causes for proteinuria need to be considered, including lower urinary tract disease, pyelonephritis, leptospirosis, tick-borne and other infectious diseases, vasculitis, inflammatory and immune-mediated diseases, neoplasia, amyloidosis, non-amyloid fibrillary deposition, genetic glomerular/renal diseases, systemic hypertension, hyperadrenocorticism, toxins (e.g. shigatoxin from ingestion of raw meat or wildlife, nephrotoxins), and other renal diseases.

Since seropositivity is a marker for tick and wildlife exposure, a search for co-infections that may cause proteinuria is warranted, especially leptospirosis, dirofilariasis, anaplasmosis, ehrlichiosis, babesiosis, bartonellosis,

Table 101.1 Diagnostic work-up for dogs with suspected Lyme nephritis [1–4,9,10].

Data	Additional detail
History	Travel? Exposure to ticks/wildlife/raw meat? Lameness? Other?
Physical examination	Complete, including retinal examination
Blood pressure measurements (BPM)	One reliable very high BPM vs persistently high BPM
CBC (including platelets)	Cytopenias may indicate co-infection or immune-mediated illness;
Chemistry profile	thrombocytopenia may be due to consumption (TE)
IRIS staging of renal disease [16]	
Possible D-dimers, TEG, AT testing	Hypercoagulopathy
DNA sample for inherited PLN	Where tests are available or for future research
Urinalysis	Sample USG before starting fluid therapy
Urine culture*	Sample urine culture before starting antimicrobials
Urine protein:creatinine ratio (UPC)	Check trend; monitor with mixture of 3 days' equal aliquots
Possible SDS-PAGE to differentiate glomerular and tubular proteinuria	Submit to IVRPS, contact Dr Mary B. Nabity, mnabity@cvm.tamu.edu
SNAP®4Dx®Plus (IDEXX):Heartworm antigen Natural exposure antibodies to:	The AccuPlex®4 (Antech) test had lower specificity/sensitivity for antibodies to *B. burgdorferi* and *A. phagocytophilum* [17]; may give false-positive results for natural infection in dogs vaccinated with bacterins that produce Lyme ospC antibodies; and may not pick up cross-reacting antibodies against *A. platys*, *E. chaffeensis* or *E. ewingii*
B. burgdorferi (qualitative C_6 test) *A. phagocytophilum/A. platys*** *E. canis/E. chaffeensis/E. ewingii***	
Lyme Quant C_6® (IDEXX), before and after (3–6 months) treatment	Lyme nephritis cases generally have high titers but so do many healthy dogs (titer height is not predictive). Posttreatment value of < 50% of prevalue may represent successful clearance and is useful as a new baseline for future comparisons (qualitative testing may be positive for many years)
Leptospirosis: PCR*, antibody titers**	*PCR testing of blood (first week of illness), urine thereafter
Other infectious diseases [9,10]:	See Chapter 200 regarding regional infectious diseases and PLN
Babesiosis	*Babesia* spp PCR* and titers for *B. canis/B. gibsoni*
Bartonellosis	*Bartonella* spp PCR*, titers, culture, and/or Western blot
Rocky Mountain spotted fever (RMSF)**	Consider RMSF only if history is acute
Hepatozoonosis	If exposure (south-eastern states) or raw meat/wildlife ingestion
Leishmaniasis	If exposure or American foxhound, spinone, cane corso, etc.
Brucellosis	For dogs at risk
Imaging	Check for neoplasia, effusion, cardiomegaly
Chest radiographs	Check for neoplasia, lower urinary tract disease, adrenal size; kidney ultrasonogram is often non-remarkable in PLN cases
Abdominal ultrasound	
Possible echocardiogram	Check for hypertensive changes (hypertrophic cardiomyopathy, left ventricular hypertrophy), pericardial effusion, other
Possible search for other causes of hypertension	Consider hyperadrenocorticism, hyperaldosteronism, pheochromocytoma, primary hypertension, etc.
Possible work-up for hyperadrenocorticism	May cause proteinuria and hypertension but usually is not associated with hypoalbuminemia
Renal biopsy [18,19]	TEM and IF are important to document immune-complex glomerulonephritis and rule out other causes of PLN; see text

*Save samples before starting antimicrobials.
**Paired (acute/convalescent) titers may be needed.
AT, antithrombin; BPM, blood pressure measurement; IF, immunofluorescence; PCR, polymerase chain reaction; PLN, protein-losing nephropathy; SDS-PAGE, sodium dodecyl sulfate polyacrylamide gel electrophoresis; TE, thromboembolism; TEG, thromboelastography; TEM, transmission electron microscopy; USG, urine specific gravity.

and, if the history is acute, Rocky Mountain spotted fever. An extended search may include rarer infections related to travel, breed predisposition, or other exposures. Response to therapy does not prove Lyme nephritis. Most dogs with Lyme arthritis respond to doxycycline quickly, but doxycycline treats many other tick-borne diseases that may cause similar signs, and has antiarthritic and anti-inflammatory properties. The in-house SNAP®4Dx®Plus (IDEXX) test offers quick confirmation of seropositive (natural exposure) status, but the clinician needs to keep an open mind and obtain the appropriate samples to rule out other causes (e.g. save whole blood in refrigerated EDTA (lavender top) tubes for PCR analysis for other agents and urine for PCR and bacterial culture before starting antimicrobials; see Table 101.1). Additional diagnostic investigations may be warranted depending on extrarenal abnormalities found, such as joint tap cytology/culture, lymph node and/or bone marrow aspirates, etc.

Renal Biopsy

Lyme nephritis is associated with immune-complex glomerulonephritis (ICGN), tubular necrosis/regeneration, and interstitial nephritis [15]. Without an experimental model, the progression is unknown, and perhaps early/mild cases have only glomerular disease without secondary tubular or interstitial involvement. Renal damage is due to deposition of Lyme-specific immune complexes in glomeruli and not spirochetal invasion of the kidney. Light microscopy can differentiate amyloidosis as a cause of PLN, but detailed examination by trained personnel with transmission electron microscopy, immunofluorescence, and thin section (3 μ) light microscopy with special stains is best to differentiate ICGN from glomerulosclerosis, hereditary nephritis, or other renal changes [18,19]. A candidate for renal biopsy is not in end-stage disease, has hypertension controlled, sufficient platelets, and has not received antithrombotics in at least 5 days.

Trained personnel should procure the samples and specimens which are then saved in glutaraldehyde, Michel's fixative, and formalin. The samples should be sent overnight with ice packs inside a styrofoam box to veterinary nephropathologists of the International Veterinary Renal Pathology Service (IVRPS) which are prepared to receive the shipments [9,10,18]. Kits for sample submission are obtained from the IVRPS (in the USA: Department of Veterinary Biosciences, Ohio State University, Columbus, OH 43210, contact Dr Rachel Cianciolo, rachel.cianciolo@cvm.osu.edu; in Europe: Utrecht Veterinary Nephropathology Service, Utrecht University, Utrecht, The Netherlands, contact Dr Astrid M. van Dongen, a.m.vandongen@uu.nl).

The finding of ICGN suggests immunosuppressive protocols may be useful in cases that are not responding to antimicrobials and standard therapy for PLN [10]. Although ICGN may be documented by biopsy, there are no validated stains to confirm that such complexes are Lyme specific, that is, they may be due to another tick-borne disease such as babesiosis [20], other infections, or neoplasia, etc. which hopefully will be recognized by the other diagnostic tests (PCR/titers, imaging, etc.) recommended (see Table 101.1) so that appropriate therapy will be given.

Treatment (Table 101.2)

Emergent care may include respiratory and intravascular volume support for dogs with hypovolemia/dehydration, thromboembolic events, hypertension, effusions/edema, and/or AKI or chronic renal disease as reviewed elsewhere (see Chapters 45, 62, 63, 94, 153). Judicious use of crystalloid therapy is warranted (if indicated at all), and colloids, diuretics, and even hemodialysis may be necessary since aggressive fluid therapy in hypoalbuminemic dogs often leads to edema/effusions, especially dogs with renal compromise (see Chapters 167, 168, 169).

Standard treatments for Lyme+PLN dogs (see Table 101.2) include long-term antimicrobials (1–3 months, or until Lyme Quant C_6® (IDEXX) wanes), angiotensin converting enzyme (ACE) inhibitors and/or other inhibitors of the renin-angiotensin-aldosterone system (RAAS), antithrombotics, antihypertensives, renal diet, omega-3 fatty acid supplement, and treatments as necessary for signs of renal failure (antiemetics, gastrointestinal protectants, antacids, phosphate binders, appetite stimulants, etc.) [16,21–23]. Immunosuppressant medication is not generally given without renal biopsy confirmation that ICGN exists, unless the case is deteriorating quickly despite standard therapy. The best protocol is unknown since there is no experimental model of Lyme nephritis and there are no validated stains to prove that immune complexes found in biopsies are Lyme specific. Thus inclusion/exclusion criteria are undefined for documented versus control cases to be studied in therapeutic trials. The current anecdotal favorite immunosuppressive is mycophenolate. Pulse steroids may be used in fulminant cases, but should be weaned as soon as possible to avoid side-effects (increased risk for thromboembolic events, hypertension, and gastric ulceration, for which these animals are already predisposed).

The prognosis for dogs admitted for intravenous fluids due to dehydration, vomiting, and moderately severe azotemia has historically been poor, but may be improving with the addition of treatments in Table 101.2; however, when dogs do well (unexpectedly), it is always

Table 101.2 Treatments for Lyme nephritis [16,21–23].

Treatment	Dose or detail (all drug doses are per os)
Antimicrobial Longer than 1 month, until Lyme Quant C_6* (IDEXX) shows at least a 50% decline	Doxycycline is first choice, 5–10 mg/kg q12h Other: amoxicillin, azithromycin, or cefovecin Duration to clear carrier status is unknown
*ACE inhibitor and/or other RAAS inhibitor** ACE inhibitor Angiotensin-receptor blocker (ARB) Aldosterone-receptor blocker	Goal for UPC < 0.5 or at least < 50% initial value Enalapril or benazepril 0.25–1.0 mg/kg q12h Telmisartan 1–2 mg/kg q24h or Losartan 0.5–1 mg/kg q24h (1/4 this dose if azotemic) Spironolactone (diuretic) 1–2 mg/kg q12h
Antithrombotic (see Chapter 71) Prevention (if renal biopsy is not planned) Treatment for existing TE events	Low-dose aspirin 1–5 mg/kg q24h or clopidogrel 1.1 mg/kg q24h
Antihypertensive (goal: < 150/95 mmHg) If hypertensive even on an ACE/RAAS inhibitor Calcium channel blocker (first choice) Beta-blocker Alpha-blocker Direct vasodilator See Chapter 63	Amlodipine 0.1–0.75 mg/kg q24h Atenolol 0.25–1.0 mg/kg q12h Prazosin, 0.5–2 mg/kg q8-12h Hydralazine 0.5–2 mg/kg q12h Acepromazine 0.5–2 mg/kg q8h
Renal diet Omega-3 fatty acid supplement	Lower in protein, phosphorus, and sodium N-3 polyunsaturated fatty acids 0.25–0.50 g/kg q24h See also Chapter 102
Fluids – colloids/crystalloids	See Chapters 94, 95, 167–169
Diuretic if necessary Aldosterone-receptor blocker Thiazide diuretic Loop diuretic	Spironolactone 1–2 mg/kg q12h Hydrochlorothiazide 2–4 mg/kg q12–24h Furosemide 1–4 mg/kg q8–24h
Antiemetics, antacids, protectants	See Chapter 102
Phosphate binders	See Chapter 102
Immunosuppressives [22] (if renal biopsy shows ICGN and case is not responding to antimicrobials and standard PLN therapy, or in cases without renal biopsy, if deteriorating quickly) [10,23]	Mycophenolate 10 mg/kg q12h Cyclophosphamide, pulse 200–250 mg/m² q3 weeks Chlorambucil 0.2 mg/kg q24–48h Azathioprine 2 mg/kg/day × 1–2 weeks; 1–2 mg/kg q48h Cyclosporine 5–20 mg/kg q12h (wax upward) Prednisone for fulminant cases: short-term pulse, 1 mg/kg q12h, wean as soon as possible
±Plasmapheresis?	Theoretically may be helpful to decrease circulating immune complexes

*An ACE inhibitor and/or ARB is standard therapy for PLN to decrease proteinuria by dilating both the afferent and efferent arterioles at the glomerulus, and should be used whether or not the dog is hypertensive.

difficult to know whether the diagnosis of Lyme nephritis was really accurate.

Monitoring

After discharge, dogs often require monitoring of arterial blood pressure, urine protein:creatinine ratio (UPC), albumin, azotemia, and other abnormalities, usually every 1–2 weeks until more stable. Since UPC values have daily variation and tend to be higher from samples obtained in the clinic [24], it is recommended that the owner collect urine samples at home each morning for 3 days; equal aliquots of the samples are then mixed and submitted to the laboratory for one UPC determination [25].

Prevention, Tick Control and Lyme Vaccination

Antimicrobial treatment of non-clinical, non-proteinuric Lyme+ dogs is controversial and reviewed elsewhere [26,27]. Whether or not a Lyme+ dog is treated, it needs continued monitoring for development of proteinuria since not all dogs are cleared of their carrier status with 1 month of antimicrobial treatment.

To avoid (re)exposure to Lyme and other vector-borne diseases, control of fleas and ticks is recommended year round, preferably including a product that prevents tick attachment (topical or collar containing permethrins or amitraz) or that kills ticks very early during feeding (oral or topical isoxazolines) in order to prevent acquiring agents that are transmitted much faster than *B. burgdorferi* [3,28]. Vaccination for Lyme disease is still controversial for both healthy and sick dogs [3,29]. There is no evidence of benefit for dogs with Lyme nephritis and vaccination may even be contraindicated lest potential deposition of circulating vaccinal antigen-antibody complexes occur in glomeruli in predisposed dogs.

References

1 Littman MP. State-of-the-Art-Review: Lyme nephritis. *J Vet Emerg Crit Care* 2013;23:163–173.

2 Littman MP, Goldstein RE, Labato MA, et al. ACVIM small animal consensus statement on Lyme disease in dogs: diagnosis, treatment, and prevention. *J Vet Intern Med* 2006;20:422–434.

3 Littman MP, Gerber B, Goldstein RE, et al. ACVIM consensus update on Lyme borreliosis in dogs and cats. *J Vet Intern Med* 2018; DOI:10.1111/JVIM.15085.

4 Littman MP. Protein-losing nephropathy in small animals. In: Acierno MJ, Labato MA, eds. Kidney Disease and Renal Replacement Therapies. *Vet Clin North Am (Small Animal)* 2011;41:31–37, special issue.

5 Tangeman LE, Littman MP. Clinicopathologic and atypical features of naturally occurring leptospirosis in dogs: 51 cases (2000–2010). *J Am Vet Med Assoc* 2013;243:1316–1322.

6 Centers for Disease Control and Prevention. Lyme Disease: Data and Statistics: Fast Facts. www.cdc.gov/lyme/stats/index.html (accessed 1 February 2018).

7 Companion Animal Parasite Council. Parasite Prevalence Maps. www.capcvet.org/parasite-prevalence-maps/ (accessed 1 February 2018).

8 Speck S, Reiner B, Streich WJ, et al. Canine borreliosis: a laboratory diagnostic trial. *Vet Microbiol* 2007;120:132–141.

9 Littman MP, Daminet S, Grauer GF, et al. Consensus recommendations for the diagnostic investigation of dogs with suspected glomerular disease. *J Vet Intern Med* 2013;27:S19–S26.

10 Goldstein RE, Brovida C, Fernandez-del Palacio MJ, et al. Consensus recommendations for treatment for dogs with serology positive glomerular disease. *J Vet Intern Med* 2013;27:S60–S66.

11 Goldstein RE, Cordner AP, Sandler JL, et al. Microalbuminuria and comparison of serologic testing for exposure to *Borrelia burgdorferi* in nonclinical Labrador and Golden Retrievers. *J Vet Diagn Invest* 2007;19:294–297.

12 Appel MJG, Allen S, Jacobson RH, et al. Experimental Lyme disease in dogs produces arthritis and persistent infection. *J Infect Dis* 1993;167:651–664.

13 Straubinger RK, Summers BA, Chang YF, et al. Persistence of *Borrelia burgdorferi* in experimentally infected dogs after antibiotic treatment. *J Clin Microbiol* 1997;35:111–116.

14 Littman MP. Emerging perspectives on hereditary glomerulopathies in canines. *Adv Genomics Genet* 2015;5:179–188.

15 Dambach DM, Smith CA, Lewis RM, et al. Morphologic, immunohistochemical, and ultrastructural characterization of a distinctive renal lesion in dogs putatively associated with *Borrelia burgdorferi* infection: 49 cases (1987–1992). *Vet Pathol* 1997;34:85–96.

16 International Renal Interest Society. IRIS Guidelines. www.iris-kidney.com/guidelines/ (accessed 1 February 2018).

17 Goldstein RE, Eberts MD, Beall MJ, et al. Performance comparison of SNAP®4Dx®Plus and AccuPlex®4 for the detection of antibodies to *Borrelia burgdorferi* and *Anaplasma phagocytophilum. Int J Appl Res Vet Med* 2014;12:141–147.

18 Cianciolo RE, Brown CA, Mohr FC, et al. Pathologic evaluation of canine renal biopsies: methods for identifying features that differentiate immune-mediated glomerulonephritides from other categories of glomerular diseases. *J Vet Intern Med* 2013;27:S10–S13.

19 Schneider SM, Cianciolo RE, Nabity MB, et al. Prevalence of immune-complex glomerulonephritides in dogs biopsied for suspected glomerular disease: 501 cases (2007–2012). *J Vet Intern Med* 2013;27:S67–S75.

20 Slade DJ, Lees GE, Berridge BR, et al. Resolution of a proteinuric nephropathy associated with *Babesia gibsoni* infection in a dog. *J Am Anim Hosp Assoc* 2011;47:e138–144.

21 Brown S, Elliott J, Francey T, et al. Consensus recommendations for standard therapy of glomerular disease in dogs. *J Vet Intern Med* 2013;27:S27–S43.

22 Segev G, Cowgill LD, Heiene R, et al. Consensus recommendations for immunosuppressive treatment of dogs with glomerular disease based on established pathology. *J Vet Intern Med* 2013;27:S44–S54.

23 Pressler B, Vaden S, Gerber B, et al. Consensus guidelines for immunosuppressive treatment of dogs with glomerular disease absent a pathologic diagnosis. *J Vet Intern Med* 2013;27:S55–S59.

24 Duffy ME, Specht A, Hill RC. Comparison between urine protein:creatinine ratios of samples obtained from dogs in home and hospital settings. *J Vet Intern Med* 2015;29:1029–1035.

25 LeVine DN, Zhang DW, Harris T, et al. The use of pooled vs serial urine samples to measure urine protein:creatinine ratios. *Vet Clin Pathol* 2010;39:53–56.

26 Littman MP, Goldstein RE. A Matter of Opinion: Should we treat asymptomatic, nonproteinuric Lyme-seropositive dogs with antibiotics? *Clinician's Brief* 2011;9:13–16.

27 Barr SC. Treating Lyme-seropositive dogs. *Clinician's Brief Sounding Board* 2012;5:8.

28 Littman MP. Tickborne and other stealth pathogen reproductive concerns. *Clin Therio* 2015;7:173–187.

29 Littman MP, Goldstein RE. Vaccinating dogs against Lyme disease: two points of view. *Today's Vet Pract* 2014;4:62–65.

102

Chronic Kidney Disease

Melisa G. Rosenthal, DVM and Mary A. Labato, DVM, DACVIM

Cummings School of Veterinary Medicine, Tufts University, North Grafton, MA, USA

Introduction

Chronic kidney disease (CKD) is a commonly recognized cause of illness in dogs and cats. The prevalence varies with the population examined, but has been estimated between 0.5% and 7% in dogs and between 1.6% and 20% in cats [1]. Given this high prevalence, it is not surprising that many cats and dogs presenting on an emergency basis suffer from CKD. One of the challenges of emergency identification of CKD is differentiating it from presentations of acute kidney injury (AKI) or concurrent CKD and AKI (acute on chronic kidney disease).

For this reason, CKD is defined as kidney damage that has persisted for greater than 3 months. This time period has been proposed because healing and resolution of azotemia may continue for several months after AKI [1]. Identification of chronicity of disease may be based on medical history, physical exam changes, historical laboratory findings, and renal structural changes, as described in Table 102.1. However, it is difficult to rule

Table 102.1 Differentiation of CKD and AKI.

Features of CKD	Features of AKI
Polyuria/polydipsia for >3 months	Recent increased or decreased urination
Inappetence for >3 months	Recent inappetence
Weight loss	Normal body condition score
Poor quality hair coat	
Small kidney size	Normal or large kidneys
Renal osteodystrophy	
Non-regenerative anemia	
History of azotemia for >3 months	Normal bloodwork in last 3 months
History of proteinuria for >3 months	Normal urinalysis in last 3 months

out a component of acute on chronic kidney disease, so many of these patients should also be treated as potential AKI cases (see Chapter 94).

Pathophysiology

Most cases of CKD in cats and dogs do not have a well-defined underlying cause. Studies of the underlying histopathology have shown that inflammatory infiltrates and fibrosis are key markers of the disease [2]. A variety of insults and predisposing factors can contribute to the development of CKD. Congenital causes such as renal dysplasia, polycystic kidney disease, and amyloidosis have been recognized. Acquired causes include the chronic perpetuation of most causes of AKI including pyelonephritis, partial obstruction from ureteroliths, glomerulonephritis, neoplasia, and renal infarctions.

Regardless of the cause, the decline in functional nephrons causes a decrease in glomerular filtration rate (GFR). Compensatory mechanisms allow for maintenance of water and electrolyte balance despite the loss of kidney function by increasing the excretory load of each surviving nephron. Ultimately, these compensatory mechanisms are insufficient to maintain adequate secretion, and the resulting decompensation manifests as hypertension, edema, hyperphosphatemia, and metabolic acidosis [1]. This loss of excretory ability also results in the gradual increase in serum uremic solutes.

A staging system for CKD has been proposed by the International Renal Interest Society (IRIS) [3]. This system is based on evaluation of the patient's serum creatinine, proteinuria, and blood pressure as measured multiple times over the course of several weeks. Therefore, staging cannot be appropriately applied in the emergency setting. In addition, it is not appropriate to stage animals who may have a component of acute disease, as

Textbook of Small Animal Emergency Medicine, First Edition. Edited by Kenneth J. Drobatz, Kate Hopper, Elizabeth Rozanski and Deborah C. Silverstein.
© 2019 John Wiley & Sons, Inc. Published 2019 by John Wiley & Sons, Inc.
Companion Website: www.wiley.com/go/drobatz/textbook

their status may improve with time. A separate clinical scoring system has been proposed for cats and dogs with AKI [4,5] (see Chapter 94).

Presentation

Cats and dogs with CKD generally present with a collection of clinical signs, including polyuria, polydipsia, weight loss, anorexia, vomiting, lethargy, halitosis, and weakness. Initial physical exam may reveal dehydration, muscle atrophy, emaciation, small and irregular kidneys, hypothermia, oral ulcers, and pallor.

Diagnostics

Laboratory Tests

The acquisition of patient samples prior to treatment is essential in determining the cause and severity of disease in these patients. Priority should be given to running a venous blood gas or other rapid analyzer of acid–base and electrolyte status, with samples for a serum chemistry panel and complete blood count also being collected at this time. Frequently identified abnormalities include azotemia and metabolic acidosis (see Chapter 107). Hypokalemia is found in 18% of cats with uremic CKD, although hyperkalemia is seen in 22% of cats with end-stage disease [6] (see Chapter 109). Calcium homeostasis is also significantly affected by CKD, with ionized hypocalcemia being reported in 56% of cats with end-stage CKD [7]. Total and ionized calcium in dogs with CKD can be decreased, normal, or elevated [8] (see Chapter 110).

The chemistry panel will typically reveal azotemia and hyperphosphatemia in addition to the electrolyte abnormalities described above. It is important to get a baseline measurement of blood urea nitrogen (BUN) and creatinine on admission in order to monitor for any improvement with correction of prerenal azotemia as targeted by initial therapy. Degree of hyperphosphatemia has been shown to be related to increased mortality in cats with CKD [9] and is correlated with worsening stage of disease in dogs [10].

The most significant finding on complete blood count for animals with CKD is anemia. This is typically a normocytic, normochromic, non-regenerative anemia (see Chapter 65). The cause of the anemia is associated with impaired production of erythropoietin (EPO), and dogs with CKD have been shown to have a relative deficiency of EPO (low or normal despite anemia) [11]. However, the anemia may be multifactorial with other causes including shortened red blood cell lifespan, poor nutrition, and gastrointestinal blood loss due to uremic gastroenteritis.

Ordering a reticulocyte count can help to further characterize the cause of the anemia in these patients.

A sterile urine sample should be acquired from all patients before starting fluid therapy. A standard urinalysis as well as a urine culture should be performed regardless of clinical signs, as cats have been shown to have positive urine cultures despite a lack of lower urinary tract signs [12] (see Chapter 96). Antibiotics should be considered until culture results are available. Other important findings on urinalysis include urine specific gravity, which should be isosthenuric in most cases of CKD, and proteinuria. Some cats (and rarely dogs) may have concentrated urine despite renal azotemia, which is suspected to be related to glomerular disease and is termed "glomerulotubular imbalance" [13]. Proteinuria is best evaluated with a urine protein:creatinine ratio (UPC) as long as there is no active sediment. Degree of UPC elevation has been shown to correlate with mortality in both cats and dogs [14,15].

Imaging

Abdominal ultrasonography is recommended for evaluation of all patients with CKD. In the emergency setting, imaging may be reserved for animals with a high suspicion of obstructive ureteral disease, such as cats with acute elevations in kidney values. At a minimum, these patients should have orthogonal abdominal radiographs taken to evaluate for the presence of ureteroliths (see Chapter 98).

Monitoring

It is important to acquire a set of baseline parameters to facilitate continued monitoring during hospitalization. Important parameters include body weight, which is essential for monitoring hydration status, and frequency of urination. In polyuric animals, placement of an indwelling urinary catheter is not necessarily required, but should be performed if there is concern regarding potential oliguria (see Chapter 95). In addition, blood pressure should be obtained in all animals presenting with CKD. Hypertension is seen in 19% of cats [16] and 31% of dogs [17] presenting with CKD and has been correlated with a worse prognosis (see Chapter 63). Urine specific gravity should not be used as a measure of hydration status in animals with CKD as their urine is typically isosthenuric despite dehydration.

Stabilization and Initial Therapy

Fluid Therapy

Cats and dogs with severe kidney disease are usually polyuric and may present with severe dehydration or hypovolemia, generally necessitating intravenous fluid therapy. Rates should be determined based on a calculation of fluid deficit (body weight (kg) × percent dehydration) and by taking into account any ongoing losses due to vomiting or diarrhea. The fluid deficit should be replaced over 6–24 hours depending on other variables that may require slower replacement (such as the identification of heart disease) or faster replacement (such as cardiovascular instability) (see Chapter 167).

Electrolyte and acid–base abnormalities are also addressed with fluid therapy. Potassium supplementation is frequently required in patients with CKD, and high rates may be required to normalize serum potassium (see Chapter 109). Metabolic acidosis is also frequently found in these patients. While this is largely corrected by improving perfusion with fluid therapy, a blood pH below 7.2 after correction of volume deficits is an indication for intravenous sodium bicarbonate supplementation [13] (see Chapter 174).

The primary risk with fluid therapy is volume overload or the development of edema. Screening for heart disease should be performed prior to high rates of fluid therapy if at all possible. In addition, animals with significant proteinuria may have hypoalbuminemia and low colloid oncotic pressure. In these patients, high rates of fluid therapy can cause fluid loss into pleural, abdominal, pulmonary, or interstitial spaces, so cautious fluid therapy rates are advised. Ideally, rates above 25 mL per kg of body weight per day should be avoided.

Management of Anemia

Patients with CKD frequently develop anemia as a consequence of an impaired ability to synthesize endogenous EPO. Typically, this anemia develops slowly as the CKD progresses, so these animals are able to tolerate more severe levels of anemia. However, if the patient is severely anemic (hematocrit less than 15%) and is displaying clinical signs of anemia such as tachycardia, tachypnea, or weakness, then a transfusion may be required. Whole blood or packed red blood cells may be used, with packed red blood cells preferred if volume overload is a concern (see Chapter 176).

If the patient is anemic but not significantly clinically affected, EPO products are recommended to stimulate erythropoiesis. Currently, darbepoietin alpha (DPO) is the preferred product due to anecdotal reports of lower risk of anti-EPO antibody development compared to the use of recombinant human EPO products. A retrospective study on DPO use in cats determined an ideal starting dose to be 1 μg/kg subcutaneously once weekly [18]. Weekly monitoring of hematocrit is recommended in order to determine when dosing frequency can be reduced to every other week or once every 3 weeks.

Target hematocrit is roughly 30–40% (closer to 30–35% for cats and 35–40% for dogs) [1,19]. DPO treatment can cause hypertension, so regular blood pressure monitoring is recommended during therapy [18].

The erythropoiesis stimulated by EPO analogues requires ready availability of iron, and iron concentrations have been shown to be low in many animals with CKD [20]. This may be due to reduced intake, iron sequestration from inflammation, or increased loss due to gastrointestinal bleeding. Therefore, iron supplementation is recommended concurrently with EPO administration. An initial intramuscular injection of iron dextran (50 mg for a cat and 50–300 mg for a dog) is recommended, and monthly dosing may be required in some animals [21].

Hypertension (see Chapter 63)

Hypertension is a common sequela to CKD, and the presence of hypertension is one of the criteria for substaging in the IRIS system [3]. However, unless systolic blood pressure exceeds 200 mmHg or there are clinical signs representative of end-organ damage (retinal lesions or neurological signs), initiation of antihypertensive therapy is not required on an emergent basis [21].

If rapid reduction of hypertension is required in an emergency setting, a calcium channel blocker such as amlodipine is recommended. Multiple studies have shown that amlodipine is an effective and safe antihypertensive agent in cats [22–24] and dogs [25,26]. Starting daily doses of 0.625–1.25 mg for cats and 0.1–0.5 mg/kg for dogs are recommended.

Management of Gastrointestinal Signs

Many animals with CKD present with decreased appetite, nausea, vomiting, and diarrhea. Antiemetics such as ondansetron, dolasetron, or maropitant are frequently warranted. Cats with CKD have been shown to have increased gastrin concentrations, suggesting a potential role of CKD in promoting gastric hyperacidity [27]. The use of histamine-2-receptor antagonists or proton pump inhibitors to suppress gastric acid secretion is often recommended, although conclusive evidence of their efficacy in reducing morbidity associated with CKD has not been established.

Management of anorexia can include the use of appetite stimulants or assisted feeding. Mirtazapine has been used to stimulate appetite in cats and dogs with CKD with recommended dosing of 15–30 mg every 24 hours in dogs and 1.875–3.75 mg every 48–72 hours in cats [19]. A pharmacokinetic study has validated every other day dosing frequency in cats with CKD [28]. Despite appetite stimulation, many animals with CKD will require supplemental feeding via placement of a feeding tube.

Placement of an esophagostomy tube is recommended since many animals will require long-term nutritional support, although nasoesophageal or nasogastric tubes can be placed for short-term supplementation. Early placement of a feeding tube is strongly recommended.

Dose Reduction

Many commonly used medications are eliminated through the kidney, and the reduced renal function associated with CKD can prolong the half-life of these medications. This can lead to drug accumulation and an increased rate of adverse reactions. Ideally, dosage reductions are made based on calculations using the patient's GFR, but this is rarely measured in veterinary patients and is never available on an emergency basis, so other methods of dose reduction have been described [1].

One option is to decrease total dose by either halving the drug dosage or doubling the dosing interval, and this is used for drugs that have low risks of toxicity. A second method is to increase the dosage interval or decrease the dosage based on the use of serum creatinine as an estimation of GFR. In this method, the dosing interval is multiplied or the dosage is divided by the patient's serum creatinine. With this method, a cut-off of serum creatinine of 5 mg/dL is recommended to avoid decreasing dose to subtherapeutic levels, as higher creatinine concentrations are not well correlated with GFR. This method is used with drugs that are more likely to be toxic. The third option is to precisely adjust doses based on calculation of the percentage reduction in GFR and is recommended for drugs that have a high risk of toxicity. Examples of drug doses that should be adjusted and the recommended methods of adjustment are shown in Table 102.2.

Prognosis and Long-Term Management

A patient with CKD is considered stable when the serum creatinine has reached a baseline and they are no longer threatened by severe anemia, hypovolemia, hypertension, or electrolyte imbalances. Longer term management includes transitioning to a restricted protein and phosphorus diet, using phosphate binders, administering subcutaneous fluids, and continuing antiemetic therapy as needed. Additional considerations include control of persistent hypertension and proteinuria. More advanced therapeutic modalities, including renal transplantation, hemodialysis, and peritoneal dialysis, are available at a small number of veterinary hospitals, but the cost and availability of these options limit the number of animals with CKD that are managed in this fashion.

Table 102.2 Drug dosage adjustments for patients with CKD (adapted from [1]). Method 1: decrease dose by half or double dosage interval. Method 2: adjust according to serum creatinine concentration. Method 3: precise dosage modification using GFR (see text for more details).

Drug	Dosage adjustment method
Amikacin	3
Amoxicillin	1 or 2
Amphotericin B	3
Ampicillin	1 or 2
Cephalexin	2
Clindamycin	None
Chloramphenicol	None
Cyclophosphamide	None
Corticosteroids	None
Doxycycline	None
Enrofloxacin	1 (increased dosing interval)
Furosemide	None
Gentamicin	3
Heparin	None
Nitrofurantoin	Contraindicated
Penicillin	1 or 2
Propranolol	None
Tetracycline	Contraindicated
Tobramycin	3
Trimethoprim/sulfamethoxazole	2

Regardless of which management strategies are employed, CKD is a progressive disease. IRIS staging has been used to provide estimates of survival time in patients with CKD. In cats, median survival time (MST) was found to be 1151 days in stage 2 (although this study only included cats on the more severe end of stage 2), 679 days in stage 3, and 35 days in stage 4 [9]. The MST in dogs with CKD is less well defined, but one study demonstrated that dogs with CKD who were fed a renal diet had a MST of 594 days, while those kept on a normal maintenance diet had a MST of 188 days [29]. Another study showed that being underweight significantly reduced survival time as well as demonstrating that dogs with IRIS stage 4 CKD had shorter survival times than dogs with stage 2 or 3 disease [30]. The magnitude of proteinuria has been associated with a reduced survival time in both dogs [15] and cats [14,31]. Hypertension has been shown to increase the risk of uremic crisis and death in dogs [17].

Overall, CKD is a serious, chronic illness that requires dedicated monitoring and treatment by the owner and rigorous follow-up with a veterinarian. Most animals with CKD will eventually succumb to the disease or its sequelae, but many can live for meaningful periods of time after diagnosis with sufficient owner dedication and supportive care.

Conclusion

In summary, cats and dogs with CKD will frequently present on an emergency basis. Initial goals in evaluating these patients are to identify azotemia as well as pinpoint life-threatening complications including hypovolemia, hypertension, metabolic acidosis, anemia, and derangements in serum potassium. Taking blood and urine samples for characterization of kidney disease is an important first step and should precede implementation of first-line therapies, including intravenous fluid administration, blood transfusion, and management of profound hypertension. While lifelong monitoring and management of CKD will be required, substantial improvement can be made in the initial emergency period of patient hospitalization.

References

1   Polzin DJ. Chronic kidney disease. In: *Textbook of Veterinary Internal Medicine*, 7th edn (eds Ettinger SJ, Feldman EC). Elsevier Saunders, St Louis, 2010, pp. 2036–2067.

2   Minkus G, Reusch C, Hörauf A, et al. Evaluation of renal biopsies in cats and dogs – histopathology in comparison with clinical data. *J Small Anim Pract* 1994;35:465–472.

3   International Renal Interest Society. IRIS CKD Guidelines. www.iris-kidney.com/guidelines/x (accessed 1 February 2018).

4   Segev G, Kass PH, Francey T, et al. A novel clinical scoring system for outcome prediction in dogs with acute kidney injury managed by hemodialysis. *J Vet Intern Med* 2008;22:301–308.

5   Segev G, Nivy R, Kass PH, et al. A retrospective study of acute kidney injury in cats and development of a novel clinical scoring system for predicting outcome for cats managed by hemodialysis. *J Vet Intern Med* 2013;27:830–839.

6   Elliott J, Barber PJ. Feline chronic renal failure: clinical findings in 80 cases diagnosed between 1992 and 1995. *J Small Anim Pract* 1998;39:78–85.

7   Barber PJ, Elliott J. Feline chronic renal failure: calcium homeostasis in 80 cases diagnosed between 1992 and 1995. *J Small Anim Pract* 1998;39:108–116.

8   Schenck PA, Chew DJ. Determination of calcium fractionation in dogs with chronic renal failure. *Am J Vet Res* 2003;64:1181–1184.

9   Boyd LM, Langston C, Thompson K, et al. Survival in cats with naturally occurring chronic kidney disease (2000–2002). *J Vet Intern Med* 2008;22: 1111–1117.

10 Cortadellas O, Fernández del Palacio MJ, Talavera J, et al. Calcium and phosphorus homeostasis in dogs with spontaneous chronic kidney disease at different stages of severity. *J Vet Intern Med* 2010;24:73–79.

11 King L, Giger U, Diserens D, et al. Anemia of chronic renal failure in dogs. *J Vet Intern Med* 1992;6:264–270.

12 Mayer-Roenne B, Goldstein RE, Erb HN. Urinary tract infections in cats with hyperthyroidism, diabetes mellitus and chronic kidney disease. *J Feline Med Surg* 2007;9:124–132.

13 Langston CE, Eatroff AE. Chronic kidney disease. In: *Small Animal Critical Care Medicine*, 2nd edn (eds Silverstein DC, Hopper K). Elsevier Saunders, St. Louis, 2015, pp. 661–666.

14 Syme HM, Markwell PJ, Pfeiffer D, et al. Survival of cats with naturally occurring chronic renal failure is related to severity of proteinuria. *J Vet Intern Med* 2006;20:528–535.

15 Jacob F, Polzin DJ, Osborne CA, et al. Evaluation of the association between initial proteinuria and morbidity rate or death in dogs with naturally occurring chronic renal failure. *J Am Vet Med Assoc* 2005;226:393–400.

16 Syme HM, Barber PJ, Markwell PJ, et al. Prevalence of systolic hypertension in cats with chronic renal failure at initial evaluation. *J Am Vet Med Assoc* 2002;220:1799–1804.

17 Jacob F, Polzin DJ, Osborne CA, et al. Association between initial systolic blood pressure and risk of developing a uremic crisis or of dying in dogs with chronic renal failure. *J Am Vet Med Assoc* 2003;222:322–329.

18 Chalhoub S, Langston CE, Farrelly J. The use of darbepoetin to stimulate erythropoiesis in anemia of chronic kidney disease in cats: 25 cases. *J Vet Intern Med* 2012;26:363–369.

19 Bartges JW. Chronic kidney disease in dogs and cats. *Vet Clin North Am Small Anim Pract* 2012;42: 669–692.

20 Cowgill LD, James KM, Levy JK, et al. Use of recombinant human erythropoietin for management of anemia in dogs and cats with renal failure. *J Am Vet Med Assoc* 1998;212:521–528.

21 Polzin DJ. Chronic kidney disease in small animals. *Vet Clin North Am Small Anim Pract* 2011;41:15–30.

22 Mathur S, Syme H, Brown CA, et al. Effects of the calcium channel antagonist amlodipine in cats with surgically induced hypertensive renal insufficiency. *Am J Vet Res* 2002;63:833–839.

Clinical Signs and Physical Examination Findings

Clinical signs may be vague and non-specific, including vomiting, anorexia or lethargy, depending on when in the course of the disease a diagnosis of uroabdomen is made. Physical examination findings may include signs of shock or impaired perfusion, a palpable fluid wave and/or abdominal distension, abdominal pain, dehydration, cardiac arrhythmias or signs of concurrent trauma such as inguinal or perineal bruising, or pelvic fractures [1,3,6,7,9,13].

It should be noted that *palpation of a seemingly intact bladder does not rule out the diagnosis of uroabdomen* [1].

Diagnosis and Laboratory Evaluation

The diagnosis of uroabdomen is made based on a combination of clinical signs, physical examination findings, laboratory assessment of peripheral blood in comparison with abdominal fluid, and imaging techniques.

Laboratory Findings

As with many emergencies, a complete blood count and serum chemistry with an electrolyte panel are invaluable in assessing the systemic health of a patient. Laboratory findings may include [1,3,5,6,9]:

- azotemia
- hyperkalemia
- hyponatremia and hypochloremia
- hyperphosphatemia
- metabolic acidosis
- hemoconcentration (if dehydrated)
- neutrophilia (+/− left shift)
- hematuria (macroscopic or microscopic).

The rise in blood urea nitrogen (BUN) may be disproportionately greater than the rise in creatinine due to the more rapid equilibration of urea between the intra-abdominal urine and the systemic circulation. In people, BUN:creatinine ratios greater than 30:1 have been reported in cases of uroabdomen, with the normal ratio being approximately 10–15:1 [14,15].

Abdominocentesis with subsequent evaluation of the fluid is arguably the most useful tool in definitively diagnosing uroabdomen, though it gives no information as to the location of the rupture (see Chapter 186). It may be performed with the guidance of ultrasound or as a blind tap. The pathophysiology of uroabdomen results in an elevated creatinine and potassium in the abdominal fluid relative to the peripheral blood. Ideally, the same serum

Table 103.1 Reported abdominal fluid potassium and creatinine to peripheral blood ratios in dogs and cats [1,2].

	Abdominal fluid: peripheral blood creatinine	Abdominal fluid: peripheral blood potassium
Dogs	>2:1 (86%, 100%)*	>1.4:1 (100%, 100%)*
Cats	>2:1**	>1.9:1**

*Sensitivity, specificity.

**Sensitivity and specificity not reported.

chemistry or electrolyte analyzer should be used for the peripheral blood as abdominal fluid to avoid confounding results. Benchtop analyzers are available, but many do not provide consistent and reliable results [16].

The published ratios consistent with uroabdomen in dogs and cats are reported in Table 103.1.

The more azotemic an animal, the lower the gradient is expected to be [2,9]. Full analysis of the abdominal fluid is also recommended, including cytology. The fluid may range from a pure transudate, modified transudate to an exudate depending on chronicity, severity, and presence of any infectious agents [17]. If the latter were found, criteria for a septic uroabdomen would be satisfied (see Chapter 87).

Imaging Findings

Ultrasound is a valuable tool in diagnosing uroabdomen. Though originally developed for use in trauma patients, the focused assessment with sonography for trauma (FAST) (see Chapter 182) examination may be useful, regardless of the etiology of the free abdominal fluid. An abdominal FAST involves evaluating four areas – caudal to the xiphoid, around the urinary bladder, and around each kidney – for presence of free fluid [18]. Contrast cystography has been described in two dogs and an *in vitro* model whereby injection of microbubbled saline allowed visualization of bladder tears with ultrasound. In this study, microbubbles were created in saline by manually injecting sterile saline and air vigorously, back and forth, between two syringes through a three-way stopcock. Larger air bubbles were expelled, and the remaining solution was infused promptly through a urinary catheter into the bladder. The presence of a bladder tear was confirmed by ultrasonographic visualization of microbubbled saline leaking outside the bladder and passing into the peritoneum [19].

Plain radiographs may show a loss of intra-abdominal serosal detail. This may be confined to the peritoneal or retroperitoneal space, or may be generalized [1,6,9,20]. The bladder or kidneys may or may not be visible [1,9]. Depending on the cause, additional abnormalities such as urinary calculi or pelvic fractures may be seen [1].

Contrast radiographic studies are easy to perform on an emergency basis and can help to definitively diagnose

Clinical Signs and Physical Examination Findings

Clinical signs may be vague and non-specific, including vomiting, anorexia or lethargy, depending on when in the course of the disease a diagnosis of uroabdomen is made. Physical examination findings may include signs of shock or impaired perfusion, a palpable fluid wave and/or abdominal distension, abdominal pain, dehydration, cardiac arrhythmias or signs of concurrent trauma such as inguinal or perineal bruising, or pelvic fractures [1,3,6,7,9,13].

It should be noted that *palpation of a seemingly intact bladder does not rule out the diagnosis of uroabdomen* [1].

Diagnosis and Laboratory Evaluation

The diagnosis of uroabdomen is made based on a combination of clinical signs, physical examination findings, laboratory assessment of peripheral blood in comparison with abdominal fluid, and imaging techniques.

Laboratory Findings

As with many emergencies, a complete blood count and serum chemistry with an electrolyte panel are invaluable in assessing the systemic health of a patient. Laboratory findings may include [1,3,5,6,9]:

- azotemia
- hyperkalemia
- hyponatremia and hypochloremia
- hyperphosphatemia
- metabolic acidosis
- hemoconcentration (if dehydrated)
- neutrophilia (+/− left shift)
- hematuria (macroscopic or microscopic).

The rise in blood urea nitrogen (BUN) may be disproportionately greater than the rise in creatinine due to the more rapid equilibration of urea between the intra-abdominal urine and the systemic circulation. In people, BUN:creatinine ratios greater than 30:1 have been reported in cases of uroabdomen, with the normal ratio being approximately 10–15:1 [14,15].

Abdominocentesis with subsequent evaluation of the fluid is arguably the most useful tool in definitively diagnosing uroabdomen, though it gives no information as to the location of the rupture (see Chapter 186). It may be performed with the guidance of ultrasound or as a blind tap. The pathophysiology of uroabdomen results in an elevated creatinine and potassium in the abdominal fluid relative to the peripheral blood. Ideally, the same serum

Table 103.1 Reported abdominal fluid potassium and creatinine to peripheral blood ratios in dogs and cats [1,2].

	Abdominal fluid: peripheral blood creatinine	Abdominal fluid: peripheral blood potassium
Dogs	>2:1 (86%, 100%)*	>1.4:1 (100%, 100%)*
Cats	>2:1**	>1.9:1**

*Sensitivity, specificity.

**Sensitivity and specificity not reported.

chemistry or electrolyte analyzer should be used for the peripheral blood as abdominal fluid to avoid confounding results. Benchtop analyzers are available, but many do not provide consistent and reliable results [16].

The published ratios consistent with uroabdomen in dogs and cats are reported in Table 103.1.

The more azotemic an animal, the lower the gradient is expected to be [2,9]. Full analysis of the abdominal fluid is also recommended, including cytology. The fluid may range from a pure transudate, modified transudate to an exudate depending on chronicity, severity, and presence of any infectious agents [17]. If the latter were found, criteria for a septic uroabdomen would be satisfied (see Chapter 87).

Imaging Findings

Ultrasound is a valuable tool in diagnosing uroabdomen. Though originally developed for use in trauma patients, the focused assessment with sonography for trauma (FAST) (see Chapter 182) examination may be useful, regardless of the etiology of the free abdominal fluid. An abdominal FAST involves evaluating four areas – caudal to the xiphoid, around the urinary bladder, and around each kidney – for presence of free fluid [18]. Contrast cystography has been described in two dogs and an *in vitro* model whereby injection of microbubbled saline allowed visualization of bladder tears with ultrasound. In this study, microbubbles were created in saline by manually injecting sterile saline and air vigorously, back and forth, between two syringes through a three-way stopcock. Larger air bubbles were expelled, and the remaining solution was infused promptly through a urinary catheter into the bladder. The presence of a bladder tear was confirmed by ultrasonographic visualization of microbubbled saline leaking outside the bladder and passing into the peritoneum [19].

Plain radiographs may show a loss of intra-abdominal serosal detail. This may be confined to the peritoneal or retroperitoneal space, or may be generalized [1,6,9,20]. The bladder or kidneys may or may not be visible [1,9]. Depending on the cause, additional abnormalities such as urinary calculi or pelvic fractures may be seen [1].

Contrast radiographic studies are easy to perform on an emergency basis and can help to definitively diagnose rigorous follow-up with a veterinarian. Most animals with CKD will eventually succumb to the disease or its sequelae, but many can live for meaningful periods of time after diagnosis with sufficient owner dedication and supportive care.

Conclusion

In summary, cats and dogs with CKD will frequently present on an emergency basis. Initial goals in evaluating

these patients are to identify azotemia as well as pinpoint life-threatening complications including hypovolemia, hypertension, metabolic acidosis, anemia, and derangements in serum potassium. Taking blood and urine samples for characterization of kidney disease is an important first step and should precede implementation of first-line therapies, including intravenous fluid administration, blood transfusion, and management of profound hypertension. While lifelong monitoring and management of CKD will be required, substantial improvement can be made in the initial emergency period of patient hospitalization.

References

1 Polzin DJ. Chronic kidney disease. In: *Textbook of Veterinary Internal Medicine*, 7th edn (eds Ettinger SJ, Feldman EC). Elsevier Saunders, St Louis, 2010, pp. 2036–2067.

2 Minkus G, Reusch C, Hörauf A, et al. Evaluation of renal biopsies in cats and dogs – histopathology in comparison with clinical data. *J Small Anim Pract* 1994;35:465–472.

3 International Renal Interest Society. IRIS CKD Guidelines. www.iris-kidney.com/guidelines/x (accessed 1 February 2018).

4 Segev G, Kass PH, Francey T, et al. A novel clinical scoring system for outcome prediction in dogs with acute kidney injury managed by hemodialysis. *J Vet Intern Med* 2008;22:301–308.

5 Segev G, Nivy R, Kass PH, et al. A retrospective study of acute kidney injury in cats and development of a novel clinical scoring system for predicting outcome for cats managed by hemodialysis. *J Vet Intern Med* 2013;27:830–839.

6 Elliott J, Barber PJ. Feline chronic renal failure: clinical findings in 80 cases diagnosed between 1992 and 1995. *J Small Anim Pract* 1998;39:78–85.

7 Barber PJ, Elliott J. Feline chronic renal failure: calcium homeostasis in 80 cases diagnosed between 1992 and 1995. *J Small Anim Pract* 1998;39:108–116.

8 Schenck PA, Chew DJ. Determination of calcium fractionation in dogs with chronic renal failure. *Am J Vet Res* 2003;64:1181–1184.

9 Boyd LM, Langston C, Thompson K, et al. Survival in cats with naturally occurring chronic kidney disease (2000–2002). *J Vet Intern Med* 2008;22:1111–1117.

10 Cortadellas O, Fernández del Palacio MJ, Talavera J, et al. Calcium and phosphorus homeostasis in dogs with spontaneous chronic kidney disease at different stages of severity. *J Vet Intern Med* 2010;24:73–79.

11 King L, Giger U, Diserens D, et al. Anemia of chronic renal failure in dogs. *J Vet Intern Med* 1992;6:264–270.

12 Mayer-Roenne B, Goldstein RE, Erb HN. Urinary tract infections in cats with hyperthyroidism, diabetes

mellitus and chronic kidney disease. *J Feline Med Surg* 2007;9:124–132.

13 Langston CE, Eatroff AE. Chronic kidney disease. In: *Small Animal Critical Care Medicine*, 2nd edn (eds Silverstein DC, Hopper K). Elsevier Saunders, St. Louis, 2015, pp. 661–666.

14 Syme HM, Markwell PJ, Pfeiffer D, et al. Survival of cats with naturally occurring chronic renal failure is related to severity of proteinuria. *J Vet Intern Med* 2006;20:528–535.

15 Jacob F, Polzin DJ, Osborne CA, et al. Evaluation of the association between initial proteinuria and morbidity rate or death in dogs with naturally occurring chronic renal failure. *J Am Vet Med Assoc* 2005;226:393–400.

16 Syme HM, Barber PJ, Markwell PJ, et al. Prevalence of systolic hypertension in cats with chronic renal failure at initial evaluation. *J Am Vet Med Assoc* 2002;220:1799–1804.

17 Jacob F, Polzin DJ, Osborne CA, et al. Association between initial systolic blood pressure and risk of developing a uremic crisis or of dying in dogs with chronic renal failure. *J Am Vet Med Assoc* 2003;222:322–329.

18 Chalhoub S, Langston CE, Farrelly J. The use of darbepoetin to stimulate erythropoiesis in anemia of chronic kidney disease in cats: 25 cases. *J Vet Intern Med* 2012;26:363–369.

19 Bartges JW. Chronic kidney disease in dogs and cats. *Vet Clin North Am Small Anim Pract* 2012;42:669–692.

20 Cowgill LD, James KM, Levy JK, et al. Use of recombinant human erythropoietin for management of anemia in dogs and cats with renal failure. *J Am Vet Med Assoc* 1998;212:521–528.

21 Polzin DJ. Chronic kidney disease in small animals. *Vet Clin North Am Small Anim Pract* 2011;41:15–30.

22 Mathur S, Syme H, Brown CA, et al. Effects of the calcium channel antagonist amlodipine in cats with surgically induced hypertensive renal insufficiency. *Am J Vet Res* 2002;63:833–839.

a uroabdomen or determine the exact location of the rupture [20]. The choice of contrast study will be determined by the suspected location of disruption. For suspected bladder or urethral tears, positive contrast cystography and urography are indicated respectively [1,20]. For renal damage or suspected ureteral rupture, excretory urography is the contrast study of choice [5,6,20]. False negatives can occur and are most commonly due to insufficient volume of contrast agent [6,9,20]. Contrast agents should be used with caution in azotemic or dehydrated patients, due to the risk of acute kidney injury [9,20] (see Chapter 94).

Advanced imaging modalities such as CT urography and MR urography are being utilized more frequently in human medicine, but limited availability and higher costs constrain their widespread application in veterinary medicine [21].

Emergent Stabilization

Initial evaluation and treatment should be directed towards achieving and/or maintaining systemic stability. Fluid therapy should be utilized as indicated to restore perfusion and normalize heart rate, pulse quality, capillary refill time, and blood pressure. These traditional endpoints of resuscitation, together with mentation and body temperature, are typically considered the standard of care, though it should be noted that ongoing oxygen debt may be sustained past normalization of these [22]. Peripheral lactate concentration, pH, base deficit, and central venous oxygen saturation may also provide valuable information about the patient's hemodynamic status (see Chapters 152 and 153).

Fluid type may depend on co-morbidities and severity of shock, and choices could include isotonic, hypertonic or colloid solutions, or combinations of the above (see Chapters 167–169). It has been suggested that avoidance of potassium-containing fluids in a hyperkalemic animal is warranted [23]. However, a study by Drobatz and Cole showed that a balanced electrolyte solution such as lactated Ringer's solution improved acid–base status after 12 hours of fluid therapy in a population of hyperkalemic cats with urethral obstructions with no difference in serum potassium, when compared to 0.9% saline, suggesting that a balanced electrolyte solution may be preferable [24].

It is important to fully evaluate the patient for concurrent injuries that may affect means of stabilization. Additionally, analgesia is an important component of initial therapy, both for the pain associated with chemical peritonitis and any concurrent orthopedic or soft tissue injuries (see Chapter 193). Opioids, specifically pure mu-agonists, are ideal due to superior pain relief and minimal risk for toxicity [25]. Non-steroidal anti-inflammatories should be avoided in patients with hemodynamic compromise and altered renal function. Ketamine should be used cautiously in these patients, since it may have a prolonged duration of action due to its excretion in urine [26,27].

Due to the potential for electrolyte derangements, particularly hyperkalemia, an electrocardiographic assessment (ECG) is warranted in all patients with diagnosed or suspected uroabdomen. ECG abnormalities reported with hyperkalemia include peaked T-waves, decreased P- and R-wave amplitude, prolonged QRS and P-R intervals, S-T segment depression, and increased Q-T intervals. With rising potassium concentration, this may progress to atrial standstill, sinoventricular rhythm, and ventricular fibrillation or asystole [10,28,29].

Symptomatic treatment (see below) of hyperkalemia is definitely warranted with ECG changes, but there is no reliable correlation between presence or absence of ECG changes and serum potassium levels [10]. Treatment has been advocated should serum potassium exceed 7.5 mmol/L, or earlier if the animal is showing any clinical signs [30].

In addition to intravenous fluid therapy, options for emergency treatment of hyperkalemia include the following [9,30–32].

- Calcium gluconate: 0.5–1.5 mL/kg of a 10% solution given slow IV (over approximately 5–10 minutes), with ECG monitoring. This does not reverse hyperkalemia but it does act as a "cardioprotectant" by raising the threshold potential in cardiomyocytes, speeding impulse propagation in the sinoatrial and atrioventricular node, and returning cardiomyocyte excitability to normal. The duration of action of calcium gluconate is 30–60 minutes.
- Drugs promoting intracellular flux of potassium.
  ○ *Regular insulin*: 0.25–0.5 U/kg IV followed by an infusion of 50% dextrose (1–2 g/unit of insulin administered) to prevent hypoglycemia. Insulin stimulates the Na+/K+/ATPase pump, which moves potassium intracellularly in exchange for sodium in a 2:3 ratio[30,31]; this effect is independent of insulin's effect on glucose. The onset of action of insulin is < 15 minutes and its effect is maximal at 30–60 minutes following a single dose [32]. Serial monitoring of blood glucose is recommended following insulin administration to monitor for hypoglycemia. Should hypoglycemia occur, dextrose supplementation (2.5–5%) in intravenous fluids can be instituted.
  ○ *Terbutaline*: 0.01 mg/kg slow IV or SC. Catecholamines activate Na+/K+/ATPase pumps through beta-2-receptor stimulation in a manner that is additive to the effect of insulin. Alternatively, nebulized albuterol may be used. The effect of beta-agonist therapy is apparent at 30 minutes and persists for at least 2 hours. Mild tachycardia is the most common side-effect of

nebulized albuterol or terbutaline. The effect of insulin is additive with that of albuterol, and a combination of the two can result in a decline in serum potassium by about 1.2 mEq/L in about 60 minutes [32].

○ *Sodium bicarbonate*: 1 mEq/kg slow IV. Sodium bicarbonate infusion can shift potassium from the extracellular to intracellular space by increasing blood pH. This therapy should be employed with caution as the possibility for paradoxical CNS acidosis and hyperosmolality from the high sodium concentration exists. There is additional risk of lowering ionized calcium which may counteract the effects of calcium gluconate administration [30]. Therefore sodium bicarbonate administration is typically considered as a last-line therapy.

Ultimately, urinary diversion or definitive repair will be required to prevent recurrence hyperkalemia.

Treatment

The two main components of treatment are urinary diversion followed by, or performed at the same time as, definitive repair of the site of rupture.

Assuming at least one of the ureters and kidneys is intact and functional, a urinary catheter should be placed into the bladder to allow emptying and prevent accumulation of urine within the abdomen [9]. In cases of urethral tears, fluoroscopic guidance may be required to facilitate correct placement [9]. Peritoneal drainage should also be performed. This may be accomplished by draining with a needle, over-the-needle catheter or placement of a peritoneal dialysis or abdominal drainage catheter [1,9] (Figure 103.1). Placement should be aseptic

Pigtail catheter placed for
peritoneal drainage of urine

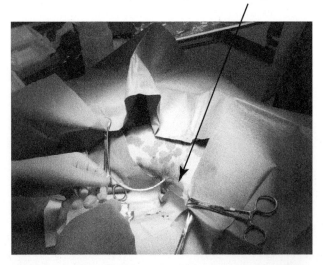

Figure 103.1 Placement of a peritoneal drainage catheter in a dog.

and the catheter should be attached to a closed collection system. A cystostomy tube may be utilized as a method of urinary diversion in cases of urethral rupture [3,9,33].

Peritoneal dialysis may be used in the preoperative period to treat severe hyperkalemia or azotemia [34]. Full discussion of this is beyond the scope of this chapter, but in brief, dialysate solution is infused into the abdominal cavity. The peritoneum acts as a selectively permeable membrane and solutes and water move between peritoneal capillaries and peritoneal fluid to equilibrate. Following a dwell time, the fluid is then removed from the peritoneal cavity and unwanted solutes can thus be eliminated [4].

Published survival rates in veterinary studies have been variable. In one study of 27 dogs and cats undergoing peritoneal dialysis, 24% survived to discharge [35]. One study evaluating dogs with leptospirosis that underwent peritoneal dialysis showed a survival rate of 80% [36]. In general, the overall survival rate with peritoneal dialysis is likely related more to the underlying disease than the actual technique of dialysis itself.

Medical management may be attempted by utilizing a urinary catheter for urethral tears, or potentially bladder rupture [9]. The urethra is reported to take 3–21 days to heal [4,37,38] (see Chapter 100), and a study by Burrows and Bovee showed healing of an iatrogenic cystotomy incision in 45 hours [11].

Surgery may be indicated for larger tears, those that have failed medical management or tears in a location that renders urinary diversion alone insufficient. Options for surgical management vary depending on the location of the tear, but include ureteronephrectomy, ureteroureterostomy, neoureterocystostomy, nephrectomy, urethral anastamosis, stent placement, subcutaneous ureteral bypass implantation, repair of bladder laceration or permanent urethrostomy [5,9,37]. For a detailed description of these techniques, the reader is referred to a surgical textbook.

Complications and Prognosis

Complications of uroabdomen include development of severe chemical peritonitis, septic peritonitis if the urine is infected, and complications associated with surgery [1,3,4,39] (see Chapter 87).

Dehiscence or delayed healing may result from urine in direct contact with recovering tissues [38]. Strictures, incontinence, ongoing urine leakage, and urinary tract infections are all possible complications that may be encountered postoperatively [1,3,4].

The published literature reports a poor outcome in 35% of dogs with urethral rupture and in 17.2–28.6% of cats [1] (see Chapter 100). In both dogs and cats, the presence of multiple traumatic injuries is associated with a higher mortality rate [3,4].

References

1 Aumann M, Worth LT, Drobatz KJ. Uroperitoneum in cats: 26 cases (1986–1995). *J Am Anim Hosp Assoc* 1998;34(4):315–324.

2 Schmiedt C, Tobias KM, Otto CM. Evaluation of abdominal fluid: peripheral blood creatinine and potassium ratios for diagnosis of uroperitoneum in dogs. *J Vet Emerg Crit Care* 2001;11(4):275–280.

3 Addison ES, Halfacree Z, Moore AH, Demetriou J, Parsons K, Tivers M. A retrospective analysis of urethral rupture in 63 cats. *J Feline Med Surg.* 2014;16(4):300–307.

4 Anderson RB, Aronson LR, Drobatz KJ, Atilla A. Prognostic factors for successful outcome following urethral rupture in dogs and cats. *J Am Anim Hosp Assoc* 2006;42(2):136–146.

5 Hamilton MH, Sissener TR, Baines SJ. Traumatic bilateral ureteric rupture in two dogs. *J Small Anim Pract* 2006;47(12):737–740.

6 Weisse C, Aronson LR, Drobatz K. Traumatic rupture of the ureter: 10 cases. *J Am Anim Hosp Assoc* 2002;38(2):188–192.

7 Klainbart S, Merchav R, Ohad DG. Traumatic urothorax in a dog: a case report. *J Small Anim Pract* 2011;52(10):544–546.

8 Osborne C, Low D, DR F. *Canine and Feline Urology.* WB Saunders, Philadelphia, 1972, pp. 343–349.

9 Chew DJ, DiBartola SP, Schenck PA. Urinary tract trauma and uroperitoneum. In: *Canine and Feline Nephrology and Urology*, 2nd edn (eds Chew DJ, DiBartola SP, Schenck PA). Elsevier Saunders, St Louis, 2011, pp. 391–408.

10 Tag TL, Day TK. Electrocardiographic assessment of hyperkalemia in dogs and cats. *J Vet Emerg Crit Care* 2008;18(1):61–67.

11 Burrows CF, Bovee KC. Metabolic changes due to experimentally induced rupture of the canine urinary bladder. *Am J Vet Res* 1974;35(8):1083–1088.

12 DiBartola SP, Autran de Morais H. Disorders of potassium: hypokalemia and hyperkalemia. In: *Fluid, Electrolyte, and Acid-Base Disorders in Small Animal Practice*, 4th edn (ed. DiBartola SP). Elsevier Saunders, St Louis, 2012, pp. 92–119.

13 Rieser TM. Urinary tract emergencies. *Vet Clin North Am Small Anim Pract* 2005;35(2):359–373.

14 Sullivan MJ, Lackner LH, Banowsky LH. Intraperitoneal extravasation of urine. BUN-serum creatinine disproportion. *JAMA* 1972;221(5):491–492.

15 Prause LC, Grauer GF. Association of gastrointestinal hemorrhage with increased blood urea nitrogen and BUN/creatinine ratio in dogs: a literature review and retrospective study. *Vet Clin Pathol* 1998;27(4): 107–111.

16 Hetzel N, Papasouliotis K, Dodkin S, Murphy K. Biochemical assessment of canine body cavity effusions using three bench-top analysers. *J Small Anim Pract* 2012;53(8):459–464.

17 Connally HE. Cytology and fluid analysis of the acute abdomen. *Clin Tech Small Anim Pract* 2003;18(1): 39–44.

18 Lisciandro GR, Lagutchik MS, Mann KA, et al. Evaluation of an abdominal fluid scoring system determined using abdominal focused assessment with sonography for trauma in 101 dogs with motor vehicle trauma. *J Vet Emerg Crit Care* 2009;19(5):426–437.

19 Coté E, Carroll MC, Beck KA, Good L, Gannon K. Diagnosis of urinary bladder rupture using ultrasound contrast cystography: in vitro model and two case-history reports. *Vet Radiol Ultrasound* 2002;43(3): 281–286.

20 Bischoff MG. Radiographic techniques and interpretation of the acute abdomen. *Clin Tech Small Anim Pract* 2003;18(1):7–19.

21 Silverman SG, Leyendecker JR, Amis ES Jr. What is the current role of CT urography and MR urography in the evaluation of the urinary tract? *Radiology* 2009;250(2):309–323.

22 Prittie J. Optimal endpoints of resuscitation and early goal-directed therapy. *J Vet Emerg Crit Care* 2006;16(4):329–339.

23 Mayhew P, Holt D. Ruptured bladder in dogs and cats. *Stand Care: Emerg Crit Care Med* 2004;6(10):6–11.

24 Drobatz KJ, Cole SG. The influence of crystalloid type on acid-base and electrolyte status of cats with urethral obstruction. *J Vet Emerg Crit Care* 2008;18(4):355–361.

25 Dyson DH. Analgesia and chemical restraint for the emergent veterinary patient. *Vet Clin North Am Small Anim Pract* 2008;38(6):1329–1352.

26 Mathews KA. Non-steroidal anti-inflammatory analgesics: a review of current practice. *J Vet Emerg Crit Care* 2002;12(2):89–97.

27 Livingston A, Waterman AE. The urinary excretion of ketamine and its metabolites in the rat. *Br J Pharmacol* 1978;64:402.

28 Ettinger PO, Regan TJ, Oldewurtel HA. Hyperkalemia, cardiac conduction, and the electrocardiogram: a review. *Am Heart J* 1974;88(3):360–371.

29 Mattu A, Brady WJ, Robinson DA. Electrocardiographic manifestations of hyperkalemia. *Am J Emerg Med* 2000;18(6):721–729.

30 Schaer M. Therapeutic approach to electrolyte emergencies. *Vet Clin North Am Small Anim Pract* 2008;38(3):513–33.

31 Parham WA, Mehdirad AA, Biermann KM, Fredman CS. Hyperkalemia revisited. *Tex Heart Inst J* 2006;33(1):40–47.

32 Weisberg LS. Management of severe hyperkalemia. *Crit Care Med* 2008;36(12):3246–3251.

33 Beck AL, Grierson JM, Ogden DM, Hamilton MH, Lipscomb VJ. Outcome of and complications associated with tube cystostomy in dogs and cats: 76 cases (1995–2006). *J Am Vet Med Assoc* 2007;230(8):1184–1189.

34 Ross LA, Labato MA. Current techniques in peritoneal dialysis. *J Vet Emerg Crit Care* 2013;23(2).

35 Crisp MS, Chew DJ, DiBartola SP. Peritoneal dialysis in dogs and cats: 27 cases (1976–1987). *J Am Vet Med Assoc* 1989;195:1262–1266.

36 Beckel N, O'Toole T, Rozanski E. Peritoneal dialysis in the management of acute renal failure in five dogs with leptospirosis. *J Vet Emerg Crit Care* 2005;15(3): 201–205.

37 Bleedorn JA, Bjorling DE. Urethra. In: *Veterinary Surgery: Small Animal*, 2nd edn (eds Tobias KM, Johnston SA). Elsevier, St Louis, 2012, pp. 1993–2010.

38 Daniel AD, Richard W. Healing responses of the lower urinary tract. *Vet Clin North Am Small Anim Pract* 1996;26(2):197–206.

39 Wagenlehner FM, Pilatz A, Naber KG, Weidner W. Therapeutic challenges of urosepsis. *Eur J Clin Invest* 2008;38:45–49.

104

Urethral Prolapse

Jennifer Carr, DVM, MS, DACVS

MedVet Medical and Cancer Center for Pets, Worthington, OH, USA

Urethral Prolapse

Urethral prolapse is a condition in male dogs where the urethral mucosa everts beyond the external urethral orifice. The mucosa is susceptible to trauma and these patients often present for blood dripping from the penis. Alternatively, patients may present for a red or purple mass located at the tip of the penis. The most common breeds affected by this condition are English bulldogs and other brachycephalic breeds. Several reports also document the condition in the Yorkshire terrier [1].

The exact cause of urethral prolapse remains unknown, but several theories exist. Respiratory difficulty, sexual excitement, urogenital or prostatic conditions such as prostatomegaly and urinary calculi, and developmental diseases have all been proposed [2]. In addition, increased abdominal pressure causing impaired venous return to the distal urethra secondary to upper airway obstruction, chronic vomiting, or dysuria has also been suggested [2].

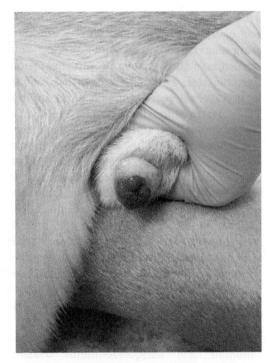

Figure 104.1 Urethral prolapse in a dog.

Diagnosis

Diagnosis of urethral prolapse is made by observation of a fleshy mass on the distal urethra through which a urinary catheter can be placed (Figure 104.1). Determining the underlying cause of urethral prolapse may be challenging diagnostically and includes bloodwork, urinalysis, urine culture, abdominal radiographs, and abdominal ultrasound. In many cases an underlying cause cannot be determined.

Treatment

Treatment of urethral prolapse in the emergent setting is directed at controlling bleeding. This can be accomplished by sedating the patient and preventing further self-trauma. Both acepromazine and butorphanol are common sedatives used for this reason [3]. There is evidence to suggest that sedation given in the perioperative period may contribute to a more optimal long-term outcome following surgery [3]. Although not reported, the author had used topical vasoconstricting agents with some success to control bleeding until surgical intervention can occur.

Definitive treatment is directed at replacing prolapsed urethral mucosa. This can be done in the emergent setting by manual reduction of the prolapsed tissue and placement of a purse-string suture. Clients should be warned that prolapse may recur over time with this method.

Textbook of Small Animal Emergency Medicine, First Edition. Edited by Kenneth J. Drobatz, Kate Hopper, Elizabeth Rozanski and Deborah C. Silverstein.
© 2019 John Wiley & Sons, Inc. Published 2019 by John Wiley & Sons, Inc.
Companion Website: www.wiley.com/go/drobatz/textbook

If a voided sample of urine is discolored due to hematuria, comparison of the sample to one obtained via cystocentesis might help to localize the source of blood. If the voided sample is hematuric and the sample obtained shortly thereafter via cystocentesis is clear, the blood is thought to originate from a source distal to the urinary bladder, such as the urethra, prostate, uterus or vulva. Cystocentesis should be performed following collection of the voided sample because of the possibility of causing iatrogenic hemorrhage. Performing cystocentesis is contraindicated when a hemostatic disorder is suspected, and relatively contraindicated when urinary bladder neoplasia is suspected.

Other tests that might help determine the cause of hematuria include urine culture, complete blood count, tests of hemostatic function, abdominal radiography or ultrasound, and cystoscopy.

Other Cells or Particles

Marked pyuria or crystalluria can lead to a turbid and discolored urine appearance that clears with centrifugation. Further examination of the urine sediment confirms the presence of WBCs, crystals, or other debris within the urine sediment.

Abnormal Urine Supernatant Color

Endogenous Pigments

Bilirubinuria

Bilirubinuria occurs in the presence or absence of hyperbilirubinemia and clinical signs of icterus. Because of its low threshold for renal excretion, bilirubinuria might be detected early in the course of disease processes before hyperbilirubinemia is evident. Trace to mild bilirubinuria is common in normal dogs, as dogs have the unique ability to conjugate bilirubin in their renal tubular cells [2]. Its presence in the urine can correspond to prehepatic (hemolysis), hepatic (hepatocellular disease), or posthepatic (biliary tract and gall bladder disease) causes of hyperbilirubinemia.

Although concentrated normal urine often has an intense yellow or amber coloration, bilirubinuria should be suspected when urine is dark yellow to brown and minimally concentrated. With prolonged storage at room temperature and/or with exposure to ultraviolet light, bilirubin becomes oxidized into biliverdin, which contributes a green color to the urine sample. Once oxidized to biliverdin, the sample will test negative for bilirubin on reagent pad analysis so the presence of bilirubin should be determined on fresh urine samples [3]. Diagnostics that might help determine the cause of bilirubinuria include plasma color inspection, complete blood count with manual differential, serum biochemistry, liver function testing, and abdominal ultrasound. A further review of hyperbilirubinemia is provided in Chapter 11.

Hemoglobinuria

The presence of free hemoglobin causes a pale pink to dark red discoloration of the urine. Unless RBCs are lysed due to *in vitro* storage conditions, true hemoglobinuria is expected to come from *in vivo* hemolysis. On urine chemistry test strips, occult blood/hemoglobin strips contain an organic peroxide [4,5] which yields a positive result in the presence of intact RBCs, free hemoglobin, and myoglobin. Examination of the urine sediment helps to exclude hematuria, but further investigation is necessary to differentiate hemoglobinuria from myoglobinuria. Hemoglobinuria is suspected when the patient's plasma or serum color is light pink to red, while serum in patients with myoglobinuria is typically colorless. Other distinguishing diagnostic findings seen in patients with myoglobinuria are found in Table 105.1 and discussed later in this chapter.

Hemolytic anemia is suspected when hemoglobinuria occurs concurrently with anemia, hemoglobinemia, and/or hyperbilirubinemia. Causes of hemolytic anemia are divided into immune-mediated (primary or secondary immune-mediated hemolytic anemia (IMHA)) and non-immune etiologies (e.g. zinc intoxication, envenomation, osmotic lysis, RBC metabolic defects, among many others). Once hemoglobinuria is confirmed, further testing is required to determine the underlying cause. A complete blood count with manual differential, examination of red blood cell morphology, and reticulocyte count are essential in the work-up of patients with hemolytic anemia. The saline agglutination test or Coombs test may aid in the differentiation of immune-mediated and non-immune-mediated causes of hemolysis. Further testing might include radiography or other diagnostic imaging, chemistry panel analysis, and serology or PCR for infectious organisms. A more detailed review of hemolytic anemia is presented in Chapter 66.

Myoglobinuria

Myoglobin, an oxygen-carrying protein present in muscle cells, causes a red to brown discoloration when present in the urine. Myoglobinuria occurs when severe muscle damage causes myoglobin to be released from the sarcoplasm of myocytes into circulation. Although there is greater understanding of conditions resulting in myoglobinuria in human medicine, etiologies reported in veterinary species include malignant hyperthermia, heat stroke, blunt trauma or crush injury, drug- and toxin-induced rhabdomyolysis, tetanus, *Babesia canis* and *Neospora caninum* infection, and snake or bee envenomation [6–11].

Seldinger technique is preferable due to the safety of a smaller access needle and improved placement stability from the wire coiled in the renal pelvis. Removal can be performed rapidly under fluoroscopic guidance after releasing the suture locking mechanism [19].

Complications

Placement of a locking loop nephrostomy tube has been shown to have infrequent complications; however, complications that do arise can be severe. In people, many complications are secondary to the percutaneous site, including pain, hemorrhage or hematoma formation, as well as hematuria, infection, urine leakage, obstruction of the tube, dislodgment, intestinal injury, septicemia, pneumothorax or hemothorax, and, rarely, loss of the kidney [21–24]. As with any surgical procedure, electrolyte and coagulation abnormalities should be addressed prior to placement. Severely uremic patients may have an acquired coagulopathy attributable to platelet dysfunction (see Chapter 70). Patients that require emergency surgical procedures have been shown to benefit from the administration of desmopressin. A recent study involving uremic people having central lines or percutaneous nephrostomy tubes placed showed that desmopressin improved platelet closure time. No patients within this study had significant hemorrhage or required any intervention due to bleeding [25].

There are few studies regarding percutaneous nephrostomy tube placement in veterinary medicine. In a retrospective study of 20 veterinary patients undergoing nephrostomy tube placement, with two feline patients having bilateral nephrostomy tubes placed, for a total of 22 kidneys, the overall rate of major complications was low, with 1/4 dogs and 1/18 cats found to have a major complication, including subcutaneous urine leakage, entrapment of other ureteral implants, dislodgment, or the need for multiple placement attempts [19]. Minor complications were also noted, including hematuria in 14 patients and bacterial infection in six patients [19].

Percutaneous Antegrade Urethral Catheterization

Indications

Urethral catheterization, as previously discussed, is the gold standard of treatment for urethral obstruction or tears due to a variety of disease processes. However, in some animals, a retrograde catheter cannot be passed due to stricture, small patient size, neoplastic obstruction, or urethral tear. Continued attempts at placement may lead to prolonged sedation, progressive urethral irritation and risk of perforation, and increase the risk of decompensation from metabolic derangements.

If a urethral catheter cannot be placed, or rupture has occurred, percutaneous antegrade urethral catheterization (PAUC) should be considered. This technique was first described in 1984 in people, and has since been described in male cats with urethral obstruction [26,27]. Animals are placed under general anesthesia, positioned in lateral recumbency, and a peripheral catheter is inserted percutaneously into the bladder for decompression, sample collection, and facilitation of a contrast cystourethrogram using fluoroscopic guidance. An angled hydrophilic guidewire is fluoroscopically guided percutaneously through the catheter into the bladder and urethra. A urinary catheter is then inserted over the wire for retrograde catheterization (Figure 106.1). Cystostomy tubes may also be indicated in this patient population, but percutaneous antegrade urethral catheterization (PAUC) can often be completed more quickly, therefore decreasing the length of general anesthesia and more rapidly relieving urethral obstruction. It also eliminates the need for a percutaneous cystostomy tube, which can be dislodged and lead to a uroabdomen (see Chapter 103).

Complications

Brief general anesthesia is required for this procedure, which is often indicated in hemodynamically unstable patients. Medical management may be required prior to induction to address severe hyperkalemia and hemodynamic compromise (see Chapter 109). Urine leakage from the cystocentesis site, bleeding, and bladder rupture are possible complications, particularly in patients with abnormal or inflamed bladder tissue from the underlying disease, severe infection, or prolonged obstruction. However, in a recent study, cystocentesis in male cats with urethral obstruction was not associated with urine leakage or rupture [28]. Other side-effects seen in human patients include contrast leakage or extravasation and anaphylactoid or anaphylactic type reactions.

Previous literature has shown high success rates in a small population of cats with feline urethral obstruction [29]. In this study, 7/9 cats were successfully catheterized with this technique. The only complication noted was inability to manipulate and pass a guidewire through the urethra in two patients due to the presence of urethral calculi and stricture. In cases where guidewire passage is not possible, conversion to cystostomy tube placement or exploratory laparotomy may be necessary to relieve the obstruction.

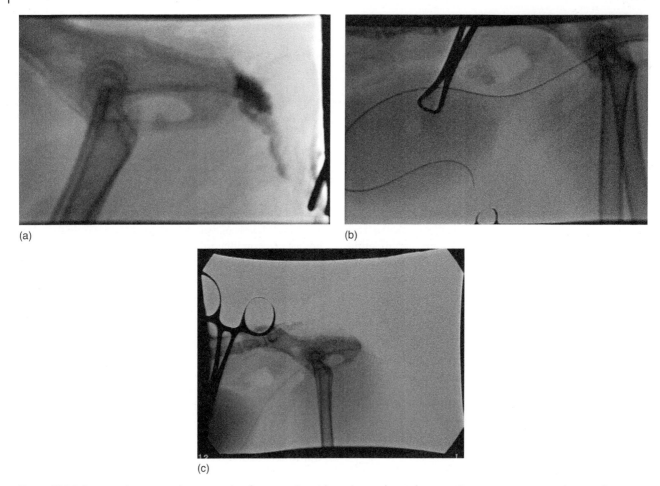

Figure 106.1 Retrograde cystourethrogram using fluoroscopic guidance in a male cat documenting contrast extravasation consistent with a urethral tear (a). Placement of a hydrophilic guidewire into the bladder and urethra via percutaneous bladder catheterization (b). Retrograde placement of a urethral catheter over the wire, bypassing the urethral tear (c).

Cystoscopy and Urethroscopy

Indications

The use of endoscopy for visualization of the urinary system has become widespread as a diagnostic tool in veterinary and human medicine. Both rigid and flexible scopes can be used to rapidly identify urethral obstructions, neoplasia, or trauma. In human patients, this can be performed under local anesthesia, though general anesthesia is required in veterinary patients. Urethroscopy can help facilitate catheterization in difficult cases using over-the-wire techniques and direct visual guidance (Figure 106.2). This may be particularly useful in small female patients, neoplastic obstructions, and those with urethral tears. Other emergent applications include fragmentation of

calculi using laser lithotripsy, ureteral stent placement or removal, assistance for urethral stent placement, and foreign body retrieval.

Complications

For cystoscopic procedures in veterinary patients, the use of general anesthesia is required due to discomfort and need for patient immobility. This may not be practical in critically ill patients. Other possible complications include irritation or trauma (including urethral or bladder perforation), hemorrhage, and lower urinary tract discomfort postoperatively. Use of cystoscopy in patients with urethral trauma can result in fluid extravasation into the surrounding soft tissues due to the pressurized saline ingress used to facilitation distension and visualization.

Figure 106.2 Appearance of the urethral papilla using rigid cystoscopy.

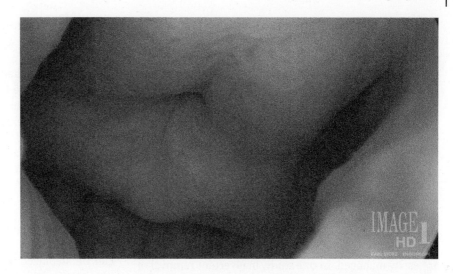

Cystostomy Tubes

Indications

Cystotomy tubes may be used for temporary or permanent purposes in both dogs and cats. Temporary indications include traumatic or iatrogenic rupture of the urinary tract, urolithiasis or other cause of urethral obstruction, and feline lower urinary tract diseases. Cystotomy tubes are often used as part of long-term management in veterinary patients with spinal cord or other neurological disease and secondary bladder dysfunction, postsurgical diversion, and obstructive neoplasia [30]. Historically, general anesthesia and surgical placement of the cystostomy

tube have been performed. With this technique, a celiotomy is carried out followed by cystotomy, tube placement, and cystopexy to the abdominal wall.

There are various types of cystotomy tubes, including Foley catheters, mushroom-tipped catheters, and low-profile gastrostomy tubes. Both a minimally invasive inguinal technique and laparoscopic techniques have been described for permanent cystostomy tube placement with relatively low complication rates [31,32].

In the emergency setting, many patients presenting with urethral obstruction are not stable enough for long periods of general anesthesia and surgery. In these patients, percutaneous cystotomy tubes or suprapubic catheterization can be performed (Figure 106.3). Often

Figure 106.3 Percutaneous locking loop catheter placed in the bladder to act as a cystotomy tube in a dog with a urethral obstruction secondary to a mineralized prostatic mass.

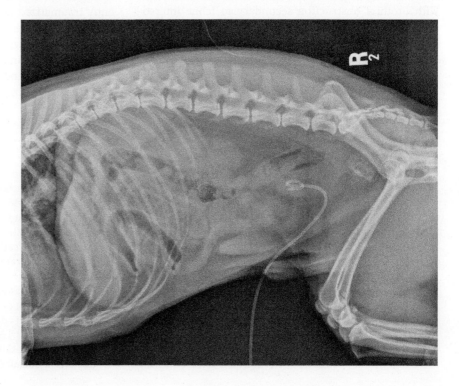

these techniques can be performed under fluoroscopic or ultrasound guidance, although the placement of a suprapubic catheter has been performed bedside without additional imaging in people with few complications using a trocar and Foley catheter method [30]. As with nephrostomy tubes, locking loop or Foley catheters can be placed quickly with injectable and local anesthesia.

Complications

Complication rates for cystotomy tube placement as high as 49% have been reported in this patient population, but rates may be lower with less invasive techniques [31,32]. Despite the high rate of occurrence, most complications are easily managed. In one study, inadvertent removal of the tube or displacement from the bladder was the most common complication, which may be reduced by the use of low-profile gastrostomy tubes. Urinary tract infection is another common complication, with one study showing that 85.7% of patients developed a bacterial infection [30]. Other risks include urine leakage or uroperitoneum, hematuria, patient trauma to the tube, breakage of a portion of the catheter during removal, subcutaneous infection at surgical site, and fistula formation after removal [30,33].

Percutaneous cystotomy tubes have been documented in human patients, with few studies describing their use in veterinary patients [34]. It has been suggested that the use of temporary cystotomy tubes may help to alleviate and prevent further obstruction to the urethra in cats with urethral obstruction secondary to feline interstitial cystitis. However, high rates of complications have been noted in a small study involving cats with urethral obstruction, including migration of the catheter allowing for urine leakage into the peritoneum, and a single incident of omental entrapment [35]. Additional studies are needed to further characterize complications, rates of complications, and potential benefits in this patient population.

Other potential adverse events that may occur during placement include hemorrhage, damage or penetration to other abdominal viscera, or bladder wall rupture, particularly in bladders that may already be diseased.

Peritoneal Drainage

Indications

Locking loop pigtail catheters may also be useful in patients with a uroabdomen. Many uroabdomen patients can be stabilized and effectively managed until definitive intervention with a urethral catheter. However, in patients with uroabdomen secondary to ureteral injury, large bladder defects, or those in which a urethral catheter cannot be placed, peritoneal drainage using a percutaneously placed abdominal locking loop catheter can be quickly placed with sedation and ultrasound guidance.

Complications

The main concern for placement of a locking loop catheter within the peritoneal cavity is injury to other abdominal structures during placement, especially the spleen and intestines, particularly when the sharp trocar supplied with the locking loop catheter system is used. Hemorrhage from the bladder or body wall, or inadvertently traumatized abdominal organs, can result during placement. In the presence of urinary tract infections, urine leakage during catheter placement can lead to intra-abdominal infection. Like other catheters in the urinary tract, ascending infections can result from external catheter contamination.

References

1 Basdani E, Papazoglou LG, Kazakos GM, Bright RM. Spontaneous urethral catheter kinking or knotting in male dogs: four cases. *J Am Anim Hosp Assoc* 2011;47(5):351–355.

2 Hugonnard M, Chalvet-Monfray K, Dernis J, et al. Occurrence of bacteriuria in 18 catheterised cats with obstructive lower urinary tract disease: a pilot study. *J Feline Med Surg* 2013;15(10):843–848.

3 Cooper ES, Lasley E, Daniels J. Incidence of urinary tract infection at presentation and after urinary catheterization in feline urethral obstruction. *J Vet Emerg Crit Care* 2013;23(S1):S13.

4 Segev G, Bankirer T, Steinberg D, et al. Evaluation of urinary catheters coated with sustained-release varnish of chlorhexidine in mitigating biofilm formation on urinary catheters in dogs. *J Vet Intern Med* 2013;27(1):39–46.

5 Bologna RA, Tu LM, Polansky M, Fraimow HD, Gordon DA, Whitmore KE. Hydrogel/silver ion-coated urinary catheter reduces nosocomial urinary tract infection rates in intensive care unit patients: a multicenter study. *Urology* 1999;54(6):982–987.

6 Ogilvie AT, Brisson BA, Singh A, Weese JS. In vitro evaluation of the impact of silver coating on Escherichia coli adherence to urinary catheters. *Can Vet J* 2015;56(5):490–494.

7 Smarick SD, Haskins SC, Aldrich J, et al. Incidence of catheter-associated urinary tract infection among dogs

in a small animal intensive care unit. *J Am Vet Med Assoc* 2004;224(12):1936–1940.

8 Trautner BW, Darouiche RO. Catheter-associated infections: pathogenesis aﬀects prevention. *Arch Intern Med* 2004;164:842–850.

9 Bubenik LJ, Hosgood GL, Waldron DR, Snow LA. Frequency of urinary tract infection in catheterized dogs and comparison of bacterial culture and susceptibility testing results for catheterized and noncatheterized dogs with urinary tract infections. *J Am Vet Med Assoc* 2007;231(6):893–899.

10 Ogeer-Gyles J, Mathews K, Weese JS, Prescott JF, Boerlin P. Evaluation of catheter-associated urinary tract infections and multi-drug-resistant Escherichia coli isolates from the urine of dogs with indwelling urinary catheters. *J Am Vet Med Assoc* 2006;229(10):1584–1590.

11 Hugonnard M, Chalvet-Monfray K, Dernis J, et al. Occurrence of bacteriuria in 18 catheterised cats with obstructive lower urinary tract disease: a pilot study. *J Feline Med Surg* 2013;15(10):843–848.

12 Lees GE, Osborne CA, Stevens JB, Ward GE. Adverse effects of open indwelling urethral catheterization in clinically normal male cats. *Am J Vet Res* 1981;42(5):825–833.

13 Barsanti JA, Shotts EB, Crowell WA, Finco DR, Brown J. Effect of therapy on susceptibility to urinary tract infection in male cats with indwelling urethral catheters. *J Vet Intern Med* 1992;6(2):64–70.

14 Berent A, Weisse C, Bagley D. Ureteral stenting for benign and malignant disease in dogs and cats. *Vet Surg* 2007;36():E1–E29.

15 Berent AC, Weisse C, Beal MW, Brown DC, Todd K, Bagley D. Use of indwelling, double-pigtail stents for treatment of malignant ureteral obstruction in dogs: 12 cases (2006–2009). *J Am Vet Med Assoc* 2011;238(8):1017–1025.

16 Zaid MS, Berent AC, Weisse C, Caceres A. Feline ureteral strictures: 10 cases (2007–2009). *J Vet Intern Med* 2011;25(2):222–229.

17 Snyder DM, Steffey MA, Mehler SJ, Drobatz KJ, Aronson LR. Diagnosis and surgical management of ureteral calculi in dogs: 16 cases (1990–2003). *N Z Vet J* 2005;53(1):19–25.

18 Hardie EM, Kyles AE. Management of ureteral obstruction. *Vet Clin North Am Small Anim Pract* 2004;34():989–1010.

19 Berent AC, Weisse CW, Todd KL, Bagley DH. Use of locking-loop pigtail nephrostomy catheters in dogs and cats: 20 cases (2004–2009). *J Am Vet Med Assoc* 2012;241(3):348–357.

20 Abdin T, Zamir G, Pikarsky A, Katz R, Landau EH, Gofrit ON. Cutaneous tube ureterostomy: a fast and effective method of urinary diversion in emergency situations. *Res Rep Urol* 2015;7():101–105.

21 Chen EH, Nemeth A. Complications of percutaneous procedures. *Am J Emerg Med* 2011;29(7):802–810.

22 Wah TM, Weston MJ, Irving HC. Percutaneous nephrostomy insertion. *Clin Radiol* 2004;59:255–261.

23 Stanley P, Diament MJ. Pediatric percutaneous nephrostomy: experience with 50 patients. *J Urol* 1986;135(6):1223–1226.

24 Barnacle AM, Wilkinson AG, Roebuck DJ. Paediatric interventional uroradiology. *Cardiovasc Intervent Radiol* 2011;34(2):227–240.

25 Kim JH, Baek CH, Min JY, Kim JS, Kim SB, Kim H. Desmopressin improves platelet function in uremic patients taking antiplatelet agents who require emergent invasive procedures. *Ann Hematol* 2015;94(9):1457–1461.

26 Lee WJ, Greenbaum R, Susi R, Khashu B, Smith AD. Percutaneous antegrade urethral catheterization of the traumatized urethra. *Radiology* 1984;151(1):250.

27 Holmes ES, Weisse C, Berent AC. Use of fluoroscopically guided percutaneous antegrade urethral catheterization for the treatment of urethral obstruction in male cats: 9 cases (2000–2009). *J Am Vet Med Assoc* 2012;241(5):603–607.

28 Hall J, Hall K, Powell LL, Lulich J. Outcome of male cats managed for urethral obstruction with decompressive cystocentesis and urinary catheterization: 47 cats (2009–2012). *J Vet Emerg Crit Care* 2015;25(2):256–262.

29 Grasso M, Beaghler M, Bagley DH, Strup S. Actively deflectable, flexible cystoscopes: no longer solely a diagnostic instrument. *J Endourol* 1993;7(6):527–530.

30 Beck AL, Grierson JM, Ogden DM, Hamilton MH, Lipscomb VJ. Outcome of and complications associated with tube cystostomy in dogs and cats: 76 cases (1995–2006). *J Am Vet Med Assoc* 2007;230(8):1184–1189.

31 Bray JP, Doyle RS, Burton CA. Minimally invasive inguinal approach for tube cystostomy. *Vet Surg* 2009;38(3):411–416.

32 Zhang JT, Wang HB, Shi J, Zhang N, Zhang SX, Fan HG. Laparoscopy for percutaneous tube cystostomy in dogs. *J Am Vet Med Assoc* 2010;236(9):975–977.

33 Stiffler KS, McCrackin Stevenson MA, et al. Clinical use of low-profile cystostomy tubes in four dogs and a cat. *J Am Vet Med Assoc* 2003;223(3):325–329, 309–310.

34 Lee MJ, Papanicolaou N, Nocks BN, Valdez JA, Yoder IC. Fluoroscopically guided percutaneous suprapubic cystostomy for long-term bladder drainage: an alternative to surgical cystostomy. *Radiology* 1993;188(3):787–789.

35 Hunt GB, Culp WT, Epstein S, Jandrey K, Ivanov M, Westropp JL. Complications of Stamey percutaneous loop cystostomy catheters in three cats. *J Feline Med Surg* 2013;15(6):503–506.

G. Acid-base, Electrolyte and Endocrine Disorders

107

Acid–Base Disorders

Kate Hopper, BVSc, PhD, DACVECC

School of Veterinary Medicine, University of California, Davis, CA, USA

Introduction

Acid–base disorders are common in emergency room patients. Identifying and understanding acid–base abnormalities can play a valuable role in diagnosis, evaluation of disease severity, and patient monitoring. There are now affordable blood gas machines that allow acid–base analysis on a very small quantity of blood, making them a very useful tool in the emergency room. This chapter will review the traditional approach to acid-base analysis. There are alternative approaches to acid-base analysis described, such as the Stewart approach and the semi-quantitative approach that may provide added insight into the mechanisms of acid-base abnormalities. These approaches do not lend themselves to rapid, patientside application and require more laboratory values than those obtained from the blood gas machine. As a result, their application in the emergency room patient may be limited.

Sample Considerations

Although there are small differences in acid–base values when arterial, central venous, and peripheral blood samples are compared in healthy research dogs, this agreement is lost in cardiovascularly unstable patients where venous PCO_2 (and hence pH) can vary greatly from arterial values [1–4]. However, there is often value in venous blood gas analysis in unstable patients, but the clinician must realize that elevated $PvCO_2$ values in the shock patient may be a product of poor cardiac output, not hypoventilation. When possible, central venous blood samples are recommended.

Acid–Base Regulation

Changes in hydrogen ion concentration can have important physiological consequences. It can alter the structure and function of proteins and nucleic acids, modify hormone and drug-binding affinities, and impair enzymatic function. By convention, the hydrogen ion concentration is expressed as pH. It is important to note that pH has an inverse relationship with hydrogen ion concentration. The normal range of hydrogen ion concentration in the extracellular fluid of a mammalian system is in the range of 35–45 nmol/L, which corresponds to a pH of 7.35–7.45.

Acid–base balance in the healthy animal is primarily affected by nature of the diet and the acid byproducts of cellular metabolism. Homeostasis is maintained by chemical buffering as well as active responses of the lungs and the kidneys to alter hydrogen ion concentration. Chemical buffering includes reactions with hemoglobin, plasma proteins, phosphate, and bicarbonate. The most important buffer system is the bicarbonate buffer system as shown in the following equation.

$$CO_2 + H_2O \longleftrightarrow H_2CO_3 \longleftrightarrow HCO_3^- + H^+$$

The Henderson–Hasselbalch equation for the bicarbonate buffer system (Table 107.1) illustrates that pH is proportional to the ratio of bicarbonate to PCO_2 (pH ~ $[HCO_3]/PCO_2$). This relationship is the basis of the traditional approach to acid–base balance. In this approach, PCO_2 represents the respiratory component of acid–base balance while bicarbonate represents the metabolic component. From this relationship, it can be appreciated that an acidemia (decrease in pH) may be due to a decrease in bicarbonate concentration, an increase in

Table 107.1 Acid–base equations.

Acid–base	Equation
pH	pH = −Log [H+]
Henderson–Hasselbalch equation	pH = 6.1 + Log [HCO$_3^-$] (0.03 × PCO$_2$)
Anion gap	AG = (Na$^+$ + K$^+$) − (HCO$_3^-$ + Cl$^-$)

Textbook of Small Animal Emergency Medicine, First Edition. Edited by Kenneth J. Drobatz, Kate Hopper, Elizabeth Rozanski and Deborah C. Silverstein.
© 2019 John Wiley & Sons, Inc. Published 2019 by John Wiley & Sons, Inc.
Companion Website: www.wiley.com/go/drobatz/textbook

PCO_2, or both. Alternatively, an alkalemia (increase in pH) may be due to an increase in bicarbonate concentration, a decrease in PCO_2, or both.

Active regulation of acid–base balance involves regulation of PCO_2 by the lungs and changes in bicarbonate handling by the kidneys in response to an abnormality in pH. These changes are known as "compensatory" responses. Compensation will return the pH towards normal, but will not completely normalize it. This is an important distinction when performing acid–base analysis (see below).

Acid–Base Analysis

A stepwise approach can simplify acid–base analysis. All acid–base analyses require comparison of the measured patient values to a reference range for that species and ideally specific to the blood gas machine in use.

Evaluate pH

If the measured pH is less than the normal range, it is categorized as acidemia (increased hydrogen ion concentration), while increases in pH are an alkalemia.

Determine the Primary Disorder

Acid–base balance is divided into the respiratory and metabolic contributions. The respiratory contribution is evaluated by PCO_2 while the metabolic contribution can be assessed by the bicarbonate concentration, total carbon dioxide (TCO_2) or base excess/base deficit. From the relationship described above, it can be appreciated that elevations in PCO_2 will decrease pH, representing a respiratory acidosis. Conversely, a decreased PCO_2 is a respiratory alkalosis.

The parameter used to assess the metabolic contribution to acid–base balance depends on what values are provided by the blood gas machine as well as the choice of the interpreter [5]. Bicarbonate concentration is a value calculated by the blood gas machine and usually not provided by chemistry analyzers. As described by the relationship above, elevations of bicarbonate concentration indicate a metabolic alkalosis while decreases in bicarbonate concentration are a metabolic acidosis. Base excess (or base deficit) is also calculated by the blood gas machine and is defined as the quantity of strong acid (or strong base) that would be needed to add to a liter of oxygenated whole blood in order to return the pH to 7.4 at a temperature of 37 °C and a PCO_2 of 40 mmHg [6]. The terms *base excess* and *base deficit* are essentially interchangeable and for the sake of simplicity, the term *base excess* will be used for the remainder of this chapter.

Bicarbonate concentration is directly altered by changes in PCO_2 whereas base excess provides a measure of the metabolic component, independent of changes in PCO_2. As such, base excess is the parameter of choice when evaluating acid–balance in animals with substantial changes in PCO_2. The algorithm for base excess used in commercial blood gas machines was derived for human patients. In the healthy human, normal base excess is 0 mmol/L (−2 to + 2 mmol/L). The normal range of base excess varies with species (due to variations in diet). Herbivores tend to have a positive value while carnivores normally have a negative base excess, when compared to humans. When interpreting base excess, values more negative than the reference range for that species represent a metabolic acidosis (the animal is missing base), while values more positive than the reference range represent a metabolic alkalosis (gain of base).

Total CO_2 is also a measure of the metabolic component. It is calculated by many blood gas machines and measured by many chemistry analyzers. Total CO_2, as the name suggests, is a measure of the total quantity of CO_2 in the blood. As the vast majority of CO_2 is carried in the blood as bicarbonate, TCO_2 is an estimation of blood bicarbonate concentration and is interpreted in a similar manner. It generally runs 1–2 mmol/L higher than the true bicarbonate concentration.

Once the contribution of the respiratory and metabolic systems has been determined, the system responsible for the abnormality in pH needs to be identified. The nature of the pH abnormality defines the disorder. So if the pH is acidemic, the system with an acidosis (respiratory or metabolic or both) is the cause. See the case example provided at the end of the chapter.

Compensation

The final step in acid–base analysis is to determine if appropriate compensation is present. When there is a single disorder in one system, then the changes in the opposing system should be evaluated to determine whether it is consistent with the degree of compensation expected, given the primary disorder. For example, if the primary disorder is metabolic in origin then it is expected that respiratory compensation will be evident at the time of acid–base analysis. The degree of respiratory compensation for a given change in bicarbonate concentration can be estimated by the values given in Table 107.2 [7]. If the measured value of PCO_2 is not similar to this estimated value, appropriate compensation is not present and the animal has two acid–base disorders (both a metabolic and a respiratory abnormality). When the primary abnormality is respiratory in origin, metabolic compensation is expected but the degree of change in bicarbonate concentration depends on the chronicity of the respiratory abnormality (see Table 107.2). Acute

Table 107.2 Expected compensatory changes to primary acid–base disorders [7].

Primary disorder	Expected compensation
Metabolic acidosis	↓ PCO_2 of 0.7 mmHg per 1 mmol/L decrease in $[HCO_3^-]$ ± 3
Metabolic alkalosis	↑ PCO_2 of 0.7 mmHg per 1 mmol/L increase in $[HCO_3^-]$ ± 3
Respiratory acidosis – acute	↑ $[HCO_3^-]$ of 0.15 mmol/L per 1 mmHg ↑ PCO_2 ± 2
Respiratory acidosis – chronic	↑ $[HCO_3^-]$ of 0.35 mmol/L per 1 mmHg ↑ PCO_2 ± 2
Respiratory alkalosis – acute	↓ $[HCO_3^-]$ of 0.25 mmol/L per 1 mmHg ↓ PCO_2 ± 2
Respiratory alkalosis – chronic	↓ $[HCO_3^-]$ of 0.55 mmol/L per 1 mmHg ↓ PCO_2 ± 2

$[HCO_3^-]$, bicarbonate concentration measured in mmol/L; PCO_2, partial pressure of carbon dioxide measured in mm Hg, ↑ increased; ↓, decreased.

respiratory acid–base disorders will have minimal metabolic compensation evident at the time of analysis.

Acid–base compensation in cats is poorly understood. There are no published guidelines at this time. There is some evidence that metabolic compensation in cats is similar to dogs but there is some suggestion in the literature that cats may not develop respiratory compensation [8–11].

Primary Versus Mixed Disorders

When there is only one acid–base abnormality present (respiratory or metabolic, but not both), and there is appropriate compensation present in the opposing system, it is considered a primary or simple acid–base disorder. When there are abnormalities present in both systems, a mixed disorder is present. If a primary disorder with appropriate compensation is not present, it is a mixed disorder. See the case examples provided at the end of the chapter.

Acid–Base Disorders

Once the acid–base diagnosis is made, the differential diagnoses for the disorder(s) should be considered for the specific patient. This will provide greater understanding of the animal's disease process and may help guide therapy.

Respiratory Alkalosis

Respiratory alkalosis is a product of increased alveolar minute ventilation generated by increased respiratory rate, increased tidal volume or both [12]. Potential causes include respiratory tract disease stimulating hyperventilation or changes to the respiratory center of the brain, altering control of alveolar ventilation. Anxiety, pain, and excitement may drive an increase in alveolar ventilation in some animals. Treatment of respiratory alkalosis is primarily focused on resolution of the underlying disease.

Respiratory Acidosis

Respiratory acidosis can be the result of decreased alveolar minute ventilation, increased CO_2 production or increases in inhaled CO_2[12]. In the cardiovascularly stable animal, venous PCO_2 will be slightly higher than arterial values. In states of shock there can be substantial increases in $PvCO_2$ that do not reflect alveolar ventilation. As a consequence, poor tissue perfusion can be a cause of an apparent respiratory acidosis when evaluating venous blood gases [13]. See Box 107.1 for a list of specific causes of respiratory acidosis.

Box 107.1 Major causes of respiratory acidosis.

Decreased alveolar ventilation
- Respiratory center depression
  - Drugs, e.g. opioids
  - Organic brain disease
- Cervical spinal cord injury or disease
- Disease of the peripheral nerves
- Disease of the neuromuscular junction
  - Generalized myasthenia gravis
  - Polyradiculoneuritis
  - Tick paralysis
  - Botulism
- Upper airway obstruction
- Lower airway obstruction

Increased CO_2 production*
- Fever
- Malignant hyperthermia

Increased inhaled CO_2 concentration
- Rebreathing (anesthesia machine or ventilator) Poor tissue perfusion
- Cause of elevated $PvCO_2$, but not $PaCO_2$

*Increased CO_2 production will only be a cause of respiratory acidosis if the animal is unable to increase alveolar ventilation appropriately (e.g. anesthetized animals).

Elevations in $PaCO_2$ will lower the alveolar PO_2, and hence lower PaO_2. This can cause hypoxemia in animals breathing room air. When severe respiratory acidosis is evident ($PCO_2 > 60\,mmHg$), oxygen therapy should be provided immediately to alleviate hypoxemia. Specific therapy to lower PCO_2 will require treatment of the underlying disease. When respiratory acidosis is severe and there is no rapidly effective therapy for the underlying disease (such as brain injury, cervical spinal cord disease or polyradiculoneuritis), mechanical ventilation is indicated in order to restore adequate alveolar ventilation.

Metabolic Alkalosis

Metabolic alkalosis is far less common than metabolic acidosis in clinical medicine [14]. The two main mechanisms of metabolic alkalosis are gain of base or loss of acid. Base can be gained by renal retention of bicarbonate or by iatrogenic administration of bicarbonate. Renal retention of bicarbonate will occur in response to chronic respiratory acidosis. The most common cause of a metabolic alkalosis in dogs and cats in one study was respiratory disease. The metabolic alkalosis in these cases was likely due to compensation for a respiratory acidosis [14].

If a patient with respiratory acidosis receives therapy to improve the PCO_2, the elevated bicarbonate from compensation will be persistent for some time, as changing renal handling of bicarbonate is a slow process. A metabolic alkalosis from loss of acid can occur from selective loss of gastric fluid or from renal loss of acid. Selective gastric acid loss can occur with pyloric outflow obstructions or proximal duodenal obstructions or with nasogastric tube aspiration. Selective gastric acid loss is usually associated with hypochloremia. Renal acid loss can occur secondary to hypokalemia and decreased effective circulating volume through the stimulation of aldosterone.

Treatment of metabolic alkalosis, like all acid–base disorders, focuses on treatment of the underlying disease. In addition, electrolyte disorders such as hypochloremia and hypokalemia must be addressed and decreases in effective circulating volume treated in order to resolve the metabolic alkalosis. Fluid therapy with 0.9% saline may be a valuable part of the treatment plan.

Metabolic Acidosis

Metabolic acidosis is considered the most common acid–base disorder in emergency room patients and it has been found to have both diagnostic and prognostic relevance [15]. Metabolic acidosis can be the result of gain of acid or loss of bicarbonate. Calculation of the anion gap (AG) may help differentiate between these two mechanisms.

Anion Gap

The AG estimates the quantity of unmeasured anions present (see Table 107.1). The majority of the cations in circulation can be readily quantitated but the total charge quantity of several anions is not easy to determine. The charge of these substances (primarily albumin and phosphorus) is estimated by calculating the AG.

The normal range for the AG will depend somewhat on the laboratory normal values for the parameters in the equation, but is generally in the range of 12–20 mmol/L [16]. In metabolic acidosis, a decreased bicarbonate concentration will need to be balanced by an increase in either chloride concentration or the AG in order to maintain electroneutrality. Diseases associated with a gain of acid will classically cause a decrease in bicarbonate concentration and an increase in AG. There are many possible gained acids that can cause a high AG metabolic acidosis but the four most common causes are diabetic ketoacidosis (DKA), uremia, ethylene glycol intoxication, and lactic acidosis. These can be remembered with the acronym DUEL (Box 107.2). Evaluation of blood glucose and lactate will allow confirmation or dismissal of DKA and lactic acidosis as potential causes. The likelihood of ethylene glycol intoxication can be further assessed with consideration of the patient history and other emergency room tests (see Chapter 131). There are many other less common causes of metabolic acidosis that can be considered if these four more common causes are ruled out.

It is very important to recognize that the AG has limitations and can be normal in some cases of acid gain. Albumin is the major contributor to the normal AG quantity. When there is a gain of acid, the anionic component of that acid accumulates and the result is an increase in AG. If the patient has hypoalbuminemia, the AG quantity will be smaller and the increase in AG associated with the

---

Box 107.2 Common causes of metabolic acidosis.

High anion gap metabolic acidosis (gain of acid)*
D = Diabetic ketoacidosis
U = Uremia
E = Ethylene glycol intoxication
L = Lactic acidosis
Hyperchloremic metabolic acidosis (loss of bicarbonate)
- Diarrhea
- Renal tubular acidosis
- Dilutional acidosis
- Hypoadrenocorticism

*Note – elevation of anion gap may not be evident in all cases of metabolic acidosis due to a gain in acid.

gain of acid may not lead to a value that is out of the reference range [17,18]. When an elevated AG is present, it tends to be a valuable tool in assessment of metabolic acidosis. A normal or decreased AG should not rule out the possibility of a gain in acid.

Treatment of metabolic acidosis due to a gain in acid is focused on resolution of the underlying cause. Bicarbonate therapy is generally considered contraindicated in the treatment of DKA and lactic acidosis [19,20]. Bicarbonate therapy may be beneficial in the management of animals with uremic acidosis (see Chapter 174).

Bicarbonate loss can occur through diarrhea or through inappropriate renal acid–base handling. Abnormal renal acid–base handling can be due to one of several defects collectively known as renal tubular acidosis. These processes of bicarbonate loss are usually associated with a concomitant gain in chloride. These animals are expected to have a normal AG, hyperchloremic metabolic acidosis. Dilutional acidosis is another cause of a normal AG metabolic acidosis and is most commonly seen following large-volume administration of IV fluids, in particular 0.9% sodium chloride [21]. Animals presenting with significant clinical signs due to hypoadrenocorticism frequently have a metabolic acidosis. This can be due to both a lactic acidosis from poor perfusion as well as impaired urine acidification [16]. Bicarbonate therapy is often indicated in the treatment of bicarbonate-losing diseases.

Acid–Base and Prognosis

Acid–base parameters have been found to have good predictive ability in human emergency room patients [22–24]. There is some evidence to support a prognostic value of acid–base abnormalities in veterinary patients, although more studies are needed to define this further in small animal patients [25,26]. Evaluation of lactate concentration in addition to acid–base analysis may provide even more valuable information.

Case Example 1

The following is the venous blood gas result from a dog on presentation to the emergency room for trauma.

Parameter	Patient value	Reference range	Interpretation
pH	7.210	7.351–7.463	Acidemia
PCO_2 mmHg	30	31–43	Respiratory alkalosis
Bicarbonate mmol/L	10	18.8–25.6	Metabolic acidosis
Base excess mmol/L	−12	−4.5 to 0.3	Metabolic acidosis
Sodium mmol/L	148	143–151	Normal
Chloride mmol/L	115	108–115	Normal
Potassium mmol/L	4	3.6–4.8	Normal
Anion gap mmol/L	27	12–20	Elevated

The acid–base disorder is defined by the pH. In this example, the pH tells us the animal has an acidemia. It is clear that the respiratory system cannot be causing this abnormality so the cause of the abnormal pH is the metabolic acidosis. The concurrent respiratory alkalosis could represent compensation. When the calculations in Table 107.2 are used, the PCO_2 value in this patient is consistent with appropriate compensation. So the final acid–base diagnosis is a simple metabolic acidosis. The elevated AG suggests this animal has a gain of acid.

Given the history of trauma, a lactic acidosis is highly likely, and direct measurement of blood lactate concentration would allow confirmation of this diagnosis.

Case Example 2

The following is the venous blood gas result from a dog on presentation to the emergency room for trauma.

Parameter	Patient value	Reference range	Interpretation
pH	7.394	7.351–7.463	Normal pH
PCO_2 mmHg	25	31–43	Respiratory alkalosis
Bicarbonate mmol/L	16	18.8–25.6	Metabolic acidosis
Base excess mmol/L	−8	−4.5 to 0.3	Metabolic acidosis

Similar to Case 1, this patient has both a respiratory alkalosis and a metabolic acidosis. Although it may be tempting to consider this a primary metabolic acidosis with very good respiratory compensation, this would break the rule that compensation will not return the pH to normal. The diagnosis is a mixed disorder with both a respiratory alkalosis and a metabolic acidosis. The animal has two acid–base abnormalities and a list of

rule-outs should be generated for each (see Boxes 107.1 and 107.2).

Case Example 3

The following is the venous blood gas results from a dog on presentation to the emergency room for trauma.

Parameter	Patient value	Reference range	Interpretation
pH	7.059	7.351–7.463	Acidemia
PCO_2 mmHg	41	31–43	Normal
Bicarbonate mmol/L	11	18.8–25.6	Metabolic acidosis
Base excess mmol/L	−17	−4.5 to 0.3	Metabolic acidosis

This case has an acidemia which is clearly due to the metabolic acidosis but there is no respiratory compensation evident. As respiratory compensation occurs soon after the onset of a metabolic acid–base abnormality, the lack of respiratory compensation is always considered abnormal. It is interesting to note that the bicarbonate concentration in this example is similar to that in Case 1, yet the pH in this example is substantially lower. This reflects the

benefits of compensation in protecting the pH from severe abnormalities. The lack of compensation in this example exposes the animal to a severe acid–base disorder. This patient therefore has two abnormalities, metabolic acidosis and a lack of respiratory compensation (something is making the PCO_2 higher than it should be). As this is a venous blood gas, hemodynamic instability is a possible cause for the PCO_2 to be higher than expected.

References

1 Ilkiw JE, Rose RJ, Martin IC. A comparison of simultaneously collected arterial, mixed venous, jugular venous and cephalic venous blood samples in the assessment of blood-gas and acid–base status in the dog. *J Vet Intern Med* 1991;5(5):294–298.
2 Middleton P, Kelly AM, Brown J, Robertson M. Agreement between arterial and central venous values for pH, bicarbonate, base excess, and lactate. *Emerg Med J* 2006;23(8):622–624.
3 Kelly AM, McAlpine R, Kyle E.Venous pH can safely replace arterial pH in the initial evaluation of patients in the emergency department. *Emerg Med J* 2001;18(5):340–342.
4 Theusinger OM, Thyes C, Frascarolo P, et al. Mismatch of arterial and central venous blood gas analysis during haemorrhage. *Eur J Anaesthesiol* 2010;27(10):890–896.
5 Davis MD, Walsh BK, Sittig SE, Restrepo RD. AARC clinical practice guideline: blood gas analysis and hemoximetry: 2013. *Respir Care* 2013;58(10):1694–1703.
6 Siggaard Andersen O. The acid–base status of the blood. *Scand J Clin Lab Invest* 1963;15:1–134.
7 de Morais HSA, DiBartola SP. Ventilatory and metabolic compensation in dogs with acid–base disturbances: *J Vet Emerg Crit Care* 1991;1:39–42.
8 Szlyk PC, Jennings DB. Effects of hypercapnia on variability of normal respiratory behavior in awake cats. *Am J Physiol* 1987;21:R538–R547.
9 Lemieux G, Lemieux C, Duplessis S, Berkofsky J. Metabolic characteristics of cat kidney: failure to adapt to metabolic acidosis. *Am J Physiol* 1990;28:R277–R281.
10 Hampson NB, Jobsis-VanderVliet FF, Piantadosi CA. Skeletal muscle oxygen availability during respiratory acid–base disturbances in cats. *Resp Physiol* 1987;70:143–158.
11 Ching SV, Fettman MJ, Hamar DW, et al. The effect of chronic dietary acidification using ammonium chloride on acid–base and mineral metabolism in the adult cat. *J Nutr* 1989;119:902–915.
12 Lumb AB. *Carbon dioxide In: Nunn's Applied Respiratory Physiology*, 7th edn. Churchill Livingston, Philadelphia, 2010, pp. 159–177.
13 Williams KB, Christmas AB, Heniford BT, Sing RF, Messick J. Arterial vs venous blood gas differences during hemorrhagic shock. *World J Crit Care Med* 2014;3(2):55–60.
14 Ha YS, Hopper K, Epstein SE. Incidence, nature and etiology of metabolic alkalosis in dogs and cats. *J Vet Intern Med* 2013;27:847–853.

15 Rice M, Ismail B, Pillow MT. Approach to metabolic acidosis in the emergency department. *Emerg Med Clin North Am* 2014;32(2):403–420.

16 DiBartola SP. Metabolic acid–base disorders. In: *Fluid, Electrolyte and Acid–Base Disorders in Small Animal Practice*, 4th edn (ed. DiBartola SP). Elsevier Saunders, St Louis, 2012, pp. 253–286.

17 Feldman M, Soni N, Dickson B. Influence of hypoalbuminemia or hyperalbuminemia on the serum anion gap. *J Lab Clin Med* 2005;146:317–320.

18 Corey HE. The anion gap (AG): studies in the nephrotic syndrome and diabetic ketoacidosis (DKA). *J Lab Clin Med* 2006;147:121–125.

19 Cooper DJ, Walley KR, Wiggs BR, Russell JA. Bicarbonate does not improve hemodynamics in critically ill patients who have lactic acidosis. A prospective, controlled clinical study. *Ann Intern Med* 1990;112:492–498.

20 Chua HR, Schneider A, Bellomo R. Bicarbonate in diabetic ketoacidosis – a systematic review. *Ann Intens Care* 2011;1:23–35.

21 Guidet B, Soni N, Della Rocca G. A balanced view of balanced solutions. *Crit Care* 2010;14(5):325.

22 Gustafson ML, Hollosi S, Chumbe JT, et. al. The effect of ethanol on lactate and base deficit as predictors of morbidity and mortality in trauma. *Am J Emerg Med* 2015;33(5):607–613.

23 Hindy-François C, Meyer P, Blanot S, et. al. Admission base deficit as a long-term prognostic factor in severe pediatric trauma patients. *J Trauma* 2009;67(6): 1272–1277.

24 Kaplan LJ, Kellum JA. Initial pH, base deficit, lactate, anion gap, strong ion difference, and strong ion gap predict outcome from major vascular injury. *Crit Care Med* 2004;32(5):1120–1124.

25 Kohen CJ, Hopper K, Kass PH, Epstein SE. Prognostic utility of lactate, base deficit, pH, and anion gap in canine and feline emergency patients. *J Vet Emerg Crit Care* 2018;28:54–61.

26 Conti-Patara A, de Araújo Caldeira J, de Mattos-Junior E, et. al. Changes in tissue perfusion parameters in dogs with severe sepsis/septic shock in response to goal-directed hemodynamic optimization at admission to ICU and the relation to outcome. *J Vet Emerg Crit Care* 2012;22(4):409–418.

108

Sodium and Water Balance

Yu Ueda, DVM, DACVECC and Kate Hopper, BVSc, PhD, DACVECC

School of Veterinary Medicine, University of California, Davis, CA, USA

Introduction

Sodium and water balance are regulated separately in the body. Sodium balance regulates the extracellular fluid (ECF) volume while abnormalities in water balance cause changes in sodium concentration. In clinical medicine, changes in serum sodium concentration are almost always a reflection of abnormal water balance. Total body water (TBW) is distributed between the intracellular (ICF) and ECF compartments.

As water moves freely across cell membranes, the distribution of water between the ICF and ECF compartments depends on the quantity of osmotically active substances in each compartment. ECF osmolality can be determined by Formula 1 shown in Box 108.1 [1–3]. As urea has high membrane permeability, it does not alter the distribution of water between the cells and the extracellular fluid, making it an ineffective osmole. Effective ECF (plasma) osmolality (P_{osm}) (Formula 2 in Box 108.1), also known as "tonicity," is mainly composed of sodium and glucose osmoles and their accompanying anions [2]. Under normal conditions, glucose contributes less than $10\,\mathrm{mOsm/kg}$ and the plasma sodium concentration is the main determinant of the effective P_{osm}. Thus, hypernatremia represents hypertonicity although hyponatremia does not always reflect hypotonicity.

The relationship of the serum sodium concentration to water balance is illustrated by the manner in which

---

Box 108.1 Formulae.

Formula 1: Calculated osmolality $(\mathrm{mOsm/kg}) = 2\,[\mathrm{Na^+}] + \dfrac{[\mathrm{Glucose}]}{18} + \dfrac{[\mathrm{BUN}]}{2.8}$

Formula 2: Calculated effective P_{osm} (Tonicity) $(\mathrm{mOsm/kg}) = 2\,[\mathrm{Na^+}] + \dfrac{[\mathrm{Glucose}]}{18}$

Formula 3: Osmol gap $(\mathrm{mOsm/kg}) = $ measured $P_{osm} - $ calculated P_{osm}

Formula 4: Na deficit $(\mathrm{mEq}) = 0.6 \times \mathrm{BW}\ (\mathrm{kg}) \times ([\mathrm{Na^+}]\ \text{normal} - [\mathrm{Na^+}]\ \text{patient})$

Formula 5: Change $[\mathrm{Na^+}]/1\mathrm{L}$ infusate $(\mathrm{mEq}) = \left(\dfrac{[\mathrm{Na^+}]\ \text{infusate} + [\mathrm{K^+}]\ \text{infusate} - [\mathrm{Na^+}]\ \text{patient}}{0.6 \times \mathrm{BW}\ (\mathrm{kg}) + 1} \right)$

Formula 6: Electrolyte-free water clearance $(\mathrm{mL}) = V_{urine}\ (\mathrm{mL}) \times \left(1 - \left[\dfrac{[\mathrm{Na^+}]\ \text{urine} + [\mathrm{K^+}]\ \text{urine}}{[\mathrm{Na^+}]\ \text{serum}} \right] \right)$

Formula 7: Water deficit $(\mathrm{L}) = 0.6 \times \mathrm{BW}\ (\mathrm{kg}) \times \left[\left(\dfrac{[\mathrm{Na^+}]\ \text{patient}}{[\mathrm{Na^+}]\ \text{normal}} \right) - 1 \right]$

$[\mathrm{Na^+}]$, $[\mathrm{K^+}]$, mEq/L; [Glucose], mg/dL; [BUN], mg/dL.

[BUN], blood urea nitrogen concentration; BW, body weight; $[\mathrm{K^+}]$, potassium concentration; $[\mathrm{Na^+}]$, sodium concentration; P_{osm}, plasma osmolality; V_{urine}, volume of urine.

Textbook of Small Animal Emergency Medicine, First Edition. Edited by Kenneth J. Drobatz, Kate Hopper, Elizabeth Rozanski and Deborah C. Silverstein.
© 2019 John Wiley & Sons, Inc. Published 2019 by John Wiley & Sons, Inc.
Companion Website: www.wiley.com/go/drobatz/textbook

the serum sodium concentration and effective P_{osm} are normally regulated by alterations in the intake and excretion of water. This regulatory response is mediated by osmoreceptors in the hypothalamus, which sense changes in the effective P_{osm} of as little as 1% [2]. When the effective P_{osm} increases, it increases water intake via thirst and decreases water excretion via the secretion of antidiuretic hormone (ADH) from the posterior pituitary gland. When the effective P_{osm} decreases, it decreases water intake and increases water excretion by excreting dilute urine in the absence of ADH. In addition, there are non-osmotic factors that can influence hypothalamic function and override the effects of osmolality. In particular, effective circulating volume (ECV) depletion is a potent stimulus for ADH release and thirst. As a result, hypovolemic patients may have persistent thirst and ADH secretion, even in the presence of hyponatremia.

The volume status also affects the rate of urinary sodium excretion, which is primarily regulated by aldosterone, angiotensin II, and natriuretic peptides [4,5]. It is important to understand the difference between osmoregulation and volume regulation. The effective P_{osm} is determined by the ratio of solutes, primarily sodium, and water, whereas the extracellular volume is determined by the absolute quantity of sodium and water present [2]. Thus, knowledge of the serum sodium concentration gives no predictable information regarding volume status, including interstitial hydration and intravascular volume status.

Hyponatremia

Etiology

Hypotonic Hyponatremia
Hyponatremia is categorized according to the concurrent effective P_{osm}. Hyponatremia with hypotonicity may be further classified based on the volume status of the patient; hypovolemic, normovolemic, or hypervolemic. Patients with hypotonic hyponatremia and hypovolemia have non-osmotic stimulation of ADH (i.e. decreased ECV), resulting in water retention and development of hyponatremia [4,5]. Hypotonic hyponatremia with normovolemia is most commonly due to inappropriate ADH secretion, psychogenic polydypsia or iatrogenic mechanisms. Hypervolemic, hyponatremia with hypotonicity is due to inadequate water excretion as evidenced by a urine osmolality >200 mOsm/kg, or decreased ECV despite increased TBW. Disease mechanisms leading to hypervolemic hyponatremia include kidney failure, nephrotic syndrome, and congestive heart failure. Figure 108.1 provides a list of causes of hyponatremia.

Isotonic Hyponatremia
Hyponatremia with normal effective P_{osm} can be an erroneous finding with severe hyperlipidemia or hyperproteinemia when serum sodium concentration is measured by a flame photometry [6].

Hypertonic Hyponatremia
Hyponatremia with hypertonicity occurs with an elevation of effective P_{osm} due to high plasma glucose or administration of hyperosmolar agents such as mannitol [4]. They retain the water content in the extracellular fluid space by a transcellular osmotic gradient and lower the serum sodium concentration by dilution. The relationship between blood glucose and serum sodium concentration has been found to be non-linear. Below glucose concentrations of 400 mg/dL, sodium concentration falls by approximately 1.6 mEq/L for every 100 mg/dL rise in the serum concentration of glucose [7]. At higher glucose concentrations, it should fall by 2.4 mEq/L for every 100 mg/dL rise in the glucose concentration [8].

Clinical Signs

The clinical signs directly attributable to hypotonic hyponatremia primarily reflect neurological dysfunction due to cerebral edema induced by hypo-osmolality [9–11]. In general, patients may develop nausea, lethargy, obtundation, seizures, and coma with severe acute hyponatremia [12,13]. In comparison, a similar degree of chronic hyponatremia results in a lower degree of cerebral edema and neurological signs. This is due to osmotic adaptation in the brain. The initial adaptation consists of the loss of potassium and sodium, followed by the loss of organic solutes such as myoinositol and amino acids [14,15]. Although less severe, chronic hyponatremia can also cause neurological signs that are likely mediated by the serum sodium concentration rather than by hypotonicity, perhaps reflecting the importance of sodium in neural function [16,17]. Overly rapid elevation of the chronic hyponatremia may also cause neurological signs; this issue will be discussed in the section on treatment. Hyponatremia associated with normal or elevated effective P_{osm} is not believed to have specific clinical signs associated with hyponatremia.

Diagnosis

The history and physical examination can provide important clues to the correct diagnosis. In addition, the initial laboratory evaluation should include measurements of serum concentrations of sodium, potassium, urea, and glucose. If hyponatremia is noted, measurement of P_{osm}, osmol gap, urine sodium concentration, and urine osmolality may help determine the cause of hyponatremia. If

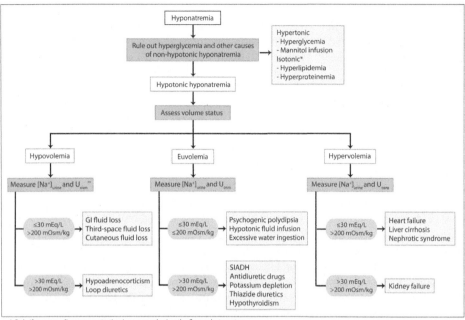

Figure 108.1 Clinical diagnostic approach to the patient with hyponatremia [72–89].

* Only if serum sodium concentration is measured using the flame photometry
** Multiplying the last two digits of the urine specific gravity by 30 - 40 gives a rough estimate of urine osmolality
$[Na^+]_{urine}$, urine sodium concentration; U_{osm}, urine osmolality; GI, gastrointestinal; SIADH, syndrome of inappropriate antidiuretic hormone secretion

the effective P_{osm} (measured P_{osm} − BUN/2.8) is normal or elevated, evaluation for hyperglycemia or existence of unmeasured osmolar agents (e.g. mannitol) should be considered. In addition, determination of the osmol gap (Formula 3 in Box 108.1) may reveal the existence of unmeasured osmolar agents in the plasma [4].

As discussed above, urinary sodium retention and excretion is one of the important regulatory mechanisms of volume status. Hyponatremia associated with decreased ECV or excess water intake should occur in conjunction with a low urine sodium concentration (≤30 mEq/L), while hyponatremia due to water retention is likely to occur in conjunction with a high urine sodium concentration (>30 mEq/L) (see Figure 108.1) [13,18]. An important exception to this may be hypoadrenocorticism and diuretic (e.g., loop diuretics) administration, which can result in decreased ECV without low urine sodium concentration [19]. Measurement of urine osmolality aids in determining the activity of ADH. Appropriate renal water excretion in the face of hyponatremia would be associated with a low urine osmolality (≤200 mOsm/kg). The presence of hyponatremia with urine osmolality >200 mOsm/kg, suggests that ADH is active and causes of appropriate or inappropriate ADH release should be considered.

Treatment

There are two basic principles involved in the treatment of hyponatremia: raising the serum sodium concentration at a safe rate and treating the underlying cause. In patients with hypertonic hyponatremia, the total body sodium content is usually normal and removal of the osmotic substance (usually glucose) from the ECF will resolve the hyponatremia. For hypotonic hyponatremia, the amount of sodium required to raise the serum sodium concentration to a desired value can be estimated from Formula 4 in Box 108.1 [4]. You can also calculate how much volume of a specific sodium-containing fluid is needed to increase the serum sodium to the normal value using Formula 5 [12,20]. However, these formulae are only estimates and serial measurement of the serum sodium concentration is necessary. In addition, these calculations do not include any ongoing losses that may occur, and thus starting with the administration of 1/4–1/3 of the calculated fluid rate using Formula 5 is suggested [21].

In patients with hypovolemic hyponatremia, restoration of euvolemia will remove the stimulus for ADH release and is usually associated with resolution of hyponatremia. In an attempt to reduce the rate of change of serum sodium concentration, use of a crystalloid fluid with a sodium concentration similar to the patient is recommended (within 10 mEq/L of the patient's serum sodium concentration). Alternatively, administering desmopressin acetate (dDAVP) to suppress water excretion into urine can be considered [22].

In patients with asymptomatic chronic (>48 hours) hyponatremia, special attention must be paid to the rate of correction. Acute elevations of the serum sodium concentration may lead to osmotic shrinkage of axons, severing their connections with the surrounding myelin sheaths. This may lead to central pontine and extrapontine demyelinating lesions, called osmotic demyelination syndrome, characterized by various neurological signs that develop within one to several days following a rapid increase in serum sodium concentration [23–28]. Experimental and clinical observations suggest that the degree of correction over the first 24 hours is much more important than the hourly rate. It thus seems advisable to raise the serum sodium concentration in asymptomatic patients by less than 10 mEq/L on the first day and less than 18 mEq/L over the first 48 hours (Box 108.2) [12,13,29,30].

If patients show neurological signs due to either acute (<48 h) or chronic hyponatremia, the risk of untreated hyponatremia is greater than the potential harm of overly rapid correction. If severe clinical signs are evident, 3% hypertonic saline (1–2 mL/kg, can be repeated 2–4 times) should be given over 10–20 minutes to raise the serum sodium concentration by 4–6 mEq/L (see Box 108.2) [13,29–31]. If the signs are mild, 3% hypertonic saline can be given at a rate of 1–3 mL/kg/h (or alternative hypertonic solution) at a correction rate of 0.5–2 mEq/L/h for 2–3 hours or until the neurological signs disappear [13,29,30]. Even with this initial rapid rate of correction, the elevation in the serum sodium concentration should not exceed 10 mEq/L in the first 24 hours [13].

There are a few reports showing that administration of hypotonic solutions or water may abate development of neurological signs when the hyponatremia is corrected more rapidly than recommended, as long as it is administered within 24 hours [32,33]. Correction of potassium depletion, if present, is another important component of therapy [34]. The exogenous potassium will primarily

---

Box 108.2 Treatment summary for hypotonic hyponatremia.

Hyponatremia with clinical signs (both acute and chronic)

- Severe clinical signs: Administer 3% hypertonic saline 1–2 mL/kg (can be repeated 2–4 times) (or alternative hypertonic saline solution at a rate calculated using Formula 5 in Box 108.1) over 10–20 min to increase $[Na]_{serum}$ by 4–6 mEq/L
- Mild clinical signs: Administer 3% hypertonic saline at a rate of 1–3 mL/kg/h (or alternative hypertonic saline solutions) at a correction rate of 0.5–2 mEq/L/h for 2–3 h or until the neurological signs are resolved
- Limit the increase in $[Na]_{serum}$ to a total of 10 mEq/L during the first 24 h and 18 mEq/L for the first 48 h, regardless of whether hyponatremia is acute or chronic
- Start cause-specific treatment and treat underlying causes
- Check the $[Na]_{serum}$ after 20–30 min, 1 h, 2 h, and every 4–8 h until hyponatremia is resolved

Acute (<48 h) hyponatremia without clinical signs

- Correct $[Na]_{serum}$ promptly by using a hypertonic crystalloid solution (no limit on the correction rate)
- Start cause-specific treatment and treat underlying causes
- Check the $[Na]_{serum}$ after 1 h, 2 h, and every 4–8 h until hyponatremia is resolved

Chronic (>48 h) hyponatremia without clinical signs

- Start treatment to increase $[Na]_{serum}$ slowly by <0.5 mEq/L/h
- Limit the increase in $[Na]_{serum}$ to a total of 10 mEq/L during the first 24 h and 18 mEq/L for the first 48 h
- Start cause-specific treatment and treat underlying causes
- Check the $[Na]_{serum}$ after 1 h, 2 h, and every 4–8 h until hyponatremia is resolved

Hyponatremia with hypovolemia

- Restore intravascular volume by administering a crystalloid solution with $[Na]_{serum}$ similar to the patient (≤10 mEq/L difference)
- Follow the treatment protocols described above depending on the presence of clinical signs and chronicity of hyponatremia.
- Check the $[Na]_{serum}$ after 10–20 min, at the end of resuscitation, and every 2–4 h until hemodynamic stability is achieved

$[Na]_{serum}$, serum sodium concentration.

enter the cells, and eletroneutrality will be maintained by shifting the sodium from the intracellular to extracellular space. The net effect is that potassium is as effective as sodium in correcting hyponatremia. Thus, administered potassium must be included when calculating the volume of fluid to be given to increase the serum sodium concentration at a safe rate using Formula 5 in Box 108.1 [12,35].

Therapy of normovolemic or hypervolemic patients with hypotonic hyponatremia is aimed at decreasing water intake and/or increasing water removal by enhancing water excretion using diuretics (e.g., loop diuretics) [13,29]. In these patients, several novel therapies, including a urea or vasopressin receptor antagonist, have been investigated as adjunctive treatment for hyponatremia, but their clinical benefits are controversial or cost prohibitive [36–39]. If clinical signs of hyponatremia develop in patients with normovolemia or hypervolemia, the serum sodium concentration can be raised by the use of a loop diuretic in combination with hypertonic saline [29,30]. No specific treatment is necessary for hyponatremia with normal to high effective P_{osm}. The serum

concentration of sodium should be normalized as the underlying cause is resolved.

Hypernatremia

Etiology

The major causes of hypernatremia are listed in Figure 108.2, and it can also be classified according to the volume status of the patient [5,40]. It must be emphasized here that the majority of patients with these conditions or diseases maintain water balance with a near normal serum sodium concentration because their thirst mechanism is intact.

Hypernatremia develops when animals cannot replace the water loss with water intake for any reason. Insensible fluid losses are usually hypotonic to plasma [40]. Any condition that increases these losses (e.g. fever, respiratory distress) predisposes toward the development of hypernatremia. Gastrointestinal losses, due to osmotic diarrhea (e.g. lactulose, sorbitol administration) can also

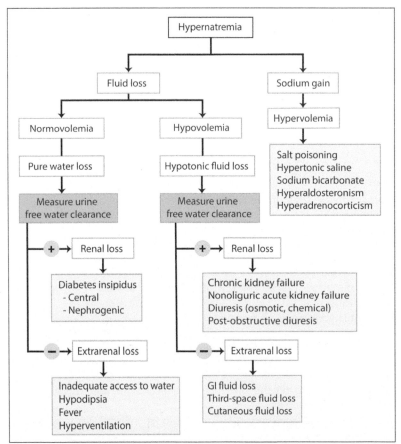

Figure 108.2 Clinical diagnostic approach to the patient with hypernatremia [43,44,90–99].

GI, gastrointestinal

produce a similar effect [41,42]. Diabetes insipidus is characterized by the complete or partial failure of ADH secretion (central diabetes insipidus (CDI)) or loss of the renal response to ADH (nephrogenic diabetes insipidus (NDI)). As a result, renal water reabsorption is inadequate or absent, and a diuresis of dilute urine ensues. Hypernatremia can also result from the ingestion or infusion of sodium salts. This problem can occur in hospital if patients are given hypertonic saline or sodium bicarbonate. There are also case reports of hypernatremia due to ingestion of sodium salts such as homemade play dough [39,43–45].

Clinical Signs

The clinical signs of hypernatremia are primarily neurological. Lethargy and weakness are commonly reported findings, which can progress to tremor, seizure, coma, and death in severe cases [5,40,46,47]. These signs are related to the movement of water out of the brain cells down the osmotic gradient created by the rise in effective P_{osm}. This cerebral dehydration may result in focal intracerebral and subarachnoid hemorrhages [48,49]. It can also result in demyelinating brain lesions similar to those associated with overly rapid correction of chronic hyponatremia [50,51].

Within several hours of the onset of hypernatremia, the brain will begin to adapt to the hyperosmolar state with an increase in brain cell osmolality, resulting in water movement back into the brain and the return of brain volume toward normal. This increase of brain cell osmolality is potentially due to sodium and potassium uptake by brain cells [14]. Intracellular osmolytes also accumulate and increase the osmolality. Because of this osmotic adaptation, patients with chronic hypernatremia may be relatively asymptomatic [52,53]. Although the evidence is less obvious than for hyponatremia, overly rapid correction of chronic hypernatremia can cause cerebral edema and possible neurological deterioration [49,53,54].

Diagnosis

As for hyponatremia, the history and physical examination can provide important information. Initial laboratory tests should include measurements of serum sodium and potassium concentrations. If hypernatremia is noted, measurement of urine osmolality, urine sodium, and urine potassium concentrations may help diagnose the cause of hypernatremia (see Figure 108.2) [40]. Using Formula 6 in Box 108.1, free water clearance into the urine can be calculated. Based on this evaluation, renal water loss can be assessed [5,55].

Treatment

Hypernatremia is considered acute if the rise in serum sodium has a documented onset within the last 48 hours [56]. If this is the case, rapid correction of hypernatremia is indicated by administering 5% dextrose solution at a rate of 3–6 mL/kg/h, or alternative hypotonic solutions (e.g. 0.45% saline) at a rate calculated using Formula 5 or 7 in Box 108.1, at a correction rate of 1–2 mEq/L/h, and complete correction within 24 hours because hypernatremia can lead to irreversible neurological injury (Box 108.3). If patients show clinical signs of acute hypernatremia, the correction rate should be increased by administering 5% dextrose solution at a rate of 7–10 mL/kg/h, or alternative hypotonic solutions, given for a correction rate of up to 2–3 mEq/L/h for the initial 2–3 hours or until the signs are resolved.

In the case of chronic hypernatremia (>48 h), osmotic adaptation has been completed and too rapid correction may result in cerebral edema [53,57]. Although no definitive trials have been performed, the maximum safe rate at which the serum sodium concentration should be lowered in chronic cases is <0.5 mEq/L/h or 10 mEq/L/day for the first 24 hours and 18 mEq/L for the first 48 hours in the absence of clinical signs [49,56]. One study suggests that excessively slow correction (<0.25 mEq/L/h) should also be avoided because of the potential increase in mortality [58].

Most cases of hypernatremia are due to water loss [5]. Gradual correction of this deficit with fluid replacement requires calculation of the water deficit using Formula 7 in Box 108.1 [40,49]. Free water can be given orally or intravenously as 5% dextrose in water. Alternatively, hypotonic solutions such as 0.45% saline can be used. The volume of water available for oral intake must be closely monitored to avoid a rapid, uncontrolled decrease in the animal's sodium concentration. Free water administration does not provide appropriate isotonic replacement of vascular volume deficits or interstitial dehydration [56]. If large-volume fluid resuscitation is needed to treat hypovolemia, it is safest to use a crystalloid with a sodium concentration that is similar to the patient (within 10 mEq/L of the patient's serum sodium concentration) (see Box 108.3). This may necessitate making a specific fluid by the addition of hypertonic saline to a commercially available crystalloid.

The most physiological therapy for treatment of CDI is exogenous ADH. This is typically achieved by the administration of dDAVP (1 drop or 1.5–4 μL in the conjunctival sac OU q8–12h) [59]. Since patients with NDI do not usually have a major response to ADH, dDAVP is ineffective. The major form of therapy for patients with NDI is the treatment of underlying causes. Thiazide diuretics, non-steroidal anti-inflammatory drugs, and a

---

Box 108.3 Treatment summary for hypernatremia.

Acute (<48h) hypernatremia

- Clinical signs present: Administer 5% dextrose solution at a rate of 7–10 mL/kg/h (or alternative hypotonic solutions at a rate calculated using Formula 5 in Box 108.1) at a correction rate of 2–3 mEq/L/h for the initial 2–3 h or until the neurological signs are resolved
- No clinical signs: Administer 5% dextrose solution at a rate of 3–6 mL/kg/h (or alternative hypotonic solutions) at a correction rate of 1–2 mEq/L/h
- Correct hypernatremia within 24 h of initial therapy
- Start cause-specific treatment and treat underlying causes
- Check the $[Na]_{serum}$ after 20–30 min, 1 h, 2 h, and every 4–8 h until hypernatremia is resolved

Chronic (>48h) hypernatremia

- Severe clinical signs present (usually acute on chronic hypernatremia): Administer 5% dextrose solution at a rate of 7–10 mL/kg/h (or alternative hypotonic solutions at a rate calculated using Formula 5 in Box 108.1) at a correction rate of 2–3 mEq/L/h for the initial 2–3 h or until the neurological signs are resolved
- No clinical signs present: start 5% dextrose solution at a rate of 1–1.5 mL/kg/h (or alternative hypotonic solutions) or oral water at a correction rate of 0.5 mEq/L/h
- Limit the decrease in $[Na]_{serum}$ to a total of 10 mEq/L during the first 24 h and 18 mEq/L for the first 48 h, regardless of whether clinical signs are present or absent
- Start cause-specific treatment and treat underlying causes
- Check the $[Na]_{serum}$ after 1 h, 2 h, and every 4–8 h until hypernatremia is resolved

Hypernatremia with hypovolemia

- Restore intravascular volume by administering a crystalloid solution with $[Na]_{serum}$ similar to the patient (≤10 mEq/L difference)
- Follow the treatment protocols described above depending on the presence of clinical signs and chronicity of hypernatremia.
- Check the $[Na]_{serum}$ after 10–20 min, at the end of resuscitation, and every 2–4 h until hemodynamic stability is achieved

$[Na]_{serum}$, serum sodium concentration.

---

low-sodium diet may decrease the severity of water loss due to NDI [40,60,61].

Therapy in patients with sodium overload is best aimed at removing the excess sodium. When renal function is normal, the sodium load will usually be excreted rapidly in the urine. This process can be facilitated by inducing a sodium and water diuresis with loop diuretics and replacing the urine output with fluid that is hypotonic to the urine [5,40]. Intravenous 5% dextrose or hypotonic crystalloid solutions can also be used in patients presenting with marked hypernatremia. However, careful monitoring is necessary, since these patients are volume expanded and the excess fluid may lead to fluid overload and pulmonary congestion or edema in susceptible cases.

Prognosis

Both hyponatremia and hypernatremia are associated with increased mortality in human patients [62–64]. More recent evidence suggests that even mild abnormalities and fluctuations in sodium values are significantly associated with poor outcome [65,66]. In dogs and cats, a retrospective study found the magnitudes of hyponatremia and hypernatremia were linearly associated with a higher mortality rate [67,68]. This was true even with the borderline to mild abnormalities. Some studies in human patients found that abnormal sodium concentration is an independent risk factor for poor prognosis and that early correction may improve outcome [69–71]. Therefore, hyponatremia and hypernatremia should be corrected carefully, but promptly.

References

1 Dugger DT, Mellema MS, Hopper K, Epstein SE. Comparative accuracy of several published formulae for the estimation of serum osmolality in cats. *J Small Anim Pract* 2013;54(4):184–189.

2 Rose B, Post T. Introduction to disorders of osmolality. In: *Clinical Physiology of Acid-Base and Electrolyte Disorders*, 5th edn (eds Wonsciewics M, McCullough K, Davis K). McGraw-Hill, New York, 2001, pp. 682–695.

3 Dugger DT, Epstein SE, Hopper K, Mellema MS. A comparison of the clinical utility of several published formulae for estimated osmolality of canine serum. *J Vet Emerg Crit Care* 2014;24(2):188–193.

4 Rose B, Post T. Hypoosmolal states-hyponatremia. In: *Clinical Physiology of Acid-Base and Electrolyte Disorders*, 5th edn (eds Wonsciewics M, McCullough K, Davis K). McGraw-Hill, New York, 2001, pp. 696–733.

5 DiBartola S. Disorders of sodium and water: hypernatremia and hyponatremia. In: *Fluid, Electrolyte, and Acid-Base Disorders in Small Animal Practice*, 4th edn (ed. DiBartola S). Saunders, St Louis, 2012, pp. 47–79.

6 Apple FS, Koch DD, Graves S, Ladenson JH. Relationship between direct-potentiometric and flame-photometric measurement of sodium in blood. *Clin Chem* 1982;28(9):1931–1935.

7 Katz MA. Hyperglycemia-induced hyponatremia – calculation of expected serum sodium depression. *N Engl J Med* 1973;289(16):843–844.

8 Hillier TA, Abbott RD, Barrett EJ. Hyponatremia: evaluating the correction factor for hyperglycemia. *Am J Med* 1999;106(4):399–403.

9 Verbalis JG, Gullans SR. Hyponatremia causes large sustained reductions in brain content of multiple organic osmolytes in rats. *Brain Res* 1991;567(2):274–282.

10 Gullans SR, Verbalis JG. Control of brain volume during hyperosmolar and hypoosmolar conditions. *Annu Rev Med* 1993;44:289–301.

11 Arieff AI. Hyponatremia, convulsions, respiratory arrest, and permanent brain damage after elective surgery in healthy women. *N Engl J Med* 1986;314(24):1529–1535.

12 Adrogue HJ, Madias NE. Hyponatremia. *N Engl J Med* 2000;342(21):1581–1589.

13 Spasovski G, Vanholder R, Allolio B, et al. Clinical practice guideline on diagnosis and treatment of hyponatraemia. *Intensive Care Med* 2014;40(3):320–331.

14 Strange K. Regulation of solute and water balance and cell volume in the central nervous system. *J Am Soc Nephrol* 1992;3(1):12–27.

15 Sterns RH, Baer J, Ebersol S, et al. Organic osmolytes in acute hyponatremia. *Am J Physiol* 1993;264(5 Pt 2):F833–F836.

16 Decaux G. Is asymptomatic hyponatremia really asymptomatic? *Am J Med* 2006;119(7 Suppl 1):S79–S82.

17 Renneboog B, Musch W, Vandemergel X, et al. Mild chronic hyponatremia is associated with falls, unsteadiness, and attention deficits. *Am J Med* 2006;119(1):71 e1–8.

18 Chung HM, Kluge R, Schrier RW, Anderson RJ. Clinical assessment of extracellular fluid volume in hyponatremia. *Am J Med* 1987;83(5):905–908.

19 Lennon EM, Hummel JB, Vaden SL. Urine sodium concentrations are predictive of hypoadrenocorticism in hyponatraemic dogs: a retrospective pilot study. *J Small Anim Pract* 2018;59(4):228–231.

20 Liamis G, Kalogirou M, Saugos V, et al. Therapeutic approach in patients with dysnatraemias. *Nephrol Dial Transplant* 2006;21(6):1564–1569.

21 Lindner G, Schwarz C, Kneidinger N, et al. Can we really predict the change in serum sodium levels? An analysis of currently proposed formulae in hypernatraemic patients. *Nephrol Dial Transplant* 2008;23(11):3501–3508.

22 MacMillan TE, Tang T, Cavalcanti RB et al. Desmopressin to Prevent Rapid Sodium Correction in Severe Hyponatremia: A Systemic Review. *Am J Med* 2015;128(12):1362.e15–24.

23 Karp BI, Laureno R. Pontine and extrapontine myelinolysis: a neurologic disorder following rapid correction of hyponatremia. *Medicine* 1993;72(6):359–373.

24 Laureno R, Karp BI. Myelinolysis after correction of hyponatremia. *Ann Intern Med* 1997;126(1):57–62.

25 O'Brien DP, Kroll RA, Johnson GC, et al. Myelinolysis after correction of hyponatremia in two dogs. *J Vet Intern Med* 1994;8(1):40–48.

26 MacMillan KL. Neurologic complications following treatment of canine hypoadrenocorticism. *Can Vet J* 2003;44(6):490–492.

27 Churcher RK, Watson AD, Eaton A. Suspected myelinolysis following rapid correction of hyponatremia in a dog. *J Am Anim Hosp Assoc* 1999;35(6):493–497.

28 Brady CA, Vite CH, Drobatz KJ. Severe neurologic sequelae in a dog after treatment of hypoadrenal crisis. *J Am Vet Med Assoc* 1999;215(2):222–225, 210.

29 Verbalis JG, Goldsmith SR, Greenberg A, et al. Diagnosis, evaluation, and treatment of hyponatremia: expert panel recommendations. *Am J Med* 2013;126(10 Suppl 1):S1–42.

30 Sterns RH, Hix JK, Silver S. Treatment of hyponatremia. *Curr Opin Nephrol Hypertens* 2010;19(5):493–498.

31 Hew-Butler T, Rosner MH, Fowkes-Godek S, et al. Statement of the Third International Exercise-Associated Hyponatremia Consensus Development Conference, Carlsbad, California, 2015. *Clin J Sport Med* 2015;25(4):303–320.

32 Gankam Kengne F, Soupart A, Pochet R, et al. Re-induction of hyponatremia after rapid overcorrection of hyponatremia reduces mortality in rats. *Kidney Int* 2009;76(6):614–621.

33 Perianayagam A, Sterns RH, Silver SM, et al. DDAVP is effective in preventing and reversing inadvertent overcorrection of hyponatremia. *Clin J Am Soc Nephrol* 2008;3(2):331–336.

34 Berl T, Rastegar A. A patient with severe hyponatremia and hypokalemia: osmotic demyelination following potassium repletion. *Am J Kidney Dis* 2010;55(4):742–748.

35 Sterns RH, Hix JK, Silver S. Treating profound hyponatremia: a strategy for controlled correction. *Am J Kidney Dis* 2010;56(4):774–779.

36 Ellison DH, Berl T. Clinical practice. *The syndrome of inappropriate antidiuresis. N Engl J Med* 2007;356(20):2064–2072.

37 Schrier RW, Gross P, Gheorghiade M, et al. Tolvaptan, a selective oral vasopressin V2-receptor antagonist, for hyponatremia. *N Engl J Med* 2006;355(20):2099–2112.

38 Decaux G, Andres C, Gankam Kengne F, et al. Treatment of euvolemic hyponatremia in the intensive care unit by urea. *Crit Care* 2010;14(5):R184.

39 Friedman B, Cirulli J. Hyponatremia in critical care patients: frequency, outcome, characteristics, and treatment with the vasopressin V2-receptor antagonist tolvaptan. *J Crit Care* 2013;28(2):219 e211–e212.

40 Rose B, Post T. Hyperosmolal states - hypernatremia. In: *Clinical Physiology of Acid-Base and Electrolyte Disorders*, 5th edn (eds Wonsciewics M, McCullough K, Davis K). McGraw-Hill, New York, 2001, pp. 746–793.

41 Donaldson C. Paintball toxicosis in dogs. *Vet Med* 2003;995–997.

42 Nelson DC, McGrew WR Jr, Hoyumpa AM Jr. Hypernatremia and lactulose therapy. *J Am Med Assoc* 1983;249(10):1295–1298.

43 Barr J, Khan S, McCullough S, et al. Hypernatremia secondary to homemade play dough ingestion in dogs: a review of 14 cases from 1998 to 2001. *J Vet Emerg Crit Care* 2004;14(3):196–202.

44 Khanna C, Boermans HJ, Wilcock B. Fatal hypernatremia in a dog from salt ingestion. *J Am Anim Hosp Assoc* 1997;33(2):113–117.

45 Pouzot C, Descone-Junot C, Loup J, et al. Successful treatment of severe salt intoxicaiton in a dog. *J Vet Emerg Crit Care* 2007;17(3):294–298.

46 Sterns RH. Disorders of plasma sodium - causes, consequences, and correction. *N Engl J Med* 2015;372(1):55–65.

47 McManus ML, Churchwell KB, Strange K. Regulation of cell volume in health and disease. *N Engl J Med* 1995;333(19):1260–1266.

48 Arieff AI, Guisado R. Effects on the central nervous system of hypernatremic and hyponatremic states. *Kidney Int* 1976;10(1):104–116.

49 Adrogue HJ, Madias NE. Hypernatremia. *N Engl J Med* 2000;342(20):1493–1499.

50 Soupart A, Penninckx R, Namias B, et al. Brain myelinolysis following hypernatremia in rats. *J Neuropathol Exp Neurol* 1996;55(1):106–113.

51 Brown WD, Caruso JM. Extrapontine myelinolysis with involvement of the hippocampus in three children with severe hypernatremia. *J Child Neurol* 1999;14(7):428–433.

52 Heilig CW, Stromski ME, Blumenfeld JD, et al. Characterization of the major brain osmolytes that accumulate in salt-loaded rats. *Am J Physiol* 1989;257(6 Pt 2):F1108–F1116.

53 Lien YH, Shapiro JI, Chan L. Effects of hypernatremia on organic brain osmoles. *J Clin Invest* 1990;85(5):1427–1435.

54 Fang C, Mao J, Dai Y, et al. Fluid management of hypernatraemic dehydration to prevent cerebral oedema: a retrospective case control study of 97 children in China. *J Paediatr Child Health* 2010;46(6):301–303.

55 Bodonyi-Kovacs G, Lecker SH. Electrolyte-free water clearance: a key to the diagnosis of hypernatremia in resolving acute renal failure. *Clin Exp Nephrol* 2008;12(1):74–78.

56 Lindner G, Funk GC. Hypernatremia in critically ill patients. *J Crit Care* 2013;28(2):216 e11–e20.

57 Pollock AS, Arieff AI. Abnormalities of cell volume regulation and their functional consequences. *Am J Physiol* 1980;239(3):F195–F205.

58 Alshayeb HM, Showkat A, Babar F, et al. Severe hypernatremia correction rate and mortality in hospitalized patients. *Am J Med Sci* 2011;341(5):356–360.

59 Rijnberk A. Diabetes insipidus. In: *Textbook of Veterinary Internal Medicine*, 7th edn (eds Ettinger S, Feldman E). Saunders, Philadelphia, 2010.

60 Libber S, Harrison H, Spector D. Treatment of nephrogenic diabetes insipidus with prostaglandin synthesis inhibitors. *J Pediatr* 1986;108(2):305–311.

61 Wesche D, Deen PM, Knoers NV. Congenital nephrogenic diabetes insipidus: the current state of affairs. *Pediatr Nephrol* 2012;27(12):2183–2204.

62 Funk GC, Lindner G, Druml W, et al. Incidence and prognosis of dysnatremias present on ICU admission. *Intensive Care Med* 2010;36(2):304–311.

63 Vandergheynst F, Sakr Y, Felleiter P, et al. Incidence and prognosis of dysnatraemia in critically ill patients: analysis of a large prevalence study. *Eur J Clin Invest* 2013;43(9):933–948.

64 Whelan B, Bennett K, O'Riordan D, et al. Serum sodium as a risk factor for in-hospital mortality in acute unselected general medical patients. *QJM* 2009;102(3):175–182.

65 Darmon M, Diconne E, Souweine B, et al. Prognostic consequences of borderline dysnatremia: pay attention to minimal serum sodium change. *Crit Care* 2013;17(1):R12.

66 Sakr Y, Rother S, Ferreira AM, et al. Fluctuations in serum sodium level are associated with an increased risk of death in surgical ICU patients. *Crit Care Med* 2013;41(1):133–142.

67 Ueda Y, Hopper K, Epstein SE. Incidence, severity and prognosis associated with hyponatremia in dogs and cats. *J Vet Intern Med* 2015;29(3):801–807.

68 Ueda Y, Hopper K, Epstein SE. Incidence, severity and prognosis associated with hypernatremia in dogs and cats. *J Vet Intern Med* 2015;29(3):794–800.

69 Lindner G, Funk GC, Schwarz C, et al. Hypernatremia in the critically ill is an independent risk factor for mortality. *Am J Kidney Dis* 2007;50(6):952–957.

70 Tzoulis P, Bagkeris E, Bouloux PM. A case-control study of hyponatraemia as an independent risk factor for inpatient mortality. *Clin Endocrinol (Oxf)* 2014;81(3):401–407.

71 Darmon M, Pichon M, Schwebel C, et al. Influence of early dysnatremia correction on survival of critically ill patients. *Shock* 2014;41(5):394–399.

72 Boag AK, Coe RJ, Martinez TA, et al. Acid-base and electrolyte abnormalities in dogs with gastrointestinal foreign bodies. *J Vet Intern Med* 2005;19(6):816–821.

73 Willard MD, Fossum TW, Torrance A, et al. Hyponatremia and hyperkalemia associated with idiopathic or experimentally induced chylothorax in four dogs. *J Am Vet Med Assoc* 1991;199(3):353–358.

74 Bissett SA, Lamb M, Ward CR. Hyponatremia and hyperkalemia associated with peritoneal effusion in four cats. *J Am Vet Med Assoc* 2001;218(10):1590–1592, 1580.

75 Feldman EC, Nelson RW. Water metabolism and diabetes insipidus. In: *Canine and Feline Endocrinology and Reproduction*, 3rd edn (eds Feldman EC, Nelson RW). Saunders, St Louis, 2004, pp. 2–44.

76 Rijnberk A, Biewenga WJ, Mol JA. Inappropriate vasopressin secretion in two dogs. *Acta Endocrinol* 1988;117(1):59–64.

77 Breitschwerdt EB, Root CR. Inappropriate secretion of antidiuretic hormone in a dog. *J Am Vet Med Assoc* 1979;175(2):181–186.

78 Kang MH, Park HM. Syndrome of inappropriate antidiuretic hormone secretion concurrent with liver disease in a dog. *J Vet Med Sci* 2012;74(5):645–649.

79 Shiel RE, Pinilla M, Mooney CT. Syndrome of inappropriate antidiuretic hormone secretion associated with congenital hydrocephalus in a dog. *J Am Anim Hosp Assoc* 2009;45(5):249–252.

80 Cameron K, Gallagher A. Syndrome of inappropriate antidiuretic hormone secretion in a cat. *J Am Anim Hosp Assoc* 2010;46(6):425–432.

81 DeMonaco SM, Koch MW, Southard TL. Syndrome of inappropriate antidiuretic hormone secretion in a cat with a putative Rathke's cleft cyst. *J Feline Med Surg* 2014;16(12):1010–1015.

82 Chastain C, Graham C, Riley M. Myxedema coma in two dogs. *Canine Pract* 1982;9:20–34.

83 Kelly M, Hill J. Canine myxedema stupor and coma. *Compend Contin Educ Pract Vet* 1984;6:1049.

84 Lee JY, Rozanski E, Anastasio M, et al. Iatrogenic water intoxication in two cats. *J Vet Emerg Crit Care* 2013;23(1):53–57.

85 Toll J, Barr S, Hickford F. Acute water intoxication in a dog. *J Vet Emerg Crit Care* 1999;9(1):19–25.

86 Brady CA. Association of hyponatremia and hyperglycemia with outcome in dogs with congestive heart failure. *J Vet Emerg Crit Care* 2004;14(3):177–182.

87 Goutal CM, Keir I, Kenney S, et al. Evaluation of acute congestive heart failure in dogs and cats: 145 cases (2007-2008). *J Vet Emerg Crit Care* 2010;20(3):330–337.

88 Hendricks HJ, de Bruijne JJ, Van den Brom WE. The clinical refractometer: a useful tool for the determination of specific gravity and osmolality of canine urine. Tijdschr Diergeneeskd 1978;103(20):1065–1068.

89 Di Bella A, Maurella C, Witt A et al. Relationship and intra-individual variation between urine-specific gravity and urine osmolarity in healthy cats. Comp Clin Path. 2014;23(3):535–538.

90 Atkins CE, Tyler R, Greenlee P. Clinical, biochemical, acid-base, and electrolyte abnormalities in cats after hypertonic sodium phosphate enema administration. *Am J Vet Res* 1985;46(4):980–988.

91 Sullivan SA, Harmon BG, Purinton PT, et al. Lobar holoprosencephaly in a Miniature Schnauzer with hypodipsic hypernatremia. *J Am Vet Med Assoc* 2003;223(12): 1778, 1783–1787.

92 Crawford MA, Kittleson MD, Fink GD. Hypernatremia and adipsia in a dog. *J Am Vet Med Assoc* 1984;184(7):818–821.

93 Hanselman B, Kruth S, Poma R, et al. Hypernatremia and hyperlipidemia in a dog with central nervous system lymphosarcoma. *J Vet Intern Med* 2006;20(4):1029–1032.

94 Morrison JA, Fales-Williams A. Hypernatremia associated with intracranial B-cell lymphoma in a cat. *Vet Clin Pathol* 2006;35(3):362–365.

95 Edwards DF, Richardson DC, Russell RG. Hypernatremic, hypertonic dehydration in a dog with diabetes insipidus and gastric dilation-volvulus. *J Am Vet Med Assoc* 1983;182(9):973–977.

96 King J, Grant D. Paintball intoxication in a Pug. *J Vet Emerg Crit Care* 2007;17(3):290–293.

97 Ash RA, Harvey AM, Tasker S. Primary hyperaldosteronism in the cat: a series of 13 cases. *J Feline Med Surg* 2005;7(3):173–182.

98 Breitschwerdt EB, Meuten DJ, Greenfield CL, et al. Idiopathic hyperaldosteronism in a dog. *J Am Vet Med Assoc* 1985;187(8):841–845.

99 Ling GV, Stabenfeldt GH, Comer KM, et al. Canine hyperadrenocorticism: pretreatment clinical and laboratory evaluation of 117 cases. *J Am Vet Med Assoc* 1979;174(11):1211–1215.

109

Potassium Disorders

Sabrina N. Hoehne, DMV, DACVECC[1] and Matthew Mellema, DVM, DACVECC[2]

[1]*William R. Pritchard Veterinary Medical Teaching Hospital, University of California, Davis, CA, USA*
[2]*School of Veterinary Medicine, University of California, Davis, CA, USA*

Introduction

Disorders of potassium homeostasis are associated with a wide range of disease types including urological, renal, toxic, and endocrine disorders. As such, altered serum potassium concentrations are considered common in both critically ill hospitalized patients and in those presenting to an emergency room. Moderate to severe hyperkalemia as well as hypokalemia can have immediately life-threatening consequences and ER clinicians must be adept at rapid recognition and correction of dyskalemias. This chapter discusses the most common causes of potassium disorders and how they may be addressed in the emergency room setting.

Potassium Homeostasis

Potassium is the major intracellular cation in mammalian cells and more than 95% of total body potassium is located within cells, predominantly in skeletal muscle cells [1,2]. Normal extracellular potassium concentration is approximately 4 mEq/L, while intracellular concentration is approximately 140 mEq/L and it is important to realize that serum potassium levels do not reflect whole-body potassium content in some settings [1,2].

The potassium concentration gradient between the intracellular and extracellular space is maintained by the active Na^+-K^+-ATPase pump that transports potassium ions into the cell and sodium out of the cell in a 3:2 ratio [3]. Potassium regulation must adapt to both the addition of potassium to the extracellular compartment by oral potassium intake in the diet and parenteral administration in intravenous fluids in hospitalized patients [2].

Two mechanisms are of great importance in maintaining a normal serum potassium concentration: the distribution of potassium between the intra- and extracellular fluid compartment (internal potassium balance), and the renal excretion of excess potassium (external potassium balance) [3]. Abnormalities in serum potassium concentrations can therefore arise from abnormal potassium intake disturbances in internal potassium balance, or abnormal external potassium balance [3].

Hypokalemia

Definition and Etiology

Normal serum potassium values for dogs and cats are expected to range from 3.5 mEq/L to 5.5 mEq/L and hypokalemia is therefore defined as serum potassium concentrations less than 3.5 mEq/L [1,2]. An abnormality in any of the processes of potassium homeostasis outlined above can lead to hypokalemia and the three general causes for hypokalemia are decreased daily potassium intake, disorders of internal potassium balance (increased intracellular shift of potassium), and disorders of external potassium balance (increased renal and, more rarely, gastrointestinal potassium losses) [1,2,4]. Box 109.1 summarizes the most common conditions associated with hypokalemia in veterinary medicine.

Due to renal adaptation and increased renal potassium reabsorption in states of low serum potassium, decreased dietary intake of potassium alone is unlikely to lead to significant hypokalemia [1,4]. Over a period of days, the kidney typically alters excretion to match intake when dietary potassium load is altered. However, an abrupt absence of dietary potassium intake in a patient that typically has a high daily intake could conceivably result in transient hypokalemia during the period when renal adaptation is yet incomplete. However, administration of intravenous fluids with an isotonic crystalloid that does not contain sufficient potassium to meet maintenance potassium needs can lead to iatrogenic hypokalemia, especially in chronically anorexic animals [1]. Potassium absorption in the gastrointestinal tract

Box 109.1 Causes of hypokalemia [1,4–21].

Decreased intake
Decreased oral intake
Intravenous administration of potassium deficient fluids
Clay ingestion (cat litter)

Disorders of internal balance (intracellular movement)
Metabolic alkalosis
Refeeding syndrome
Hypokalemic periodic paralysis
Hypothermia
Rattlesnake envenomation
Insulin excess (endogenous and exogenous)
Beta-adrenergic agonism

Disorders of external balance (renal and gastrointestinal losses)
Gastrointestinal losses
  Vomiting
  Diarrhea
Urinary losses
  Chronic kidney disease (cat > dog)
  Postobstructive diuresis
  Diuretics
  Renal tubular acidosis
  Diabetic ketoacidosis
  Hyperaldosteronism
  Hyperadrenocorticism
  Dialysis

can rarely be impaired by chronic ingestion of clay in humans, and hypokalemia in a cat due to the ingestion of clay cat litter containing bentonite has also been reported [5,6].

An increased flux of potassium into cells can lead to hypokalemia, as observed with metabolic or respiratory alkalosis, refeeding syndrome, periodic hypokalemic paralysis, hypothermia, rattle snake envenomation, or activation of the Na^+-K^+-ATPase pump due to increased endogenous or exogenous insulin, increased endogenous catecholamines, or beta-adrenergic agonist therapy or toxicosis [1,7–12].

Increased gastrointestinal and urinary losses are the most important causes of hypokalemia due to increased potassium loss in small animals [1,2]. An overview of conditions most commonly leading to urinary and gastrointestinal losses of potassium can be found in Box 109.1 [1,4,13].

Symptoms

The severity of symptoms resulting from hypokalemia usually correlates with the degree of hypokalemia and symptoms are generally not seen until potassium

concentrations reach 3.0 mEq/L to 2.5 mEq/L [4]. Hypokalemia can have a major effect on acid–base balance and glucose metabolism, neuromuscular function, cardiovascular, and renal function, and abnormalities induced by hypokalemia can therefore be divided into those four categories [1,2,4].

In dogs, acute potassium depletion leads to metabolic acidosis, which is reversible as soon as potassium is reintroduced to the diet [22]. Similar effects have been shown in cats with chronic potassium depletion [23]. Hyperglycemia is another adverse metabolic effect of total body potassium depletion and is thought to occur secondary to impaired beta-cell insulin release [24].

Hypokalemia can induce skeletal muscle weakness or paralysis, as well as cardiac arrhythmias and conduction disturbances. The mechanisms by which alterations in cell membrane excitability occur are complex but ascribed to the fact that potassium is necessary to maintain a normal resting membrane potential in skeletal and cardiac muscle [1,4,25]. Clinically, pelvic limb weakness can be observed in hypokalemic dogs and cats [1]. In cats specifically, hypokalemic myopathy frequently manifests as ventroflexion of the neck and head and occurs most commonly with chronically decreased dietary potassium intake and increased urinary potassium excretion [26,27]. Feline hyperaldosteronism has also been recognized as a cause of marked hypokalemia and associated muscle weakness [13,28]. In severe cases, respiratory muscle fatigue can require ventilatory support until hypokalemia and associated polymyopathy have resolved [29].

A variety of electrocardiographic (ECG) changes and cardiac arrhythmias have been observed in hypokalemic dogs and cats. The mechanisms by which arrhythmias develop is incompletely understood, but might be similar to the enhanced automaticity described in skeletal muscle of dogs with severe hypokalemia [4,25]. Hypokalemia also delays ventricular repolarization, prolonging the ventricular refractory period and predisposing the heart to re-entry arrhythmias [1,4]. Arrhythmias and ECG changes in hypokalemic dogs are less predictable than in dogs with hyperkalemia but can include atrial and ventricular tachyarrhythmias, ST segment depression, decreased amplitude of T-waves, prolongation of the QT interval, and the appearance of U-waves [1,30,31]. Increased P-wave amplitude and prolongation of the QRS complex have also been described [4]. Hypokalemia leaves the myocardium refractory to the effects of class I antiarrhythmic agents (e.g. lidocaine) and serum potassium concentrations should be corrected in patients with ventricular arrhythmias non responsive to therapy [1].

Potassium depletion can interfere with several renal functions. Polyuria and polydipsia along with decreased urinary concentration ability have been described in hypokalemic patients, which are thought to be due to decreased renal ADH responsiveness in states of potassium depletion [1,4].

Treatment

The main goal in managing patients with hypokalemia is to correct the primary disease process and to rapidly decrease the risk of hypokalemia-associated adverse events.

Potassium deficits should be corrected, but immediate correction of the full deficit is not commonly urgent and monitoring of the clinical consequences of potassium depletion (e.g. ECG changes and muscle strength) should guide the rate of initial potassium replacement. Potassium replacement can generally be administered as enteral forms of potassium or parenteral.

Parenterally administration of potassium solutions (e.g. potassium chloride, potassium phosphate) is indicated in patients with moderate (2.5–3.4 mEq/L) to severe (<2.5 mEq/L) hypokalemia [1,2]. The rate of intravenous potassium administration should generally not exceed 0.5 mEq/kg/h of potassium to avoid potential life-threatening effects of iatrogenic hyperkalemia [1]. In profoundly hypokalemic patients, the rate can cautiously be increased to 1.0–1.5 mEq/kg/h long as close ECG monitoring is available [2]. In human patients, it is recommended that the concentration of potassium in intravenous fluids administered through a peripheral vein should not exceed 60 mEq/L due to the risk of pain associated with administration and peripheral venous sclerosis [4]. It is unknown if these issues are relevant to dogs and cats. Furthermore, administration of infusions containing high potassium concentrations through a central venous line should be performed with caution due to the risk for direct effects on cardiac conduction [4].

Guidelines for potassium supplementation based on degree of hypokalemia are provided in Table 109.1 [32]. Potassium supplementation should be conservative and closely monitored in patients suffering from oligoanuria, hypoaldosteronism, or those in which potassium-sparing diuretics are administered concurrently (e.g. spironolactone), as these conditions can predispose patients to development of hyperkalemia [2]. Patients that present in shock or dehydrated should be resuscitated or rehydrated with isotonic crystalloid fluids prior to the addition of potassium so as not to exceed a rate of 0.5 mEq/kg/h of potassium at the high necessary fluid rates [2].

Only in severely hypokalemic animals should potassium repletion be started at the time of rehydration. This can be achieved by staying within safe margins for potassium supplementation (<0.5 mEq/kg/h) or by an infusion containing potassium supplementation separate from the isotonic crystalloid used for rehydration

Table 109.1 Guidelines for intravenous potassium supplementation in dogs and cats [32].

Serum potassium concentration (mEq/L)	mEq KCL to add to 250 mL fluid	mEq KCL to add to 1 L fluid	Maximal fluid rate (mL/kg/h)
<2.0	20	80	6
2.1 to 2.5	15	60	8
2.6 to 3.0	10	40	12
3.1 to 3.5	7	28	18
3.6 to 5.0	5	20	25

KCL, potassium chloride.

[2]. Similarly, the administration of sodium bicarbonate and insulin to patients in diabetic ketoacidosis should be delayed until rehydration is achieved and serum potassium levels are >3.5 mEq/L, as sudden correction of acidemia and insulin replacement can worsen hypokalemia by enhancing intracellular potassium shifts [2,4]. In a subset of hypokalemic patients, simultaneous correction of magnesium deficits is likely to allow for more rapid and thorough correction of potassium deficit [33].

When supplementing flexible intravenous fluid bags, extreme care must be taken to sufficiently mix the content of the bag to avoid inadvertent administration of fluids containing life-threateningly high potassium concentrations [34]. The clinician must also bear in mind that reduced insulin release in hypokalemic patients can lead to reduced Na^+-K^+-ATPase activity, which in turn leads to elevated intracellular sodium concentrations. As potassium is provided and pump activity increases, sodium export from the cell will increase. Thus, in the initial stages of potassium repletion, parallel increases in serum sodium concentration may be observed.

Oral potassium most commonly is administered in the form of potassium gluconate powder or tablets with food. The recommended dose is 0.5 mEq/kg body weight orally once to twice daily and should be titrated to effect [35]. Oral potassium substitution is limited to patients experiencing mild hypokalemia (serum potassium concentration >3.4 mEq/L) and patients that voluntarily intake food or can be fed by esophageal or gastroenteral feeding tubes.

Hyperkalemia

Definition and Etiology

Hyperkalemia is defined as serum potassium concentrations that exceed 5.5 mEq/L and can be life-threatening at concentrations greater than 7.5 mEq/L [1]. As outlined above, potassium intake occurs orally, by intravenous infusion, or by increased potassium release from intracellular sites. Initially, most excess potassium is taken up and transiently stored intracellularly and then excreted primarily by the kidneys [3]. Therefore, an abnormality in any process of potassium intake or generation, translocation from cells into extracellular fluid, or decreased renal excretion can lead to hyperkalemia [3]. Box 109.2 lists the most common causes of hyperkalemia in veterinary patients. In chronic, persistently hyperkalemic patients, reduced renal excretion is nearly always the underlying mechanism. However, such reductions in potassium clearance can be the result of extrarenal (e.g. hypoaldosteronism, urethral obstruction) or intrinsic renal (e.g. CKD) causes.

Hyperkalemia occurs more commonly due to excessive potassium supplementation in intravenous fluids (by addition of potassium chloride or potassium phosphate) than with increased oral intake. However, the authors have observed severe, yet transient hyperkalemia during oral potassium bromide loading in small animal patients. Patients with impaired renal potassium excretion due to any of the causes listed in Box 109.2 are at an increased risk of hyperkalemia secondary to increased

---

Box 109.2 Causes of hyperkalemia [1,34,36–41,43, 45–75].

Increased intake
Oral
Intravenous potassium-containing fluids
Packed red blood cell transfusions

Disorders of internal balance (extracellular movement)
Metabolic acidosis
Insulin deficiency with ketoacidosis or hyperosmolarity
Tissue catabolism
Reperfusion injury (e.g. aortic thromboembolism)

Pseudohyperkalemia
Thrombocytosis or leukocytosis
In vitro hemolysis in Japanese breed dogs

Disorders of external balance (decreased renal excretion)
Anuric or oliguric renal failure
Ureteral obstruction
Urethral obstruction
Uroabdomen
Decreased effective circulating volume
　Cavitary effusions with drainage
Hypoadrenocorticism
Pseudohypoaldosteronism
　Gastrointestinal disease (trichuriasis)

---

potassium intake [36]. Rapid rates of intravenous fluid administration as well as inadequate mixing when preparing potassium-supplemented intravenous fluid bags can lead to inadvertent potassium overdose and hyperkalemia [34,37]. To avoid adverse effects, administration of intravenous potassium should not exceed 0.5 mEq/kg/h [1].

Increased potassium concentrations in the supernatant of stored human red blood cell products is recognized and can lead to potentially fatal hyperkalemia during blood transfusions. The majority of adult canine and feline erythrocytes lack Na^+-K^+-ATPase pump activity and intracellular potassium concentration is low. Newborn puppies of all breeds still have the Na^+-K^+-ATPase present in their red blood cells (RBC) membranes, as do reticulocytes in adult dogs. The Asian dog breeds retain the transporter in adult RBC membranes even into adulthood. However, since puppies and Asian dog breeds rarely serve as blood donors, it is unlikely that significant potassium accumulation occurs in canine and feline stored blood products. Nonetheless, one case of potential transfusion-related hyperkalemia has been reported in a dog [41,42].

Hyperkalemia occurs frequently in patients with chronic kidney disease and has been described to persist in a subset of dogs even after initiation of feeding of a commercial renal diet [43]. Potassium-reduced diets specifically formulated by a veterinary nutritionist have been shown to be an effective alternative to correct persistent hyperkalemia [43].

Transcellular shift of potassium out of cells is another common cause of hyperkalemia in which the rise in plasma potassium is too rapid to be corrected by increased renal excretion. Metabolic acidosis due to inorganic acid accumulation (uremic acids, respiratory acidosis, hydrogen chloride, or calcium chloride infusions) results in buffering of excess hydrogen ions intracellularly and, in exchange, an extracellular shift of potassium occurs in order to maintain electroneutrality [2,36,44]. Release of potassium from the intracellular space can further occur when the rate of tissue breakdown is increased such as in severe exercise (especially with concurrent hypothyroidism), trauma (rarely; hypokalemia more common), heat stroke, administration of cytotoxic agents or radiation therapy to patients with malignant lymphoma (tumor lysis syndrome), and during spontaneous reperfusion of the limbs or following treatment with thrombolytic agents in cats that suffer from aortic thromboembolism [41,45–53]. Treatment with or accidental ingestion of angiotensin converting enzyme inhibitors, beta-adrenergic blockers (e.g. atenolol, propranolol), or Na^+-K^+-ATPase pump inhibitors such as digitalis can also lead to hyperkalemia [54].

Diabetic ketoacidosis and non-ketotic states of hyperglycemia and hyperosmolarity in patients with insulin deficiency can further lead to shift of potassium in the extracellular space [1]. Hyperkalemia occurs due to a decreased uptake of potassium intracellularly secondary to a decreased Na^+-K^+-ATPase pump activity in the absence of insulin, while hyperosmolar states lead to water shifts out of the cell which raise the intracellular potassium concentration and promote a favorable gradient for passive potassium exit out of the cell [3,36]. Additionally, frictional forces from water leaving the cell to the hyperosmolar extracellular space can result in potassium being carried along ("solvent drag") [36].

It is important to realize that total body potassium stores in states of insulin deficiency are commonly depleted and the extracellular hyperkalemia is a relative hyperkalemia. Correction of concurrent acidemia as well as insulin replacement enables relocation of the potassium to the intracellular space and can lead to severe hypokalemia [2,4].

Pseudohyperkalemia is an artifactual increase in serum potassium in which potassium shifts out of the cells during or after blood sample acquisition [36]. Potassium can be released from several different circulating blood cells (e.g. blood platelets, leukocytes, and erythrocytes) and pseudohyperkalemia is seen most commonly in patients with severe thrombocytosis [55]. Akita dogs and other dogs of Japanese origin have a functional erythrocyte membrane Na^+-K^+-ATPase and therefore high intracellular potassium concentrations and artifactual hyperkalemia can be observed if hemolysis occurs during or following blood sampling [56,57]. Pseudohyperkalemia due to thrombocytosis or leukocytosis can be confirmed by comparison of plasma potassium levels with the initially acquired serum potassium levels [36]. Plasma potassium levels should not be affected by thrombocytosis and leukocytosis as the extracellular fluid gets separated from the cells before coagulation has occurred and intracellular potassium is released. Reducing the time plasma is in contact with red cells in Japanese breed dogs prior to potassium measurement can help reduce the occurrence of pseudyhyperkalemia [57].

Renal potassium excretion is usually so efficient that an increase in potassium intake alone will not cause hyperkalemia in a normal subject [1]. For hyperkalemia to develop, urinary excretion of potassium must be reduced and prerenal (e.g. decreased effective circulating volume), renal (e.g. acute or chronic renal disease, hypoaldosteronism), and postrenal diseases (e.g. ureteral obstruction, urethral obstruction, uroabdomen) are the most common causes for persistent hyperkalemia in companion animals [1,3]. Effective circulating volume depletion such as from excessive fluid losses or third spacing of fluid into a non-circulating body cavity will

lead to reduced distal renal tubular flow and decreased urinary potassium excretion [3]. Urinary potassium excretion can be improved by restoring effective circulating volume, renal perfusion, and urine output. By reducing effective circulating volume, chylothorax, non-chylous pleural effusion, and peritoneal effusion, especially when managed with intermittent drainage, can result in hyperkalemia and hyponatremia [58–63]. In renal failure, adequate potassium excretion is maintained by increased potassium excretion per functioning nephron, which is dependent on aldosterone and enhanced Na^+-K^+-ATPase activity and maintained urine flow rate and, therefore, the ability to excrete potassium decreases once oliguria develops [36].

Most commonly, oliguria and anuria are associated with acute insults to the kidneys leading to tubular damage, but oliguria and subsequent hyperkalemia can also occur with end-stage chronic kidney disease [64–66]. Hyperkalemia has been reported due to decreased potassium excretion in feline and canine uroabdomen, ureteral, and urethral obstruction [67–71].

Hyperkalemia in conjunction with hyponatremia and sodium to potassium ratios of < 27:1 are highly suggestive of hyperkalemia due to hypoaldosteronism (Addison's disease) and hyperkalemia has been reported in the majority of canine and feline patients suffering from hypoaldosteronism [72,73]. Natriuresis, vomiting, and anorexia in hypoaldosteronism patients commonly worsen the ability to excrete sufficient amounts of potassium in the face of inadequate endogenous mineralocorticoids by decreasing effective circulating volume and distal tubular flow rate [1]. Initial therapy aimed at restoring effective circulating volume often can decrease potassium concentrations into the normal range [1]. Treatment with exogenous mineralocorticoids (e.g. desoxycorticosterone) is begun immediately after a presumptive diagnosis of hypoaldosteronism is made, but definitive diagnosis is achieved by measuring resting cortisol levels and adrenocorticotropin hormone (ACTH) stimulation test [1,2].

Pseudohypoaldosteronism with a reduced sodium to potassium ratio of < 27:1 can be found in dogs with gastrointestinal disease, especially patients suffering from trichuriasis, salmonellosis, and perforated duodenal ulcers [74,75].

Symptoms

The clinical manifestations of hyperkalemia are limited to skeletal muscle weakness and abnormal cardiac conduction and reflect the physiological effect of potassium on resting membrane potential as well as cell membrane excitability [1,36]. Skeletal muscle weakness can develop

Table 109.2 Electrocardiographic changes secondary to hyperkalemia [82].

Serum potassium concentration	Electrocardiographic change
>5.5 mEq/L	Peaked, narrow T-wave
>6.5 mEq/L	Prolonged QRS complex and PR interval
	Depressed R-wave amplitude
	Depressed ST segment
>7 mEq/L	Depressed P-wave amplitude
>8.5 mEq/L	Atrial standstill
	Sinoventricular rhythm
>10 mEq/L	Biphasic QRS complex
	Ventricular flutter
	Ventricular fibrillation
	Asystole

in hyperkalemic states, usually when serum potassium concentration exceeds 8.0 mEq/L [1]. Severe hyperkalemia can lead to atrial standstill, bradycardia, and ventricular asystole due to impaired membrane excitability of the cardiac conduction system [36]. Rarely, wide complex tachycardia can be seen in cats with severe hyperkalemia [76]. The electrocardiographic changes caused by hyperkalemia have been studied in experimental dogs and cats and typically follow a similar pattern, but do not always correlate with serum potassium concentrations in the critically ill patient [1,77–80].

One must bear in mind that the manifestation of hyperkalemia at any given serum potassium level will be dependent on other factors as well (e.g. ionized calcium). The progressions of waveform and conduction changes are summarized in Table 109.2.

Treatment

The most appropriate treatment for hyperkalemia is dependent on the degree of hyperkalemia, the timeframe of onset, and the underlying cause.

An ECG should be performed in every patient with moderate to severe hyperkalemia as rapid onset of even moderate hyperkalemia can cause cardiac arrhythmias [1,2]. Animals capable of normal urine potassium excretion (i.e. with normal urine output) and without clinical signs associated with hyperkalemia in the range of 5.5–6.5 mEq/L might not require immediate treatment, but exogenous potassium administration should be discontinued and the cause for the hyperkalemia investigated [1]. Potassium-free (e.g. 0.9% NaCl) or potassium-deficient fluids (e.g. lactated Ringer's) can be administered to patients with normal urinary output to promote diuresis and may be sufficient to decrease serum potassium concentrations to normal ranges.

The goals of treatment of patients suffering from severe hyperkalemia or exhibiting clinical signs associated with hyperkalemia are aimed at restoring the resting membrane potential of cells, normalizing cardiac action potential conduction velocities, and ultimately lowering the serum potassium concentration. Ten percent calcium gluconate antagonizes the effect of hyperkalemia on myocardial resting membrane potential, but will not lower the potassium concentration [1]. Regular insulin with dextrose to prevent hypoglycemia or the sole administration of dextrose solutions to increase endogenous insulin levels, sodium bicarbonate, and beta-adrenergic agonists can all be successfully used to decrease serum potassium concentrations by promoting increased intracellular shifts of potassium [2,81]. A summary of treatments for life-threatening hyperkalemia is provided in Table 109.3.

Table 109.3 Treatment of severe hyperkalemia [1,2,81].

Drug	Dosage	Mechanism of action	Comment
10% Calcium gluconate	0.5–1.5 mL/kg IV over 5–10 min with ECG monitoring	Reduces cardiac excitability by re-establishing the normal gradient between the resting membrane and threshold potentials	Cardioprotective but will not lower serum potassium concentration
Insulin and 50% Dextrose	Regular insulin 0.5 U/kg IV with dextrose 2 g/U of insulin (4 mL of 50% dextrose)	Promotes intracellular shift of potassium through activation of Na^+-K^+-ATPase	
50% Dextrose	0.7–1 g/kg IV over 3–5 min	Same as above	
Sodium bicarbonate	1–2 mEq/kg IV slowly over 15 min	Increases extracellular pH and promotes intracellular shift of potassium in exchange for H^+ ions	
Terbutaline	0.01 mg/kg IV slowly	Promotes intracellular shift of potassium through activation of Na^+-K^+-ATPase	

References

1 DiBartola SP, DeMorais HA. Disorders of potassium: hypokalemia and hyperkalemia. In: *Fluid, Electrolyte, and Acid–Base Disorders in Small Animal Practice*, 4th edn (ed. DiBartola SP). Saunders-Elsevier, St Louis, 2012.

2 Riordan LL, Schaer M. Potassium disorders. In: *Small Animal Critical Care Medicine* (eds Silverstein DC, Hopper K). Elsevier, St Louis, 2015.

3 Rose B, Post T. Potassium homeostasis. In: *Clinical Physiology of Acid–Base and Electrolyte Disorders*, 5th edn (eds Rose B, Post T). McGraw-Hill, New York, 2001.

4 Rose B, Post T. Hypokalemia. In: *Clinical Physiology of Acid–Base and Electrolyte Disorders*, 5th edn (eds Rose B, Post T). New York: McGraw-Hill, 2001.

5 Gonzalez JJ, Owens W, Ungaro PC, Werk EE, Wentz PW. Clay ingestion: a rare cause of hypokalemia. *Ann Intern Med* 1982;97(1):65–66.

6 Hornfeldt CS, Westfall ML. Suspected bentonite toxicosis in a cat from ingestion of clay cat litter. *Vet Hum Toxicol* 1996;38(5):365–366.

7 Adrogué HJ, Madias NE. Changes in plasma potassium concentration during acute acid-base disturbances. *Am J Med* 1981;71(3):456–467.

8 Armitage-Chan EA, O'Toole T, Chan DL. Management of prolonged food deprivation, hypothermia, and refeeding syndrome in a cat. *J Vet Emerg Crit Care* 2006;16(s1):S34–S41.

9 Julius TM, Kaelble MK, Leech EB, et al. Retrospective evaluation of neurotoxic rattlesnake envenomation in dogs and cats: 34 cases (2005–2010): neurotoxic rattlesnake envenomation in dogs and cats. *J Vet Emerg Crit Care* 2012;22(4):460–469.

10 Malik R, Musca FJ, Gunew MN, et al. Periodic hypokalaemic polymyopathy in Burmese and closely related cats: a review including the latest genetic data. *J Feline Med Surg* 2015;17(5):417–426.

11 Matos MJ, Jenni S, Fischer N, Bienz H, Glaus MT. Myokardschädigung und paroxysmale ventrikuläre tachykardie bei einem hund nach albuterolintoxikation. *Schweiz Arch Tierheilkd* 2012;154(7):302–305.

12 McCown JL, Lechner ES, Cooke KL. Suspected albuterol toxicosis in a dog. *J Am Vet Med Assoc* 2008;232(8):1168–1171.

13 Ash RA, Harvey AM, Tasker S. Primary hyperaldosteronism in the cat: a series of 13 cases. *J Feline Med Surg* 2005;7(3):173–182.

14 Boag AK, Coe RJ, Martinez TA, Hughes D. Acid-base and electrolyte abnormalities in dogs with gastrointestinal foreign bodies. *J Vet Intern Med* 2005;19(6):816–821.

15 Bruskiewicz KA, Nelson RW, Feldman EC, Griffey SM. Diabetic ketosis and ketoacidosis in cats: 42 cases (1980–1995). *J Am Vet Med Assoc* 1997;211(2):188–192.

16 Burrows CF, Bovée KC. Characterization and treatment of acid-base and renal defects due to urethral obstruction in cats. *J Am Vet Med Assoc* 1978;172(7):801–805.

17 Cobb M, Michell AR. Plasma electrolyte concentrations in dogs receiving diuretic therapy for cardiac failure. *J Small Anim Pract* 1992;33(11):526–529.

18 Breitschwerdt EB, Meuten DJ, Greenfield CI, et al. Idiopathic hyperaldosteronism in a dog. *J Am Vet Med Assoc* 1985;187(8):841–845.

19 Elliott J, Barber PJ. Feline chronic renal failure: clinical findings in 80 cases diagnosed between 1992 and 1995. *J Small Anim Pract* 1998;39(2):78–85.

20 Rose SA, Kyles AE, Labelle P, et al. Adrenalectomy and caval thrombectomy in a cat with primary hyperaldosteronism. *J Am Anim Hosp Assoc* 2007;43(4):209–214.

21 DiBartola SP, Rutgers HC, Zack PM, Tarr MJ. Clinicopathologic findings associated with chronic renal disease in cats: 74 cases (1973–1984). *J Am Vet Med Assoc* 1987;190(9):1196–1202.

22 Garella S, Chang B, Kahn S. Alterations of hydrogen ion homeostasis in pure potassium depletion: studies in rats and dogs during the recovery phase. *J Lab Clin Med* 1979;93(2):321–331.

23 Dow SW, Fettman MJ, Smith KR, et al. Effects of dietary acidification and potassium depletion on acid-base balance, mineral metabolism and renal function in adult cats. *J Nutr* 1990;120(6):569–578.

24 Rowe JW, Tobin JD, Rosa RM, Andres R. Effect of experimental potassium deficiency on glucose and insulin metabolism. *Metabolism* 1980;29(6):498–502.

25 Bilbrey GL, Herbin L, Carter NW, Knochel JP. Skeletal muscle resting membrane potential in potassium deficiency. *J Clin Invest* 1973;52(12):3011–3018.

26 Dow SW, Fettman MJ, LeCouteur RA, Hamar DW. Potassium depletion in cats: renal and dietary influences. *J Am Vet Med Assoc* 1987;191(12):1569–1575.

27 Dow SW, LeCouteur RA, Fettman MJ, Spurgeon TI. Potassium depletion in cats: hypokalemic polymyopathy. *J Am Vet Med Assoc* 1987;191(12):1563–1568.

28 Shiel R, Mooney C. Diagnosis and management of primary hyperaldosteronism in cats. *In Pract* 2007;29(4):194–201.

29 Hammond TN, Holm JL. Successful use of short-term mechanical ventilation to manage respiratory failure secondary to profound hypokalemia in a cat with hyperaldosteronism. *J Vet Emerg Crit Care* 2008;18(5):517–525.

30 Felkai F. Electrocardiographic signs in ventricular repolarization of experimentally induced hypokalaemia and appearance of the U-wave in dogs. *Acta Vet Hung* 1985;33(3-4):221–228.

31 Hanton G, Yvon A, Provost J-P, Racaud A, Doubovetzky M. Quantitative relationship between plasma potassium levels and QT interval in beagle dogs. *Lab Anim* 2007;41(2):204–217.

32 Greene RW, Scott RC. Lower urinary tract disease. In: *Textbook of Veterinary Internal Medicine* (ed. Ettinger SJ). Saunders, Philadelphia, 1975.

33 Hamill-Ruth RJ, McGory R. Magnesium repletion and its effects on potassium homeostasis in critically ill adults: results of a double-blind, randomized, controlled trial. *Crit Care Med* 1996; 24(1):38–45.

34 Hoehne SN, Hopper K, Epstein SE. Accuracy of potassium supplementation of fluids administered intravenously. *J Vet Intern Med* 2015;29(3):834–839.

35 Papich MG. *Saunders Handbook of Veterinary Drugs: Small and Large Animal.* Elsevier-Saunders, Philadelphia, 2011.

36 Rose B, Post T, editors. Hyperkalemia. In: *Clinical Physiology of Acid–Base and Electrolyte Disorders*, 5th edn (eds Rose B, Post T). McGraw-Hill, New York, 2001.

37 Lankton JW, Siler JN, Neigh JL. Letter: Hyperkalemia after administration of potassium from nonrigid parenteral-fluid containers. *Anesthesiology* 1973;39(6):660–661.

38 Lawson DH. Adverse reactions to potassium chloride. *Q J Med* 1974;43(171):433–440.

39 Shapiro S. Fatal drug reactions among medical inpatients. *J Am Med Assoc* 1971;216(3):467.

40 Williams RH. Potassium overdosage: a potential hazard of non-rigid parenteral fluid containers. *Br Med J* 1973;1(5855):714–715.

41 Nickell JR, Shih A. Anesthesia case of the month: administration of aged packed RBCs. *J Am Vet Med Assoc* 2011;239(11):1429–1431.

42 Obrador R, Musulin S, Hansen B. Red blood cell storage lesion. *J Vet Emerg Crit Care* 2015;25(2):187–199.

43 Segev G, Fascetti AJ, Weeth LP, Cowgill LD. Correction of hyperkalemia in dogs with chronic kidney disease consuming commercial renal therapeutic diets by a potassium-reduced home-prepared diet: hyperkalemia in dogs with CKD. *J Vet Intern Med* 2010;24(3):546–550.

44 Abrams WB. The effect of acidosis and alkalosis on the plasma potassium concentration and the electrocardiogram of normal and potassium depleted dogs. *Am J Med Sci* 1951;222(5):506–515.

45 Borgeat K, Wright J, Garrod O, Payne JR, Fuentes VL. Arterial thromboembolism in 250 cats in general practice: 2004–2012. *J Vet Intern Med* 2014;28(1):102–108.

46 Calia CM, Hohenhaus AE, Fox PR, Meleo KA. Acute tumor lysis syndrome in a cat with lymphoma. *J Vet Intern Med* 1996;10(6):409–411.

47 Henry CJ, Lanevschi A, Marks SI, et al. Acute lymphoblastic leukemia, hypercalcemia, and pseudohyperkalemia in a dog. *J Am Vet Med Assoc* 1996;208(2):237–239.

48 Fuentes VL. Arterial thromboembolism risks, realities and a rational first-line approach. *J Feline Med Surg* 2012;14(7):459–470.

49 Laing EJ, Fitzpatrick PJ, Binnington AG, et al. Half-body radiotherapy in the treatment of canine lymphoma. *J Vet Intern Med* 1989;3(2):102–108.

50 Schaafsma IA, van Emst MG, Kooistra HS, et al. Exercise-induced hyperkalemia in hypothyroid dogs. *Domest Anim Endocrinol* 2002;22(2):113–125.

51 Teichmann S, Turković V, Dörfelt R. Hitzschlag bei hunden in Süddeutschland. *Tierärztl Prax Kleintiere* 2014;42(4):213–222.

52 Welch KM, Rozanski EA, Freeman LM, Rush JE. Prospective evaluation of tissue plasminogen activator in 11 cats with arterial thromboembolism. *J Feline Med Surg* 2010;12(2):122–128.

53 Ookuma T, Miyasho K, Kashitani N, et al. The clinical relevance of plasma potassium abnormalities on admission in trauma patients: a retrospective observational study. *J Intensive Care* 2015;3(1):37.

54 Perazella MA. Drug-induced hyperkalemia: old culprits and new offenders. *Am J Med* 2000;109(4):307–314.

55 Reimann KA, Knowlen GG, Tvedten HW. Factitious hyperkalemia in dogs with thrombocytosis. *J Vet Intern Med* 1989;3(1):47–52.

56 Battison A. Apparent pseudohyperkalemia in a Chinese Shar Pei dog. *Vet Clin Pathol* 2007;36(1):89–93.

57 Degen M. Pseudohyperkalemia in Akitas. *J Am Vet Med Assoc* 1987;190(5):541–543.

58 Bell, R, Mellor, DJ, Ramsey, I, Knottenbelt C. Decreased sodium:potassium ratios in cats: 49 cases. *Vet Clin Pathol* 2005;34(2):110–114.

59 Lamb WA, Muir P. Lymphangiosarcoma associated with hyonatraemia and hyperkalaemia in a dog. *J Small Anim Pract* 1994;35(7):374–376.

60 Willard MD, Fossum TW, Torrance A, Lippert A. Hyponatremia and hyperkalemia associated with idiopathic or experimentally induced chylothorax in four dogs. *J Am Vet Med Assoc* 1991;199(3):353–358.

61 Schaer M, Halling KB, Collins KE, Grant DC. Combined hyponatremia and hyperkalemia mimicking acute hypoadrenocorticism in three pregnant dogs. *J Am Vet Med Assoc* 2001;218(6):897–899.

62 Thompson MD, Carr AP. Hyponatremia and hyperkalemia associated with chylous pleural and peritoneal effusion in a cat. *Can Vet J* 2002;43(8):610–613.

63 Zenger E. Persistent hyperkalemia associated with nonchylous pleural effusion in a dog. *J Am Anim Hosp Assoc* 1992;28:411–413.

64 Polzin DJ. Chronic kidney disease in small animals. *Vet Clin North Am Small Anim Pract* 2011;41(1):15–30.

65 Vaden SL, Levine J, Breitschwerdt EB. A retrospective case-control of acute renal failure in 99 dogs. *J Vet Intern Med* 1997;11(2):58–64.

66 Worwag S, Langston CE. Acute intrinsic renal failure in cats: 32 cases (1997–2004). *J Am Vet Med Assoc* 2008;232(5):728–732.

67 Aumann M, Worth L, Drobatz K. Uroperitoneum in cats: 26 cases (1986–1995). *J Am Anim Hosp Assoc* 1998;34(4):315–324.

68 Berent AC. Ureteral obstructions in dogs and cats: a review of traditional and new interventional diagnostic and therapeutic options. *J Vet Emerg Crit Care* 2011;21(2):86–103.

69 Garcia de Carellan Mateo A, Brodbelt D, Kulendra N, Alibhai H. Retrospective study of the perioperative management and complications of ureteral obstruction in 37 cats. *Vet Anaesth Analg* 2015;42(6):570–579.

70 Gerber B, Boretti FS, Kley S, et al. Evaluation of clinical signs and causes of lower urinary tract disease in European cats. *J Small Anim Pract* 2005;46(12):571–577.

71 Lee JA, Drobatz KJ. Characterization of the clinical characteristics, electrolytes, acid–base, and renal parameters in male cats with urethral obstruction. *J Vet Emerg Crit Care* 2003;13(4):227–233.

72 Peterson ME, Greco DS, Orth DN. Primary hypoadrenocorticism in ten cats. *J Vet Intern Med Am Coll Vet Intern Med* 1989;3(2):55–58.

73 Peterson ME, Kintzer PP, Kass PH. Pretreatment clinical and laboratory findings in dogs with hypoadrenocorticism: 225 cases (1979–1993). *J Am Vet Med Assoc* 1996;208(1):85–91.

74 Malik R, Hunt GB, Hinchliffe JM, Church DB. Severe whipworm infection in the dog. *J Small Anim Pract* 1990;31(4):185–188.

75 DiBartola SP, Johnson SE, Davenport DJ, et al. Clinicopathologic findings resembling hypoadrenocorticism in dogs with primary gastrointestinal disease. *J Am Vet Med Assoc* 1985;187(1):60–63.

76 Norman BC, Côté E, Barrett KA. Wide-complex tachycardia associated with severe hyperkalemia in three cats. *J Feline Med Surg* 2006;8(6):372–378.

77 Cohen HC, Gozo EG, Pick A. The nature and type of arrhythmias in acute experimental hyperkalemia in the intact dog. *Am Heart J* 1971;82(6):777–785.

78 Coulter DB, Duncan RJ, Sander PD. Effects of asphyxia and potassium on canine and feline electrocardiograms. *Can J Comp Med* 1975;39(4):442–449.

79 Surawicz B. Arrhythmias and electrolyte disturbances. *Bull N Y Acad Med* 1967;43(12):1160–1180.

80 Surawicz B. Relationship between electrocardiogram and electrolytes. *Am Heart J* 1967;73(6):814–834.

81 Stafford JR, Bartges JW. A clinical review of pathophysiology, diagnosis, and treatment of uroabdomen in the dog and cat. *J Vet Emerg Crit Care* 2013;23(2):216–229.

82 Tilley LP. *Essentials of Canine and Feline Electrocardiography: Interpretation and Treatment*, 2nd edn. Lea and Febiger, Philadelphia, 1985.

110

Calcium, Magnesium, and Phosphorus Disorders

Matthew Mellema, DVM, DACVECC

School of Veterinary Medicine, University of California, Davis, CA, USA

Introduction

The term *minerals* refers to all forms of inorganic nutrients. However, the most physiologically abundant of these elements (sodium, potassium, chloride) all nearly completely dissociate in water and are thus generally categorized as electrolytes and discussed separately from other minerals.

This chapter focuses on three minerals, calcium, magnesium, and phosphorus, (Ca, Mg, and P), that share several important features including hormonal regulation, renal excretion, abundant divalent forms, predominance of non-exchangeable mass, and extensive protein/macromolecule binding. The importance of mineral disorders in the veterinary emergency room setting is likely to be comparable to what is observed in human medicine (with the exception of alcohol-related disorders). A retrospective study of 1447 human emergency room (ER) patient records revealed the following: 17.6% of these patients had one or more abnormalities in Ca, Mg, and/or P, 0.3% required treatment in the ER, and 5.1% were treated only after hospital admission [1]. The authors also concluded that significant treatments were largely administered to just three main types of patients: diabetics, alcoholics, and patients with renal failure. They further recommended that STAT testing be largely restricted to those patient categories.

In veterinary medicine, ER clinicians are far more likely to encounter acute kidney injury (a largely hospital-acquired condition in humans), urinary tract obstruction, and poorly regulated diabetics than their MD counterparts. From this, one might predict that mineral disorders may, in fact, be slightly more common in a veterinary ER setting than in a human emergency department. This chapter discusses the most common causes of Mg, Ca, and P disorders and how they may be addressed in the emergency room setting.

Phosphorus Homeostasis

Phosphorus is essential to the function of lipid bilayer cell membranes. Mammalian lipid bilayers are constructed of phospholipids such as phosphatidylcholine, phosphatidylserine, phosphatidylethanolamine, and sphingomyelin [2]. The phosphorylation of the lipid glycerol head is essential to the creation of a hydrophilic subregion and to the assembly of oriented bilayers. Phosphorylation is central to the processes of glycolysis and the generation of the high-energy compounds used to redistribute free energy (e.g. ATP, phosphocreatine) in living systems [3,4]. Phosphates play a key role in the activation of clotting factors (V and X) and platelet aggregation [5]. Phosphate moieties are extensively utilized to alter protein function. It has been estimated that up to 30% of all mammalian proteins have at least one phosphorylation site [6]. Phosphate is also a co-factor for many co-enzymes and is essential for the formation of 2-3 diphosphoglycerate (2-3DPG), which is utilized to modify hemoglobin's oxygen affinity within the erythrocytes of some mammals (not cows or cats) [7].

Eighty percent of whole-body phosphorus is complexed in (hydroxy)apatite biomineral in the skeleton, whereas 19–20% is found in the intracellular compartment where it is the most abundant anion. Less than 1% is found in the plasma where it may be bound to organic macromolecules or unbound in its ionic form. At normal physiological pH (i.e. 7.4), 80% of the unbound phosphate will be in its divalent (HPO_4^{2-}) form and the remaining 20% in its univalent ($H_2PO_4^-$) form. Clinical laboratories typically only measure the unbound portion of serum phosphate and thus the main screening test used to assess phosphate in the clinical setting is examining but a fraction of whole-body stores.

Ingested phosphate is taken up by the small bowel via both passive and active transport. Intestinal uptake of both phosphorus and calcium is enhanced by vitamin D [8]. Parathyroid hormone (PTH), vitamin D, and calcitonin regulate the mobilization (or storage) of phosphorus in skeletal biomineral deposits [9]. At the level of the kidney, phosphate excretion is regulated by both PTH and fibroblast growth factor-23 (FGF-23) [10]. FGF-23 is secreted by osteoblasts in response to increases in phosphorus intake. In a negative feedback loop, FGF-23 inhibits the production and stimulates the degradation of 1,25-dihydroxyvitamin D, while promoting a concurrent increase in urinary phosphorus excretion in a manner independent of both PTH and vitamin D [10].

The renal tubular Na-PO4 co-transporter is the predominant site of regulation for phosphate excretion [10]. This co-transporter is inhibited by metabolic acidosis [11]. Elevated serum phosphate or PTH promotes removal of this membrane co-transporter via endocytosis. Conversely, insertion of the transporter into the renal tubular membrane is stimulated by acute reductions in serum phosphate, whereas chronic hypophosphatemia promotes the synthesis of new transporters [11].

Hypophosphatemia

Definition and Etiology

Normal serum phosphate values for dogs and cats are expected to range from approximately 3.0 mg/dL up to 5.0 mg/dL (canine) or 6.0 mg/dL (feline). Assuming a Gaussian distribution of values from both diseased and non-diseased patients, one can assume that there will be overlap between serum phosphate concentrations obtained from these two groups [12]. This author typically views values that lie 15–20% above or below the reference interval to be reliably abnormal (and not due to the nature of reference interval generation). Hypophosphatemia may therefore be broadly defined as serum phosphate concentrations less than 2.5 mg/dL in both dogs and cats. An abnormality in any of the processes of phosphate homeostasis (as outlined above) can lead to hypophosphatemia. The three general causes for hypophosphatemia are internal redistribution/transcellular shifts, decreased intake or absorption, and increased urinary excretion [12–16]. Box 110.1 summarizes the most common conditions associated with hypophosphatemia in small animal practice.

Significant redistribution/intracellular shifts of phosphate are a common cause of hypophosphatemia. Respiratory alkalosis (hyperventilation, hypocapnia) has a potent effect, and can abruptly lower serum concentrations below the reference interval [16]. Refeeding syndrome, wherein insulin release in the face of a pre-existing phosphate deficiency causes phosphate (as well as potassium and magnesium) to be taken up intracellularly, can also cause a significant abrupt decline in serum phosphate

---

Box 110.1 Causes of hypophosphatemia.

Decreased gastrointestinal absorption
Vitamin D deficiency
Malabsorption
Vomiting and diarrhea
Phosphate binder administration
Antacids

Increased renal excretion
Diabetes mellitus
Diabetic ketoacidosis
Renal tubular defects
Diuretic administration
Hyperadrenocorticism
Eclampsia
Hyperaldosteronism
Early hypercalcemia of malignancy

Transcellular shifts
Insulin administration
Parenteral glucose administration
Bicarbonate administration
Total parenteral nutrition administration
Refeeding syndrome
Hypothermia
Respiratory alkalosis

---

concentrations [17]. The so-called "hungry bone syndrome" can potentially occur following parathyroidectomy or parathyroid ablation for chronic hyperparathyroidism, as the previously substrate-limited osteoblasts quickly resume their uptake of phosphate, although this is atypical and postoperative hyperphosphatemia has been described in this setting as well [18–20].

The restoration of effective insulin signaling during the treatment of diabetic ketoacidosis (DKA) will commonly reduce serum phosphate concentrations within the first 24 hours after insulin therapy is begun [20–23]. Serum phosphate levels should begin to return to the healthy steady-state values once the factors driving the translocation have been rectified. Treatment should generally be initiated if the serum phosphate concentration is below 1.5 mg/dL or if it is below 2.5 mg/dL and the patient is exhibiting compatible clinical signs [24].

Care must be taken with severe DKA patients. Patients with blood glucose concentrations of greater than 250 mg/dL *must* have a significant reduction in glomerular filtration rate (or their blood glucose would not be able to persist that far above the renal threshold) [22]. In this setting, serum phosphate may be markedly elevated due to impaired renal excretion. The author has cared for a DKA dog whose pretreatment serum phosphate was 22.6 mg/dL (in the absence of renal injury). Pre-emptively administering phosphate supplementation to such a patient would only serve to drive the calcium-phosphorus product even further above the *in vivo* solubility saturation point and promote metastatic calcification of soft tissues. Phosphorus supplementation should be reserved for those cases in which recent total calcium and serum phosphate measurements are available for review.

Clinical Signs

The severity of symptoms resulting from hypophosphatemia often correlates weakly with the degree of the reduction and is generally not evident until phosphate concentrations reach 1.5–2.0 mg/dL [25–28]. Moderate hypophosphatemia (1.5–2.5 mg/dL) does not obligate correction if clinical signs are absent. The exception to this guideline would be patients on mechanical ventilation in whom even moderate hypophosphatemia may prevent successful weaning [25].

In dogs and cats, the clinical signs associated with hypophosphatemia are highly variable and include many organ systems [12,26]. Table 110.1 details the clinical signs associated with hypophosphatemia (and hyperphosphatemia which is covered below). Several of these complications can severely alter the path towards recovery for a patient whose primary problem is otherwise resolving. Prompt correction of hypophosphatemia has the potential to avoid serious complications and reduce reliance on expensive life support measures such as transfusion, hemodialysis, oxygen therapy, and mechanical ventilation.

Treatment

The main goal in managing patients with hypophosphatemia is to correct the primary disease process and rapidly decrease the risk of hypophosphatemia-associated adverse events. Phosphate deficits should be

Table 110.1 Clinical signs associated with extreme elevations or reductions in serum phosphorus concentrations (subcategorized by organ system).

Organ system	Clinical signs observed with:	
	Severe hypophosphatemia (<1.5 mg/dL)	**Severe hyperphosphatemia (>8–10 mg/dL)**
Central nervous system	Confusion	Decreased mentation
	Paresthesias	Seizures
	Seizure	
	Coma	
Cardiovascular	Congestive heart failure	Dysrhythmias
	Dysrhythmias	Q-T interval prolongation
Pulmonary	Acute respiratory failure	
	Tissue hypoxia	
Musculoskeletal	Myalgias	Weakness
	Weakness	Cramping
	Rhabdomyolysis	Hyperreflexia
		Tetany
Renal	Acute kidney injury	Renal injury
	Metabolic acidosis	Progression of pre-existing chronic kidney disease
Hematological	Hemolysis	
	Platelet dysfunction	
	Leukocyte dysfunction	
Gastrointestinal	Persistent ileus	Anorexia
	Nausea	Nausea
	Vomiting	Vomiting
Ocular		Reduced visual acuity
		Conjunctivitis
Dermatological		Pruritus

corrected, but immediate correction of the full deficit commonly is not urgent and monitoring of the visually apparent clinical consequences of phosphate depletion (e.g. seizures, muscle weakness, pigmenturia, ileus, hemolysis) should guide both the total quantity and rate of initial phosphate replacement. Phosphate replacement can generally be administered as enteral forms (mild to moderate) or through parenteral administration (moderate with clinical signs and severe).

Enteral phosphate supplementation in humans is typically in the range of 15–45 mg/kg/day. While well-established guidelines for oral supplementation in dogs and cats are lacking, staying well below the dose at which renal interstitial mineralization has been shown to occur (108 mg/kg/day) is advised [29]. Parenteral administration of phosphate solutions (e.g. potassium phosphates, sodium phosphates, or Glycophos) is indicated in patients with moderate (1.5–2.5 mg/dL) to severe (<1.5 mg/dL) hypophosphatemia [24]. For moderate hypophosphatemia, administration rates of 0.01–0.03 mmol PO4/kg/h have been recommended, whereas in severe hypophosphatemia rates of 0.03–1.2 mmol PO4/kg/h may be required [30,31]. Reassessment of serum phosphate concentrations every 8–12 hours while supplementation is ongoing is advised.

Hyperphosphatemia

Definition and Etiology
Hyperphosphatemia may be broadly defined as serum phosphate concentrations greater than 6 mg/dL (dogs) or 7 mg/dL (cats). An abnormality in any of the processes of phosphate homeostasis can lead to hyperphosphatemia. The three general causes for hyperphosphatemia are increased endogenous release, increased exogenous uptake, and decreased urinary excretion [32–40]. Box 110.2 summarizes the most common conditions associated with hyperphosphatemia in small animal practice.

Symptoms
The clinical manifestations of hyperphosphatemia are dependent on the severity of the elevation and the rate at which it has increased. Similar to hypophosphatemia, the clinical signs associated with hyperphosphatemia are highly variable and include many organ systems [32–34,36]. Table 110.1 details the clinical signs associated with hyperphosphatemia. Several of these complications can severely alter the path towards recovery for a patient whose primary problem is otherwise resolving. Prompt correction of hyperphosphatemia is often only achievable by extracorporeal therapies (e.g. hemodialysis) or by the prompt restoration of renal excretion.

Box 110.2 Causes of hyperphosphatemia.

Increased gastrointestinal absorption
Vitamin D toxicosis
  Cholecalciferol
  Calcipotriene
Phosphate enemas

Decreased renal excretion
Azotemia
  Prerenal
    Hypoadrenocorticism
  Renal
    Acute kidney injury
    Chronic kidney injury
  Postrenal
    Uroabdomen
    Obstructive uropathies
Hypoparathyroidism
Acromegaly
Hyperthyroidism

Transcellular shifts
Hemolysis
Tumor lysis syndrome
Crush injury/rhabdomyolysis

Physiological
Young, rapidly growing dogs
Postprandial

Treatment
Hyperphosphatemia is best addressed by treating the underlying disorder. In situations of increased intracellular phosphate release such as rhabdomyolysis and tumor lysis syndrome, the administration of calcium-poor fluids can accelerate renal excretion of phosphate. Loop diuretics such as furosemide may also promote phosphate excretion. Renal excretion is generally so efficient in patients with adequate renal function that balance can be maintained with only a minimal rise in serum phosphorus concentration even for a relatively large phosphorus load. Therefore, acute hyperphosphatemia usually resolves within a few hours if renal function is sufficiently preserved. Patients with chronic kidney disease (CKD) and mild asymptomatic hyperphosphatemia can be treated by reducing dietary protein intake and reducing intestinal absorption with phosphate-binding salts of aluminum, magnesium, or calcium. However, these agents have little role or no role to play in the emergency setting. Emergency room patients are often anorexic and dietary intake is of little concern in the immediate future.

Hemodialysis or peritoneal dialysis may be required to correct hyperphosphatemia in AKI or CKD patients and some have proposed that phosphate be a determining factor in timing the initiation of hemodialysis support [41].

Calcium Homeostasis

Calcium ion is an essential chemical factor in several essential body functions such as muscle contraction, nerve conduction, neurotransmitter release, hormone secretion, cell division and motility, enzyme activity, blood coagulation, action potentials, and pacemaker automaticity. Calcium homeostasis refers to the regulation of the concentration of calcium ions in the extracellular fluid environment (ECF_{Ca2+}). Quite different mechanisms regulate the abundance and distribution of ionized and complexed calcium within the intracellular environment. Intracellular calcium ion is a major second messenger system and cytoplasmic levels must be tightly controlled to avoid cytotoxicity [42].

Extracellular calcium ion concentration is also tightly controlled due to the adverse effects of both elevations and decreases in this parameter. ECF_{Ca2+} greatly impacts the function of voltage-gated ion channels (VGIC). Decreases in ECF_{Ca2+} (hypocalcemia) lead to VGIC opening that is too easily triggered or spontaneous in nature. Clinically, this effect manifests as nerve and muscle dysfunction such as hypocalcemic tetany. Conversely, increases in ECF_{Ca2+} (hypercalcemia) can prevent or reduce VGIC opening and clinical manifestations include many types of depressed nervous system function. Due to its ability to form insoluble particulates with phosphate ions, increases in ECF_{Ca2+} can also lead to excessive accumulation of mineral deposits within soft tissues or within third spaces such as the bladder lumen or renal collecting system.

The regulation of ECF_{Ca2+} is complex and involves the interplay of several organ systems. However, ultimately [ECF_{Ca2+}] depends on three main factors [42,43]:

- the absorption of dietary calcium
- the extent of ECF_{Ca2+} excretion by the kidney

- the relative rate of release and uptake of ECF_{Ca2+} from the bony skeleton which contains a massive reservoir of 99% of ECF_{Ca2+}. The mobilization of even a tiny portion of this skeletal reservoir can have major impacts on [ECF_{Ca2+}].

The major humoral factors and their roles in calcium homeostasis are outlined in Figure 110.1. The three major hormonal mediators are PTH, calcitriol, and calcitonin. PTH typically serves a key role in minute-to-minute regulation of ECF_{Ca2+} while calcitriol plays the central role in day-to-day ECF_{Ca2+} regulation. Calcitonin plays a relatively minor role involving the control of bone mineral mobilization and fine-tuning PTH release.

Hypocalcemia

Definition and Etiology
Hypocalcemia is defined as an abnormal reduction in the concentration of calcium in the extracellular fluid compartment. The recognition of such a reduction and the cut-off values used in identifying hypocalcemia will depend heavily on the means by which calcium is measured. Plasma calcium is present in three major forms: (1) ionized (~55% of total calcium present), (2) non-ionized chelated (~10% of total calcium present), and protein (largely albumin) bound (~35% of total calcium present) [42]. As just under half of the total calcium present in plasma is not in the form that is physiologically regulated, reductions in total calcium cannot always be assumed to be coincident with reductions in the ionized fraction. Reductions in ionized calcium are best identified by direct measurement rather than inference methods. The absolute value at which one will identify ionized hypocalcemia will vary between institutions but will typically be characterized as below the range of 1.0–1.2 mmol/L. When total calcium is used to identify

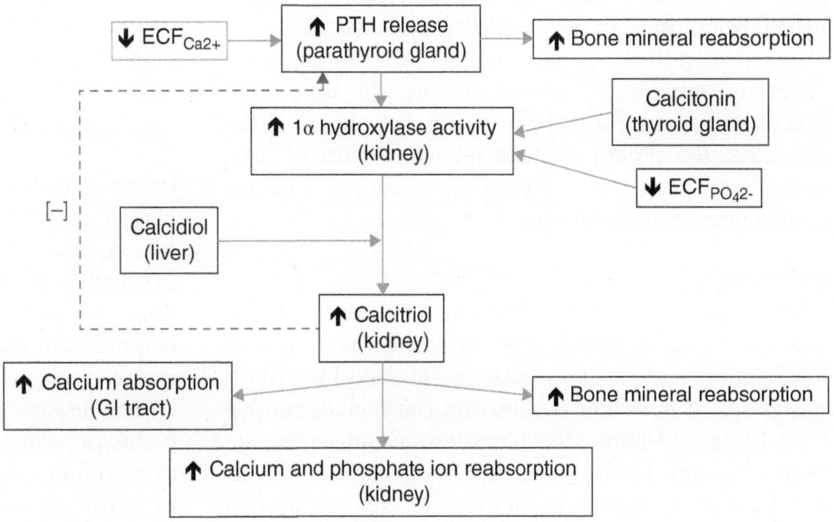

Figure 110.1 Calcium homeostasis overview.

Box 110.3 Causes of hypocalcemia.

Common
Hypoalbuminemia
Chronic kidney disease
Eclampsia
Acute kidney injury
Acute pancreatitis

Occasional
Soft tissue trauma/rhabdomyolysis
Hypoparathyroidism
Ethylene glycol intoxication
Phosphate enema administration
Bicarbonate administration

Uncommon
Lab/anticoagulant error
Rapid IV phosphate administration
Dilutional
Intestinal malabsorption
Hypovitaminosis D
Blood transfusions
Hypomagnesemia
Intralipid infusion

---

hypocalcemia (not advised), cut-off values of < 8 mg/dL are often used in the clinical setting.

Causes of hypocalcemia are outlined in Box 110.3. These causes have been broken down into three categories of common, uncommon, and rare for the reader; however, the relative prevalence of these underlying causes may vary by region and/or practice type. Among the causes of hypocalcemia considered common by this author, hypoalbuminemia is considered to be the least likely to result in concurrent ionized hypocalcemia and thus clinical signs reflecting nerve and muscle dysfunction. Both acute and chronic injury to the kidneys can result in hypocalcemia due to direct and indirect mechanisms. Eclampsia can be considered the cause of hypocalcemia most likely to be recognized due to its direct effects on muscle and nerve function. The hypocalcemia of acute pancreatitis has long been attributed to the saponification of peripancreatic fat but evidence of more widespread disruptions of calcium homeostasis in this setting bears consideration.

Clinical Signs

Clinical signs due to hypocalcemia may be subcategorized as due to muscle dysfunction, nervous system dysfunction, and cardiovascular dysfunction [42]. Manifestations of muscular dysfunction can include muscle tremors, fasciculation, twitching, and sustained contractions or tetany. Ineffective contractions may also manifest, as seen in some forms of dystocia. Nervous system

dysfunction manifestations can include disorientation, restlessness, parasthesias (particularly facial pruritus), panting, and hyperthermia. The CNS may also play a role in hypocalcemia-related arrhythmogenesis, but local effects on the cardiac tissue likely play a larger role. Cardiovascular manifestations of hypocalcemia include the aforementioned arrhythmias as well as arterial hypotension (see Chapter 53).

Treatment

Treatment options are based on addressing the underlying cause of the hypocalcemia and supplementing calcium in either enteral or parenteral form for an appropriate duration of time. When ionized hypocalcemia has been identified then treatment is advised if the $[iCa^{2+}] < 0.7-0.9$ mmol/L. If ionized hypocalcemia is to be inferred from total calcium measurements then treatment when the total Ca < 6–7 mg/dL could be justified if suitable clinical signs are evident.

Acute treatment typically involves the administration of parenteral calcium gluconate (10%). Dose ranges of the order of 0.5–1.5 mL/kg of 10% calcium gluconate administered over 1–5 minutes are generally required. Rechecking $[Ca^{2+}]$ before readministration is advised. For persistent hypocalcemia, a maintenance constant rate infusion at doses of 0.25–1.0 mL/kg/h of 10% calcium gluconate are often sufficient. Long-term supplementation often takes the form of calcium carbonate, which is inexpensive and widely available. In some instances, calcium citrate or oyster shell calcium may be preferable. Dosing requirements are widely variable and should be titrated based on individual patient responses to supplementation. Treatment precautions during any form of calcium supplementation include avoidance of extravasation of parenteral calcium solutions (particularly calcium chloride which can lead to local tissue necrosis), making every attempt to avoid a calcium × phosphate product of greater than 70, and the creation of a monitoring plan sufficiently intensive so as to avoid iatrogenic hypercalcemia.

Hypercalcemia

Definition and Etiology

Hypercalcemia is an abnormal increase in ECF_{Ca2+}. Increases in ionized calcium, total calcium, or both may be identified. The common causes of hypercalcemia in dogs and cats are summarized in Box 110.4. The most common causes of hypercalcemia in dogs are hypercalcemia of malignancy, hypoadrenocorticism, and chronic kidney disease. In cats, hypercalcemia of malignancy is highly prevalent, but idiopathic hypercalcemia is nearly as common (see Chapters 72 and 73). Renal causes of hypercalcemia are also quite common in feline patients.

Box 110.4 Causes of hypercalcemia.

More common (dogs)
Hypercalcemia of malignancy
Hypoadrenocorticism
Chronic kidney disease

More common (cats)
Hypercalcemia of malignancy
Idiopathic
Chronic kidney disease

Less common (both)
Primary hyperparathyroidism
Hypervitaminosis D
Osteolysis
Iatrogenic
Granulomatous disease
Thiazide diuretics

Mechanisms underlying hypercalcemia often involve the overactivity of PTH or a hormonally active-related peptide. Bony destruction due to neoplasia, extensive bone inflammation, or infection can also cause persistent hypercalcemia. Certain medications (thiazides) and toxins (vitamin D analogue rodenticides) (see Chapter 130) are also causes of hypercalcemia that may be encountered in small animal practice [42].

Clinical Signs

The consequences of persistent hypercalcemia may be linked to calcium's role in determining cellular threshold potential and its ability to form relatively insoluble mineral complexes with phosphate ion. Hypercalcemia results in threshold potential becoming a less highly negative voltage. This shift increases the voltage gap between resting and threshold potentials and makes cells less excitable and more difficult to polarize. Hypercalcemia also increases muscle contractile state and increases ATP utilization while decreasing ATP production.

Clinical signs relating to CNS functions include obtundation, seizures, and lethargy. Cardiovascular signs of hypercalcemia include increased arteriolar tone (which may elevate arterial pressure in some patients), poor diastolic function, and arrhythmias. Muscle tremors or muscle weakness may be noted. Polyuria due to diminished urine concentrating ability can also occur in hypercalcemic patients.

In cases of chronic hypercalcemia, additional clinical manifestations may be noted. Gastric hyperacidity and vomiting are not uncommon in this setting. Calciuresis, urolithiasis, renal injury, and soft tissue mineralizations are also encountered in this clinical setting.

Treatment

Treatment of the underlying cause is always a priority in hypercalcemic patients. Thus, identification of the underlying etiology is a high priority in such cases. Options for non-specific treatment of hypercalcemia include the following [42]:

- ECF volume expansion and saline diuresis
- loop diuretics such as furosemide
- avoidance or discontinuation of thiazide diuretics
- bicarbonate administration (transient effect)
- corticosteroids (particularly in cases of hypoadrenocorticism, neoplasia, or granulomatous disease.

In cases of severe life-threatening hypercalcemia, additional treatment measures should be considered, including:

- calcium-chelating agents
- calcium channel blockers
- extracorporeal therapies such as hemodialysis or continuous renal replacement therapy
- bisphosphonate agents such as pamidronate.

For longer-term therapy, agents such as calcitonin and the antineoplastic antibiotic mithramycin may be employed.

Magnesium Homeostasis

The mechanisms underlying magnesium regulation are complex, poorly understood at present, and incompletely defined. The majority of the major transcellular transport proteins for magnesium have only recently been identified and our understanding of their regulation is an area of ongoing active research. While hormones do play a role in magnesium homeostasis, that role is quite minor when compared to their central importance in calcium homeostasis. Like calcium, magnesium is a divalent cation that can be found in ionized, complexed, or protein-bound forms.

The majority of body magnesium in found in the intracellular compartment where it is the second most abundant cation after potassium [44]. Much is often made of the fact that ionized magnesium is the most "biologically active" form. This is true of all electrolytes and is in no way unique to magnesium. Moreover, an argument can be made that it is in fact the common complexed form (i.e. Mg-ATP) that is the most biologically important form.

Magnesium homeostasis involves uptake of dietary magnesium. Magnesium is found in abundance in green plant matter as it is the central cation in chlorophyll, much as iron is in hemoglobin. In humans, enteral absorption of magnesium occurs in the small intestine, whereas fistula studies suggest that the major site of magnesium uptake in dogs is the colon. The site of feline magnesium uptake has not yet been defined.

Uptake of dietary magnesium follows a biphasic pattern. When whole-body magnesium stores are sufficient, magnesium uptake is limited and passive in nature. When whole-body magnesium is depleted, active uptake of magnesium from the bowel lumen becomes the predominant mechanism of absorption. Magnesium excretion occurs via the kidney with a minor contribution from the large bowel in certain circumstances. Fine-tuning of magnesium homeostasis occurs at the level of the distal convoluted tubule. As uptake of dietary magnesium is limited and passive when deficiency is absent, it is not surprising that reduced glomerular filtration is the principal cause for sustained elevations in plasma magnesium concentrations [44,45].

Hypomagnesemia

Definition and Etiology

The definition of hypomagnesemia is somewhat controversial. Many authors feel strongly that hypomagnesemia should only be defined by reductions in ionized magnesium [iMg] concentrations. Indeed, in the acute setting, [iMg] is an invaluable indicator of magnesium losses and shifts between the intracellular and extracelluar compartments. However, in situations of chronic magnesium deficiency, [iMg] is not an ideal monitoring tool. In chronic deficiency, decreases in total serum magnesium [tMg] are large and [iMg] often remains within the reference interval. It has been suggested that in the setting of chronic inadequate magnesium intake, [tMg] is decreased in an attempt to preserve [iMg]. The mechanism most often proposed is down-regulation of an as yet unidentified magnesium-binding protein. In this author's practice, [tMg] is used as an initial screening test and [iMg] is used to further define magnesium imbalances in select patients. Causes of hypomagnesemia are outlined in Box 110.5 [44,45].

Clinical Signs

Magnesium is involved in over 300 enzymatic reactions as an essential co-factor. Surprisingly, the clinical signs are often associated (perhaps incorrectly) with only four major body systems: ECF composition (hypokalemia, hypocalcemia), neuromuscular, neurological, and cardiovascular, as shown in Box 110.6. This author would add additional hemostatic, respiratory, and gastrointestinal clinical signs as well. Specifically, magnesium acts as an endogenous calcium channel blocker and hypomagnesemia is a well-known cause of platelet activation secondary to increased cytosolic calcium. In addition, hypomagnesemia has been reported to cause weakness of accessory respiratory muscles and has been linked to sleep apnea manifestations. Lastly, hypomagnesemia can be associated with severe gastrointestinal ileus that is unresponsive to therapies other than enteral magnesium supplementation.

Box 110.5 Causes of hypomagnesemia.

Gastrointestinal
Malnutrition
Malabsorption
Chronic diarrhea
Nasogastric suction
Proton pump inhibitors

Renal
Congenital/heritable magnesium wasting syndromes
Postobstructive diuresis
Diuretic phase of acute kidney injury
Loop and thiazide diuretics
Cisplatin
Aminoglycosides
Cyclosporine A
Tacrolimus

Endocrine
Hyperparathyroidism
Hyperthyroidism
Syndrome of inappropriate antidiuretic hormone
    secretion
Hyperaldosteronism

Redistribution
Hungry bone syndrome
Acute pancreatitis
Blood transfusions
Insulin therapy

Miscellaneous
Diabetes mellitus
Chronic or recurrent hypercapnia (e.g brachycephalic
    syndrome)

Treatment

Treatment of hypomagnesemia is also an area where an understanding of the underlying physiology is essential. Uptake of enteral magnesium is passive unless whole-body deficiency is present. As such, excessive administration of enteral magnesium to patients without a magnesium deficit is likely to lead to a laxative effect with minimal alteration in serum magnesium concentrations. In addition, cellular uptake of magnesium is quite slow and cells may take 24 hours or more to equilibrate with ECF magnesium. As such, parenteral magnesium administration given as a single bolus is unlikely to alter intracellular magnesium concentrations. This author advises that bolus administration of magnesium (typically $MgSO_4$) be followed by constant infusions of at least 24 hours duration to address intracellular magnesium deficits. Total per day doses required in this setting are typically of the order of 0.5 g for small dogs/cats, 1 g for dogs 6–20 kg, and 2 g for larger dogs.

Box 110.6 Clinical signs associated with hypomagnesemia.

Alterations in ECF composition
Hypokalemia
Hypocalcemia

Neuromuscular signs
Muscle cramps
Fasiculations
Tetany
Muscle weakness

Neurological signs
Nystagmus
Hemiparesis
Obtundation

Cardiovascular signs
Arrhythmias
Arterial hypertension

Hemostatic alterations
Increased platelet activation

Gastrointestinal signs
Ileus

Respiratory signs
Accessory muscle weakness
Reduced upper airway patency

maintenance doses are typically of the order of 200 mg per day for patients less than 20 kg, and 400 mg per day for larger patients. Magnesium excretion follows a diurnal rhythm and supplementation is likely to have greater impact if given with breakfast than with the evening meal.

Hypermagnesemia

Definition and Etiology
Hypermagnesemia is defined as an increase in [iMg], [tMg], or both. Most often, elevations in serum magnesium are due to reductions in renal function and glomerular filtration rate. Due to the nature of magnesium uptake from the bowel, dietary excess is an infrequent and unlikely cause of hypermagnesemia. However, iatrogenic causes should be considered, such as administration of magnesium salts or certain magnesium-containing antacids and laxatives.

Clinical Signs
As hypermagnesemia is most often found in the setting of azotemia, the signs associated with it are often obscured by the underlying disorder. In cases of iatrogenic hypermagnesemia, clinical signs such as weakness, hypotension, and respiratory difficulty have been reported. In rare cases of severe acute hypermagnesemia, asystole may occur, likely due to the calcium channel-blocking properties of magnesium.

Treatment
The restoration of glomerular filtration rate with fluids and diuretics is the mainstay of treatment for hypermagnesemia. Insulin and dextrose can also help to accelerate the uptake of magnesium by cells. Parenteral calcium gluconate (10%), as described above in the section on treatment of hypocalcemia, can also be employed in patients experiencing severe signs.

Enteral supplementation of magnesium also requires some forethought. Not all forms of magnesium supplement are equally absorbable or bioavailable. The common Epsom salt ($MgSO_4$) is poorly absorbed and is thus often used as a cathartic and laxative. This author preferentially uses magnesium oxide and has observed no such laxative effect. Oral

References

1 Rose WD. Calcium, magnesium and phosphorus; emergency department testing yield. *Acad Emerg Med* 1997;4(6):559–563.
2 Dowhan W. The role of phospholipids in cell function. In: *Advances in Lipobiology*, vol. 2 (ed. Gross R). Elsevier, St Louis, 1997, pp. 79–107.
3 Subramanian R, Khardori R. Severe hypophosphatemia: pathophysiologic implications, clinical presentations, and treatment. *Medicine* 2000;79:1–8.
4 Polancic JE. In: Clinical Chemistry: Principles,Procedures, Correlations, 4th edn (ed. Bishop ML). Lippincott Williams and Wilkins, Philadelphia, 2000, pp. 314–316.
5 Travers RJ, Smith SA, Morrissey JH. Polyphosphate, platelets, and coagulation. *Int J Lab Hematol* 2015;37 Suppl 1:31–35.
6 Sharma K, D'Souza R, Tyanova S, et al. Ultradeep human phosphoproteome reveals a distinct regulatory nature of Tyr and Ser/Thr-based signaling. *Cell Rep* 2014;8(5):1583–1594.
7 Bunn HF. Differences in the interaction of 2,3-diphosphoglycerate with certain mammalian hemoglobins. *Science* 1971;172(3987):1049–1050.
8 Dittmer KE, Thompson KG. Vitamin D metabolism and rickets in domestic animals: a review. *Vet Pathol* 2011;48(2):389–407.

9 Harada S, Rodan GA. Control of osteoblast function and regulation of bone mass. *Nature* 2003;423(6937):349–355.

10 Martin A, David V, Quarles LD. Regulation and function of the FGF23/klotho endocrine pathways. *Physiol Rev* 2012;92(1):131–155.

11 Murer H, Biber J. Phosphate transport in the kidney. *J Nephrol* 2010;23 Suppl 16:S145–151.

12 Kita MW. Drawing conclusions from test results. *J Insur Med* 1990;22:270–278.

13 Subramanian R, Khardori R. Severe hypophosphatemia: pathophysiologic implications, clinical presentations, and treatment. *Medicine* 2000;79:1–8.

14 Miller DW, Slovis CM. Hypophosphatemia in the emergency department therapeutics. *Am J Emerg Med* 2000;18:457–461.

15 Rutecki GW, Whittier FC. Life-threatening phosphate imbalance: when to suspect, how to treat. *J Crit Illness* 1997;12:699–704.

16 Weisinger JR, Bellorin-Font E. Magnesium and phosphorus. *Lancet* 1998;352:391–396.

17 Marik PE, Bedigian MK. Refeeding hypophosphatemia in critically ill patients in an intensive care unit: a prospective study. *Arch Surg* 1996;131:1043–1047.

18 Malvin RL, Lotspeich WD. Relation between tubular transport of inorganic phosphate and bicarbonate in the dog. *Am J Physiol* 1956;187:51–56.

19 Solomon SM, Kirby DF. The refeeding syndrome: a review. *J Parent Ent Nutr* 1990;14:90–97.

20 Reinhart JM, Nuth EK, Byers CG, et al. Pre-operative fibrous osteodystrophy and severe, refractory, post-operative hypocalcemia following parathyroidectomy in a dog. *Can Vet J* 2015;56(8):867–871.

21 Milovancev M, Schmiedt CW. Preoperative factors associated with postoperative hypocalcemia in dogs with primary hyperparathyroidism that underwent parathyroidectomy: 62 cases (2004–2009). *J Am Vet Med Assoc* 2013;242(4):507–515.

22 Bruskiewicz KA, Nelson RW, Feldman EC, Griffey SM. Diabetic ketosis and ketoacidosis in cats: 42 cases (1980–1995). *J Am Vet Med Assoc* 1997;211(2):188–192.

23 Hume DZ, Drobatz KJ, Hess RS. Outcome of dogs with diabetic ketoacidosis: 127 dogs (1993–2003). *J Vet Intern Med* 2006;20(3):547–555.

24 Marinella MA. The refeeding syndrome and hypophosphatemia. *Nutr Rev* 2003;61(9):320–323.

25 Wiseman MJ, Viberti GC, Keen H. Threshold effect of plasma glucose in the glomerular hyperfiltration of diabetes. *Nephron* 1984;38(4):257–260.

26 Amanzadeh J, Reilly RF Jr. Hypophosphatemia: an evidence-based approach to its clinical consequences and management. *Nat Clin Pract Nephrol* 2006;2: 136–148.

27 Lentz RD, Brown DM, Kjellstrand CM. Treatment of severe hypophosphatemia. *Ann Intern Med* 1978;89:941–944.

28 Buell JF, Berger AC, Plotkin JS, Kuo PC, Johnson LB. The clinical implications of hypophosphatemia following major hepatic resection or cryosurgery. *Arch Surg* 1998;133(7):757–761.

29 Harris WH, Heaney RP, Davis LA, Weinberg EH, Coutts RD, Schiller AL. Stimulation of bone formation in vivo by phosphate supplementation. *Calcif Tissue Res* 1976;22(1):85–98.

30 Willard MD, Zerbe CA, Schall WD, Johnson C, Crow SE, Jones R. Severe hypophosphatemia associated with diabetes mellitus in six dogs and one cat. *J Am Vet Med Assoc* 1987;190(8):1007–1010.

31 Nichols R, Crenshaw KL. Complications and concurrent disease associated with diabetic ketoacidosis and other severe forms of diabetes mellitus. *Vet Clin North Am Small Anim Pract* 1995;25(3):617–624.

32 Rutecki GW, Whittier FC. Life-threatening phosphate imbalance: when to suspect, how to treat. *J Crit Illness* 1997;12:699–704.

33 Weisinger JR, Bellorin-Font E. Magnesium and phosphorous. *Lancet* 1998;352:391–396.

34 Perlman JM. Fatal hyperphosphatemia after oral phosphate overdose in a premature infant. *Am J Health Syst Pharm* 1997;54:2480–2490.

35 Rose BD. *Clinical Physiology of Acid-Base and Electrolyte Disorders*, 4th edn. McGraw-Hill, New York, 1994, pp. 737–762.

36 Vachvanichsanong P, Maipang M, Dissaneewate P, et al. Severe hyperphosphatemia following acute tumor lysis syndrome. *Med Pediatr Oncol* 1995;24:63–66.

37 Orias M, Mahnensmith RL, Perazella MA. Extreme hyperphosphatemia and acute renal failure after a phosphorous-containing bowel regimen. *Am J Nephrol* 1999;19:60–63.

38 Escalante CP, Weisser MA, Finkel K. Hyperphosphatemia associated with phosphorous-containing laxatives in a patient with chronic renal insufficiency. *South Med J* 1997;90:240–242.

39 Peterson ME, Fluegeman K. Cholecalciferol. *Top Compan Anim Med* 2013;28(1):24–27.

40 Murphy LA, Coleman AE. Xylitol toxicosis in dogs. *Vet Clin North Am Small Anim Pract* 2012;42(2):307–312.

41 Lu YA, Lee SY, Lin HY, et al. Serum phosphate as an additional marker for initiating hemodialysis in patients with advanced chronic kidney disease. *Biomed J* 2015;38(6):531–537.

42 Schenck PA, Chew DJ, Nagode LA, Rosol TJ. Disorders of calcium: hypercalcemia and hypocalcemia. In: *Fluid, Electrolyte, and Acid–Base Disorders*, 4th edn (ed. DiBartola SP). Elsevier-Saunders, St Louis, 2012.

43 Moe SM. Calcium homeostasis in health and in kidney disease. *Compr Physiol* 2016;6(4):1781–1800.

44 Bateman S. Disorders of magnesium: magnesium deficit and excess. In: *Fluid, Electrolyte, and Acid–Base Disorders*, 4th edn (ed. DiBartola SP). Elsevier-Saunders, St Louis, 2012.

45 Hoorn EJ, Zietse R. Disorders of calcium and magnesium balance: a physiology-based approach. *Pediatr Nephrol* 2013;28:1195–1206.

111

Hypoglycemia

Anthony L. Gonzalez, DVM, DACVECC[1] and Deborah C. Silverstein, DVM, DACVECC[2]

[1]ACCESS Specialty Animal Hospitals, Los Angeles, CA, USA
[2]University of Pennsylvania, Philadelphia, PA, USA

Introduction

Glucose, the breakdown product from carbohydrates, is an important source of energy in the animal body. It is the main energy source in cells such as red blood cells and the brain, so feedback mechanisms are in place to maintain normal glucose levels in the bloodstream (Figure 111.1). Small animals presenting to the emergency room frequently suffer from hypoglycemia. Hypoglycemia is associated with an increased risk of death in critically ill human patients [1].

Pathophysiology

Glucose homeostasis requires a balance between absorption, production, and utilization. Glucose becomes available to the body via intestinal digestion and absorption of carbohydrates, the breakdown of glycogen via glycogenolysis, or the production of glucose via gluconeogenesis. Over

80% of the carbohydrate metabolism end-products are glucose; the remainder are fructose and galactose [2]. These are subsequently converted into glucose in the liver, leaving glucose as the final product of carbohydrate digestion.

Postprandially, glucose is stored in the liver as glycogen, a large polymer of glucose. As the only direct storage form of glucose, glycogen can be stored in all cells. However, most is stored in the liver and skeletal muscle. The amount of glycogen stored in the liver rarely exceeds 10% of the total weight of the liver in humans; it is assumed to be similar in dogs and cats [3]. The remainder of glucose is oxidized via glycolysis to form two molecules of pyruvate for each molecule of glucose. Pyruvate is converted to acetyl-CoA in the mitochondria and utilized in the Krebs cycle for final energy production. Alternatively, it can be converted to fatty acids for fat storage when intake of glucose exceeds demand.

Several key hormones play a role in the body with regard to glucose regulation. Insulin is produced via the beta-cells of the pancreas and is released when blood

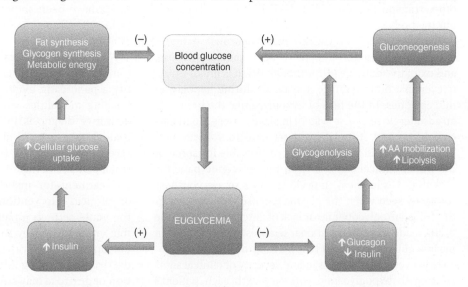

Figure 111.1 Positive (+) and negative (−) feedback mechanisms to maintain normoglycemia.

glucose levels begin to increase. The counterregulatory hormones are released when glucose levels begin to decrease; they include glucagon, catecholamines, cortisol, and growth hormone. Glucagon is produced by the alpha-cells of the pancreas and stimulates glycogenolysis in the liver via cyclic AMP production and subsequent phosphorylation of glycogen phosphorylase. Epinephrine is released via sympathetic stimulation of the adrenal medulla and serves to potentiate glucagon's activation of phosphorylase.

Glycogenolysis by itself can only sustain the body's glucose demands for 6–12 hours [2]. The production of glucose via gluconeogenesis occurs in times of prolonged or increased demands. This process involves using the end-products of glycolysis, including lactic acid, pyruvate, glycerol and amino acids, to form glucose.

Cortisol helps mobilize proteins and adipocytes to ensure that amino acids and fatty acids are available for glucose production. Close to 60% of amino acids in the body can be converted to glucose [2]. Cortisol, along with growth hormone, also serves to inhibit the actions of insulin and potentiate the effects of glucagon and epinephrine in the liver. The kidney also has limited glucose production capabilities and can contribute up to 40% of total glucose production under certain conditions (ex. hepatic insufficiency) [4].

Clinical Signs

Normally, the central nervous system is entirely dependent on plasma glucose as a source of energy. Glucose concentrations in the brain are up to 30% lower compared to plasma and special facilitative glucose transporters are required for entry into the brain cells [5]. GLUT 1 is the predominant transporter in the brain vasculature, with other transporters (GLUT 1–GLUT 5) found throughout the body.

Hypoglycemia can cause severe neuronal damage, including a reduction in cerebral ATP, cellular swelling, and oxidative damage [6]. Although death is uncommon, irreversible brain damage may occur during hypoglycemic episodes. In the face of hypoglycemia, the brain has an adrenergic response system in place to raise blood glucose levels and stimulate counterregulatory hormones. This sympathoadrenal system is responsible for some of the initial clinical signs seen in hypoglycemic patients, including restlessness, muscle tremors or nervousness (typically seen when the plasma glucose level is < 68 mg/dL) [6]. Neuroglycopenia, or lack of glucose supply to the brain, leads to lethargy, ataxia, seizures, and coma when plasma glucose levels fall below 18 mg/dL [6].

However, the progression and severity of clinical signs relating to hypoglycemia will vary with each patient's rate of development, duration, and severity of the underlying disease process. Patients that have acclimated to a lower glucose level may not display the expected clinical signs of hypoglycemia.

Causes of Hypoglycemia

The differential diagnoses for hypoglycemia can be categorized into excess secretion of insulin or insulin-like factors, decreased glucose production, excess glucose consumption, drug-associated causes, and spurious causes (Box 111.1).

Excess Secretion of Insulin or Insulin-Like Factors

Insulinoma

Although rare, functional beta-cell tumors of the pancreas, known as insulinomas, are one of the most common neuroendocrine tumors in dogs [7]. These are malignant tumors which commonly metastasize to local lymph nodes and the liver. Middle-aged medium- to large-breed dogs are most commonly affected. Clinical signs commonly follow meals (due to increased insulin release) or exercise and can include seizures, weakness, collapse, ataxia, and muscle fasciculations.

Bloodwork may show hypokalemia (due to insulin-induced intracellular shifts) and elevated liver values, but hypoglycemia (<70 mg/dL) is the most consistent finding. Fructosamine levels are typically low in canines with an insulinoma [8–10]. Measuring insulin levels may be helpful in making the diagnosis as normal to elevated insulin values present in the face of hypoglycemia are abnormal. An amended insulin:glucose ratio (AIGR) of > 30 is supportive of an insulinoma, but other causes such as sepsis and non-pancreatic neoplasia have been shown to produce an elevated AIGR [4,11–13]. Thus an amended AIGR should not be used as a sole diagnostic.

Abdominal imaging via an ultrasound, computed tomography (CT) or scintigraphy has been used to identify a pancreatic mass. However, the accuracy of these imaging modalities varies and may or may not give a definitive diagnosis in cases of suspected insulinoma. Radiographs can be utilized to image the thorax and screen for metastasis, but are not helpful in identifying small pancreatic masses.

Treatment for insulinomas involves either medical or surgical intervention, or a combination of both. In the acute setting, a patient presenting in a hypoglycemic crisis secondary to a suspected insulinoma should be supplemented with 50% dextrose and continued on dextrose-containing intravenous fluids. The administration of dextrose may stimulate additional insulin release,

Box 111.1 Causes of hypoglycemia in dogs and cats [16,43].

Excess secretion of insulin or insulin-like factors
Insulinoma
Islet cell hyperplasia
Paraneoplastic syndrome
  Hepatocellular carcinoma
  Hepatoma
  Leiomyosarcoma
  Leiomyoma
  Oral melanoma
  Hemangiosarcoma
  Lymphoma
  Pulmonary, mammary and salivary carcinoma

Decreased glucose production
Hypoadrenocorticism
Hypopituitarism
Growth hormone deficiency
Hepatic disease
  Acute hepatic failure
  Portosystemic shunt
  Chronic fibrosis
  Cirrhosis
  Glycogen storage disease
Renal failure*
Neonates and toy breeds
Fasting

Excess glucose consumption
Sepsis
Babesia
Hunting dog hypoglycemia
Pregnancy

Drug-associated causes
Insulin
Beta-receptor antagonists
Xylitol
Sulfonylurea

Spurious
Manual error
Equipment error
Polycythemia
Leukocytosis

* Has not been reported in cats and dogs.

causing a rebound hypoglycemia. The emergency clinician should remember that the goal of treatment is to administer enough dextrose to alleviate any clinical signs but not necessarily normalize the blood glucose level. Glucocorticoids will antagonize the effects of insulin and a constant-rate infusion of glucagon to promote gluconeogenesis and glycogenolysis may also prove beneficial. Long-term management involves the use of glucocorticoids and diet modifications; frequent, low simple sugar-containing meals are recommended.

Other possible therapies include diazoxide (benzothiadiazine diuretic, potassium channel activator), octreotide (synthetic somatostatin analogue) and streptomycin as a chemotherapeutic agent. Surgical removal of the tumor is not usually curative as metastatic disease is suspected at the time of diagnosis in most cases of canine insulinoma [4].

Prognosis and survival time vary with each patient and the extent of disease. Survival times were reported as 12–14 months in dogs that underwent partial pancreatectomy [14,15]. A study comparing surgical versus medical management reported a median survival time of 381 days in dogs undergoing partial pancreatectomy

and 74 days in dogs with medical management only [14]. Another recent study reported a median survival time of 785 days with partial pancreatectomy, 196 with only medical management and 1316 with a combination of both [15]. Postoperative hypoglycemia was found to be a negative prognostic indicator [16].

Paraneoplastic Syndrome
Neoplastic tumors may produce hormones, growth factors, and cytokines, causing various effects in the body. Hepatomas, hepatocellular carcinoma, leiomyoma, leiomyosarcoma, and hemangiosarcoma are some of the most common tumors associated with the production of insulin-like growth factors or peptides causing paraneoplasic hypoglycemia [17] (see Chapters 72 and 73).

Decreased Glucose Production

Hypoadrenocorticism (see Chapter 115)
Hypoadrenocorticism, also known as Addison's disease, is a common endocrine disease found in young to middle-aged dogs. Often called "the great pretender" for its broad spectrum of general clinical signs, Addison's

disease involves a deficiency of cortisol and mineralo-corticoids. Atypical cases have been seen in which only cortisol deficiency is detected. Patients may present with waxing and waning lethargy, diarrhea, inappetence, weight loss or in an Addisonian crisis with severe hypovolemic shock. Hypoglycemia occurs due to decreased cortisol production causing a decrease in gluconeogenesis. Although classic electrolyte changes are suggestive of the disease (Na : K ratio < 27 : 1), an ACTH stimulation test remains the gold standard for diagnosis. A resting cortisol level has also been shown to be diagnostic, with one study reporting a basal cortisol concentration of < 1 mg/dL having a 100% sensitivity and 98.2% specificity for diagnosing hypoadrenocorticism in dogs [18]. Treatment involves mineralocorticoid and glucocorticoid supplementation and generally carries an excellent prognosis.

Hepatic Disease (see Chapter 90)
Various etiologies can lead to hepatic dysfunction, including portosystemic shunts, chronic fibrosis, cirrhosis or hepatopathy (e.g. glycogen storage disease). Signs secondary to hepatic dysfunction vary but may include lethargy, inappetence, fever, weight loss, jaundice, increased or decreased thirst, and abnormal bowel movements. Hepatic dysfunction is characterized by hypoalbuminemia, hypoglycemia, hypocholesteremia, and low blood urea nitrogen (BUN). Liver function testing often reveals hyperammonemia and elevated postprandial bile acids.

Neonates and Toy Breeds (see Chapter 120)
Neonates have been shown to have a decreased liver glycogen content and limited body fat reserves, thus predisposing them to developing hypoglycemia. Toy and miniature-breed dogs may also have hypoglycemic episodes associated with an alanine deficiency [19]. Due to their small size and fragility, adequate nutrition must be provided to neonates and small-breed puppies.

Excess Glucose Consumption

Sepsis
Sepsis, defined as the clinical syndrome caused by infection and the host's systemic inflammatory response to it, can cause severe hemodynamic compromise and vasodilatory shock in critically ill patients. While hyperglycemia is noted in some septic patients, contributing factors to hypoglycemia include depleted glycogen stores, impaired gluconeogenesis, and increased peripheral glucose utilization [20]. Patients suspected of or diagnosed with sepsis should have immediate stabilization and treatment protocols started (see Chapter 159).

Canine pregnancy-associated hypoglycemia is caused by blunting of the normal counterregulatory responses to hypoglycemia [21,22]. Hypoglycemia is also a common complication of canine babesiosis and is a poor prognostic indicator on admission [23].

Drug-Associated Causes

Insulin
Exogenous insulin therapy is most commonly used in animals with diabetes mellitus. Insulin overdose resulting in hypoglycemia is more common in obese cats than in dogs, and in cats receiving insulin doses greater than 6 units per injection [24]. The duration of severity of hypoglycemia does not correlate with the dose and type of insulin used [24]. Animals with inappetence or inconsistent meals and regular insulin administration often develop hypoglycemia. Insulin therapy may need to be temporarily discontinued and restarted at a 25–50% reduced dose until the patient's glucose is stabilized [25]. Other medications such as sulfonylureas and beta-blockers have also been demonstrated to induce hypoglycemia [26,27].

Xylitol
Xylitol is a 5-carbon sugar-alcohol sweetener that is most commonly associated with chewing gum. However, it is found in many other products such as toothpaste and "low carb" snacks like syrups, candies, and cookies. In contrast to humans, xylitol causes stimulation of insulin release from the pancreas in dogs [28]. Hypoglycemia has been associated with a 100 mg/kg exposure and hepatotoxicity with greater than a 500 mg/kg exposure [29].

Spurious

Besides operator and machine error in processing samples, polycythemia and leukocytosis have both been associated with artifactual hypoglycemia via increased cellular metabolism [30,31].

Diagnosis

Hypoglycemia is defined as a blood glucose concentration of less than 60 mg/dL. Whipple's triad was originally developed in 1935 as criteria for the diagnosis of insulinomas, but its lack of specificity allows it to be applied to numerous causes of hypoglycemia [4]. The triad consists of hypoglycemia, clinical signs consistent with hypoglycemia, and resolution of clinical signs with correction of hypoglycemia.

Point-of-care glucometers (POCGs) are routinely used in veterinary medicine as they provide a quick and cost-effective method of evaluating blood glucose concentrations in dogs and cats. Variable degrees of accuracy have been noted when using POCGs designated for humans [32–34]. AlphaTRAK 2 is a POCG marketed for veterinary patients which takes into account species differences between free and hemoglobin-bound glucose [34]. The measurement of glucose using serum and plasma, as opposed to whole blood, by POCGs has been shown to more accurately reflect the serum glucose concentration when compared to biochemical analyzers [35].

Depending on the underlying etiology, continuous glucose monitoring may be required. Repeated venipuncture is not desirable for the patient, so the placement of a sampling line is recommended. The use of a continuous interstitial glucose monitoring system (CGMS), which measures the interstitial glucose concentration as an estimation of blood glucose, may also be an option for some patients. This technology was recently validated for use in dogs and cats, and studies have shown it to be useful and accurate in rats, rabbits, dogs, cats, and humans [36,37]. Additional diagnostics, including a complete cell count, chemistry, urinalysis, and imaging, should be performed to determine the underlying etiology of the hypoglycemia. Further bloodwork such as ammonia levels, pre- and postprandial bile acids, insulin levels, and cortisol levels should be performed when appropriate.

Treatment of a Hypoglycemic Crisis

Historically, it has been recommended for owners at home to administer karosyrup, honey or maple syrup to the gums of pets suspected of suffering from hypoglycemic episodes. However, studies show the limited effect of buccal absorption which renders these methods ineffective unless the syrups are actually swallowed by the patient [38–40]. Thus a veterinarian should evaluate any pet suspected of suffering from a suspected hypoglycemic episode.

In hospital, the goal of stabilization is not necessarily to correct the blood glucose to a normal range but rather to eliminate clinical signs. Dextrose is given at 0.25–0.5 g/kg diluted 1:3 with sterile water for injection

Table 111.1 Treatment of hypoglycemia.

Dextrose 50%	Adults: 0.5 g/kg IV diluted 1:3 in 0.9% NaCl
	Neonates: Dextrose 1.0 ml/kg of 12.5% dextrose (50% dextrose diluted 1:3 in 0.9% NaCl)
Glucagon	50 ng/kg IV, followed by CRI of 5–40 ng/kg/min IV to effect
Dexamethasone	0.1–0.2 mg/kg IV followed by 0.05–0.1 mg/kg IV q12
Prednisone/Prednisolone	HA: 1–2 mg/kg IV followed by 0.5–1 mg/kg IV q8
	Insulinoma: 0.25–0.5 mg/kg PO q12

or 0.9% NaCl as a slow intravenous bolus. In cases of suspected insulinoma, large boluses of dextrose up to 1 g/kg should be avoided as they can stimulate insulin release. Instead, small boluses should be administered and repeated as needed. Neonates require a more dilute bolus of dextrose (see Box 111.1). The patient should subsequently be placed on a constant-rate infusion of 2.5–5% dextrose-containing fluids. The concentration may be increased based on individual need. Dextrose concentrations greater than 5–7% should be administered through a central line as phlebitis due to high tonicity can occur if given via peripheral catheter administration. D5W should be avoided as the sole intravenous fluid choice for glucose supplementation as it can cause severe to life-threatening hyponatremia [41].

Adjunctive therapy involving glucocorticoids to stimulate gluconeogenesis and antagonize insulin release can be used. A constant-rate infusion of glucagon to stimulate glycogenolysis and increase hepatic glucose production has also been utilized in cases of insulin or insulin-like peptide-secreting tumors [42]. Table 111.1 presents information on dosing. When the patient is conscious and alert, small frequent meals should be provided as an additional source of simple sugars. Blood glucose levels should be monitored and treatments modified to avoid iatrogenic hyperglycemia. Animals with suspected cerebral edema should be treated with 0.25–0.5 g/kg of 25% mannitol intravenously over 10–20 minutes (an in-line filter is recommended).

References

1 Finfer S, Liu B, Chittock DR, et al. Hypoglycemia and risk of death in critically ill patients. *N Engl J Med* 2012;367:1108–18.
2 Guyton AC, Hall JE. Metabolism of carbohydrates, and formation of adenosine triphosphate. In: *Textbook of Medical Physiology*, 11th edn (eds Guyton AC, Hall JE). Elsevier Saunders, Philadelphia, 2006, pp. 961–977.
3 Cunningham JG, Klein BG. *Textbook of Veterinary Physiology*, 4th edn. Elsevier Saunders, St Louis, 2007.

4 Feldman EC, Nelson RW. Beta cell neoplasia: insulinoma. In: *Canine and Feline Endocrinology and Reproduction*, 3rd edn (eds Feldman EC, Nelson RW). Elsevier Saunders, St Louis, 2004, pp. 616–644.

5 Loose NL, Rudloff E, Kirby R. Hypoglycemia and its effect on the brain. *J Vet Emerg Crit Care* 2008;18: 223–234.

6 Dwyer DS. Glucose metabolism in the brain, In: *International Review of Neurobiology*, vol. 51 (ed. Dwyer DS). Elsevier Science, Philadelphia, 2002, pp. 1–100, 164–176, 421–436.

7 Goutal CM, Brugmann BL, Ryan KA. Insulinoma in dogs: a review. *J Am Anim Hosp Assoc* 2012;48 (3): 151–163.

8 Mellanby RJ, Herrtage ME. Insulinoma in a normoglycaemic dog with low serum fructosamine. *J Small Anim Pract* 2002;43(11):506–508.

9 Loste A, Marca MC, Pérez M, et al. Clinical value of fructosamine measurements in non-healthy dogs. *Vet Res Commun* 2001;25(2):109–115.

10 Thoresen SI, Aleksandersen M, Lønaas L, et al. Pancreatic insulin-secreting carcinoma in a dog: fructosamine for determining persistent hypoglycaemia. *J Small Anim Pract* 1995;36(6): 282–286.

11 Caywood DD, Klausner JS, O'Leary TP, et al. Pancreatic insulin-secreting neoplasms: clinical, diagnostic and prognostic features in 73 dogs. *J Am Anim Hosp Assoc* 1988;24:577–584.

12 Leifer CE, Peterson ME, Matus RE. Insulin-secreting tumor: diagnosis and medical and surgical management in 55 dogs. *J Am Vet Med Assoc* 1986;188(1):60–64.

13 Edwards DF. It's time to unamend the insulin-glucose ratio. *J Am Vet Med Assoc* 1986;188:951–953.

14 Tobin RL, Nelson RW, Lucroy MD, et al. Outcome of surgical versus medical treatment of dogs with beta cell neoplasia: 39 cases (1990–1997). *J Am Vet Med Assoc* 1999;215(2):226–230.

15 Polton GA, White RN, Brearley MJ, et al. Improved survival in a retrospective cohort of 28 dogs with insulinoma. *J Small Anim Pract* 2007;48(3):151–156.

16 Hess RS. Insulin secreting islet cell neoplasia. In: *Textbook of Veterinary Internal Medicine*, 6th edn (eds Ettinger SJ, Feldman EC). *Elsevier Saunders*, Philadelphia, 2005, pp. 1560–1563.

17 Gaschen FP, Teske E. Paraneoplastic syndrome. In: *Textbook of Veterinary Internal Medicine*, 6th edn (eds Ettinger SJ, Feldman EC). Elsevier Saunders, Philadelphia, 2005, pp. 789–795.

18 Lennon EM, Boyle TW, Hutchins RG, et al. Use of basal serum or plasma cortisol concentrations to rule out a diagnosis of hypoadrenocorticism in dogs: 123 cases (2000–2005). *J Am Vet Med Assoc* 2007;231:413–416.

19 Chew DJ, et al. Hyperglycemia and hypoglycemia. In: *Quick Reference to Veterinary Medicine* (ed. Klenner WR). JB Lippincott, Philadelphia, 1982, p. 432.

20 Miller SI, Wallace RJ, Musher DM, et al. Hypoglycemia as a manifestation of sepsis. *Am J Med* 1980;68:5.

21 Johnson CA. Glucose homeostasis during canine pregnancy: insulin resistance, ketosis, and hypoglycemia. *Theriogenology* 2008;70(9):1418–1423.

22 Connolly CC, Aglione LN, Smith MS, et al. Pregnancy impairs the counterregulatory response to insulin-induced hypoglycemia in the dog. *Am J Physiol Endocrinol Metab* 2004;287:E480–E488.

23 Keller N, Jacobson LS, Nel M, et al. Prevalence and risk factors of hypoglycemia in virulent canine babesiosis. *J Vet Intern Med* 2004;18:265–270.

24 Whitley N, Drobatz K, Panciera D. Insulin overdose in dogs and cats: 28 cases (1986–1993), *J Am Vet Med Assoc* 1997;211:326.

25 Mcintire DK. Emergency therapy of diabetic crisis: insulin overdose, diabetic ketoacidosis, and hyperosmolar coma. *Vet Clin North Am Small Anim Pract* 1995;25:639.

26 Fonseca VA. Effects of beta-blockers on glucose and lipid metabolism. *Curr Med Res Opin* 2010;26(3):615–629.

27 Hanchard B, Boulouffe C, Vanpee D. Sulfonylurea-induced hypoglycemia: use of octreotide. *Acta Clin Belg* 2009;64(1):56–58.

28 Kuzuya T, Kanazawa Y, Hayashi M, et al. Species differences in plasma insulin responses to intravenous xylitol in man and several mammals. *Endocrinol Jpn* 1971;18:309–320.

29 Dunayer EK. New findings on the effects of xylitol ingestion in dogs. *Vet Med* 2006;12:791–796.

30 Paul A, Shiel RE, Juvet F, et al. Effect of hematocrit on accuracy of two point-of-care glucometers for use in dogs, *Am J Vet Res* 2011;72(9):1204.

31 Latimer KS (ed.). *Duncan and Prasse's Veterinary Laboratory Medicine Clinical Pathology*, 5th edn. Wiley-Blackwell, Hoboken, 2011.

32 Cohen TA, Nelson RW, Kass PH, et al. Evaluation of six portable blood glucose meters for measuring blood glucose concentration in dogs. *J Am Vet Med Assoc* 2009;235:276–280.

33 Johnson BM, Fry MM, Flatland B, et al. Comparison of a human portable blood glucose meter, veterinary portable blood glucose meter, and automated chemistry analyzer for measurement of blood glucose concentrations in dogs. *J Am Vet Med Assoc* 2009;235:1309–1313.

34 Zini E, Moretti S, Tschuor F, et al. Evaluation of a new portable glucose meter designed for use in cats. *Schweiz Arch Tierheilkd* 2009;151:448–451.

35 Tauk BS, Drobatz KJ, Wallace KA, et al. Correlation between glucose concentrations in serum, plasma, and whole blood measures by a point-of-care glucometer and serum glucose concentration measured by an automated biochemical analyzer for canine and feline blood samples. *J Am Vet Med Assoc* 2015;246(12):1327–1333.

36 Rebrin K, Steil GM, van Antwerp WP, et al. Subcutaneous glucose predicts plasma glucose independent of insulin: implications for continuous monitoring. *Am J Physiol* 1999;277(3 part 1):E561–E571.

37 Reineke EL, Fletcher DJ, King LG, Drobatz KJ. Accuracy of a continuous glucose monitoring system in dogs and cats with diabetic ketoacidosis. *J Vet Emerg Crit Care* 2010;20:303–312.

38 Chlup R, Zapletalova J, Peterson K, et al. Impact of buccal glucose spray, liquid sugars and dextrose tables on the evolution of plasma glucose concentration in healthy persons. *Biomed Pap Med Fac Univ Palacky Olomouc Czech Repub* 2009;153(3):205.

39 Gunning RR, Garber AJ. Bioactivity of instant glucose. Failure of absorption through oral mucosa. *JAMA* 1978;240(15):1611.

40 Manning AS, Evered DF. The absorption of sugars from the human buccal cavity. *Clin Sci Mol Med* 1976;51(2):127.

41 Koenig A. Hypoglycemia. In: *Small Animal Critical Care Medicine*, 2nd edn (eds Silverstein DC, Hopper K). Elsevier Saunders, St Louis, 2015, pp. 352–356.

42 Fischer JR, Smith SA, Harkin KR. Glucagon constant rate infusion: a novel strategy for the management of hyperinsulinemic-hypoglycemic crisis in the dog. *J Am Animal Hosp Assoc* 2000;36:27.

43 Cote E. *Clinical Veterinary Advisor: Dogs and Cats*, 2nd edn. Elsevier Saunders, St Louis, 2011, pp. 1401.

112

Hyperglycemia

Gideon Daniel, DVM, DACVIM[1] and Alex Lynch, BVSc (Hons), DACVECC, MRCVS[2]

[1] *Friendship Hospital for Animals, Washington, DC, USA*
[2] *North Carolina State University, Raleigh, NC, USA*

Introduction

Hyperglycemia is frequently encountered in dogs and cats presented for emergency care (Box 112.1). Animals may be presented for signs directly associated with hyperglycemia (e.g. polyuria/polydipsia) or it may be stumbled upon incidentally. Stress-induced hyperglycemia and diabetes mellitus are the most common reasons for hyperglycemia in animals [1]. Diabetes mellitus occurs associated with an absolute or relative insulin insufficiency. Alternative explanations for insulin deficiency include animals with exocrine pancreatic insufficiency and those that have undergone partial pancreatectomy. Severely systemically compromised animals may also develop hyperglycemia associated with massive catecholamine release (e.g. after severe traumatic brain injury) [2]. A careful drug history is important in the emergency setting to ensure that there is no iatrogenic explanation for hyperglycemia (e.g. glucocorticoids, progestins) [1]. Hyperglycemia may also develop in a smaller

proportion of hospitalized animals that were initially normoglycemic with potential negative impact on morbidity and mortality [3].

Stress Hyperglycemia

A transient period of hyperglycemia is common in cats in the hospital setting associated with catecholamine release. This may also be noted in dogs, albeit less frequently. Hyperlactatemia may also have an additive effect on the degree of hyperglycemia noted in animals associated with increased hepatic glucose production. In this setting, blood glucose concentrations are typically in the range of 200–400 mg/dL [1].

It is important to consider the influence that stress may be playing on the severity of hyperglycemia in diabetic animals being examined in the hospital. Disparate results may be seen in the hospital compared to those achieved from obtaining blood glucose measurements at home by owners. More profound hyperglycemia (associated with catecholamine excess) may mislead the clinician into assuming worse overall glycemic control than is likely present. Reflex changes in insulin prescription (e.g. increasing dose or frequency) should be avoided based on these data alone. It can be clinically challenging to separate stress-associated hyperglycemia from other disease-associated causes of hyperglycemia. The clinician should use historical clues (e.g. presence or absence of polyuria and polydipsia, weight loss despite polyphagia) along with other pieces of clinicopathological data (e.g. ketonuria, ketonemia) to reasonably distinguish incidentally identified stress hyperglycemia from other causes.

The hyperglycemia associated with traumatic brain injury is likely associated with catecholamine discharge. The severity of brain injury is associated with the degree of hyperglycemia [2]. The requirement for specific

---

Box 112.1 Causes of hyperglycemia in dogs and cats.

Diabetes mellitus

Stress

Postprandial

Traumatic brain injury

Hyperadrenocorticism

Hypersomatotropism

Diestrus

Drug therapy (glucocorticoids, progestins)

Parenteral nutrition

Glucose-containing fluid administration

Textbook of Small Animal Emergency Medicine, First Edition. Edited by Kenneth J. Drobatz, Kate Hopper, Elizabeth Rozanski and Deborah C. Silverstein.
© 2019 John Wiley & Sons, Inc. Published 2019 by John Wiley & Sons, Inc.
Companion Website: www.wiley.com/go/drobatz/textbook

management of hyperglycemia (e.g. via insulin) is seldom necessary.

Diabetes Mellitus

Animals with diabetes mellitus are commonly seen in the emergency setting. Animals may be presented for assessment of signs associated with previously unrecognized diabetes mellitus. Alternatively, previously diagnosed diabetics may be examined for new issues that could be considered a recognized complication in diabetics (e.g. bacterial cystitis) or be apparently coincidental (e.g. heart failure). For animals without a prior diagnosis of diabetes mellitus, identification of the hallmarks of the disease (i.e. PU/PD, polyphagia, weight loss) along with persistent fasting hyperglycemia with concurrent glucosuria is usually straightforward.

Glucose undergoes filtration by the kidney, with almost all the glucose in the glomerular filtrate being reabsorbed in the proximal tubules. It is therefore not usual to identify glucose in the urine of dogs and cats. Glucosuria is seen if blood glucose concentration exceeds the renal threshold (approximately 180 mg/dL in dogs and 300 mg/dL in cats) [4]. Most dipstick tests use a colorimetric test based on an enzymatic reaction (glucose oxidase). Diabetes mellitus is the most common cause of glucosuria but other conditions may occasionally be recognized (e.g. stress, excitement, administration of glucose-containing fluids, primary renal glucosuria, Fanconi syndrome) [4].

Longer term glycemic control can be gauged via serum fructosamine assessment. An increased fructosamine supports sustained hyperglycemia. This is typically a send-out test, limiting its utility in the emergency setting and lending itself more to the chronic monitoring of diabetic animals receiving insulin.

The emergency clinician should be aware that previously unrecognized diabetic animals may present severely compromised with collapse, severe dehydration, acid–base disturbances, and electrolyte derangements. In some cases, this may be the first overt clinical manifestation of issues. In such cases, the classic historical clues of diabetes outlined above may have been overlooked or their significance underappreciated. This is especially relevant for cats where urinating and drinking habits may be less obvious to owners.

For the systemically compromised diabetic animal, two major scenarios are encountered: the ketotic animal with or without metabolic acidosis, and the non- (or minimally) ketotic hyperosmolar pet. The ability to estimate blood ketones in urine or serum is therefore helpful in the emergency setting. The nitroprusside reagent present in dipstick tests reacts with acetone and acetoacetate, but not beta-hydroxybutyrate. False-negative results from urine

ketone measurements and whole-blood or plasma ketone measurements are more accurate in detection of ketonemia in diabetic animals [5,6]. Ketosis implies an absolute or relative insulin deficiency promoting lipolysis. Ketosis is very common in newly diagnosed diabetic animals. Many of these cases will be only mildly systemically compromised, with retention of their appetite and thirst. Other animals with evidence of ketosis will have concurrent metabolic acidosis (i.e. diabetic ketoacidosis) and benefit from intensive hospitalized care. In these cases, it is important to search for concurrent conditions that may trigger insulin resistance (see below). Fundamentally, exogenous insulin administration is necessary to reverse ketosis and is a major component of the treatment for DKA.

Animals that develop hyperglycemic hyperosmolar diabetes mellitus, on the other hand, have sustained an insult leading to a marked reduction in glomerular filtration rate. In this setting, the ability to excrete glucose in urine is compromised, leading to abnormal retention of glucose in the blood and subsequent hyperosmolality. Profound hyperglycemia is usually present but without ketosis. In this scenario, restoration of glomerular filtration is high priority compared to the provision of insulin. In these animals, careful fluid resuscitation with the judicious use of insulin to slowly reduce hyperglycemia and correct hyperosmolality is necessary. For further information on management of diabetes mellitus see Chapter 113.

Insulin Deficiency and Insulin Resistance

Absolute insulin deficiency (analogous to type 1 diabetes mellitus) is likely present in most dogs with diabetes mellitus. Genetic predisposition with immune-mediated destruction of pancreatic islet cells leads to significantly reduced insulin production. Exogenous insulin supplementation will enable maintenance of normoglycemia, especially when combined with appropriate diet and exercise in the long term. Other situations where insulin insufficiency may be noted include dogs with exocrine pancreatic insufficiency and animals that have undergone a partial pancreatectomy. Partial pancreatectomy is most commonly performed in dogs with insulinoma. Following surgery, exogenous insulin administration may be necessary, depending on the beta-cell mass remaining in the dog. In this situation, appreciation of a reduced insulin requirement over time may be misinterpreted as a positive development. In reality, it may be an indication of increased endogenous insulin production associated with tumor recurrence or metastasis.

It is also important to consider if insulin resistance may have an additive effect in diabetic dogs.

Insulin resistance may occur in situations where counterregulatory hormones like cortisol, epinephrine, growth hormone or progesterone are elevated [1,4]. Clinical situations where this may occur include hyperadrenocorticism, hypersomatotropism, diestrus, hyperlipidemia, and hypothyroidism. The use of diabetogenic drugs (e.g. glucocorticoids, progestins) may also induce insulin resistance. Insulin resistance exerts a negative influence on insulin sensitivity at the level of the insulin receptor or insulin signaling cascade [4]. This response results in a number of alterations in carbohydrate metabolism, including insulin resistance, increased hepatic glucose production, impaired peripheral glucose utilization, and relative insulin deficiency. Epinephrine stimulates glucagon secretion and inhibits insulin release by pancreatic beta-cells. High cortisol levels increase hepatic glucose production and stimulate protein catabolism and increased gluconeogenesis.

Any sick diabetic dog should be screened for concurrent diseases, especially pancreatitis and occult sources of sepsis, despite the genetic and immune-mediated components of their disease. Diabetes mellitus in cats has increased similarities with type 2 diabetes in people. This typically is characterized by insulin resistance rather than immune-mediated beta-cell destruction. Dietary changes and oral antihyperglycemic drugs have been investigated in the management of diabetic cats. Exogenous insulin administration is the mainstay of therapy however, with evidence that intensified insulin therapy early in the disease course may lead to clinical diabetic remission [7]. Concurrent endocrinopathies should be considered plausible in all diabetic pets, especially those proving to be difficult to control. In dogs, hyperadrencorticism is the most likely culprit, while hypersomatotropism and hyperadrenocorticism may be present in cats.

The development of hyperglycemia leads to generation of reactive oxygen species and elevated inflammatory markers. The release of proinflammatory cytokines (TNF-alpha, IL-6, and IL-1-beta) contributes to the insulin-resistant state. Increasing evidence suggests that TNF-alpha interferes with insulin receptor signaling, as well as the synthesis and/or translocation of the glucose transport GLUT-4 to the plasma membrane [8]. Hyperglycemia has been shown to impair leukocyte function and limit phagocytosis, chemotaxis, and bacterial destruction. Hyperglycemia limits neovascularization and collagen synthesis, restricting the body's ability to generate new and healthy tissue at the surgical site. The presence of inflammatory cytokines and state of relative insulin resistance promote lipolysis, increasing the release of free fatty acids (FFAs). Elevated FFAs have detrimental effects on the cardiovascular system by increasing catecholamine concentrations and mean arterial blood pressure. They are also associated with malignant cardiac dysrhythmia, increased myocardial oxygen consumption and presence of ischemic stroke [8]. Hyperglycemia also results in increased platelet aggregation and prothrombotic state. An overproduction of reactive oxygen species can result in direct cellular damage, vascular and immune dysfunction. NF-kappa-B activation and the production of inflammatory cytokines like TNF-alpha, IL-6, and plasminogen activator inhibitor-1 (PAF-1) increase vascular permeability and activate both leukocytes and platelets.

Specific guidelines are instituted for hyperglycemic patients recovering from surgery or critical illness in people. These are typically a combination of basal (long-acting such as glargine) insulin and fast-acting insulin (such as lispro, aspart or glulisine) [8]. These negative effects of hyperglycemia appear to occur in small animal patients also with respect to hospitalization and certain complications (e.g. sepsis) [3]. These patient should be closely monitored during their hospitalization. With increased recognition, similar guidelines for treatment can be established for veterinary patients as well.

References

1 Ettinger SJ, Feldman ED (eds). *Textbook of Veterinary Internal Medicine*, 7th edn. WB Saunders, St Louis, 2010, pp. 1782–1796.
2 Syring RS, Otto CM, Drobatz KJ. Hyperglycemia in dgos and cats with head trauma: 122 cats (1997–1999). *J Am Vet Med Assoc* 2001;218(7):1124–1129.
3 Torre DM, deLaforacade AM, Chan DL. Incidence and clinical relevance of hyperglycemia in critically ill dogs. *J Vet Intern Med* 2007;21:971–975.
4 Feldman E, Nelson R. *Canine and Feline Endocrinology and Reproduction*, 3rd edn. WB Saunders, St Louis, 2004, pp. 486–580.
5 Zeugswetter F, Pagitz M. Ketone measurements using dipstick methodology in cats with diabetes mellitus. *J Small Anim Pract* 2009;50(1):4–8.
6 Di Tommaso M, Aste G, Rocconi F, et al. Evaluation of a portable meter to measure ketonemia and comparison with ketonuria for the diagnosis of canine diabetes ketoacidosis. *J Vet Intern Med* 2009;23(3): 466–471.
7 Sparkes AH, Cannon M, Church D, et al. ISFM consensus guidelines on the practical management of diabetes mellitus in cats. *J Feline Med Surg* 2015;17(3):235–250.
8 Jafar N, Edriss H, Nugent K, et al. The effect of short-term hyperglycemia on the innate immune system. *Am J Med Sci* 2015;251(12):201–211.

113

Complicated Diabetes Mellitus

Amie Koenig, DVM, DACVIM (SAIM), DACVECC

College of Veterinary Medicine, University of Georgia, Athens, GA, USA

Introduction

Complicated diabetes mellitus takes one of two forms: diabetic ketoacidosis (DKA) or hyperglycemic hyperosmolar syndrome (HHS). Criteria for diagnosing diabetic ketoacidosis include presence of hyperglycemia, glucosuria, and ketonemia or ketonuria with a metabolic acidosis. HHS criteria include severe hyperglycemia (>600 mg/dL), minimal or absent serum or urine ketones, and severe hyperosmolality (>350 mOsm/kg).

Pathogenesis

In both forms of diabetic crisis, insulin deficiency promotes gluconeogenesis and glycogenolysis and reduces cellular utilization of glucose, all of which cause hyperglycemia. Activity of hormone-sensitive lipase is stimulated and free fatty acids (FFA) are released from adipocytes to be used as an energy source. FFA are metabolized to triglycerides, carbon dioxide (CO_2) and water, or the ketone bodies: acetoacetate, beta-hydroxybutyrate, and acetone. In the uncomplicated diabetic, triglyceride production predominates and the small amounts of ketones that are produced are completely metabolized for energy [1]. Counterregulatory hormones (glucagon, epinephrine, cortisol, and growth hormone) are released in response to a concurrent physiological stressor, and this contributes to glucose production, insulin resistance, and protein catabolism. The counterregulatory hormones also stimulate lipolysis, which increases the amount of circulating FFA available for ketone formation [1].

Diabetic ketoacidosis occurs once the quantity of ketoacids overwhelms the metabolic pathways that normally convert ketones to energy, as well as the buffering systems that normally mitigate the effects of ketones on acid–base status. In HHS, ketosis is prevented by small quantities of circulating insulin and hepatic glucagon resistance that inhibit lipolysis [2,3]. The primary result is hyperglycemia, progressive osmotic diuresis, dehydration, and subsequent decrease in GFR, which is required to achieve the massive blood glucose increase associated with HHS [4,5]. Therefore, the lower the GFR, the higher the blood glucose concentration [4].

History and Physical Examination

Animals with DKA and HHS can present with various historical and clinical findings, since any concurrent disease can stimulate stress hormone release and progression to diabetic crisis. Classic historical findings in diabetic patients include polyuria, polydipsia (PU/PD), polyphagia, and weight loss. Dehydration is seen in both disease processes due to osmotic diuresis, lack of intake, and additional losses via the gastrointestinal tract. Dogs and cats with DKA typically manifest lethargy, mental depression, anorexia, vomiting, diarrhea, weakness, and ketone breath. HHS patients manifest hyporexia, lethargy, vomiting, and weakness. Some animals with HHS also have neurological signs such as circling, pacing, mentation changes (from depression to coma), abnormal pupillary light reflexes, or seizures, which are thought to develop due to hyperosmolality-induced cerebral dehydration [6–10].

Signs of hypovolemia (see Chapter 153) can accompany both crises; findings may include tachycardia, bradycardia (cats), tachypnea, hypothermia, pallor, prolonged capillary refill time, poor pulse quality, and hypotension. Tachypnea and increased respiratory effort may be consistent with hyperosmolality, acidosis, infection, primary respiratory disease or heart failure, which commonly accompany HHS [7]. Many dogs with HHS have a history of recent steroid administration [8].

Textbook of Small Animal Emergency Medicine, First Edition. Edited by Kenneth J. Drobatz, Kate Hopper, Elizabeth Rozanski and Deborah C. Silverstein.
© 2019 John Wiley & Sons, Inc. Published 2019 by John Wiley & Sons, Inc.
Companion Website: www.wiley.com/go/drobatz/textbook

Diagnostic Evaluation in the Emergency Room

Triage Panel

The first indication that a patient is in a diabetic crisis may be discovered on an emergency blood panel which includes a minimum of "the big 4" (PCV/TP, glucose, azostix) or, preferably, a more comprehensive panel including a (venous) blood gas, glucose, electrolytes, lactate, and BUN/creatinine. Sick animals with a previous history of DM, those with hyperglycemia identified on the emergency panel, or patients with a metabolic acidosis of undetermined cause should be screened for HHS and DKA.

Measure Blood Glucose Concentration

Extremely high blood glucose concentrations may surpass the upper limit of glucose analyzers. Obtaining a definitive glucose measurement is important for developing a therapeutic plan that reduces risk of an overly rapid decrease in blood glucose. If glucose concentration is too high to measure, the sample can be diluted, reanalyzed, and the glucose concentration calculated. If diluting samples and using a whole-blood point-of-care glucometer, packed cell volume must be taken into account when interpreting these measurements, as hemodilute or anemic blood can result in falsely elevated plasma glucose readings [11,12].

Measure Ketones and Assess Degree of Acidemia

Ketones can be identified using a ketone meter or urine dipstick [13–17]. Ketone meters are more sensitive than urine dipsticks [15], but presence of ketones on either would support a diagnosis of DKA. If urine is unavailable at admission, another highly sensitive way to identify ketonemia is by placing serum or plasma from a spun hematocrit tube on the urine dipstick ketone pad [16,17].

Blood gas analysis can clarify the magnitude of acidemia arising from ketoacidosis, lactic acidosis, uremia, and possibly hyperchloremia; however, acid–base abnormalities cannot be used to differentiate between the two crises.

Quantify Degree of Hyperosmolality

Normal serum osmolality is 290–310 mOsm/kg and neurological signs have been documented in animals when osmolality exceeds 340 mOsm/kg [18]. There are many ways to estimate serum osmolality [19,20]. BUN is an ineffective osmole and effects of potassium on osmolality are minimal, so using a modified equation may better reflect the effects of osmolality on the patient: Effective osm = 2(Na+) + (glucose÷18). Glucose is measured in mg/dL and Na+ in mEq/L.

Assess Electrolyte Abnormalities

Profound electrolyte abnormalities often develop in patients with DKA and HHS. While the initial measured blood concentrations of these electrolytes can be normal, decreased, or increased, the total body content is typically reduced and deficiencies become evident with the onset of insulin therapy. It is important to obtain baseline electrolyte concentrations in order to develop the optimal therapeutic plan. Failure to address electrolyte deficiencies prior to initiating insulin therapy can lead to complications that can be life threatening.

Sodium

Hyperglycemia and hyperosmolality exert an osmotic force that pulls water into the extracellular (includes vascular space) space. This increase in plasma water dilutes sodium and causes a pseudohyponatremia, a falsely decreased sodium measurement [21]. As the blood glucose level decreases, the osmotic gradient is also diminished, and the excess water leaves the vasculature and interstitium and returns to the intracellular space, causing the measured serum sodium level to rise. An estimate of the actual sodium level can be calculated using the equation:

$$Na^+_{(corrected)} = 1.6 \times [(\text{measured glucose} - \text{normal glucose})/100] + Na^+_{(measured)}$$

Potassium, Magnesium, and Phosphorus (see Chapter 110) Multiple mechanisms influence the initial measured potassium concentration in patients with DKA and HHS. Glucosuria and ketonuria induce osmotic diuresis, and electrolytes are excreted along with the ketoacids to maintain electroneutrality [1]. Potassium concentrations are further influenced by insulin deficiency, which decreases the amount of potassium co-transported into cells; acidemia, which causes potassium to shift out of cells in exchange for hydrogen ions; severe hyperosmolality [22], which leads to a shift of potassium out of cells; hypovolemia-induced hyperaldosteronism [23], which increases renal potassium loss; poor renal perfusion or renal dysfunction, which can increase potassium; and decreased intake and gastrointestinal losses which contribute to a decrease in potassium concentration [1]. Regardless of the initial measurement, serum potassium concentration will decrease with therapy as insulin induces transport of glucose and potassium into cells and, as the acidemia improves, shifting potassium into cells in exchange for hydrogen.

Magnesium and phosphorus concentrations are influenced by similar mechanisms. With insulin therapy, magnesium and phosphorus levels will also decrease as they shift back into cells and are utilized for ATP production. The decline in phosphorus and magnesium has been shown to directly correlate with decline in blood glucose and hydrogen ions [24].

Stabilization and Emergency Treatment

Therapeutic goals for HHS and DKA are to restore effective circulating volume, provide rehydration and maintenance fluids, supplement electrolytes to correct and prevent deficiencies, initiate insulin therapy to help reduce glucose levels and reverse ketone production, and identify and treat underlying diseases.

Restore Effective Circulating Volume (see Chapter 153)

Hypovolemia and severe dehydration are consequences of osmotic diuresis, gastrointestinal and renal water losses, and lack of water intake. In humans, the fluid deficit for an HHS patient is estimated to be twice that of DKA patients and as much as 12–15% of body weight [25–28]. Failure to normalize vascular volume can lead to cardiovascular collapse and contributes to a high mortality rate [25–31]. As long as the patient is not in congestive heart failure, restoration of vascular volume should begin with an intravenous fluid bolus of approximately 15 mL/kg (cat) to 20–30 mL/kg (dog) of an isotonic replacement crystalloid (such as lactated Ringer's solution, Plasmalyte A, Normosol R, or 0.9% NaCl) over 15–20 minutes (see Chapter 167). This dose can be repeated if resuscitation endpoints have not been met (see Chapter 153).

Provide Ongoing Fluid Therapy

Once the patient is volume resuscitated, fluids should then address the patient's dehydration, ongoing losses, and maintenance needs (see Chapters 167 and 172). The patient must frequently be reassessed to ensure the plan is optimal and that rapid changes in body weight and other signs of fluid deficit or overload are not developing. Ongoing losses should be recalculated, typically every 4–6 hours, and fluid rate adjusted accordingly. In patients with heart disease, rehydration must be done carefully, as parenteral fluids can exacerbate pulmonary congestion and subsequent edema. Nasoesophageal (NE) tubes can be effectively used to provide enteral fluids while minimizing risk of fluid overload.

For most patients, a buffered balanced isotonic replacement crystalloid (e.g. lactated Ringer's, Normosol-R, Plasmalyte-A) or 0.9% NaCl is a good initial choice for replacing fluid deficits and ongoing losses (see Chapter 167). Maintenance (half-strength) solutions can be used to provide the maintenance fluid needs or extra free water for treating hypernatremia. Compared to DKA patients receiving a balanced buffered replacement crystalloid, those receiving 0.9% NaCl solution have been shown to have higher chloride and lower bicarbonate concentrations, which can delay resolution of acidemia [32,33]. Improved urine output and blood pressure have also been identified in DKA patients receiving a balanced replacement crystalloid compared to saline [33]. Ultimate fluid composition is based on patient electrolytes. In severely hypernatremic patients, care should be taken to correct serum sodium slowly, with a decrease of no more than 1 mEq/L/h to prevent cerebral edema [34] (see Chapter 108). Fluid therapy reduces blood glucose and ketone concentrations via dilution, an increase in urinary excretion, and decrease in circulating catecholamines [30,35,36]. Acidemia is also improved as enhanced tissue blood flow decreases lactate production and improves GFR.

Treat Electrolyte Abnormalities

Regardless of the measured blood concentrations, whole-body deficits in potassium, magnesium, and phosphorus are usually present and insulin administration will further decrease these electrolyte concentrations (see Chapter 110). Failure to address electrolyte deficiencies before and during insulin administration can precipitate life-threatening complications. Electrolytes are usually added to the fluids used for rehydration and maintenance (Table 113.1). Once electrolytes increase to within reference range and potassium is at least 3.5 mEq/L, insulin therapy should commence. Electrolytes should be monitored frequently (q4–6h, initially) and fluids and electrolyte content should be altered as necessary. As the patient normalizes, intervals between electrolyte measurements can be extended. If electrolytes cannot be tested on site, referral to a practice with in-hospital electrolyte measuring capability should be considered.

Patients initially manifesting hyperkalemia should be monitored closely and potassium supplementation should begin once the concentration drops within the reference range.

Bicarbonate therapy is rarely indicated in the treatment of diabetic crises (see Chapter 174). Sodium bicarbonate can worsen hypokalemia, ionized hypocalcemia, and hyperosmolality, cause hypernatremia, or induce paradoxical central nervous system acidosis. In patients with DKA, bicarbonate may increase acetoacetate levels,

Table 113.1 Electrolyte supplementation guide for diabetic ketoacidosis and hyperglycemic hyperosmolar syndrome.

Electrolyte	Form	Dose for supplementation		Consequence of severe deficiency
Potassium	Potassium chloride (KCl) (can also use potassium phosphate, see below)	Serum potassium (mEq/L)	Potassium added to bag (mEq/L)*	Hypotension, arrhythmias, weakness, cervical ventroflexion, hypoventilation, respiratory paralysis, and death
		3.5–5	20	
		3.0–3.4	30	
		2.5–2.9	40	
		2–2.4	60	
		<2	80–100	
			Not to exceed 0.5 mEq K+/kg/h	
Phosphorus	Potassium phosphate (KPhos)	0.01–0.2 mmol/kg/h OR give 25–50% of potassium as KPhos and 50–75% as KCl		Hemolysis, weakness, obtundation, myocardial depression, arrhythmias, seizures
Magnesium	Magnesium sulfate (MgSO$_4$)	0.5–1 mEq/kg given as constant-rate infusion over 24 hours		Refractory hypokalemia, hypotension, obtundation, seizures, weakness, arrhythmias, possible insulin resistance

*Recommended amounts of potassium are recommended for fluids running at a maintenance fluid rate. Caution should be exercised when using higher fluid rates.

delay resolution of ketoacidosis [37], and worsen cerebral edema [38]. Dogs with DKA administered bicarbonate had a poorer outcome than those that did not, although it was unclear whether the outcome was due to the bicarbonate or the severity of disease prompting bicarbonate therapy [6]. Bicarbonate is generally reserved for patients with ongoing severe acidemia (pH < 7.1, bicarbonate < 8 mmol/L) with refractory hypotension, arrhythmias, insulin resistance or presence of stupor or coma despite adequate and appropriate fluid and electrolyte therapy.

Initiate Insulin Therapy

Prior to starting insulin, it is imperative that the patient is fluid resuscitated and electrolyte deficiencies are corrected. Early insulin therapy can worsen hypovolemia by rapidly decreasing blood glucose and osmolality, which causes water to move out of the vascular space. A rapid decrease in the blood glucose concentration can also contribute to cerebral edema formation [39,40]. Insulin therapy will also worsen deficiencies of potassium, magnesium, and phosphorus, which can cause life-threatening complications or death.

The primary goal of insulin therapy for DKA is reversal of ketogenesis, and the secondary goal is reduction of blood glucose concentration. Most commonly, successful treatment is obtained with a short-acting regular insulin administered using either an intermittent intramuscular (IM) or intravenous (IV) continuous-rate infusion (CRI) protocol (Table 113.2) [41,42]. Absorption of subcutaneous (SC) insulin injections may be poor or unpredictable in a dehydrated or hypotensive DKA or HHS patient. Newer insulin products, such as glargine, aspart

Table 113.2 Regular insulin protocols for treating diabetic ketoacidosis (DKA) and hyperglycemic hyperosmolar syndrome (HHS).

Insulin protocol type	Initial dose for DKA	Initial dose for HHS	Subsequent management
IV regular insulin CRI	Dilute 1.1–2.2 U/kg of regular insulin in 250 mL 0.9% NaCl. Start this solution at 5–10 mL/h	Dilute 0.5–1.0 U/kg of regular insulin in 250 mL 0.9% NaCl. Start this solution at 5–10 mL/h	Check blood glucose q2h and adjust CRI rate as necessary (see Table 113.3). Goal is to reduce blood glucose by 50–70 mg/dL/h
Intermittent IM regular insulin	0.2–0.25 U/kg of regular insulin, then 0.1 U/kg q2–4h	0.1 U/kg of regular insulin, then 0.05 U/kg q2–4h	Check blood glucose q4h. Goal is to reduce blood glucose by 50–70 mg/dL/h. Subsequent insulin doses are increased or decreased by ~25% to meet this goal. Add dextrose to fluids when glucose < 250 mg/dL

CRI, continuous rate infusion; IM, intramuscular; IV, intravenous.

and lispro, have prompted evaluation of other protocols [43–46], some of which show promise and may be used more commonly after additional study and refinement.

The primary goal for treating HHS patients is steady reduction of glucose concentration. Compared to DKA, in which insulin is critical for reversing ketogenesis, insulin is less critical for resolution of HHS because most of the syndrome is improved by replacing fluid deficit. In the non-ketotic HHS patient, insulin can be withheld until the patient is volume resuscitated and better hydrated, and the glucose concentrations are no longer adequately declining (<50 mg/dL/h) with appropriate fluid therapy alone [36]. The optimal treatment protocol for HHS has not been identified for humans or animals [47]. Compared to DKA protocols, insulin doses are usually decreased by 50% to facilitate a slow decline in blood glucose and reduce the risk of cerebral edema and development of neurological signs [36]. The recommended rate for an IV CRI of regular insulin is 0.025–0.05 U/kg/h [36,48]. For the IM protocol, 0.1 U/kg of regular insulin is administered, followed by 0.05 U/kg q2h until the glucose is less than 300 mg/dL, then q4–6 h.

With both DKA and HHS protocols, the goal is to decrease glucose by 50–75 mg/dL/h [36,39,48]. Blood glucose should be measured every 1–2 hours and the insulin dose adjusted to achieve the desired rate of decline (Table 113.3). If the glucose is dropping too rapidly, the insulin dosage should be decreased by 25–50%.

Identify and Treat Concurrent Diseases

Once cardiovascularly stable, diabetics experiencing DKA or HHS warrant a comprehensive battery of diagnostic tests looking for other conditions that may have contributed to the development of the diabetic crisis. Concurrent treatment of these co-morbidities is necessary for successful outcome of DKA and HHS patients.

A complete blood count (CBC), comprehensive biochemical profile, and urinalysis with culture are indicated for all patients. Other diagnostic tests, such as radiographs of the chest and abdomen, abdominal ultrasound, echocardiography, electrocardiogram, FeLV/FIV screening, endocrine testing (most often of the thyroid or adrenal glands), heartworm testing, and pancreatic lipase measurement may be indicated based on historical, clinical, or physical examination findings.

Abnormalities identified by clinicopathological data are not specific for DKA or HHS and will vary with concurrent disease processes. CBC may reveal anemia or hemoconcentration. Stress or inflammatory leukograms are common in response to physiological stress, infection, or inflammation. Azotemia and hyperphosphatemia may reflect hypovolemia, dehydration, or concurrent primary renal dysfunction. Elevated liver enzyme activities and cholesterol occur commonly with diabetes mellitus, but may also reflect shock, concurrent pancreatitis or hepatobiliary disease, or concurrent endocrine dysfunction, such as hyperadrenocorticism. Hyperbilirubinemia, hypercholesterolemia, and hypertriglyceridemia are more commonly identified in cats with DKA than those with HHS [7].

Urinalysis assesses for presence of ketones and infection. Diabetics have impaired migration of white blood cells to sites of infection, so failure to find an inflammatory sediment does not preclude infection. Urine culture should always be submitted since urinary tract infection was reported in 20% of dogs with DKA [6].

Post-crisis Therapy for Diabetes Mellitus

Regular insulin protocols should be continued until the animal is eating, at which time the patient is transitioned to a long-acting insulin regimen. The recovered DKA/HHS patient is then managed as a "new" diabetic with special attention given to vigilant monitoring, insulin titration, and diagnosis and treatment of any concurrent problems as a means of preventing recurrence of DKA and HHS.

Outcome

Death and euthanasia rate for veterinary DKA patients has been reported to be 7–30% [6,9,42]. In one study, azotemia, metabolic acidosis, and hyperosmolality were more severe in cats that died [9]. In dogs, non-survivors had lower ionized calcium concentration, hematocrit and venous pH; base deficit was associated with outcome such that each 1 mEq/L increase in base deficit yielded a 9% increase in likelihood of discharge from the hospital [6]. Recurrence rate for DKA in cats has been reported to be as high as 42% [9].

Table 113.3 Insulin constant-rate infusion (CRI) adjustment chart for diabetic ketoacidosis and hyperglycemic hyperosmolar syndrome.

Blood glucose (mg/dL)	Insulin CRI rate (mL/h) (see Table 113.2 for details)	Maintenance/ replacement fluid composition
>250	10	As is
200–250	7	plus 2.5% dextrose
150–199	5	plus 2.5% dextrose
100–149	5	plus 5% dextrose
<100	0	plus 5% dextrose

Mortality rate for HHS in people is consistently 15–17% [49–51] and has been documented as high as 72% in children [52]. In animals, mortality rate for HHS is also high: 65% of cats and 38% of dogs died or were euthanized prior to discharge and only 12% of cats sur-vived > 2 months [7,8]. There are no consistent predictors of survival for dogs and cats, although long-term feline survivors had curable concurrent diseases [6] and dogs with abnormal mental status and low venous pH had a poorer outcome [7].

References

1 Hall JE (ed.). *Guyton and Hall Textbook of Medical Physiology*, 12th edn. Saunders, Philadelphia, 2011.

2 McGarry JD, Woeltje KF, Kuwajima M, et al. Regulation of ketogenesis and the renaissance of carnitine palmitoyltransferase. *Diabetes Metab Rev* 1989;5:271–284.

3 Chupin M, Charbonnel B, Chupin F. C-peptide blood levels in keto-acidosis and in hyperosmolar non-ketotic diabetic coma. *Acta Diabetolol Lat* 1981;18:123–128.

4 Kandel G, Aberman A. Selected developments in understanding of diabetic ketoacidosis. *Can Med Assoc J* 1983;128:392–397.

5 Owen OE, Licht JH, Sapir DG. Renal function and effects of partial rehydration during diabetic ketoacidosis. *Diabetes* 1981;30:510–518.

6 Hume DZ, Drobatz KJ, Hess RS. Outcome of dogs with diabetic ketoacidosis: 127 dogs (1993–2003). *J Vet Intern Med* 2006;20:547–555.

7 Koenig A, Drobatz KJ, Beale AB, et al. Hypergylcemic, hyperosmolar syndrome in feline diabetics: 17 cases (1995–2001). *J Vet Emerg Crit Care* 2004;14:30–40.

8 Trotman TK, Drobatz KJ, Hess RS. Retrospective evaluation of hyperosmolar hyperglycemia in 66 dogs (1993–2008). *J Vet Emerg Crit Care* 2013;23:557–564.

9 Bruskiewicz KA, Nelson RW, Feldman EC, et al. Diabetic ketosis and ketoacidosis in cats: 42 cases (1980–1995). *J Am Vet Med Assoc* 1997;211:188–192.

10 Nichols R, Crenshaw KL. Complications and concurrent disease associated with diabetic ketoacidosis and other severe forms of diabetes mellitus. *Vet Clin North Am Small Anim Pract* 1995;25:617–624.

11 Lane SL, Koenig A, Brainard B. Formulation and validation of a predictive model to correct blood glucose concentrations obtained using a veterinary point-of-care glucometer in hemodilute and hemoconcentrated canine samples. *J Am Vet Med Assoc* 2015;246:307–312.

12 Paul AE, Shiel RE, Juvet F, et al. Effect of hematocrit on accuracy of two point-of-care glucometers for use in dogs. *Am J Vet Res* 2011;72:1204–1208.

13 Hoenig M, Dorfman M, Koenig A. Use of a hand-held meter for the measurement of blood beta-hydroxybutyrate in dogs and cats. *J Vet Emerg Crit Care* 2008;18:86–87.

14 Zeugswetter F, Pagitz M. Ketone measurements using dipstick methodology in cats with diabetes mellitus. *J Small Anim Pract* 2009;50:4–8.

15 DiTommaso M, Aste G, Rocconi F, et al. Evaluation of a portable meter to measure ketonemia and comparison with ketonuria for the diagnosis of canine diabetic ketoacidosis. *J Vet Intern Med* 2009;23:466–471.

16 Hendey GW, Schwab T, Soliz T. Urine ketone dip test as a screen for ketonemia in diabetic ketoacidosis and ketosis in the emergency department. *Ann Emerg Med* 1997;29:735–738.

17 Brady MA, Dennis JS, Wagner Mann C. Evaluating the use of plasma hematocrit samples to detect ketones utilizing urine dipstick colorimetric methodology in diabetic dogs and cats. *J Vet Emerg Crit Care* 2003;13:1–6.

18 Chrisman C. *Problems in Small Animal Neurology*, 2nd edn. Lea and Febiger, Philadelphia, 1991.

19 Dugger DT, Mellema MS, Hopper K, Epstein SE. A comparison of the clinical utility of several published formulae for estimated osmolality of canine serum. *J Vet Emerg Crit Care* 2014;24:188–193.

20 Dugger DT, Epstein SE, Hopper K, Mellema MS. Comparative accuracy of several published formulae for the estimation of serum osmolality in cats. *J Small Anim Pract* 2013;54:184–189.

21 Katz MA. Hyperglycemia-induced hyponatremia: calculation of expected serum sodium depression. *N Engl J Med* 1973;289:843–844.

22 Montolieu J, Revert L. Lethal hyperkalemia associated with severe hyperglycemia in diabetic patients with renal failure. *Am J Kidney Dis* 1985;5:47–48.

23 Wolfsdorf J, Glaser N, Sperling MA. Diabetic ketoacidosis in infants, children and adolescents. *Diabetes Care* 2006;29:1150–1159.

24 Ionescu-Tirgoviște C, Bruckner I, Mihalache N, Ionescu C. Plasma phosphorus and magnesium values during treatment of severe diabetic ketoacidosis. *Med Interne* 1981;19:63–68.

25 Kitabchi AE, Umpierrez GE, Murphy MB, et al. Management of hyperglycemic crises in patients with diabetes. *Diabetes Care* 2001;24:131–153.

26 Nugent BW. Hyperosmolar hyperglycemic state. *Emerg Med Clin North Am* 2005;23:629–648.

27 Kitabchi AE, Umpierrez GE, Fisher JN, Murphy MB, Stentz FB. Thirty years of personal experience in hyperglycemic crises: diabetic ketoacidosis and hyperglycemic hyperosmolar state. *J Clin Endocrinol Metab* 2008;93:1541–1552.

28 Kitabchi AE, Nyenwe EA. Hyperglycemic crises in diabetes mellitus: diabetic ketoacidosis and

hyperglycemic hyperosmolar state. *Endocrinol Metabol Clin North Am* 2006;35:725–751.

29 Delaney MF, Zisman A, Kettyle WM. Diabetic ketoacidosis and hyperglycemic hyperosmolar nonketotic syndrome. *Endocrinol Metab Clin North Am* 2000;29:683–705.

30 Ellis EN. Concepts of fluid therapy in diabetic ketoacidosis and hyperosmolar hyperglycemic nonketotic coma. *Pediatr Clin North Am* 1990;37:313–321.

31 Delaney MF, Zisman A, Kettyle WM. Diabetic ketoacidosis and hyperglycemic hyperosmolar nonketotic syndrome. *Endocrinol Metab Clin North Am* 2000;29:683–705.

32 Mahler SA, Conrad SA, Wang H, Arnold TC. Resuscitation with balanced electrolyte solution prevents hyperchloremic metabolic acidosis in patients with diabetic ketoacidosis. *Am J Emerg Med* 2011;29:670–674.

33 Chua HR, Venkatesh B, Stachowski E, et al. Plasma-lyte 148 vs 0. 9% saline for fluid resuscitation in diabetic ketoacidosis. *J Crit Care* 2012;27:138–145.

34 Kahn A, Brachet E, Blum D, Controlled fall in natremia and risk of seizures in hypertonic dehydration. *Intens Care Med* 1979;5:27–31.

35 West ML, Marsden PA, Singer GG, Halperin ML. Quantitative analysis of glucose loss during acute therapy for hyperglycemic, hyperosmolar syndrome. *Diabetes Care* 1986;9:465–471.

36 Zeitler P, Haqq A, Rosenbloom A, Glaser N. Hyperglycemic hyperosmolar syndrome in children:pathophysiological considerations and suggested guidelines for treatment. *J Pediatr* 2011;158:9–14.

37 Okuda Y, Adrogue HJ, Field JB, Nohara H, Yamashita K. Counterproductive effects of sodium bicarbonate in diabetic ketoacidosis. *J Clin Endocrinol Metab* 1996;81:314–320.

38 Rose KL, Pin CL, Wang R, Fraser DD. Combined insulin and bicarbonate therapy elicits cerebral edema in a juvenile mouse model of diabetic ketoacidosis. *Pediatr Res* 2007;61:301–306.

39 Arieff AI, Kleeman CR. Studies on mechanisms of cerebral edema in diabetic comas. Effects of hyperglycemia and rapid lowering of plasma glucose in normal rabbits. *J Clin Invest* 1973;52:571–583.

40 Silver SM, Clark EC, Schroeder BM, Sterns RH. Pathogenesis of cerebral edema after treatment of diabetic ketoacidosis. *Kidney Int* 1997;51:1237–1244.

41 Macintire DK. Treatment of diabetic ketoacidosis in dogs by continuous low-dose intravenous infusion of insulin. *J Am Vet Med Assoc* 1993;202:1266–1272.

42 Claus MA, Silverstein DC, Shofer FS, Mellema MS. Comparison of regular insulin infusion doses in critically ill diabetic cats: 29 cases (1999–2007). *J Vet Emerg Crit Care* 2010;20:509–517.

43 Marshall RD, Rand JS, Gunew MN, Menrath VH. Intramuscular glargine with or without concurrent subcutaneous administration for treatment of feline diabetic ketoacidosis. *J Vet Emerg Crit Care* 2013;23:286–290.

44 Gallagher BE, Mahony OM, Rozanski EA, Buob S, Freeman LM. A pilot study comparing a protocol using intermittent administration of glargine and regular insulin to a continuous rate infusion of regular insulin in cats with naturally occurring diabetic ketoacidosis. *J Vet Emerg Crit Care* 2015;25:234–239.

45 Sears KW, Drobatz K, Hess R. Use of lispro insulin for treatment of diabetic ketoacidosis in dogs. *J Vet Emerg Crit Care* 2012;22:211–218.

46 Walsh ES, Drobatz KJ, Hess RS. Use of intravenous insulin aspart for treatment of naturally occurring diabetic ketoacidosis in dogs. *J Vet Emerg Crit Care* 2016;26:101–7.

47 Pasquel FJ, Umpierrez GE. Hyperosmolar hyperglycemic state: a historic review of the clinical presentation, diagnosis, and treatment. *Diabetes Care* 2014;37:3124–3131.

48 Wagner A, Risse A, Brill H, et al. Therapy of severe diabetic ketoacidosis zero mortality under very-low-dose insulin application. *Diabetes Care* 1999;22: 674–677.

49 Pinies JA, Cairo G, Gaztambide S, Vazquez JA. Course and prognosis of 132 patients with diabetic nonketotic hyperosmolar state. *Diabetes Metab* 1994;20:43–48.

50 Hamblin PS, Topliss DJ, Chosich N, et al. Deaths associated with diabetic ketoacidosis and hyperosmolar coma: 1973–1988. *Med J Aust* 1989;151:439–444.

51 Fadini GP, de Kreutzenberg SV, Rigato M, et al. Characteristics and outcomes of the hyperglycemic hyperosmolar non-ketotic syndrome in a cohort of 51 consecutive cases at a single center. *Diabetes Res Clin Pract* 2011;94:172–179.

52 Cochran JB, Walters S, Losek JD. Pediatric hyperglycemic hyperosmolar syndrome: diagnostic difficulties and high mortality rate. *Am J Emerg Med* 2006;24:297–301.

114

Adrenal Gland Disorders

Jonathan D. Dear, DVM, DACVIM[1] and Guillaume L. Hoareau, DVM, PhD, DACVECC, DECVECC[2]

[1] *School of Veterinary Medicine, University of California, Davis, CA, USA*
[2] *Clinical Investigation Facility, Travis Air Force Base, Fairfield, CA, USA*

Introduction

The adrenal glands are paired endocrine organs adjacent to the kidneys within the retroperitoneum. The adrenal cortex is composed of three distinct layers: the zona glomerulosa, zona fasciculata, and zona reticularis. These zones produce and secrete mineralocorticoids, glucocorticoids, and sex hormones, respectively, and are under the control of the juxtaglomerular apparatus (JGA) (as part of the renin-angiotensin-aldosterone system (RAAS) for mineralocorticoids) and the pituitary gland (for glucocorticoid regulation). The adrenal medulla secretes and produces catecholamines and is regulated by the autonomic nervous system. Disease can arise from either excess or deficiency of the hormones produced by the adrenal gland.

Pheochromocytoma

Pheochromocytomas are catecholamine-producing tumors predominantly arising from the adrenal medulla. Similarly, extra-adrenal pheochromocytomas, or paragangliomas, are neuroendocrine chromaffin cells tumors that oversecrete catecholamines. In humans, paragangliomas account for 10% of pheochromocytomas [1]. It has only been reported in two canine patients [2,3]. Since paragangliomas are rare, the rest of this section will focus on pheochromocytoma.

Incidence

In canine patients with an adrenal mass undergoing surgical treatment, 13–31% had a confirmed diagnosis of pheochromocytoma [4–8]. In dogs with non-traumatic adrenal gland rupture and associated hemoabdomen, 2/4 dogs suffered from a pheochromocytoma [9]. In larger reports of canine acute non-traumatic hemoabdomen, in the subgroup of dogs with hemorrhage due to malignant neoplasia, the incidence of pheochromocytoma ranged from 0% to 4% [10,11].

Pathophysiology

Intermittent production of supraphysiological levels of catecholamines results in clinical signs associated with high sympathetic tone (tachycardia, tachyarrhythmias, and/or hypertension). While tachyarrhythmias are most common, there are reports of pheochromocytoma-associated atrioventricuar blocks [12]. While rare, decreased conduction abnormalities can be attributed to chronic myocardial injury [13] (see Chapter 53). Chronic severe hypertension can lead to target organ damage such as renal, ocular, or brain injury (see Chapter 63).

Tumor progression can be associated with intravascular invasion or thrombus formation and ascites. Caval thrombus formation is a common co-morbidity in patients with pheochromocytoma, leading to thrombectomy in 35–55% of patients undergoing adrenalectomy [4,6,14]. Approximately 50–66% of those tumors are locally invasive or have metastasized at the time of diagnosis [14,15].

Clinical Signs and Physical Examination

Middle-aged to older dogs are overrepresented [15]. Presenting complaint and clinical signs can be attributed to catecholamine secretion, vascular invasion, metastasis, or tumor rupture. In one canine report, owners reported weakness (62%), polyuria-polydipsia (PU/PD) (29%), collapse (29%), vomiting (24%), panting/dyspnea (19%), anorexia (19%), weight loss (14%), and seizures (5%) [15]. With intravascular tumor invasion or thrombus formation, patients might develop a Budd-Chiari-like syndrome marked by ascites accumulation [16]. Upon physical examination, patients may present signs of hypovolemic shock, along with abdominal enlargement and pain, especially if significant abdominal hemorrhage is present (see Chapter 84).

Textbook of Small Animal Emergency Medicine, First Edition. Edited by Kenneth J. Drobatz, Kate Hopper, Elizabeth Rozanski and Deborah C. Silverstein.
© 2019 John Wiley & Sons, Inc. Published 2019 by John Wiley & Sons, Inc.
Companion Website: www.wiley.com/go/drobatz/textbook

Diagnostic Results

If pheochromocytoma is suspected, an electrocardiogram should be performed in order to rule out the presence of tachyarrhythmias. Blood pressure should also be measured in order to rule out a hypertensive crisis, as this was reported in 43–86% of patients [14,15]. In patients with confirmed or suspected hemoabdomen, a packed cell volume along with a serum total protein measurement will help guide resuscitative efforts.

Abdominal ultrasound allows for evaluation for the presence of a mass, detection of potential caval thrombi, peritoneal fluid accumulation, local invasion or metastasis. Three-dimensional imaging such as computed tomography (CT) provides additional information of benefit for surgical planning: local invasion, metastasis, vascular invasion, and thrombus formation [8,17]. Thoracic imaging (radiographs or CT) should be performed in order to rule out metastasis.

Fine needle aspiration of adrenal masses for cytological examination allowed for reliable differentiation between medullar and cortical tumor origin in dogs and cats but was associated with serious complications such as hemorrhage or massive catecholamine release [18,19]. However, impression of surgical specimen following mass resection can be used for cytology.

Numerous studies have investigated the use of catecholamines' and their metabolites' concentrations in plasma and urine in order to diagnose pheochromocytomas [20–25]. Urinary normetanephrine-to-creatinine ratio proved to be superior to epinephrine-, norepinephrine-, or metanephrine-to-creatinine ratios [22]. Dogs with hypercortisolism may also have elevated circulating levels of catecholamines and their metabolites. The urinary normetanephrine-to-creatinine ratio outperformed plasma normetanephrine in differentiating pheochromocytoma patients from those with hypercortisolism [25]. It is prudent to recommend standardizing sampling conditions for those tests and allow the patients to have 30 minutes of rest prior to sampling [26] or consider collecting urine at home (which can be impractical due to the need for sample acidification shortly after collection) [27]. The utility of the clonidine suppression test remains unknown in canine patients [28]. Definitive diagnosis requires histopathology.

Treatment

Patients in need of emergent therapy should be stabilized, in particular those with clinical signs of hypovolemic shock due to abdominal hemorrhage (see Chapters 84 and 170). Patients with serious tachyarrhythmias should receive appropriate antiarrhythmic therapy (see Chapter 53). Hypertensive crisis should be addressed if present (see Chapter 63).

Medical therapy in stable patients aims at controlling the effect of excessive catecholamine secretion. Phenoxybenzamine, an alpha-adrenergic antagonist, at a median dose of 0.6 mg/kg PO q12h for a median period of 20 days prior to surgical removal, lowered the mortality rate from 48% to 13% in patients undergoing adrenalectomy [29]. This finding was not repeated in a more recent but smaller study [7]. The use of beta-blockers has not been reported in veterinary pheochromocytoma patients and should be initiated only after proper alpha-blockade is achieved.

Definitive treatment is obtained by surgery either via an open celiotomy or, for non-invasive masses in stable patients, laparoscopy [30,31].

Surgical Outcome and Prognostic Factors

The immediate postoperative period can be accompanied with significant morbidity and mortality; 18–31% of canine patients that underwent adrenalectomy for pheochromocytoma removal did not survive to the postoperative period [4,29]. Of interest to the emergency clinician, 50% of dogs with acute hemoabdomen due to adrenal tumor rupture died in the perioperative period [5]. Patients with pheochromocytoma had worse short- and long-term survival when compared to those with adrenocortical carcinoma (48% versus 79%). Reported median survival time for those patients was 364 days [32]. Another study presented 1-, 2-, and 3-year survival rates of 83%, 60%, and 60% in dogs with pheochromocytoma undergoing adrenalectomy. Negative prognostic indicators include vena cava invasion and extent of invasion (short but not long term) [7], older age, intraoperative arrhythmias, and prolonged surgical time [29].

Hyperaldosteronism

Aldosterone is a steroid hormone with mineralocorticoid activity produced mainly from the zona glomerulosa of the adrenal cortex. In physiological conditions, aldosterone is secreted in response to angiotensin II release following activation of the RAAS as a consequence of decreased renal arterial perfusion or hyperkalemia. Aldosterone acts within the nephron and vascular endothelial cells to restore fluid volume and increase systemic vascular resistance to maintain systemic arterial blood pressure [33].

Secondary hyperaldosteronism can result from decreased renal perfusion or, rarely, due to excessive renin production from the JGA due to neoplasia or decreased JGA blood flow. Primary hyperaldosteronsim (PHA) refers to autonomous secretion of aldosterone from the adrenal cortex and is the most commonly diagnosed form of the disease. The remainder of this section will focus on this condition.

Incidence

Primary hyperaldosteronism is more frequently diagnosed in cats, but there have been case reports of dogs with the disease [34]. Historically, the prevalence in humans was estimated between 0.01% to 3% of hypertensive patients, but more recent studies have shown the true prevalence to be 5.9% of all hypertensive patients [35] and up to 11.3% of patients with refractory hypertension [36].

Pathophysiology

Primary hyperaldosteronism is caused by autonomous secretion of aldosterone due to adrenocortical adenomas, carcinomas or bilateral adrenocortical hyperplasia. Approximately 63% of the documented cases in cats due to adrenal masses have been attributed to malignant neoplasia. Since definitive diagnosis relies on histopathological evaluation, which rarely occurs in patients without an adrenal mass, the incidence of hyperplastic change is likely underreported [37].

In cases of neoplastic PHA, hyperaldosteronism occurs in the presence of hyporeninism. Due to the effects of aldosterone, the nephron retains both sodium and, consequently, free water, resulting in an increased intravascular volume and systemic hypertension. Despite an absolute increase in total body sodium, these patients generally appear to be normonatremic due to the dilutional effect of the retained water. The potassium-wasting properties of mineralocorticoids often lead to hypokalemia, though 10–12% of feline patients with PHA may remain normokalemic [33,38].

Clinical Signs and Physical Examination

The most common clinical sign is muscle weakness associated with a hypokalemic polymyopathy (including plantigrade stance, cervical ventroflexion, and flaccid paralysis) although severity of clinical signs does not always correlate with severity of electrolyte disturbances. Cats with severe hypertension may present for mydriasis or apparent blindness [39,40]. Cats with PHA and concurrent adrenocortical hormone excess (progesterone or other sex hormones) may present clinical signs as a result of diabetes mellitus or hyperadrenocorticism [41,42].

Diagnostic Results

Most cats with PHA will have normal sodium concentrations but are typically hypokalemic. Complete blood counts and routine biochemical analysis are generally unrewarding other than for evaluation of serum potassium concentration. There is an increasing reported incidence of adrenal hyperplasia and these cats tend to have normo- to mild hypokelamia. Cats with bilateral hyperplasia are more likely to be azotemic but often remain normophosphatemic [37]. Measurement of systemic arterial blood pressure reveals hypertension in the majority of patients.

Abdominal imaging plays a central role in the investigation of any cat with unexplained hypertension or hypokalemia and ultrasonography is a reliable, quick, and non-invasive technique to document the size and architecture of both adrenal glands and kidneys [43]. Sonography should also be used to evaluate for metastatic disease, tumor invasion or evidence of thrombus formation.

Definitive diagnosis is achieved by documentation of elevated plasma aldosterone concentration or aldosterone:renin ratio. The lack of suppression of aldosterone in a fludrocortisone suppression test can be used to confirm hyperaldosteronism [44].

Treatment and Prognosis

Definitive treatment relies on adrenalectomy, which can be performed by either laparotomy or laparoscopy [39,46]. Intraoperative complications include hemorrhage and hypotension, while postoperative complications include pancreatitis, hypoadrenocorticism, and acute kidney injury. Survival rates range from 70% to 77%, with highest mortality in the perioperative period [39,40].

Prior to surgery, medical management should be instituted in order to manage the effects of PHA (hypokalemia and hypertension). Amlodipine besylate should be started at 0.625 mg/cat PO once daily. Its dose should be escalated to achieve a systolic or mean arterial blood pressure less than 150 or 130 mmHg, respectively [45]. To address hypokalemia, both oral potassium supplementation (potassium gluconate 2 mEq/cat twice daily) and mineralocorticoid antagonists (spironolactone, initially 2 mg/kg twice daily) can be combined. Although resolution of the hypokalemia may not occur, its severity generally improves and associated myopathy resolves [40].

Hyperadrenocorticism

Hyperadrenocorticism suggests excessive production of hormones from the adrenal cortex, but in most cases specifically refers to glucocorticoid excess (iatrogenic, pituitary dependent or adrenal dependent). Glucocorticoids are produced by the zona fasciculata and reticularis under the control of the anterior pituitary; their release is regulated by secretion of adrenocorticotropic hormone (ACTH), which is under negative feedback control.

Pathophysiology

Hypercortisolism can occur due to either exogenous administration of glucocorticoids or endogenous overproduction of glucocorticoids. In dogs and cats, approximately 80–85% of the cases are due to pituitary adenoma (either micro- or macroadenomas), leading to hypersecretion of ACTH [47]. Most cases of neurological signs relating to a pituitary tumor are caused by macroadenomas [48]. Approximately 15% of cases of naturally occurring hypercortisolism are caused by functional adrenal tumors, which are malignant roughly half of the time [49]. Rarely, concurrent pituitary and adrenal pathologies are identified [50].

Regardless of the etiopathogenesis, clinical signs primarily relate to glucocorticoid excess. A small population of dogs with functional adrenal tumors will develop clinical signs referable to the presence of an abdominal mass (hemoabdomen or Budd-Chiari-like syndrome).

The mechanisms of thromboembolic disease (such as a pulmomary thromboembolism) in patients with hypercortisolism are not well understood [51] (see Chapter 62).

Clinical Signs and Physical Examination

The clinical signs displayed by animals with Cushing's syndrome are a consequence of the immunosuppressive, catabolic, and anti-inflammatory effects of glucocorticoids. The most common clinical signs include PU/PD, polyphagia, and exercise intolerance or muscle weakness. Other clinical signs in the dog include panting, a pot belly or dermatological manifestations (truncal alopecia, pyoderma, and cutaneous atrophy). In the cat, dermatological abnormalities are the most frequent reason for presentation; cutaneous atrophy can be more severe and patients may present with severe skin lacerations and degloving injuries. Often, cats with Cushing's syndrome have previously been diagnosed with diabetes mellitus and are presented for poorly controlled disease [52].

Most clinical signs of hypercortisolism in the dog are slowly progressive, but rarely they might present in acute respiratory distress due to pulmonary thromboembolic disease. Similarly, thromboemboli can affect other critical systems such as the brain, kidneys, pancreas, or gut [53] (see Chapter 62).

Dogs with moderate to severe disease may present with marked muscle atrophy, abdominal distension, changes to the coat, including bilateral, symmetrical truncal alopecia, as well as evidence of chronic pyoderma, bruising, or calcinosis cutis.

Diagnostic Results

Diagnosis of hypercortisolism is dependent on the presence of appropriate clinical signs and documentation of inappropriate glucocorticoid secretion. Routine laboratory tests may reveal thrombocytosis, elevated alkaline phosphatase activity, hypercholesterolemia, hyperglycemia, or low urine specific gravity, but none of these findings alone confirms its diagnosis. The low-dose dexamethasone suppression test (LDDST) is considered the optimal screening test for Cushing's disease in dogs [54]. In many cases, the clinician may choose to perform a urine cortisol:creatinine ratio (UC:Cr) initially as this test only requires a single urine sample (as opposed to three blood samples, 4 hours apart). These tests rely on a systemically well, calm dog since stress and excitation can lead to false-positive results. As a consequence, neither the LDDST nor UC:Cr should generally be performed in the emergency room setting.

The finding of bilateral adrenomegaly or a solitary adrenal tumor via diagnostic imaging is supportive of the presence of adrenal disease, but should not be the sole criterion upon which a search for endocrine disease is based. Adrenal "incidentalomas" are a common finding in dogs and human meta-analyses suggest that they are unlikely to be a significant finding in patients lacking clinical signs [55], although size greater than 20 mm in a canine study was associated with malignant disease [56].

Thromboelastography, PFA-100 closure times, and fibrinogen activity have been shown to be affected in dogs with Cushing's syndrome [57,58]. Unfortunately, none of these parameters appears to normalize with treatment, even though well-controlled dogs appear to be at lower risk for thromboembolic disease [51].

Treatment and Prognosis

Treatment for the stable dog with hypercortisolism relies on suppression of glucocorticoid synthesis (trilostane, mitotane), adrenalectomy (for patients with functional adrenal tumors) or, potentially, hypophysectomy. Treated dogs generally respond well and have an improved quality of life. In cases of functional adrenal masses, laparoscopic adrenalectomy has been shown to carry a low risk of complications with shorter hospitalization when compared to open approaches [59].

Prognosis for dogs with thromboembolic disease is guarded to grave and treatment is usually empiric (see Chapter 42).

References

1 Rangaswamy M, Kumar SP, Asha M, et al. CT-guided fine needle aspiration cytology diagnosis of extra-adrenal pheochromocytoma. *J Cytol* 2010;27(1):26–28.

2 Wey AC, Moore FM. Right atrial chromaffin paraganglioma in a dog. *J Vet Cardiol* 2012;14(3):459–464.

3 Yanagawa H, Hatai H, Taoda T, et al. A canine case of primary intra-right atrial paraganglioma. *J Vet Med Sci* 2014;76(7):1051–1053.

4 Kyles AE, Feldman EC, De Cock HE, et al. Surgical management of adrenal gland tumors with and without associated tumor thrombi in dogs: 40 cases (1994–2001). *J Am Vet Med Assoc* 2003;223(5):654–662.

5 Lang JM, Schertel E, Kennedy S, et al. Elective and emergency surgical management of adrenal gland tumors: 60 cases (1999–2006). *J Am Anim Hosp Assoc* 2011;47(6):428–435.

6 Massari F, Nicoli S, Romanelli G, et al. Adrenalectomy in dogs with adrenal gland tumors: 52 cases (2002–2008). *J Am Vet Med Assoc* 2011;239(2):216–221.

7 Barrera JS, Bernard F, Ehrhart EJ, et al. Evaluation of risk factors for outcome associated with adrenal gland tumors with or without invasion of the caudal vena cava and treated via adrenalectomy in dogs: 86 cases (1993–2009). *J Am Vet Med Assoc* 2013;242(12):1715–1721.

8 Gregori T, Mantis P, Benigni L, et al. Comparison of computed tomographic and pathologic findings in 17 dogs with primary adrenal neoplasia. *Vet Radiol Ultrasound* 2015;56(2):153–159.

9 Whittemore JC, Preston CA, Kyles AE, et al. Nontraumatic rupture of an adrenal gland tumor causing intra-abdominal or retroperitoneal hemorrhage in four dogs. *J Am Vet Med Assoc* 2001;219(3):329–333.

10 Pintar J, Breitschwerdt EB, Hardie EM, et al. Acute nontraumatic hemoabdomen in the dog: a retrospective analysis of 39 cases (1987–2001). *J Am Anim Hosp Assoc* 2003;39(6):518–522.

11 Aronsohn MG, Dubiel B, Roberts B, et al. Prognosis for acute nontraumatic hemoperitoneum in the dog: a retrospective analysis of 60 cases (2003–2006). *J Am Anim Hosp Assoc* 2009;45(2):72–77.

12 Mak G, Allen J. Simultaneous pheochromocytoma and third-degree atrioventricular block in 2 dogs. *J Vet Emerg Crit Care* 2013;23(6):610–614.

13 Edmondson EF, Bright JM, Halsey CH, et al. Pathologic and cardiovascular characterization of pheochromocytoma-associated cardiomyopathy in dogs. *Vet Pathol* 2015;52(2):338–343.

14 Gilson SD, Withrow SJ, Wheeler SL, et al. Pheochromocytoma in 50 dogs. *J Vet Intern Med* 1994;8(3):228–232.

15 Barthez PY, Marks SL, Woo J, et al. Pheochromocytoma in dogs: 61 cases (1984-1995). *J Vet Intern Med* 1997;11(5): 272–278.

16 Schoeman JP, Stidworthy MF. Budd–Chiari-like syndrome associated with an adrenal phaeochromocytoma in a dog. *J Small Anim Pract* 2001;42(4):191–194.

17 Schultz RM, Wisner ER, Johnson EG, et al. Contrast-enhanced computed tomography as a preoperative indicator of vascular invasion from adrenal masses in dogs. *Vet Radiol Ultrasound* 2009;50(6):625–629.

18 McCorkell SJ, Niles NL. Fine-needle aspiration of catecholamine-producing adrenal masses: a possibly fatal mistake. *Am J Roentgenol* 1985;145(1):113–114.

19 Bertazzolo W, Didier M, Gelain ME, et al. Accuracy of cytology in distinguishing adrenocortical tumors from pheochromocytoma in companion animals. *Vet Clin Pathol* 2014;43(3):453–459.

20 Francis RC, Pickerodt PA, Salewski L, et al. Detection of catecholamines and metanephrines by radio-immunoassay in canine plasma. *Vet J* 2010;183(2):228–231.

21 Kook PH, Grest P, Quante S, et al. Urinary catecholamine and metadrenaline to creatinine ratios in dogs with a phaeochromocytoma. *Vet Rec* 2010;166(6):169–174.

22 Quante S, Boretti FS, Kook PH, et al. Urinary catecholamine and metanephrine to creatinine ratios in dogs with hyperadrenocorticism or pheochromocytoma, and in healthy dogs. *J Vet Intern Med* 2010;24(5):1093–1097.

23 Gostelow R, Bridger N, Syme HM. Plasma-free metanephrine and free normetanephrine measurement for the diagnosis of pheochromocytoma in dogs. *J Vet Intern Med* 2013;27(1):83–90.

24 Green BA, Frank EL. Comparison of plasma free metanephrines between healthy dogs and 3 dogs with pheochromocytoma. *Vet Clin Pathol* 2013;42(4):499–503.

25 Salesov E, Boretti FS, Sieber-Ruckstuhl NS, et al. Urinary and plasma catecholamines and metanephrines in dogs with pheochromocytoma, hypercortisolism, nonadrenal disease and in healthy dogs. *J Vet Intern Med* 2015;29(2):597–602.

26 Pappachan JM, Raskauskiene D, Sriraman R, et al. Diagnosis and management of pheochromocytoma: a practical guide to clinicians. *Curr Hypertens Rep* 2014;16(7):442.

27 Kook PH, Boretti FS, Hersberger M, et al. Urinary catecholamine and metanephrine to creatinine ratios in healthy dogs at home and in a hospital environment and in 2 dogs with pheochromocytoma. *J Vet Intern Med* 2007;21(3):388–393.

28 Van Berkel A, Lenders JW, Timmers HJ. Diagnosis of endocrine disease: biochemical diagnosis of phaeochromocytoma and paraganglioma. *Eur J Endocrinol* 2014;170:R109–119.

29 Herrera MA, Mehl ML, Kass PH, et al. Predictive factors and the effect of phenoxybenzamine on outcome in dogs undergoing adrenalectomy for pheochromocytoma. *J Vet Intern Med* 2008;22(6):1333–1339.

30 Mayhew PD, Culp WT, Hunt GB, et al. Comparison of perioperative morbidity and mortality rates in dogs with noninvasive adrenocortical masses undergoing laparoscopic versus open adrenalectomy. *J Am Vet Med Assoc* 2014;245(9):1028–1035.

31 Pitt K, Mayhew PD, Steffey M, et al. Laparoscopic adrenalectomy for removal of unilateral non-invasive pheochromocytomas in dogs. *Vet Surg* 2016;44:E62.

32 Schwartz P, Kovak JR, Koprowski A, et al. Evaluation of prognostic factors in the surgical treatment of adrenal gland tumors in dogs: 41 cases (1999–2005). *J Am Vet Med Assoc* 2008;232(1):77–84.

33 Djajadiningrat-Laanen S, Galac S, Kooistra H. Primary hyperaldosteronism: expanding the diagnostic net. *J Feline Med Surg* 2011;13:641–650.

34 Donnelly K, DeClue AE, Sharp CR. What is your diagnosis? 12-year-old spayed female Labrador Retriever with a history of polyuria and polydipsia. *J Am Vet Med Assoc* 2012;240:1283–1285.

35 Fogari R, Preti P, Zoppi A, et al. Prevalence of primary aldosteronism among unselected hypertensive patients: a prospective study based on the use of an aldosterone/renin ratio above 25 as a screening test. *Hypertens Res* 2006;30:111–117.

36 Douma S, Petidis K, Doumas M, et al. Prevalence of primary hyperaldosteronism in resistant hypertension: a retrospective observational study. *Lancet* 2008;371:1921–1926.

37 Javadi S, Djajadiningrat-Laanen SC, Kooistra HS, et al. Primary hyperaldosteronism, a mediator of progressive renal disease in cats. *Domest Anim Endocrinol* 2005;28:85–104.

38 Lo AJ, Holt DE, Brown DC, et al. Treatment of aldosterone-secreting adrenocortical tumors in cats by unilateral adrenalectomy: 10 cases (2002–2012). *J Vet Intern Med* 2014;28:137–143.

39 Daniel G, Mahony OM, Markovich JE, et al. Clinical findings, diagnostics and outcome in 33 cats with adrenal neoplasia (2002–2013). *J Feline Med Surg* 2016;18:77–84.

40 Ash RA, Harvey AM, Tasker S. Primary hyperaldosteronism in the cat: a series of 13 cases. *J Feline Med Surg* 2005;7:173–182.

41 DeClue AE, Breshears LA, Pardo ID, et al. Hyperaldosteronism and hyperprogesteronism in a cat with an adrenal cortical carcinoma. *J Vet Intern Med* 2005;19:355–358.

42 Briscoe K, Barrs VR, Foster DF, et al. Hyperaldosteronism and hyperprogesteronism in a cat. *J Feline Med Surg* 2009;11:758–762.

43 Combes A, Stock E, van der Vekens E, et al. Ultrasonographical examination of feline adrenal glands: intra- and inter-observer variability. *J Feline Med Surg* 2014;16:937–942.

44 Matsuda M, Behrend EN, Kemppainen R, et al. Serum aldosterone and cortisol concentrations before and after suppression with fludrocortisone in cats: a pilot study. *J Vet Diagn Invest* 2015;27:361–368.

45 Brown, S., Atkins, C., Bagley, R., Carr, A., Cowgill, L., Davidson, M., . . . Stepien, R. (2007). Guidelines for the identification, evaluation, and management of systemic hypertension in dogs and cats. *J Vet Intern Med*, 21(3), 542–558.

46 Smith RR, Mayhew PD, Berent AC. Laparoscopic adrenalectomy for management of a functional adrenal tumor in a cat. *J Am Vet Med Assoc* 2012;241:368–372.

47 Feldman EC. Distinguishing dogs with functioning adrenocortical tumors from dogs with pituitary-dependent hyperadrenocorticism. *J Am Vet Med Assoc* 1983;183:195–200.

48 Nelson RW, Ihle SL, Feldman EC. Pituitary macroadenomas and macroadenocarcinomas in dogs treated with mitotane for pituitary-dependent hyperadrenocorticism: 13 cases (1981–1986). *J Am Vet Med Assoc* 1989;194:1612–1617.

49 Reusch CE, Feldman EC. Canine hyperadrenocorticism due to adrenocortical neoplasia – pretreatment evaluation of 41 dogs. *J Vet Intern Med* 1991;5:3–10.

50 Greco DS, Peterson ME, Davidson AP, et al. Concurrent pituitary and adrenal tumors in dogs with hyperadrenocorticism: 17 cases (1978–1995). *J Am Vet Med Assoc* 1999;214:1349–1353.

51 Pace SL, Creevy KE, Krimer PM, et al. Assessment of coagulation and potential biochemical markers for hypercoagulability in canine hyperadrenocorticism. *J Vet Intern Med* 2013;27:1113–1120.

52 Valentin SY, Cortright CC, Nelson RW, et al. Clinical findings, diagnostic test results, and treatment outcome in cats with spontaneous hyperadrenocorticism: 30 cases. *J Vet Intern Med* 2014;28:481–487.

53 Coelho MC, Santos CV, Vieira Neto L, et al. Adverse effects of glucocorticoids: coagulopathy. *Eur J Endocrinol* 2015;173:M11–21.

54 Behrend EN, Kooistra HS, Nelson R, et al. Diagnosis of spontaneous canine hyperadrenocorticism: 2012 ACVIM consensus statement (small animal). *J Vet Intern Med* 2013;27:1292–1304.

55 Loh HH, Yee A, Loh HS, et al. The natural progression and outcomes of adrenal incidentaloma: a systematic review and meta-analysis. *Minerva Endocrinol* 2017;42:77–87.

56 Cook AK, Spaulding KA, Edwards JF. Clinical findings in dogs with incidental adrenal gland lesions determined by ultrasonography: 151 cases (2007–2010). *J Am Vet Med Assoc* 2014;244(10):1181–1185.

57 Park FM, Blois SL, Abrams-Ogg AC, et al. Hypercoagulability and ACTH-dependent hyperadrenocorticism in dogs. *J Vet Intern Med* 2013;27:1136–1142.

58 Kol A, Nelson RW, Gosselin RC, et al. Characterization of thrombelastography over time in dogs with hyperadrenocorticism. *Vet J* 2013;197:675–681.

59 Mayhew PD, Culp WTN, Hunt GB, et al. Comparison of perioperative morbidity and mortality rates in dogs with noninvasive adrenocortical masses undergoing laparoscopic versus open adrenalectomy. *J Am Vet Med Assoc* 2014;245:1028–1035.

115

Hypoadrenocorticism
Søren Boysen, DVM, DACVECC

Faculty of Veterinary Medicine, University of Calgary, Calgary, AB, Canada

Etiology and Pathogenesis

Anatomy and Pathophysiology

The adrenal glands are located at the craniomedial poles of the kidneys. They are composed of an outer cortex (90%) surrounding the inner medulla (10%). The cortex consists of three distinct layers, which from the serosal surface inward include the zona glomerulosa, zona fasiculata, and zona reticularis. The cortex secretes mineralocorticoids (aldosterone) from the zona glomerulosa, glucocorticoids (cortisol) from the zona fasiculata, and androgens (e.g. androstenedione, dehydroepiandrosterone) from the zona reticulara. Hypoadrenocorticism involves all three zones of the adrenal cortex, with clinical signs most attributable to loss of mineralocorticoid and glucocorticoid activity. It is reported that up to 90% of the adrenal cortex must be destroyed before clinical signs become evident (Web Figure 115.1a and 115.1b) [1,2].

There are two general categories of hypoadrenocorticism: primary and secondary. Primary hypoadrenocorticism is much more common in dogs than cats (>95% of cases). In dogs, it is believed to result from immune-mediated damage to all three layers of the adrenal cortex (Table 115.1) [1]. Nova Scotia duck tolling retrievers, standard poodles, bearded collies, and Portuguese water dogs have been identified as having a genetic predisposition [3–5]. Primary hypoadrenocorticism is also over-represented in the Great Dane, West Highland white terrier, St Bernard, wheaten terrier, leonberger, basset hound, Airdale terrier, springer spaniel, and rottweiler [1,6,7]. Females tend to be more commonly affected (70% of cases) and the median age of onset in dogs is 4 years (range 4 months to 14 years) [1]. Dogs and cats with primary hypoadrenocorticism (70–90%) will have both glucocorticoid and mineralocorticoid deficiencies and will present with electrolyte abnormalities [1,2]. Primary

Table 115.1 Causes of hypoadrenocorticism in dogs.

Primary causes	Secondary causes
Most common:	**Most common:**
Immune mediated	Iatrogenic secondary to withdrawal of exogenous corticosteroid administration (rarely causes clinical signs)
Uncommon:	**Uncommon:**
Iatrogenic drug induced (e.g. mitotane or trilostane)	Idiopathic
Rare causes:	**Rare causes:**
Granulomatous destruction (e.g. blastomycosis, histoplasmosis, cryptococcosis)	Surgical induced
Amyloidosis	Head trauma
Hemorrhagic infarction (secondary to trauma, infection, necrosis, or coagulopathy)	
Metastatic neoplasia (lymphoma and bilateral anaplastic neoplasia)	
Bilateral abscessing adrenalitis	
Adrenal suppressors (e.g. ketoconazole, etomidate)	

hypoadrenocorticism resulting in only glucocorticoid deficiency and the absence of electrolyte imbalances is uncommon, but has been reported in dogs [6].

Secondary hypoadrenocorticism is much less common (<5% of canine and feline cases) and results from abnormal pituitary gland (a lack of ACTH secretion) or hypothalamic function (a lack of corticotropin-releasing hormone (CRH) secretion). Examples of secondary hypoadrenocorticism include trauma and neoplasia of the pituitary gland or hypothalamus (see Table 115.1). Secondary hypoadrenocorticism tends to result in a lack

Textbook of Small Animal Emergency Medicine, First Edition. Edited by Kenneth J. Drobatz, Kate Hopper, Elizabeth Rozanski and Deborah C. Silverstein.
© 2019 John Wiley & Sons, Inc. Published 2019 by John Wiley & Sons, Inc.
Companion Website: www.wiley.com/go/drobatz/textbook

of cortisol production while mineralocorticoid levels are preserved (due to atrophy of the zona fasciculata and zona reticularis, with the zona glomerulosa remaining unaffected) [1,2,8]. Therapy differs between primary and secondary causes so it is important to differentiate the two conditions (see Table 115.1).

Mineralocorticoid Deficiency

Aldosterone is vital to maintaining normal sodium, potassium, and water homeostasis through sodium, chloride, and water reabsorption and potassium excretion. The primary site of action is the renal tubule, although aldosterone also plays a role in regulating the gastrointestinal (GI) tract as well as the salivary and sweat glands.

Sodium, Chloride, and Water Homeostasis
Aldosterone deficiency causes increased loss of sodium, chloride, and water via the urine. This contributes to dehydration, prerenal azotemia, unconcentrated urine, hypovolemia, weakness, and shock. Specifically, aldosterone acts on the principal cells of the collecting tubules of the kidney to increase the absorption of sodium. When sodium is reabsorbed via tubular epithelial cells, negative ions such as chloride move with sodium due to electrical potentials. Water is reabsorbed passively as it follows the concentration gradients between the tubular lumen and renal interstitium created by the reabsorption of sodium and chloride [9]. Aldosterone also plays an important role in sodium absorption in the GI tract, particularly in the colon [10,11]. Aldosterone deficiency impairs GI sodium absorption, which also leads to a decrease in chloride and water absorption from the GI lumen. Decreased absorption of GI electrolytes and water contributes to diarrhea, which is often accompanied by vomiting, both of which can further exacerbate extracellular fluid losses and hypovolemia.

With ongoing extracellular fluid loss, intravascular volume can eventually become depleted, leading to hypoperfusion and shock. Death occurs in the untreated patient 4 days to 2 weeks following a complete cessation of mineralocorticoid secretion [9].

Potassium Homeostasis
Aldosterone deficiency can lead to marked hyperkalemia, which is further exaggerated by hypovolemia and decreased glomerular filtration rate (GFR). Plasma potassium concentration is primarily regulated by the action of aldosterone on the renal excretion of potassium and the movement of potassium between extracellular and intracellular compartments [9]. Acidosis is also common in patients with hypoadrenocorticism, which will shift potassium out of cells, contributing to hyperkalemia [12]. One of the more serious sequelae of

hyperkalemia is abnormal cardiac conduction leading to prolonged refractory periods of the cardiac action potential, which can lead to clinically significant bradycardia, atrial standstill, decreased cardiac output, and in severe cases ventricular fibrillation and death (see Chapter 109) [13,14].

Acid–Base Homeostasis
Aldosterone plays a role in the secretion of hydrogen ions (in exchange for sodium) by the intercalated cells of the cortical collecting tubules of the kidneys [9]. In the absence of confounding factors, a mild acidosis develops secondary to aldosterone deficiency. However, during an adrenal crisis in a patient with hypoadrenocorticism, the absence of aldosterone in conjunction with lactic acidosis and decreased GFR (secondary to hypoperfusion) can lead to a marked acidosis (see Chapter 107).

Glucocorticoid Deficiency

Cortisol plays an important role in numerous homeostatic processes. The role of cortisol in regulating blood pressure, blood volume, and blood glucose concentration contributes to some of the more serious complications in patients with hypoadrenocorticism. Cortisol stimulates the release of vasoactive substances, sensitizes blood vessels to the effects of catecholamine, and decreases blood vessel permeability [9]. Cortisol also plays an important role in gluconeogenesis. In the absence of cortisol, intravascular volume decreases, blood pressure falls, and hypoglycemia can develop [9]. Cortisol deficiency may also contribute to GI ileus, further exacerbating diarrhea and vomiting [10].

Cortisol also contributes to sodium homeostasis along with aldosterone [13]. There are reports of hypoadrenocorticism being associated with hyponatremia when mineralocorticoid activity is normal [15]. Cortisol inhibits the release of antidiuretic hormone (ADH). In the absence of cortisol, ADH levels are elevated, causing increased water resorption at the kidneys, which subsequently dilutes the plasma sodium concentration [13].

Patient Evaluation

History and Physical Examination Findings

The history in patients with hypoadrenocorticism can be non-specific and may include vomiting, diarrhea, melena, polyuria/polydipsia, ataxia, tremors or seizures, lethargy, anorexia, weight loss, and inactivity (Tables 115.2 and 115.3). These clinical signs may wax and wane over time. Many dogs will have a history of primary GI signs that may have previously responded to fluid and/or

Table 115.2 Most common findings in canine patients with hypoadrenocorticism.

History	Physical exam findings	Laboratory/diagnostic findings
Lethargy 95%	Depression 95%	**Complete blood count:**
Inappetence 90%	Weakness 75%	Lack of stress leukogram 92%
Weakness 75%	Dehydration 45%	Neutrophilia 32%
Vomiting 75%	Bradycardia%	Non-regenerative anemia 25–27%
Diarrhea 40%	Hypothermia 35%	Eosinophilia 20%
Weight loss 50%	Collapse 35%	Lymphocytosis 10%
Waxing and waning course 40%	Prolonged capillary refill time 30%	**Chemistry:**
Prior response to therapy 35%	Melena 20%	Sodium:potassium ratio <27 95%
Shivering and/or muscle stiffness 25%	Weak pulses 20%	Hyperkalemia 85–95%
Polyuria 25%	Bradycardia 18%	Azotemia 85–88%
Polydipsia 25%	Painful abdomen 8%	Hyponatremia 81–82%
		Hypochloremia 40–68%
		Hyperphosphataemia 68%
		Acidosis (low bicarbonate) 40–57%
		Elevated liver enzymes 30–50%
		Hypercalcemia 18–40%
		Hypoalbuminemia 6–39%
		Hypoglycemia 10–30%
		Hypocalcemia 25%
		Hyperglycemia 18%
		Elevated lactate 14%
		Hypocholesterolemia 7%
		Urine specific gravity <1.030 60%

Source: Adapted from Feldman et al. [48], Peterson et al. [7], Adler et al. [16], Kintzer and Peterson [2].

Table 115.3 Most common findings in feline patients with primary hypoadrenocorticism.

History	Physical exam findings	Laboratory/diagnostic findings
Lethargy 100%	Dehydration 86%	**Complete blood count:**
Anorexia/decreased appetite 95%	Weakness 73%	Anemia 27%
Weight loss 77%	Hypothermia 68%	Lymphocytosis 27%
Vomiting 55%	Weak pulse 45%	Eosinophilia 9%
Waxing-waning course 32%	Slow capillary refill time 41%	**Chemistry:**
Prior response to therapy 27%	Bradycardia 23%	Sodium-to-potassium ration <27 100%
Polyuria and polydipsia 27%	Collapse/inability to rise 23%	Hyponatremia 95%
Dysphagia 4%	Constipation 9%	Hyperkalemia 91%
	Painful abdomen 4%	Azotaemia 82%
		Hypochloremia 73%
		Hyperphosphatemia 68%
		Low total CO_2 (metabolic acidosis) 26%
		Elevated liver enzymes 25%
		Hypercalcemia 23%
		*Hypoglycemia: 7%
		Urine specific gravity < 1.030 74%

* Low normal glucose concentrations are often reported in cats with hypoadrenocorticism.

Source: Adapted from Peterson et al. [43], Kasabalis et al. [44], Sicken and Neiger [45], Spalla et al.[46], and Woolcock and Ward [47].

glucocorticoid therapy. A precipitating stressful event may also be evident in some cases. The duration of illness is reportedly longer (average 4 months) in dogs with only glucocorticoid deficiency compared to those with both mineralocorticoid and glucocorticoid deficiency (average 1 month) [6]. Hypothermia, bradycardia, weak pulses, dehydration, ataxia, collapse, and abnormal respiratory pattern may be noted in some cases (see Tables 115.2 and 115.3). Clinical signs tend to be milder in dogs with only glucocorticoid deficiency that maintain normal electrolytes (secondary hypoadrenocorticism or a small number of cases with primary hypoadrenocorticism) [6].

Shock is more likely in dogs with both glucocorticoid and mineralocorticoid deficiency than cases with just glucocorticoid deficiency [6]. Patients presenting in shock with concurrent bradycardia should prompt consideration of diseases leading to hyperkalemia, including hypoadrenocorticism.

Feline Hypoadrenocorticism

Hypoadrenocorticism is extremely rare in cats, with fewer than 50 cases having been reported in the literature. Clinical findings in cats are similar to those in dogs and humans, with lethargy, anorexia, and weight loss being the most common signs reported by owners and depression, dehydration, weakness, and hypothermia being the most common physical exam findings (see Table 115.3).

Diagnosis

Emergency Cage-Side Tests and Imaging

An emergency minimum database should be collected in patients presenting with an acute adrenal crisis and shock. This may vary by patient but typically includes blood pressure measurement, biochemistry (glucose, urea, creatinine, lactate, electrolytes, total solids, packed cell volume), acid–base status, electrocardiogram (ECG), and abdominal and thoracic focused assessment with sonography to detect free fluid in the abdominal and thoracic cavities, respectively. Imaging is often undertaken in patients with GI signs or undifferentiated shock. Patients with hypoadrenocorticism may have bilateral adrenal atrophy noted on abdominal sonography (in cases of primary hypoadrenocorticism), but a finding of normal-sized adrenal glands on ultrasound should not preclude a diagnosis of hypoadrenocorticism [16,17]. Radiographs are often unremarkable or may show evidence of hypovolemia, including microcardia, decreased pulmonary vessel vasculature, and a narrowed caudal vena cava (Figure 115.1). Rarely, megesophagus will be

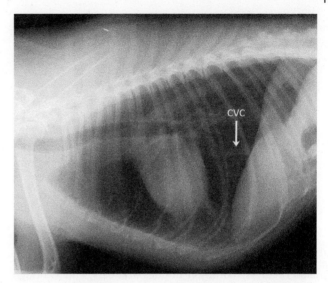

Figure 115.1 Left lateral thoracic radiograph of a collie cross dog with hypoadrenocorticism. Note the marked microcardia and narrowing of the caudal vena cava (CVC, *white arrow*), consistent with marked hypovolemia.

noted on thoracic radiographs, which is reversible with medical therapy of hypoadrenocorticism.

Complete Blood Count (CBC)

The absence of a stress leukogram (neutrophilia, lymphopenia, monocytosis, and eosinopenia) in a sick patient should prompt consideration of hypoadrenocorticism, but most dogs and cats with hypoadrenocorticism will have variable leukocyte counts [1,6–8,18]. It has been reported that the lymphocyte count is the most reliable CBC parameter in dogs with hypoadrenocorticism and the presence of lymphocytosis in the sick dog should prompt consideration of hypoadrenocorticism [18]. Similarly, eosinophilia or lymphocytosis in a sick cat should prompt consideration of hypoadrenocorticism in the absence of another explanation.

Serum Chemistry Panel

The most frequent findings on the serum chemistry profile in dogs and cats with hypoadrenocorticism include hyperkalemia, hyponatremia, and azotemia (see Tables 115.2 and 115.3) [2,6,16]. Although the sodium:potassium ratio of <27 is considered very sensitive and specific for hypoadrenocorticism, some dogs with hypoadrenocorticism will have ratios >27, particularly in rare cases of glucocorticoid deficiency without concurrent mineralocorticoid deficiency [16,18]. Other conditions including GI disease, parasitic infection (e.g. *Trichuris vulpus*), third space losses, congestive heart failure, and diabetes mellitus can also result in sodium:potassium ratios <27 in both dogs and cats. However, a ratio <27 should raise suspicion for hypoadrenocorticism and ratios of ≤20 are very suggestive of hypoadrenocorticism, warranting strong consideration of ACTH stimulation testing [16,18].

Azotemia is most likely prerenal in origin as a result of hypovolemia, hypoperfusion, and decreased renal perfusion. Patients should be monitored during fluid resuscitation and rehydration to ensure that azotemia is resolving and that renal insufficiency is not present. Urine specific gravity cannot be relied on to differentiate prerenal from renal causes of azotemia as many patients with hypoadrenocorticism will have medullary washout secondary to hyponatremia, which results in an inappropriately low USG in the face of azotemia (see Tables 115.2 and 115.3).

Hypoproteinemia and hypoalbuminemia are relatively common in dogs as a result of increased GI protein losses and decreased hepatic synthesis. Hypercalcemia is also relatively common in dogs and cats, and although the exact cause of hypercalcemia is uncertain, it tends to resolve quickly following glucocorticoid therapy [2]. In very rare cases, hypoglycemia associated with hypoadrenocorticism may result in seizures in both dogs and cats but tends to resolve quickly following IV dextrose and glucocorticoid therapy. Hypocholesterolemia, increased liver enzymes, and metabolic acidosis have also been reported (see Tables 115.2 and 115.3). Non-specific biochemical changes including anemia, hypocholesterolemia, hypercalcemia, hypoglycemia, and hypoalbuminemia in patients with vague clinical signs should prompt consideration of glucocorticoid deficiency.

Resting or Basal Serum Cortisol Levels

Measurement of resting cortisol level is rapid and inexpensive to perform. Only 1% of dogs with hypoadrenocorticism have values >2 μg/dL, which makes the diagnosis very unlikely when the resting cortisol is >2 μg/dL. However, 21% of dogs with non-adrenal disease may have values <2 μg/dL [19,20], so an ACTH stimulation test should be performed to confirm the diagnosis in patients with resting cortisol <2 μg/dL.

ACTH Stimulation Testing

Adrenocorticotropin hormone (ACTH) stimulation testing is the definitive test for hypoadrenocorticism. A serum cortisol concentration ≤2 μg/dL pre- and 1 hour post ACTH administration in dogs (30 minutes post for cats) is considered diagnostic of hypoadrenocorticism in the absence of exposure to exogenous corticosteroids or mitotane [6].

Protocols for ACTH administration vary between product manufacturers and it is important to read manufacturer directions when performing ACTH stimulation testing. Liquid formulations and sterile powders requiring reconstitution with sterile saline have been used with equivocal results [21–23]. Several authors have recommended avoiding ACTH gel preparations as they do not produce reliable ACTH stimulation test results [24,25]. Numerous studies have demonstrated that 5 μg/kg (or lower) doses given IV (check product routes of administration) produce reliable adrenal stimulation in dogs, and current recommendations are to administer ACTH at 5 μg/kg IV (up to a maximum dose of 250 μg) [21,24,26]. Current recommendations in cats are to use a single 125 μg dose IV.

Most exogenous glucocorticoids falsely elevate cortisol assays so administration of these medications should be avoided until after ACTH stimulation testing is performed. The exception is dexamethasone, which does not interfere with cortisol assays and should be used if emergency glucocorticoid therapy is required prior to ACTH stimulation testing. It has been suggested to wait 24–48 hours before performing an ACTH stimulation test if short-acting glucocorticoids (with the exception of dexamethasone) have been administered, or longer (up to several weeks) if glucocorticoids have been used chronically [1,24].

It may be helpful to perform ACTH stimulation testing in dogs and cats with vague non-specific symptoms in which another cause cannot be found, particularly if GI signs are present. Particularly in dogs, it is reasonable to perform ACTH stimulation testing to rule out hypoadrenocorticism before more invasive testing such as endoscopy and exploratory laparotomy is undertaken.

Cortisol-to-Adrenocorticotropic Hormone Ratio

Recent studies suggest that the cortisol-to-adrenocorticotropic hormone ratio (CAR) could potentially be used in place of the ACTH stimulation test for diagnosis of hypoadrenocorticism [27,28]. The advantage of the CAR compared to ACTH stimulation testing is the need for only a single blood sample from which both serum cortisol and plasma ACTH concentrations can be measured. However, differentiation between dogs with hypoadrenocorticism and those with diseases mimicking hypoadrenocorticism is not 100% [28]. In addition, the reliability of the CAR in diagnosing secondary hypoadrenocorticism requires further investigation.

Primary Versus Secondary Hypoadrenocorticism

Primary and secondary causes of hypoadrenocorticism cannot be differentiated based on results of ACTH stimulation testing. When electrolyte imbalances are present, it is highly probable that the patient has primary hypoadrenocorticism, indicating that mineralocorticoid therapy will be required for chronic management. In cases where there are no electrolyte imbalances, it is difficult to determine whether the cause is primary or secondary and whether the patient is likely to require mineralocorticoid therapy in the future. Secondary causes are unlikely to develop electrolyte imbalances and therefore unlikely to require mineralocorticoid therapy, while many primary cases will progress to develop electrolyte imbalances and eventually need mineralocorticoid therapy.

To differentiate primary from secondary causes, endogenous plasma ACTH concentrations must be evaluated; plasma endogenous ACTH concentration is high in primary hypoadrenocorticism due to loss of feedback inhibition from cortisol on pituitary function, while plasma endogenous ACTH concentration is low in secondary hypoadrenocorticism due to decreased release of ACTH from the pituitary gland.

Consultation with the local reference laboratory is recommended regarding the best way to collect and handle sampling for endogenous plasma ACTH concentration.

Treatment

The most life-threatening presentation in animals with hypoadrenocorticism is shock. Initial therapy should involve improving tissue perfusion via restoration of intravascular volume, correction of life-threatening arrhythmias, correcting electrolyte imbalances, correcting hypoglycemia, and administering rapid-acting intravenous glucocorticoids (see Chapter 153). Once the patient is stable, differentiating primary from secondary hypoadrenocorticism and correcting any underlying causes should be undertaken. It should be noted that although dogs generally tend to respond quickly to therapy for acute adrenal crisis, cats may take 3–5 days before they show improvement despite appropriate therapy.

Fluid Therapy

Intravenous fluid resuscitation should be initiated when shock is first identified and should not be delayed until a definitive diagnosis of hypoadrenocorticism is confirmed (see Chapter 153 for treatment of hypovolemic shock). Early aggressive fluid therapy in patients with hypoadrenocorticism helps to address hypovolemic shock and can help rapidly correct hyperkalemia through plasma dilution and increased renal excretion of potassium. A small proportion of dogs [29] that develop gastrointestinal hemorrhage (present in roughly 15% of dogs with hypoadrenocorticism) [7] will have severe anemia, which may require a blood transfusion depending on the hematocrit and response to fluid therapy (see Chapter 176).

Isotonic crystalloids are a reasonable initial fluid choice in patients with hypoadrenocorticism (see Chapter 167).

There are no studies in veterinary medicine that demonstrate a benefit of one particular isotonic crystalloid over another for treating hypoadrenocorticism. Any commercially available balanced isotonic crystalloid solution will decrease potassium levels through dilution, help correct acid–base imbalances, and improve renal perfusion. Historically, normal saline was the fluid of choice to correct hypovolemia, hyperkalemia, and hyponatremia in veterinary patients with hypoadrenocorticism because it restores intravascular volume, does not contain potassium, and is relatively high in sodium compared to other isotonic crystalloids [12,14]. However, due to the risk of central pontine myelinolysis, which has been reported in dogs that are markedly hyponatremic [30–33], isotonic crystalloids that are lower in sodium concentration (e.g. lactated Ringer's solution or Plasma-Lyte 148) may be a better alternative in the initial management of patients with hypoadrenocorticism. An initial bolus of normal saline followed by boluses of another isotonic crystalloid can also be used if the patient has marked hyperkalemia.

Strong evidence to support a maximal rate of increase in sodium concentration to prevent central pontine myelinolysis is lacking, but it has been suggested that the rate of increase in sodium should not be faster than 0.5 mEq/L/h. To ensure sodium levels do not increase too rapidly, electrolytes should be monitored frequently and fluid therapy adjusted in accordance with the rate of change in electrolytes.

Hyperkalemia

Fluid resuscitation is essential in correcting hyperkalemia through dilution of serum potassium concentration, increased GFR, and correction of acidosis. The vast majority of hyperkalemic patients with hypoadrenocorticism will respond well to fluid therapy alone, and do not require additional therapy to address the hyperkalemia. However, in patients with relevant ECG changes consistent with hyperkalemia (absent P-wave, spiked T-waves, prolonged QRS complexes, bradycardia, atrial standstill, and sinoventricular complexes) [13,14] to the point where cardiac output is decreased and contributing to hypoperfusion, additional therapy for hyperkalemia is warranted (see Chapter 109). This consists of antagonizing the effects of hyperkalemia on myocardial cells concurrent with efforts to reduce the serum potassium concentration.

Calcium gluconate (10% solution) given IV (0.5–1.0 mL/kg to effect over 5–10 min) does not decrease serum potassium levels but will antagonize the cardiotoxic effects of hyperkalemia for 30–60 minutes. The advantage of calcium gluconate is that its cardioprotective effects occur very rapidly and much sooner than other therapies can decrease serum potassium levels.

Patients should be monitored closely with an ECG during administration of calcium gluconate, and calcium gluconate administration should be discontinued if the heart rate falls or if other significant ECG findings (ST segment elevation or arrhythmias) develop. Restarting the infusion at a slower rate once the ECG changes resolve can be attempted [34]. The goal of calcium gluconate therapy is to stabilize cardiac function long enough to allow other therapies to decrease the serum potassium concentration [35].

A dextrose bolus alone (0.5–1.0 mL/kg 50% dextrose dilute to <25% with isotonic crystalloids) or in combination with insulin (regular crystalline insulin 0.1–0.2 U/kg IV) can be administered to decrease serum potassium levels. Intravenous dextrose administration increases endogenous insulin secretion from the pancreas and will shift potassium intracellularly, decreasing serum potassium concentrations up to 0.5–1 mEq/L within an hour [13,14]. The effects can last up to 6 hours. Administering IV insulin along with dextrose produces a more pronounced and rapid decrease in serum potassium levels. Insulin should only be given with an accompanying IV dextrose bolus and an IV CRI of dextrose (add 50% dextrose to IV fluids to make a 2.5–5% solution) for at least 6 hours to prevent iatrogenic hypoglycemia. Ideally, the serum glucose concentration should be measured hourly for at least 6 hours following IV insulin administration.

Alternatively, sodium bicarbonate (1–2 mEq/L) IV can be used to decrease serum potassium by shifting potassium intracellularly in exchange for hydrogen ions (see Chapter 174). The disadvantage of sodium bicarbonate is that it takes longer to decrease serum potassium concentrations compared to the administration of dextrose and regular insulin. It is also important to ensure patients have sufficient ventilation when giving sodium bicarbonate to avoid development of paradoxical central nervous system acidosis. Other concerns associated with administration of sodium bicarbonate include a transient decline in mean arterial pressure after rapid intravenous administration, decreased ionized calcium concentration (which may affect left ventricular contractility), and decreased oxygen delivery caused by decreased unloading of oxygen from hemoglobin at the tissue level (e.g. Bohr effect) [36–39]. In addition, overshoot alkalosis may occur when lactate is metabolized (which results in bicarbonate production) following other resuscitative efforts. There is also evidence to suggest sodium bicarbonate is less effective at decreasing serum potassium concentration in human patients with hyperkalemia when compared to other treatment modalities [40]. For this reason, it is becoming less common in human ICUs as a monotherapy or as part of a combination therapy to treat hyperkalemia [40].

Nebulized albuterol has been prescribed in people for therapy of hyperkalemia, particularly in renal failure patients receiving hemodialysis (10–20 mg monotherapy can reduce K+ by 0.6–1.0 mEq/L [41] or 1.2 mEq/L when a 20 mg dose is combined with insulin) [42]. Studies investigating the use of inhaled or IV albuterol in hyperkalemic veterinary patients are lacking although the use of terbutaline has been described in a cat.

In most cases, the combination of IV fluid boluses, calcium gluconate, and IV dextrose with regular insulin will be sufficient to decrease hyperkalemia without the need for sodium bicarbonate or albuterol.

Acidosis

The acidosis seen with an acute adrenal crisis tends to be the result of hypoperfusion (causing decreased renal perfusion and lactic acidosis) rather than the direct effect of aldosterone deficiency on hydrogen excretion by the kidney. Therefore, most cases of acidosis will resolve following initial fluid resuscitation and rarely require treatment with sodium bicarbonate.

Glucocorticoids

Patients presenting in an acute adrenal crisis should have rapid-acting IV glucocorticoids administered as soon as possible. In veterinary medicine, dexamethasone (0.2–0.25 mg/kg IV q12–24h) is probably the most commonly used glucocorticoid as it can be given IV, is fast acting, and does not interfere with ACTH stimulation testing. Dexamethasone should be started concurrent with or as soon as possible following IV catheter placement and fluid resuscitation in patients with an acute adrenal crisis. Other glucocorticoids including prednisone, prednisolone, and hydrocortisone interfere with ACTH stimulation testing and should therefore be avoided until after a diagnosis is confirmed or stimulation testing has been performed.

There is no rapid-acting IV mineralocorticoid for treatment of an adrenal crisis and most animals in an adrenal crisis respond well to fluid therapy, correction of hyperkalemia, and IV dexamethasone. Mineralocorticoid therapy is not generally required until electrolytes have been corrected and the animal is stable following initial therapy. Mineralocorticoid administration should generally be avoided early in the course of treatment while serum sodium concentrations are still low, because they may increase sodium concentrations more quickly and predispose the patient to central pontine myelinolysis.

Chronic Management

Patients diagnosed with hypoadrenocorticism and classic electrolyte imbalances require lifelong glucocorticoid and mineralocorticoid therapy. Patients with normal electrolytes diagnosed with primary hypoadrenocorticism require glucocorticoid therapy and close electrolyte monitoring as they are very likely to progress and require mineralocorticoid therapy. Patients with secondary hypoadrenocorticism will require lifelong glucocorticoid therapy but are very unlikely to need mineralocorticoid therapy.

Long-term mineralocorticoid supplementation in dogs can be provided by oral administration of fludrocortisone (0.02 mg/kg PO q24h or divided and given twice daily with a daily increase of 0.05–0.1 mg increments until serum electrolyte concentrations are stable). Fludrocortisone does have some glucocorticoid activity but some dogs may still need additional prednisone supplementation, particularly in stressful situations [14]. Alternatively, mineralocorticoid supplementation can be provided to dogs with an injection of deoxycorticosterone pivalate (DOCP; 2 mg/kg SC or IM q25 days) [35]. DOCP does not possess any glucocorticoid activity so prednisone (0.22 mg/kg PO SID) is often required concurrently. Cats are generally treated with DOCP (2.2 mg/kg or 12.5 mg/cat) SQ q3–4 weeks) and daily oral prednisone (0.22 mg/kg q24h) [43]. If cat owners are having difficulty with oral medications then methylprednisolone acetate (Depo-Medrol; 10 mg/cat SC every 3–4 weeks) has been suggested by some authors to replace oral prednisone therapy [14,43].

Complications

Major complications of an acute adrenal crisis are rare, but central pontine myelinolysis and acute renal failure have been reported [24,30,31]. Central pontine myelinolysis results in neurological signs and is more likely in cases of severe chronic hyponatremia (>48 h) that is corrected too rapidly. Neurological signs may not occur until days to weeks after the crisis. Diagnosis of central pontine myelinolysis can be difficult, because it requires MRI and lesions may not be detectable with MRI for up to 4 weeks after an adrenal crisis.

There is no specific treatment for the condition and neurological abnormalities may be irreversible. There is evidence in humans that dexamethasone may be protective against the development of central pontine myelinolysis if administered early (within 3 hours of starting fluid therapy). Correcting sodium, no faster than 0.5 mEq/L/h, may also decrease the chances of occurrence. Acute renal failure is likely the result of hypoperfusion secondary to hypovolemia and decreased cardiac function leading to renal ischemia. Early aggressive therapy to improve hypoperfusion and close monitoring of renal parameters are recommended to decrease the likelihood of developing acute renal failure and to help differentiate the condition from prerenal azotemia that often accompanies an acute adrenal crisis.

Outcome

Prognosis for patients with hypoadrenocorticism is good to excellent following successful management of an acute adrenal crisis. Most dogs with hypoadrenocorticism die from unrelated diseases and a normal quality of life and life expectancy have been reported [24,43]. However, lifelong therapy is required and an increase in glucocorticoid therapy is often necessary during periods of stress (e.g. travel, surgery, etc.).

References

1 Scott-Moncrieff CJ. Hypoadrenocorticism. In: *Canine and Feline Endocrinology*, 4th edn (eds Feldman E, Nelson R, Reusch C, et al.). Elsevier, St Louis, 2015, pp. 485–516.
2 Kintzer PP, Peterson ME. Hypoadrenocorticism. In: *Kirk's Current Veterinary Therapy XIV* (eds Bonagura JD, Twedt DC). Elsevier, St Louis, 2009, pp. 231–235.
3 Oberbauer AM, Benemann KS, Belanger JM, et al. Inheritance of hypoadrenocorticism in bearded collies. *Am J Vet Res* 2002;63:643–647.
4 Famula TR, Belanger JM, Oberbauer AM. Heritability and complex segregation analysis of hypoadrenocorticism in the standard poodle. *J Small Anim Pract* 2003;44:8–12.
5 Hughes AM, Nelson RW, Famula TR, et al. Clinical features and heritability of hypoadrenocorticism in Nova Scotia duck tolling retrievers:25 cases (1994–2006). *J Am Vet Med Assoc* 2007;231:407–412.
6 Thompson AL, Scott-Moncrieff JC, Anderson JD. Comparison of classic hypoadrenocorticism with glucocorticoid-deficient hypoadrenocorticism in dogs: 46 cases (1985–2005). *J Am Vet Med Assoc* 2007;230:1190–1194.
7 Peterson ME, Kintzer PP, Kass PH. Pretreatment clinical and laboratory findings in dogs with hypoadrenocorticism: 225cases (1979–1993). *J Am Vet Med Assoc* 1996;208:85–91.
8 Tyler J, Lathan P. Canine hypoadrenocorticism: pathogenesis and clinical features. *Compend Cont Educ Pract* 2005;27:110–120.
9 Guyton AC, Hall JE. Adrenocortical hormones. In: *Textbook of Medical Physiology*, 12th edn (eds Guyton AC,

Hall JE). Elsevier Saunders, Philadelphia, 2010, pp. 1695–1720.

10 Valenzula GA, Smalley WE, Schain DC, et al. Reversibility of gastric dysmotility in cortisol deficiency. *Am J Gastroenterol* 1987;82:1066–1068.

11 Sandle GI, McGlone F. Acute effects of dexamethasone on cation transport in colonic epithelium. *Gut* 1987;28:701–706.

12 Meeking S. Treatment of acute adrenal insufficiency. *Clin Tech Small Anim Pract* 2007;22(1):36–39.

13 Rose BD, Post T. Hyperkalemia. In: *Clinical Physiology of Acid–Base and Electrolyte Disorders*, 5th edn. McGraw-Hill, New York, 2001, pp. 696–930.

14 Greco DS. Hypoadrenocorticism in small animals. *Clin Tech Small Anim Pract* 2007;22(1):32–35.

15 Shulman DI, Palmert MR, Kemp SF, et al. Adrenal insufficiency:still a cause of morbidity and death in childhood. *Pediatrics* 2007;119(2):e484–494.

16 Adler JA, Drobatz KJ, Hess RS Abnormalities of serum electrolyte concentrations in dogs with hypoadrenocorticism. *J Vet Intern Med* 2007;21:1168–1173.

17 Hoerauf A, Reusch C. Ultrasonographic evaluation of the adrenal glands in six dogs with hypoadrenocorticism. *J Am Anim Hosp Assoc* 1999;35:214–218.

18 Seth M, Drobatz KJ, Church DB, et al. White blood cell count and the sodium to potassium ratio to screen for hypoadrenocorticism in dogs. *J Vet Intern Med* 2011;25:1351–1356.

19 Lennon EM, Boyle TE, Hutchins RG, et al. Use of basal serum or plasma cortisol concentrations to rule out a diagnosis of hypoadrenocorticism in dogs: 123 cases (2000–2005). *J Am Vet Med Assoc* 2007;231:413–416.

20 Bovens C, Tennant K, Reeve J, et al. Basal serum cortisol concentration as a screening test for hypoadrenocorticism in dogs. *J Vet Intern Med* 2014;28:1541–1545.

21 Cohen TA, Feldman EC. Comparison of IV and IM formulations of synthetic ACTH for ACTH stimulation tests in healthy dogs. *J Vet Intern Med* 2012;26:412–414.

22 Watson AD, Church DB, Emslie DR, et al. Plasma cortisol responses to three corticotrophic preparations in normal dogs. *Aust Vet J* 1998;76:255–257.

23 Behrend EN, Kemppainen RJ, Bruyette DS, et al. Intramuscular administration of a low dose of ACTH for ACTH stimulation testing in dogs. *J Am Vet Med Assoc* 2006;229:528–530.

24 Van Lanen K, Sande A. Canine hypoadrenocorticism: pathogenesis, diagnosis, and treatment. *Top Compan Anim Med* 2014;29(4):88–95.

25 Kemppainen RJ, Behrend EN, Busch KA. Use of compounded adrenocorticotropic hormone (ACTH) for adrenal function testing in dogs. *J Am Anim Hosp Assoc* 2005;41:368–372.

26 Lathan P, Moore GE, Zambon S, et al. Use of a low-dose ACTH stimulation test for diagnosis of hypoadrenocorticism in dogs. *J Vet Intern Med* 2008;22:1070–1073.

27 Lathan P, Scott-Moncrieff JC, Wills RW. Use of the cortisol-to-ACTH ratio for diagnosis of primary hypoadrenocorticism in dogs. *J Vet Intern Med* 2014;28:1546–1550.

28 Boretti FS, Meyer F, Burkhardt WA, et al. Evaluation of the cortisol-to-ACTH ratio in dogs with hypoadrenocorticism, dogs with diseases mimicking hypoadrenocorticism and in healthy dogs. *J Vet Intern Med* 2015;29(5):1335–1341.

29 Medinger TL, Williams DA, Bruyette DS. Severe gastrointestinal tract hemorrhage in three dogs with hypoadrenocorticism. *J Am Vet Med Assoc* 1993;202:1869–1872.

30 Brady CA, Vite CH, Drobatz KJ. Severe neurologic sequelae in a dog after treatment of hypoadrenal crisis. *J Am Vet Med Assoc* 1999;215:222–225.

31 Churcher RK, Watson ADJ, Eaton A. Suspected myelinolysis following rapid correction of hyponatremia in a dog. *J Am Anim Hosp Assoc* 1999;35:493–497.

32 O'Brien DP, Kroll RA, Johnson GC, et al. Myelinolysis after correction of hyponatremia in two dogs. *J Vet Intern Med* 1994;8(1):40–48.

33 Burkitt JM. Hypoadrenocorticism. In: *Small Animal Critical Care Medicine*, 2nd edn (eds Silverstein DC, Hopper K). Elsevier Saunders, St Louis, 2015, pp. 380–383.

34 Klein SE, Peterson ME. Canine hypoadrenocorticism: Part II. *Can Vet J* 2010;51:179–184.

35 Lathan P, Tyler J. Canine hypoadrenocorticism: diagnosis and treatment. *Compend Contin Educ Pract Vet* 2005;27(2):121–132.

36 Chiasson JL, Aris-Jilwan N, Belanger R, et al. Diagnosis and treatment of diabetic ketoacidosis and the hyperglycemic hyperosmolar state. *Can Med Assoc J* 2003;168(7):859–866.

37 Forsythe SM, Schmidt G. Sodium bicarbonate for the treatment of lactic acidosis. *Chest* 2000;118:882–884.

38 Heseby JS, Gumprecht DG. Hemodynamic effects of rapid bolus hypertonic sodium bicarbonate. *Chest* 1981;79:552–554.

39 Lang RM, Fellner SK, Neumann A, et al. Left ventricular contractility varies directly with blood ionized calcium. *Ann Intern Med* 1988;108:524–529.

40 Fordjour KN, Walton T, Doran JJ. Management of hyperkalemia in hospitalized patients. *Am J Med Sci* 2014;347(2):93–100.

41 Allon M, Dunlay R, Copkney C. Nebulized albuterol for acute hyperkalemia in patients on hemodialysis. *Ann Intern Med* 1989;110:426–429.

42 Allon M, Copkney C. Albuterol and insulin for treatment of hyperkalemia in hemodialysis patients. *Kidney Int* 1990;38:869–872.

43 Peterson ME. Feline hypoadrenocorticism. In: *BSAVA Manual of Canine and Feline Endocrinology*, 4th edn (eds Mooney CT, Peterson ME). British Small Animal Veterinary Association, Gloucester, 2012, pp. 213–217.

44 Kasabalis D, Bodina E, Saridomichelakis MN. Severe hypoglycaemia in a cat with primary

hypoadrenocorticism. *J Feline Med Surg* 2012;14(10):755–758.

45 Sicken J, Neiger R. Addisonian crisis and severe acidosis in a cat: a case of feline hypoadrenocorticism. *J Feline Med Surg* 2013;15(10):941–944.

46 Spalla I, Spinelli D, Lucatini C, et al. ECG of the month. *J Am Vet Med Assoc* 2014;1:45.

47 Woolcock A, Ward C. Successful treatment of a cat with primary hypoadrenocorticism and severe hyponatremia with desoxycorticosterone pivalate (DOCP). *Can Vet J* 2015;56:1158–1160.

48 Feldman E, Nelson R, Reusch C, et al. (eds). *Canine and Feline Endocrinology*, 4th edn. Elsevier, St Louis, 2015.

116

Thyroid Disorders

Jonathan D. Dear, DVM, DACVIM

School of Veterinary Medicine, University of California, Davis, CA, USA

Introduction

Thyroid hormones are critical to the regulation of physiological homeostasis. Their activities directly affect the cellular functions of the entire body, including regulation of the basal metabolic rate, as well as the cardiopulmonary, musculoskeletal, nervous, and reproductive systems. Thyroid dysfunctions are the most commonly diagnosed endocrinopathies of small animals and their clinical sequelae vary widely from mild to severe disease.

Thyroid Physiology

The thyroid is a paired endocrine gland adjacent to the trachea and larynx. A set of parathyroid glands are closely associated with each thyroid within the cranial and caudal poles. Thyroid hormones are made within thyroid follicles where thyroid peroxidase iodinates thyroglobulin molecules to produce biologically active iodothyronines: tri-iodothyronine (T3) and tetraiodothyronine (T4). Inactive reverse tri-iodothyronine is produced in smaller amounts within the thyroid follicles. Thyroid hormone secretion relies on thyroid-stimulating hormone (TSH), which is released by the posterior pituitary under the negative feedback of T3 and T4. Disease states and drugs, such as glucocorticoids, can also cause negative feedback on the posterior pituitary (reducing secretion of TSH).

Thyroid hormones act by crossing into the cell and increasing synthesis of proteins involved with cellular metabolism. Despite being the biologically active form, T3 is only produced in small amounts (roughly 10%) by the thyroid. Most T3 is formed within target cells or through peripheral conversion of T4 by organs (liver, kidneys, and skeletal muscle). Tyrosine-specific deiodinases cleave iodine moieties from T4 to produce active T3. T4 is the major thyroid hormone in plasma and can be measured as either free, unbound T4 (fT4) or total (free and protein bound) T4 (tT4).

Once formed, iodothyronines are stored within the lumen of the follicle in a substance known as colloid. Following release from the thyroid, most hormones remain protein bound within peripheral circulation. The high affinity for protein binding buffers concentrations of these hormones that can result from acute change in thyroid function. This binding also helps to prevent urinary loss.

Thyroid-stimulating hormone affects all aspects of thyroid production and regulation. In normal states, thyroid hormones have little diurnal fluctuation. However, illness can cause reduced production of thyroid hormones due to the increased plasma glucocorticoid concentrations. This can also serve to retain resources in times of disease when the catabolic effects of thyroid hormones could be detrimental.

Non-thyroidal conditions can affect thyroid production and measurement. Breed and age variations are well documented; geriatric dogs and sighthounds have been shown to have lower thyroid hormone concentrations than control populations. Euthyroid sick syndrome refers to a condition in which thyroid hormone production is reduced due to concurrent non-thyroidal illness. The degree of inhibition is often related to the severity of disease. Non-thyroidal illness including renal, hepatic, endocrine, cardiac, neurological, neoplastic, and inflammatory diseases have all been documented as causes of euthyroid sick syndrome. Euthyroid sick syndrome has been well documented in many species, including both dog and human [1–4].

Thyroid Testing

The diagnosis of thyroid dysfunction can be challenging due to the effect of non-thyroidal illness on circulating thyroid hormone concentrations. There are many

Textbook of Small Animal Emergency Medicine, First Edition. Edited by Kenneth J. Drobatz, Kate Hopper, Elizabeth Rozanski and Deborah C. Silverstein.
© 2019 John Wiley & Sons, Inc. Published 2019 by John Wiley & Sons, Inc.
Companion Website: www.wiley.com/go/drobatz/textbook

hormones involved with thyroid function and commercial assays are available for most. Despite not being the most biologically active, T4 remains the most sensitive indicator of thyroid dysfunction. This is because roughly 90% of the extracellular pool of thyroid hormones is stored as T4. T4 can be measured as either total T4 or free T4. Testing of total T4 tends to be more cost-effective and rapid in turnround, although it is also more affected by non-thyroidal illness as decreases in thyroid-binding proteins often reflect systemic disease rather than endocrine dysfunction.

Thyroid-stimulating hormone can be measured in both dogs and cats, although its utility in the diagnosis of feline hyperthyroidism remains questionable [4]. T3 is an unreliable indicator of thyroid function as it is mostly an intracellular hormone and is degraded rapidly in circulation.

Hyperthyroidism

Hyperthyroidism refers to the excessive release of thyroid hormones. In most cases this is a result of primary disease (autonomous secretion) due to hyperplasia or neoplasia. Hyperthyroidism is the most common endocrinopathy of geriatric cats and is generally caused by either a single adenoma or, more often, bilateral hyperplasia or adenomatous hyperplasia. The pathogenesis leading to feline hyperthyroidism is not well understood and studies investigating nutritional and environmental risk factors have yet to find compelling evidence of its etiology [5–7]. Canine hyperthyroidism is rare and usually the result of thyroid carcinoma, excessive iatrogenic supplementation or dietary intake [8,9].

Hypothyroidism

Hypothyroidism refers to an insufficient production of thyroid hormones and may result from decreased TSH stimulation (secondary hypothyroidism) or decreased production of thyroxine within the thyroid gland due to destructive or infiltrative disease (primary hypothyroidism). Naturally occurring hypothyroidism is most often a result of immune-mediated destruction of the thyroid (lymphoplasmacytic thyroiditis). Hypothyroidism is the most frequently diagnosed endocrinopathy of dogs though it is quite rare in cats.

Clinical Presentations

Hyperthyroidism

Clinical Signs
The clinical signs common to hyperthyroidism reflect the increased metabolic demands of excessive thyroid

hormone concentrations. These include polyphagia with weight loss, polyuria/polydipsia, restlessness or altered behavior, vomiting, and diarrhea. Hyperthyroid cats may appear to seek out cool areas, be less interactive with others, and groom sporadically.

Diagnosis
Diagnosis of hyperthyroidism is established by suspicion of disease along with documentation of elevated thyroid values. fT4 and tT4 measurements both have good sensitivity for disease, although tT4 appears to be more specific. TSH is not generally measured in cats with hyperthyroidism since its concentration might fall below the limit of detection [4].

All cats with hyperactive thyroid tissue will have an enlarged thyroid, although it is not always palpable in cases of ectopic disease, metastatic disease or in large adenomas, which sink into the thoracic inlet.

Treatment
Treatment of hyperthyroidism is aimed at restoration of normal thyroid hormone production either by mitigation or destruction of the overactive thyroid tissue. Medical, surgical, and radiation therapies have been shown to be effective in restoration of this balance [10].

Methimazole, a reversible inhibitor of thyroid peroxidase, has been demonstrated to be effective in the control of both hyperthyroid dogs and cats and can be administered by mouth or topically (usually on the ear pinna) [11]. The starting dose is typically 1.25–2.5 mg per cat once to twice daily. Dosing should be adjusted based on clinical response and follow-up measurement of tT4. Although it is highly effective, side-effects are encountered in up to 44% of cats who receive this medication [12]. Most side-effects relate to the gastrointestinal tract and may be transient in nature, but more severe sequelae such as hepatotoxicity, myelotoxicity, dermatitis, and neuromuscular blockade have been reported [12–14]. These effects are idiosyncratic and do not appear to be dose dependent [14].

A diet deficient in dietary iodide (Hill's Prescription y/d Diet) has been approved and marketed for the treatment of hyperthyroidism in cats. By eliminating dietary intake of iodide, the hyperfunctional thyroid gland is unable to produce excessive thyroid hormones which allows for restoration of more normal values [15]. Unfortunately, ingestion of even a small amount of iodine-containing food can undermine this treatment, so appropriate case selection and client education are critical to the success of this therapy.

Permanent resolution of hyperthyroidism can be achieved via surgical thyroidectomy or administration of radioactive iodine[131].

Hypertensive Retinopathy

Acute blindness is a common opthalmic reason for presentation of cats and dogs to the general practitioner or emergency clinician. Hypertensive retinopathy is the most common reason for acute blindness in the geriatric cat. Upon diagnosis of systemic hypertension, rapid diagnosis of the underlying pathology and pharmacological intervention to control hypertension should be initiated as vision loss is often irreversible and likely inevitable beyond 10–14 days. See Chapters 12 and Chapter 63 for further information.

Physical Examination

Patients with hypertensive retinopathy typically present with mydriasis, although the anterior chamber is generally unaffected. Fundic examination reveals retinal separation, hemorrhage or tortuous vasculature. Some patients might present with hyphema.

Diagnosis

The combination of systemic hypertension and retinal changes described above confirms the diagnosis of hypertensive retinopathy. The practitioner should focus on the diagnosis of the cause of systemic hypertension (Table 116.1).

Treatment

Rapid initiation of antihypertensive medications is indicated. Most often, amlodipine (0.625 mg/cat or 0.1–0.3 mg/kg PO once daily) is effective in controlling systemic hypertension. In refractory cases, acepromazine or hydralazine can be considered.

Thyroid Storm

Thyroid storm or thyrotoxicosis is a rare consequence of uncontrolled hyperthyroidism in human patients that has not been well described in cats. Clinical signs of thyroid storm reflect an acute exacerbation of hyperthyroidism, including fever and perturbations of the cardiovascular, gastrointestinal, and central nervous systems. Although the pathogenesis of thyrotoxicosis is unknown,

there is evidence to suggest that its incidence is more closely correlated to rapid increases in thyroid hormone concentrations rather than absolute values [16,17].

Thyroid storm may occur due to either thyroidal or non-thyroidal disease. Thyroidal causes include I-131 administration, thyroid surgery or abrupt withdrawal of antithyroid medication. Non-thyroidal causes include non-thyroidal surgery, infection, stress or trauma.

Clinical Signs

The clinical signs associated with a thyroid storm are similar to those seen with hyperthyroidism although, as a consequence of thyrotoxicosis, are likely more severe. Cats may become profoundly tachycardic and tachypneic, resulting in decreased systolic function and respiratory fatigue. Fever has also been reported in cats suspected of having a thyroid storm [18].

Diagnosis

No guidelines exist for the diagnosis of feline thyroid storm; its diagnosis is based on the presence of compelling clinical signs, documentation of elevated thyroid hormone concentrations, and evidence of an event or events leading to its occurrence. Hormone levels cannot be used to determine its severity as evidence in human medical literature suggests a lack of correlation between hormone concentration and severity of clinical signs.

Treatment

The goals of treatment are to reduce thyroid hormone production, decrease the effects of systemic thyroid hormones, and identify (or preferably eliminate) the factor leading to its occurrence.

Methimazole is a highly effective drug; its activity inhibits the iodination of tyrosine into thyroid hormones. It can be administered by mouth, transdermal or per rectum. Beta-blockers and antihypertensives (such as amlodipine or hydralazine) can be effective in reducing sympathetic tone and restoring normal blood pressure (see Chapter 63). Crystalloids should be administered judiciously to patients who appear volume depleted; close monitoring is essential to avoid fluid overload as the cardiotoxic effects of thyroid hormone predispose to hypertrophic changes and may result in cardiomyopathy (see Chapter 167).

Iatrogenic Hyperthyroidism

Hyperthyroidism can result from inadvertent oversupplementation of thyroid hormone either by supplementation of thyroid hormones or ingestion of thyroid-containing offal [8,9]. In many instances, patients with iatrogenic hyperthyroidism lack clinical signs of the disease. Diagnosis of this condition stems from identification and

Table 116.1 Common differentials for systemic hypertension.

Dog	Dog or cat	Cat
Hyperadrenocorticism	Diabetes mellitus	Hyperaldosteronism
Pheochromocytoma	Renal insufficiency	Hyperthyroidism
	Idiopathic	

withdrawal of the causative agent, leading to resolution of the thyroid hormone imbalance.

Hypothyroidism

Clinical Signs
Clinical signs of hypothyroidism are often mild and non-specific and include lethargy, weight gain, decreased appetite or stamina. Dermatological findings such as endocrine (bilateral, truncal, and non-pruritic) alopecia or rat tail are common. Intact animals may lack libido or have increased rates of reproductive failure. Less common signs include neurological disease such as seizures, vestibular disease, stupor or coma.

Diagnosis
Diagnosis of true hypothyroidism can be challenging due to the influence of other systemic disorders on the pituitary-thyroid axis. Since the common clinical signs of hypothyroidism mimic those of other metabolic diseases which cause euthyroid sick syndrome, the clinician must be careful to not overinterpret a single low thyroid hormone concentration [2]. In order to raise the suspicion of disease, the clinician must initially identify compatible clinical signs. Only these patients should have thyroid testing as routine testing of healthy animals will lower the predictive value of these tests. Identification of other clinicopathological features such as a mild, non-regenerative anemia or hyperlipidemia may also provoke evaluation of thyroid function.

Total T4 is the most commonly measured thyroid hormone used in the diagnosis of hypothyroidism and remains the most sensitive indicator of disease. Unfortunately, due to the effects of protein binding related to systemic disease, it lacks specificity. However, a low tT4 in a dog with compelling clinical signs, physical examination findings and clinicopathological changes might be sufficient for diagnosis [19]. In other patients with co-morbidities that could affect thyroid function or hormone concentration, measurement of fT4, TSH, and thyroglobulin autoantibodies can be helpful in the diagnosis of true hypothyroidism [20].

Treatment
Treatment of hypothyroidism, whether primary or secondary, involves thyroid hormone replacement therapy. Levothyroxine is administered by mouth at a dose of 0.01–0.02 mg/kg twice daily. Dosing should be adjusted based on response to therapy and recheck measurement of tT4. Side-effects of levothyroxine are rare, although there are anecdotal reports of brand names being more effective than generic formulations. Thyro-tabs (Lloyd Inc, Shenandoah, IA) are the only FDA-approved oral thyroid supplementation for use in dogs.

Myxedema Coma

Myxedema, or cutaneous mucinosis, is a severe consequence of protracted, untreated hypothyroidism that leads to hyaluronic acid accumulation within the dermis. This leads to accumulation of extracellular fluid and skin thickening. Dogs with myxedema are described as having a "tragic facial expression" characterized by ectropion and a puffy face. When left untreated, this condition may progress to generalized weakness, bradycardia, hypothermia, and, eventually, coma or death. Myxedema may be triggered by the development of concurrent disease [21].

Treatment
Treatment of myxedema relies on parenteral supplementation of thyroid hormone, stabilization of the patient including fluid resuscitation, controlled warming and, in some cases, mechanical ventilation [21]. Since myxedema is often precipitated by concurrent non-thyroidal illness, quick identification and diagnosis of co-morbidities is essential in its treatment. Unfortunately, many dogs with myxedema die due to lack of diagnosis or severity of concurrent disease precluding their stabilization and resuscitation.

References

1 Mooney CT, Shiel R, Dixon R. Thyroid hormone abnormalities and outcome in dogs with non-thyroidal illness. *J Small Anim Pract* 2008;49(1):11–16.
2 Nelson RW, Ihle S, Feldman S, et al. Serum free thyroxine concentration in healthy dogs, dogs with hypothyroidism, and euthyroid dogs with concurrent illness. *J Am Vet Med Assoc* 1991;198(8):1401–1407.
3 Lee S, Farwell AP. Euthyroid sick syndrome. *Compr Physiol* 2016;6(2):1071–1080.
4 Peterson ME, Guterl J, Nichols R, et al. Evaluation of serum thyroid-stimulating hormone concentration as a diagnostic test for hyperthyroidism in cats. *J Vet Intern Med* 2015;29(5):1327–1334.
5 Chow K, Hearn L, Zuber M, et al. Evaluation of polybrominated diphenyl ethers (PBDEs) in matched cat sera and house dust samples: investigation of a potential link between PBDEs and spontaneous feline hyperthyroidism. *Environ Res* 2015;136:173–179.
6 Edinboro CH, Scott-Moncrieff JC, Glickman LT. Feline hyperthyroidism: potential relationship with iodine supplement requirements of commercial cat foods. *J Feline Med Surg* 2010;12(9):672–679.

7 Wakeling J, Everard A, Brodbelt D, et al. Risk factors for feline hyperthyroidism in the UK. *J Small Anim Pract* 2009;50(8):406–414.

8 Broome MR, Peterson M, Kemppainen R, et al. Exogenous thyrotoxicosis in dogs attributable to consumption of all-meat commercial dog food or treats containing excessive thyroid hormone: 14 cases (2008–2013). *J Am Vet Med Assoc* 2015;246(1):105–111.

9 Kohler, B, Stengel C, Neiger R. Dietary hyperthyroidism in dogs. *J Small Anim Pract* 2012;53(3):182–184.

10 Carney HC, Ward C, Bailey S, et al. 2016 AAFP Guidelines for the Management of Feline Hyperthyroidism. *J Feline Med Surg* 2016;18(5):400–416.

11 Boretti FS, Sieber-Ruckstuhl N, Schafer S, et al. Transdermal application of methimazole in hyperthyroid cats: a long-term follow-up study. *J Feline Med Surg* 2014;16(6):453–459.

12 Trepanier LA, Hoffman S, Kroll M, et al. Efficacy and safety of once versus twice daily administration of methimazole in cats with hyperthyroidism. *J Am Vet Med Assoc* 2003;222(7):954–958.

13 Bell ET, Mansfield CS, James FE. Immune-mediated myasthenia gravis in a methimazole-treated cat. *J Small Anim Pract* 2012;53(11):661–663.

14 Peterson ME, Kintzer P, Hurvitz A. Methimazole Treatment of 262 cats with hyperthyroidism. *J Vet Intern Med* 1988;2(3):150–157.

15 Hui TY, Bruyette D, Moore G, et al. Effect of feeding an iodine-restricted diet in cats with spontaneous hyperthyroidism. *J Vet Intern Med* 2015;29(4):1063–1068.

16 McDermott MT, Kidd G, Dodson L, et al. Radioiodine-induced thyroid storm. *Case report and literature review. Am J Med* 1983;75(2):353–359.

17 Mandel SH, Magnusson A, Burton B, et al. Massive levothyroxine ingestion. Conservative management. *Clin Pediatr* 1989;28(8):374–376.

18 Ward CR. Feline thyroid storm. *Vet Clin North Am Small Anim Pract* 2007;37(4):745–754, vii.

19 Dixon M, Mooney C. Evaluation of serum free thyroxine and thyrotropin concentrations in the diagnosis of canine hypothyroidism. *J Small Anim Pract* 1999;40(2):72–78.

20 Kantrowitz LB, Peterson M, Melian C, et al. Serum total thyroxine, total triiodothyronine, free thyroxine, and thyrotropin concentrations in dogs with nonthyroidal disease. *J Am Vet Med Assoc* 2001;219(6):765–769.

21 Henik RA, Dixon R. Intravenous administration of levothyroxine for treatment of suspected myxedema coma complicated by severe hypothermia in a dog. *J Am Vet Med Assoc* 2000;216(5):713–717, 685.

117

Diabetes Insipidus

Jamie M. Burkitt Creedon, DVM, DACVECC

School of Veterinary Medicine, University of California, Davis, CA, USA

Introduction

Diabetes insipidus (DI) causes polyuria (PU) due to inadequate free water reabsorption in the kidney in dogs and cats. It is an uncommon disease in small animals, and is rarely the primary diagnosis in a dog or cat seen on an emergency basis. Occasionally, a patient may present for an unrelated problem, and pre-existing, undiagnosed DI may be uncovered during a hospital stay. Alternatively, newly acquired DI may develop as a result of another condition. The purpose of this chapter is to help the clinician recognize DI in emergency patients and treat it appropriately in the short term.

Pathophysiology

Arginine vasopressin (AVP), also called antidiuretic hormone (ADH), is produced by the supraoptic and paraventricular nuclei of the hypothalamus and released from the posterior pituitary gland. It acts on the principal cells of the renal collecting tubules to allow electrolyte-free water reabsorption in this normally water-impermeable region of the nephron. Arginine vasopressin is released due to either plasma hyperosmolality or ineffective circulating volume. A plasma osmolality as little as 1–2% above an individual's set-point stimulates central chemoreceptors and leads to AVP secretion [1].

After AVP is released, it binds vasopressin 2 (V_2) receptors on the basolateral membrane of the renal collecting tubule's principal cells. Stimulation of the V_2 receptor activates a G-protein coupled to adenylyl cyclase, which is stimulated to increase intracellular cyclic AMP, leading to protein kinase A activation and resultant insertion of specialized water channels into the collecting tubule cell's luminal membrane. These water channels are composed of aquaporin-2 molecules, which are stored in cytosolic vesicles until this AVP-dependent cascade

leads to their translocation to the luminal membrane. Aquaporin-2 water channels allow electrolyte-free water to be reabsorbed from the ultrafiltrate in the nephron's tubular lumen into the relatively hypertonic medulla, which decreases plasma osmolality back toward normal.

When AVP is produced in inadequate amounts or not at all, or when AVP is ineffective at its target cell, the patient is unable to reabsorb water adequately in the kidney. As a result, a large volume of very dilute urine is produced and the animal drinks excessively to compensate for the water loss. This problem is called diabetes insipidus. Diabetes insipidus may be due to pituitary disease, in which case it is called "central," or due to disease at the level of the collecting tubule cell, in which case it is called "nephrogenic." Nephrogenic DI is usually due to a problem with the V_2 receptor or aquaporin-2 water channel [2]. Both central and nephrogenic DI can be either congenital ("primary") or acquired ("secondary"), although congenital nephrogenic DI has not been reported in the cat [3]. Reported causes of acquired DI in dogs and cats, many of which are seen in the emergency room, are listed in Table 117.1. Finally, DI may be "complete," which implies a complete lack of AVP production or responsiveness, or "partial," which indicates that AVP production or responsiveness is present but inadequate. Animals with complete DI are more severely clinically affected than those with partial DI.

Recognizing Diabetes Insipidus in the Emergency Patient

Diabetes insipidus is rarely seen in the emergency room. In this author's experience, when DI is seen in this setting, it is most often an incidental or secondary finding. Diabetes insipidus may have been a pre-existing condition that the client did not recognize, particularly if the pet lives outdoors or is largely unattended. In such

Textbook of Small Animal Emergency Medicine, First Edition. Edited by Kenneth J. Drobatz, Kate Hopper, Elizabeth Rozanski and Deborah C. Silverstein.
© 2019 John Wiley & Sons, Inc. Published 2019 by John Wiley & Sons, Inc.
Companion Website: www.wiley.com/go/drobatz/textbook

Table 117.1 Causes of acquired diabetes insipidus.

Central	Nephrogenic
Traumatic brain injury [4–9]	Paraneoplastic – intestinal leiomyosarcoma in the dog [2,10]
Neoplasia [11–14]	Hypercalcemia [2,3]
Pituitary surgery [15,16]	Hypokalemia [2,3]
Post cardiopulmonary arrest [17]	Leptospirosis [18]
Inflammation [19,20]	Ureteral obstruction [2]
Idiopathic	Kidney failure [2]
Drugs [3]:	Drugs [3]:
Alpha-adrenergics	Alpha-adrenergics
Glucocorticoids	Barbiturates
Ethanol	Glucocorticoids
Phenytoin	Tetracyclines
	Vinca alkaloids
Parasite migration	*E. coli* endotoxin [3]

cases, DI may be uncovered once PU, polydipsia (PD), or hypernatremia is noted during hospitalization. Alternatively, newly acquired DI may appear secondary to a separate, new condition such as traumatic brain injury, intracranial neoplasia, electrolyte imbalance, or medication (see Table 117.1).

History

Polyuria is the most prominent and reliable clinical sign in patients with DI. The PU is generally profound, although its degree depends on whether the DI is complete or partial and, if partial, how severe. Patients with access to water and able to drink will also be polydipsic. Clients may not appreciate that their pet's urination and drinking habits are abnormal, or the DI may be acquired due to a new problem; thus, lack of reported historical PU/PD does not rule out the diagnosis. Dogs with DI often also have urinary incontinence [14].

As shown in Table 117.1, there are many causes of acquired DI seen in emergency room patients. Therefore, DI should be considered in the patient with any of these conditions that develops PU, PD, inappropriately low urine specific gravity (USG), or hypernatremia. Figure 117.1 provides a diagnostic algorithm for the recognition of DI.

Physical Examination

Compensated DI does not produce physical examination abnormalities because patients drink water to offset their excessive urinary losses. However, if water intake is inadequate, marked hypernatremia can develop and cause central nervous system signs such as obtundation, head pressing, or seizures. Clinical interstitial dehydration

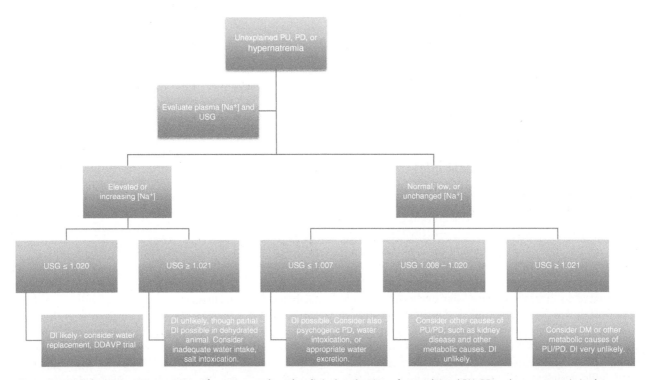

Figure 117.1 Schematic representation of one approach to the clinical evaluation of unexplained PU, PD, or hypernatremia in the acutely ill animal.

may be seen in decompensated patients. However, most patients with DI have no specific physical examination abnormalities attributable to the disease.

Clinicopathological Abnormalities

The patient with DI generally has hyposthenuric to isosthenuric USG due to excessive free water in the urine, although partial DI patients that are ≥5% dehydrated may have a USG as high as 1.020 or greater. [3]. Urine osmolality is generally iso-osmolar to plasma (280–310 mOsm/kg), although dehydrated patients with partial DI may be able to achieve urine osmolalities ≥600 mOsm/kg [3]. Patients with DI that do not take in enough water to compensate for their urinary water loss develop hypernatremia, although normally compensated individuals allowed to drink water freely may be normo- or even hyponatremic [14]. Emergency room and hospitalized patients with DI can develop clinically important hypernatremia in just a few hours, particularly if their DI is severe, because they are often either unable or disallowed to drink water. This hypernatremia can occur regardless of physical examination hydration findings or blood volume status, and thus must be found by blood electrolyte monitoring. Electrolytes should be evaluated in any animal with unexplained PU, and hypernatremia should increase the suspicion for DI.

One investigation found that 24% of dogs with central DI whose urine was cultured had bacterial cystitis [14].

Definitive Diagnosis

When DI occurs in an emergency setting, a formal definitive diagnosis often cannot be made. The two most common methods for diagnosis, response to exogenous AVP and the modified water deprivation test, often require more time than is practical in the emergency room.

Response to Exogenous AVP

Patients with central DI show improvement in polyuria and hypernatremia with administration of exogenous AVP, usually in the form of desmopressin acetate (DDAVP). Thus, a DDAVP trial may help in diagnosis. Injectable DDAVP can be given at 5 μg SC and the urine evaluated 2 and 4 hours later. Injectable synthetic aqueous vasopressin can be given at 0.2–0.4 U/kg up to a maximum of 5 U/kg IM; urine is evaluated 30, 60, and 120 minutes following injection [3].

Another option is the intranasal desmopressin acetate preparation, which can be administered subconjunctivally to dogs and cats at a dose of 1–2 drops OU every 12–24 hours.

An increase in USG of ≥50% after exogenous AVP administration is consistent with a diagnosis of central DI

[3]. Although it may take patients with decreased renal medullary tonicity ("medullary washout") many days to respond to exogenous AVP, a subconjunctival DDAVP trial has been described as a fairly quick diagnostic method for central DI in a critically ill dog [17]. Patients with nephrogenic DI generally do not respond to AVP, so response to exogenous AVP cannot be used to rule out that disease.

Modified Water Deprivation Test

The traditional test for DI is the modified water deprivation test, in which a pet is not allowed any intake (oral, intravenous, or otherwise) until it loses 3% of its body weight in urine, at which time USG is measured and the animal is administered exogenous vasopressin to evaluate for response with injectable AVP as described above. The test can be used to distinguish partial from complete and central from nephrogenic DI. Full details of this test are available elsewhere [3].

For obvious reasons, the modified water deprivation test is not appropriate for emergency room patients. Additionally, it can be dangerous even in stable animals, and can lead to misdiagnoses [21].

Although a formal, definitive diagnosis often cannot be made in this setting, recognition and supportive care for DI in the emergency room are critical. In the sick, hospitalized patient, DI is strongly suspected when a combination of polyuria with lower than expected USG (generally ≤1.020, commonly <1.008) [3] and hypernatremia is present. In this author's experience, it is usually progressive hypernatremia on routine, serial blood work that initially suggests DI. The patient is then treated for hypernatremia and polyuria.

Treatment

Emergency room patients with DI usually have hypernatremia because they have an obligate urinary free water loss and are not drinking enough water to compensate for it, either because of their illness or because water is being withheld.

Water Replacement

Hypernatremia should be treated, even if it is not causing obvious clinical signs. Treatment involves free water administration, usually in the form of intravenous 5% dextrose in water or oral water intake. The dose and rate of water administration need to be carefully determined. A full discussion of the treatment of hypernatremia is provided in Chapter 108. During treatment, plasma [Na$^+$] should be measured no less often than every 4 hours and the fluid administration rate adjusted accordingly, to ensure an appropriate rate of correction.

AVP Administration

Once the plasma [Na$^+$] reaches a safe value (probably the high end of the reference interval), initiation of subconjunctival DDAVP at 1–2 drops OU every 12–24 hours is reasonable. Starting DDAVP when the patient is still hypernatremic can be done, but this method risks an overly rapid drop in plasma [Na$^+$], which can cause cerebral edema. Oral DDAVP can also be used; reported doses are 0.1–0.2 mg in dogs [3] and 0.025–0.05 mg in cats [4] every 8–12 hours.

Complications of Treatment – Cerebral Edema

Overly rapid correction of plasma [Na$^+$] can cause cerebral edema due to water shifting into comparatively hyperosmolar brain tissue. Patients with hypernatremia should be monitored for obtundation, head pressing, seizures, or other central nervous system abnormalities. If the patient develops such signs, plasma [Na$^+$] should be measured to confirm that it is less than when treatment was initiated. This step is important because the clinical signs of progressive hypernatremia can be similar to signs of overzealous correction. If plasma [Na$^+$] has dropped, the patient should be treated with mannitol 0.5–1 g/kg IV or 7.2% NaCl at 3–5 mL/kg over 20–30 minutes. Administration should ideally be through a central vein, and if the first dose is ineffective, a second dose or other

medication may be tried. Hypertonic saline should not be administered rapidly because it can cause vasodilation and hypotension when given as a rapid bolus.

Patient Discharge

If signs persist beyond hospital discharge, the pet should be referred to its general practitioner or an internal medicine specialist for definitive testing for DI. In the meantime, free access to ample fresh water must be provided once the pet returns home, and the client should be warned about expected polyuria.

Prognosis

The prognosis for DI varies by etiology. Patients with congenital central DI are often successfully treated with DDAVP. Patients with congenital nephrogenic DI can be treated with sodium restriction and thiazide diuretics [3,22], but marked PU/PD usually persists and so these patients generally require lifelong ample free water access and tolerant owners. Patients with acquired DI may see resolution if the underlying cause can be eliminated. However, one study found that dogs with acquired central DI often have underlying brain neoplasia, which commonly leads to euthanasia or death within months of diagnosis [14].

References

1 Rose BD, Post TW. Regulation of plasma osmolality. In: *Clinical Physiology of Acid–Base and Electrolyte Disorders*, 5th edn. McGraw-Hill, New York, 2001, pp. 285–298.

2 Cohen M, Post GS. Water transport in the kidney and nephrogenic diabetes insipidus. *J Vet Intern Med* 2002;16(5):510–517.

3 Nelson RW. Water metabolism and diabetes insipidus. In: *Canine and Feline Endocrinology*, 4th edn (eds Feldman EC, Nelson RW, Reusch CE, et al.). Elsevier Saunders, St Louis, 2015, pp. 1–36.

4 Aroch I, Mazaki-Tovi M, Shemesh O, Sarfaty H, Segev G. Central diabetes insipidus in five cats: clinical presentation, diagnosis and oral desmopressin therapy. *J Feline Med Surg* 2005;7(6):333–339.

5 Campbell FE, Bredhauer B. Trauma-induced central diabetes insipidus in a cat. *Aust Vet J* 2005;83(12):732–735.

6 Mellanby RJ, Jeffery ND, Gopal MS, Herrtage ME. Secondary hypothyroidism following head trauma in a cat. *J Feline Med Surg* 2005;7(2):135–139.

7 Oliveira KM, Fukushima FB, Oliveira CM, et al. Head trauma as a possible cause of central diabetes insipidus in a cat. *J Feline Med Surg* 2013;15(2):155–159.

8 Smith JR, Elwood CM. Traumatic partial hypopituitarism in a cat. *J Small Anim Pract* 2004;45(8):405–409.

9 Foley C, Bracker K, Drellich S. Hypothalamic-pituitary axis deficiency following traumatic brain injury in a dog. *J Vet Emerg Crit Care* 2009;19(3):269–274.

10 Cohen M, Post GS. Nephrogenic diabetes insipidus in a dog with intestinal leiomyosarcoma. *J Am Vet Med Assoc* 1999;215(12):1818–1820.

11 Goossens MM, Rijnberk A, Mol JA, Wolfswinkel J, Voorhout G. Central diabetes insipidus in a dog with a pro-opiomelanocortin-producing pituitary tumor not causing hyperadrenocorticism. *J Vet Intern Med* 1995;9(5):361–365.

12 Nielsen L, Thompson H, Hammond GJ, Chang YP, Ramsey IK. Central diabetes insipidus associated with primary focal B cell lymphoma in a dog. *Vet Rec* 2008;162(4):124–126.

13 Simpson CJ, Mansfield CS, Milne ME, Hodge PJ. Central diabetes insipidus in a cat with central nervous system B cell lymphoma. *J Feline Med Surg* 2011;13(10):787–792.

14 Harb MF, Nelson RW, Feldman EC, Scott-Moncrieff JC, Griffey SM. Central diabetes insipidus in dogs: 20 cases (1986–1995). *J Am Vet Med Assoc* 1996;209(11): 1884–1888.

15 Hanson JM, van 't HM, Voorhout G, Teske E, Kooistra HS, Meij BP. Efficacy of transsphenoidal hypophysectomy in treatment of dogs with pituitary-dependent hyperadrenocorticism. *J Vet Intern Med* 2005;19(5):687–694.

16 Teshima T, Hara Y, Taoda T, Teramoto A, Tagawa M. Central diabetes insipidus after transsphenoidal surgery in dogs with Cushing's disease. *J Vet Med Sci* 2011;73(1):33–39.

17 Bellis T, Daly M, Davidson B. Central diabetes insipidus following cardiopulmonary arrest in a dog. *J Vet Emerg Crit Care* 2015;25:745–750.

18 Etish JL, Chapman PS, Klag AR. Acquired nephrogenic diabetes insipidus in a dog with leptospirosis. *Irish Vet J* 2014;67(1):7.

19 Meij BP, Voorhout G, Gerritsen RJ, Grinwis GC, Ijzer J. Lymphocytic hypophysitis in a dog with diabetes insipidus. *J Compar Pathol* 2012;147(4):503–507.

20 Rudinsky AJ, Clark ES, Russell DS, Gilor C. Adrenal insufficiency secondary to lymphocytic panhypophysitis in a cat. *Aust Vet J* 2015;93(9):327–331.

21 Goldstein RE. Diabetes insipidus. In: *Small Animal Critical Care Medicine*, 2nd edn (eds Silverstein DC, Hopper K). Elsevier Saunders, St Louis, 2015, pp. 357–362.

22 Takemura N. Successful long-term treatment of congenital nephrogenic diabetes insipidus in a dog. *J Small Anim Pract* 1998;39(12):592–594.

H. Reproductive Disorders

118

Dystocia

Liam Donaldson, BVSc[1] and Philip Thomas, BVSc, PhD, FANZCVS, DACT[2]

[1] University of Melbourne, Melbourne, Australia
[2] Queensland Veterinary Specialists, Queensland, Australia

Female Reproductive Anatomy and the Physiology of Parturition

Anatomy

The genital organs of the bitch and queen consist of two ovaries, two fallopian (ovarian) tubes, a bicornuate uterus, a single cervix, the vagina, the vulva, and the mammary glands [1].

The bitch and the queen have a long vagina, short uterine body, and long uterine horns. The ovaries and ovarian tubes receive blood supply from the ovarian arteries, whereas the vagina receives blood supply via the vaginal artery. The major blood supply of the uterus is via the uterine artery, but the cranial and caudal aspects of the uterus receive some blood supply via the ovarian and vaginal arteries respectively [2].

The female reproductive tract is innervated by both sympathetic and parasympathetic nerve fibers. Sympathetic innervation of the ovary runs concurrently with the ovarian artery, while sympathetic innervation of the uterus and vagina forms plexuses both within the respective organs and within the broad ligament (having arisen from retroperitoneal pelvic tissue) [3]. Parasympathetic nerve fibers arise from the pelvic nerves and innervate via the pelvic plexus [3].

Physiology of Parturition

The progesterone required to maintain pregnancy in the bitch is secreted by the corpus luteum [2]. Progesterone concentration is not markedly different between pregnant bitches and non-pregnant bitches [4,5]. Peak progesterone levels are reached at approximately day 20–30 of pregnancy, ranging between 15 and 80 ng/mL. After this time, progesterone levels steadily decline. In order to

maintain pregnancy, progesterone concentration must be maintained above a minimum concentration of 2 ng/mL [4,5].

The signal for parturition is thought to be fetal. Maturation of the fetal adrenal cortices results in cortisol release from the fetal adrenal gland [5] which in turn results in increased estrogen secretion by ovarian tissue through day 45–60 of pregnancy [6]. Estrogen stimulates the upregulation of genes encoding myometrial contraction-associated proteins, and promotes prostaglandin release from the uteroplacental complex (now thought to be primarily trophoblastic cells) [7,8]. Prostaglandin E2 (PGE2) produced is luteolytic, resulting in corpus luteum regression and a reduction in circulating progesterone [9]. As a result of the luteolytic effect of PGE2, progesterone concentration rapidly drops from a range of 4–10 ng/mL to approximately 2 ng/mL over a 12–24-hour period toward the end of pregnancy [5]. Falling progesterone is believed to cause a rise in circulating prolactin, and subsequently lactation [5]. Parturition occurs 24–48 hours following the rapid decline in circulating progesterone [5].

Prostaglandin F2-alpha plays a key role in increasing the sensitivity of the myometrium to oxytocin. This in turn facilitates smooth muscle contraction, and softening of the cervix [5].

Oxytocin also plays a role in parturition. Oxytocin is secreted via the posterior pituitary gland in response to increased pressure placed upon the cervix. Oxytocin release results in activation of a sensory pathway that ultimately terminates in the proventricular nucleus of the hypothalamus. Neural impulses are then sent to the posterior pituitary resulting in the release of oxytocin. Oxytocin in turn increases myometrial contractility.

Textbook of Small Animal Emergency Medicine, First Edition. Edited by Kenneth J. Drobatz, Kate Hopper, Elizabeth Rozanski and Deborah C. Silverstein.
© 2019 John Wiley & Sons, Inc. Published 2019 by John Wiley & Sons, Inc.
Companion Website: www.wiley.com/go/drobatz/textbook

Estimating Expected Date of Parturition

Using mating date as the basis for estimating parturition date in the bitch is unreliable, with parturition possible at any point 57–72 days post mating [10]. Causes for variation in expected parturition date include the variable time at which a bitch may stand to be mated relative to time of ovulation, prolonged life of the oocyte and the length of time spermatozoa can survive in the reproductive tract of the bitch [10,11].

Vaginal cytology and endocrinology can give a better indicator of expected parturition date. Parturition occurs 57+/– 3 days following the onset of cytological diestrus in the bitch [11,12]. Onset of cytological diestrus is indicated through a sudden shift from primarily superficial cornified cells (>90%) (seen throughout estrus) to approx 50% non-cornified parabasal and intermediate cells within 24 hours of onset of diestrus [13]. Serum luteinizing hormone or progesterone can be used as markers to predict parturition. Parturition typically occurs 65 days after a peak in LH [11,12]. At the time of ovulation, progesterone concentration typically measures 4–10 ng/mL. Parturition occurs 63 days (+/–1) following the date of ovulation [12].

Transabdominal ultrasonography can be used to predict parturition date. There is relatively good predictive accuracy when at least two fetal parameters (fetal crown rump length and body diameter) are measured on more than two fetuses between day 30 and 39 of pregnancy [14,15].

There can be large variation in expected parturition date in the queen if date of mating is used as the marker for expected date of parturition. Parturition in the queen can range from 52 to 74 days depending on whether gestation was timed from the first or the last date of breeding.

Stages of Parturition

There are three distinct stages of parturition (Table 118.1). Literature regarding expected duration of each stage of parturition is anecdotal. Whether a clinician should intervene with parturition should be based upon indicators of dystocia and the patient, rather than anecdotal expectations.

Dystocia

Dystocia is defined as an inability to expel the fetus(es) from the uterus or birth canal [17].

Risk Factors

Brachycephalic and chondrodysplastic canine breeds are generally overrepresented with respect to dystocia,

Table 118.1 Stages of parturition.

Stage of parturition	Expected duration	Characterized by
Stage 1	6–12 hours (bitch and queen)	Nesting behavior [10,12,16]
		Subclinical uterine contractions
		Dilation of the cervix
		Uterine contractions
Stage 2	2–12 hours (bitch) Up to 24 hours (queen)	Overt abdominal contractions
		Expulsion of fetus(es) from vaginal canal
Stage 3	Varies with stage 2 parturition	Placental expulsion [1,2,4]
		Uterine involution

as are brachycephalic (e.g. Persian and British shorthair) and dolichocephalic (e.g. Siamese and Cornish rex) breeds in cats [18,19]. The underlying cause for the overrepresentation of these breeds is likely the result of congenitally narrowed birth canals and maternal–fetal disproportion [10].

Other risk factors for dystocia include small litter size, excessive litter size, increased age of the bitch, and underlying metabolic disease resulting in uterine inertia [20–22].

Literature is devoid of studies exploring a potential cause for a perceived high probability of dystocia in singleton pregnancies. It is proposed that the fetal signal required to initiate parturition is insufficient, perhaps resulting in a failure of production of luteolytic hormone and subsequently no prepartum drop in progesterone. As such, dams fail to demonstrate some premonitory signs of parturition (for instance, no lactation prior to parturition), have delayed parturition or may fail to enter stage 1 or stage 2 of parturition.

Classifying Dystocia

Dystocia can be classified by the manner of presentation (clinical category), or by underlying etiology.

In divergence from previous literature that is extrapolated from large animal obstetrics studies, we propose a new manner of classifying small animal dystocia based upon the clinical presentation of the patient [23]. The manner of presentation of a patient suffering dystocia can be classified into four clinical categories (Box 118.1).

The aetiology for dystocia is best divided into maternal and fetal causes (Table 118.2). Dystocia has been found to be of maternal origin in 13% of cases, fetal in 37% of cases, and attributable to small litter size in 17% of cases [18]. Approximately one-third of dystocia cases do not have a clear underlying cause attributed even after surgical intervention [18].

The majority of fetal causes of dystocia are the result of malpresentation [22]. The presentation of the fetus in the birth canal is categorized three ways.

- *Presentation*: anterior, posterior or transverse.
- *Position*: the positioning of the fetal spine in relation to the dam's pelvis.
- *Posture*: how the fetus' limbs and head are positioned in relation to the body.

Up to 40% of canine fetuses are born in a posterior presentation [24]. Causes of malpresentation can include but are not limited to transverse presentations, an anterior presentation with retention of the forelimbs, a posterior presentation with retention of the hindlimbs, or lateral or ventroflexion of the neck.

When is Examination of the Bitch or Queen Warranted?

Owners frequently call with concerns during parturition. The challenge is to determine if there is a reason for

Table 118.2 Attributable causes of dystocia.

Physiological	Anatomical
Maternal	
Primary uterine inertia	Primary:
Secondary uterine inertia	Abnormal pelvic canal size
Stress/environmental factors	Secondary:
Reduced abdominal muscle tone (high body condition score, old age)	Pelvic fracture
Hereditary/genetic	Uterine torsion
Estrogen/progesterone abnormalities	Uterine prolapse
Hypocalcaemia	Vaginal mass
Inadequate oxytocin release	Vaginal stricture
Fetal	
Malpresentation	
Fetal oversize	
Anasarca and other fetal malformation	
Fetal death and subsequent reduced cortisol release	

the dam to be transported to the veterinary facility for examination. Unneccessary transport of the dam may be disruptive to normal parturition and should be avoided if possible.

Examination is indicated under specific conditions as outlined in Box 118.2.

Clinical Examination

History
History should include expected whelping date, previous diagnostics (e.g. endocrinology or vaginal cytology at time of mating), breed of sire, parity, expected litter size, and underlying medical conditions.

Physical Examination
The physical should encompass assessment of vital signs, mucous membrane colour and refill, femoral and metatarsal pulse quality, thoracic auscultation, abdominal palpation, and, mammary, vaginal, and rectal examination.

Diagnostics

Diagnostics should consist of blood biochemistry and hematology, blood gas (including ionized calcium), and electrolytes. Assessing serum progesterone is warranted if the whelping date has been exceeded and the female fails to demonstrate signs of active labor. Radiography is warranted to confirm pregnancy, ensure cessation of parturition, or to assess for abnormalities such as gas in the uterus, or a fetus positioned in transverse presentation.

Sonography is the modality of choice for dystocia. Ultrasound can diagnose fetal distress via assessment of fetal heart rate. Normal fetal heart rate should be in the range of 200–220 beats per minute. Fetal bradycardia is a sign of fetal distress and warrants intervention. If fetal heart rate is below 180 beats per minute, intervention may be indicated [10,25,26].

Indicators for Intervention

Veterinary intervention is warranted if:

- there is obstruction (diagnosed on vaginal examination, radiography or sonography) (Figure 118.1)
- the bitch/queen has not entered labor, and progesterone is <2 ng/mL
- the bitch/queen is systemically ill
- fetal heart rate is deemed bradycardic (<160 to 180 beats per minute) at term
- there is suspicion of uterine rupture or torsion.

Medical Management of Dystocia

Medical management of dystocia is controversial; the use of ecbolics such as oxytocin is often contraindicated, and can result in poor outcomes. Medical management in the bitch typically results in a parturition success rate of approximately 30% [20]. Finding an appropriate medical candidate in itself is difficult (Box 118.3).

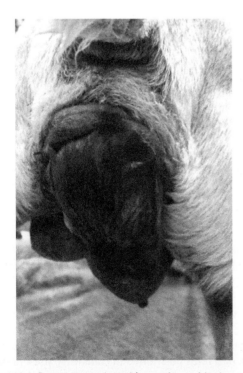

Figure 118.1 Puppy presenting with anterior positioning and retainment of forelimbs, resulting in obstruction of the birth canal.

Box 118.3 Prerequisites for a candidate to be treated via medical means [16,25].

Labor has not been prolonged
Cervix is dilated
Fetal size is within limits for vaginal delivery
Obstructive causes of dystocia have been ruled out

If medical management is chosen, electrolyte or acid–base abnormalities should be corrected prior to administering supplemental calcium or glucose. If the bitch is found to have low ionized calcium, 10% calcium gluconate 0.2 mL/kg can be administered IV [27]. Intravenous calcium should be administered as a constant-rate infusion (CRI) over a matter of minutes, while heart rate and rhythm are monitored with ECG and concurrent thoracic auscultation [16,27].

Hypoglycemia can be corrected with dextrose at a dose rate of 0.25–0.5 g/kg, diluted 1:2 with 0.9% NaCl. This should be administered over a 10-minute period as a CRI [28].

If the criteria for medical management are met, oxytocin can be administered at a dose rate of 0.5–2 IU SC or IM [29]. Oxytocin is best used in conjunction with calcium gluconate, with oxytocin stimulating smooth muscle contraction and calcium gluconate increasing the force of smooth muscle contraction [30]. Repeated use of oxytocin is controversial.

If medical management fails to result in parturition, surgical intervention is necessary.

Surgical Management

Prior to surgery, the patient should have an intravenous catheter placed, intravenous fluid administration started, and flow-by oxygen administered [31]. The abdomen should be clipped and scrubbed prior to induction. Premedication of the bitch or queen is not warranted [18,31]. Alfaxalone at 2 mg/kg IV to effect or propofol at 2–6 mg/kg IV to effect for induction, and maintenance on low-level isoflurane are widely recommended anaesthetic protocols [18,31,32] (see Section 7). For maintenance of intravenous fluids, balanced crystalloids at 5 mL/kg/h is recommended during the procedure.

A ventral midline approach to the abdomen is made. The incision is extended from slightly cranial to the umbilicus to just cranial to the pubic bone [25]. The linea alba is visualized, and care is taken to lift the linea alba from the underlying abdominal structures before an incision is made. The uterus is easily identifiable; uterine horns are lifted and exteriorized from the abdomen (ensuring that not too much tension is placed on the uterus) and placed on moistened laparotomy sponges overlying the abdominal cavity. A small, single, uterine incision is then made

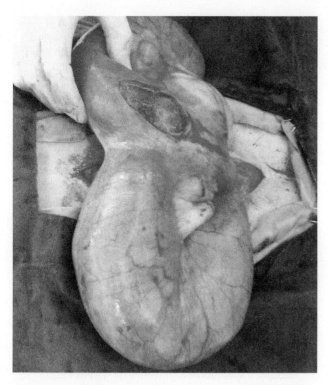

Figure 118.2 Incision through the uterine wall, with subsequent exposure of the chorioallantois.

over the base of one of the uterine horns with a scalpel (Figure 118.2). This is extended with Metzenbaum scissors to a size allowing the passage of the fetus(es) out of the uterine body. Each fetus is manipulated toward the incision site, and on presentation to the site of the uterine incision, the chorioallantois is broken with hemostats to allow delivery of the neonate from the uterus [32]. The amnion is also ruptured and the resultant umbilicus is clamped and tied. If the chorioallantois fails to separate from the uterine wall when the neonate is delivered, it can be gently separated from the endometrium.

Prior to closing the surgical site careful visual and digital examination of the anterior vagina, cervix and both uterine horns must be performed. This is to ensure all neonates have been delivered. The uterine incision is closed with a single layer of 2-0 or 3-0 absorbable suture in the Utrecht (modified Cushing) pattern [18,33].

Following closure of the uterus, oxytocin is administered at 0.5–1.0 IU/kg SC, the abdomen is lavaged with warm saline, and closed in three layers. Skin should be closed with a simple interrupted pattern (horizontal mattress or cruciate patterns are commonly used), or alternatively, the surgeon may wish to close with intradermal sutures. Postoperative analgesia upon recovery often consists of a single injection of non-steroidal anti-inflammatory drugs (meloxicam 0.2 mg/kg SC for bitches or meloxicam 0.1 mg/kg SC for queens), assuming there is no underlying renal or gastrointestinal compromise.

Postoperative Care and Management

Postoperative care of the bitch or queen and the neonate(s) is vital. Dams, especially maidens, are prone to mismothering after a cesarean. The owner must be made aware of the risk of mismothering, and the importance of monitoring neonatal weights to ensure continued growth in the days after birth. Pups should be weighed every 12 hours for the first 2 weeks of life. Over the initial 24 hours, it is normal for weight to decrease but over the coming fortnight, a growth rate of 2–4 g per day per expected kilogram of adult weight should be expected [34]. The bitch or queen should be fed a concentrated, high-quality food several times daily during lactation to ensure she maintains a healthy body condition score and the puppies/kittens receive adequate nutrition. Calcium supplementation is not recommended unless the bitch or queen demonstrates clinical signs of eclampsia [34]. Neonates should be fed soon after parturition to ensure transfer of maternal antibodies through colostrum. Supervised feeding of the puppies or kittens (with the owner assisting attachment to the teat if needed) should occur every 2–3 hours for the first days. Neonates should be kept separate from the bitch or queen until normal mothering is confirmed.

References

1 Sisson S. *The Anatomy of Domestic Animals*, 4th edn. WB Saunders, Philadelphia, 1966, p. 606.

2 Reece W. *Functional Anatomy and Physiology of Domestic Animals*, 4th edn. Wiley-Blackwell, Ames, 2009, p. 458.

3 Dyce K, Sack W, Wensing C. *Textbook of Veterinary Anatomy*, 3rd edn. Saunders, Philadelphia, 2002, p. 199.

4 Concannon P, Castracane V, Temple M, et al. Endocrine control of ovarian function in dogs and other carnivores. *Anim Reprod* 2009;6: 172–193.

5 Verstegen-Onclin K, Verstegen J. Endocrinology of pregnancy in the dog: a review. *Therio* 2008;70: 291–299.

6 Concannon P, Hansel P, Visek W. The ovarian cycle of the bitch: plasma estrogen, *LH and progesterone. Biol Reprod* 1975;13:112–121.

7 Mesian S, Welsh TN. Steroid hormone control of myometrial contractility and parturition. *Semin Cell Dev Biol* 2007;18:321–331.

8 Kowalewski M, Beceriklisov H, Pfarrer C, et al. Canine placenta: a source of prepartal prostaglandins during normal and antiprogestin-induced parturition. *Reproduction* 2010;139:655–664.

9 Kowalewski M, Mutembei H, Hoffman B. Canine prostaglandin E2 synthase (PGES) and its receptors (EP2 and EP4): expression in the corpus luteum during dioestrus. *Anim Reprod Sci* 2008;109:319–329.

10 Jukowitz LA. Reproductive emergencies. *Vet Clin Small Anim* 2005;35:397–420.

11 Concannon P, England G, Verstegen J. Canine Pregnancy: Predicting Parturition and Timing Events of Gestation. International Veterinary Information Service. Available at: http://people.upei.ca/lofstedt/public/chromosome.puzzle/images%20for%20chromosomes/private/pdf.files.not.in.courses/pregnacy.concannon.pdf (accessed 3 February 2018).

12 Johnson C. False pregnancy, disorders of pregnancy and parturition, and mismating. In: *Small Animal Internal Medicine*, 4th edn (eds Nelson RW, Couto CG). Mosby Elsevier, St Louis, 2009, p. 926.

13 Johnson C. Disorders of the estrous cycle. In: *Small Animal Internal Medicine*, 4th edn (eds Nelson RW, Couto CG). Mosby Elsevier, St Louis, 2009, pp. 885–910.

14 Kutzler M, Yeager A, Mohammed H, et al. Accuracy of canine parturition date prediction using fetal measurements obtained by ultrasonography. *Therio* 2003;60:1309–1317.

15 Kim Y, Travis A, Meyers-Wallen V. Parturition prediction and timing of canine pregnancy. *Therio* 2007;68: 1177–1182.

16 Pretzer SD. Medical management of canine and feline dystocia. *Therio* 2008;70:332–336.

17 Biddle D, Macintire DK. Obstetrical emergencies. *Clin Tech Small Anim Pract* 2000;15:88–93.

18 Ayers SE, Thomas PGA. Population characteristics of 453 bitches undergoing 510 caesarian section procedures between 1999 and 2009: a retrospective study. *Clin Therio* 2001;2:451.

19 Gunn-Moore DA, Thrusfield MV. Feline dystocia – prevalence, and association with cranial conformation and breed. *Vet Rec* 1995;136:350–353.

20 Darvelid AW, Linde-Forsberg C. Dystocia in the bitch – a retrospective study of 182 cases. *J Small Anim Pract* 1994;35:402–407.

21 Linde-Forsberg C, Eneroth A. Abnormalities in pregnancy, parturition and the periparturient period. In *Textbook of Veterinary Internal Medicine*, 5th edn (Ettinger S, Feldman E) Saunders, St Louis, 2000, p. 1527.

22 Johnson C. False pregnancy, disorders of pregnancy and parturition, and mismating. In: *Small Animal Internal Medicine*, 4th edn (eds Nelson RW, Couto CG). Mosby Elsevier, St Louis, 2009, p. 931.

23 Nakahara N, Thomas PGA. Proposal of a new classification of canine dystocia based on clinical presentation. Paper presented at the Science Week of Australian and New Zealand College of Veterinary Scientists 2015, August 9, Gold Coast, Australia.

24 Greer ML. *Canine Reproduction and Neonatology. Teton Newmedia, Jackson Hole*, 2014.

25 Traas AM. Surgical management of canine and feline dystocia. *Therio* 2008;70:337–342.

26 Smith FO. Challenges in small animal parturition – timing elective and emergency caesarean sections. *Therio* 2007;68:348–353.

27 Schweizer CM, Meyers-Wallen VN. Medical management of dystocia and indications for caesarean section in the bitch. In: *Kirk's Current Veterinary Therapy*, 13th edn (eds Bonagura JD, Twedt DC). Elsevier Saunders, Philadelphia, 1999, p. 933.

28 Linde-Forsberg C. Abnormalities in pregnancy, parturition, and the periparturient period. In: *Textbook of Veterinary Internal Medicine*, 6th edn (eds Ettinger S, Feldman E). Elsevier Saunders, Philadelphia, 2005, p. 1655.

29 Davidson AP. Frustrating case presentations in canine theriogenology. *Vet Clin North Am Small Anim Pract* 2001;31:411–420.

30 Davidson AP. Dystocia management. In: *Kirk's Current Veterinary Therapy*, 15th edn (eds Bonagura JD, Twedt DC). Elsevier Saunders, Philadelphia, 2013, p. 1343.

31 Doebeli A, Michel E. Bettschart R, et al. Apgar score after induction of anaesthesia for canine caesarean section with alfaxalone versus propofol. *Therio* 2013;80:850–854.

32 Fossum T. *Small Animal Surgery Textbook*, 3rd edn. Elsevier, St Louis, 2006.

33 Haysom L, Thomas PGA. Effect of prior caesarean on bitches presented for caesarean section. Paper presented at the Science Week of Australian and New Zealand College of Veterinary Scientists, 2012, Gold Coast, Australia.

34 Cline J. Kennel management and nutrition of the bitch and her offspring. In: *Management of Pregnant and Neonatal Dogs, Cats and Exotic Pets* (ed. Lopate C). John Wiley and Sons, Hoboken, 2012, pp. 1–13.

119

Eclampsia

Michelle A. Kutzler, DVM, PhD, DACT

Oregon State University, Corvallis, OR, USA

Introduction

Eclampsia is a life-threatening condition first described nearly 100 years ago [1]. It results from an acute depletion of ionized calcium in the extracellular compartment during the peripartum period.

Etiopathogenesis

Eclampsia occurs more frequently in bitches than queens with young, primiparous bitches at greatest risk [2]. Eclampsia most frequently occurs 2–4 weeks postpartum (peak time of lactation) but can occur during late pregnancy [3] or parturition [4] or more than 45 days postpartum (time of weaning), which is especially true in cats [5,6]. Although not reported in the literature, the author has managed one case of eclampsia that developed in a small-breed dog with an overt false pregnancy and significant galactorrhea. Bitches with large litters or a large litter size to body weight ratio [7] are at the greatest risk. Although eclampsia can occur in any breed, small- and toy-breed dogs are overrepresented. Eclampsia is very rare in large-breed bitches [8], with the exception of the German short-haired pointer [9]. There does not appear to be a breed predisposition in cats [10].

Mechanistically, eclampsia develops from the inability of calcium homeostatic mechanisms (increased gastrointestinal absorption, decreased renal excretion, increased osteolysis) to compensate for the loss of calcium through lactation, and to a lesser extent from fetal skeletal ossification [11–13]. Therefore, additional predisposing factors include inappropriate prepartum calcium supplementation as well as improper or inadequate perinatal nutrition [7]. Excessive prenatal calcium supplementation or insufficient dietary magnesium inhibits parathyroid hormone release and can promote parathyroid gland atrophy. In addition, excessive prenatal calcium supplementation stimulates thyroid calcitonin secretion, which then acts to decrease the rate of bone resorption of calcium. Through both of these actions, normal physiological mechanisms to mobilize and conserve adequate calcium stores as well as utilize dietary calcium sources are reduced.

Ionized serum calcium in dogs is normally about 55% of total serum calcium concentration [3]. However, prolonged hyperpnea during labor or dystocia can promote or exacerbate hypocalcemia as the resulting alkalosis favors protein binding of calcium, thereby decreasing ionized calcium (the biologically active form of calcium). It is important to mention that total serum calcium concentration is not affected by changes in pH. However, the equilibrium between ionized calcium and protein-bound calcium is affected by pH and an alkalotic animal may show signs of eclampsia yet have a normal total serum calcium concentration [14]. For this reason, albumin, bicarbonate, and anion gap measurements should be simultaneously interpreted [7,15].

Diagnosis

A presumptive diagnosis of eclampsia is often made based upon history and the presenting clinical signs. The onset of clinical signs of eclampsia in dogs is usually rapid with a predictable progression (Table 119.1) [3,16].

Early clinical signs include anxiety, restlessness, pacing, whining, and lack of interest in offspring. Facial pruritus of variable intensity and biting at the feet have also been reported [3]. Neuromuscular transmission is directly proportional to the calcium to magnesium ion ratio in the extracellular fluid [17,18]. In dogs and cats, decreased extracellular calcium ion levels increase nerve cell membrane permeability to sodium ions, especially in peripheral nerves, which has an excitatory

Textbook of Small Animal Emergency Medicine, First Edition. Edited by Kenneth J. Drobatz, Kate Hopper, Elizabeth Rozanski and Deborah C. Silverstein.
© 2019 John Wiley & Sons, Inc. Published 2019 by John Wiley & Sons, Inc.
Companion Website: www.wiley.com/go/drobatz/textbook

Table 119.1 Progression of eclampsia stages in dogs with corresponding clinical signs.

Stage	Clinical signs
I	Anxiety, restlessness, pacing, whining, hypersalivation, anorexia, polyuria, polydipsia, vomiting, diarrhea ± facial pruritus of variable intensity and biting at the feet
II	Ataxia, staggering, muscle tremors, mydriasis with diminished pupillary light reflexes, behavioral changes associated with lack of interest in offspring
III	Muscle stiffness and hyperesthesia, hyperthermia secondary to tetanic muscle contractions, panting, tachycardia, behavior changes associated with aggression
IV	Tonic-clonic muscle spasms in all four limbs (tetany), collapse with opisthotonos, labored respiration, behavior changes associated with disorientation
V	Arrhythmia (premature ventricular complexes) and seizures (musculoskeletal signs are often exaggerated with tactile stimulus); death may ensue

effect [18,19]. This allows for spontaneous discharge of nerve fibers to induce contraction of skeletal muscles and alteration of central nervous system function [3]. As a result, neuromuscular clinical signs quickly progress from generalized muscle fasciculations and stiffness to spasms and tetany [4,8,18–21]. Bitches showing signs of tetany usually have ionized calcium levels <0.6–0.8 mmol/L [7,11]. Extreme hypocalcemia can also cause low myocardial contractility and subsequent low cardiac output [21]. As the symptoms worsen, seizures and death may ensue [4,21].

Clinical signs of eclampsia in queens are similar to dogs and include acute lethargy, anorexia, weakness, bradycardia, hypersalivation, tachypnea progressing to dyspnea, and muscle fasiculations progressing to seizures [3,10,22–24].

Because total calcium concentrations fluctuate with serum protein concentration, acid–base status, and other electrolyte alterations, total serum calcium concentrations do not reliably correlate with ionized calcium [25–29]. Clinical manifestations of eclampsia correlate with both the absolute decrease in ionized calcium concentrations (<2.4–3.2 mg/dL or <0.6 mmol/L) and the rate and progression of ionized calcium decrease [11,14]. In queens, eclampsia occurs when serum ionized calcium concentrations fall below 1.0 mmol/L [30].

Hypoglycemia is a common sequela of eclampsia and can arise secondarily due to energy demands of tetany. But it is important to remember that severe primary hypoglycemia can also result in seizures [31] and must be ruled out with additional primary seizure causes (e.g. meningoencephalitis and strychnine toxicity) [20].

Treatment (Box 119.1)

In cases of eclampsia, treatment should not be delayed for laboratory confirmation. Response to treatment is dramatic and often a gratifying diagnostic tool.

Treatment is primarily aimed at correcting ionized calcium concentrations. Initial treatment includes slow intravenous administration of organic calcium compounds (20% calcium borogluconate or 10% calcium gluconate) at a rate of 1–1.5 mL/kg for dogs and 2.5 mL/kg for cats over a 10–30-minute period or until resolution of clinical signs [3,4,32]. Calcium chloride should be avoided due to the corrosive perivascular effects if extravasation occurs. Vomiting during intravenous calcium administration has been reported [20]. Careful cardiac monitoring via auscultation or electrocardiography is critical during calcium administration to prevent serious cardiac effects, including asystole [33]. Development of bradycardia, QT shortening, or arrhythmias indicates that the rate of calcium administration is too rapid and it must be temporarily discontinued and then restarted at a slower rate [4].

Response to initial treatment may last for only a short period (2 hours) and the animal must be monitored for signs of relapse. The original dose may be repeated [14]. The IV dose of calcium gluconate (not chloride) required to resolve clinical signs can be diluted 1:1 in a normal (0.9%) saline solution or 5% dextrose for subcutaneous administration divided into three equal doses over 24–48 hours to prevent immediate relapse. A continuous-rate infusion (CRI) of elemental calcium can be delivered at 1–3 mg/kg/h to maintain normal calcium levels in severe cases [14]. To avoid precipitation of calcium salts, solutions containing sulfate, phosphate, or bicarbonate should not be infused with calcium.

Secondary hypoglycemia and seizuring must be treated if present. Administration of a 10% dextrose solution is recommended in cases of co-existing hypoglycemia [4]. To control seizure activity, barbiturates or diazepam can be administered [3,5,34]. Because cerebral

---

Box 119.1 Emergency treatment for eclampsia.

5–15 mg/kg of elemental calcium slow IV
10% calcium gluconate or 20% calcium borogluconate

- Dogs: 1–1.5 mL/kg slow IV
- Cats: 2.5 mL/kg slow IV

Note: if other calcium salts or concentrations are used, the volume of administration will need to be changed accordingly.

Calcium administration should take place over 10–30 minutes with close monitoring via auscultation or ECG.

edema can occur from uncontrolled seizures, mannitol may be indicated for potential cerebral edema [34]. If severe hyperthermia (>104 °F, > 40 °C) exists, this should be controlled with active cooling. Magnesium deficiency or alkalosis should be corrected if present [14].

Prognosis after treatment is favorable, but relapses can occur through the end of lactation and with a subsequent pregnancy [20]. The offspring should be removed from the dam and hand-fed a milk supplement for 24–36 hours to reduce the risk of a relapse [4,32,35]. The lactating dam which experienced eclampsia should be orally supplemented with calcium carbonate or calcium lactate at 100 mg/kg body weight per day, divided with meals [4,23,32]. Vitamin D metabolites should be started early if hypocalcemia is expected to persist, as it takes several days for intestinal calcium transport to be upregulated. Calcitriol is the preferred active vitamin D metabolite, given its quick onset of action, short plasma half-life, and relatively short biological half-life; thus, discontinuing the drug will rapidly correct iatrogenic hypercalcemia, if it occurs. Calcitriol is administered at a dose of 20–30 ng/kg once daily for 3–4 days for induction, then 5–15 ng/kg once daily for maintenance therapy, titrated to desired serum calcium concentration [14].

If the offspring are 4 weeks old or more, they should be weaned [4]. If puppies are weaned to stop lactation, monitor the dam for self-milking (licking own mammary glands, which can induce milk letdown). Wrapping the mammary glands with a bandage for part of the day and then releasing the bandage an hour or so before replacing it may help in some cases. Alternatively, lactation cessation can be achieved using an antiprolactinic drug (cabergoline 5 μg/kg orally once daily for 7 days) [36,37]. Historical literature includes the use of glucocorticoids (e.g. prednisolone) to reduce the risk of eclampsia relapse [38]. However, glucocorticoids are contraindicated as they decrease intestinal calcium absorption, enhance renal excretion of calcium, and impair osteoclasia [13,34].

Prevention

A number of authors have speculated that eclampsia is a nutritionally related disorder of pregnancy or lactation resulting from either the overfeeding of high calcium-containing animal protein (egg or meat) or the feeding of dog foods containing cereals with phytate (because phytate binds ionized calcium, making it biologically unavailable) [5,9,39]. As a result, recommendations to prevent eclampsia involve feeding a balanced (puppy or kitten) formula commercial pet food without additional vitamin or mineral supplementation during the second half of gestation. This gestational diet should contain between 1.0% and 1.8% calcium and 0.8% and 1.6% phosphorus. Dietary supplementation with any dairy products during gestation should be avoided as they disrupt normal calcium-phosphorus-magnesium balance in the diet and may promote the development of eclampsia. The postpartum diet should be balanced for all lifestages, including lactation, and contain at least 1.4% calcium, with a calcium:phosphorus ratio of 1:1.3 [34]

References

1 Carlstrøm B. Studies of the etiology of eclampsia in the bitch. *Sv Vet T* 1929;34:101.

2 Martin BW, De Silva AS, Da Adbuchi A, Gannan J Jr. Eclampsia in the dog and cat. *Actualid Vet Brazil* 1973;2:14.

3 Wiebe VJ, Howard JP. Pharmacologic advances in canine and feline reproduction. *Top Compan Anim Med* 2009;24(2):71–99.

4 Wallace MS. Management of parturition and problems of the periparturient period of dogs and cats. *Semin Vet Med Surg Small Anim* 1994;9:28–37.

5 Mayer P. Eclampsia in the carnivore. *Wien Tierärtzl Mschr* 1968;55:592.

6 Biddle D, Macintire DK. Obstetrical emergencies. *Clin Techn Small Anim Pract* 2000;15(2):88–93.

7 Drobatz KJ, Casey KK. Eclampsia in dogs: 31 cases: 1995–1998. *J Am Vet Med Assoc* 2000;217: 216–219.

8 Mudaliar ASR, Hussain MM. Puerperal tetany in a bitch. *Indian Vet J* 1967;44(9):804–805.

9 Nesvadba J. Clinical symptomatology and prophylaxis of eclampsia in the bitch. *Kleintier Prax* 1971;16:56.

10 Edney ATB. Lactational tetany in the cat. *J Small Anim Pract* 1969;10:231–236.

11 Feldman EC, Nelson RW. Periparturient diseases. In: *Canine and Feline Endocrinology and Reproduction*, 3rd edn. WB Saunders, Philadelphia, 2004, pp. 829–831.

12 Aroch I, Ohad DG, Baneth G. Paresis and unusual electrocardiographic signs in a severely hypomagnesemic, hypocalcemic lactating bitch. *J Small Anim Pract* 1998;39:299–302.

13 Smith FO. Reproductive tract emergencies. In: *Veterinary Emergency and Critical Care Medicine* (eds Murtaugh RJ, Kaplan PM). Mosby, St Louis, 1992, pp. 420–426.

14 Groman RP. Acute management of calcium disorders. *Topics Compan Anim Med* 2012;27:167–171.

15 Johnson CA. Postpartum and mammary disorders. In: *Small Animal Internal Medicine*, 5th edn (eds Nelson RW, Couto GC). Mosby, St Louis, 2009, pp. 944–949.

16 Wallace MS, Davidson AP. Abnormalities in pregnancy, parturition and the periparturient period. In: *Textbook of Veterinary Internal Medicine: Diseases of the Dog and the Cat*, 4th edn (eds Ettinger SJ, Feldman ED). WB Saunders, Philadelphia, 1995, p. 1620.

17 Iggo A. Activity of peripheral nerves and junctional regions. In: *Dukes' Physiology of Domestic Animals*, 10th edn (ed. Swenson MJ). Comstock/Cornell University Press, Ithaca, pp. 612–614.

18 Rosol TJ, Capen CC. Calcium-regulating hormones and diseases of abnormal mineral (calcium, phosphorus, magnesium) metabolism. In: *Clinical Biochemistry of Domestic Animals*, 5th edn (eds Keneko JJ, Harvey JW, Bruss ML). Academic Press, San Diego, 1997, pp. 619–702.

19 Schaer M. Endocrine and metabolic causes of weakness. In: *Current Veterinary Therapy XI: Small Animal Practice* (eds Kirk RW, Bonagura JD). WB Saunders, Philadelphia, 1992, pp. 301–309.

20 Austad R, Bjerkas E. Eclampsia in the bitch. *J Small Anim Pract* 1976;17:793–798.

21 Aroch I, Srebro H, Shpigel NY. Serum electrolyte concentrations in bitches with eclampsia. *Vet Rec* 1999;145:318–320.

22 Bjerkås E. Eclampsia in the cat. *J Small Anim Pract* 1974;15:411–414.

23 Adeyanju JB. Eclampsia in a cat. *Vet Rec* 1984;114: 196–197.

24 Carolan MG. Eclampsia in a cat. *Vet Rec* 1984;114(2):303.

25 Sharp CR, Kerl ME, Mann FA. A comparison of total calcium, corrected calcium, and ionized calcium concentrations as indicators of calcium homeostasis among hypoalbuminemic dogs requiring intensive care. *J Vet Emerg Crit Care* 2009;19:571–578.

26 Taylor B, Siebald WJ, Edmonds MW, et al. Ionized hypocalcemia in critically ill patients with sepsis. *Can J Surg* 1978;21:429–433.

27 Drop LJ, Laver MB. Low plasma ionized calcium and response to calcium therapy in critically ill man. *Anesthesiology* 1975;43:300–306.

28 Zaloga GP, Chernow B, Cook D, et al. Assessment of calcium homeostasis in the critically ill surgical patient. The diagnostic pitfalls of the McLean-Hastings nomogram. *Ann Surg* 1985;202:587–594.

29 Broner CW, Stidham GL, Westenkirchner DF, et al. Hypermagnesemia and hypocalcemia as predicators of high mortality in critically ill patients. *Crit Care Med* 1990;18:921–928.

30 Nelson RW. Electrolyte imbalances. In: *Small Animal Internal Medicine*, 5th edn (Nelson RW, Couto GC). Mosby/Elsevier, St Louis, 2009, pp. 864–883.

31 Irvine CHG. Hypoglycemia in the bitch. *N Z Vet J* 1964;12:40.

32 Smith FO. Postpartum diseases. *Vet Clin North Am Small Anim Pract* 1986;16(3):521–524.

33 Kadar E, Rush JE, Wetmore L, Chan DL. Electrolyte disturbances and cardiac arrhythmias in a dog following pamidronate, calcitonin, and furosemide administration for hypercalcemia of malignancy. *J Am Anim Hosp Assoc* 2004;40:75–81.

34 Davidson AP. Reproductive causes of hypocalcemia. *Topics Compan Anim Med* 2012;27:165–166.

35 Wikstrøm B. Eclampsia in the bitch. *Sv Vet T* 1974;26:34.

36 Jöchle W, Arbeiter K, Post K, Ballabio R, d'Ver AS. Effects on pseudopregnancy, pregnancy and interestrous interval of pharmacological suppresion of prolactin secretion in female dogs and cats. *J Reprod Fertil Suppl* 1989;39:199–207.

37 Jöchle W, Ballbio R, di Salle E. Inhibition of lactation in the Beagle bitch with the prolactin inhibitor cabergoline (FCE 21336): dose response and aspects of long-term safety. *Theriogenology* 1987;27:799–811.

38 Kallfelz FA. In: *Current Veterinary Therapy III* (ed. Kirk RW). WB Saunders, Philadelphia, 1968, p. 64.

39 Resnick S. Hypocalcemic tetany in the dog. *J Am Vet Med Assoc* 1964;44:1115.

120

Neonatal Resuscitation

Carol A. Margolis, DVM, DACT and Margret L. Casal, DVM, MS, PhD

School of Veterinary Medicine, University of Pennsylvania, Philadelphia, PA, USA

Physical Examination

The physical examination should be performed quickly and Apgar scores obtained, paying particular attention to keeping the neonate warm and stimulated to breathe at all times.

The neonate should be assessed for the presence of a cleft palate, open fontanelle, umbilical hernia, patent urachus, hair coat and limb conformation, and patency of urogenital openings. The mucous membranes should be pink and moist, the umbilicus should not have surrounding erythema, the hair coat should be complete, and the limbs should have normal conformation with moderate muscle tone. Thoracic auscultation should reveal normal vesicular breath sounds and the lack of a heart murmur, although physiological murmurs may be possible. Normal heart and respiratory rates at birth in neonatal puppies and kittens are 200–220 beats per minute and 10–18 breaths per minute, respectively. The abdomen will be less haired than in an adult and should be pliant and not painful. Many neurological reflexes are not present at this age but the suckling, righting, rooting, and dorsal stimulation reflexes should be present within an hour after birth (Table 120.1). Observation of meconium staining indicates high stress *in utero*.

The Apgar evaluation parameters are assessed, scored, and the sum is taken (Table 120.2). Puppies with scores of 7–10 are classified as no distress, with significantly better survival than those with scores of 4–6 (moderate distress) or 0–3 (severe distress). Using the Apgar score in conjunction with the findings of a complete physical examination, an informed decision can be made as to how aggressive the resuscitation efforts should be [1].

Umbilical cord care should take place after the neonate is resuscitated; clamping is best 2+ cm from the body wall, which reduces traction and iatrogenic umbilical hernia. The umbilicus of the neonate should be treated with 2% tincture of iodine immediately after

Table 120.1 Neonatal reflexes. Assessment of the following four reflexes in a neonate helps to determine vigor.

Reflex	Response
Dorsal stimulation	A neonate is rubbed strongly over the dorsal lumbar area and should move vigorously and/or squeal in response
Righting reflex	The neonate is placed on its back and should then immediately turn itself over into ventral recumbency
Suckling reflex	A finger, bottle or the dam's nipple is offered to the neonate that should then begin suckling
Rooting reflex	The neonate should push its muzzle into a cupped hand or against its mother's mammaries in search of milk

birth to reduce contamination and prevent ascent of bacteria into the peritoneal cavity (omphalitis-peritonitis). Alcohol-based tincture of iodine is superior to aqueous povidone-iodine, which does not promote umbilical desiccation as quickly.

Table 120.2 Apgar scores.

Parameter	Score		
	0	1	2
Heart rate (bpm)	<180	180–220	>220
Respiratory effort: breaths per minute	No crying; <6	Mild crying; 6–15	Crying; >15
Reflex irritability	Absent	Grimace	Vigorous
Mobility	Flaccid	Some flexions	Active motion
Mucous membrane color	Cyanotic	Pale	Pink

bpm, beats per minute.
Source: Adapted from Johnson and Casal [1]. Reproduced with permission of John Wiley and Sons.

Textbook of Small Animal Emergency Medicine, First Edition. Edited by Kenneth J. Drobatz, Kate Hopper, Elizabeth Rozanski and Deborah C. Silverstein.
© 2019 John Wiley & Sons, Inc. Published 2019 by John Wiley & Sons, Inc.
Companion Website: www.wiley.com/go/drobatz/textbook

Respiratory Concerns

Normal respiratory rate in the neonate ranges from 10–18 breaths per minute at 1 day of age to 16–32 breaths per minute by 1 week of age [2]. If respiratory distress is encountered at birth, it may indicate pulmonary hypertension, decreased surfactant levels (prematurity), aspiration of meconium, or excess fluid in the airways. Congenital defects may cause persistent pulmonary hypertension and respiratory distress that is refractory to treatment [3].

Neonates should never be "swung" in a downward arc to remove fluid as this has been documented to cause intracranial trauma [4]. Airways are established by removing fetal membranes from the face followed by gentle suction with a bulb syringe or aspirator, prior to umbilical clamping. Systems capable of generating greater negative pressure than a bulb syringe should be used with caution, as they may cause airway injury and laryngospasm.

Cleaning and drying of the neonate stimulates respiration, crying, and movement. Stimulating genital and umbilical areas induces reflex respiration in neonates [2]. Another method to stimulate respiration is use of the Jen Chung acupuncture point (GV 26), in which a needle is inserted into the nasal philtrum at the base of the nares and rotated when cartilage/bone is contacted. Drying the muzzle and the Jen Chung acupuncture point likely stimulates respiratory neuroreceptors present in the muzzle that are functional at birth [5].

If respiratory distress is evident, oxygen can be supplied via face mask. If no improvement is noted after 1 minute, positive pressure ventilation with a snugly fitting mask should be initiated. Initial ventilation rates should be 40–60 breaths per minute during the first 30 seconds, then the rate should be decreased to 12–20 bpm [3]. Endotracheal intubation and use of a rescue breathing bag (using a 2 mm endotracheal tube or a 12–16 gauge intravenous catheter) is feasible but there is more potential for trauma of the upper airway. Administering 30–40 breaths per minute, with FIO_2 less than 40–60% and approximately 10 cmH$_2$O pressure, is advised [5]. Excessive insufflation using a mask can cause aerophagia, and overventilation is associated with higher mortality. Doxapram acts as a central stimulant and its effect is diminished by brain hypoxemia [6]. The use of doxapram as a respiratory stimulant is unlikely to improve hypoxemia associated with hypoventilation and is not recommended [5].

Cardiac Concerns

The two most common causes of neonatal bradycardia or asystole are hypoxia and hypothermia [1,5]. During the first 4 days of life, bradycardia is not vagally mediated and is considered to be indicative of hypoxia [2]. When hypothermia (below 96 °F/35.5 °C) is identified, normal cardiac function is not likely to resume. If not corrected with oxygen and ventilation alone, external chest compression can be initiated [3,5], done with the thumb and forefinger on either side of the thorax with approximately 100–120 compressions per minute.

There are multiple causes of ventricular tachycardia, including hypoxia, pain, ischemia, sepsis, electrolyte changes, trauma, and primary cardiac disease. Treatment of the underlying cause should be attempted first. Cardiopulmonary arrest requires rapid identification and intervention. Positive pressure ventilation and chest compressions should be started immediately. Cardiopulmonary resuscitation of the neonate follows the general CPR guidelines (see Chapter 150). Intravenous drug administration may not be feasible. Intratracheal administration can be considered but the intraosseous route is recommended. Atropine is not indicated, as neonatal bradycardia is not vagally mediated and anticholinergic-induced tachycardia will exacerbate myocardial oxygen deficits [2,5]. ECG evaluation may aid in guiding resuscitation. If ventricular fibrillation is identified, defibrillation is the ideal treatment but providing appropriate defibrillation doses for a neonate may not be possible.

Glucose is the main energy substrate of the neonatal brain and myocardium and should be monitored frequently. Sodium bicarbonate or calcium administration is not recommended [3].

Hypothermia

Newborn puppies and kittens cannot regulate their body temperature until about 4 weeks of age and are thus dependent on outside sources of heat (maternal care, heat lamps, etc.). Normal body temperature in puppies is 96 °F (35.5 °C) to 97 °F (36 °C) for the first 1–2 weeks of life. Normal body temperature in kittens is 98 °F (36.7 °C) at birth and increases to 100 °F (37.8 °C) by the end of the first week. For orphaned puppies, it has been recommended to maintain an environmental temperature of 80–90 °F (26.7–32.2 °C).

Hypothermia has been shown to have a negative impact on immunity, nursing, and digestion. In addition, it decreases food intake and exacerbates dehydration, hypoglycemia, bradycardia and ileus, decreasing the willingness to nurse and predisposing tube-fed puppies to aspiration and subsequent pneumonia [2]. Chilled neonates must be rewarmed slowly (minimum 30 minutes), avoiding peripheral vasodilation, to a maximum of 32.7 °C (99 °F) in neonates up to 7 days old [7]. During resuscitation, placing a chilled neonate's body into a warm water bath (95–99 °F) can improve core temperature. Resuscitation efforts can continue while a neonate is being actively warmed.

Exogenous heat is best supplied in the form of an overhead heat lamp. Heating pads may burn neonates incapable of moving away [5]. Neonates have a behavioral heat-seeking response [2]. Neonates lying separately may be too hot, vocalize loudly when too warm, then quickly fatigue and stop crying. Neonates that are too cold also quit vocalizing and become inactive; kittens are almost always quiet to begin with, making subjective observation of euthermia more difficult [1]. Studies in neonatal kittens have shown that rapid rewarming in the face of hypoxia may result in relative hyperthermia [8]. The response of the respiratory chemoreflex decreases at the same time as the ventilation decreases due to the decrease in metabolism, predisposing to apnea [9].

Dehydration and Fluid Therapy

Dehydration in the neonate is most commonly associated with diarrhea, vomiting, or decreased fluid intake. Low urine specific gravity (1.006–1.0017) is normal, as is the detection of protein, glucose, and amino acids because of immaturity of the proximal tubules during the first 2 weeks of life. The value of skin turgor as an assessment of hydration status is less than ideal in the neonate due to difference in body water content [10]. Checking mucous membranes is a better method of assessing the neonate's hydration state. Tacky mucous membranes indicate 5–7% dehydration and any increase in dehydration beyond that will result in dry mucous membranes and decreased skin elasticity.

Neonates have greater water requirements and greater insensible water loss than adults [11], and because neonatal canine kidneys have minimal capacity to conserve water before 40 days of age [12], dehydration will occur in any instance of decreased milk intake. Therefore, neonates are more prone than older animals to develop water and electrolyte imbalances, either excess or deficit, during fluid therapy [1].

Maintenance fluid requirements are reported to be 80–100 mL/kg/day [6]. When neonates are found to be dehydrated but normovolemic, fluids should be administered for correction over 6–8 hours to decrease the chances of inadvertent overload. In normovolemia, subcutaneous administration is often used to replace the fluid deficit if the patient is not severely compromised, if only a small volume is needed or there are financial concerns. In the face of moderate dehydration, a bolus of 30–40 mL/kg is recommended, followed by a constant-rate infusion of 80–100 mL/kg/day of warmed crystalloids. In cases of hypovolemia or shock, recommended rates are up to 40–45 mL/kg/h [6], with serial monitoring of mucous membrane color, pulse quality, extremity temperature, lactate levels, and mentation [3]. Lactated Ringer's solution may be ideal, since lactate is the preferred metabolic fuel in the neonate during times of hypoglycemia [3]. Signs of fluid overload include increased respiratory rate or effort, restlessness, serous nasal discharge, subcutaneous edema, ascites, or excessive weight gain within less than 24 hours.

Fluids are administered through the cephalic or jugular vein in these smallest of patients using small (22–25 G) and short (0.5 inch) IV catheters. Fluids may also be administered via the intraosseous (IO) route if IV access is not possible. Options for IO catheter placement include the femur, humerus or tibia, depending on the size of the patient. Typically, 18–22 G spinal needles or 18–25 G hypodermic needles will be used. This portal can be used for fluid boluses, emergency drug administration, and blood transfusions. Sterile preparation is required for IO placement, with the catheter inserted parallel to the long axis and into the marrow space. Gentle aspiration will ensure placement and patency followed by suturing in place for security. Intravenous access should then be established as soon as possible, and the IO catheter should be removed to minimize the possibility of osteitis or sepsis [3].

For quick drug administration but not large volumes of fluids, the umbilical vein may be considered if it has not already thrombosed.

Hypoglycemia

Clinical signs associated with hypoglycemia include weakness, flaccidity, seizure, and coma. The goal is to restore a euglycemic range without causing hyperglycemia. Because the neonatal kidney is ineffective at conserving water in the face of osmotic diuresis, dehydration may result from hyperglycemia [1]. Resolution of clinical signs of hypoglycemia is a poor indicator of treatment response, as there are several similar non-specific clinical signs, such as hypothermia, metabolic errors, and seizures, which may also be seen with hypoglycemia.

Clinical hypoglycemia is characterized by blood glucose levels less than 30–40 mg/dL. It can be treated with a dextrose solution given either IV or IO, at a dose of 0.5–1.0 g/kg body weight using a 5–10% dextrose solution (1 to 2 ml/100g weight). Subcutaneous administration of dextrose is undesirable due to the potential for abscessation at the site [5]. Dextrose at 50% must be diluted for IV administration to avoid phlebitis. However, this concentration may be applied to the mucous membranes but if severe hypovolemia or dehydration is present, the neonate's circulation may not be adequate for absorption, so IO administration is preferable. If the neonate is too weak to nurse, a mixture of warmed 4.5% saline with 2.5% dextrose can be administered via a stomach tube at

0.1–0.5 mL/30 g body weight every 15–30 minutes until suckle capability returns. However, if available, colostrum from the dam is superior to this mixture [5].

There are some cases of neonates with refractory hypoglycemia, which may only respond to hourly boluses of dextrose in addition to IV CRI crystalloid with dextrose supplemented. If no positive responses are noted within 24 hours, the neonate should be assessed for inborn errors of metabolism.

Sepsis

Bacterial sepsis is a common contributor to neonatal mortality. The most commonly cultured organisms associated with sepsis are *Escherichia coli*, streptococci, staphylococci, and *Klebsiella* spp. Sudden death may be the only clinical sign observed; a decrease in weight gain or net loss with failure to suckle may be the first indication of infection. Other clinical signs may include hematuria, decreased urine output, persistent diarrhea, unusual vocalization, abdominal distension and pain, cold limbs or body, possible sloughing of extremities.

Empirical therapy includes use of the antibiotic ceftiofur at a dose of 2.5 mg/kg SC every 12 hours for no longer than 5 days [1,2,13]. It alters normal intestinal flora minimally and is usually effective against the causative organisms. Alternatively, amoxicillin/clavulanic acid is a safe, broad-spectrum antibiotic that can be given at 20 mg/kg orally twice daily.

Septic patients can have increased capillary permeability and vasodilation and may require aggressive fluid resuscitation. It has been demonstrated that using fresh or frozen plasma from a well-vaccinated adult dog might augment immunity, and may be administered either via CRI or subcutaneously [14]. Because puppies less than 48 hours old have reduced thrombin levels, presumptive therapy with vitamin K1 may be used (0.01–1.0 mg subcutaneously per puppy) [5].

When to Stop Resuscitation Efforts

Deciding when to stop attempts at resuscitation can be difficult. Some helpful guidelines include discontinuing after 30 minutes of effort with no response or continued bradycardia with agonal respirations despite resuscitation attempts. Cessation of attempts should also be considered in the face of a serious congenital defect. This may include but is not limited to a cleft palate, loud murmur, large umbilical hernia, large omphalocele, large open fontanelle, anasarca, anogenital defects, and severe vertebral or limb abnormalities not compatible with a good quality of life.

References

1 Johnson CA, Casal ML. Neonatal resuscitation: canine and feline. In: *Management of Pregnant and Neonatal Dogs, Cats, and Exotic Pets* (ed. Lopate C). Wiley, New York, 2012, pp. 77–92.
2 Grundy SA. Clinically relevant physiology of the neonate. *Vet Clin North Am Small Anim Pract* 2006;36(3):443–459.
3 McMichael MA. Emergency and critical care issues. In: *Small Animal Pediatrics: The First 12 Months of Life* (eds Peterson M, Kutzler M). Saunders Elsevier, St Louis, 2011, pp. 73–81.
4 Grundy SA, Liu S, Davidson A, et al. Intracranial trauma in a dog due to being "swung" at birth. *Topics Compan Anim Medic* 2009;24:100–103.
5 Davidson, AP. Neonatal resuscitation, improving the outcome. *Vet Clin North Am Small Anim Pract* 2014;44:191–204.
6 Moon PF, Massat B, Pascoe P. Neonatal critical care. *Vet Clin North Am Small Anim Pract* 2001;31(2):343–376.
7 Lawler DF. Neonatal and pediatric care of the puppy and kitten. *Theriogenology* 2008;70:384–392.
8 Rohlicek CV, Saiki C, Matsuoka T, et al. Cardiovascular and respiratory consequences of body warming during hypoia in conscious newborn cats. *Pediatr Res* 1996;40:1–5.
9 Watanabe T, Kumar P, Hanson M. Effect of ambient temperature on respiratory chemoreflex in unanaesthetized kittens. *Respir Physiol* 1996;106:239–246.
10 Hardy RM, Osborne C. Water deprivation test in the dog: maximal normal values. *J Am Vet Med Assoc* 1979;174:479–483.
11 Fettman MJ, Allen T. Developmental aspects of fluid an electrolyte metabolism and renal function in the neonates. *Compend Contin Educ Pract Vet* 1991;13:392–403.
12 Horster M, Valtin H. Postnatal development of renal function: micropuncture and clearance studies in the dog. *J Clin Invest* 1971;50:779–795.
13 Davidson AP. Approaches to reducing neonatal mortality in dogs. Available at: www.researchgate.net/publication/267937790_Approaches_to_Reducing_Neonatal_Mortality_in_Dogs_19-Mar-2003 (accessed 4 February 2018).
14 Poffenbarger EM, Olson P, Chandler M, et al. Use of adult dog serum as a substitute for colostrum in the neonatal dog. *Am J Vet Res* 1991;52:1221–1224.

121

Diseases of the Neonate

Andrea Hesser, DVM, DACT[1] and Autumn P. Davidson, DVM, MS, DACVIM[2]

[1]*Advanced Care Veterinary Hospital, Sapulpa, OK, USA*
[2]*School of Veterinary Medicine, University of California, Davis, CA, USA*

Introduction

Neonatal dogs and cats are defined here as being less than 4 weeks of age, prior to weaning, which normally occurs at 5–6 weeks. Orphan puppies and kittens present unique sets of disorders related to their immaturity at birth, dependence on acquisition of colostrum, small size, and fragility. Neonatal patients are most commonly presented to the emergency veterinarian due to failure to thrive or to an acute onset of signs of illness. Clinical signs are most commonly due to historical dystocia, congenital anomalies, infectious disease, and environmental trauma.

Epizootiology

Average reported neonatal mortality rates (greatest during the first week of life) vary, ranging from 9% to 26%. Most puppies and kittens that fail to survive to weaning are stillborn or die within the first 3–7 days of life [1]. Prudent veterinary intervention in the prenatal, parturient, and postpartum periods can increase neonatal survival by controlling or eliminating factors contributing to puppy morbidity and mortality. Poor prepartum condition of the dam, dystocia, prematurity, congenital malformations, genetic defects, injury, environmental exposure, malnutrition, parasitism, and infectious disease all contribute to neonatal morbidity and mortality. Optimal husbandry affects neonatal survival favorably by managing labor and delivery to reduce stillbirths, controlling parasitism and reducing exposure to infectious disease, preventing injury and harmful environmental exposure, and optimizing nutrition of the dam and neonates. Proper genetic screening for selection of breeding animals minimizes inherited congenital defects.

Low birth weight is the most significant risk factor for neonatal puppy and kitten death. Birth weights of puppies are breed dependent; normal birth weights for the smaller breeds can range from 75 g to 350 g, medium breeds 200–300 g and the larger breeds from 400 g up to 800 g. The average birth weight of surviving kittens is 100 ± 10 g [2]. Morbid puppies and kittens may be smaller at birth, with reduced weight gain or even weight loss. The cause of low birth weight or poor growth is usually difficult to determine but may include prematurity, inborn errors of metabolism, birth defects, infections, nutritional deficiencies, and maternal neglect.

Risk of neonatal loss was also associated with obese dams, singleton litters, and for the first neonate born in a litter. A higher rate of death of the first neonate born could reflect an inexperienced dam. The breeder's level of knowledge about whelping may also play a key role in neonatal survival. Delaying nursing until the entire litter is born or until the dam is awake from anesthesia for a cesarean section subjects neonates to delayed colostral intake. Neonatal survival is directly related to the quality of labor (avoidance of dystocia). Extended or difficult labor may result in birth trauma, in neonates that are too weak to nurse, or in ill or exhausted dams that are unable to care for their offspring.

Physiology

Post resuscitation, or within the first 24 hours of a natural delivery, a complete physical examination should be performed by a veterinarian, technician, or knowledgeable breeder. Body temperature ranges from 95 °F to 99 °F (35.5–36.5 °C). The oral cavity, hair coat, limbs, umbilicus, and urogenital structures should be visually inspected. Normal hydration is evidenced by normal skin turgor. The mucous membranes should be pink and moist, a suckle reflex present, the coat full and clean, the urethra and anus patent. Urination and defecation are easily elicited by gentle stimulation with a cotton ball

Textbook of Small Animal Emergency Medicine, First Edition. Edited by Kenneth J. Drobatz, Kate Hopper, Elizabeth Rozanski and Deborah C. Silverstein.
© 2019 John Wiley & Sons, Inc. Published 2019 by John Wiley & Sons, Inc.
Companion Website: www.wiley.com/go/drobatz/textbook

moistened with warm water. A normal umbilicus is dry without surrounding erythema. The thorax should be ausculted; vesicular breath sounds and a lack of murmur are normal. If a murmur is detected, auscultation should be repeated in 48–72 hours; innocent physiological murmurs will disappear. Respiration is regular, 15–35 breaths per minute, and no fluid should be ausculted over the lung fields. Minimal clear nasal discharge can be evident. The heart rate is rapid, usually 180–250 beats per minute. The abdomen should be pliant and not painful. A normal neonate will squirm and vocalize when examined, but will sleep quietly or nurse when returned to the dam. Normal neonates will attempt to right themselves and orient by rooting toward their dam. Daily examination of each neonate for vigor and recording of weight is critical.

The signs of distress or disease in neonates are usually non-specific, most commonly including continuous vocalization, ineffective nursing, and restlessness. Failing neonates can become disoriented, stranded, limp, and hypothermic.

Puppies and kittens lack adult thermoregulatory mechanisms until 3–4 weeks of age, so the ambient temperature must be high enough to facilitate maintenance of a body temperature of at least 97 °F (36 °C). Typically, the dam and littermates will provide adequate warmth in a draft-free box indoors with an ambient room temperature of 70–75 °F, resulting in adequate thermal support to the neonates (Box 121.1). Hypothermia negatively affects immunity, nursing, and digestion. Low-birth weight neonates are most susceptible to chilling. Exogenous heat should be supplied as indicated (i.e. in the absence of the dam), best in the form of an overhead infrared heat lamp. Heating pads run the risk of burning neonates incapable of moving away from excessively hot surfaces. Hyperthermia is to be avoided; dams will avoid the box, resulting in reduced nursing and mothering behavior. Excessive exogenous heat results in vocalization and

restlessness. Neonates typically pile up together in the absence of the dam to maintain body heat.

Chilled neonates must be rewarmed slowly (30 minutes) to avoid peripheral vasodilation and dehydration. Tube feeding should be delayed until the neonate is euthermic, as hypothermia induces ileus and regurgitation, and aspiration can result.

Neonates are inefficient at gluconeogenesis, and have low glycogen storage capabilities. Glycogen stores are depleted shortly after birth, making adequate nourishment from nursing vital. Even minimal fasting can result in hypoglycemia. In addition, neonates have poor glucose absorption from the kidneys.

Incompletely developed immune systems during the first 10 days of life make neonates vulnerable to systemic infection (most commonly bacterial and viral) [2].

Neonatal Disorders in the Immediate Postpartum Period

Disorders of Metabolism

Pathophysiology
Inborn errors of metabolism, lysosomal storage disorders, and mucopolysaccharidoses occur in dogs and cats. Congenital hypoglycemia and intracellular accumulation of deleterious substrates will occur.

Clinical Presentation
Disorders of metabolism are suspected in neonates that appear normal at birth, but display progressive lethargy, poor nursing, persistent vomiting and eventually central nervous system signs. No infectious or traumatic etiology can be identified.

Diagnostics
The history of a related animal having a documented inborn metabolic disorder is of interest. Specific genetic tests are available for some disorders [3,4].

Therapy
The prognosis is usually hopeless for veterinary patients, as gene therapy is indicated.

Anasarca

Pathophysiology
Anasarca, a lethal congenital edema, can occur with or without concurrent cardiovascular abnormalities. Congenital hereditary lymphedema causes edema of the extremities and sometimes head, and is associated with morphological lymphatic abnormalities. The genetics are not known; the trait is thought to be inherited as an autosomal dominant trait.

Box 121.1 Normal neonatal body temperatures by age and ambient room temperature required to maintain this.	
Neonatal normal body temperature (rectal)	
Week 1	95–99 °F
Week 2–3	97–100 °F
At weaning	99–101 °F
Environmental warmth required at level of neonates	
Week 1	84–89 °F
Week 2–3	80 °F
Week 4	69–75 °F

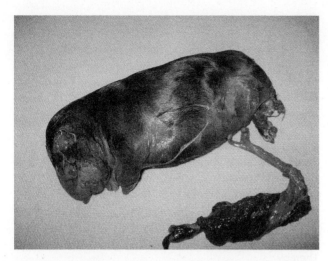

Figure 121.1 Anasarca. Stillborn Labrador retriever; obstructive dystocia resulted in emergency cesarean section.

Clinical Presentation

Generalized subcutaneous edema, with intrathoracic and intraperitoneal fluid accumulation, is present. Anasarca puppies are commonly a cause of dystocia due to oversize, and can be stillborn. Anasarca is a problem common in bulldogs, but recognized in other breeds as well. It is suspected to have a heritable component (Figure 121.1).

Diagnostics

Prepartum ultrasonographic evaluation of the fetuses can be used to screen for this disorder, especially in breeds at risk. On radiographic evaluation, the skeleton may appear of appropriate size for natural delivery, but generalized edema often prevents passage through the birth canal.

Therapy

There are multiple anecdotal remedies, none proven or reported in the scientific literature. Diuretic therapy can sometimes slightly normalize affected neonates, but euthanasia is usually indicated if the neonate is not stillborn. Environmental, dietary, and pharmacological contributory factors are not scientifically defined.

Ciliary Dyskinesia

Pathophysiology

Abnormal mucociliary transport and neutrophil function result in chronic rhinitis, tracheobronchitis, and bronchopneumonia. Situs inversus can be present.

Clinical Presentation

Primary ciliary dyskinesia, the extremely rare immotile cilia syndrome, should be suspected in neonates exhibiting persistent mucopurulent nasal discharge, coughing, and abnormal breath sounds without other demonstrable cause (i.e. cleft palate).

Diagnostics

The diagnosis is most easily made if semen can be acquired and evaluated for motility in the postpubertal individual; confirmation of the diagnosis requires pulmonary electron microscopy in prepubertal puppies.

Therapy

The long-term prognosis, even with supportive therapy, is poor.

Hydrocephalus

Pathophysiology

Neonatal neurological disorders can be inherited or can result from intrauterine teratogens or trauma during parturition. Morphological neurological abnormalities occur most frequently. Aqueduct atresia, birth trauma, or meningoencephalitis can also cause the development of (acquired) hydrocephalus [5].

Clinical Presentation

A domed calvarium, open fontanelle, and prominent suture lines are often present. Clinical signs vary from inapparent to progressively debilitating neurological changes. Hydrocephalus has an increased frequency in toy and brachycephalic breeds, and can occur in cats. Early clumsy, weak, or ataxic ambulation can indicate a neurological or musculoskeletal abnormality.

Diagnostics

Neonatal patients with focal, partial, or grand mal seizures for which no metabolic or toxic etiology can be identified can benefit from intracranial ultrasound. Scanning the brain through the fontanelle, usually partially open in pediatric patients, permits non-invasive evaluation of the ventricles. Evaluation of a normal littermate facilitates recognition of excessive cerebral spinal fluid accumulation by serving as a control. CT scanning or MRI can confirm the diagnosis.

Therapy

Omeprazole decreases CSF movement into the ventricles via proton pump inhibition. Corticosteroids and diuretics can offer some relief. Ventriculoperitoneal shunting has been described in puppies [6]. Neurological abnormalities noted on physical exam may be permanent.

Umbilical Herniation

Pathophysiology

A developmental anomaly resulting in extrusion of a portion of the gastrointestinal tract outside of the body wall, occurring within the umbilical canal (omphalocele) or lateral to the umbilical canal (gastroschisis), has been reported in humans and occurs in both dogs and cats.

Clinical Presentation

Umbilical herniation is noted on physical examination of a neonate (Web Figure 121.1).

Diagnostics

The diagnosis is made antepartum in humans with abdominal ultrasound, based on the recognition of fetal gastric wall (rugal) structures or intestinal contents in an abnormal location, and is theoretically possible in veterinary patients.

Therapy

The condition is usually hopeless in small veterinary patients presented to the veterinarian hours after birth; however, a 30–70% survival rate is reported in humans with immediate postpartum surgical intervention. The prognosis for omphalocele is worse than gastroschisis. Earlier surgical intervention before inevitable septic contamination occurs may improve the prognosis in veterinary patients; clients should be educated as to its recognition postpartum and timely presentation to a veterinarian.

Bowel Malformation: Agenesis or Duplication

Pathophysiology

Agenesis is most common at the terminal colon, but can occur anywhere in the intestinal tract. Duplication is rare, but again can occur anywhere in the intestinal tract.

Clinical Presentation

The clinical signs may be non-specific. Enteric agenesis usually results in severe clinical signs in the neonatal period (failure to defecate, abdominal distension, vomiting).

Diagnostics

Enteric duplication or agenesis can be confirmed ultrasonographically in neonatal patients. A fluid-filled juxtaintestinal formation with variable peristalsis and contents can be seen. Ultrasonographic findings usually include marked fluid and gas distension of bowel proximal to the defect.

Therapy

Surgical repair of rectal agenesis is possible if the defect is diagnosed in a timely manner; fecal incontinence can result.

Patent Urachus

Pathophysiology

The urachus permits the flow of urine from the bladder into the allantoic sac of the fetus, and normally atrophies at birth.

Clinical Presentation

A persistent patent urachus in the neonate is characterized clinically by urine dribbling from the umbilicus. If an incompletely patent urachus is present, a urachal diverticulum may result. Urachal diverticula can predispose the bladder to recurrent infection because of abnormal urinary flow in the region.

Diagnostics

Patent urachus is apparent on physical examination. The fluid-filled urachus can be identified ultrasonographically, extending cranially from the cranioventral bladder wall. A urachal diverticulum is seen as a divot in the apex of the bladder.

Therapy

Ligation of the urachus is indicated if spontaneous closure does not occur. Surgical excision of a diverticulum can be indicated in the future if urinary tract infection occurs.

Cleft Palate

Pathophysiology

Congenital palate defects occur in dogs with an incidence of up to 25%. Secondary cleft palate is a congenital oronasal fistula resulting in incomplete closure of the hard and soft palate. Cleft palate occurs alone or in combination with a primary cleft palate involving the lip and premaxilla. Cleft palate results from incomplete fusion of the palatine shelves, most critical at 25–28 days gestation. Palatal defects are attributed to genetic (recessive or incompletely dominant polygenic inheritance), teratogenic (drugs, supplements), nutritional (folic acid deficiency) or infectious (viral) factors [7].

Clinical Presentation

Ineffective nursing and suckling result; these neonates fail to thrive, developing aspiration pneumonia and rhinitis. Milk may be seen coming from the nares during or after nursing.

Diagnostics

Affected neonates are diagnosed by visual inspection of the face and oral cavity (Figure 121.2).

Therapy

Feeding by orogastric tube is indicated until the puppy reaches a size permitting oral surgery, traditionally advised at 8–12 weeks of age. Palatoplasty in such young puppies remains difficult due to patient size and anticipated postoperative orofacial growth, often necessitating multiple operations. Esophagostomy or gastrostomy tube placement can facilitate feeding over time,

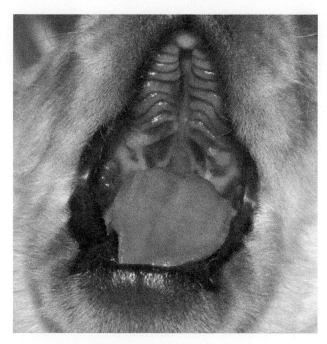

Figure 121.2 Cleft palate in a 3-day-old Labrador retriever puppy; no craniofacial defect is present.

but requires significant client commitment and can still result in aspiration. Palatal prostheses are problematic.

Methods to improve survival of pet puppies with cleft palates are sought by motivated clients. Following the postpartum diagnosis of cleft palate, feeding the dam's colostrum for 24 hours followed by artificial bitch milk replacer by intermittent orogastric tube can be instituted. At 4 weeks of age, transition to a dry (not soft soaked) commercial pediatric dog food should be made, facilitating swallowing without ingesta becoming misplaced into the nasal cavity. Water should be made available through an overhead ballpoint tube cap system. This permits dogs with secondary cleft palate to attain adult size before reconstructive surgery, which may not be necessary due to closure of the defect with maturity.

Neonatal Isoerythrolysis (see Chapter 66)

Pathophysiology
Neonatal isoerythrolysis occurs in kittens after initial colostral ingestion. The disease occurs as a result of the dam's and kitten's blood types being different, and the kitten ingesting antibodies against its own blood type. Type B cats with type A kittens are the most likely to produce this condition, as type B cats carry strong anti-A antibodies [8].

Clinical Presentation
The most common breeds with high numbers of type B cats include the Cornish rex, Devon rex, and British short-hair. Kittens show signs of anemia, such as lethargy, tachycardia, tachypnea, and pale mucous membranes, and are often icteric. Extreme presentation may also show necrosis of the tail tips and other extremities due to ischemia.

Diagnostics
The diagnosis is based on the findings of anemia and icterus with no evidence of blood loss or hemoparasites.

Therapy
Treatment depends on severity. All affected kittens should be removed immediately from the dam. Transfusion of cross-matched donor blood or washed type B from the dam may be used. Blood products can be transfused at a rate of 10–20 mL/kg over a 4-hour period via intravenous or intraosseous catheter. The prognosis is poor in kittens showing any degree of clinical signs. Prevention is achieved by avoiding mating type B queens to type A toms. Breeding animals should be blood typed, ideally with A bred to A and B bred to B. Another strategy is to collect umbilical blood from kittens before nursing, and determine if the type is the same as the dam's before nursing is allowed.

Immunodeficiency

Pathophysiology
Neonatal dogs and cats are born immunocompetent but immunodeficient due to minimal transplacental acquisition of maternal antibodies. Adequate ingestion of colostrum must occur promptly postpartum for puppies to acquire passive transfer of immunity. Neonates should be encouraged to suckle promptly after birth once resuscitation is completed; this usually necessitates close monitoring after a cesarean section as the dam is still groggy from anesthesia. The intestinal absorption of IgG generally ceases by 24 hours after parturition.

Clinical Presentation
Neonates which have failed to nurse adequately can present with signs of hypoglycemia, excessive vocalization due to hunger, or lethargy; subsequent signs of infectious disease occur. Orphans should be considered to be colostrum deprived.

Diagnostics
Failing to observe colostrum ingestion is key to the diagnosis. Neonates should show weight gain after nursing in the immediate postpartum period. The diagnosis is usually presumptive. Snap tests for semi-quantitative antibody measurement do not exist for dogs or cats currently.

Therapy

Failure to acquire colostrum within 24 hours of birth should prompt administration of adult conspecific plasma to a neonate; if >24 hours of age, parenteral administration is indicated (SC or IP). Colostrum-deprived kittens given adult cat serum at a dose of 150 mL/kg (0.15 mL/g) developed serum IgG levels comparable with suckling littermates, but colostrum-deprived puppies given 40 mL/kg (0.40 mL/g) adult dog serum orally and parenterally failed to match suckling littermates' IgG levels. Puppies likely require as much as 100 mL/kg (0.10 mL/g). The dose should be divided over several administrations within a 12-hour period due to the volume [9,10].

Neonatal Ophthalmia

Pathophysiology

Neonatal ophthalmia is an acute, mucopurulent infection of the conjunctiva which occurs before the eyelids separate (~14 days of age). Both gram-positive and gram-negative bacteria have been causal.

Clinical Presentation

Accumulation of fluid associated with ophthalmia produces noticeable swelling over the eye(s).

Diagnostics

The condition is apparent on physical examination and confirmed by intervention (Web Figure 121.2).

Therapy

Opening the eyelid by gentle manipulation with a gauze sponge or sterile mosquito forceps will allow cytology and culture of the fluid. The conjunctival space should be irrigated with sterile saline. Ten to14 days of topical antibiotic is indicated. Ocular lubrication can be advisable as normal tear production is diminished until 10–14 days of life. Damage to the eye can occur if the condition is not recognized and treated.

Limb Deformities: Amelia, Hemimelia (Absence of a Limb or Distal Portion of a Limb), Pelvic Limb Hyperextension

Pathophysiology

Limb deformities are commonly idiopathic; in some cases they are suspected to be heritable defects.

Clinical Presentation

Neonates with pelvic limb hyperextension are not as mobile as normal littermates and may not nurse effectively or competitively. The pelvic limbs are hyperextended and commonly rotated laterally.

Diagnostics

The defects are apparent in the physical examination. (Web Figure 121.3).

Therapy

Pelvic limb hyperextension can be corrected if addressed early in the neonatal period. Physical therapy (flexing and rotating medially) and gentle binding of the limbs can correct the defect in 3–4 days (Web Figure 121.4).

Neonatal Disorders in the Later Postpartum Period

Orphans

Pathophysiology

Kittens and puppies under 3 weeks of age lack voluntary elimination without external stimulation, normally provided by the dam. The lack of nursing can result in hunger-driven suckling of littermates.

Clinical Presentation

Neonates with distended abdomen, vocalization, and restlessness can indicate constipation or urine retention. Focal areas of petechiation can be evident from littermate suckling.

Diagnostics

The diagnosis is made from the history of orphaning and physical examination.

Therapy

The micturition and defecation reflexes are stimulated using a cotton ball with lubrication on the anogenital area after each feeding. Periodic separation of the neonates in an orphaned litter may be necessary until solid food is introduced. Tube feeding is often the easiest and safest option for continued nutritional maintenance in orphan neonates until bottle feeding is well accepted. Neonates should receive multiple small feedings to achieve acceptable daily weight gain, approximately every 2 hours. For any patient receiving meals via tube feeding, care should be taken that the feeding tube is placed into the esophagus, not the trachea. The easiest way to ensure that placement is correct is to witness vocalization while the tube is in place, or to initiate it by pinching a toe or the scruff of the neck. If vocalization is heard, the tube is presently in the esophagus. When bottle feeding or tube feeding, the neonate's body should be sternal in orientation, with the skull planes parallel to the body.

In the first day of life, each puppy or kitten may lose or maintain the birth weight or even lose weight, but subsequently should steadily be gaining 5–10% of their body weight daily. Neonates should gain weight steadily from the first day after birth (a transient mild loss from birth weight is acceptable on day 1) – puppies gaining 1–3 g per day per kilo (2.2 lb) of anticipated adult weight and kittens 50–100 g weekly.

The neonatal caloric requirement is 133 calories/kg/day during the first week of life, 155 calories/kg/day for the second, 175–198 calories/kg/day for the third, and 220 calories/kg/day for the fourth [2]. Commercially manufactured milk replacement formulae (Esbilac, Pet-Ag Inc., Elgin, IL; Puppy Milk Replacer Formula, Eukanuba, Iams Co., Dayton, OH; Veta-Lac Powder for Puppies, Vet-A-Mix, Shenandoah, IA; KMR, Pet-Ag Inc., Elgin, IL) are usually superior to home-made versions; recent studies have shown that none is equal to a bitch's milk and none is perfect. The use of milk obtained from the dam can be considered if available. An osmotic diarrhea (usually yellow, curdled stool appearance) can result from overfeeding formula, necessitating dilution of the product by 50% with water or a balanced crystalloid such as lactated Ringer's solution.

Aspiration Pneumonia

Pathophysiology
Aspiration pneumonia is a common disease of neonatal puppies and kittens. The disease often presents concurrently with the presence of cleft palate, but can occur spontaneously during nursing, bottle feeding, or tube feeding. Overfeeding causing overdistension of the stomach and placing a feeding tube in the trachea are the most common causes of aspiration.

Clinical Presentation
Aspiration pneumonia can present as an acute respiratory problem, but can also present with a history of the neonate or others in the litter wheezing or coughing, often accompanied with poor weight gain or fever. Other causes of dyspnea include congenital peritoneopericardial diaphragmatic hernias and trauma.

Diagnostics
Mucous membranes may be gray or blue in severely affected neonates. Auscultation of the chest will yield the presence of crackles and/or wheezes which may be distributed in all fields, or may be focal in nature. Puppies or kittens are often febrile due to infectious process. The neonate will often be unthrifty and small in appearance if the disease has been chronic. Thoracic radiographs can be performed if the patient is stable enough to tolerate room air or flow-by oxygen as well as restraint techniques. Radiographs can indicate how extensive the pneumonia is, which can be important in prognosis and monitoring improvement during treatment.

Therapy
Puppies and kittens with marked dyspnea should be immediately transferred to an oxygen cage (see Chapter 181), and handled within that environment until the animal is eupneic on room air. Some neonates that are more mildly dyspneic or tachypneic may tolerate flow-by oxygen during initial evaluation.

Empirical antibiotic therapy should be initiated. Clavulanic acid-potentiated beta-lactam antibiotics are often implemented initially, as they are among those safest to administer to neonates [11]. Initially parenteral administration is advised. Transtracheal washing for culture samples in a tiny neonate is rarely attempted, but may be applicable in neonates that do not respond to empirical treatment. Fluid and nutrient support are indicated.

If the animal becomes stable in oxygen and appears to have improved, slow tapering of the environmental oxygen can be initiated, monitoring for respiratory changes as the environmental oxygen is reduced. The patient should be comfortable breathing room air consistently for at least 12–24 hours prior to release. Oral liquid preparations of the antibiotic are preferable for home administration with proper instruction.

Swimmer Puppies

Pathophysiology
Swimmer puppies fail to develop normal ambulation by 10–14 days of life, moving instead on their ventrum by paddling their limbs laterally and caudally. Obese puppies from small litters, commonly raised on relatively slippery surfaces, are predisposed.

Clinical Presentation
A failure to ambulate normally is evident upon physical examination. Compression and deformation of the sternum and thorax occur concurrently.

Diagnostics
The defect is apparent on physical examination.

Therapy
Treatment should be instituted immediately upon diagnosis, consisting of caloric restriction, physical therapy, and improved traction in the nest box. Refractory cases can require body harnessing to keep the limbs under the trunk (Web Figure 121.5). If diagnosed early (3–5 weeks of age), the condition is reversible.

Juvenile Cellulitis

Pathophysiology
Juvenile cellulitis (puppy strangles) is a progressive, granulomatous, pustular disorder of puppies, most commonly

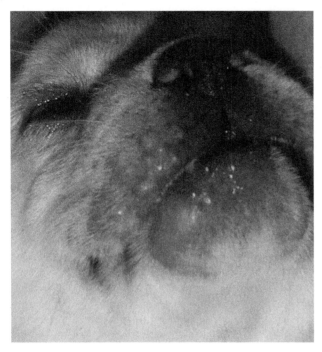

Figure 121.3 Juvenile cellulitis in a 4-week-old Labrador retriever. Pustules at the oral mucocutaneous junction.

in dogs younger than 4 months of age but occasionally reported in dogs up to 4 years of age.

Clinical Presentation

The eyelids, pinnae, lips, chin, muzzle, paws, abdomen, thorax, vulva, prepuce, and anus can be affected with lesions that fistulate, drain, and crust (Figure 121.3). Lymphadenomegaly, most commonly mandibular and superficial cervical, can be distant from the affected skin sites and is often painful. Pyrexia, anorexia, sterile suppurative painful arthritis, and an inflammatory hemogram can occur. Severe pyoderma, necessitating only antibiotic therapy, can have a similar appearance.

Diagnostics

Pustules and lymph nodes are usually sterile when cultured. Superficial cutaneous flora can be cultured from open, draining lesions. The diagnosis is confirmed by histopathological evaluation, but is commonly made on the basis of clinical appearance, especially if no response to antibiotic therapy occurs. The predominant inflammatory cell in juvenile cellulitis, characterized by light and electron microscopy and immunohistochemical staining, is an epithelioid macrophage.

Therapy

Juvenile cellulitis requires aggressive immunosuppressive therapy early in the course of the disease for resolution and to avoid the sequelae of cicatricial lesions.

Traditionally, puppies have been placed on immunosuppressive doses of prednisone (2.2 mg/kg/day), causing concerns with immunization efforts. Griseofulvin therapy offers an apparently effective treatment without the side-effects associated with corticosteroid administration, enabling discontinuation of corticosteroids sooner in the course of the disease. It has been reported to be effective as sole immunomodulatory therapy (14.2–34 mg/kg PO q12h). Griseofulvin is postulated to induce downregulatory signals within the lesions. The use of griseofulvin as sole therapy could be attempted in early cases [12].

Vaccination of puppies undergoing immunosuppressive therapy is not advised and they must be strictly isolated from sources of infectious disease.

Bacterial Overgrowth Syndrome-Associated Diarrhea

Pathophysiology

Persistent diarrhea can occur in otherwise healthy neonates due to bacterial overgrowth associated with overfeeding. Symbiotic colonic bacteria assist digestion. The upper GI tract was once believed to be sterile, but normal colonization of the duodenum, jejunum, and ileum is now appreciated. Bacterial overgrowth syndrome (BOS) occurs when the normally low bacterial colonization in the upper GI tract significantly increases. Neonates lack propulsive peristaltic action; gut motility results only from aboral pressure from nursing. Diminished gut motility promotes bacterial overgrowth. Gastric acid normally reduces the proximal small intestinal bacteria. Neonates have reduced gastric acidity. Malabsorption of bile acids, fats, carbohydrates, proteins, and vitamins causes many of the symptoms of diarrhea and weight loss associated with BOS. Bacteria deconjugate bile acids, promoting further carbohydrate malabsorption and producing an osmotic diarrhea.

Clinical Presentation

Otherwise healthy, vigorous, and often overweight neonates have persistently soft, sometimes malodorous stools.

Diagnostics

Fecal examination for parasites is negative, although prepatency can mask infection. A direct smear can support BOS.

Therapy

Treatment is aimed at reducing the damage caused by malabsorption and restoring nutritional health and normal gut flora. The antimicrobials of choice for therapy of BOS-associated diarrhea are ampicillin, amoxicillin or metronidazole; the latter is less preferable in neonates due to the potential for CNS signs with overdosage and the neonatal diminished capacity for hepatic metabolism. Probiotics can be helpful to normalize beneficial gut flora populations. Enterocolitis from intestinal parasites can be severe in pediatric patients with high worm burdens. Prophylactic deworming with a broad-spectrum anthelmintic such as pyrantel pamoate should be instituted at 2, 4, and 6 weeks of age, before identification of infestation is possible with fecal examination.

Urinary Ectopia

Pathophysiology
Urinary ectopia is considered a heritable congenital condition more common in females. Ectopic placement of the distal ureter into the urethra, vestibule or vagina is usually associated with ureteral dilation with or without renal pelvic dilation. A ureterocele is an uncommon congenital dilation of the ureter near the bladder, appearing as a cystic structure within the bladder lumen or wall. The ureterocele occurs most commonly in association with an ectopic ureter. Hydronephrosis can eventually result from an uncorrected ectopic ureter due to flow impedance at the abnormal site of insertion. Urinary tract infection is commonly associated with ectopia, due to accompanying urethral sphincter mechanism anomalies and, if not detected and treated, can progress to pyelonephritis and ureteritis. Infection and its associated inflammation in the tract can cause further damage.

Clinical Presentation
The most common sign of ectopia of the urinary tract is incontinence. Astute breeders can identify incontinence in neonates; ectopia should be ruled out. Urine scalding in the perivulvar area can be evident.

Diagnostics
Abdominal ultrasound offers an excellent initial screening tool. Visualization of a non-vascular fluid-filled structure with a hyperechoic wall passing dorsal to the urinary bladder, or obvious insertion of the structure into the proximal urethra, suggest the diagnosis. Visualization of the ureteral jets in the bladder suggests normalcy, but some ectopic ureters insert initially into the bladder and additionally tunnel distally to terminate in an abnormal site. Visualization of the dilated ureter usually occurs near the urinary bladder. Visualization of the bladder neck and proximal urethra may be obscured by pubic bone, making identification of such termination difficult. Contrast-enhanced computed tomography is the most sensitive and specific modality for the diagnosis of ectopia but, like double contrast radiography, requires anesthesia, making initial evaluation with ultrasound desirable when ectopia is suspected clinically.

Therapy
Repair is delayed until adequate patient size is achieved and can be surgical or by endoscopically facilitated laser technique. Control of infection and urine scalding is advised in the meantime.

Hypoglycemia

Pathophysiology
Previously described neonatal limited gluconeogenesis, glycogenolysis, glycogen reserves and dependence on frequent feeding predispose puppies and kittens to clinical hypoglycemia. Hypoglycemia can also result from endotoxemia, septicemia, portosystemic shunts, and glycogen storage abnormalities. Extreme or prolonged hypoglycemia can result in permanent neurological changes due to brain injury.

Clinical Presentation
A hypoglycemic neonate may be weak and have poor responsiveness to stimulation, but may alternatively be crying and restless.

Diagnostics
Acquisition of blood and evaluation of glucose using table-top testing is most efficient and appropriate given the available blood volume. A value of 70 mg/dL is considered normal in neonatal life, and a value <50 mg/dL is an indication of hypoglycemia [13].

Therapy
If possible, parenteral dextrose is preferred over oral sources. Clinical hypoglycemia can be treated with dextrose solution intravenously or intraosseously, at a dose of 0.5–1.0 g/kg using a 5–10% solution, or a dose of 2–4 mL/kg of a 10% dextrose solution. Single administration of parenteral glucose is adequate if the puppy can then be fed or nurses. Fifty percent dextrose solution should only be applied to the mucous membranes because of the potential for phlebitis if administered intravenously; however, circulation must be adequate for absorption from the mucosa. Neonates administered dextrose should be monitored for hyperglycemia because of immature metabolic regulatory mechanisms. If a neonate is too weak to nurse or suckle, a mixture of a warmed, balanced crystalloid (1/2 strength) saline solution and 5% dextrose may be administered subcutaneously at a dose of 1 ml per 30 g of body weight, until the pup can be fed or nurses. A balanced warmed nutrient-electrolyte solution can be administered orally by stomach tube every 15–30 minutes until the neonate is capable of suckling. Oral fluid and glucose replacement may be preferable if the puppy has an adequate swallowing reflex and is not clinically compromised.

Fading Puppy Syndrome: Neonatal Bacterial Septicemia and Herpes Infection (CHV-1)

Pathophysiology

The fading puppy syndrome refers to neonatal death secondary to systemic infection. *In utero* or postpartum viral infection with canine distemper, canine parvovirus, canine adenovirus, canine and feline herpes, feline infectious peritonitis, feline immunodeficiency virus, panleukopenia, and feline leukemia virus cause neonatal mortality. Bacterial causes of neonatal infection include *Brucella canis* (canine), *Campylobacter*, *Salmonella*, *Klebsiella*, streptococci and staphylococci, and *Leptospira* (canine); *Neospora* (canine) and *Toxoplasma gondii* (canine and feline) are potential protozoal pathogens. Mycotic infection is rare.

Incompletely developed immune systems and inadequate thermoregulatory capacity during the first days of life make neonates vulnerable to systemic infection (both bacterial and viral).

Exposure of a naive bitch to CHV-1 during the last 3 weeks of gestation can result in either late term abortion of a litter or neonatal deaths within their first few weeks of life, because inadequate periparturient maternal antibodies exist to allow passive immunity to be acquired by the neonates. Transmission of CHV-1 to neonates can occur subsequent to contact with infectious vaginal fluids during whelping or with vulvar or oronasal secretions in the postpartum period. Puppies born to a naive bitch may also come into significant, infectious contact with CHV-1 from another dog shedding the organism. The recently infected brood bitch generally has no other clinical signs. Healthy recently infected adult dogs of either gender can show signs of a mild upper respiratory infection (sneezing, serous oculonasal discharge) for a few days, but are otherwise usually unremarkable.

The incubation period of CHV is 6–10 days. The virus replicates in the epithelial cells of the oronasal and pharyngeal mucosa and the regional lymphatics. The lower (<38°C or 100°F) body temperature normal in canine neonates permits the virus to actively replicate and spread.

Clinical Presentation

Factors that reportedly predispose a puppy to septicemia include endometritis in the bitch, a prolonged delivery/dystocia, feeding of replacement formulae, the use of ampicillin, stress, low birth weight (<350 g for a medium-sized breed), and chilling with body temperature < 96°F [14]. Commonly, a decrease in weight gain, failure to suckle, hematuria, persistent diarrhea, unusual vocalization, abdominal distension and pain, and sloughing of the extremities indicate bacterial septicemia may be present. Neonatal bacterial septicemia can cause rapid deterioration resulting in death if not recognized and treated promptly.

In CHV-1, puppies often present as individuals, but the disease often has affected or will later present similarly in the littermates. Although reported to cause fetal loss and resorption, the classic presentation is a high rate of stillborns in a litter, followed by the remaining live puppies dying due to systemic effects of herpesvirus. Classic signs in the neonate are not specific and include incessant vocalization, anorexia (with poor weight gain), dyspnea, abdominal pain, incoordination, diarrhea, serous to hemorrhagic nasal discharge, and petechiation of the mucous membranes. The mortality rate in litters infected *in utero* or during birth can approach 100%, with deaths occurring during the first few days to a week of life [15].

Diagnostics

Premortem diagnosis can be challenging, and clinical signs may not be noted due to sudden death. Necropsy with identification of viral inclusion bodies or positive PCR testing confirm the diagnosis of CHV-1. Gross histopathology of bacterial septicemia and canine herpes infection can be very similar. PCR profiles for abortion and neonatal death are commercially available.

Prevention

The umbilicus of neonates should be treated with tincture of iodine immediately after birth to reduce contamination and prevent ascent of environmental bacteria into the peritoneal cavity (omphalitis-peritonitis).

Minimal transplacental transfer of immunity occurs in the dog. Adequate ingestion of colostrum must occur promptly postpartum for puppies to acquire passive immunity. The transmission of protective immunity (placental or colostral antibodies) between a bitch and her puppies depends upon the prior existence of adequate serum maternal antibodies. Therefore, breeding bitches with exposure to CHV-1 earlier in life have the best opportunity to seroconvert and develop protective antibodies. This commonly occurs in kennels or at crowded canine events such as dog shows and trials. Documentation of positive CHV-1 serology generally indicates adequate maternal antibodies. Bitches who are naive to CHV-1 during pregnancy must be strictly isolated from potential exposure during gestation and for at least 6 weeks postpartum to prevent transmission of the virus to her fetuses or neonates. Subsequent litters of the infected pregnant or postpartum bitch are usually normal, having acquired resultant maternal antibodies.

A vaccine is available in Europe, but not currently in the United States. Efficacy studies for use of the vaccine are limited. The vaccine is recommended only in female breeding dogs with a perceived risk of CHV-1 infection (exposure in a pregnant naive bitch) to prevent neonatal disease and mortality.

Therapy

Therapy with broad-spectrum, bactericidal antibiotics, improved nutrition via supported nursing, tube feeding or bottle feeding, maintenance of body temperature, and appropriate fluid replacement are indicated. The third-generation cephalosporin antibiotic ceftiofur sodium (Naxcel; Pharmacia and Upjohn) is an appropriate choice for neonatal bacterial septicemia as it alters normal intestinal flora minimally and is usually effective against the causative organisms. Ceftiofur sodium should be administered at a dose of 2.5 mg/kg SC q12h for no longer than 5 days. Because puppies less than 48 hours old have reduced thrombin levels, presumptive therapy with vitamin K1 may be used (0.01–1.0 mg SC per puppy).

Failure to respond to antibiotic therapy for neonatal septicemia should prompt consideration of CHV-1 infection.

Specific antiviral therapy, if instituted in a timely manner, has been reported to reduce mortality from CHV-1. Aciclovir is an antiviral agent with activity against a variety of viruses, including herpes simplex. Aciclovir is preferentially taken up by susceptible viruses and converted into the active triphosphate form, inhibiting viral DNA replication. Aciclovir is poorly absorbed after oral administration and is primarily hepatically metabolized. It can increase the toxicity of nephrotoxic drugs. The half-life in humans is approximately 3 hours. Its use in veterinary medicine is not well established and it should be used with caution and only in situations where indicated. The safety and effectiveness in humans less than 2 weeks of age are not established. The dose (20 mg/kg PO q6h × 5 days) is currently extrapolated from that for humans. Providing ambient exogenous heat to raise the neonatal body temperature above 101°F can reduce viral replication [16].

Trauma

Pathophysiology

Trauma of a variety of causes can result in emergency presentation. Trauma can result from the dam's manipulation of her litter (Web Figure 121.6). Sometimes trauma can be intentional, and more commonly so in the bitch than the queen. First-time mothers can sometimes become aggressive or cannibalistic towards a litter. Also, trauma may present due to improper handling by the owner or children in the home. Breeders who "swing" puppies to clear fluid from the lungs after delivery can cause intracranial trauma resulting in neurological signs [17].

Clinical Presentation

Pain, dyspnea, abdominal distension, contusions/lacerations, hemorrhage, weakness, and seizures can occur with trauma.

Diagnostics

Physical examination reveals signs of trauma. Ultrasound of the abdomen and whole-body radiography are useful.

Therapy

Therapy is dictated by the nature of the injury. Special aspects of neonatal anesthesia (local or general) should be taken into consideration.

References

1 Davidson AP. Approaches to reducing neonatal mortality in dogs. Available at: www.researchgate.net/publication/267937790_Approaches_to_Reducing_Neonatal_Mortality_in_Dogs_19-Mar-2003 (accessed 5 February 2018).

2 Grundy SA. Clinically relevant physiology of the neonate. *Vet Clin North Am Small Anim Pract.* 2006;36(3):443–459.

3 Lyons LA. Feline genetics: clinical applications and genetic testing. *Top Compan Anim Med* 2010;25(4).

4 Metallinos DL. Canine molecular genetic testing. *Vet Clin North Am Small Anim Pract* 2001;31(2):421–431.

5 Lavely JA. Pediatric neurology of the dog and cat. *Vet Clin North Am Small Anim Pract* 2006;36:475–501.

6 Shihab N, Davies ES, Kenny P, Loderstedt S, Volk HA. Treatment of hydrocephalus with ventriculoperitoneal shunting in twelve dogs. *Vet Surg* 2011;40(4):477–484.

7 Davidson AP, Gregory C, Dedrick P. Successful management permitting delayed operative revision of cleft palate in a labrador retriever. *Vet Clin North Am Small Anim Pract* 2015;44(2):325–329.

8 Silvestre-Ferreira AC, Pastor J. Feline neonatal isoerythrolysis and the importance of feline blood types. *Vet Med Int* 2010; article 753726.

9 Levy JK, Crawford PC, Collante WR. Use of adult cat serum to correct failure of passive transfer in kittens. *J Am Vet Med Assoc* 2001;219(10):1401–1405.

10 Poffenbarger EM, Olson PN, Chandler ML, Seim HB, Varman M. Use of adult dog serum as a substitute for colostrum in the neonatal dog. *Am J Vet Res* 1991;52(8):1221–1224.

11 Wiebe VJ. Neonatal infections. In: *Canine and Feline Infectious Diseases* (ed. Sykes JE). Elsevier, St Louis, 2014, pp. 859–870.

12 Shibata K, Nagata M. FC-20 Efficacy of griseofulvin for juvenile cellulitis in dogs. *Vet Dermatol* 2004;15:26.

13 Linde-Forsberg C. Abnormalities in pregnancy, parturition and the periparturient period. In: *Textbook of Veterinary Internal Medicine*, 6th edn (eds Ettinger SJ, Feldman EW). WB Saunders, Philadelphia, 2005.

14 Lelli JL, Drongowski RA, Coran AG, et al. Hypoxia-induced bacterial translocation in the puppy. *J Pediatr Surg* 1992;27:974–982.

15 Morresey P. Reproductive effects of canine herpesvirus. *Compendium* 2004;4:804.

16 Davidson AP, Grundy SA, Foley JE. Successful medical management of neonatal canine herpesvirus: a case report. *Commun Theriogenol* 2003;3:1–5.

17 Grundy SA, Liu SM, Davidson AP. Intracranial trauma in a dog due to being "swung" at birth. *Top Compan Anim Med* 2009;24(2):100–103.

122

Metritis and Mastitis

Sophie A. Grundy, GVSc (Hons), MANZCVSc, DACVIM

IDEXX Laboratories, Westbrook, ME, USA

Metritis

Metritis in the bitch and queen is predominantly a postpartum condition that results from an ascending bacterial infection in association with parturition. It is hormonally distinct from pyometra as it occurs during a time when the serum progesterone concentration is low, and is a primary event rather than secondary to underlying uterine pathology such as cystic endometrial hyperplasia–pyometra complex (see Chapter 123). Predisposing factors for the development of metritis include abortion, dystocia, obstetric manipulation, retained fetal or placental tissue, and uterine prolapse [1]. The bitch is more frequently represented than the queen. A diagnosis of metritis in the postpartum dam may be made with consideration of history, clinical signs, clinical pathology data, and imaging.

Clinical Signs

Clinical signs of metritis vary, and range in severity, depending on the degree of endotoxemia and systemic involvement (Figure 122.1) [1–3]. Vaginal discharge may be considered a key clinical marker for metritis but it is not always easy to objectively define what is normal during the postpartum period.

Figure 122.1 Range of clinical signs of metritis in the bitch and queen.

Increasing severity of bacterial infection/systemic →

- Neonate neglect
- Lack of appetite, depression
- Agalactia
- Vaginal discharge – malodorous, copious, sanguinous
- Fever (>103.5 °F)
- Dehydration
- Injected membranes, tachycardia, collapse

Any sick dam presented within 7 days of parturition should be evaluated for metritis. A malodorous serosanguinous vaginal discharge is not abnormal *per se* for the bitch during the postpartum period. However, as a general rule, the combination of voluminous, hemorrhagic, and/or putrid-smelling postpartum vaginal discharge should raise concern for metritis [4]. Unless postparturition imaging is known to have been completed prior to presentation, the possibility of a dead retained fetus should always be considered. Untreated, a dam with a persistent retained dead fetus(es) may rapidly develop sepsis.

Diagnostics

Initial diagnostics should include a complete blood count, biochemical analysis, and abdominal imaging. Ultrasound-guided cystocentesis is the preferred method for urine collection. Cases presenting with signs of sepsis or peritonitis may benefit from evaluation for disorders of coagulation (see Chapter 70).

Classically, metritis is associated with a leukocytosis and left shift. Biochemical parameters are variable, but may include alterations in serum proteins, renal function consistent with dehydration, and sepsis [1,2]. A single report of hypercalcemia has been described [5]. Coagulation changes may be present in cases with sepsis. The majority of cases are associated with *Escherichia coli* but other pathogens such as *Staphylococcus* and *Streptoccus* are also encountered [1,6]. Guarded culture and sensitivity of the cranial vaginal discharge may be considered to confirm bacterial populations and obtain sensitivity and minimum inhibitory concentration data. If a speculum is not available, an empty 1 or 3 mL sterile syringe case may be introduced into the caudal vaginal canal to act as a guard for the introduction of a sterile cotton tip applicator to the cranial vaginal vault for culture.

Diagnostic imaging is required to identify any retained fetus(es). Radiographs may be helpful for the rapid

Textbook of Small Animal Emergency Medicine, First Edition. Edited by Kenneth J. Drobatz, Kate Hopper, Elizabeth Rozanski and Deborah C. Silverstein.
© 2019 John Wiley & Sons, Inc. Published 2019 by John Wiley & Sons, Inc.
Companion Website: www.wiley.com/go/drobatz/textbook

identification of a retained fetus, but ultrasound is the diagnostic imaging of choice as it permits evaluation of the uterine contents [2]. The urinary bladder provides an acoustic window for the body of the uterus and predicts the location of the uterine body. The normal postpartum uterus is prominent, and retained fetuses can be readily identified and lack of heart beat confirmed [7]. From days 1 to 4 post partum, the normal canine uterus is enlarged and echogenic with irregular uterine walls that may be difficult to distinguish from uterine contents. Uterine diameter varies and is report to range from 1.1 to 3.8 cm at placental sites, and 0.5 to 1.4 cm in between [8]. The typical mean uterine diameter in the queen changes from 16.6 mm at day 1 to 6.2 mm at day 14 post partum [9]. Normal variations in uterine diameter during the period of involution make confirmation of metritis based on a single-timepoint ultrasound evaluation challenging. The most complete clinical evaluation includes serial ultrasonographic evaluation of the uterus and uterine content, in conjunction with clinical pathology data and clinical parameters [7].

As metritis is clinically distinct from pyometra based on the timing of presentation (postpartum), evaluation of serum progesterone is rarely, if ever, indicated.

Treatment

Treatment priorities include rehydration, antimicrobial therapy, and administration of an ecbolic agent. Pending culture and sensitivity, antimicrobial choice should be based on efficacy towards *Escherichia coli* with consideration of whether or not continued nursing of neonates is planned (see Chapter 200). The decision regarding whether or not to remove neonates and hand raise them depends predominantly on the health of the dam. Enrofloxacin, amikacin, and second-generation cephalosporins are good initial choices for *E. coli*; the addition of amoxicillin is of benefit for streptococcal cover [10,11]. While amoxicillin/clavulanic acid is generally considered neonate safe, and a good choice when treating genital *E. coli* infections in the dog and cat, recent data suggests increasing resistance [12,13]. Based on susceptibility changes, trimethoprim-sulfonamides may be the preferred empirical oral treatment however, its use would preclude continued nursing as it is excreted in milk [12].

PGF2-alpha (Lutalyse) is the first choice for an ecbolic agent and may be used at 250 μg/kg SC q24h until uterine evaluation has occurred. More frequent PGF2-alpha administration (q8h) in conjunction with repeated imaging and in-house monitoring may be used to evacuate a single dead fetus in the bitch [4]. Caution is advised if more than one dead fetus is present. An intravaginal PGF2-alpha protocol has been described in the literature but is not routinely used [14]. Due to changes in oxytocin receptor expression that are not well defined for the dog

and cat, the use of oxytocin as an ecbolic agent is not advised more than 24 hours post partum.

For the majority of patients with mild clinical signs, medical treatment can be administered as an outpatient within a few hours. Follow-up treatment can typically be provided within 24 hours by the regular veterinarian. More severe cases requiring intensive supportive care and/or surgery typically require separation of the neonate and dam. As metritis is not associated with an underlying uterine pathology, the prognosis for return to fertility is considered to be good.

Mastitis

Mastitis typically occurs in the postpartum period and covers a wide range of presentations from non-septic galactostasis through gangrenous mastitis and sepsis [2,3]. One or multiple glands may be affected as connective tissue separates each gland sinus system [3]. In the postpartum period, mastitis is typically associated with ascending infection and environmental hygiene may be a factor in its development. As neonates are also susceptible to adverse environmental conditions, basic husbandry should be evaluated.

Mastitis may also occur during pseudopregnancy in the bitch and with inflammatory mammary adenocarcinoma [3]. In the dog, mastitis has also been reported with systemic blastomycosis and *Mycobacterium* [15,16]. In the queen, there is very little mammary tissue in the non-lactating female and clinical cases of mastitis are typically limited to the postpartum period [17].

Clinical Signs

Presentation is generally during the first 2 weeks post partum. Mild cases of mastitis are accompanied by discomfort, pain, and swelling of one or more gland. More severe cases may present with fever (>103.5 °F), depression, anorexia, and failure to care for neonates, or failure of neonates to thrive. The most severe cases present with signs of septic shock, mammary abscess formation, or gangrene. Milk from the affected gland(s) is not always grossly abnormal but green, reddish brown, or hemorrhagic discoloration should raise suspicion for mastitis.

Diagnostics

Initial diagnostics should include a complete blood count, biochemical analysis, and urinalysis. Classically, mastitis is associated with a leukocytosis and left shift. Biochemical parameters are variable but are typically normal for mild cases, and consistent with dehydration, and sepsis for severe cases. Color Doppler imaging is described for evaluation of central lobar vascular supply for cases progressing to gangrene and tissue necrosis, but B-mode ultrasound alone does not appear to predict treatment outcome [18]. Cytology of milk from the affected gland(s) may be helpful to identify abundant bacteria, but it is worth noting that normal milk may contain some bacteria [3]. Milk white blood cells are not an indicator of mastitis and vary greatly from gland to gland [19].

A milk sample should ideally be submitted for bacterial culture and sensitivity and measurement of pH to help guide antimicrobial selection. Typical bacterial isolates associated with bacterial mastitis include *E.coli*, *Streptococcus* and *Staphylococcus* spp [1–3,17].

For those cases presenting outside the postpartum period, thoracic radiographs and fine needle aspirate cytology should be considered for any mass lesions associated with the mammary gland [15].

Treatment

Dams with non-septic milk stasis and mild discomfort are typically not systemically ill and may be treated with warm compress application, analgesia, and monitoring. Nursing of the affected glands should continue as galactostasis will contribute to the disease process. Dams with signs of fever and peripheral leukocyte changes benefit from antimicrobial therapy and supportive care (see Chapter 200). The degree of intervention will vary depending on the severity of their clinical signs. Whether or not to remove neonates from the dam and hand raise the litter is a decision that should be based on the condition of the bitch, the age of the neonates, and the availability of nursing care. If neonates are to be removed, cabergoline (5 µg/kg PO q24h for 5 days) may be used to decrease milk production [1].

Selection of antimicrobials based on milk pH has been described to improve distribution into the mammary gland [2]. Under normal circumstances, milk is slightly more acidic than serum and antimicrobial agents that are weak bases with good activity against *E. coli* may be advantageous (such as trimethoprim-sulfonamides). However, milk may become more alkaline with bacterial infection and under those circumstances amoxicillin-clavulanic acid or cephalosporins may be preferred. Enrofloxacin may be used regardless of milk pH, and in patients that continue nursing if the benefits outweigh the risk of cartilage abnormalities.

For cases that progress to mammary abscessation or gangrenous mastitis despite treatment, neonates should be removed from the dam and the affected glands removed or surgically debrided.

References

1 Kutzler MA. Canine post partum disorders. In: *Kirk's Current Veterinary Therapy XIV* (eds Bonagura J, Twedt D). Saunders Elsevier, St Louis, 2009, pp. 999–1002.

2 Feldman E. Periparturient diseases. In: *Canine and Feline Endocrinology and Reproduction* (ed. Nelson F). Saunders, St Louis, 2004, pp. 808–834.

3 Johnston SD, Olson PN. Periparturient disorders in the bitch. In: *Canine and Feline Theriogenology*. WB Saunders, Philadelphia, 2001, pp. 129–145.

4 Grundy SA, Davidson AP. Theriogenology question of the month. Acute metritis secondary to retained fetal membranes and a retained nonviable fetus. *J Am Vet Med Assoc* 2004;224(6):844–847.

5 Hirt RA, Kneissl S, Teinfalt M. Severe hypercalcemia in a dog with a retained fetus and endometritis. *J Am Vet Med Assoc* 2000;216(9):1423–1425.

6 Watts JR, Wright PJ, Lee CS, Whithear KG. New techniques using transcervical uterine cannulation for the diagnosis of uterine disorders in bitches. *J Reprod Fertil Suppl* 1997;51:283–293.

7 Davidson AP, Baker TW. Reproductive ultrasound of the bitch and queen. *Top Compan Anim Med* 2009;24(2):55–63.

8 Yeager AE, Concannon PW. Serial ultrasonographic appearance of postpartum uterine involution in beagle dogs. *Theriogenology* 1990;34(3):523–535.

9 Ferretti LM, Newell SM, Graham JP, Roberts GD. Radiographic and ultrasonographic evaluation of the normal feline postpartum uterus. *Vet Radiol Ultrasound* 2000;41(3):287–291.

10 Henriques S, Silva E, Lemsaddek A, Lopes-da-Costa L, Mateus L. Genotypic and phenotypic comparison of Escherichia coli from uterine infections with different outcomes: clinical metritis in the cow and pyometra in the bitch. *Vet Microbiol* 2014;170(1–2):109–116.

11 Hombach M, Bloemberg GV, Bottger EC. Effects of clinical breakpoint changes in CLSI guidelines 2010/2011 and EUCAST guidelines 2011 on antibiotic susceptibility test reporting of Gram-negative bacilli. *J Antimicrob Chemother* 2012;67(3):622–632.

12 Thungrat K, Price SB, Carpenter DM, Boothe DM. Antimicrobial susceptibility patterns of clinical Escherichia coli isolates from dogs and cats in the United States: January 2008 through January 2013. *Vet Microbiol* 2015;179(3–4):287–295.

13 Grobbel M, Lubke-Becker A, Alesik E, et al. Antimicrobial susceptibility of Escherichia coli from swine, horses, dogs and cats as determined in the BfT-GermVet monitoring program 2004–2006. *Berl Munch Tierarztl Wochenschr* 2007;120(9–10):391–401.

14 Gabor G, Siver L, Szenci O. Intravaginal prostaglandin F2 alpha for the treatment of metritis and pyometra in the bitch. *Acta Vet Hung* 1999;47(1):103–108.

15 Ditmyer H, Craig L. Mycotic mastitis in three dogs due to Blastomyces dermatitidis. *J Am Anim Hosp Assoc* 2011;47(5):356–358.

16 Murai A, Maruyama S, Nagata M, Yuki M. Mastitis caused by Mycobacterium kansasii infection in a dog. *Vet Clin Pathol* 2013;42(3):377–381.

17 Johnston SD, Olson PN. The postpartum period in the cat. In: *Canine and Feline Theriogenology*. WB Saunders, Philadelphia, 2001, pp. 438–446.

18 Trasch K, Wehrend A, Bostedt H. Ultrasonographic description of canine mastitis. *Vet Radiol Ultrasound* 2007;48(6):580–584.

19 Olson PN. Cytologic evaluation of canine milk. *Vet Med Small Anim Clin* 1984;79:641.

123

Pyometra

Grayson B. Wallace, DVM[1] and Margret L. Casal, DVM, MS, PhD[2]

[1]*North Oatlands Veterinary Hospital, Leesburg, VA, USA*
[2]*School of Veterinary Medicine, University of Pennsylvania, Philadelphia, PA, USA*

Signalment, Clinical Presentation, and Associated Disease

Pyometra is a reproductive disorder of mature, intact bitches and queens. However, previous exposure to reproductive hormonal therapy and congenital abnormalities of the genital tract, such as vaginal strictures, predispose younger bitches and queens to developing pyometra [1–4]. Dramatic variation in the incidence of pyometra between different breeds suggests a genetic component in both bitches and queens. In bitches, the mean age of pyometra diagnosis is 7.25 years with a range of as early as 4 months to 16 years [5]. Fewer data are available in queens, as the incidence is lower, presumably due to less cumulative uterine exposure to progesterone when compared to the bitch.

The majority of pyometra cases present with a history of recent estrus, and pyometra is preceded by cystic endometrial hyperplasia (CEH). In bitches, the classic time frame is 1–4 months after estrus [6], while queens typically present within 4 weeks (2–5 weeks range) [7]. In any ill intact bitch or queen, pyometra should be considered as a differential and a thorough reproductive history taken (noting parity, last estrus, and any prior hormonal therapy). The most common clinical findings of pyometra in bitches are vaginal discharge (80%), pyrexia (47%), polyuria/polydipsia (<50%), and emesis [8,9]. Non-specific findings include lethargy and anorexia and in more advanced cases, signs of shock such as tachycardia, tachypnea, hypotension, and pale or injected mucous membranes. Careful abdominal palpation may reveal large tubular organ/uterine enlargement and may elicit pain. Queens classically present with milder signs that can include purulent vaginal discharge, anorexia, lethargy, emesis, unkempt appearance, and a palpable uterine enlargement/abdominal distension [7,10,11]. The cervical patency determines the presence or absence of vaginal discharge and is an important consideration in case management. Open-cervix pyometra typically results in milder systemic signs. In contrast, closed-cervix pyometra cases typically present without overt vaginal discharge and generally marked clinical signs of illness due to sepsis. Vaginal discharge can range from purulent to hemorrhagic to mucoid.

The pathogen predominantly associated with pyometra is *Escherichia coli* (>70% of cases), but other vaginal commensal bacteria (*Staphylococcus aureus, Enterobacter, Pseudomonas, Klebsiella, Proteus,* and *Streptococcus* spp) have been recovered [12–15]. The majority *E. coli* strains isolated in pyometra contain specific uropathogenic virulence factors (UVF) that enhance endometrial adherence [16] and may produce lipopolysaccharide (LPS), leading to serious systemic disease in the patient. Pyometra can lead to the development of the systemic inflammatory response syndrome (SIRS) (see Chapter 159). SIRS has been reported in up to 50% of bitches with pyometra and has been associated with a poor prognosis and increased duration of hospitalization [15,17]. In cases of pyometra-induced sepsis, serum concentrations of inflammatory markers such as C-reactive protein (CRP), serum amyloid A (SAA), and prostaglandin F2 metabolites (PGFM) have been shown to significantly increase [15,17,18]. Pyometra can lead to severe sepsis and multiple organ dysfunction syndrome [19].

Diagnostics

Cranial vaginal cytology, culture, and vaginal speculum visualization may aid in the diagnosis of pyometra.

Textbook of Small Animal Emergency Medicine, First Edition. Edited by Kenneth J. Drobatz, Kate Hopper, Elizabeth Rozanski and Deborah C. Silverstein.
© 2019 John Wiley & Sons, Inc. Published 2019 by John Wiley & Sons, Inc.
Companion Website: www.wiley.com/go/drobatz/textbook

For aerobic culture and susceptibility, a sample of the cranial vaginal discharge is obtained using a guarded swab and speculum. In the majority of pyometra cases, a large number of degenerate neutrophils and intra- or extracellular bacteria are typically seen on cytology. However, the diagnosis of pyometra should not be made on vaginal cytology alone, as large numbers of neutrophils with some bacteria are normal during diestrus.

The diagnosis of pyometra is primarily made by ultrasound. Typical ultrasonographic findings consistent with pyometra include uteromegaly, thickened uterine walls, proliferative endometrial changes, fluid-distended convoluted tubular horns, and anechoic to hyperechoic luminal fluid [20,21]. Uterine fluid in pyometra is usually homogenous, but can be flocculent with slow swirling patterns [22]. Ultrasound can differentiate pyometra from other soft tissue causes of uterine distension, and is imperative for evaluation of the presence of cystic endometrial hyperplasia and integrity of the endometrium. Moderate to advanced CEH can be reliably diagnosed as 1–4 mm anechoic cysts within a thickened endometrium [8]. Severe CEH may be associated with a poorer response to medical therapy [8]. If uterine torsion or rupture is suspected, ultrasound can also be used to evaluate the presence of peritonitis (see Chapter 87).

Pyometra classically presents with a marked leukocytosis characterized by monocytosis and a severe neutrophilia with a left shift and toxic changes. The leukocytosis is typically more severe in closed-cervix pyometra cases [12]. A mild to moderate normocytic, normochromic, non-regenerative anemia of chronic disease may be present. Up to 25% of pyometra cases can have a normal complete blood cell count (CBC), especially if pyometra is detected early in its course on ultrasonographic examination [9].

Patients with pyometra may have variable changes in their serum chemistry values. The most common abnormalities include azotemia, increased liver enzymes, hyperbilirubinemia, hypercholesterolemia, hyperglobulinemia, hypoalbuminemia, and hyperproteinemia [12]. Azotemia may be present (12–37%) in affected bitches and can be due to prerenal dehydration and/or endotoxin-induced (*E. coli*) renal tubular damage [23]. These renal changes are typically transient and reversible with treatment. However, a blood urea nitrogen of over 60 mg/dL has been associated with acute kidney injury and a poor prognosis [24] (see Chapter 94). Some strains of *E. coli* produce cytotoxic necrotizing factors, which in conjunction with dehydration can cause reversible hepatocellular damage or hypoxia [24]. Urinalysis may reveal dilute urine, bacteriuria, glucosuria, and/or proteinuria.

Treatment

Stabilization

Due to the insidious onset and non-specific signs of pyometra, many patients present in the advanced stage of the disease and may require stabilization prior to initiating definitive therapy. Full evaluation of cardiovascular, respiratory, and metabolic systems is required and stabilization provided as indicated prior to anesthesia (see Chapter 2). If the patient is stable, surgical and anesthetic risk may be reduced and stability improved by initiating medical therapy to lyze the corpus luteum, dilate the cervix, and facilitate evacuation of the purulent uterine fluid [25].

Antibiotic Therapy

Broad-spectrum antibiotic therapy should be started immediately upon presentation in all pyometra cases (see Chapter 200). Empiric antibiotic selection initially should target *E. coli* and have good uterine penetration. A combination of a fluoroquinolone and extended-spectrum penicillin is preferred [26]. Other appropriate antibiotic choices in pyometra include trimethoprim-sulfonamide and third-generation cephalosporins [27]. Long-term antibiotic therapy should be based on the results of a bacterial culture and sensitivity profile of the purulent exudate, and should be continued for 2 weeks (in surgical cases) to 1 month (with medical management).

Surgical Versus Medical Management

The severity of clinical presentation and breeding potential of the animal direct the decision to pursue medical or surgical management to address the underlying cause of pyometra. Historically, surgical ovariohysterectomy (OHE) was the only treatment for pyometra and still is the treatment of choice in most cases (especially in non-breeding animals). Surgery directly removes the source of the purulent exudate and endotoxin release. With the advances made over the last 20 years, medical management is a viable alternative to surgery in pyometra cases in which the owner wishes to preserve fertility. Medical management should be considered in valuable breeding bitches/queens (<6 years). However, if the patient's condition deteriorates or if significant clinical improvement is not seen within 2 days of initiating medical therapy, surgical management may need to be reconsidered. If peritonitis or uterine torsion is suspected, medical management is contraindicated (see Chapter 87).

Surgical Management

Once the patient has been stabilized, antibiotic therapy instituted, and surgical risk minimized, surgery can be performed. Pyometra OHE surgery is similar to spay surgery except the uterus is grossly enlarged and can be quite friable. After careful removal of the uterine stump, the remaining small amount of uterine lumen should be lavaged with warm isotonic saline and omentalized. Afterwards, the peritoneal cavity should be copiously lavaged, and a sample of the uterine fluid should be obtained for culture and susceptibility [25]. If peritonitis is present, a closed active suction drainage system should be placed [28]. Surgical management of uterine stump pyometra is similar and requires exploratory laparotomy with surgical excision of all remaining uterine and remnant ovarian tissue.

All surgically managed pyometra cases should be intensively monitored for 24–48 hours postoperatively. Signs of sepsis, hypovolemia, azotemia, anemia, hypoglycemia, hyperproteinemia, liver or renal dysfunction, and acid–base derangement should be immediately addressed [25]. Supportive treatments and intravenous fluids should be continued for at least 24 hours until the patient is eating and drinking on their own. Serum biochemistry and CBC should be followed postoperatively until abnormalities resolve (typically within 5 days). Appropriate surgical treatment of pyometra should cause the marked inflammatory response to subside, so monitoring of serum SAA, CRP, and hepatoglobin may be useful in postoperative detection of complications (ongoing infection) and resolution [29].

Peritonitis is the most common complication followed by anorexia, pyrexia, vomiting, renal insufficiency, and hepatic disease (see Chapter 87). Most complications resolve within 2 weeks [25]. After surgery, 92% of bitches survive, suggesting a good prognosis [23]. Renal status (pre- and postoperatively) is the best prognostic indicator. Other factors that affect prognosis for pyometra include cervical patency, dehydration status, uterine rupture (septic peritonitis), and significant co-morbidities [25].

Medical Management

Medical treatment (Table 123.1) involves the use of prostaglandin F2-alpha (PGF2-alpha), dopamine agonists, and progesterone receptor antagonists (antiprogestins), either alone or in combination. Although many protocols have been described for the medical management of pyometra, their goals are essentially the same.

The first goal is to remove the effects of progesterone to facilitate cervical relaxation, myometrial contractions, and improved local uterine immunity. These changes allow natural expulsion of purulent uterine contents and bacteria through an open cervix. This goal can be accomplished by the use of prostaglandins (alone or in combination with dopamine agonists) and/or progesterone receptor antagonists. The second goal of medical management is prevention of bacterial proliferation through appropriate antibiotic therapy. In animals with advanced CEH, the final goal of medical management is to facilitate endometrial regeneration (thus preserving fertility) by prolonging the anestrus period. This can be accomplished by the use of androgen receptor agonists, such as mibolerone. Owners should be warned of possible future recurrence after treatment and potential reduction in fertility.

Prostaglandin F2-alpha and Prostaglandin Agonists

Success in the treatment of pyometra has been reported with the use of PGF2-alpha therapy alone or in combination (off-label). Repeated dosing of PGF2-alpha induces luteolysis, directly decreasing progesterone levels, which leads to cervical opening and decreased glandular secretions [30,31]. Additionally, prostaglandins directly promote uterine contractions, which with a patent cervix permit expulsion of uterine discharge. Therapeutic PGF2-alpha is available in a natural form (dinoprost tromethamine) and a synthetic form (cloprostenol or alfaprostol).

Treatment with PGF2-alpha can have significant dose-dependent side-effects, especially at higher doses. Side-effects include panting, emesis, hypersalivation, hypothermia, diarrhea, urination, anxiety/shivering, ataxia, and abdominal contractions. Additional side-effects seen specifically in queens were vocalization, grooming, kneading, mydriasis, and lordosis [10]. PGF2-alpha has a narrow therapeutic index and in rare cases (especially with higher doses and a closed cervix), shock and death may result [25]. Therefore, administration of low doses through subcutaneous or intramuscular injections is recommended. Adverse effects typically develop within 20–30 minutes and should abate within another 30 minutes. Tolerance develops quickly and reduction of side-effects generally occurs with each subsequent dose. Hospitalization, at least at the onset of PGF2-alpha therapy, is recommended due to frequency of side-effects and dosing and potential toxicity. Suggested doses are given in Table 123.1. The use of ecbolics is contraindicated in a closed cervix pyometra in both bitches and queens unless the cervix opens spontaneously or is induced medically [5,9,10,25,30].

Clinical improvement is expected within 48 hours of initiating prostaglandin treatment. Copious vaginal discharge is typically observed for at least 48 hours then gradually diminishes. A rapid reduction in uterine diameter on ultrasound should be evident within 24–48 hours [32]. Following the progression of uterine evacuation by ultrasound every few days is important to determine the duration and efficacy of therapy. Resolution of pyometra is characterized

Table 123.1 Suggested medical management protocols for pyometra.

Protocols	Drug(s) and dosing	Side-effects and indications	References
Low-dose PGF2-alpha	**Dinoprost trimethamine** (low dose): 20–25 µg/kg SC q2–4h daily until uterine evacuation/luteolysis	May require hospitalization due to high dosing frequency	[45]
		This dosing regimen minimizes side-effects of PGF2-alpha	[46]
Titrating dose PGF2-alpha	**Dinoprost trimethamine** (titrating dose): 10 µg/kg SC for 3–5 doses on day 1; 25 µg/kg SC for 3–5 doses on day 2; 50 µg/kg SC for 3–5 doses on days 3–10 (or until resolution of vaginal discharge)	This dosing regimen minimizes side-effects of PGF2-alpha	[9]
High-dose PGF2-alpha (>0. mg/kg q24h)	**Dinoprost trimethamine** (high dose): 250–500 µg/kg SC q24h × 3 days	Worse PGF2-alpha side-effects Increased risk of uterine rupture	[30]
		Contraindicated in closed-cervix pyometra (due to risk of peritonitis/rupture)	
Intravaginal infusion of PGF2-alpha	**Dinoprost trimethamine** (intravaginally): 150 µg/kg topically (as a vaginal infusion at 0.3 mL/kg) q12h × 3–12 days (until resolution)	Better results in treatment of open-cervix pyometra	[44]
		Intravaginal adminstration helps minimize systemic side-effects of PGF2-alpha	
PGF2-alpha in queens *	**Dinoprost trimethamine** (medium dose): 100 µg/kg SC q12–24 h × 3–5 days	Side-effects of PGF2-alpha dosing (especially with first doses)	[10]
	OR		
	Dinoprost trimethamine (titrating dose): 10–15 µg/kg SC q8h on day 1; 25 µg/kg SC q8h on day 2; 50 mg/kg SC q8h for day 3–10 (or until complete uterine emptying)	This dosing regimen minimizes side-effects of PGF2-alpha	[25]
PGF2-alpha analogue**	**Cloprostenol** (synthetic PGF agonist): 1–5 µg/kg SC q24h × until resolution	Treatment may need to be continued for 7–10 days or until complete uterine emptying is observed [17,43,44]	[5] [45]
PGF2-alpha analogue + dopamine agonist	**Cloprostenol** (PGF2-alpha analogue): 1 µg/kg SC q24h × 7 days	Dosing protocol is similar in both bitches and queens	[36]
	WITH	Dopamine agonist should be given for at least 7 days or until resolution when used in combination with PGF2-alpha	[25]
	Cabergoline (dopamine agonist): 5 µg/kg PO q24h × up to 14 days		
	OR	Bromocriptine is less popular since it must be given TID with food and is associated with emesis	
	Bromocriptine (dopamine agonist): 10–20 µg/kg PO q8h × up to 14 days		
Antiprogestin	**Aglepristone:** 10 mg/kg SC once only on days 1, 2, 8, 15, and 30 (after dosing on day 8, evaluate treatment efficacy weekly prior to additional doses)	Very few adverse effects, but aglepristone is contraindicated with compromised hepatic or renal function	[38] [32]
		Negligible uterotonic effects, so can be used with open- or closed- cervix pyometras	
		Reported resolution rates of 45% by 28 days to 60% by 90 days	

Protocols	Drug(s) and dosing	Side-effects and indications	References
Antiprogestin + PGF2-alpha analogue	**Aglepristone** (antiprogestin): 10 mg/kg SC once on days 1, 3, 8, and 15 WITH	100% resolution rates reported when protocol used on open-cervix pyometras	[37]
	Cloprostenol (PGF2-alpha analogue): 1 µg/kg SC once on days 3 and 8 (OR once on days 3, 5, 8, 10, 12, and 15) (after dosing on day 15, than weekly doses until complete resolution on US)	With closed-cervix pyometra, PGF2-alpha therapy should be commenced 24–48 h after initial aglepristone dose (to allow cervical opening by aglepristone prior to PGF2-alpha induction of uterine contractions)	[38]

*In queens, the early corpora lutea are more refractory to PGF2-alpha-induced luteolysis, therefore a higher daily dosing of PGF2-alpha may be required for a longer period in early diestrus [25].

**Synthetic PGF2-alpha analogues have been associated with prolonged activity, enhanced specificity for uterine smooth muscle, and reduced observable side-effects (especially emesis). However, they have reduced ability to stimulate uterine contractions so are not as effective as natural PGF2-alpha for uterine emptying [9].

by complete uterine emptying observed on ultrasound and cessation of vaginal discharge [24].

Future fertility with prostaglandin therapy is reported to be 75–87% in bitches [33,34]. Variable recurrence of pyometra after PGF2-alpha treatment has been reported: between 5% recurrence for bitches that became pregnant on their next heat to as high as 70% recurrence in all treated bitches followed over a period of 27 months [34,35].

Dopamine Agonists
Dopamine agonists, such as cabergoline or bromocriptine, can be used (off-label) in combination with PGF2-alpha therapy to treat pyometra. Dopamine agonists have antiprolactin activity and cause luteolysis indirectly through decreasing prolactin levels as early as 25 days after the luteinizing hormone (LH) peak. In the bitch, prolactin is one of the major supporters in the long-term maintenance of a functional corpus luteum. When used synergistically in conjunction with PGF2-alpha, dopamine agonists can potentiate luteolysis, leading to rapid progesterone decrease and cervical patency within 24–48 hours [36].

Progesterone Receptor Antagonists (Antiprogestins)
Antiprogestins, such as aglepristone, can be successfully used alone or in combination with PGF2-alpha for medical management of pyometra [37]. Since it has negligible uterotonic effects, aglepristone can be used relatively safely regardless of cervical patency [38]. When used to convert a closed-cervix pyometra into an open-cervix case, aglepristone (administration on day 1 and 2) safely perpetuates cervical opening with minimal uterine contractions by 25 hours (range 4–48 hours) after the first injection [38]. Cervical opening is associated clinically with voiding of copious amount of purulent discharge and significant improvement and increased appetite. Recurrence

of pyometra on subsequent heat cycles after treatment with aglepristone is generally thought to be lower, from no occurrence within a year to around 18% [32,37,39]. The use of aglepristone in combination with prostaglandin therapy results in better recovery rates for pyometra due to their synergistic actions, with reported success rates of 72–100% in bitches and 90% in queens [37,40,41].

Follow-Up Care, Monitoring Medical Management, and Recurrence Rates
After the initiation of medical therapy for pyometra, certain parameters should be closely monitored. A dramatic increase in vaginal discharge should be noted within 24–36 hours and generally lasts 7–10 days with medical therapy. Weekly CBCs are recommended to monitor decreasing neutrophilia. The left shift should resolve within the first week, and the neutrophilia should completely resolve within 10–15 days after starting medical management [16]. Any biochemistry abnormalities on presentation should be assessed until resolution as well. Serial uterine ultrasounds are recommended to assess response to treatment, and a visible reduction in luminal diameter should be noted in 5–7 days. The animal should be re-evaluated 10–20 days after recovery to assess the need for additional treatment and continuation of antibiotics [42].

With medical management, the rate of pyometra recurrence within 2 years is reported as 20–70% in bitches and slightly lower at 14% in queens [10,30,36], and 40–70% of bitches whelp normally [5,30]. Since pregnancy is considered protective, it is recommended the bitch or queen be bred on her next heat cycle. Treatment with prophylactic antibiotics may be considered during her subsequent proestrus and estrus period. Fertility is generally better in younger animals or those that develop pyometra as the result of exogenous hormone administration.

References

1 Von Berky A, Townsend WL. The relationship between the prevalence of uterine lesions and the use of medroxyprogesterone acetate for canine population control. *Aust Vet J* 1994;70:249.

2 Bowen RA, Olson PN, Behrendt MD, Wheeler SL, Husted PW, Net TM. Efficacy and toxicity of estrogens commonly used to terminate canine pregnancy. *J Am Vet Med Assoc* 1985;186:783–788.

3 Sutton DJ, Geary MR, Bergman JGHE. Prevention of pregnancy in bitches following unwanted mating: a clinical trial using low dose oestradiol benzoate. *J Reprod Fertil Suppl* 1997;51:239–243.

4 Pretzer SD. Clinical presentation of canine pyometra and mucometra: a review. *Theriogenology* 2008;70: 359–363.

5 Johnston SD, Kustritz MVR, Olson PNS. Disorders of the canine uterus and uterine tubes (oviducts). In: *Canine and Feline Theriogenology* (eds Johnston SD, Root Kustritz MV, Olson P). WB Saunders, Philadelphia, 2001, pp. 206–224.

6 Smith FO. Canine pyometra. *Theriogenology* 2006;66:610–612.

7 Kenney KJ, Matthiesen DT, Brown NO, et al. Pyometra in cats: 183 cases (1979–1984). *J Am Vet Med Assoc* 1987;191:1130–1132.

8 Bigliardi E, Parmigiani E, Cavirani S, et al. Ultrasonography and cystic hyperplasia- pyometra complex in the bitch. *Reprod Domest Anim* 2004;39:136.

9 Verstegen J, Dhaliwal G, Verstegen-Onclin K. Mucometra, cystic endometrial hyperplasia, and pyometra in the bitch: advances in treatment and assessment of future reproductive success. *Theriogenology* 2008;70:364–374.

10 Davidson AP, Feldman EC, Nelson RW. Treatment of pyometra in cats, using prostaglandin F2-a: 21 cases (1982–1990). *J Am Vet Med Assoc* 1992;200:825.

11 Van Haaften B, Taverne MAM. Sonographic diagnosis of a mucometra in a cat. *Vet Rec* 1989;124:346–347.

12 Fransson B, Lagerstedt AS, Hellmen E, Jonsson P. Bacteriological findings, blood chemistry profile and plasma endotoxin levels in bitches with pyometra or other uterine diseases. *Zentralbl Veterinarmed A* 1997;44:417–426.

13 Chen YMM, Wright PJ, Lee CS, Browning GF. Uropathogenic virulence factors in isolates of Escherichia coli form clinical cases of canine pyometra and feces of healthy bitches. *Vet Microbiol* 2003;94: 57–69.

14 Hagman R, Kuhn I. Escherichia coli strains isolated from the uterus and urinary bladder of bitches suffering from pyometra: comparison by restriction enzyme digestion and pulsed-field gel electrophoresis. *Vet Microbiol* 2002;84:143–153.

15 Hagman R, Kindahl H, Lagerstedt AS. Pyometra in bitches induces elevated plasma endotoxin and prostaglandin F2a metabolites levels. *Acta Vet Scand* 2006;47:55–68.

16 Krekeler N, Marenda MS, Browning GF, Holden KF, Charles JA, Wright PJ. Uropathogenic virulence factor FimH facilitates binding of uteropathogenic Escherichia coli to canine endometrium. *Comp Immunol Microbiol Infect Dis* 2012;35:461–467.

17 Fransson BA, Ragle CA. Canine pyometra: an update on pathogenesis and treatment. *Compend Cont Educ Pract Vet* 2003;25:602–612.

18 Jitpean S, Pettersson A, Hoglund OV, Holst BS, Olsson U, Hagman R. Increased concentrations of Serum amyloid A in dogs with sepsis caused by pyometra. *BMC Vet Res* 2014;10:273.

19 Hagman R. Clinical and molecular characteristics of pyometra in female dogs. *Reprod Dom Anim* 2012;47:323–325.

20 Voges AK, Neuwirth L. Ultrasound diagnosis- cystic uterine hyperplasia. *Vet Radiol Ultrasound* 1996;37:131–132.

21 Fayrer-Hosken RA, Mahaffey M, Miller-Liebl D, Candle AB. Early diagnosis of canine pyometra using ultrasonography. *Vet Radiol* 1991;32:287–289.

22 Nyland TG, Mattoon JS. Ovaries and uterus. In: *Small Animal Diagnostic Ultrasound*, 2nd edn (ed. Nyland TG). Saunders, Philadelphia, 2002, pp. 231–249.

23 Jutkowitz LA. Reproductive emergencies. *Vet Clin North Am Small Anim Pract* 2005;35:397.

24 Crane BM. Pyometra. In: *Small Animal Critical Care*, 2nd edn (eds Silverstein DC, Hopper K). Elsevier Saunders, St Louis, 2015, pp. 667–671.

25 Krekler N, Hollinshead F. Pyometra. In: *Small Animal Soft Tissue Surgery* (ed. Monnet E). Wiley-Blackwell, Ames, 2013, pp. 625–634.

26 Brown SA. Fluoroquinolones in animal health. *J Vet Pharmacol Ther* 1996;19:1–14.

27 Lee S, Cho J, Shin N, et al. Identification and antimicrobial susceptibility of bacteria from the uterus of bitches with pyometra. *Korean J Vet Res* 2000;40:763–767.

28 Halfacree Z. Optimising the treatment of the pyometra patient. *Presented at the British Small Animal Veterinary Conference*, 2014.

29 Dabrowski R, Kostro K, Lisiecka U, et al. Usefulness of C-reactive protein, serum amyloid A, and haptoglobin determinations in bitches with pyometra for monitoring early post-ovariohysterectomy complications. *Theriogenology* 2009;72(4):471–476.

30 Meyers-Wallen V, Goldschmidt M, Flickinger G. Prostaglandin F2α treatment of canine pyometra. *J Am Vet Med Assoc* 1986;189:1557.

31 Renton JP, Boyd JS, Harvey MJA. Observations on the treatment and diagnosis of open pyometra in the bitch (*Canis familiaris*). *J Reprod Fertil* 1993;47:465–469.

32 Fieni F, Topie E, Gogny A. Medical treatment for pyometra in dogs. *Reprod Dom Anim* 2014;49:28–32.

33 Burke TJ (ed.). *Small Animal Reproduction and Infertility: A Clinical Approach to Diagnosis and Treatment.* Lea and Febiger, Philadelphia, 1986, pp. 279–283.

34 Feldman EC, Nelson RW (eds). Cystic endometrial hyperplasia/pyometra complex. In: *Canine and Feline Endocrinology and Reproduction*, 3rd edn. WB Saunders, Philadelphia, 2004, pp. 852–867.

35 Memon MA, Mickelsen WD. Diagnosis and treatment of closed-cervix pyometra in the bitch. *J Am Vet Med Assoc* 1993;203:509–512.

36 Corrada Y, Arias D, Rodriguez R, et al. Combination of dopamine agonist and prostaglandin agonist treatment of cystic endometrial hyperplasia-pyometra complex in the bitch. *Theriogenology* 2006;66:1557.

37 Gobello C, Castex G, Klima L, et al. A study of two protocols combining aglepristone and cloprostenol to treat open cervix pyometra in the bitch. *Theriogenology* 2003;60:901.

38 Fieni F. Clinical evaluation of the use of aglepristone, with or without cloprostenol, to treat cystic endometrial hyperplasia-pyometra complex in bitches. *Theriogenology* 2006;66:1550–1556.

39 Jurka P, Max A, Hawrynska K, Snochowski M. Age related pregnancy results and further examination of bitches after aglepristone treatment of pyometra. *Reprod Dom Anim* 2010;45:525–529.

40 Fukuda S. Incidence of pyometra in colony-raised Beagle dogs. *Exp Anim* 2001;50:325.

41 Nak D, Nak Y, Tuna B. Follow-up examinations after medical treatment of pyometra in cats with the progesterone-antagonist aglepristone. *J Feline Med Surg* 2009;11(6):499–502.

42 Threlfall WR. Diagnosis and medical management of pyometra. *Semin Vet Med Surg (Small Anim)* 1995;10:21.

43 Sridevi P, Balasubramanian S, Devanathan TG, et al. Low dose prostaglandin F2 alpha therapy in treatment of canine pyometra. *Indian Vet J* 2000;77:889–890.

44 Gabor G, Siver L, Szenci O.: Intravaginal prostaglandin F2alpha for the treatment of metritis and pyometra in the bitch. *Acta Vet Hung* 1999;47:103–108.

45 Romagoli S. Canine pyometra: pathogenesis, therapy and clinical cases. Proceedings of the 27th World Small Animal Veterinary Association Congress, 2002.

46 Arnold S, Hubler M, Casal M, et al. Use of a low-dose prostaglandin for the treatment of canine pyometra. *J Small Anim Pract* 1988;29:303.

124

Prostatic Disease

Autumn P. Davidson, DVM, MS, DACVIM (SAIM)

School of Veterinary Medicine, University of California, Davis, CA, USA

Introduction

Prostatic disease is common in dogs but rare in cats. In the dog, prostatic disease is the most common disease of the male reproductive tract. Diseases of the prostate gland include benign hyperplasia (BPH), cystic benign hyperplasia (CBPH), squamous metaplasia (SM), paraprostatic cysts (PPCs), infectious prostatitis/prostatic abscessation (IP), and prostatic neoplasia (PN). BPH, CBPH, and IP are more common in intact dogs. PN is more common in neutered dogs compared to intact dogs, and is a disease of aged dogs. SM is associated with endogenous or exogenous estrogenic exposure. PPCs are more common in intact dogs and rare in cats [1,2].

Anatomy

The prostate gland is the only accessory sex gland in the dog; it surrounds the urethra just caudal to the urinary bladder and is normally easily palpated per rectum as a bilobed oval gland with a median septum. The prostate gland of the cat has four lobes and is located dorsal to the proximal urethra. The prostate gland in both species is primarily corpus (external to the urethra); the disseminate prostate (within the pelvic urethral wall) is vestigial. Additionally, the cat has bilobed bulbourethral glands found near the ischial arch on either side of the urethra.

Diagnostics

Multiple diagnostic techniques exist for evaluation of the prostate gland; most are more feasible in the dog than the cat. Obtain a thorough history including general health, diet, supplements, and present and past medications; specific inquiry should also be made concerning urination, defecation, preputial discharge, and outcome of breedings (if any) or time of neutering.

Physical examination of the prostate includes transabdominal and rectal palpation which can require analgesia/sedation if painful. Evaluation of the size, symmetry, firmness, presence of pain or compression of the colon or urethra should be made. Careful examination of the testes, prepuce, preputial discharge, and penis should also be performed. Note signs of any orthopedic or abdominal pain. Most dogs under evaluation for prostatic disorders should minimally have a complete blood count, serum chemistry panel, urinalysis with culture (cystocentesis), and *Brucella canis* screen (slide or tube agglutination). Cytology of semen permits evaluation of the prostatic portion (first and third fractions) of the ejaculate, but can be too painful in an emergency presentation [3]. Additionally, culture of ejaculated semen requires special considerations for the presence of urethral and preputial normal flora; >100 000/mL organisms suggests a pathogen [4].

Ultrasound-guided fine needle aspiration (FNA) of the prostate under appropriate sedation/analgesia offers an alternative method of evaluation [5]. Prostatic massage, urethral catheterization, and urethroscopy are usually reserved for sampling urethral masses when concern about tumor seeding (transitional cell carcinoma (TCC)) exists. Surgical (open) biopsies are performed as indicated, usually when surgical intervention (marsupialization, excision) is planned. Radiography remains important for evaluation of anatomical sites not amenable to ultrasound (gas-filled) metastasis checks; computed tomography and magnetic resonance imaging provide more precise evaluations.

Textbook of Small Animal Emergency Medicine, First Edition. Edited by Kenneth J. Drobatz, Kate Hopper, Elizabeth Rozanski and Deborah C. Silverstein.
© 2019 John Wiley & Sons, Inc. Published 2019 by John Wiley & Sons, Inc.
Companion Website: www.wiley.com/go/drobatz/textbook

Prostatic Disorders

Benign Prostatic Hyperplasia and Cystic Benign Prostatic Hyperplasia

Pathophysiology

Dihydrotestosterone (DHT) causes symmetrical, progressive, eccentric prostatic parenchymal enlargement (BPH), which can become cystic (CBPH). Prostatic cell hyperplasia and hypertrophy are both contributory, but hyperplasia predominates. BPH occurs predictably in all intact dogs after the age of 5 years, and can be present as early as 2.5 years. An age-associated alteration in the intraprostatic estrogen:androgen ratio potentiates the hyperplastic response to DHT.

Clinical Findings

Benign prostatic hyperplasia and CBPH occur in the dog. Prostatic hyperplasia can occur without any clinical signs. Because prostatic enlargement in canine BPH is eccentric, urethral compression, as seen in men with concentric hyperplasia, is unlikely. Tenesmus secondary to colonic compression from marked prostatomegaly can be seen in advanced cases. The most common clinical signs of BPH and CBPH are blood (of prostatic origin) dripping from the urethra/prepuce, hemospermia, and hematuria, which can be alarming to clients, prompting an emergency presentation. Hemospermia is limited to the prostatic portion of the ejaculate. Semen quality is not affected; the sperm count, sperm cell morphology, and motility are not altered. Urinary outflow compromise, prostatic or lumbar pain, or semen quality deterioration should prompt closer evaluation for more serious prostatic disorders/disease.

Diagnostics

The physical examination is unremarkable; the prostate is not painful upon palpation but is usually prominent, sometimes with mild asymmetry. When physical examination findings and semen evaluation are normal (other than hemospermia), an aggressive diagnostic evaluation is not indicated. The CBC and chemistry panel should be normal. An abdominal ultrasound is prudent to evaluate the appearance of the prostate gland and guide the acquisition of a urine sample by cystocentesis to rule out urinary tract infection.

Benign prostatic hyperplasia and CBPH have a characteristic ultrasonographic appearance; a symmetrical parenchymal striation with increased echogenicity is apparent with variable hypoechoic to anechoic intraparenchymal cystic structures evident. The cystic structures vary in size. No associated lymphadenomegaly is evident. Urinalysis is normal other than hematuria and urine culture is negative.

Cytology from a prostatic parenchymal fine needle aspirate, intraprostatic cyst aspirate, or actual prostatic biopsy for histopathology can be used to confirm the diagnosis if ultrasound is not characteristic. BPH and CBPH can accompany infectious prostatitis or more serious prostatic disorders in older dogs, making ultrasonographic conclusions difficult. Fluid aspirated from prostatic cysts should always be submitted for cytology, culture, and sensitivity.

Therapy

Castration is curative and the most effective treatment. Atrophy of the prostate gland is noticeable in 2 weeks and maximizes in 4 months. Failure of such atrophy following castration suggests concurrent prostatic disease. In valuable stud dogs, medical antiandrogen therapy is an option, indicated if defecation is difficult or if the owners find the clinical signs of BPH/CBPH objectionable [6].

Squamous Metaplasia

Pathophysiology

Squamous metaplasia occurs as a consequence of hyperestrogenism, either of endogenous (functional Sertoli cell tumor, adrenal gland dysfunction) or exogenous (therapy for BPH, inadvertent exposure to transdermal hormone replacement therapy in human) origin. Prostatic epithelial squamous metaplasia is accompanied by secretory stasis; intraprostatic cysts can form.

Clinical Findings

The prostate gland enlarges and is firm on palpation. Compression of the urethra and colon can cause dysuria and tenesmus, prompting an emergency presentation. Other physical findings typical of hyperestrogenism can be present: attractiveness to males, gynecomastia, symmetrical alopecia, hyperpigmentation, testicular atrophy or dissymmetry (if a mass is present) and a pendulous prepuce. The presence of an abdominal (cryptorchid) testis should be ruled out when two scrotal testes are not present. Estrogen toxicity to bone marrow can cause pale mucous membranes (anemia), petechiation or hemorrhage (thrombocytopenia), and fever (secondary to neutropenia) (see Chapters 64, 65, and 67).

Diagnostics

A careful history should be taken concerning possible exposure to transdermal hormone replacement therapies in humans in contact with the dog, or past purposeful therapy with estrogen for prostatomegaly.

A complete blood count, serum chemistry panel, and urinalysis/culture should be performed to evaluate for myelotoxicity and metabolic status. Changes are variable and dependent upon exposure duration and dose, and the time delay between insult and testing. Generally, in the initial 2–3 weeks both thrombocytopenia and thrombocytosis may be noted with progressive anemia and leukocytosis (WBC count may exceed 100 000/μL). After 3 weeks, pancytopenia and aplastic anemia may be noted. Hematuria may occur secondary to thrombocytopenia or due to blood of prostatic origin in the urine.

In an intact dog, semen collection will show deterioration of semen quality (primarily sperm count; oligospermia or azoospermia); squamous epithelial cells can be present in the prostatic fluid, and can often be sampled from the preputial mucosa. If a scrotal testicular mass is palpable (or discovered with ultrasound), a fine needle aspirate can reveal cytological evidence of a functional testicular neoplasia. Ultrasound will reveal enlarged prostate with hyperechoic parenchyma, often with cavitations; the typical striations of BPH are lacking. In a neutered dog with no scrotal testes, abdominal ultrasound should be performed to screen for a cryptorchid, malignantly transformed testis [7]. If negative, a serum luteinizing hormone (LH, Zoetis) screen can support the presence of a gonad; serum antimullerian hormone assay (AMH, MOFA) would be positive. Cytology from a fine needle aspirate or biopsy of the prostate can be performed to support suspicions.

Therapy

Therapy is dictated by the clinical findings: discontinuation of exogenous estrogen exposure or therapy or castration if functional testicular neoplasia is present. Concurrent prostatic infection or abscessation can be present and should be treated appropriately.

Paraprostatic Cysts

Pathophysiology

Paraprostatic cysts are fluid-filled structures adjacent and attached to the prostate gland, which can be patent or not. They can be prostatic in origin or remnants of the uterus masculinus in both dogs and cats. They have been diagnosed in both intact and neutered dogs.

Clinical Findings

The chronicity and size of PPC dictate the clinical signs, which can be minimal to marked. Large cysts can encroach on the urethra or colon, causing dysuria, incontinence or tenesmus, abdominomegaly or perineal swelling, prompting an emergency presentation.

Diagnostics

Other than hematuria, the CBC, chemistry panel, and urinalysis are generally unremarkable. Ultrasound identifies a fluid-filled structure adjacent to the urinary bladder. Ultrasound-guided centesis of the PPC provides fluid for cytology and culture.

Therapy

Ultrasound-guided cyst drainage can relieve emergent clinical signs until surgical removal is performed. Castration is recommended. Antibiotic therapy is dictated by culture and sensitivity and tailored for likely prostatic involvement (see Chapter 96).

Infectious Prostatitis

Pathophysiology

Infectious prostatitis occurs most commonly with bacterial organisms; mycotic prostatitis has been reported. Infection of the prostate gland can be acute and fulminant or chronic and progressive. Prostatic abscessation can occur. The most common route of infection is the ascension of urethral flora, but the hematogenous route of infection is also possible. The organisms most commonly isolated from the infected prostate are *E. coli* and *Staphylococcus*, *Streptococcus*, and *Mycoplasma* spp. Occasionally, *Proteus* spp, *Pseudomonas*, or anaerobic organisms are found. Mycotic prostatitis is uncommon and usually limited to endemic regions [8]. CBPH predisposes dogs to IP. This alteration of the normal architecture of the prostate gland predisposes to bacterial colonization by interfering with normal defense mechanisms and by providing an environment that supports bacterial growth; infectious agents gain access to intraparenchymal cysts, flourish, and can encapsulate to form abscesses.

Infectious prostatitis occurs most commonly in intact male dogs, but can occur in dogs neutered after infection is in place without appropriate antimicrobial therapy. Acute septic prostatitis can result in the later development of chronic septic prostatitis.

Clinical Findings

Clinical signs of IP can be mild to fulminant. Evaluation of the prostate is indicated in any male dog presenting with signs of lumbar or abdominal pain, lethargy, fever or tenesmus. The prostate is painful on palpation; sublumbar lymphadenomegaly can be present. Hemorrhagic and purulent urethral discharge, excessive preputial licking, dysuria, constipation and tenesmus can be present. Dogs are commonly febrile, anorexic, and lethargic, exhibiting pain on ambulation and kyphosis. Ejaculation can be painful, and affected dogs may be reluctant to breed or be collected. Peritonitis can cause nausea and abdominal discomfort.

Recurrent urinary tract infections imply chronic septic prostatitis. Chronic septic prostatitis may be asymptomatic, with deteriorating semen quality the only sign.

The prostate may be painful, firm, and irregular on palpation. Ultrasonographic findings are non-specific but typically will be of mixed echotexture with hyperechoic areas reflecting fibrosis. The ultrasonographic appearance can be similar to that of prostatic neoplasia. Additionally, multiple prostatic pathologies can be present in an individual patient.

Diagnostics

Septic prostatitis is best diagnosed on the basis of the findings from physical examination followed by ultrasonography and cytology and culture of urine and the prostate, with specific attention to any cystic structures within the parenchyma (Web Figure 124.1).

If IP is mild, semen collection can be attempted. Semen is typically abnormal, with suppurative inflammation, hemospermia, pyospermia, necrospermia, and decreased prostatic fluid volume evident. Because prostatic fluid normally refluxes into the urinary bladder, urinary tract infection is usually present whenever there is bacterial prostatitis (see Chapter 96). Culture of semen is not ideal as normal urethral flora will be acquired. Quantitating urethral versus prostatic ejaculate organisms can help differentiate normal flora from pathogens but is expensive and laborious. Prostatic massage/wash requires sedation and also will collect urethral flora. Pyuria and bacteriuria should always prompt evaluation of the prostate in any intact male dog.

A complete blood count reflects systemic inflammation. Chemistries can be normal or reflect prerenal azotemia, hepatopathy, nephrogenic diabetes insipidus, sepsis or peritonitis. The urinalysis and urine culture reflect an infectious etiology.

Ultrasound provides the best opportunity for sampling IP with appropriate analgesia/sedation. IP is characterized by both hypoechoic and hyperechoic non-homogenous parenchyma and if abscessed, hypoechoic to isoechoic thick irregular-walled cystic structures in the parenchyma. Sublumbar lymphadenomegaly can be present.

The diagnosis of chronic septic prostatitis requires cytological and microbiological examination of urine and prostatic tissue, which may be obtained by ultrasound-guided fine needle aspiration.

Therapy

Acute PI is a serious disorder and can lead to sepsis and death. Treatment must be prompt and aggressive. Fluid therapy is necessary to correct dehydration and shock (see Chapters 153, 155, and 159). Large prostatic abscesses are treated most effectively by surgical drainage and omentalization once stabilized. Abscesses may also be drained by FNA under ultrasound guidance if the dog is not stable.

Pending the results of culture and susceptibility, treatment with a fluoroquinolone and potentiated amoxicillin should be initiated. Antibiotic penetration in acute prostatitis is not as problematic as inflammation alters the blood–prostate barrier, allowing most antibiotics to penetrate. A negative culture of the urine or prostate should be obtained once therapy has been initiated to confirm effectiveness. Antibiotic treatment for acute prostatitis should be continued for a minimum of 4 weeks. Urine or prostatic fluid acquired via ultrasound guidance should be recultured a week after discontinuing antibiotic therapy and again 2–4 weeks later to be certain the infection has resolved.

Castration should be considered. Medical castration with finasteride is an acceptable alternative if the dog stabilizes rapidly and is valuable for breeding (finasteride does not affect spermatogenesis). Relapse is common, and can be diminished with the use of finasteride chronically.

Prostatic Neoplasia

Pathophysiology

Transitional cell carcinoma (TCC) and prostatic adenocarcinoma (ACA) are the most common primary prostatic malignancies. TCC is more common; regional lymphatic and distant pulmonary or bone metastasis occurs in <20% of cases. Scottish Terriers (18-fold), Shetland Sheepdogs, Beagles, Wirehaired Fox Terriers, and West Highland White Terriers are the breeds most commonly affected by TCC. It occurs in middle-aged to older dogs with a reported mean age of 11 years. ACA is locally invasive and metastasizes to regional lymphatics, lungs and the skeleton in 24–42% cases. There is an increased incidence in medium- to large-breed dogs >10 years of age, neutered early in life. Squamous cell carcinoma, fibrosarcoma, leiomyosarcoma, hemangiosarcoma, and lymphoma can occur in the prostate gland [9,10].

Clinical Findings

Malignant prostatomegaly commonly causes signs of tenesmus and constipation due to compression of the rectum accompanied by sublumbar lymphadenomegaly, overdistension of the urinary bladder due to urethral compression, lumbar pain from invasion into the lumbar vertebrae and nerve roots, and lower urinary tract signs of stranguria, dysuria, pollakiuria, and hematuria. Concurrent urinary tract infection is not uncommon. Pelvic limb ataxia and paresis or paralysis can occur. Physical examination findings commonly include prostatomegaly, sublumbar lymphadenomegaly, abdominal pain, and gait abnormalities. The prostate is unusually enlarged for a neutered dog. Anorexia and associated weight loss reduce body condition.

Diagnostics

Complete blood count and chemistry panel findings reflect chronic disease and inflammation. Postrenal azotemia can be present with obstructive masses. An elevation of alkaline phosphatase occurs in ~50% of cases. Hematuria, pyuria, bacteriuria, and atypical transitional cells can be found in the urinalysis. Malignant transitional cells appear similar to reactive transitional cells, making biopsy important.

Thoracic radiographs are indicated to screen for pulmonary metastasis. Lumbar spinal radiographs can show vertebral metastasis. Mineralization in the enlarged prostate and sublumbar lymphadenomegaly are suggestive of a malignant disease.

Abdominal ultrasound is the most useful diagnostic tool, permitting evaluation of the prostatic parenchyma, regional lymphatics, extension into the urinary bladder, urethral obstruction, and presence of hydroureter and hydronephrosis. Focal or multifocal hyperechoic prostatic parenchyma with asymmetry and irregular capsule outline and mineralization are common findings (Web Figure 124.2). Cavitary regions of necrosis and hemorrhage can be present. Sublumbar lymphadenomegaly can be marked.

Definitive diagnosis requires histopathological examination of affected tissues and can help differentiate between TCC and ACA or other malignancies. Tissue samples are usually obtained by surgical biopsy. If the mass extends into the urinary bladder, cystoscopic biopsy is possible. Transabdominal ultrasound-guided biopsy is straightforward, but TCCs are very exfoliative and seed readily, making the procedure risky for iatrogenic spread [11].

Therapy

Poor quality of life is common with prostatic neoplasia; most dogs are euthanized within 2 months of the diagnosis. Castration has little benefit. Prostatectomy could be considered with local, intracapsular disease, but is associated with incontinence. Palliative radiation can relieve clinical signs for some time. Urethral stenting can relieve urethral obstruction but is associated with incontinence and dislodgment.

The use of NSAIDs is associated with prolonged survival with prostatic carcinomas. Concurrent use of gastric protectants is advised. Oral analgesics that can be combined with NSAIDs can be helpful in controlling pain. Stool softeners are indicated if tenesmus is present. Intravenous bisphosphonates such as pamidronate can help with pain relief from skeletal metastases. Chemotherapy can result in partial, short-term clinical responses. Agents used include mitoxantrone, vinblastine, carboplatin, gemcitabine, and cisplatin (TCC), and carboplatin, cisplatin, doxorubicin, and gemcitabine (ACA). Piroxicam in combination with mitoxantrone, carboplatin or gemcitabine improves success rates. Consultation with a veterinary oncologist is advised.

References

1 Purswell BJ, Parker NA, Forrester SD. Prostatic diseases in dogs: a review. *Vet Med* 2000;95:315–321.
2 Smith J. Canine prostatic disease: a review of anatomy, pathology, diagnosis, and treatment. *Theriogenology* 2008;70:375–383.
3 Rijsselaere T. New techniques for the assessment of canine semen quality: a review. *Theriogenology* 2005;64:706.
4 Root Kustritz M. Relationship between inflammatory cytology of canine seminal fluid and significant aerobic bacterial, anaerobic bacterial or Mycoplasma cultures of canine seminal fluid: 95 cases (1987–2000). *Theriogenology* 2005;64:1333.
5 Davidson AP, Baker TW. Reproductive ultrasound of the dog and tom. *Top Compan Anim Med* 2009;24:64.
6 Sirinarumitr K, Johnston SD, Kustritz MR. Effects of finasteride on size of the prostate gland and semen quality in dogs with benign prostatic hypertrophy. *J Am Vet Med Assoc* 2001;218(8):1275–1280.
7 Pettersson A. Age at surgery for undescended testis and risk of testicular cancer. *N Engl J Med* 2007;356:1835.
8 Bjurström L. Long-term study of aerobic bacteria in the genital tract in stud dogs. *Am J Vet Res* 1992;53:670.
9 Withrow SJ, Vail DM. *Withrow and MacEwen's Small Animal Clinical Oncology*, 4th edn. Saunders Elsevier, St Louis, 2007, pp. 649–657.
10 Grieco V, Riccardi E, Greppi GF. Canine testicular tumors: a study on 232 dogs. *J Comp Pathol* 2008;138:86–89.
11 Mutsaers AJ, Widmer WR, Knapp DW. Canine transitional cell carcinoma. *J Vet Intern Med* 2003;17:136–144.

125

Uterine and Vaginal Prolapse

Michelle A. Kutzler, DVM, PhD, DACT

Oregon State University, Corvallis, OR, USA

Uterine Prolapse

Etiopathogenesis

Uterine prolapse is a very rare reproductive disorder in the dog and rare in the cat [1–3]. The condition occurs most commonly during parturition or in the immediate postpartum period because the cervix must be dilated for the uterus to prolapse through it [1]. Rare cases of uterine prolapse in parturient dogs have been reported in which one horn prolapsed while fetuses were still present in the other horn [4]. In addition, there has been one report of uterine prolapse in a dog with functional ovarian cysts [5].

Predisposing factors for the development of uterine prolapse in the bitch and queen include severe tenesmus during or after parturition, dystocia, incomplete placental separation, large litters, an atonic, flaccid, usually diseased uterus, chronic coughing, advanced age or excessive relaxation of the pelvic and perineal region [4,6–8] but it can also occur following normal parturition [3].

Diagnosis

Uterine prolapse can either be complete (involving both uterine horns; Figure 125.1) or partial (with either one entire horn or part of one horn involved), with the latter being more common [1]. Diagnosis is based on physical examination, visual examination of the protruding mass, and careful digital examination of the vagina. Physical examination findings include acute abdominal distension, pain and splinting, tachycardia, tachypnea and vocalization, hemorrhagic vulvar discharge, excessive vulvar licking ± devitalized prolapsed tissue. Dogs with uterine prolapse generally present in an extremely hypotensive state secondary to

hemorrhage following the tear of a uterine or ovarian artery during the prolapse.

Treatment

The primary treatment goal is to replace the uterus and prevent uterine infection once supportive treatment for shock is implemented and the patient is stabilized [9].

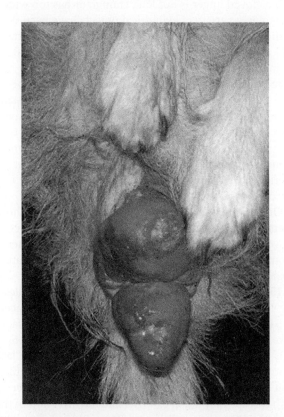

Figure 125.1 Uterine prolapse in a 9-year-old mixed-breed dog. Notice the two uterine horns protruding from the vulva. Reproduced with permission of John Wiley & Sons.

Textbook of Small Animal Emergency Medicine, First Edition. Edited by Kenneth J. Drobatz, Kate Hopper, Elizabeth Rozanski and Deborah C. Silverstein.
© 2019 John Wiley & Sons, Inc. Published 2019 by John Wiley & Sons, Inc.
Companion Website: www.wiley.com/go/drobatz/textbook

Exposed tissues should be covered with warm, saline-soaked towels, and the tissues should be cleaned and lubricated. Hyperosmotic agents (e.g. 50% dextrose) may help slightly in reducing the size of the edematous tissue but in this author's experience, hyperosmotic agents have offered little, if any, benefit.

In simple, uncomplicated cases, the manual reposition under general anesthesia is the preferred method [3]. If the uterus is still viable, it should be cleaned gently and manual reduction should be attempted [9]. Replacement of the prolapsed uterus has been achieved using gloved fingers and copious obstetrical lubricant [1,10]. Performing an episiotomy may improve chances for a successful manual reduction [11]. Routine closure of an episiotomy is performed in four layers: mucosa, muscular and subcutaneous tissues, and skin. The mucosa is closed in a simple interrupted or continuous pattern of 3-0 monofilament absorbable sutures. The muscular and subcutaneous tissues can be closed together or separately, depending on the size of the animal, using a simple continuous pattern of 3-0 or 4-0 absorbable sutures. The skin edges can be closed with sutures (simple interrupted or cruciates) or surgical staples.

If a gloved finger is not long enough or has too wide a diameter, a variety of cylindrical objects have been used in the successful reduction of uterine prolapses in bitches and queens. Inserting a 6 mL syringe case [2], a 10 mL syringe followed by an insemination tube [12], a test tube [13], a sterile swab [14], or an endotracheal tube [6] into the uterine horn or infusing saline under pressure have all successfully been used in accomplishing inversion of a complete prolapse. Using the endotracheal tube technique, sterile physiological saline (5–10 mL) can be administered through the free end of the tube so that the uterine horns can be slowly distended and recede into the pelvic and abdominal cavities [6].

Once completely reduced without any uterine horn eversion remaining, the prolapse does not usually recur. However, placing a purse-string suture in the perineum around the vulva (bitch) [9] or a single mattress suture through the perineal skin to close the vulva (queen) [1,15] is typically performed for the first 48 hours following reduction. Once the uterus is *completely* replaced, 3–5 IU of oxytocin should be administered IM to facilitate rapid uterine involution and cervical closure [16].

If the prolapse cannot be completely reduced, a laparotomy will need to be performed. Using cranial traction from the abdomen by gently grasping the cervix with forceps may aid in external manual inversion of the prolapsed tissue and allow the uterus to be drawn back into the abdomen [13,17]. If the uterus is still viable after reduction and the female is still intended for breeding, a hysteropexy should be performed, in which the vagina and uterus are sutured to the ventrolateral abdominal wall to prevent prolapse from recurring [7,13]. If the uterus is no longer viable or the female will be retired from breeding, ovariohysterectomy can be performed in conjunction with prolapse reduction.

An *en bloc* amputation of the prolapsed uterus is suggested if the patient is not stable enough to undergo a laparotomy with complete ovariohysterectomy at that time. To amputate the uterus, a smooth, cylindrical object should be placed into the uterine lumen and four stay sutures placed at equidistant points around the prolapsed uterus. All the layers of the uterus are incised to the inserted object, one quadrant at a time. Immediately after incising one quadrant, the inner and outer layers of the prolapsed uterus are anastomosed with simple interrupted absorbable sutures before incising the next quadrant. This process is repeated until the entire uterus is amputated [3,6,18]. Care must be taken to ligate the uterine arteries separately and the urethra must be catheterized and carefully protected [13,19]. Broad-spectrum systemic antibiotics for 7–14 days are warranted to reduce the risk of peritonitis following correction of a uterine prolapse (see Chapter 200).

Vaginal Prolapse

Vaginal prolapse has been reported in virtually all domestic mammals. True vaginal prolapses are rare in bitches and very rare in queens. However, vaginal fold prolapses of varying severity are the most common vaginal mass in the bitch [20].

True Vaginal Prolapse

Etiopathogenesis
Although the most severe form of vaginal fold prolapse can present as a true vaginal prolapse, the etiopathogenesis of a true vaginal prolapse is distinct from that of a vaginal fold prolapse. A true vaginal prolapse mainly occurs near parturition, as the concentration of serum progesterone declines and that of serum estrogen increases [21–24]. Excess prepartum pelvic relaxation and increased intra-abdominal pressure are believed to contribute to the development of a true vaginal prolapse [25]. Vaginal prolapse occurs less commonly in diestrus and normal pregnancy [21,22,26]. In the event of dystocia, extreme tenesmus may also predispose to this disorder. The reported incidence of periparturient true vaginal prolapse ranges from 8% [27] to 12% [28] of all vaginal prolapse cases.

Diagnosis
Although a true vaginal prolapse involves the entire vaginal wall, it may vary in appearance depending upon the duration of the prolapse (Figure 125.2 and Figure 125.3)

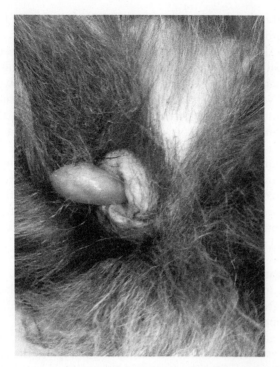

Figure 125.2 True vaginal prolapse in a 4-year-old Chihuahua 2 weeks prepartum. The prolapse was gently replaced and retained with a purse-string suture until parturition. Reproduced with permission of Matthew H. Goetz.

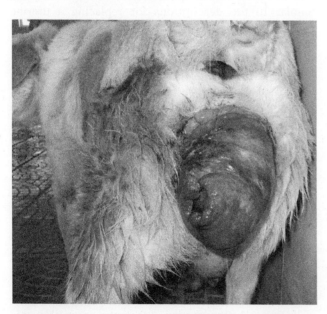

Figure 125.3 True vaginal prolapse in a 5-year-old mixed-breed dog following a dystocia. Notice the severe edema and tissue excoriation from the prolonged duration. Reproduced with permission of Elsevier.

as well as the involvement of other organs (e.g. urinary bladder, uterine body, and/or distal part of the colon) within the prolapse [29]. The cervix may or may not be exteriorized with a true vaginal prolapse [30].

Treatment

Jones and Joshua [31] reported that in most cases of vaginal prolapse that arise just prior to whelping, there is usually no need for any intervention and parturition can proceed normally. However, there is the possibility that the prolapse may prohibit normal parturition by narrowing the birth canal [32]. Konig and colleagues [23] reported on a case of a true vaginal prolapse that developed during the last weeks of gestation and caused no problem during delivery except for the last puppy. In cases in which the prolapse occurs a number of days before parturition, the outcome may depend upon the severity of swelling and tissue damage.

An alternative to the benign neglect approach is surgical correction by hysteropexy before delivery ± resection of the prolapsed tissue. Recurrence after surgical excision is uncommon but can occur. If surgery is not performed, following parturition the prolapsed tissue undergoes significant and rapid reduction in size until self-cure has been achieved. If the female is no longer intended as a breeding animal, ovariectomy or ovariohysterectomy should prevent further recurrence of the condition.

Vaginal Fold Prolapse (Canine Only)

Etiopathogenesis and Diagnosis

Vaginal fold prolapse is initiated by the protrusion of edematous vaginal tissue into the vestibule (type I) and then through the opening of the vulva (type II; Figure 125.4), which can progress to a true vaginal prolapse (type III) (Table 125.1). Reduction in venous and lymphatic circulation and inflammation secondary to exposure of the mucosa contribute to the progression from type II to type III [31].

Vaginal fold prolapses occur primarily during proestrus or early estrus [33]. During these stages of the canine estrous cycle, the vaginal mucosa becomes edematous and hyperplastic under the influence of estrogen [21]. In addition to its effects on the vaginal mucosa, estrogen may be responsible for relaxation of the vulvar and perivulvar musculature and associated tissues, predisposing to vaginal fold prolapse [29]. A vaginal fold prolapse was iatrogenically induced following estrogen administration for canine estrus induction [34]. Other suspected causes of vaginal fold prolapse include constipation, trauma from forced separation during coitus [35], size discrepancy between breeding animals [4,29,36], and vaginal tumors [37]. These factors, combined with a possible inherited weakness of the perivaginal tissue, may initiate or contribute to vaginal fold prolapse [29].

The reported incidence of vaginal fold prolapse ranges from 73% [28] to 86% [27] of all vaginal prolapse cases. Vaginal fold prolapse is more common in large-breed dogs, but may occur in small breeds [27,28,38]. The condition may be seen in families of pure-bred dogs,

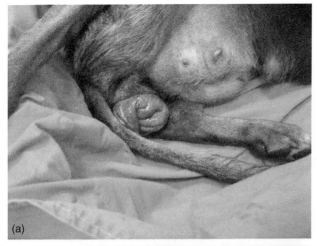

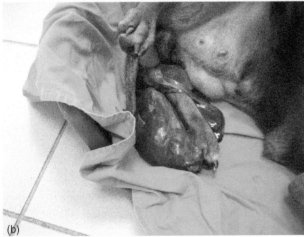

Figure 125.4 Type II vaginal fold prolapse in a 1.5-year-old Greek hound dog that occurred during late gestation.
Reproduced with permission of Elsevier.

suggesting a hereditary predisposition [4,27,28,30]. Breeds predisposed to vaginal fold prolapse include American Pit Bull Terrier, Boxer, Bulldog, Chesapeake Bay Retriever, Dalmatian, German Shepherd Dog,

Table 125.1 Three-stage classification scheme for vaginal prolapse in the dog, described by Schutte [38].

Type	Description
I	Slight-to-moderate eversion of vaginal mucosa originating from the vaginal floor cranial to the urethral opening but confined to the vestibulum. This appears as a bulge at the perineum
II	A well-developed swelling of the vaginal floor that may include the lateral vaginal walls with protrusion of the vaginal mucosa through the vulvar labia. This incomplete prolapse appears dome shaped
III	Complete protrusion of the entire circumference of the vaginal wall through the vulvar lips. This complete prolapse appears donut shaped

Labrador Retriever, Mastiff, Springer Spaneil, St Bernard, Walker Hound and Weimeraner.

Although somewhat similar in appearance, the etiopathogenesis as well as the urgency and method of treatment vary between a uterine prolapse and the types of vaginal prolapse. Uterine prolapse is a rare parturient condition typically associated with dystocia that requires immediate shock-supporting therapy in addition to replacement of the prolapsed tissue. While rare in queens, some types of vaginal prolapse are common in intact bitches and occur in association with elevated estrogen concentrations during proestrus. Most of these cases reduce spontaneously during diestrus but efforts should be made to keep prolapsed tissues moist, clean, and free from self-mutilation.

Treatment

In mild-to-moderate cases, the vaginal fold prolapse regresses spontaneously during diestrus [29]. It is important that the prolapsed tissue stay moist and clean and does not fall prey to self-mutilation. General anesthesia is required if attempting to replace the prolapsed mucosa. The prolapsed tissue should be cleaned with a mild antiseptic solution or saline. If the edema is severe, manual compression to the mucosal surface may decrease its size, therefore facilitating reduction. Similar to the descriptions for replacing a uterine prolapse, a lubricated plastic syringe can be used to reduce the vaginal fold prolapse. An episiotomy may be necessary to provide better exposure for reduction. Reduction can also be assisted by traction on the uterus via a ventral abdominal approach. Once the vagina is reduced, reprolapse can be minimized by suturing the uterine body or the broad ligament to the abdominal wall. A urinary catheter should be placed at the time of the episiotomy and maintained until the vaginal swelling resolves.

Dogs with long-standing prolapses may have secondary necrosis, infection, or hemorrhage of the prolapsed tissues. These dogs should be evaluated and treated as necessary for hypotension and/or sepsis (see Chapters 155 and 159). Surgical resection of the devitalized tissues is indicated in these patients to prevent further sepsis and self-mutilation. A stepwise full-thickness circumferential incision should be made through the vaginal wall. Then, a 1–2 cm section of the outer mucosal layer is incised, followed by resection of the inner non-inverted mucosal layer. Horizontal mattress sutures are used to close the incision edges. Hemorrhage can be significant and should be controlled with cautery and ligation. This is continued circumferentially in small sections until the entire prolapsed tissue is resected.

In a follow-up study of 13 bitches, vaginal fold prolapse recurred in all 13 during the second and third subsequent estrous cycles [28]. Although more studies are needed to ascertain the hereditary aspect of the vaginal prolapse in dogs [33], it has been recommended that affected bitches should not be bred [28]. Furthermore, as the recurrence rate in affected bitches is high, ovariectomy or ovariohysterectomy will fully eliminate the incidence of recurrence [30].

References

1 Maxson FB, Krausnick KE. Dystocia with uterine prolapse in a Siamese cat. *Vet Med Sm Anim Clin* 1969;64(12):1065–1066.

2 Biddle D, Macintire DK. Obstetrical emergencies. *Clin Tech Small Anim Pract* 2000;15(2):88–93.

3 Van der Kolk FR. Uterine inversion and prolapse in a cat. *Tijdschr Diergeneeskd* 1984;109(18):702–707.

4 Roberts SJ. *Veterinary Obstetrics and Genital Diseases*, 3rd edn. Edwards Brothers Inc., Ann Arbor, 1986, pp. 216–221.

5 Ragni RA. What is your diagnosis? *J Small Anim Pract* 2006;47:625–627.

6 Wilson FD. Bicornual uterine prolapse and its novel reduction. *Indian Vet J* 1965;42(9):707–709.

7 Whitehead JE. *Feline Medicine and Surgery*. American Veterinary Publications Inc, Santa Barbara, 1964, pp. 285–286.

8 Luckhurst J. Prolapse of the uterus in the cat. *Vet Rec* 1961;73(29):728.

9 Egger EL. Uterine prolapse in a cat. *Fel Pract* 1978;8:34–37.

10 Herbert CR. Prolapsed uterus in the cat. *Vet Rec* 1979;104(2):42.

11 Roberts DD, Straw RC. Uterine prolapse in a cat. *Comped Contin Educ Pract Vet* 1988;10:1294–1296.

12 Wallace LJ, Henry JD Jr, Clifford JH. Manual reduction of uterine prolapse in a domestic cat. *Vet Med Small Anim Clin* 1970;65(6):595–596.

13 Knight GC. Dystocia and surgical procedures. In: Reproduction in the Dog (ed Harrop AE). Bailliere, Tindall & Cox, London, 1960, pp. 120–145.

14 Vaughan L, McGucklin S. Uterine prolapse in cat. *Vet Rec* 1993;132(22):568.

15 Davies JE. Prolapsed uterus in the cat. *Vet Rec* 1978;103(25):567.

16 Macintire DK. Emergencies of the female reproductive tract. *Vet Clin North Am Small Anim Pract* 1994;24: 1173–1188.

17 Grundy AM. Partial uterine prolapse in a bitch. *Vet Rec* 1980;106(18-20):420–421.

18 Vanderhurst SR. Bicornuate uterine prolapse in a cat. *Vet Med Small Anim Clin* 1975;70(6):681.

19 Bruinsma DL. Feline uterine prolapse. *Vet Med Small Anim Clin* 1981;76(1):60.

20 Manothaiudom K, Johnston SD. Clinical approach to vaginal/vestibular masses in the bitch. *Vet Clin North Am Small Anim Pract* 1991;21:509–521.

21 Johnston SD, Root Kustritz MV, Olson PN. Disorders of the canine uterus and uterine tubes. In: *Canine and Feline Theriogenology* (eds Root Kustritz MV, Olson PN, Johnston SD). WB Saunders, Philadelphia, 2001, pp. 206.

22 Johnston SD, Root Kustritz MV, Olson PN. Disorders of the feline uterus and uterine tubes. In: *Canine and Feline Theriogenology* (eds Root Kustritz MV, Olson PN, Johnston SD). WB Saunders, Philadelphia, 2001, p. 463.

23 Konig GJ, Handler J, Arbeiter K. Rare case of a vaginal prolapse during the last third of pregnancy in a Golden Retriever bitch. *Kleintierpraxis* 2004;49:299.

24 Rani RU, Kathiresan D, Sivaseelan S. Vaginal fold prolapse in a pregnant bitch and its surgical management. *Indian Vet J* 2004;81:1390–1391.

25 Markandeya NM, Patil AD, Bhikane AU. Pre-partum vaginal prolapse in a dog. *Indian Vet J* 2004;81:449.

26 Schaefers-Okkens AC. Vaginal edema and vaginal fold prolapse in the bitch, including surgical management. Available at: www.ivis.org/advances/Concannon/schaefers/IVIS.pdf?q=ivis (accessed 15 February 2018).

27 Johnston SD. Vaginal prolapse. In: *Current Veterinary Therapy X* (ed. Kirk RW). WB Saunders, Philadelphia, 1989, pp. 1302–1305.

28 Trager CP. Vaginal prolapse in the bitch. *Mod Vet Pract* 1970;51:39–41.

29 McNamara PS, Harvey HJ, Dykes N. Chronic vaginocervical prolapse with visceral incarceration in a dog. *J Am Hosp Assoc* 1997;33:533–536.

30 Wykes PM. Diseases of the vagina and vulva in the bitch. In: *Current Therapy in Theriogenology* (ed Morrow DA). WB Saunders Co, London, 1986, pp. 476–481.

31 Jones DE, Joshua JO. *Reproductive Clinical Problems in the Dog*. Wright PSG, Bristol, 1982, pp. 22–28.

32 Alan M, Cetin Y, Sendag S, Eski, F. True vaginal prolapse in a bitch. *Anim Rep Sci* 2007;100:411–414.

33 Memon MA, Pavletic MM, Kumar MSA. Chronic vaginal prolapse during pregnancy in a bitch. *J Am Vet Med Assoc* 1993;202:295–297.

34 Sarrafzadeh-Rezaei F, Saifzadeh S, Mazaheri R, Behfar M. First report of vaginal prolapse in a bitch treated with oestrogen. *Anim Reprod Sci* 2008;106(1-2):194–199.

35 Arbeiter K, Bucher A. Traumatically caused prolapse of the vaginal mucosa and retroflexion of the bladder in the bitch. *Tierarztl Prax* 1994;22:78–79.

36 Purswell BJ. Vaginal disorders. In: *Textbook of Veterinary Internal Medicine* (eds Ettinger SJ, Feldman EC). WB Saunders, London, 2000, pp. 1566–1571.

37 Williams JH, Birrell J, Wilpe E. Lymphangiosarcoma in a 3.5-year-old Bullmastiff bitch with vaginal prolapse, primary lymph node fibrosis and other congenital defects. *J S Afr Vet Assoc* 2005;76:165–171.

38 Schutte AP. Vaginal prolapse in the bitch. *J S Afr Vet Assoc* 1967;38(2):197–203.

126

Penile, Preputial, and Testicular Disease

James Lavely, DVM, DACVIM[1] and Autumn P. Davidson, DVM, MS, DACVIM (SAIM)[2]

[1]*VCA Animal Care Center, Rohnert Park, CA, USA*
[2]*School of Veterinary Medicine, Davis, CA, USA*

Priapism

Pathophysiology

Priapism is a persistent penile erection lasting greater than 4 hours, without sexual stimulation. Priapism is infrequently reported in dogs and cats. Idiopathic, neurological, traumatic, neoplastic. and infectious causes have been reported [1]. Neurological causes have included spinal injury, canine distemper virus, post hemilaminectomy and lumbosacral stenosis; priapism has occurred in a dog with a syringohydromyelia in the lumbar spine and a concurrent meningomyelocele in the cauda equina [1,2].

A dysregulatory hypothesis has been considered. Dyssynergic stimulation of inflow and outflow penile blood vessels causes prolonged vascular and smooth muscle spasms. Dysregulation may occur within the penis or at other neurological regulatory centers of penile erection [3]. The pelvic nerve (S1–S2) is composed of parasympathetic fibers and mediates the canine erection. Pelvic nerve stimulation dilates penile arteries, partially inhibits venous drainage, and increases penile blood pressure, thus resulting in an erection. The pudendal nerve (S1–S3) stimulates contraction of the extrinsic penile muscles. Sympathetic chain fibers inhibit erection by decreasing venous resistance, decreasing corpus cavernosal pressure, and increasing arterial resistance. Sympathetic inhibition of erection is mediated by the alpha-1 adrenergic system [1].

Anesthesia or perioperative medications, including alpha-adrenergic antagonists, such as phenothiazine drugs can cause priapism in people and horses. In horses, this risk is due to the retractor penis muscle being solely controlled by alpha-adrenergic fibers. In dogs, intracorporeal chlorpromazine injection caused consistent erection but intravenous chlorpromazine injections were not shown to result in erection [1].

Priapism in people is differentiated between ischemic (veno-occlusive or low flow) and non-ischemic (arterial or high flow) types. Recurrent episodes of ischemic priapism can occur and is termed stuttering priapism. Identifying the type of priapism is essential. Ischemic priapism is most common in people and treatment is considered an emergency, recommended within 4 hours. Delayed treatment can result in diminished therapeutic success and irreversible corporal fibrosis. Histological changes occur within 12 hours of ischemic priapism. Ischemic priapism lasting greater than 48 hours is highly likely to result in fibrosis and permanent erectile dysfunction [4].

Clinical Presentation

Ischemic priapism has been reported in cats and a dog (Web Figures 126.1 and 126.2). A traumatic cause is common, with priapism often developing during mating attempts or after castration. Ischemic priapism occurred in a cat with feline infectious peritonitis and an idiopathic cause has been suspected in other cats. Siamese cats have been overrepresented thus far [1,5].

Diagnostics

Clinical examination can help differentiate ischemic from non-ischemic priapism. The examination findings of ischemic priapism include a rigid and painful corpora cavernosa, while the glans and corpus spongiosum are soft. In non-ischemic priapism, the corpora cavernosa are tumescent but not rigid or painful and the glans and corpus spongiosum are soft or partially tumescent [4].

Aspiration of blood from the corpus cavernosum may differentiate non-ischemic and ischemic priapism. Cavernous blood gas evaluation in ischemic priapism typically results in a pH <7.25, a $PO_2 <30$ mmHg and a $PCO_2 >60$ mmHg, while non-ischemic priapism typically

Textbook of Small Animal Emergency Medicine, First Edition. Edited by Kenneth J. Drobatz, Kate Hopper, Elizabeth Rozanski and Deborah C. Silverstein.
© 2019 John Wiley & Sons, Inc. Published 2019 by John Wiley & Sons, Inc.
Companion Website: www.wiley.com/go/drobatz/textbook

Table 126.1 Features of ischemic versus non-ischemic priapism.

	Ischemic	Non-ischemic
Pain?	Usually	Uncommon
Corpora cavernosa fully rigid	Usually	Uncommon
Cavernous blood gas	Abnormal	Normal
pH	<7.25	7.4
PO_2	<30	>90
PCO_2	>60	<40

results in pH 7.4, PO_2 >90 mmHg and PCO_2 <40 mm Hg [3,4] (Table 126.1).

Ultrasound of the penis confirms tumescence (Web Figure 126.3). Ultrasonography may also detect anatomical abnormalities such as emboli, neoplasia, and other obstructive causes. Ultrasonography of the perineum and then the entire penile shaft should be done. Perineal portions of the corpora cavernosa may be abnormal in trauma. Color flow Doppler ultrasonography can detect high systolic flow into the cavernosal artery or can help evaluate for an arterial to cavernosum fistula. Retrograde urethrography can also be used to evaluate for urethral obstruction that may be related to the priapism [1].

Therapy

In the cat, penile amputation and perineal urethrostomy has been the most common treatment, due to penile damage and infection [1,5]. Successful surgical treatment has been reported in a cat via small bilateral incisions in the tunica albuginea of the corpora cavernosa penis and portions of the corpora cavernosa. The corpora cavernosa were then irrigated with heparinized saline. Skin sutures were placed, but the tunica albuginea was not sutured. Similarly, a dog was treated successfully via bilateral incisions to the longa glandis and the tunica albuginea. Blood was pressed out and heparinized saline irrigation was carried out until red blood flow returned. The tunica albuginea was then sutured [6].

Guidelines for the treatment of priapism in people have been established [7,8]. First-line management in the treatment of ischemic priapism is decompression of the corpora cavernosa via penile aspiration with a 19 gauge butterfly needle or a 16–18 gauge angiocatheter. The catheter is placed in the corpora cavernosa on either lateral aspect of the proximal penile shaft. Blood is evacuated until fresh red blood is obtained. Saline irrigation may be done in conjunction with aspiration. The use of two catheters or two butterfly needles can be helpful, with one used for saline irrigation and the other for aspiration.

If priapism returns after aspiration then intracavernosal injection of a sympathomimetic agent such as

phenylephrine is done. The phenylephrine is diluted with normal saline to 100–500 μg/mL and given in 1 mL doses every 5 minutes. A maximum dose of 1 mg for no more than an hour is used in people. Lower dosages are used in patients with cardiovascular risks. Careful monitoring is recommended when giving phenylephrine. The penis may be semi-rigid following intracavernosal injections due to residual edema. This can make it challenging to determine if the priapism has been successfully treated.

Aspiration +/− saline irrigation is about 30% successful in people. Success increases up to 80% with concomitant use of intracavernosal injection of a sympathomimetic agent. A longer duration of ischemic priapism (>12 hours) prior to first-line treatment is thought to decrease the chance of success. When drug-induced priapism is of short duration, a single injection of a sympathomimetic agent on each side of the penis may be attempted. "Milking" or massaging the penis after the injection can help distribute the sympathomimetic agent [4].

When first-line management is not successful then surgical therapy may be pursued. This consists of shunting blood via a surgically created vent that allows blood to exit the corpora cavernosa. The vent is anticipated to close spontaneously following resolution of priapism. Surgical intervention can cause erectile dysfunction [4].

Treatment of stuttering priapism in people is directed toward prevention of episodes. Various systemic medications have been used. Hormonal therapies are most commonly used, such as gonadotropin-releasing hormone agonists, estrogen and androgen receptor antagonists. Baclofen, pseudoephedrine, terbutaline, gabapentin, hydroxyurea, and phosphodiesterase type 5 inhibitors have also been used [7,9].

Non-ischemic priapism is less urgent in people and thus conservative management is recommended. Applying ice to the perineum and compression may be used [8]. Monitoring is typically recommended in people with non-ischemic priapism as 62% have spontaneous resolution [3,7]. Embolization procedures and surgical ligation of cavernous fistulae may be considered, but carry the risk of erectile dysfunction. Blood aspiration is diagnostic, but not carried out for treatment of non-ischemic priapism. Alpha-adrenergic antagonists are not recommended due to the potential for severe adverse effects [7,8].

Non-ischemic priapism in dogs has been treated with pseudoephedrine (from 0.86 mg/kg q8-12 h to 1.74 mg/kg PO q12 h) with possible success [1]. Terbutaline sulfate is available as tablets in strengths of 2.5 mg and 5 mg; terbutaline is also available as an injectable medication and may be administered subcutaneously or intramuscularly. In both dogs and cats, the typical dose of terbutaline as an injectable is 0.01 mg/kg every 4 to 6 hours prn. In tablet form for dogs, the typical dose is 1.25 to 5 mg per dog every 8 hours. In tablet form for cats, the dose is 0.1

to 0.2 mg/kg every 12 hours [10]. Very few controlled data exist to evaluate systemic therapies in people. The limited number of reported cases in dogs and cats and the possibility of spontaneous resolution make evaluation of systemic therapies difficult.

The pathophysiology and histopathology findings of priapism in people and dogs are similar so following similar algorithms is likely reasonable. Distinguishing ischemic from non-ischemic priapism, identifying and treating the underlying cause are important. Veterinary patients likely have a longer duration of signs at presentation so success may be diminished. Protecting the integrity of penile tissue with lubrication and an Elizabethan collar is important. Surgical incisions in the tunica albuginea, longa glandis or corpora cavernosa to evacuate accumulated blood, followed by saline irrigation, may be considered if initial therapy is not successful. Penile amputation and perineal urethrostomy may be indicated if penile tissue damage is significant.

If non-ischemic priapism is present then cold compresses, monitoring, and possible systemic therapy are reasonable provided that the medication is not contraindicated and adverse effects are monitored for. Protecting penile integrity via lubrication + /− an Elizabethan collar is essential. Self-trauma may necessitate antibiotic therapy or surgical intervention.

Paraphimosis

Pathophysiology

Paraphimosis could be confused with priapism. With paraphimosis, the typically non-erect penis cannot be ensheathed within the prepuce and can become edematous from exposure. Paraphimosis can be caused by trauma, inadequate length of the prepuce, weakened preputial muscles or too small a preputial orifice compared to the size of the penis during detumescence. Paraphimosis can occur after manual semen collection as the erect penis is exposed to air rather than being encased within the vulva of a bitch until detumescence. Dry mucous membranes, long preputial hair, and enfolding of the preputial orifice then prevent normal detumescence. Entrapment of the distal tip of the penis can then induce severe edema (in moments) which exacerbates the problem. Chronic infolding can result in desiccation of the tip of the penis.

Clinical Presentation

Penile enlargement with paraphimosis is a result of failure of detumescence exacerbated by edema, rather than a chronic erection. Typically, dogs with paraphimosis are uncomfortable, attempting to groom the penis and not

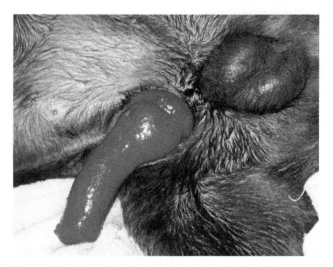

Figure 126.1 Paraphimosis in an 11-month-old Cane Corso mastiff after breeding. The penis is severely edematous and cannot be returned into the prepuce.

enthusiastic about ambulating. Dogs can be presented after breeding or manual semen collection.

Diagnostics

The diagnosis is made on the basis of physical examination. Priapism is the main differential. Acute paraphimosis usually presents with the penis completely extruded from the prepuce (Figure 126.1). Chronic paraphimosis presents with only partial extrusion and excoriation and scarring of the distal penis. Usually a history of sexual stimulation exists (even in neutered dogs) such as an estrual bitch, actual breeding or masturbation.

Therapy

Treatment of paraphimosis consists of saline irrigation and generous lubrication as the penis is manipulated back into the prepuce (Web Figure 126.4). Diuretics do not significantly reduce penile swelling. The use of topical osmotic agents has been helpful in some cases. Temporary purse-string sutures can be beneficial in some cases but interference with urination must be avoided. Surgical correction of underlying preputial anatomical abnormalities may be required if the penis cannot be ensheathed in the prepuce, if the problem recurs repeatedly or becomes chronic (Web Figure 126.5). The most common surgery required is a revision of the preputial opening. Antibiotic and anti-inflammatory therapy, prevention of mutilation, and pain management should be used as clinically indicated. Castration can be helpful if the dog is not valuable for breeding, but neutered male dogs can still achieve erection and ejaculation if stimulated and habitually masturbating.

Phimosis

Pathophysiology

Phimosis is a condition in which the penis is trapped within the preputial cavity. It usually occurs as a congenital defect in which the preputial opening is abnormally small and the penis, even when not erect, cannot protrude or be extruded manually. Phimosis can occur from the presence of a persistent penile frenulum. It can also occur as a consequence of erection without prior extrusion of the penis during manual semen collection.

Clinical Presentation

Phimosis is uncommon in dogs and rare in cats. It may be recognized in young dogs as a cause of partial urinary tract outflow obstruction resulting in dribbling of urine that has accumulated in the preputial cavity. Phimosis may be recognized in a postpubertal affected dog when he is unable to copulate (or have manual semen collection) due to a small preputial opening. The preputial hair of long-coated cats may entangle the preputial orifice, causing clinical signs similar to phimosis.

Diagnostics

Phimosis is diagnosed by physical examination of the prepuce and penis. Preputial endoscopy and ultrasound of the prepuce can be performed to rule out other causes of penile entrapment such as a hematoma, ruptured tunica albuginea or penile mass lesion.

Therapy

Phimosis is treated by conservatively surgically enlarging the preputial orifice. Exposure of penile mucosa can result if the opening is too large.

Persistent Penile Frenulum

Pathophysiology

Under the influence of androgens, the surfaces of the glans penis and the preputial mucosa normally separate before or within weeks of birth. If this separation does not occur, connective tissue persists between the penis and the prepuce. In dogs, the persistent penile frenulum is usually located on the ventral midline of the penis.

Clinical Presentation

A persistent penile frenulum may cause no clinical signs, or it may be associated with preputial discharge or excessive licking of the prepuce. Persistent frenulum may cause the penis to deviate ventrally or laterally so that the dog is unable or unwilling to mate, or it may interfere with normal tumescence.

Diagnostics

The diagnosis is made by visual examination.

Therapy

Treatment is surgical excision, which can often be done using just sedation with local anesthesia as the frenulum tends to be a sheer, avascular membrane.

Balanoposthitis

Pathophysiology

Balanoposthitis is inflammation or infection of the preputial cavity and penis. The causative organisms are usually members of the normal preputial flora, although overgrowth of one organism or a predominance of *Pseudomonas* spp can occur [11]. Lymphoid follicular hyperplasia is commonly also present and thought to develop as a result of chronic irritation.

Clinical Presentation

Balanoposthitis is common in dogs and rare in cats. It usually causes no clinical signs other than a purulent preputial discharge that is quite variable, from a scant white smegma to a copious green pus, and excessive licking. The discharge associated with balanoposthitis is not sanguineous unless the cause is neoplasia or accumulated foreign material.

Diagnostics

The diagnosis of balanoposthitis is made by physical examination of the penis and preputial cavity all the way to the fornix, in a search for foreign material, neoplasia, ulceration, or inflammatory nodules. Cultures and cytological studies are rarely helpful unless a mycotic infection or neoplastic process is suspected.

In persistent or refractory cases, cytology, culture, and endoscopic examination of the prepuce and urethra should be considered. Preputial discharge from benign prostatic hyperplasia, prostatitis, urethritis or cystitis should be ruled out if the penis and prepuce appear normal. Penile mass lesions can cause excessive preputial discharge. Transmissible venereal tumor (TVT) is the most commonly reported penile tumor in dogs.

Cytological evaluation of TVT is supportive; biopsy is diagnostic. The macroscopic appearance of TVT and penile papilloma virus may be similar.

Therapy

The treatment of balanoposthitis is usually conservative. The hair should be clipped from the preputial orifice and the surrounding area if discharge has been accumulating there. Flushing the preputial cavity with very dilute, gentle antiseptic solutions (e.g. chlorhexidine, povidone-iodine) can be helpful. Topical antibacterial or combination corticosteroid antibacterial medications may be instilled into the preputial cavity. Penile warts often resolve spontaneously after biopsy of the lesion.

Urethral Prolapse (see Chapter 104)

Pathophysiology

Eversion of the urethral mucosa at the distal tip of the penis results in focal refractory hemorrhage. The condition is associated with the increased intra-abdominal pressure associated with the brachycephalic syndrome [12].

Clinical Presentation

Urethral prolapse occurs most commonly in bulldogs and Boston terriers, and is likely familial.

Diagnostics

Urethral prolapse is evident upon physical examination. Urethral obstruction due to urolithiasis and a urethral mass are rule-outs.

Therapy

Surgical revision is indicated as the condition will not resolve spontaneously. Preventing erection with sedation during recovery is important; breeding these dogs can cause relapse, and castration should be suggested.

Penile Trauma

Pathophysiology

Laceration of the penis and prepuce can occur secondary to trauma (most commonly in hunting dogs on rough terrain or through barbed wire fencing), dog fights or in animal abuse cases (Web Figures 126.6 and 126.7).

Rupture of the tunica albuginea and fracture of the os penis can occur from blunt trauma in the dog (Web Figure 126.8). Self-trauma can be significant from urolithiasis, priapism or paraphimosis.

Clinical Presentation

Because of the vascularity of the penis, trauma usually results in impressive hemorrhage.

Diagnostics

Physical examination with sedation and analgesia is indicated. Radiography can identify a fractured os penis. Ultrasound of the penis can identify internal hematomas, thrombi, uroliths, and loss of linear integrity of the os in the case of a fracture [13,14]. Evaluation of the integrity of the urethra with contrast radiography should be made as indicated (see Chapter 100).

Therapy

Surgical repair of lacerations has a good prognosis if significant tissue devitalization is not present (Web Figure 126.9). Temporary catheterization (3–7 days) can enable healing of urethral tears if not extensive. Amputation of the penis and permanent urethrostomy are indicated in severe cases.

Infectious Orchitis and Epididymitis

Pathophysiology

Bacterial orchitis and epididymitis not associated with brucellosis (canine) can occur separately or in concert. Bacterial contamination of the testis or epididymis can originate hematogenously, by extension from other genitourinary organs or by injection (bite wounds) [11].

Clinical Presentation

Male dogs and cats are typically presented because their owners noticed an enlarged scrotum. Scrotal enlargement can be due to scrotal neoplasia, scrotal dermatitis, scrotal edema, intrascrotal effusion or hemorrhage, testicular enlargement or epididymal enlargement. Testicular or epididymal enlargement can be due to an acute infectious process or infiltrative disease, which can be granulomatous or neoplastic. Foreign bodies such as grass awns can be a cause of infection of the testes or epididymis. Animals with infectious orchitis/epididymitis are typically painful and febrile.

Diagnostics

Brucellosis should always be ruled out in the dog. A careful palpation of the scrotum and contents with appropriate analgesia and sedation can differentiate the source of enlargement; ultrasound evaluation is very helpful in identifying pathology and localizing the cause of enlargement. Ultrasound-guided sampling will permit cytology and culture/sensitivity to be performed.

Therapy

Dogs or cats should be treated with appropriate antibiotic therapy based on culture and sensitivity profiles, and keeping in mind penetration into the prostate gland (dog) if suspected to be involved (see Chapters 96 and 200). Appropriate antimicrobial therapy should continue for a minimum of 2–8 weeks, longer in the case of chronic bacterial prostatitis. The prognosis for fertility is guarded (but not hopeless), even with therapy; thermal damage from heat associated with inflammation affects spermatogenesis, and the potential for sperm autoantibody formation exists following such an inflammatory process. Males not valuable for breeding can be castrated to hasten recovery [12].

Testicular Torsion

Pathophysiology

Other than malignant transformation, the most common complication of uncorrected cryptorchidism in the dog is testicular torsion, which occurs with an increased incidence in neoplastic intra-abdominal testes [15]. Intrascrotal testicular torsion is rare.

Clinical Presentation

Cryptorchid testicular torsion presents as an acute abdomen. The dog can appear to be neutered when actually cryptorchid. Intrascrotal testicular torsion presents as acute, severe scrotal pain.

Diagnostics

Ultrasound is commonly performed in dogs with acute abdominal distress. Cryptorchid testes can be positioned anywhere between the ipsilateral kidney and the inguinal canal, but tend to gravitate to the midventral abdomen when enlarged by neoplasia. Testicular torsion can appear similar to orchitis with a diffuse hypoechoic appearance to the testis; malignant transformation and

gangrenous change can make their appearance less recognizable. Doppler examination reveals aberrant blood flow [13,14].

Therapy

Stabilization and immediate surgical intervention for removal are indicated.

Scrotal Dermatitis

Pathophysiology

Scrotal dermatitis most commonly results from superficial irritants, contact or insect bite hypersensitivity, ophitoxemia (snake envenomation; Web Figure 126.10), thermal insult (heat or cold), excessive grooming/clipping, or trauma. Self-excoriation often complicates the initial insult. Cutaneous neoplasia, most commonly mast cell tumors, can also produce scrotal dermatitis. Uncommonly, a varicocele can produce scrotal dermatitis. Heat from inflammation of the scrotum can damage spermatogenesis; this may not be apparent for days to weeks.

Clinical Presentation

Scrotal dermatitis is most common in intact dogs. The scrotum can be markedly edematous, erythemic, and ulcerated. Affected dogs are painful with an abnormal gait.

Diagnostics

The diagnosis is based on physical examination and palpation of the scrotum under adequate sedation/analgesia. Differentiation of scrotal enlargement secondary to a testicular mass, orchitis/epididymitis, intrascrotal testicular torsion or entrapment of tissue through an inguinal hernia should be made. Ultrasound can be helpful in identifying the origin of scrotal enlargement [13].

Therapy

Prevention of further excoriation by the use of an Elizabethan collar is important. Treatment depends on the etiology identified. Non-specific dermatitis should be treated with systemic antibiotics, analgesics, and anti-inflammatories as indicated. Gentle cleansing of the scrotum with saline is advised, avoiding antiseptics with irritant potential.

References

1 Lavely JA. Priapism in dogs. *Top Compan Anim Med* 2009;24:49–54.

2 Payan-Carreira R, Colaco B, Rocha C, et al. Priapism associated with lumbar stenosis in a dog. *Reprod Dom Anim* 2013;48:58–64.

3 Burnett AL, Bivalacqua TJ. Priapism: current principles and practice. *Urol Clin North Am* 2007;34:631–642.

4 Burnett AL, Sharlip ID. Standard operating procedures for priapism. *J Sex Med* 2013;10:180–194.

5 Gunn-Moore DA, Brown PJ, Holt PE, et al. Priapism in seven cats. *J Small Anim Pract* 1995;36:262–266.

6 Orima H, Tsutsui T, Waki T, et al. Surgical treatment of priapism observed in a dog and a cat. *Nippon Juigaku Zasshi* 1989;51:1227–1229.

7 Montague DK, Jarow J, Broderick GA, et al. American Urological Association guideline to the management of priapism. *J Urol* 2003;170:1318–1324.

8 Salonia A, Eardley I, Giuliano F, et al. European Association of Urology guidelines on priapism. *Eur Urol* 2014;65:480–489.

9 Yuan J, DeSouza R, Westney L, et al. Insights of priapism mechanism and rationale treatment for recurrent priapism. *Asian J Androl* 2008;1:88–101.

10 Cassutto BH. Using drug therapy to treat priapism in two dogs. *Vet Med* 2012;107:220–225.

11 Bjurström L, Linde-Forsberg C. Long-term study of aerobic bacteria in the genital tract in stud dogs. *Am J Vet Res* 1992;53:670.

12 Davidson AP. Clinical conditions of the dog and tom. In: *Small Animal Internal Medicine*, 5th edn (eds Nelson RW, Couto CG). Mosby, St Louis, 2015.

13 Davidson AP, Baker TW. Reproductive ultrasound of the dog and tom. *Top Compan Anim Med* 2009;24:64.

14 Davidson AP. Clinical theriogenology, *Vet Clin North Am* 2001;31:2.

15 Peters MAJ, de Jong F, Teerds K, et al. Aging, testicular tumours and the pituitary-testis axis in dogs. *J Endocrinol* 2000;166:153.

I. Common Toxins

127

Decontamination and Toxicological Analyses of the Poisoned Patient

Justine A. Lee, DVM, DACVECC, DABT

Animal Emergency and Referral Center of Minnesota, St Paul, MN, USA

Introduction

The goal of decontamination in the poisoned veterinary patient is to "inhibit or minimize further toxicant absorption and to promote excretion or elimination of the toxicant from the body" [1,2]. When treating the poisoned patient, the clinician should have an understanding of the toxic dose (if available), the pharmacokinetics (including absorption, distribution, metabolism, and excretion), the underlying mechanism of action, and the potential clinical signs that can be observed with the toxicant [2]. This will help determine appropriate decontamination and therapy for the patient. If this information is not readily available, the reader is advised to contact the ASPCA Animal Poison Control Center (APCC) (888-426-4435) for life-saving, 24/7 advice.

There are several methods of decontamination for use in the poisoned patient. While the gastrointestinal (GI) route is the most common type of decontamination used in veterinary medicine, other types include ocular, dermal, inhalation, injection, forced diuresis, blood purification (see Chapter 129), or surgical removal of the toxicant (Table 127.1) [1,2]. Additionally, lipid therapy is now recognized as a potentially useful treatment for lipophilic drug intoxications (see Chapter 128).

Gastrointestinal Decontamination

Gastrointestinal decontamination can be safely performed at home by the pet owner (for dogs) or by the veterinary professional. Keep in mind that the medical recommendation to decontaminate a pet at home must be thoroughly evaluated by the veterinarian, veterinary staff, or the ASPCA APCC first. Prior to inducing emesis, one should be aware that there is a narrow time frame to perform decontamination. Also, note that the effectiveness of emesis induction is dependent on several factors (Box 127.1) [1–6]. Lastly,

decontamination is contraindicated in certain circumstances (Table 127.2).

Prior to emesis induction, a complete history should be obtained from the pet owner. Particular information that should be obtained includes the time frame since ingestion, confirmation of the active ingredient, the amount of toxicant ingested (in order to calculate the toxic dose), the presence of clinical signs, previous medical history, and the toxin's potential to cause severe illness.

Emesis induction should only be performed with recent ingestion of a toxicant or unknown time of ingestion in an *asymptomatic* patient. The sooner that emesis induction can be performed, the greater the amount of gastric contents that will be recovered [2]; the gastric recovery volumes decrease as time passes. Studies have shown that gastric recovery within 1 hour after toxin ingestion was approximately 17–62% [1,3–6]. When emesis was induced within an even shorter time span (within 11–30 minutes), mean recovery of gastric contents was approximately 49% (range 9–75%) [1,3]. If several hours have elapsed since ingestion, the contents have likely moved out of the stomach and emesis may no longer be of benefit [1,2]. That said, induction of emesis can be performed in *asymptomatic* patients up to 1–2 hours post ingestion, particularly with certain toxicants [1,2].

Emetic Agents

Veterinary professionals should recommend or use safe, effective emetic agents, as several agents have fallen out of favor. Many home or internet remedies are used without success and have the potential of causing further harm.

Emetic agents work by causing local gastric irritation, stimulating the central nervous system (CNS) chemoreceptor trigger zone (CRTZ), or a combination of the two [1,2]. Emetic agents are not effective if an antiemetic

Textbook of Small Animal Emergency Medicine, First Edition. Edited by Kenneth J. Drobatz, Kate Hopper, Elizabeth Rozanski and Deborah C. Silverstein.
© 2019 John Wiley & Sons, Inc. Published 2019 by John Wiley & Sons, Inc.
Companion Website: www.wiley.com/go/drobatz/textbook

Table 127.1 Other routes of decontamination [1,2].

Type of decontamination	Treatment	Treatment	Avoid
Ocular	With ocular exposure to a corrosive or caustic toxicant, the pet owner should attempt to copiously flush the eyes at home with tepid water or physiological saline (e.g. contact lens solution *without* any soaps or cleaners), ideally for 15–20 minutes, prior to seeking veterinary attention	Elizabethan collar Immediate veterinary evaluation	Prevent rubbing/scratching Avoid contact lens chemicals (e.g. cleaners, soaps, etc.)
Dermal	Prevent pet from grooming (which can result in secondary re-exposure)	Prevent exposure to pet owner (e.g. protective gear) Wash with tepid or lukewarm water and mild, gentle, degreasing liquid dish soap (e.g. Dawn, Palmolive, etc.)	Avoid scrubbing or pressurized sprays which can result in further dermal injury Avoid "neutralizing" agents on the skin (e.g. an alkaline for an acid exposure); this may cause a chemical or thermal reaction, resulting in additional injury
Inhalation	Prompt removal from environment	Humidified oxygen source Immediate veterinary evaluation Monitoring of oxygenation and ventilation	
Injection	The stinger or venom sac should be gently and carefully removed from the patient's skin	Immediate veterinary evaluation	Pet owners and veterinary professionals should avoid the following with a snake bite: making an incision and "sucking" the affected area; applying cold or hot compresses; applying a tourniquet
Forced diuresis	The concurrent use of aggressive intravenous fluids and concurrent diuretic therapy Used ideally for certain toxicants that have a high level of excretion through the kidney including salicylates, phenobarbital, bromide, amphetamines, lithium, etc.	Monitor for electrolyte abnormalities, acid–base disturbances, and fluid overload	Avoid fluid overload Consider urinary catheterization to remove urine and quantify output
Surgical removal	For certain toxicants that result in a FBO, bezoar, or life-threatening, acute abdomen (e.g. unbaked yeast bread dough, di-isocyanate glues, bone meal, etc.), surgery may be required	Gastric lavage should be attempted first to help break up the potential toxicant (e.g. bezoar). If the toxicant cannot be removed by gastric lavage, or if it is sharp, surgical removal may be necessary	Immediate surgical intervention (following radiographs) is warranted with di-isocyanate glues (Gorilla Glue), due to rapid formation of a FBO

FBO, foreign body obstruction.

(e.g. ondansetron, maropitant, etc.) has been previously administered. Currently, the only home recommendation for dog owners is 3% hydrogen peroxide [1,2,7]. There is no safe at-home emetic agent that is recommended for cats; anecdotally, 25% of cats can develop a severe hemorrhagic gastritis secondary to hydrogen peroxide administration and deaths have rarely been reported (personal communication, ASPCA APCC, Urbana, USA) [8].

Methods that are no longer recommended for emesis induction include digital induction of emesis (e.g. stimulation of the gag reflex), syrup of ipecac, liquid dishwashing detergent, liquid soaps, dry mustard powders, and table salt (sodium chloride) [1,2,9]. Digital induction of emesis often results in physical injury to the pet owner (dog bite), or injury to the pet's throat and soft palate. Syrup of ipecac has historically been recommended to

Box 127.1 Factors affecting the effectiveness of emesis induction [11,12].

When recommending or performing emesis induction, keep in mind that the following factors affect gastric recovery of the toxicant [1,2].

- What type of emetic agent was used
- Time since last meal fed (e.g. presence of gastric acid or amount of gastric contents)
- How much time has passed since time of ingestion of the toxicant
- The texture or physical characteristics of the toxicant ingested (e.g. gel caps are rapidly absorbed, etc.)
- Whether the toxicant affects gastric emptying (e.g. opioids, salicylates, tricyclic antidepressants, etc.)
- The amount ingested (e.g. massive ingestions which can result in concretions or bezoars, causing delayed gastric emptying)

induce emesis, but is no longer the standard of care. Its cardiotoxic potential and tendency to result in prolonged vomiting, lethargy, hematemesis, depression, and diarrhea have caused it to fall out of favor in both human and veterinary medicine [1,2]. Soaps, mustard powders, and table salt are not reliable as emetic agents and may be detrimental (e.g. resulting in further complications such as hypernatremia) [9].

Common veterinary emetic agents include apomorphine (e.g. tablets, capsules, or injectable) for dogs and alpha-2 adrenergic agonist agents (e.g, dexmedetomidine, xylazine) for cats [10–12]. Hydrogen peroxide is commonly used by veterinarians as an emetic agent in dogs and is equally effective as apomorphine [7]; however, it has been recently associated with gastrointestinal inflammation and ulceration even in dogs [13]. See Table 127.3 for more information.

Gastric Lavage

Gastric lavage, while less commonly performed than emesis induction, is still indicated in certain situations or with certain ingested toxicants in the veterinary patient. Gastric lavage should be performed when emesis induction is unproductive or contraindicated, yet the toxicant is still thought to be present in the stomach; the goal is to assist in removal of gastric contents and ease of administration of activated charcoal.

Table 127.2 Emesis induction: indications and contraindications [1,2].

Indications to induce emesis	Contraindications to inducing emesis
Following a recent toxicant ingestion (<1–2h) in an asymptomatic patient	Following ingestion of caustic or corrosive toxicants (e.g. batteries, ultra-bleach, lye, oven cleaning chemicals) or when emesis induction may result in further injury to the oropharynx, esophagus, and gastrointestinal tract when these agents are expelled
With unknown time of toxicant ingestion in an asymptomatic patient	Following ingestion of petroleum distillates or hydrocarbons (e.g. kerosene, gasoline, motor oil, transmission fluid, etc.); these toxicants can be easily aspirated into the respiratory system and result in severe aspiration pneumonitis
Following ingestion of a product known to stay in the stomach for a long time period in an asymptomatic patient (e.g. bezoar, massive ingestions, grapes/raisins, chocolate, wads of xylitol gum, foreign body, etc.)	In symptomatic patients that have a decreased gag reflex (e.g. sedation, coma, hypoglycemia, etc.) or a lowered seizure threshold (e.g. tremoring, seizuring, etc.) that may be unable to protect their airway, resulting in aspiration pneumonitis
	In patients with underlying medical conditions that may predispose them towards aspiration pneumonitis or complications associated with emesis induction (e.g. megaesophagus, history of aspiration pneumonia, upper airway disease, laryngeal paralysis)
	Brachycephalic breeds (e.g. English bulldog, pug, shih-tzu) with an elongated soft palate, everted saccules, a hypoplastic trachea, or stenotic nares may be better candidates for sedation, intubation, and gastric lavage rather than emesis induction due to the risks of aspiration
	Species that anatomically cannot vomit or cannot safely have emesis chemically induced such as birds, rabbits, ruminants (e.g. sheep, cattle, llamas, and goats), horses, and rodents (e.g. chinchillas, rats, gerbils)

Table 127.3 Drug doses for common emetic agents and their reversal agents [1,2,7,10–12].

Drug	Mechanism of action	Dose
Apomorphine (available as tablets, capsules or injectable)	Acts on the CRTZ	Dose: dogs, 0.02–0.04 mg/kg IV or IM; can also apply the tablet or capsule contents directly into subconjuctival sac [1,2,10]
		Generally not used in cats as not effective
		If administered via the subconjunctival route, flush well after emesis, or eye irritation and protracted vomition can occur
		If emesis does not occur, a second dose of apomorphine can be used. The author does not recommend additional dosing thereafter; rather, an oral dose of hydrogen peroxide may be beneficial, if needed (dogs only)
3% Hydrogen peroxide	Acts as a direct gastric irritation on the stomach	1–2 mL/kg, PO once; repeat if needed [1,2]
	In dogs, effective for at-home or veterinary use. [7] Due to the risk of GIT irritation and ulceration, antacid therapy should be used (e.g., famotidine, sucralfate X 5-7 days) [13]	Maximum dose: 50–150 mL/large dog [1,2]
	Not recommended for use in cats due to risks of hemorrhagic gastritis and rarely, death [8]	
Atipamezole (Antisedan)	Alpha-2 adrenergic antagonists	0.1 mg/kg IM, IV [10]
	Reverses the effects of dexmedetomidine and xylazine	
Dexmedetomidine	Used as an emetic for cats due to alpha-2 adrenergic agonist properties	7-10 mcg/kg IM, SC [11,12]
		Adverse effects from dexmedetomidine include respiratory depression, hypotension, and excessive sedation
Liquid dish detergent (e.g. Dawn, Palmolive, Joy)	Acts as a direct gastric irritant	Dose: 10 mL/kg of a mixture of 3 tablespoons of detergent to 8 ounces of water [1,2]
	Generally not recommended, due to the increased effectiveness and wider margin of safety of hydrogen peroxide (for dogs)	Can take longer to result in emesis; as hydrogen peroxide has a faster onset of action as an emetic agent, dish detergent is rarely used or recommended any more
	Eco-friendly products (without phosphate) are anecdotally not as effective as an emetic agent	NOTE: When counseling pet owners on how to decontaminate a pet at home (e.g. whether for emesis induction or for dermal decontamination), appropriate detailed communication must occur; one should not use corrosive products used for automatic dishwashers (e.g. Cascade)
Table salt	Acts as an emetic by direct gastric irritation	Dose: 1–3 teaspoons orally [1,2]
	While readily available within the household, the use of salt is *no longer* recommended as an emetic due to potential side-effects	Emesis induction typically occurs within 10–15 min [2]
	Rare reports of electrolyte disturbances (e.g. hypernatremia, hyperchloremia); hematemesis, and persistent emesis can be seen [9]	In children treated with salt as an emetic, hypernatremia, secondary cerebral edema, and neurological complications have been seen [1,2]. Rarely, death has been reported [9]
7% Syrup of ipecac	Syrup of ipecac contains the alkaloid compounds cephaeline and emetine, which act as a direct gastric irritant and stimulate the CRTZ [1,2]	Dose: dogs, 1–2 mL/kg PO; cats, 3.3 mL/kg; cumulative dose in either species is not to exceed 15 mL [1,2]
	Due to the availability of safer emetic agents, the use of syrup of ipecac or ipecac fluid extract (which is more potent) is *no longer* recommended in either human and veterinary medicine [1,2]	Emesis induction typically occurs within 10–30 min [1,2]
		Several adverse effects can be seen with syrup of ipecac including cardiotoxicity, lethargy, diarrhea, weakness, diarrhea, protracted vomiting, hematemesis, hypersalivation, distaste (cats), ineffectiveness, and delayed onset of action (which can take up to 1 hour) [1,2]

Drug	Mechanism of action	Dose
Xylazine hydrochloride	Used as an emetic for cats due to alpha-2 adrenergic agonist properties Due to the availability of more effective, safer emetic agents in dogs (e.g. hydrogen peroxide, apomorphine), xylazine is not recommended in this species.	Dose: cats, 0.44 mg/kg, IM or SC [10,11,12] In the author's experience, only 50% of cats given xylazine have effective emesis Delayed emesis may be seen following administration Adverse effects from xylazine include respiratory depression, hypotension, and excessive sedation
Yohimbine	Alpha-2 adrenergic antagonists Reverses the effects of xylazine	0.1 mg/kg IM, SC, or IV slowly [10]

CRTZ, chemoreceptor trigger zone; IM, intramuscular; IV, intravenous; PO, by mouth (*per os*); SC, subcutaneous.

Human studies have shown minimal gastric lavage recoveries (range 29–38%) when gastric lavage was performed within 15–20 minutes after toxicant ingestion [1–5,14]. Gastric lavage recoveries drop even further to 8.6–13% when lavage is performed at 60 minutes post ingestion [1–5,14]. In the veterinary scenario, most poisoned patients are presented to the veterinary clinic more than 60 minutes post ingestion, making the clinical usefulness of gastric lavage debatable [1,2]. Knowing that gastric lavage can be labor intensive and may yield low gastric recovery, veterinarians are often hesitant to perform this potentially life-saving procedure [1,2]. That said, the use of gastric lavage is warranted in the following situations [2].

- When the patient is already significantly affected by the toxicant, thereby predisposing the patient to aspiration if emesis induction is performed (e.g. unconscious, excessively sedate, tremoring, seizuring, etc.).
- With toxicants that have a narrow margin of safety that may still require decontamination with a controlled airway (e.g. baclofen, macrocyclic lactones, metaldehyde, marijuana, organophosphates, carbamates, calcium channel blockers, beta-blockers, etc.).
- With toxicants that can result in a bezoar formation or concretion (e.g. massive ingestions, unbaked yeast bread dough, prenatal iron tablets, bone meal, etc.).
- With ingestions approaching the LD_{50}.

Rare complications may occur when performing gastric lavage, including aspiration pneumonitis, complications from sedation, hypoxemia secondary to aspiration pneumonia, hypercapnia from sedation or anesthesia, laryngospasm, fluid and electrolyte abnormalities, or mechanical injury to the mouth, oropharynx, esophagus, or stomach [1,2,14].

Contraindications for gastric lavage include ingestion of sharp objects (e.g. sewing needles, etc.), corrosive agents (where perforation to the oropharynx, esophagus, and stomach can occur during orogastric tube placement), petroleum distillates or hydrocarbons (e.g. low-viscosity liquids that can result in severe aspiration pneumonia), or in patients with underlying pathology that could increase the risk of esophageal or gastric perforation or hemorrhage [1,2].

Many veterinarians may not feel comfortable performing gastric lavage, but it can be easily accomplished when organized with the appropriate supplies and a team-oriented approach. Box 127.2 gives a step-by-step guide on how to perform this important procedure [1,2].

Lastly, whole-bowel irrigation (WBI) is listed in the literature as a means of decontaminating the gastrointestinal tract (GIT) by removing toxins and normal intraluminal GI contents. This is typically done by the enteral administration of large amounts of polyethylene glycol electrolyte solution (PEG-ES or PEG, e.g. Golytely) until effluent (e.g. stool) is clear. Anecdotally, this is rarely indicated for the management of the poisoned veterinary patient. The reader is referred to another toxicology source for more information on this technique [1,2].

Activated Charcoal

Activated charcoal (AC) has been used for over 100 years for the treatment of toxic ingestions [15]. Activated charcoal is created by controlled pyrolysis of petroleum, coconut shells, lignite (coal), peat, and wood, which then produces charcoal [1,15]. Once charcoal is created, it is activated by heating at high temperatures (600–900 °C) with steam, air, or carbon dioxide [1,2,15]. This results in a small particle size, a large surface area (950–2000 m²/g), and a highly developed internal pore structure which contributes to adsorptive properties and extent of adsorption at equilibrium [15].

Activated charcoal works by adsorbing poison in the GIT and decreasing the extent of systemic absorption of the poison [1,10,15]. In order for AC to work, it must physically contact the toxicant. To maximize AC absorption of the toxicant, the administration of

Box 127.2 Performing gastric lavage [1,2].

- While gastric lavage can be labor-intensive and require several assistants, it can be potentially life saving for the poisoned patient.
- Prepare the following materials in advance:
  - IV catheter supplies
  - Sedatives and an anti-emetic (predrawn and labeled appropriately)
  - Endotracheal tube (ETT)
  - Syringe to inflate the ETT cuff
  - Gauze (to secure the ETT in place)
  - Anesthetic machine and appropriate monitoring
  - Orogastric tube
  - 2" roll of white tape
  - Mouth gag
  - Lubrication (for orogastric tube)
  - Empty bucket
  - Warm lavage water in a bucket
  - Bilge or stomach pump; alternatively a funnel can be used with gravity assistance
  - Step stool
  - Activated charcoal predrawn in the appropriate dose in 60 mL syringes ready for administration
  - Sedation reversal agents
  - Oxygen supplementation
  - Monitoring equipment
- After placing an IV catheter, preoxygenate patient, then sedate and intubate. Ensure the airway is protected. Connect to an oxygen ± inhalant anesthesia source. Place in either sternal (clinician preference) or right lateral recumbency.
- Administer a potent antiemetic to prevent secondary aspiration pneumonia (e.g. maropitant, ondansetron).
- Prepare an appropriately sized orogastric tube and premeasure to the outside of the patient's body (to the last rib); mark this location with white tape so you know how far to insert the tube.
- Lubricate the orogastric tube, and gently pass it through the oropharynx, down the esophagus, and into the stomach. Simultaneous inflation (e.g. blowing into the orogastric tube) and using gentle, twisting motions of the tube will help with passage of the tube into the stomach.
- Confirm appropriate placement of the orogastric tube. This can be done by palpating the tracheal region for two "tubes," by blowing into the tube while simultaneously ausculting over the stomach region (to listen for gurgling or bubbling), and by the presence of gastric gas coming from the end of the tube. Once in the stomach, infuse tepid or warm water through the orogastric tube via the bilge/stomach pump. The volume of the stomach is estimated to be approximately 60 mL/kg; therefore, copious amounts of fluid can be used to gavage. Some sources recommend using 10 mL/kg per gavage, and performing 15–20 gavage cycles [1].
- The stomach should be frequently palpated during gavage to prevent overdistension.
- Aggressive agitation and palpation of the stomach can be performed by an assistant to help break up the gastric contents to enhance gastric lavage recovery.
- Once all the gavage liquid is removed, activated charcoal can be administered via the orogastric tube and flushed into the stomach (to clear the tube).
- Gastric lavage fluid can be saved for toxicological testing at a veterinary diagnostic laboratory as needed. The clinician should physically evaluate the gastric lavage contents to look for the presence of the toxicant(s).
- The orogastric tube must be kinked off prior to removal to prevent lavage fluid from being accidentally aspirated from the oropharynx.
- Recover the patient in a sternal position with the head elevated to prevent aspiration. The patient should be kept intubated until a strong gag reflex is present, allowing for extubation.
- A video example of gastric lavage can be found here: http://vetgirlontherun.com/veterinary-continuing-education-how-perform-gastric-lavage-dog-vetgirl-video/

AC should be implemented as soon as possible, as delayed administration reduces its effectiveness [15]. Non-polar compounds bind to AC well [2] while heavy metals and alcohols (e.g. ethylene glycol, sugar alcohols, etc.) [16] are not adsorbed by AC [2,15]. In general, *in vitro* adsorption to AC reaches equilibrium in less than 30 minutes [1,15]. While desorption of toxicants to AC can occur, as binding to AC is a reversible process, this clinical effect is not known or well described [1,2,15]. For this reason, a cathartic should be given with the first dose of AC to enhance fecal expulsion of the bound AC and toxicant [1,2].

Over the past few decades, the use of AC has fallen out of favor in human medicine. The American Academy of Clinical Toxicology (AACT) and European Association of Poisons Centres and Clinical Toxicologists (EAPCCT) created a position paper in 1997 (revised again in 2004) which clearly stated that "single-dose AC should not be administered routinely in the management of poisoned patients ... [as] ... there is no evidence that administration of AC improves clinical outcome" [15]. Since then, the use of AC in human medicine has continued to decline, according to the American Association of Poison Control Centers Toxic Exposure Surveillance System (from 7.7% to 5.9% in 2003) [15].

That said, the administration of AC is still considered part of the mainstay of treatment for GI decontamination in the veterinary poisoned patient [1,2]. Current recommended dosing for single-dose AC is 1–5 g AC/kg with a cathartic (e.g. sorbitol) [1,2]. Likewise, AC can be administered with food, but ideally small amounts should be used to prevent interference with absorptive properties [17].

Multidose Activated Charcoal

Certain situations or toxicities warrant the administration of multiple doses of AC including ingestion of sustained- (SR), extended- (XR), or long-acting (LA) release products; drugs undergoing enterohepatic recirculation; drugs with a long half-life (e.g. naproxen; 72 hours), or drugs that diffuse from the systemic circulation back into the GIT down the concentration gradient [2]. When administering multiple doses of AC, the use of a one-time dose of a cathartic is recommended to help promote GIT motility [1,2]; however, continued use of cathartics can result in profound dehydration, fluid losses, and hypernatremia due to water moving into the GIT. While veterinary studies are lacking, there is likely an added benefit from multidosing AC, provided the patient is well hydrated and monitored appropriately. Current recommended dosing for multiple doses of AC is 1–2 g AC *without a cathartic* per kg of body weight, PO, every 6 hours for 24 hours.

Complications

In both human and veterinary medicine, there are relatively rare reports of AC-related adverse events, especially when considering the widespread use of AC [1,2,15]. Complications include vomiting [1], fluid, electrolyte, and acid–base abnormalities (including hypernatremia, hypokalemia, hypermagnesemia, and metabolic acidosis) [1,2,15], respiratory complications (e.g. aspiration pneumonia) [15], difficult endoscopy (due to the presence of AC in the GIT), constipation, and, rarely, corneal abrasions (if accidental contact with the eye occurs). In humans given multidose AC, complications of ileus and small intestinal obstruction (from charcoal bezoars) requiring surgical intervention have been reported [15]. When AC is used appropriately in a hydrated patient, the majority of adverse events are not directly related to AC; rather, they may be due to the cathartic effects or pulmonary complications (e.g. aspiration into the lungs) [15].

Administration of Charcoal

Prior to administration of AC with or without a cathartic, the patient's hydration status should be assessed carefully. Appropriate fluid supplementation (SC, IV) should be administered to prevent dehydration and hypernatremia. In addition, the concurrent use of parenteral antiemetics (e.g. maropitant, dolasetron, etc.) should be considered due to the high incidence of vomiting from cathartic administration (or from the emetic agent which was previously used to decontaminate the patient); this will also allow for rapid return to oral water and help minimize the risks of hypernatremia and aspiration pneumonia. Cathartics should not be used in the dehydrated poisoned patient due to the risks of free water loss into the GIT and subsequent hypernatremia [2]. For patients receiving multiple doses of AC with or without cathartics, serum sodium levels should be monitored daily, along with hydration status (personal communication, ASPCA APCC, Urbana, USA). Patients with underlying diseases that may affect hydration status and water balance (e.g. renal disease, diabetes mellitus, psychogenic polydipsia, diabetes insipidus, etc.) may have an increased risk for the development of significant, clinical hypernatremia secondary to AC and/or cathartic administration.

Toxicological Analyses

In certain situations, routine and advanced diagnostic testing for toxicological analyses may be indicated in the poisoned veterinary patient. Routine testing may include a complete blood count, biochemistry panel, venous or arterial blood gas, coagulation testing (e.g.

prothrombin (PT), activated partial thromboplastin time (aPTT)), and urinalysis. For example, hepatotoxicants (e.g. acetaminophen, sago palm, xylitol, etc.) may result in increased liver enzymes, bile acids, bilirubin, and prolonged coagulation times. With nephrotoxicants (e.g. NSAIDs, grapes, ethylene glycol (EG), *Lilium* or *Hemerocallis* spp, etc.), elevated SDMA, BUN and creatinine, metabolic acidosis, electrolyte abnormalities, along with presence of isosthenuria, crystalluria, or urinary casts may be seen. With anticoagulant rodenticides (e.g. bromadiolone, brodifacoum, etc.), prolongation of PT/aPTT may be seen at 36 hours post exposure. Electrolyte changes may also be seen with calcium-related toxicants (e.g. vitamin D, calcipotriene, etc.), cardiac glycoside-containing plants, calcium channel blocker medications, albuterol, etc.

Keep in mind that certain in-house diagnostic tests commonly used in veterinary medicine have limitations.

The results of rapid in-house tests for certain toxicants (e.g. EG, anticoagulant rodenticide, urine illicit drug testing) must be interpreted carefully and appropriately based on limitations of the test (e.g. false-positive or negative results) and the pharmacokinetics of the toxicant (e.g. mechanism of action, metabolism of the toxicant, half-life). For example, over-the-counter (OTC) urine illicit drug screening tests (designed for humans) are often utilized by emergency veterinarians. These commonly test for heroin, cocaine, tetrahydrocannabinol (THC), methamphetamines, and phencyclidine (PCP). The clinician must be aware that these OTC qualitative tests have limitations. False positives can occur with exposure to opioids, lidocaine, amphetamines, tramadol, trazodone, diphenhydramine, NSAIDs, etc. Dogs often test false negative for THC, due to an altered metabolite (e.g. 8-OH-Δ^9-THC versus 11-OH-Δ^9-THC). For this reason, the author does not routinely advocate

Table 127.4 Drug doses for common medications used to treat the poisoned patient [1,2,10].

Drug	Use	Dose
Activated charcoal	To minimize toxicant absorption from the GIT	1–5 g/kg PO once. If multiple doses are used, dose at 1–2 g/kg orally q6h × 24 h, without a cathartic
Atropine	Competes with both acetylcholine and muscarine at cholinergic muscarinic receptor sites; used for muscarine mushroom toxicosis	0.02-0.2 mg/kg, divided IV and IM
Diazepam	Anticonvulsant	0.25–0.5 mg/kg IV PRN
Dolasetron	Antiemetic	0.6 mg/kg, SC, IM, IV q24h
Maropitant	Antiemetic	1 mg/kg SC or IV q24h
Metoclopramide	Prokinetic Antiemetic	0.2–0.5 mg/kg, SC, IM q6–12 h; or CRI at 1–2 mg/kg/day IV Generally less effective than maropitant or ondansetron, but provides gastric emptying and a prokinetic effect
N-acetylcysteine	Hepatoprotectant; used for hepatotoxicants (e.g. *Amanita* mushrooms, acetaminophen, xylitol, blue-green algae, sago palm, etc.)	140–280 mg/kg IV* or PO once, followed by 70 mg/kg IV or PO q6h × 48–72 h as needed
Ondansetron	Antiemetic	0.1–1.0 mg/kg, SC, IM, IV q6–12 h
Phenobarbital	Anticonvulsant	4–20 mg/kg IV as needed
Plasma (as fresh frozen plasma or frozen plasma)	Used to treat coagulopathy secondary to hepatoxicants	10–20 mL/kg IV PRN if coagulopathic
S-adenosylmethionine	Hepatoprotectant	18–20 mg/kg PO q24h
Silibinin	Hepatoprotectant	50 mg/kg IV, 5 h and 24 h after *A. phalloides*exposure. Alternatively 2–5 mg/kg PO q24h
Vitamin K1	Used to treat coagulopathy secondary to vitamin K-dependent factors inactivated during hepatic injury or anticoagulant rodenticide toxicosis	2.5–5 mg/kg PO, SC q12h

*Intravenous route preferred to prevent interaction with activated charcoal.

CRI, constant-rate infusion; GIT, gastrointestinal tract; IM, intramuscular; IV, intravenous; PO, by mouth (*per os*); PRN, as needed (*pro re nata*); SC, subcutaneous.

the use of this testing method without careful interpretation. When in doubt, the use of a human or veterinary diagnostic laboratory should be considered for more accurate testing.

Advanced diagnostic testing can be performed with a reputable human or veterinary diagnostic laboratory. Toxicological analysis may include broad-spectrum screening tests utilizing gas chromatography, mass spectrometry, immunological technology, ELISA testing, quantitative analysis, necropsy, etc. [18]. While this is less commonly performed, toxicological analysis is particularly important with the unknown, suspected, or malicious poisoning situation. For example, the most accurate way of detecting EG toxicosis in dogs and cats is by submitting a quantitative serum EG level. Likewise, acetaminophen levels can be easily measured at a human hospital. Unfortunately, the cost of testing and delay in results (which can take several days to weeks) often preclude clinical utility in the veterinary poisoned patient.

If a necropsy is performed, the following necropsy specimen tissue samples are recommended for collection.

- Brain (with half frozen and half submitted in formalin)
- Ocular fluid
- Injection site (if applicable)
- Gastrointestinal contents (e.g. stomach, intestinal and colonic contents)
- Kidney
- Liver
- Urine (with half frozen and half chilled)

For more information on toxicological analyses, readers are referred to a veterinary toxicology book or consultation directly with a human or veterinary diagnostic laboratory.

Conclusion

In veterinary medicine, the primary treatment for toxicant exposure should be decontamination and detoxification of the patient to inhibit or minimize further toxicant absorption and promote excretion or elimination of the toxicant from the body [1,2]. Aggressive decontamination and detoxification of the poisoned patient are imperative and still considered the mainstay therapy in veterinary medicine. As the majority of toxicants do not have an antidote, treatment of the poisoned patient should be aimed at decontamination and symptomatic supportive care, including fluid therapy, GI support (e.g. antiemetics, gastric protectants, etc.), cardiovascular support, neurological support (e.g. muscle relaxants, anticonvulsants, etc.), miscellaneous therapy (e.g. hepatoprotectants, reversal agents, vitamin K1, intravenous lipid emulsion, etc.), and antidotal therapy, when available (Table 127.4). The clinician should feel well versed in how to appropriately decontaminate the poisoned veterinary patient.

References

1 Peterson ME. Toxicological decontamination. In: *Small Animal Toxicology*, 3rd edn (eds Peterson ME, Talcott PA). Elsevier Saunders, St Louis, 2013, pp. 73–85.
2 Lee JA. Decontamination and detoxification of the poisoned patient. In: *Blackwell's Five-Minute Veterinary Consult Clinical Companion Small Animal Toxicology* (eds Osweiler GD, Hovda LR, Brutlag AG, Lee JA). Wiley-Blackwell, Ames, 2011, pp. 5–19.
3 Arnold FJ, Hodges JB Jr, Barta RA Jr. Evaluation of the efficacy of lavage and induced emesis in treatment of salicylate poisoning. *Pediatrics* 1959;23:286–301.
4 Abdallah AH, Tye A. A comparison of the efficacy of emetic drugs and stomach lavage. *Am J Dis Child* 1967;113:571–575.
5 Corby DG, Lisciandro RC, Lehman RW, et al. The efficacy of methods used to evacuate the stomach after acute ingestions. *Pediatrics* 1967;40:871–874.
6 Teshima D, Suzuki A, Otsubo K, et al. Efficacy of emetic and United States Pharmacopoeia ipecac syrup in prevention of drug absorption. *Chem Pharm Bull* 1990;38:2242–2245.
7 Khan SA, McLean MK, Slater M, et al. Effectiveness and adverse effects of the use of apomorphine and 3% hydrogen peroxide solution to induce emesis in dogs. *J Am Vet Med Assoc* 2012;241(9):1179–1184.
8 Obr TD, Fry JK, Lee JA, et al. Necroulcerative hemorrhagic gastritits in a cat secondary to the administration of 3% hydrogen peroxide as an emetic agent. *J Vet Emerg Crit Care* 2017;27(5):605–608.
9 Türk EE, Schulz F, Koops E, et al. Fatal hypernatremia after using salt as an emetic – report of three autopsy cases. *Leg Med (Tokyo)* 2005;7(1):47–50.
10 Plumb DC. *Veterinary Drug Handbook*, 7th edn. Blackwell Publishing, Ames, 2011.
11 Thawley VJ, Drobatz KJ. Assessment of dexmedetomidine and other agents for emesis induction in cats: 43 cases (2009–2014). *J Am Vet Med Assoc* 2015;247(12):1415–1418.
12 Willey JL, Julius TM, Claypool SPA, et al. Evaluation and comparison of xylazine hydrochloride and dexmedetomidine hydrochloride for the induction of emesis in cats: 47 cases (2007–2013). *J Am Vet Med Assoc* 2016;248(8):923–928.

13 Niedzwecki AH, Book BP, Lewis KM, et al. Effect of oral 3% hydrogen peroxide used as an emetic on the gastroduodenal mucosa of healthy dogs. *J Vet Emerg Crit Care* 2017;27(2):178–184.

14 American Academy of Clinical Toxicology and European Association of Poisons Centres and Clinical Toxicologists. Position paper: gastric lavage. *J Toxicol* 2004;42(7):933–943.

15 American Academy of Clinical Toxicology and European Association of Poisons Centres and Clinical Toxicologists. Position paper: single-dose activated charcoal. *Clin Toxicol* 2005;43:61–87.

16 Cope RB. A screening study of xylitol binding in vitro to activated charcoal. *Vet Human Tox* 2004;46:336–337.

17 Wilson HE, Humm KR. In vitro study of the effect of dog food on the adsorptive capacity of activated charcoal. *J Vet Emerg Crit Care* 2013;23(3):263–267.

18 Osweiler G. Laboratory diagnostics for toxicology. In: *Blackwell's Five-Minute Veterinary Consult Clinical Companion Small Animal Toxicology* (eds Osweiler GD, Hovda LR, Brutlag AG, Lee JA). Wiley-Blackwell, Ames, 2011, pp. 50–56.

128

Lipid "Rescue" Therapy

Kathryn Benavides, DVM[1] and Jonathan Babyak, MS, DVM, DACVECC[2]

[1]*Veterinary Specialists and Emergency Service of Rochester, Rochester, NY, USA*
[2]*Cummings School of Veterinary Medicine, Tufts University, North Grafton, MA, USA*

Introduction

Intravenous lipid emulsion (ILE) has been routinely used in human and veterinary medicine for decades as a component of partial or total parenteral nutrition (PN) as well as a vehicle for certain drugs (e.g. propofol). The first documented successful use for the treatment of local anesthetic systemic toxicity was in 2006 when it was used to treat seizures and subsequent cardiopulmonary arrest (CPA) in a patient following a local anesthetic protocol of bupivacaine and mepivacaine after standard resuscitation efforts failed to result in return of spontaneous circulation (ROSC) [1]. Since then, ILE has been more frequently used in human medicine as a treatment for local anesthetic systemic toxicities and more recently as a treatment for various lipophilic drug toxicities.

This application is clinically useful in veterinary medicine where lipophilic medications make up a large portion of reported exposures to the ASPCA Animal Poison Control Center (APCC) [2]. While further evaluation is needed to fully understand the mechanism of action, efficacy, and potential safety concerns associated with ILE therapy when used as an antidote, current case studies and anecdotal reports suggest clinical efficacy of ILE in the treatment of various lipophilic drug toxicities, especially where morbidity and mortality may be high and no known antidote or alternative is available.

Available Formulations

Intravenous lipid emulsion is commonly composed of medium- to long-chain triglycerides found in various oils (soybean oil, safflower oil, etc.), a phospholipid emulsifier, and glycerin [2]. The various formulations are classified by droplet size and the available compositions used in PN or for antidotal therapy are similar in size to endogenous chylomicrons and are thought to be eliminated by the body tissues in a similar fashion. These molecules are typically cleared by skeletal muscle, splanchnic viscera, myocardial cells, and subcutaneous tissues where they are broken down into glycerol, free fatty acids, and choline to be used as energy by the tissues [3].

The most commonly used commercial product is Intralipid 20% which is a 20% fat emulsion and is the formulation used in dosing strategies. This is the preferred formulation due to the lower proportion of free phospholipids as higher free phospholipids may be associated with adverse effects due to interference with lipoprotein lipase activity and decreased clearance [2]. Stored correctly at room temperature, the shelf-life of ILE is typically up to 2 years. Once opened, strict aseptic technique is required when handling to reduce the risk of bacterial contamination [4]. Unused product must be refrigerated between uses and should be discarded after 24 hours. An emulsion of 20% or less is isotonic and can be administered through a peripheral catheter. Emulsions of 30% are intended to be combined with other components for PN and are not to be administered alone.

Historical Use in Human Medicine

As mentioned previously, ILE therapy was first used in the treatment of CPA secondary to local anesthetic systemic toxicity that was not responsive to traditional resuscitative efforts after 20 minutes [1]. As resuscitation continued, the patient was given a bolus of ILE followed by a constant rate infusion. Shortly after, return of spontaneous circulation (ROSC) with a normal sinus rhythm on EKG was achieved.

Another instance was in a patient treated for bupropion and lamotrigine intoxication where conventional life support measures were unsuccessful for 52 minutes. Treatment with ILE resulted in ROSC [5]. In this case, plasma concentrations of both drugs were measured serially. Peak plasma concentrations of bupropion occurred after ILE administration, which supports the "lipid sink" theory mechanism of action to be described later. Similar results were not seen with lamotrigine, a less lipophilic medication, suggesting that the beneficial clinical effects of ILE therapy may be dependent on the lipid solubility of the toxic agent.

Various other case studies are available in the human medical literature highlighting the successful use of ILE in treatment of local anesthetic systemic toxicities. Due to the nature of the cases in which ILE therapy is warranted in human medicine, randomized controlled clinical trials are not possible. However, there is an effort by investigators to collaborate by contributing case reports and anecdotal accounts. These are available at www.lipidrescue.org – a web resource established by Dr Guy Weinberg [6].

Use in Veterinary Medicine

Although considered safe in people, ILE is reserved for patients with severe toxicity and life-threatening clinical signs and only after conventional methods of treatment and resuscitation have failed. Conversely, extra-label use of ILE therapy in veterinary patients for lipophilic drug toxicities has been initiated early in the course of treatment to mitigate severe clinical signs and shorten the anticipated clinical course. This strategy may be particularly beneficial for patients in which conventional supportive care, including intensive nursing care, prolonged hospitalization, and mechanical ventilation, may be a barrier to further treatment.

When ILE therapy is considered as an antidote for lipophilic drug toxicities, it should always be in addition to reasonable and appropriate medical management and supportive care and should not be initiated prior to addressing appropriate emergency treatment (i.e. fluid therapy, oxygen, etc.). This is particularly important because ILE, in the face of hypoxia, can potentially result in a negative myocardial inotropy and subsequent decreased contractility and cardiac output [2].

The majority of research on the use of ILE in animal patients is from experimental animal studies, beginning in 1974 when ILE was evaluated for the treatment of chlorpromazine toxicity in a rabbit model. ILE-pretreated rabbits survived and all control animals died [7]. Dr Guy Weinberg has contributed a large portion of the research done with ILE therapy. A seminal study was published in 1998 in which ILE reduced the LD_{50} by 48% in rats with bupivacaine-induced asystole [8]. He also evaluated ILE resuscitation in a bupivacaine-induced CPA model in 12 dogs. All dogs treated with ILE in addition to cardiopulmonary resuscitation survived compared to 100% mortality in the control group [9].

There are multiple reports of ILE therapy for lipophilic toxicities, including moxidectin toxicity in a Jack Russell terrier puppy [10], ivermectin toxicity in a border collie not affected by the MDR-1 gene mutation [11], and lidocaine toxicity in a cat undergoing wound closure [12]. ILE use in these instances has remained controversial due to the inability to establish a causal relationship between ILE therapy and the outcome. Additionally, there have been two experimental studies in a porcine model which showed that ILE failed to result in reversal of cardiotoxicity of bupivacaine; however, there is concern that the cardiac effects of the anesthetic drugs administered prior to the bupivacaine overdose contributed to these results [13,14]. Currently, there is a single prospective, randomized, controlled study evaluating the use of ILE as a treatment for permethrin toxicosis in cats [15]. The study established a reliable algorithm for staging toxicosis ranging from stage A (no clinical signs) to stage F (grand mal seizures). Cats receiving ILE achieved lower clinical stages (B or A) earlier, but there was no significant difference in duration of hospitalization between the groups. Further controlled trials are necessary to fully evaluate the efficacy and safety of ILE as a first-line therapy for various lipophilic drug toxicities.

Currently, ILE therapy has promise in the treatment of the following toxicities in veterinary medicine: local anesthetics, calcium channel blockers, macrolytic lactones, muscle relaxants, cyclic antidepressants, and psychotropic drugs. The ASPCA APCC also reported its successful use in the following intoxications: amlodipine, baclofen, benzocaine, bromethalin, bupropion, CCNU, chlorpyrifox, diltiazem, doramectin, endosulfan, ivermectin, moxidectin, minoxidil, marijuana, permethrin, and phenobarbital [4].

Mechanism of Action

The exact mechanism of action by which ILE therapy decreases recovery time and ameliorates clinical signs is unknown, but multiple theories have been proposed based on the available studies and the pathophysiology of lipid metabolism. The two most widely accepted theories are improved myocardial performance and the "lipid sink" theory [2–4] and there may be multiple mechanisms at play in the way ILE exerts its beneficial effects.

Intravenous lipid emulsion therapy is thought to improve myocardial performance by delivering free fatty acids (FFA) to the myocardium as this is the preferred substrate. Bupivacaine inhibits the mitochondrial use of FFA by blocking carnitine acylcarnitine translocase and preventing movement of FFA into the mitochondria. It is thought that rapid infusion of ILE overcomes this inhibition of the mitochondria either by competitive inhibition or some other unknown mechanism of action. The influx of FFA also stimulates the voltage-gated calcium channels and results in an increase in intracellular calcium and increased myocardial function. This may be particularly helpful when cardiac dysfunction is secondary to calcium channel blocker toxicity.

The "lipid sink" mechanism of action involves the creation of an expanded lipid phase within the plasma that acts to sequester various lipophilic compounds and reduce the effective concentration at the target tissues. The pull into this compartment may be strong enough to pull lipophilic toxins out of brain and heart tissue into the intravascular space, thereby decreasing the clinical signs and accelerating clearance of the toxin. This is supported by the previously mentioned study where peak plasma levels of bupropion were identified after treatment with ILE [5]. If this is the predominant mechanism of action, the variable response of different toxins to therapy with ILE may be due to differences in lipid solubility and therefore the pull that the "lipid sink" exerts on these compounds. The lipophilicity is related to the log P value where P is a partition coefficient and is the measure of the solubility of a compound between two solvents – one hydrophilic (water) and one lipophilic (typically octanol). A compound is considered to be lipophilic if log P is >1.0, but the higher the log P value, the more lipophilic the compound is. For a list of lipophilic drugs which may be amenable to treatment with ILE therapy and their corresponding log P values, see the review by Fernandez et al. [3].

Recommended Dosing

There is no single recommended dosing strategy in veterinary medicine and all values are extrapolated from human data. Use in veterinary medicine of ILE as an antidote is considered extra-label. The current human resources include *Guidelines for the Management of Severe Local Anesthetic Toxicity* as provided by the Association of Anaesthetists of Great Britain and Ireland [16] and recommendations by Dr Guy Weinberg available on his website www.lipidrescue.org [6].

Dosing is based on the use of lipid emulsion in PN with a maximum not to exceed 10 mL/kg/day of a 20% emulsion. A commonly published dosing strategy using the 20% emulsion is a rapid 1.5 mL/kg IV bolus over 1–3 minutes followed by a constant-rate infusion (CRI) at 0.25–0.50 mL/kg/min for 30–60 minutes [4]. Serial serum evaluation for lipemia should be performed if multiple doses are considered. If the serum is not lipemic, the bolus and CRI dosing may be repeated as needed if clinical signs have not improved for up to 24 hours; however, ILE therapy should be discontinued

if no improvement is seen following three total doses. In some human protocols, continued intermittent bolus dosing of 1.5 mL/kg every 4–6 hours until clinical signs improve is advocated, but again not to exceed 24 hours. There are no safety studies available for the use of ILE in this manner, so caution should be exercised with careful monitoring and risk assessment for all patients undergoing antidotal treatment with ILE.

Potential Complications

As with any therapy, particularly in the somewhat novel use of ILE as an antidote for lipophilic drug toxicity, there are potential adverse effects and complications that must be considered prior to administering this therapy to any patient. A safety study performed in rats identified an LD_{50} of 67.7 mL/kg in rats for a 20% soybean oil emulsion. Few adverse effects have been reported and the majority are associated with more chronic lipid emulsion infusion such as that associated with long-term PN, including immunological, pulmonary, and hepatic dysfunction. Clinical signs may include nausea, vomiting, fever, or respiratory distress. The significant difference between the two uses of ILE therapy is the administration rate. PN is a slower infusion over a prolonged period of time versus a high volume given over a short period of time as an antidote, so further safety studies are necessary to evaluate its use in this manner.

Aseptic technique and cautious handling are crucial to avoid bacterial contamination which could result in local or systemic infection, venous irritation, and subsequent thrombophlebitis. This is more likely with PN due to the length of treatment. Patients may also have a hypersensitivity reaction to the components of the emulsion (often egg phospholipid or soybean oil), developing clinical signs such as fever, nausea, dyspnea, cyanosis, arrhythmias, hypotension, and cardiovascular collapse. Lipemia can interfere with certain laboratory tests, including showing a false hyperglycemia on certain analyzers. If lipemia is persistent, pancreatitis is a theoretical sequela, particularly in patients with a history of pancreatitis, though no cases have been reported in veterinary medicine when using ILE as an antidote.

In patients with acute respiratory distress syndrome (ARDS) or other severe inflammatory diseases, ILE therapy has been shown to decrease the arterial partial pressure of oxygen to fraction of inspired oxygen ratio (PaO_2:FiO_2). Pulmonary lipid emboli have been reported in children, but similar lesions have not been reproduced when using ILE as an antidote. The final reported complication associated with ILE for PN in people is "fat overload syndrome" which is typically due to high volume or excessive administration rates that overwhelm the lipid clearance mechanisms and lead to hyperlipidemia, hepatomegaly, icterus, splenomegaly, thrombocytopenia, abnormal clotting times, and hemolysis [2–4]. This syndrome has not yet been reported in animals.

Further investigation is needed to evaluate the safety and determine the efficacy of ILE therapy when used as an antidote, but given the case reports and case series, it can be considered in certain lipophilic drug toxicities where morbidity and mortality may be high and no known antidote or alternative is available.

References

1 Rosenblatt MA, Abel M, Fischer GW, et al. Successful use of a 20% lipid emulsion to resuscitate a patient after a presumed bupivacaine-related cardiac arrest. *Anesthesiology* 2006;105(1):217–218.

2 Kaplan A, Whelan M. The use of IV lipid emulsion for lipophilic drug toxicities. *J Am Anim Hosp Assoc* 2012;48:221–227.

3 Fernandez AL, Lee JA, Rahilly L, et al. The use of intravenous lipid emulsion as an antidote in veterinary toxicology. *J Vet Emerg Crit Care* 2001;21(4):309–320.

4 Gwaltney-Brant S, Meadows I. Use of intravenous lipid emulsions for treating certain poisoning cases in small animals. *Vet Clin Small Anim* 2012;42:251–262.

5 Sirianni AJ, Osterhoudt KC, Calello DP, et al. Use of lipid emulsion in the resuscitation of a patient with prolonged cardiovascular collapse after overdose of bupropion and lamotrigine. *Ann Emerg Med* 2008;51(4):412–415.

6 Weinberg G. Lipid rescue: resuscitation for drug toxicity. Available at: www.lipidrescue.org (accessed 7 February 2018).

7 Krieglstei J, Meffert A, Niemeyer DH. Influence of emulsified fat on chlorpromazine availability in rabbit blood. *Experientia* 1974;30(8):924–926.

8 Weinberg GL, VadeBoncouer T, Ramaraju GA, et al. Pretreatment or resuscitation with a lipid infusion shifts the dose-response to bupivacaine-induced asystole in rats. *Anesthesiology* 1998;88(4):1071–1075.

9 Weinberg G, Ripper R, Feinstein DL, et al. Lipid emulsion infusion rescues dogs from bupivicaine-induced cardiac toxicity. *Reg Anesth Pain Med* 2003;28(3):198–202.

10 Crandell DE, Weinberg GL. Moxidectin toxicosis in a puppy successfully treated with intravenous lipids. *J Vet Emerg Crit Care* 2009;19(2):181–186.

11 Clarke DL, Lee JA, Murphy LA, et al. Use of intravenous lipid emulsion to treat ivermectin toxicosis in a Border Collie. *J Am Vet Med Assoc* 2011;239(10):1328–1333.

12 O'Brien TQ, Clarke-Price SC, Evans EE, et al. Infusion of a lipid emulsion to treat lidocaine intoxication in a cat. *J Am Vet Med Assoc* 2010;237(12):1455–1458.

13 Mayr VD, Mitterschiffthaler L, Neurauter A, et al. A comparison of the combination of epinephrine and vasopressin with lipid emulsion in a porcine model of asphyxia cardiac arrest after intravenous injection of bupivacaine. *Anesth Analg* 2008;106(5):1566–1571.

14 Heavner JE, Dryden CF Jr, Sanghani V, et al. Severe hypoxia enhances central nervous system and cardiovascular toxicity of bupivacaine in lightly anesthetized pigs. *Anesthesiology* 1992;77(1):142–147.

15 Jourdan G, Boyer G, Raymond-Letron I, et al. Intravenous lipid emulsion therapy in 20 cats accidentally overdosed with ivermectin. *J Vet Emerg Crit Care* 2015;25(5):667–671.

16 Association of Anaesthetists of Great Britain and Ireland. AAGBI Safety Guidelines: Management of severe local anaesthetic toxicity. Available at: www. aagbi.org/sites/default/files/la_toxicity_2010_0.pdf (accessed 7 February 2018).

129

Blood Purification Techniques for Intoxications

Carrie Palm, DVM, DACVIM

William R. Pritchard School of Veterinary Medicine, University of California, Davis, CA, USA

Introduction

Extracorporeal therapies involve the removal of blood from a patient's circulation with subsequent processing of the blood before it is returned to the patient. Processing of blood or "blood purification" can include removal of endogenous substances (e.g. BUN, creatinine or malignant antibodies) and exogenous substances (e.g. drugs and intoxicants). Extracorporeal therapies utilized in veterinary medicine include hemodialysis (HD) (both intermittent and continuous modalities), hemoperfusion (HP), and apheresis [1]. Peritoneal dialysis, which is not an extracorporeal therapy because blood is not removed from patient circulation, utilizes the peritoneum as a semi-permeable membrane for solute removal and is the least effective for treatment of intoxications of the therapies above.

This chapter will focus on the use of extracorporeal therapies for the removal of intoxicants and poisons in the emergency setting, with a focus on the decision-making process for pursuing use of these technologies and concurrent medical therapy. As specific information regarding the role of blood purification for many individual toxins is lacking, the clinician must use their understanding of the nature of the toxic substance to determine which, if any, blood purification technique is appropriate.

Intermittent Hemodialysis

Hemodialysis is an extracorporeal therapy, where blood is removed from the patient and is passed through a hemodialyzer or "artificial kidney." The hemodialyzer is composed of thousands of small semi-permeable tubes with microscopic pores that are too small for the passage of blood cells and proteins, but do allow the passage of many small molecular weight molecules. As blood passes through the lumens of these tubes, the tubes are bathed in a specifically prescribed dialysate. Specific solutes, such as ethylene glycol (EG) in an intoxicated patient, move down their respective concentration gradient across the semi-permeable dialyzer membrane from the blood and into the dialysate. This *diffusion* is the primary method that allows for toxin removal via intermittent HD, where a toxin moves from the blood down its concentration gradient into the dialysate and subsequently down the drain. Likewise, for an intoxicant such as EG, where ethanol is a specific antidote to prevent breakdown of EG into its toxic components, the ethanol is placed into the dialysate, where it moves down a concentration gradient and then into patient circulation [2,3].

There are several characteristics of drugs and toxins that allow for the most efficient removal via diffusion. Small molecular weight substances (less than 500 Da) can readily move across the dialysis membrane, allowing for efficient removal; newer, more efficient dialyzers allow passage of larger molecules and can therefore provide efficient removal of larger molecular weight poisons (Table 129.1). Albumin is too large to fit through dialyzer pores, so significant protein binding of the toxin prevents efficient removal with HD.

Since HD removes substances directly from the vascular space, drugs and toxins with large volumes of distribution (i.e. into the interstitial and intracellular compartments) are less efficiently removed. This can be overcome by performing longer HD sessions and/or repeat treatments. This extra time allows for redistribution of toxins into the vascular space (as they move down their concentration gradient), where removal can occur via extracorporeal therapies (see Chapter 167, Figure 167.1). High water solubility increases ease of toxin removal, as toxins distributed into lipids do not readily pass into the intravascular space. HD has been utilized in the removal of poisons, such as ethylene glycol and barbiturates, as well as many others.

Textbook of Small Animal Emergency Medicine, First Edition. Edited by Kenneth J. Drobatz, Kate Hopper, Elizabeth Rozanski and Deborah C. Silverstein.
© 2019 John Wiley & Sons, Inc. Published 2019 by John Wiley & Sons, Inc.
Companion Website: www.wiley.com/go/drobatz/textbook

Table 129.1 General characteristics of toxins suited to extracorporeal therapy (ECT) with examples of toxins treated at the authors institution with ECT.

Therapy	Remarks
Hemodialysis	Drugs less than 500 Da, moderate to large volume of distribution, minimal protein binding Examples: • Ethylene glycol • Antibiotics ○ Enrofloxacin* • Barbiturates*
Hemoperfusion	Intoxicant size and protein binding do not affect efficiency (provided charcoal has the highest affinity for the compound), moderate to large volume of distribution

Combined hemodialysis/ hemoperfusion	Intoxicants
	
	Examples:
	• Non-steroidal anti-inflammatory drugs
	  ○ Acetaminophen
	  ○ Ibuprofen*
	  ○ Carprofen*
	  ○ Deracoxib
	• Barbiturates
	  ○ Phenobarbital*
	• Caffeine*
	• Theobromine*
	• Chemotherapeutics
	  ○ Vincristine

Apheresis (total plasma exchange)	Small volume of distribution, efficiency unaffected by protein binding and size Examples: • Chemotherapeutics ○ Vincristine • *Amanita* intoxication

Note: Scientific evidence regarding definitive benefits of ECT for various intoxicants is currently lacking. The decision to pursue ECT for treatment of intoxications should be based on individual patient and intoxicant data and should be instituted immediately following ingestion. Note that there are many additional intoxications that may be benefit from ECT.

*Anecdotal evidence (based on clinical outcome and serial drug levels) that a benefit was incurred by ECT. Note that for intoxicants treated with combined HD/HP, serial drug levels were not always collected, so it is difficult to discern the individual contribution for each therapy.

Prolonged Intermittent HD and Continuous Therapies

For drugs with a high volume of distribution or significant enterohepatic recirculation, therapies can be extended to provide continued prolonged treatment (hours to days), whereby constant removal from the intravascular space occurs as the toxin or poisoning redistributes there. This prolonged treatment can be done by prolonging therapy with an intermittent platform (up to 8 hours) or by using a continuous renal replacement platform, which can allow treatment to be extended for days. By definition, continuous therapies are meant to allow for slow, continual solute removal, which may not be ideal for treatment of intoxications; however, treatment prescriptions can be altered to allow for more rapid removal [4]. The application for such a prolonged therapy does require a trained treatment team to be available for the entire treatment period. At the author's institution, when prolonged therapy is indicated, repeated prolonged intermittent treatments are performed, rather than continuous therapy.

Another treatment modality for toxin removal is removal of large volumes of plasma water by convection (alone or in combination with diffusive therapy). This technology is available on many of the machines designed for continuous renal replacement therapy. With this method, specifically designed filters allow for significant volumes of plasma water to be removed by hydrostatic pressures and this can aid in toxin removal. This may allow for removal of larger compounds (up to 50 kDa) than can be achieved with diffusive dialysis, but does not remove protein-bound drugs.

Hemoperfusion

Hemoperfusion is an extracorporeal therapy where large volumes of blood are exposed to an adsorbent (typically activated charcoal/carbon) that binds toxic substances. The removal of toxins by HP is dictated by the affinity of the activated charcoal for the toxin (see Table 129.1). As opposed to HD, molecular weight and protein binding of the toxin do not decrease removal efficiency with HP, provided that the affinity of the charcoal for the toxin is high enough. In contrast to HD, where there is a constant supply of fresh dialysate allowing for continuous toxin removal by diffusion, charcoal-binding sites can become saturated over time, preventing further toxin removal unless a new cartridge is used. Since online blood testing for most toxins is not available, previous experience and educated estimations are used to determine when therapy should be finished or a new cartridge be replaced.

Combination Hemodialysis/Hemoperfusion

An optimal treatment in many cases is to combine HD and HP (see Table 129.1). When performing these two modalities in combination, blood is pumped through the HP cartridge and then into the dialyzer. The advantages of this combination include more efficient toxin removal, as both diffusion and charcoal binding are utilized, as well as normalization of blood through the dialyzer before it is returned to the patient. For example, glucose, which can be bound by the charcoal, is returned to the extracorporeal blood through the dialysate before return to the patient.

One disadvantage of this combined therapy is the increased volume of blood in the circuit and outside the patient, when both a dialyzer and charcoal cartridge are used. This can limit the size of patient that can be safely treated with HP, although an experienced team can often make alterations to the prescription that allow for treatment of smaller patients. Figures 129.1 and 129.2 show dogs receiving combined HD and HP. In the author's institution, HP is always combined with HD.

Apheresis

Apheresis is an extracorporeal therapy in which blood is removed from the circulation, separated into components and one or more of the components is removed or processed. For treatment of intoxications, apheresis in the form of therapeutic plasma exchange (TPE) is most commonly utilized. During this therapy,

as the blood is separated, the plasma component (containing toxic substances) is removed, discarded and replaced with plasma, colloids, and other fluids. TPE can allow for efficient removal of toxins that have a small volume of distribution and are limited primarily to the intravascular space, because only the intravascular volume is treated (see Table 129.1) [5]. In addition, because all plasma components are removed, intoxicants with significant protein binding will also be removed.

Of the extracorporeal therapies available, apheresis is the newest technology being evaluated in veterinary patients, and the indications and outcomes of this therapy are still unknown for many intoxications. At the author's institution, apheresis has been used for treatment of advanced stages of *Amanita* mushroom intoxications with minimal success. As in human medicine, earlier intervention of patients with *Amanita* poisoning may allow for better outcomes [6–8].

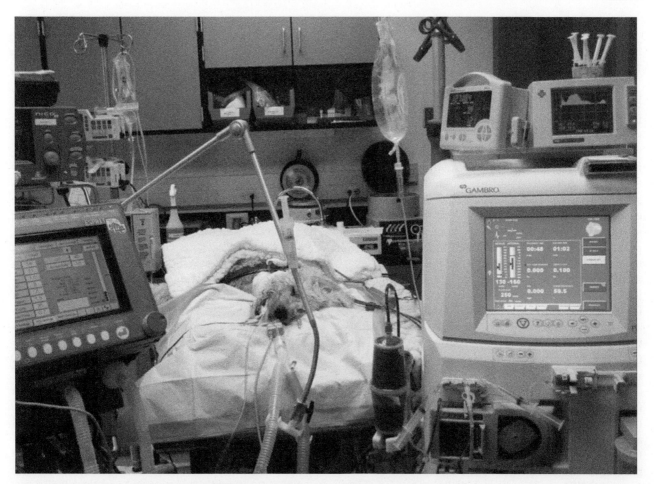

Figure 129.1 A dog with life-threatening caffeine and theobromine intoxication that is receiving mechanical ventilation for drug-induced respiratory arrest, while combined hemodialysis and hemoperfusion is performed. The hemoperfusion activated charcoal canister can be seen in line with the hemodialysis circuit. This dog was discharged with mild neurological deficits 4 days after initial presentation.

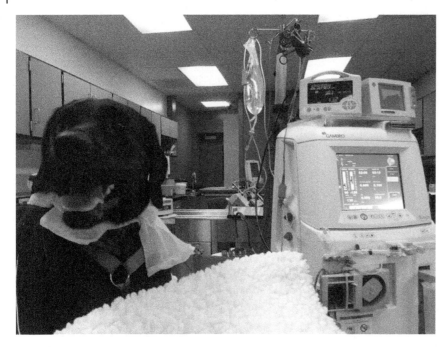

Figure 129.2 A dog receiving combined hemodialysis and hemoperfusion for ibuprofen ingestion (2000 mg/kg). She was presented immediately after ingestion, was stable at the time of presentation and remained stable during hospitalization. She received medical management in conjunction with hemodialysis and hemoperfusion and never developed any adverse clinical manifestations of intoxication. She remains normal 2 years post treatment.

Indications for the Use of Extracorporeal Therapies in Treatment of Poisoning

Before extracorporeal therapies are employed, several factors should be considered. Considerations for treatment of intoxications with extracorporeal therapies include the associated morbidity and mortality of the intoxication, treatment outcome with traditional medical therapies, patient characteristics (co-morbidities, patient size, dose of intoxication, time of exposure), endogenous clearance of the intoxicant, and characteristics of the intoxicant (molecular weight, volume of distribution, protein binding, solubility, and half-life). It is important to ensure (as far as possible) that benefits from the treatment outweigh the potential risks. In the author's opinion, any intoxication with severe adverse consequences for the patient should be considered for treatment with an extracorporeal therapy, provided that the characteristics of the patient and the intoxicant support its potential use, especially if the treatment is carried out by an experienced team.

It is critical to obtain a thorough history of ingestion from the owner. Owners may be able to provide information concerning the type and amount of toxin ingested, as well as the time of ingestion. Knowing this information can improve the ability of the treating clinician to provide an accurate prognosis and determine if an extracorporeal therapy is indicated. If toxin ingestion was days before presentation, an extracorporeal therapy is likely not indicated, as the toxin will have been metabolized and/or excreted. It is also important to determine

specific characteristics of the toxin, such as molecular weight and pharmacokinetics, so that informed decisions can be made. If the patient has not already vomited, ingestion was recent (within 1–2 hours) and there are no contraindications, such as a comatose patient or ingestion of a caustic substance, vomiting should be induced (see Chapter 127). If a large amount of the ingested material is eliminated during vomiting, extracorporeal therapy may not be necessary; however, this can be very difficult to judge. If the consequences of intoxication are life threatening, then it still may be reasonable to consider pursuing an extracorporeal therapy.

For many intoxicants, information regarding drug metabolism in veterinary patients is limited, and in these cases, extrapolation from human and other animal studies is often performed. In addition, in cases of massive overdose, volume of distribution may increase beyond what has been reported with therapeutic dosing. For example, with a massive overdose of a highly protein-bound compound, protein-binding sites may become saturated, and unbound drug may therefore distribute into interstitial and possibly intercellular spaces (beyond what occurs with therapeutic dosing).

Rapid initiation of an extracorporeal therapy is critical for successful treatment of intoxications. The location of facilities that are capable of performing HD and HP or apheresis must therefore be considered, and referral and transfer should occur quickly. In addition, initiation of medical management (see below) must be instituted immediately, and not delayed while making final decisions regarding benefits of an extracorporeal therapy. If other treatments (other than extracorporeal therapies) are available, these should be considered as a sole therapy or in conjunction with an extracorporeal therapy. Figure 129.1 shows a dog with caffeine intoxication that required mechanical ventilation as part of its supportive care while HD/HP were performed.

Finally, when making decisions regarding extracorporeal therapy for intoxications, patient size should be a consideration. The volume of the extracorporeal circuit can be variable, depending on the machines and cartridges used, but can range from 70 ml to several hundred milliliters. While variations can be made to the extracorporeal circuit, treatment of very small patients can be more complicated. Nonetheless, use of blood priming (filling the extracorporeal circuit with cross-matched compatible blood) can allow for treatment of almost any patient size.

Hemodialysis and HP procedures are not inexpensive. In many cases, however, rapid removal of the toxin via HD/HP can lead to much shorter hospital stays, compared with traditional medical management. Clients need to be properly informed of potential risks. In addition, it is important to note that controlled veterinary studies evaluating the efficacy of HD/HP treatment for treatment of many poisonings are lacking.

Medical Management for Intoxications

Decontamination may be indicated prior to initiation of HD/HP (see Chapter 127). As discussed above, induced emesis may be performed in alert patients that have ingested non-caustic substances or patients that have recently ingested toxins. Gastric lavage may be performed in selected cases. Cathartics such as sorbitol may be indicated. Depending on the timing of toxin ingestion, activated charcoal may be indicated, and can be given either orally or rectally in obtunded patients. Repeat dosing may be necessary for drugs with significant enterohepatic circulation, whereby a drug concentrated in bile is re-excreted into the intestines where further absorption can occur [9]. Forced diuresis via administration of intravenous fluids may increase renal tubular flow and decrease reabsorption of toxin in the distal tubule.

In certain cases where the toxin was recently ingested and the owner knows the ingested toxin, antidotes may be considered. For example, the administration of ethanol or fomepizole (4-methypyrazole) is indicated in cases of EG ingestion to prevent formation of toxic metabolites. For cases of suspected EG ingestion, early administration of alcohol can be life saving and should be started immediately.

It is critical for the treating clinician to have a solid knowledge base regarding optimal medical management for each intoxication encountered. While medical management is mandatory, it is ideal to minimize trauma to jugular veins when possible, so that appropriate catheters can be placed rapidly for initiation of extracorporeal therapy.

Manipulation of urinary pH, typically via alkalinization, can be used to force certain toxins into an ionized form. Ionized substances do not readily cross cell membranes, so ionization may prevent reabsorption across the tubular membrane with subsequent excretion in urine. This process is known as "ion trapping."

Since many toxins have volumes of distributions beyond the vascular space, these compartments are not as readily cleared of toxin and can redistribute following a HD/HP treatment, leading to recurrence of clinical signs or ongoing adverse effects. This phenomenon may necessitate repeat treatments of HD and HP. Additionally, medical management may need to be prolonged and combined with these extracorporeal therapies to optimize outcomes.

Conclusion

In conclusion, extracorporeal therapies can be life-saving treatments for poisonings. Use of these therapies can improve patient outcome and may decrease hospitalization time. It is essential to inform owners of the available treatment options and prognosis associated with certain toxins. Cost and risks of extracorporeal therapies must also be discussed. Clinicians should consider both medical management strategies and extracorporeal therapies, and it is critical to recognize that these two therapies may need to be combined. At our institution, HD and/or combined HD/HP have been used to treat poisonings of EG, non-steroidal anti-inflammatory drugs, chemotherapeutics, caffeine, barbiturates, and antibiotics. At this time, many of the extracorporeal therapies used for the treatment of poisonings are based on human studies and small veterinary case series, but current research into the utility of these therapies for various intoxications is ongoing.

References

1 Fertel BS, Nelson LS, Goldfarb DS. Extracorporeal removal techniques for the poisoned patient: a review for the intensivist. *J Intens Care Med* 2010;25:139–148.

2 Keno LA, Langston CE. Treatment of accidental ethanol intoxication with hemodialysis in a dog. *J Vet Emerg Crit Care* 2011;21:363–368.

3 Schweighauser A, Francey T. Ethylene glycol poisoning in three dogs: importance of early diagnosis and role of hemodialysis as a treatment option. *Schweiz Archiv Tierheilkunde* 2016;158:109–114.

4 Goodman JW, Goldfarb DS. The role of continuous renal replacement therapy in the treatment of poisoning. *Semin Dialysis* 2006;19:402–407.

5 Nenov VD, Marinov P, Sabeva J, et al. Current applications of plasmapheresis in clinical toxicology. *Nephrol Dialysis Transplant* 2003;18 Suppl 5:v56–58.

6 Garcia J, Costa VM, Carvalho A, et al. Amanita phalloides poisoning: mechanisms of toxicity and treatment. *Food Chem Toxicol* 2015;86:41–55.

7 Jander S, Bischoff J. Treatment of Amanita phalloides poisoning: I. Retrospective evaluation of plasmapheresis in 21 patients. *Therapeut Apheresis* 2000;4:303–307.

8 Jander S, Bischoff J, Woodcock BG. Plasmapheresis in the treatment of Amanita phalloides poisoning: II. *A review and recommendations. Therapeut Apheresis* 2000;4:308–312.

9 Koenigshof AM, Beal MW, Poppenga RH, et al. Effect of sorbitol, single, and multidose activated charcoal administration on carprofen absorption following experimental overdose in dogs. *J Vet Emerg Crit Care* 2015;25:606–610.

130

Rodenticide Toxicity

Jesse Bullock, DVM¹ and Alex Lynch, BVSc (Hons), DACVECC, MRCVS²

¹College of Veterinary Medicine, University of Florida, Gainesville, FL, USA
²North Carolina State University, Raleigh, NC, USA

Introduction

Rodenticide ingestion is a common concern in dogs, and clinical signs vary widely depending on the type and amount ingested. Cats rarely present with known or suspected rodenticide ingestion, but many of the same principles for case identification and management apply in this species [1]. As with all toxicities, a known dose and time frame of toxin ingestion can be extremely helpful in determining which signs to monitor for, and over what time period monitoring is necessary. Data available from the ASPCA Animal Poison Control Center identify a downward trend in anticoagulant rodenticides and an upward trend in neurotoxic rodenticide exposures from 2008 to 2014 (Figure 130.1). This trend correlates with EPA legislate changes that restricted use of second-generation anticoagulant rodenticides availability to consumers, increasing exposure to other types of compounds.

As practitioners, it is important to be aware of all types of rodenticides as many different compounds are packaged nearly identically. Any pet that produces teal or blue-green pigmented feces or vomitus should be examined and monitored for various potential rodenticide toxicities; paint ball toxicity would be another important consideration.

Decontamination

If a known toxic dose or unknown dose of any rodenticide is ingested within 4 hours of presentation and the animal is mentally appropriate, decontamination is the most appropriate first action (see Chapter 127). Inducing emesis with intravenous apomorphine is preferred to other methods (0.03–0.04 mg/kg IV, which may be repeated once). Apomorphine can also be applied conjunctivally and rinsed out following successful emesis.

Xylazine (0.4-1.1 mg/kg IM or SC) and dexmedetomidine (7 mcg/kg IM, 3.5 mcg/kg IV) are first-line emetics in cats although the likelihood of rodenticide ingestion is low. If veterinary treatment is delayed by transport time, or owners are unable to bring the dog to the clinic, hydrogen peroxide 3% solution may be used (1 mL/lb or 2.2 mL/kg), but this induces emesis by means of physical gastric irritation. Hydrogen peroxide is unlikely to induce emesis in cats. If mental status is significantly affected, gastric lavage is recommended over induction of emesis.

Caution should be exercised if zinc phosphide ingestion is known as the vomitus produced is likely to contain noxious gases that can affect staff and owners. Emesis for these patients should be performed in a well-ventilated room or an outdoor location in accordance with AVMA guidelines [2]. If an unknown rodenticide is ingested, activated charcoal is recommended at 1 g/kg PO every 6–8 hours for the first 24 hours as some rodenticides are enterohepatically recirculated.

Anticoagulant Rodenticides

Anticoagulant rodenticides all inhibit physiological recycling of vitamin K by inhibiting vitamin K epoxide reductase in the liver [3]. First-generation (chlorphacinone, diphacinone, dicoumarol, warfarin) and second-generation anticoagulants (brodifacoum, bromadiolone, difenacoum, difethialone) both inhibit vitamin K synthesis, but the second-generation products are more acutely toxic and have longer half-lives [4]. Many concentrations and preparations (pellets, blocks, powders, etc.) are available for consumers to purchase, so it can be very helpful to have access to the rodenticide package during patient evaluation.

Clinical signs may range from no visible or clinically appreciable abnormalities (within the first 72 hours) to animals presenting with hemorrhagic shock from

Textbook of Small Animal Emergency Medicine, First Edition. Edited by Kenneth J. Drobatz, Kate Hopper, Elizabeth Rozanski and Deborah C. Silverstein.
© 2019 John Wiley & Sons, Inc. Published 2019 by John Wiley & Sons, Inc.
Companion Website: www.wiley.com/go/drobatz/textbook

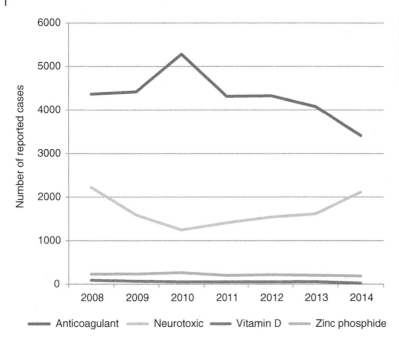

Figure 130.1 ASPCA reported rodenticide exposures by year. Rodenticide exposures are displayed by category of rodenticide and year. Note the recent downward trend in anticoagulant rodenticides and the upward trend in neurotoxic rodenticides.

internal or external blood loss. Dyspnea, lethargy, coughing, and hemoptysis are the most common presenting signs, but signs may vary depending on the location of bleeding for each pet [3]. Anticoagulant rodenticide ingestion classically results in conspicuous large-volume bleeding events (e.g. hemothorax, hemarthrosis) rather than surface mucosal bleeds that are more consistent with a primary hemostatic disorder (e.g. severe thrombocytopenia).

If no clinical signs are apparent and ingestion is uncertain, gastrointestinal decontamination should be considered, including the administration of a single dose of activated charcoal (as these compounds do not undergo enterohepatic recirculation). Prothrombin time should be measured in 48 hours to confirm diagnosis prior to administration of vitamin K1. The likelihood of coagulopathy development, as assessed by prolongation of prothrombin time, is low after timely gastrointestinal decontamination in dogs that have recently ingested anticoagulant rodenticide [5]. Administration of vitamin K1 will mask clinical signs of rodenticide toxicity until all administered vitamin K is inactivated.

Coagulopathies are not routinely apparent for 48–72 hours after ingestion. Vitamin K is required for the post-translational carboxylation of clotting factors II, VII, IX, and X required for functional activation. Vitamin K is also necessary for function of the antithrombotic factors C, S, and Z (Figure 130.2). Clinical signs of hemorrhage will not become apparent until bodily stores of these factors are depleted. In order, protein C levels, one-stage prothrombin time (OSPT, factor VII), prothrombin time

(PT, factor VII), activated partial thromboplastin time (aPTT, factor IX), and activated clotting time (ACT, factor IX) are all affected after a toxic dose of anticoagulant rodenticide and each test can be used for diagnosis in combination with other baseline testing [6]. Protein C estimation has the potential to be the earliest clinical indicator of clinically relevant anticoagulant rodenticide ingestion [7] but is uncommonly available to the emergency practitioner. In clinical cases, these coagulation tests are typically markedly prolonged (e.g. out of range high), which may differ from other causes of coagulopathy (e.g. disseminated intravascular coagulation).

Anticoagulant rodenticide screening panels are available to help characterize whether hemorrhagic tendency is due to rodenticide ingestion or an alternative diagnosis. Patients with severe coagulopathies that tested negative on anticoagulant rodenticide screening had a worse outcome compared to dogs that were coagulopathic associated with anticoagulant rodenticide ingestion [8]. The major limitation of these panels is the test turnround time, since few centers offer this test routinely, usually necessitating sending out samples to remote laboratories. Point-of-care anticoagulant rodenticide tests for dogs have been of limited clinical utility to date [9].

Management of anticoagulant rodenticide ingestion will vary depending on the presence or absence of severe coagulopathy. In the dog with known or suspected ingestion but no evidence of coagulopathy, management is focused on decontamination initially. Vitamin K1 can be started prophylactically at this point, being continued for 30 days, or alternatively held off until laboratory evidence

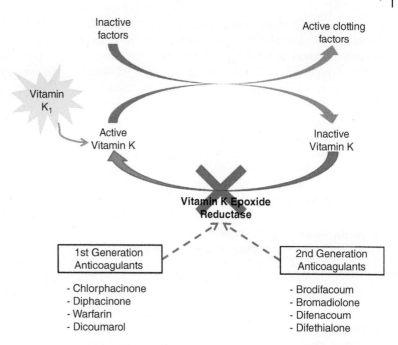

Figure 130.2 Vitamin K rodenticide mechanism of action. Inactive clotting factors include antithrombotic factors C, S, and Z and clotting factors II, VII, IX, and X. Administration of vitamin K1 restores normal function by providing fresh influx of active vitamin K.

of coagulopathy is rechecked at 48 hours. If the dog has a normal hemostatic profile at this point, no further treatment is necessary, while dogs with evidence of coagulopathy can then be started on a 30-day course of vitamin K1. Coagulation tests should be repeated 48 hours following cessation of vitamin K1 therapy to ensure no residual coagulopathy remains.

In the case of the clinically affected animal with severe coagulopathy and bleeding, treatment is focused on vitamin K1 administration and clotting factor replacement via either fresh frozen plasma or frozen plasma transfusion (see Chapter 176). If the dog has evidence of impaired oxygen delivery due to anemia, red cell supplementation may be necessary, as packed red blood cell transfusion. Fresh whole blood could be administered alternatively as an efficient means of administering both red cells and clotting factors. Coagulopathies resolve rapidly after the administration of vitamin K1 and plasma in these cases, with the expectation that the coagulopathy should not recur. If an animal develops recurrent coagulopathy or fails to correct its coagulopathy, alternative differential diagnoses for coagulopathy should be considered. Despite rapid laboratory improvement in coagulopathy, some clinical consequences of bleeding that have already occurred may still take days to resolve (e.g. resorption of hemorrhagic pleural effusion).

If the animal can tolerate oral administration of vitamin K1, this route is preferred, and as a fat-soluble vitamin, it is best absorbed with food. If oral administration is not tolerated, subcutaneous administration is recommended. Intramuscular administration is likely to cause increased bleeding and pain relative to subcutaneous

administration. Intravenous administration should be avoided as it may cause serious anaphylactic reactions.

Prognosis for anticoagulant rodenticide ingestion ranges from excellent (up to 98.7% in one study [8]) to guarded, depending on the severity of clinical signs at presentation and the promptness of instituting appropriate therapy.

Neurotoxic Rodenticides

With the decline in production of second-generation rodenticides, neurotoxic rodenticides are becoming increasingly common (see Figure 130.1). Bromethalin, the active ingredient in these rodenticides, is a neurotoxin that uncouples oxidative phosphorylation, decreasing adenosine triphosphate (ATP) production [10]. Most bromethalin is sold as one ounce 0.01% blocks, with each block containing 2.84 mg bromethalin. Clinical signs depend heavily on ingested dose and may be seen at 10% of the LD_{50} (which constitutes a lethal dose in 50% of exposed animals) [11]. The LD_{50} for bromethalin is reported as low as 0.3 mg/kg in cats and 2.4 mg/kg in dogs [11].

The onset of clinical signs is associated with severity of toxicosis: low doses may not show signs for up to 5 days, but larger doses may present as quickly as 2 hours after ingestion. Clinical signs initially manifest as hindlimb ataxia and weakness, and may progress to include lethargy, depressed mentation, seizures, coma, respiratory paralysis, and death. There are no distinguishing findings on routine laboratory tests, and there is no specific screening test available.

Unfortunately, there is also no antidote available for treatment of bromethalin intoxication, so very early decontamination is crucial in these cases. Emesis and gastric lavage are unlikely to be useful after 1.5 hours of ingestion as the toxin is very rapidly absorbed [11]. Repeated doses of activated charcoal are recommended at 1 g/kg every 4–6 hours for 48–72 hours as bromethalin undergo enterohepatic recirculation [11]. Intravenous lipid emulsion therapy is also a possible consideration, as it reduced blood levels significantly in one case report [13]. In affected animals, supportive care is recommended, including intravenous fluids, nutritional support, hypertonic saline or mannitol administration, antiepileptic medications, and mechanical ventilation if necessary. Prognosis is guarded to poor if clinical signs develop.

Cholecalciferol Rodenticides

Ingestion of cholecalciferol (vitamin D3) rodenticides induces potentially fatal hypercalcemia and hyperphosphatemia. Cholecalciferol is rapidly absorbed and converted to calcifediol in the liver. Calcifediol is then converted to calcitriol (active vitamin D, 1-25-dihydroxycholeciferol) in the proximal convoluted tubule of the kidney. Excess levels of active vitamin D cause increased absorption of calcium and phosphorus from the GI tract, bone, and kidneys. Metastatic mineralization of tissues can occur at calcium–phosphorus products over 60 (mg/dL), and can affect many tissues throughout the body irreversibly. Most cholecalciferol rodenticides are sold as 0.075% (0.75 mg/kg of product) baits. Clinical signs may be seen with doses as low as 0.5 mg/kg, and fatalities have been reported with doses of 2 mg/kg in dogs [12].

Clinical signs are related to the effects of hypercalcemia and hyperphosphatemia and can affect the GI, renal, and CNS systems most noticeably. Patients often present for inappetence, vomiting, diarrhea, polyuria, polydipsia, lethargy, depression, muscle tremors, and seizures, depending on which systems are most affected. Acute renal failure and irreversible GI tract mineralization are primary contributors to the morbidity and mortality of cholecalciferol rodenticides.

Initial laboratory testing should include a biochemical profile, complete blood count, and urinalysis. Hyperphosphatemia generally precedes hypercalcemia, and ionized calcium is the most clinically relevant form of calcium. Confirmatory testing for cholecalciferol exposure consists of increased serum calcium, increased serum phosphorus, and decreased serum parathyroid hormone levels. Important differentials include other sources of cholecalciferol (jasmine, vitamin D supplements or creams) and other causes of hypercalcemia (see Chapter 110). As calcifediol has a functional half-life of 29 days [12], both short- and long-term treatment plans must be formulated for affected patients.

Decontamination by emesis or gastric lavage is only warranted if rodenticide has been ingested in the prior 2 hours, as cholecalciferol is rapidly absorbed (see Chapter 127). Activated charcoal is recommended every 4–6 hours for 24 hours as cholecalciferol undergoes significant enterohepatic recirculation. Cholestyramine resin administration (0.3–1 g/kg PO q8h for 4 days, between charcoal administrations) is also recommended to help decrease GI absorption. Chemistry profiles should be monitored daily until calcium and phosphorus levels decrease and stabilize.

Additional supportive care for hypercalcemia includes IV fluid support with 0.9% saline diuresis (4–6 mL/kg/h, or twice maintenance), furosemide (0.66 mg/kg loading dose, then 0.66 mg/kg/h CRI), and steroid administration (2–3 mg/kg/day prednisone or 1 mg/kg/day dexamethasone SP) until calcium levels decrease appropriately. Close monitoring for seizures or tremors is warranted. In very severe cases, treatment with bisphosphonates may be warranted (pamidronate 1.05–2 mg/kg IV diluted in saline and given over 2 hours) [14], although this will result in less immediate reduction in hypercalcemia compared to the aforementioned options. Control of hyperphosphatemia involves use of phosphate binders once the patient is eating or able to be medicated enterally.

Short-term goals are aimed at controlling calcium levels, and this may take days to weeks in the hospital setting. Once calcium levels are controlled, patients may be released for at-home monitoring over the coming weeks with twice-weekly biochemical profiles recommended. Return of clinical signs warrants immediate re-evaluation.

Prognosis is good to guarded depending on severity and duration of clinical signs, degree of renal insufficiency and tissue mineralization, and client commitment to long-term care.

Phosphide Rodenticides

Zinc and aluminum phosphide are relatively uncommon rodenticides that elicit toxicity by several potential mechanisms [15]. These salts produce phosphine, the active agent, that may inhibit cytochrome C oxidase, disrupt the mitochondrial membrane, and generate free radicals that peroxidize lipids. Phosphine has rapid, directly toxic effects on the heart, adrenal glands, and kidneys, and is a corrosive agent. Death may result from a combination of cardiogenic and non-cardiogenic pulmonary edema, neurological consequences, acid–base disturbances, and renal failure.

Zinc phosphide rodenticides are available in various strengths and preparations (pellets, paste, tablets, powders, etc.). The lowest reported lethal dose in dogs and cats is 40 mg/kg, but the LD_{50} for most other animals is listed at 20 mg/kg [16]. The phosphide component reacts with water and acid to release phosphine gas, which is then absorbed across the gastric mucosa. Phosphine gas may be odorless or may have a garlic or rotten fish odor. Exposure to phosphine gas may result in fatigue, headaches, vomiting, dizziness, and shortness of breath in people if exposure doses are high enough. Emesis should therefore be induced in a well-ventilated area or outdoors, and owners should be cautioned about vomitus produced or induced at home. Consult AVMA guidelines regarding zinc phosphide for additional information [2].

According to the AVMA zinc phosphide guidelines, common presenting clinical signs include vomiting, hematemesis, depression, abdominal pain, diarrhea, convulsions, paralysis, coma, and death within minutes to hours of exposure. Liver and kidney injury may develop within 48–72 hours, if the patient survives initial exposure. As there is no antidote, supportive care is recommended based on initial presenting signs. Activated charcoal is not indicated as the active compound is a gas, mental status is likely to deteriorate rapidly, and addition of liquid components to the GI tract increases rate of production of the toxic gas.

Prognosis is guarded to grave if clinical signs are present from phosphide salt ingestion.

Aldicarb Rodenticide

"Tres Pasitos" is an uncommon rodenticide whose name quite accurately implies that death happens so quickly that only "three little steps" can happen after ingestion. This rodenticide may be imported illegally, and its active ingredient, aldicarb, is a carbamate that acts as a reversible inhibitor of acetylcholinesterase, preventing breakdown of acetylcholine in the synapse [17,18]. It is often sold in poorly labeled plastic baggies and looks like a brown grain, occasionally mistaken for a food product. This rodenticide is unfortunately still used in South America and South Africa in intentional pet poisonings.

Common clinical signs include those of an acute cholinergic crisis: dyspnea, vomiting, diarrhea, seizure, and/or acute death. If presented in time, treatment with atropine may slightly improve clinical signs by blocking muscarinic receptors, but ventilation and intense supportive care are also necessary to prevent respiratory arrest as there is no antidote to prevent stimulation of the nicotinic receptors. Prognosis is grave in symptomatic patients.

References

1 Kohn B, Weingart C, Giger U. Haemorrhage in seven cats with suspected anticoagulant rodenticide intoxication. *J Feline Med Surg* 2003;5:295–304.

2 AVMA Zinc Phosphide Guidelines. Available at: www.avma.org/KB/Resources/Reference/Pages/Phosphine-product-precautions.aspx (accessed 6 February 2018).

3 Sheafor SE, Couto CG. Anticoagulant rodenticide toxicity in 21 dogs. *J Am Anim Hosp Assoc* 1999;35:38–46.

4 Walker LA, Turk A, Long SA, et al. Second generation anticoagulant rodenticides in tawny owls (Strix aluco) from Great Britain. *Science Total Environ* 2008;392:93–98.

5 Pachtinger GE, Otto CM, Syring RS. Incidence of prolonged prothrombin time in dogs following gastrointestinal decontamination for acute anticoagulant rodenticide ingestion. *J Vet Emerg Crit Care* 2008;18(3):285–291.

6 Woody BJ, Murphy MJ, Ray AC, Green RA. Coagulopathic effects and therapy of brodifacoum toxicosis in dogs. *J Vet Intern Med* 1992;6:23–28.

7 Babyak J, Rozanski EA, Sharp C, de Laforcade AM. Protein C activity in dogs with anticoagulant rodenticide induced coagulopathy. *J Vet Emerg Crit Care* 2013;1 Suppl:s4.

8 Waddell LS, Poppenga RH, Drobatz KJ. Anticoagulant rodenticide screening in dogs: 123 cases (1996–2003). *J Am Vet Med Assoc* 2013;242:516–521.

9 Istvan SA, Marks SL, Murphy LA, et al. Evaluation of a point-of-care anticoagulant rodenticide test for dogs. *J Vet Emerg Crit Care* 2014;24(2):168–173.

10 Dorman DC, Simon J, Harlin KA, Buck WB. Diagnosis of bromethalin toxicosis in the dog. *J Vet Diagn Invest* 1990;2:123–128.

11 Peterson, ME. Bromethalin. *Topics Compan Anim Med* 2013;28:21–23.

12 Peterson ME, Fluegeman K. Cholecalciferol. *Topics Compan Anim Med* 2013;28:24–27.

13 Hegel-Perry B, McMichael M, O'Brien M, et al. Intravenous lipid emulsion therapy for bromethalin toxicity in a dog. *J Am Anim Hosp Assoc* 2016;52:265–268.

14 Hostutler RA, Chew DJ, Jaeger JQ, et al. Uses and effectiveness of pamidronate disodium for treatment of dogs and cats with hypercalcemia. *J Vet Intern Med* 2005;19(1):29–33.

15 Proudfoot AT. Aluminium and zinc phosphide poisoning. *Clin Toxicol* 2009;47:89–100.

16 www.vin.com/Members/Associate/Associate.plx?DiseaseId=870

17 Anastasio JD, Sharp CR. Acute aldicarb toxicity in dogs: 15 cases (2001–2009). *J Vet Emerg Crit Care* 2011;21(3):253–260.

18 De Siqueira A, Salvagni FA, Yoshida AS, et al. Poisoning of cats and dogs by the carbamate pesticides aldicarb and carbofuran. *Res Vet Sci* 2015;102:142–149.

131

Ethylene Glycol Intoxication

Rachel B. Davy-Moyle, DVM, DACVECC[1] and Leo Londoño, DVM, DACVECC[2]

[1]*Austin Veterinary Emergency and Specialty Center, Austin, TX, USA*
[2]*College of Veterinary Medicine, University of Florida, Gainesville, FL, USA*

Introduction

Ethylene glycol (EG) is a sweet-tasting, odorless substance extremely toxic to humans and animals. Antifreeze is the most common source of exposure for small animals and contains the highest concentration of EG at greater than 95% in some products. EG can also be found in a variety of other household items, including paint, adhesives, wood stain, and windshield deicers. As little as 6.6 mL/kg of EG is fatal for dogs and only 1.5 mL/kg in cats [1].

Ethylene glycol is absorbed from the GI tract as rapidly as 30 minutes after ingestion and metabolized primarily in the liver, with the remainder being eliminated unchanged in the urine. Within the liver, EG is oxidized by alcohol dehydrogenase (ADH) to glycoaldehyde, then to glycolic acid and then to glyoxylic acid (Figure 131.1). EG itself is a CNS depressant and can also cause direct

gastrointestinal irritation. However, EG's metabolites are primarily responsible for the acute kidney injury (AKI) and metabolic acidosis that are hallmarks of this toxicosis. Glycoaldehyde is thought to be the principal metabolite responsible for the CNS signs. Glycolic acid accumulation results in severe metabolic acidosis and elevations in the anion gap. Circulating calcium binds to oxalic acid, resulting in calcium oxalate crystalluria, as well as calcium oxalate crystal deposits in multiple organs; hypocalcemia may develop due to utilization during crystal formation. AKI, the most severe consequence of EG intoxication, is caused by the direct toxic effects of glycolic acid on the renal tubular epithelium as well as calcium oxalate crystal deposition within the tubular lumen [2]. Mortality rates are reported as high as 96–100% in cats, and 59–70% in dogs [3,4].

Clinical Signs

The clinical signs of EG toxicosis can vary depending on the amount of toxin ingested and the time after toxin exposure. EG toxicosis is classically described as occurring in three phases.

The first phase occurs within several hours of ingestion; clinical signs may include vomiting, lethargy, paresis, ataxia, and muscle fasciculations, and may progress to seizures and coma. These signs are attributed to the direct effects of EG on the GI and CNS systems. Polyuria and polydipsia may also develop, driven by increases in serum osmolality and osmotic diuresis. In dogs, neurological signs can resolve after 12 hours, falsely suggesting recovery. Cats do not typically show recovery from the CNS phase of the toxicosis. The second phase occurs approximately 12–24 hours after ingestion. During this time, CNS signs abate and cardiopulmonary signs can develop, including tachyarrhythmias and tachypnea due to severe metabolic acidosis, and hypocalcemia if

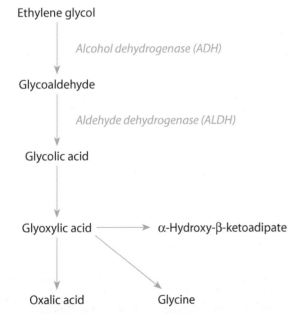

Figure 131.1 Metabolism of ethylene glycol.

present. Oliguric or anuric AKI then develops during the third phase of toxicosis, approximately 24–72 hours following ingestion in dogs and 12–24 hours in cats. Clinical signs of AKI at this stage may include lethargy, anorexia, vomiting, oral ulceration, ptyalism, coma, and seizures.

Diagnostic Testing

Since clinical signs of EG can vary depending on the amount of metabolite accumulation, bloodwork abnormalities and other diagnostic test results can also vary depending on the stage of intoxication. One of the earliest biochemical changes identified is a rise in the osmolal gap, which is the difference between the patient's measured and calculated osmolality. Increases in the osmolal gap indicate the presence of unmeasured osmotically active particles, such as mannitol, acetone, propylene glycol, and ethylene glycol [5]. A rise in serum osmolality can occur as early as 1 hour after EG ingestion, facilitating early recognition and treatment if recognized. The osmolal gap peaks at 6 hours after ingestion, but remains elevated for up to 18 hours after ingestion. Measurement of osmolality can be performed using freezing point osmometry or vapor pressure osmometry. These tests are rarely available in general practice and may delay diagnosis and treatment when sent out to laboratories. Calculated osmolality can be obtained using the equation $2(Na + K) + [glucose/18]$ [BUN /2.8], and the normal osmolal gap using this formula in dogs is $< 10 \, mOsm/L$ [6,7].

Blood gas analysis should be performed in all patients with suspected EG toxicity. Glycolic acid accumulation results in a profound normochloremic metabolic acidosis characterized by a decreased plasma bicarbonate concentration, and an increased anion gap due to the presence of unmeasured anions. The anion gap rises within 3 hours after ingestion and peaks at 6 hours, but remains elevated for approximately 48 hours [1]. Electrolyte abnormalities include hyperphosphatemia due to decreased glomerular filtration, hyperkalemia due to oliguria and anuria, and hypocalcemia. Serum biochemistry may reveal hypocalcemia in approximately 50% of patients due to binding of calcium to oxalic acid, and hyperglycemia is seen in 50% of cases due to inhibition of glucose metabolism by aldehyde metabolites of ethylene glycol [1]. An erroneous hyperlactatemia may be reported by enzymatic point-of-care (POC) machines and can be attributed to the measurement of glycolate, a chemically similar metabolite of EG [8]. As lactic acidosis also results in a high anion gap metabolic acidosis, this could result in a missed diagnosis of EG intoxication.

Urinalysis can also aid in the diagnosis of EG intoxication during its early stages. Isosthenuria is observed

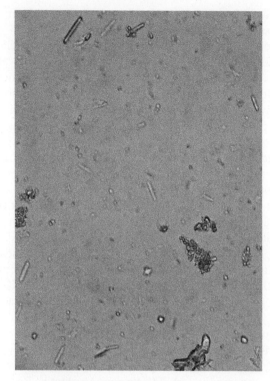

Figure 131.2 Calcium monohydrate crystals in a dog with antifreeze toxicity.

as soon as 3 hours post ingestion secondary to osmotic diuresis and polydipsia. Patients remain hyposthenuric as renal dysfunction develops. Calcium oxalate crystalluria is commonly seen, developing within 3–6 hours after ingestion. Calcium oxalate monohydrate crystals are the most common type observed and have a distinct appearance, looking like long, clear, six-sided or "picket fence" shaped structures, versus the square envelope shape of the dihydrate crystals (Figure 131.2). Other urinalysis findings may include decreased pH, hematuria, proteinuria, glucosuria, casts, white blood cells, and red blood cells.

Examination of the urine, mouth or paws with a Wood's lamp to look for fluorescence can be performed as many antifreeze solutions are made with sodium fluorescein dye in order to detect radiator leaks. Since this is not found in all solutions, and is only excreted in the urine for 6 hours following ingestion of antifreeze [9], a negative test does not exclude the diagnosis of EG intoxication.

Abdominal radiographs may reveal signs of renomegaly and renal mineralization late in the toxicity. Abdominal ultrasound can show increased renal cortical echogenicity, which combined with areas of lesser echo intensity in the medulla is referred to as a "halo sign" [10].

Complete blood count findings are non-specific in EG intoxication, and typically relate to dehydration (i.e.

elevated hematocrit and elevated plasma protein); a stress leukogram can be identified.

Specific tests for detection of EG are commercially available and vary in respect to their specificity and sensitivity, as wells as their ability to make a diagnosis in dogs versus cats. EG levels peak within 1–6 hours following ingestion, and are typically not detectable in serum or urine 48–72 hours after ingestion, so testing for EG is only successful early on in the toxicosis. The gold standard for testing for EG is gas chromatography. This is performed in human medicine but is not a POC test so is not as readily available.

There are several commercially available POC test kits for EG detection that have been evaluated in veterinary medicine. A semi-quantitative POC test (Kacey EG Test Strips, Kacey Inc, Asheville, NC) is available for use on canine or feline plasma, with a lower limit of detection at 20 mg/dL, which is the lethal dose for cats. The Kacey EG Test Strips were compared to a second qualitative POC test in dogs, the VetSpec Qualitative Reagent Test Kit (Catachem Inc, Oxford, CT) [11]. In this study, the semi-quantitative Kacey EG Test Strips had 100% sensitivity and 100% specificity and good agreement between those reading the test. The VetSpec Qualitative Reagent Test Kit was both less sensitive (65–95%) and less specific (40–70%), with less agreement between those reading the test, suggesting for dogs that the Kacey EG Test Strips were more accurate as well as being easy to use. Additionally, it was found that the Kacey EG Test Strips showed good agreement with measurements via gas chromatography, the gold standard for EG measurement.

However, when evaluated in cats, the Kacey EG Test Strips had a large number of false negatives and false positives at varying EG concentrations, indicating that the results of this test should be interpreted cautiously and it should not be used as a stand-alone test in cats [12]. Additionally, this test can cross-react with ethanol, glycerol, and propylene glycol. Propylene glycol can be found as a carrier in several medications, including diazepam, and as an ingredient in activated charcoal. A quantitative test, designed as an add-on test on the Hitachi-P chemistry analyzer (Roche Diagnostics, Indianapolis, IN), has been evaluated in both dogs and cats, and was found to be both highly accurate and precise, correlating well with measurements via gas chromatography (Quantitative Ethylene Glycol Assay, Catachem Inc, Oxford, CT) [13]. Additionally, unlike the POC tests, it does not cross-react with propylene glycol.

Treatment

Decontamination procedures, including induction of emesis and/or gastric lavage, as well as administration of activated charcoal are typically of little benefit in patients with EG intoxication due to its rapid absorption (see Chapter 127). For that reason, the mainstay of treatment of EG intoxication is preventing its metabolism in the liver and increasing its excretion. Preventing metabolism of EG is accomplished by competitively inhibiting the function of alcohol dehydrogenase (ADH) with ethanol or fomepizole (4-methyl-1H-pyrazole, or 4-MP). These two antidotes have a higher affinity for the enzyme than EG, which allows excretion of the toxin unchanged into the urine. If EG has already been metabolized, administration of ethanol or fomepizole may be of minimal to no benefit. In fact, these antidotes increase the half-life of EG and thus if renal damage has already occurred then EG may not be effectively eliminated. Therefore, antidotal therapy should be administered as quickly as possible after ingestion. In human toxicology, fomepizole is the preferred antidote as it effectively inactivates ADH without the adverse effects of ethanol, but evidence supporting benefits in mortality or morbidity rates between the two antidotes is lacking [14].

The recommended 4-MP dose in dogs is 20 mg/kg 5% IV initially, followed by 15 mg/kg IV at 12 and 24 hours and 5 mg/kg IV at 36 hours. In cats, a higher dose is required at 125 mg/kg IV initially, then 31.25 mg/kg IV at 12, 24, and 36 hours. This dose was safe and effective in cats with EG intoxication, being more effective than treatment with ethanol, and preventing AKI when initiated within 3 hours of ingestion [15,16]. Ethanol is more readily available and less costly than fomepizole, but it compounds the CNS depressant effects of EG, increases serum osmolality, and induces diuresis.

Because of ethanol's short half-life, ideally it should be administered as a CRI with a 1.3 mL/kg IV bolus of 30% ethanol followed by a CRI of 0.42 mL/kg/h for 48 hours [17]. Intermittent bolus dosage recommendations in dogs include 5.5 mL/kg of 20% ethanol IV every 4 hours for five treatments and then every 6 hours for four additional treatments, and 5 mL/kg of 20% ethanol IV every 6 hours for five treatments and then every 8 hours for four additional treatments in cats [17]. Ethanol can also be given orally when IV therapy cannot be provided, although this is less ideal due to its emetogenic properties and neurological status of the animal; one suggested dose is 2–3 mL/lb of an 80 proof (40% ethanol) alcoholic beverage [1].

Concurrent fluid therapy is recommended to enhance renal excretion of EG and its metabolites, correct dehydration, and increase tissue perfusion. Additional therapy includes treatment of seizure activity and arrhythmias, and correction of electrolyte imbalances.

Hemodialysis

The use of hemodialysis for treatment of EG toxicity is two-fold: *early* during the toxicity (first 12–24 hours), in order to remove EG and its metabolites from the system and prevent AKI, and/or *late* (after 24–48 hours) once AKI has occurred (see Chapter 129). Because of its low molecular weight and lack of protein-binding capacity, approximately 90–100% of EG and its metabolites can be removed from circulation with a single treatment of intermittent hemodialysis [18,19].

Ethylene glycol and methanol poisoning in people are amongst the most common toxin indication for extracorporeal treatments (ECTR) [20]. Despite this, a low percentage of reported EG and methanol intoxications in people are treated with ECTR. The current recommendations for ECTR use versus ADH antagonism in less severely intoxicated people are limited by regional differences in price and availability of fomepizole and possible complications associated with either technique [21].

In veterinary medicine, no guidelines are available for the use of ECTR in animal intoxications. Similar limitations such as availability of fomepizole, complications associated with ADH antagonism and the small number of veterinary dialysis centers are likely to affect the choice of treatment for small animals. In the authors' experience, if EG toxicity is recognized early (within 24 hours), referral to a dialysis center may provide partial to complete removal of the toxin from circulation, correct any acid–base and electrolyte disturbances, prevent AKI, and decrease hospitalization time. Administration of fomepizole or ethanol, whichever is available, is recommended before transportation and while preparing the patient for hemodialysis in order to inhibit metabolism of EG.

Once metabolism of EG has occurred and AKI has developed, treatment with supportive care and ADH antagonism is likely to be ineffective. Therefore, hemodialysis is indicated for the removal of any remaining EG and metabolites, as well as management of AKI. The prognosis for these cases varies depending on the timing of diagnosis and initiation of dialysis. In one study, 3/9 cats with AKI secondary to EG toxicosis and managed with intermittent hemodialysis alone survived to discharge; an average number of 12 treatments were required [22]. Another study showed a more negative outcome with only 8% survival, but fewer dialysis treatments were provided in these animals [23]. In dogs managed with hemodialysis for AKI, EG toxicosis was associated with a worse outcome when compared to other identified etiologies [24].

References

1 Thrall MA, Connally HE, Grauer GF, Hamar DW. Ethylene glycol. In: *Small Animal Toxicology*, 3rd edn (ed. Peterson M). Elsevier, St Louis, 2013, pp. 551–567.

2 De Water R, Noordermeer C, van der Kwast TH, et al. Calcium oxalate nephrolithiasis: effect of renal crystal deposition on the cellular composition of the renal interstitium. *Am J Kidney Dis* 1999;33:761–771.

3 Barton J, Oehme FW. The incidence and characteristics of animal poisonings seen at Kansas State University from 1975 to 1980. *Vet Hum Toxicol* 1981;23:101–102.

4 Rowland J. Incidence of ethylene glycol intoxication in dogs and cats seen at Colorado State University Veterinary Teaching Hospital. *Vet Hum Toxicol* 1987;29:41–44.

5 Lynd LD, Richardson KJ, Purssell RA, et al. An evaluation of the osmole gap as a screening test for toxic alcohol poisoning. *BMC Emerg Med* 2008;8:5–15.

6 Dugger DT, Epstein SE, Hopper K, Mellema MS. A comparison of the clinical utility of several published formulae for estimated osmolality of canine serum. *J Vet Emerg Crit Care* 2014;24:188–193.

7 Barr JW, Pesillo-Crosby A. Use of the advanced micro-osmometer model 3300 for validation of a normal osmolality and evaluation of different formulas for calculated osmolarity and osmole gap in adult dogs. *J Vet Emerg Crit Care* 2008;18:270–276.

8 Hopper K, Epstein SE. Falsely increased plasma lactate concentration due to ethylene glycol poisoning in 2 dogs. *J Vet Emerg Crit Care* 2013;23:63–67.

9 Winter ML, Ellis MD, Snodgrass WR. Urine fluorescence using a Wood's lamp to detect the antifreeze additive sodium fluorescein: a qualitative adjunctive test in suspected ethylene glycol ingestions. *Ann Emerg Med* 1990;19:663–667.

10 Adams WH, Toal RL, Breider MA. Ultrasonographic findings in dogs and cats with oxalate nephrosis attributed to ethylene glycol intoxication: 15 cases (1984–1988). *J Am Vet Med Assoc* 1991;199:492–496.

11 Creighton KJ, Koenigshof AM, Weder CD, et al. Evaluation of two point-of-care ethylene glycol tests for dogs. *J Vet Emerg Crit Care* 2014;24:398–402.

12 Acierno MJ, Serra VF, Johnson ME, et al. Preliminary validation of a point-of-care ethylene glycol test for cats. *J Vet Emerg Crit Care* 2008;18:477–479.

13 Scherk JR, Brainard BM, Collicutt NB, et al. Preliminary evaluation of a quantitative ethylene glycol test in dogs and cats. *J Vet Diagn Invest* 2013;25:219–225.

14 Beatty L, Green R, Magee K, Zed P. A systematic review of ethanol and fomepizole use in toxic alcohol ingestions. *Emerg Med Int* 2013; article 638057.

15 Connally HE, Thrall MA, Hamar DW. Safety and efficacy of high-dose fomepizole compared with ethanol as therapy for ethylene glycol intoxication in cats. *J Vet Emerg Crit Care* 2010;20:191–206.

16 Tart KM, Powell LL. 4-Methylpyrazole as a treatment in naturally occurring ethylene glycol intoxication in cats. *J Vet Emerg Crit Care* 2011;21:268–272.

17 Rollings C. Ethylene glycol. In: *Small Animal Critical Care Medicine* (eds Silverstein DC, Hopper K). Elsevier, St Louis, 2009, pp. 330–334.

18 Langston CE, Poeppel K, Mitelberg E. *Veterinary Dialysis Handbook. Extracorporeal Renal Replacement Therapies: Intermittent Hemodialysis and Continuous Renal Replacement Therapy*, version 4. Animal Medical Center, New York, 2014, p. 105.

19 Palm CA, Kanakubo K. Blood purification for intoxications and drug overdose. In: *Small Animal Critical Care*, 2nd edn (eds Silverstein DC, Hopper K). Elsevier Saunders, St Louis, 2015, pp. 392.

20 Ghannoum M, Lavergne V, Gosselin S, et al. Practice trends in use of extracorporeal treatments for poisoning in four countries. *Semin Dialysis* 2016;29:71–80.

21 Roberts D, Yates C, Megarbane B, et al. Recommendations for the role of extracorporeal treatments in the management of acute methanol poisoning: a systemic review and consensus statement. *Crit Care Med* 2015;43:461–472.

22 Langston CE, Cowgill LD, Spano JA. Applications and outcome of hemodialysis in cats: a review of 29 cases. *J Vet Intern Med* 1997;11:348–355.

23 Segev G, Nivy R, Kass PH, Cowgill LD. Retrospective study of acute kidney injury in cats and development of a novel clinical scoring system for predicting outcome for cats managed by hemodialysis. *J Vet Intern Med* 2013;27:830–839.

24 Segev G, Kass PH, Francey T, Cowgill LD. A novel clinical scoring system for outcome prediction in dogs with acute kidney injury managed by hemodialysis. *J Vet Intern Med* 2008;22:301–308.

132

Acetaminophen Intoxication

Amanda Thomer, VMD, DACVECC[1] and Lesley G. King, MVB, DACVECC, DACVIM (Internal Medicine)[†2]

[1]*ACCESS Specialty Animal Hospitals, Culver City, CA, USA*
[2]*Matthew J. Ryan Veterinary Hospital, University of Pennsylvania, Philadelphia, CA, USA*

Introduction

Acetaminophen is an analgesic and antipyretic that has been used in human medicine since 1893 [1]. It is an over-the-counter drug and can be found in many medications. Dogs and cats are exposed to acetaminophen through accidental ingestion or following administration by well-intentioned owners.

Pharmacokinetics and Toxicokinetics

Acetaminophen (APAP) appears to exert its analgesic effects via central cyclo-oxygenase (COX) inhibition. APAP crosses the blood–brain barrier and inhibits the central COX enzyme pathway, with only weak peripheral COX inhibition [2,3]. Other theories of APAP's mechanism of action include blockade of substance P's nociceptive actions via N-methyl-D-aspartate inhibition and activation of serotonergic nociception pathways centrally [2]. COX enzymes are important for prostaglandin production [4]. Prostaglandins are important in the regulation of many bodily functions, including gastric mucosal integrity and kidney function [4]. Non-steroidal anti-inflammatory drugs (NSAIDs) are known to inhibit peripheral COX enzymes and are associated with adverse effects such as gastric irritation, including ulceration, and renal insufficiency, among others [4]. Since APAP primarily inhibits central COX enzymes, it lacks the adverse local gastric and renal effects of NSAIDs.

Acetaminophen is metabolized by the liver [2,3] (Figure 132.1). Glucuronidation is the main metabolic pathway in dogs, followed by sulfuric acid conjugation [2,3]. In contrast, cats primarily use the sulfation pathway [5,6]. If the glucuronidation and sulfation pathways are saturated, residual APAP is metabolized by CYP2E1 and CYP1A2 (cytochrome p450) oxidation to the toxic compound N-acetyl-p-benzoquinone imine (NAPQI), which is converted into non-toxic metabolites by glutathione [2,3]. These metabolites are further converted into cysteine and mercapturic acid conjugates that are excreted in urine along with APAP-glucuronide and APAP-sulfate in dogs and cats respectively [2,5]. Peak plasma APAP levels occur within 4 hours of ingestion [5,7] and correlate with the dose ingested [5]. In mice, some APAP is metabolized by CYP2E1 in the proximal tubules of the kidney, causing NAPQI formation [8].

If glutathione stores are depleted to less than 70% of normal, NAPQI remains in its toxic form and binds to hepatic cell membranes, causing necrosis and hepatotoxicity [2,3,5,7,9]. Glutathione depletion also leads to oxidative damage to the heme in red blood cells, causing methemoglobinemia in dogs and cats and Heinz body anemia in cats [7,10]. It is theorized that subcutaneous edema can occur due to anoxia and increased capillary wall permeability secondary to methemoglobinemia [11]. Methemoglobin levels peak within 4 hours of APAP ingestion [12]. When renal glutathione stores in mice are depleted, NAPQI damages renal proteins and cell death ensues [8]. This is likely the underlying pathophysiology of APAP-induced nephrotoxicity in dogs and cats.

Cats are more sensitive to APAP as they lack a specific form of glucuronyl transferase, hepatic acetaminophen-directed uridine 5′-diphosphate [13], which is needed to conjugate APAP to glucuronic acid [9,10,12]. Cat erythrocytes are also more susceptible to oxidative damage by NAPQI due to the increased number of sulfhydryl groups on feline heme compared to other species [9,10,14].

It has been suggested that a metabolite other than NAPQI, para-aminophenol (PAP), may cause methemoglobinemia in dogs and cats [15]. PAP is metabolized by N-acetyltransferase. *In vitro*, dog and cat erythrocytes are more susceptible to oxidative injury (causing methemoglobin) by PAP than NAPQI [15]. Dogs and cats accumulate higher levels of PAP in erythrocytes compared

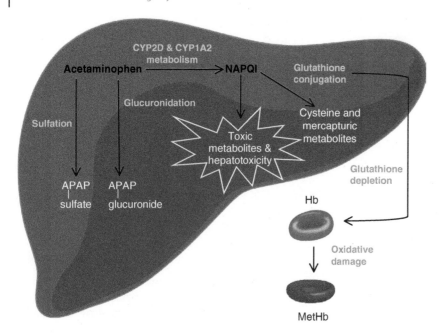

Figure 132.1 Acetaminophen metabolism in the liver and mechanism of toxic effects.

to other species, as canine erythrocytes do not contain N-acetyltransferase and feline erythrocytes only contain one N-acetyltransferase enzyme [15].

Toxic Doses

Therapeutic doses of APAP exist in dogs and range from 10 to 15 mg/kg every 8–12 hours [7,16]. Dogs usually do not show clinical signs of acetaminophen toxicity until over 100 mg/kg of acetaminophen has been ingested [5].

There is no therapeutic APAP dose in cats. Toxic doses in cats tend to occur with ingestion of 50–100 mg/kg, which represents one regular strength OTC human tablet (325 mg) [9]. However, there are reports of cats developing clinical signs after ingestion of as little as 10 mg/kg [10].

Clinical Signs

Common clinical signs in dogs and cats presenting with acetaminophen toxicity include depression, vomiting, lethargy, anorexia, icterus, cyanosis, muddy or brown mucous membranes, hypothermia, hyperthermia, tachycardia, tachypnea, respiratory distress, pigmenturia, and facial, paw, or forelimb edema [1,5–7,10,12,14,17]. The severity of clinical signs is correlated with the dose ingested [5].

Gross and Histological Lesions

Dogs develop centrilobular hepatic necrosis [5,18,19] that may or may not be accompanied by gross lesions of hepatic congestion and hemorrhage. Liver necrosis is less common in cats; instead, cats may have histological evidence of peripheral hepatocyte degeneration [5]. Gross hepatic lesions may include a nutmeg appearance, or a pale and mottled or edematous liver [5].

Renal cortex and medullary congestion, proteinaceous tubular casts, nephrosis, jejunal hemorrhages, and hemoglobin imbibition throughout other organs can also be seen [5]. Studies in humans show that upper gastrointestinal complications, such as ulceration, can occur at increasing doses of APAP [20,21]. Although weak, APAP does inhibit COX enzymes and, in theory, high doses could affect gastrointestinal mucosal integrity.

Diagnosis

The diagnosis of APAP toxicity is usually based on a patient's history of exposure to APAP, clinical signs, and laboratory abnormalities [7]. Plasma levels of acetaminophen can be measured at some human hospitals [7]. Laboratory evidence of hepatotoxicity is not seen until 24–36 hours after acetaminophen ingestion [7].

Bloodwork abnormalities in dogs include elevated values for alanine aminotransferase (ALT) [5,18], serum alkaline phosphatase (ALP) [5], total bilirubin and ammonia, and decreased serum concentrations of albumin and cholesterol [18]. Ingestion of higher doses of acetaminophen in dogs can cause nephrotoxicity [5,7], with an increase in BUN and creatinine, and decreased glomerular filtration rate (GFR) [7]. Abnormalities in cats include increased ALT, aspartate transaminase (AST), lactate dehydrogenase (LDH), and total bilirubin, as well as Heinz body anemia [10,14,22], low cholesterol, and low albumin [10].

Treatment

The goals of treatment are to decrease acetaminophen absorption, increase its elimination, limit NAPQI formation, supplement glutathione stores, and provide supportive care [13] (Figure 132.2).

Patients presented for acetaminophen ingestion should have emesis induced if the ingestion was recent (within < 1–3 hours) [23], unless contraindicated (see Chapter 127) [7]. Contraindications include CNS depression, underlying conditions placing the patient at risk of aspiration pneumonia, and concurrent ingestion of a corrosive, caustic, or volatile substance [23]. If emesis is contraindicated, gastric lavage may be a safer alternative for detoxification [7]. Activated charcoal at a dose of 1–3 g/kg should be administered to bind any remaining APAP in the gastrointestinal tract [7]. Contraindications for activated charcoal administration are the same as for emesis induction [23]. Since APAP undergoes enterohepatic recirculation, activated charcoal administration should be repeated [7]. Repeated doses should be administered every 4–8 hours for 2–3 days at half of the original dose [23]. Repeat doses should not contain cathartics.

In addition to specific treatments listed below, supportive care includes correcting dehydration, electrolyte, and acid–base abnormalities. Depending on clinical signs and hematocrit, some patients may need transfusion with packed red blood cells (pRBC). Patients clinical for methemoglobinemia may require oxygen supplementation.

N-Acetylcysteine

Administration of N-acetylcysteine (NAC) is currently the best treatment for APAP toxicity in dogs and cats. NAC is a glutathione precursor [7,10,14,17,24] and it binds with APAP metabolites, making them inactive [10,14], and it can increase sulfate conjugation by being a sulfur donor [12,14]. In dogs, NAC administration has been proven to increase acetaminophen elimination [24]. In cats, NAC administration decreased methemoglobinemia and Heinz body formation [6]. A loading dose of 140 mg/kg should be administered IV or PO followed by 70 mg/kg IV or PO every 4 hours for 3–7 treatments [7,10,17,24]. Intravenous use of NAC is off-label [7] and when administered by this route it should be diluted with 5% dextrose [25] to a 5% solution and administered slowly over 15–20 minutes [7]. If oral NAC is administered, it should be given 2–3 hours apart from activated charcoal [7].

Ascorbic Acid

Ascorbic acid reduces methemoglobin to hemoglobin, but its effectiveness in patients with acetaminophen toxicity is questionable [7,10]. Recommended doses include 10 mg/kg PO or IV every 6–12 hours [7] or 30 mg/kg IV every 6 hours [10].

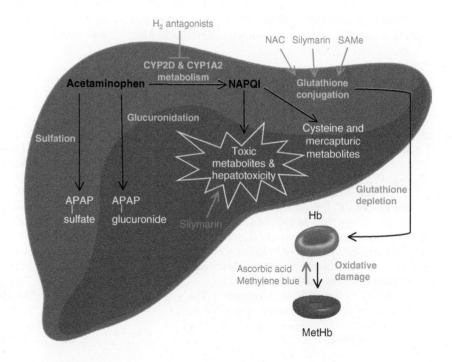

Figure 132.2 Acetaminophen intoxication treatment locations based on acetaminophen metabolism pathways. Hb, hemoglobin; metHb, methemoglobin; NAC, N-acetylcysteine; SAMe, s-adenosyl methionine.

Silymarin

Silymarin is a milk thistle extract composed of an anti-oxidant flavonoid complex. It is used non-specifically to treat liver disease by scavenging free radicals, stabilizing membrane permeability via lipid peroxidation, and preventing liver glutathione depletion [22]. A study showed that 30 mg/kg PO in cats administered at the time of APAP ingestion or 4 hours after ingestion had a similar hepatoprotective effect as NAC [22].

Histamine Receptor Antagonists

Cimetidine is an H2 antagonist that decreases APAP metabolism by inhibiting the cytochrome p450 oxidation system, but its ability to prevent hepatotoxicity is controversial [7,10,14]. Recommended doses are 5–10 mg/kg PO, IM, or IV every 6–8 hours in dogs and cats [7].

Ranitidine is an H2 antagonist that at high concentrations binds to cytochrome p450 and prevents oxidation of acetaminophen [18]. One study showed that a high dose (120 mg/kg) of ranitidine was protective against hepatotoxicity.

S-Adenosyl Methionine

S-adenosyl methionine (SAMe) initiates transmethylation and transulfuration pathways in hepatocytes and in theory should help prevent hepatotoxicity from APAP ingestion [13]. A study comparing cats treated with SAMe for APAP toxicity versus no treatment did not show a significant difference in the amount of Heinz body formation between the groups, but did show that the SAMe group cleared Heinz bodies faster than the control group [26]. SAMe may be considered a benign therapeutic option in dogs. There is one case report of administration of SAMe (40 mg/kg given PO then 20 mg/kg PO SID for 1 week) to a dog with severe APAP toxicity (ingestion of over 500 mg/kg) that survived [13].

Methylene Blue

Methylene blue reduces methemoglobin to hemoglobin but it should be used cautiously in cats as a treatment for APAP toxicosis [27]. At high doses, it has the potential to induce methemoglobinemia by oxidizing heme [27]. Methylene blue is generally not recommended as a treatment for methemoglobinemia in cats [10], although one study showed that one or two doses did not induce hemolytic anemia in cats [28]. Another study compared methylene blue alone, NAC alone, and NAC plus methylene blue as treatments for APAP toxicosis in cats; results showed that methylene blue decreased the plasma APAP half-life better than NAC alone in female cats but prolonged the plasma APAP half-life in the male cats [12]. The cause for this gender difference is unknown [12].

Prognosis

The prognosis varies from guarded to good for dogs and cats with APAP toxicosis, depending on the time between ingestion and treatment. The earlier treatment is implemented, the better the prognosis. One study of APAP toxicosis in cats showed that four of five non-survivors did not receive treatment for 17 hours after ingestion, but the 10 survivors received treatment within 14 hours of ingestion. One cat in the non-survivor group ingested as little at 10 mg/kg, and one cat in the survivor group ingested 400 mg/kg [10].

References

1 Finco DR, Duncan J, Schall W, Prasse K. Acetaminophen toxicosis in the cat. *J Am Vet Med Assoc* 1975;166:469–472.

2 Duggan ST, Scott LJ. Intravenous paracetamol (acetaminophen). *Drugs* 2009;69:101–113.

3 Jahr JS, Lee VK. Intravenous acetaminophen. *Anesthesiology* 2010;28:619–645.

4 Mathews, Karol A. Nonsteroidal anti-inflammatory analgesics. In: *Textbook of Veterinary Internal Medicine*, 7th edn (eds Ettinger SJ, Feldman EC). Saunders, St Louis, 2010, pp. 608–611.

5 Savides M, Oehme F, Nash S, Leipold H. The toxicity and biotransformation of single doses of acetaminophen in dogs and cats. *Toxicol Appl Pharmacol* 1984;74:26–34.

6 Gaunt SD, Baker D, Green R. Clinicopathologic evaluation of n-acetylcysteine therapy in acetaminophen toxicosis in the cat. *Am J Vet Res* 1981;42:1982–1984.

7 Richardson JA. Management of acetaminophen and ibuprofen toxicoses in dogs and cats. *J Vet Emerg Crit Care* 2000;10:285–291.

8 Schnellman RG. Toxic response of the kidney. In: *Casarett and Doull's Toxicology: The Basic Science of Poisons*, 8th edn (ed. Klaassen CD). McGraw-Hill, New York, 2013, p. 683.

9 Allen AL. The diagnosis of acetaminophen toxicosis in a cat. *Can Vet J* 2003;44:509–510.

10 Aronson LR, Drobatz K. Acetaminophen toxicosis in 17 cats. *J Vet Emerg Crit Care* 1996;6;65–69.

11 Leyland A. Probable paracetamol toxicity in a cat. *Vet Rec* 1974;94:104–105.

12 Rumbeiha WK, Lin Y, Oehme F. Comparison of n-acetylcysteine and methylene blue, alone or in combination, for treatment of acetaminophen toxicosis in cats. *Am J Vet Res* 1995;56.1529–1533.

13 Wallace KP, Center S, Hickford F, et al. S-adenosyl-l-methionine (SAMe) for the treatment of acetaminophen toxicity in the dog. *J Am Anim Hosp Assoc* 2002;38:246–254.

14 Ilkiw JE, Ratcliffe RC. Paracetamol toxicosis in a cat. *Aust Vet J* 1987;64:245–247.

15 McConkey SE, Grant D, Cribb A. The role of para-aminophenol in acetaminophen-induced methemoglobinemia in dogs and cats. *J Vet Pharamcol Ther* 2009;32:585–595.

16 Villar D, Buck WB. Ibuprofen, aspirin, and acetaminophen toxicosis and treatment in dogs and cats. *Vet Human Toxicol* 1998;40:156–162.

17 Omer V, McKnight ED. Acetylcysteine for treatment of acetaminophen toxicosis in the cat. *J Am Vet Med Assoc* 1980;176:911–913.

18 Francavilla A, Makowka L, Polimeno L, et al. A dog model of acetaminophen-induced fulminant hepatic failure. *Gastroenterology* 1989;96:470–478.

19 Ortega L, Landa Garcia J, Torres Garcia A, et al. Acetaminophen-induced fulminant hepatic failure in dogs. *Hepatology* 1985;5:673–676.

20 Rodríguez L, Hernández-Díaz S. Relative risk of upper gastrointestinal complications among users of acetaminophen and nonsteroidal anti-inflammatory drugs. *Epidemiology* 2001;12:570–576.

21 Cryer B, Feldman M. Cyclooxygenase-1 and cyclooxygenase-2 selectivity of widely used nonsteroidal anti-inflammatory drugs. *Am J Med* 1998;104:413–421.

22 Avizeh R, Najafzadeh H, Razijalali M, Shirali S. Evaluation of prophylactic and therapeutic effects of silymarin and N-acetylcysteine in acetaminophen-induced hepatoxicity in cats. *J Vet Pharmacol Ther* 2009;33:95–99.

23 DeClementi C. Prevention and treatment of poisoning. In: *Veterinary Toxicology*, 2nd edn (ed. Gupta RC). Elsevier, London, 2012, pp. 1361–1368.

24 Omer V, Mohammad FK. Effect of antidotal N-acetylcysteine on the pharmacokinetics of acetaminophen in dogs. *J Vet Pharmacol Ther* 1984;7:277–281.

25 Cumberland Pharmaceuticals Inc. Acetadote˚ (acetylcysteine) Injection (package insert). Nashville, TN: Cumberland Pharmaceuticals Inc., 2015.

26 Webb CB, Twedt D, Fettman M, Mason G. S-adenosylmethionine (SAMe) in a feline acetaminophen model of oxidative injury. *J Feline Med Surg* 2003;5:69–75.

27 Clifton J II, Leikin JB. Methylene blue. *Am J Therapeut* 2003;10:289–291.

28 Rumbeiha WK, Oehme F. Methylene blue can be used to treat methemoglobinemia in cats without inducing Heinz body hemolytic anemia. *Vet Hum Toxicol* 1992;34:120–122.

133

Non-Steroidal Anti-Inflammatory Drug Intoxications

Angela Borchers, DVM, DACVIM, DACVECC

William R. Pritchard Veterinary Medical Teaching Hospital, University of California, Davis, CA, USA

Mechanism of Action

Non-steroidal anti-inflammatory drugs (NSAIDs) are a class of drugs whose actions are typified by the inhibition of cyclo-oxygenase (COX). This drug class includes aspirin. Acetaminophen is not considered a traditional NSAID as it has only minimal anti-inflammatory activity so it is excluded from further discussion in this chapter unless stated otherwise (see Chapter 132).

Non-steroidal anti-inflammatory drugs exert their analgesic, antipyretic, and anti-inflammatory actions by direct inhibition of COX by competing with arachidonic acid (AA) for the active site of the enzyme [1]. All NSAIDs other than aspirin cause reversible inhibition of COX. The COX pathway uses AA, which is released from membrane phospholipids during trauma, infection, inflammation or platelet aggregation, to produce prostaglandins and thromboxane (PGD_2, PGE_2, PGF_{2alpha}, PGI_2, TXA_2) [1–3]. Prostaglandins are local, bioactive hormones with a short half-life of seconds to minutes. They are important for many physiological functions in the body as well as promotion and resolution of inflammation [3].

There are two isoforms of COX enzymes that are responsible for synthesis of prostaglandins and thromboxane [2]. COX-1 is a constitutive enzyme, responsible for prostaglandin production for many normal physiological functions such as renal and gastric blood flow [4]. COX-1 is mainly found in the stomach, kidney, endothelium, and platelets. COX-2 is a mostly inducible enzyme, synthesized in response to inflammation by macrophages, monocytes, fibroblasts, and chondrocytes after stimulation by cytokines and other mediators of inflammation [4]. Many currently marketed NSAIDs have higher COX-2 selectivity with the goal of providing analgesia and suppressing inflammation while sparing

physiologically important COX-1-mediated prostaglandins [2–5]. However, COX-2 appears to be constitutive in canine pyloric and duodenal mucosa, where COX-2 enzyme products are important for healing of gastroduodenal ulcers [6]. It appears that both COX-1 and COX-2 play a role in prostaglandin synthesis and maintenance of gastric mucosal integrity. COX-2 appears to play a "back-up" role by alleviating prostaglandin deficiency induced by COX-1 inhibition [7]. Hence, newer NSAIDs can still produce gastrointestinal adverse effects.

Aspirin (acetylsalicylic acid) is a non-selective, irreversible dual COX inhibitor that has more COX-1 selectivity at low doses [4]. By acetylating COX, aspirin irreversibly inhibits TXA_2 and PGI_2. Platelets are unable to synthesize new COX enzymes as they lack a nucleus. As a result, COX inhibition following aspirin exposure will persist for the lifespan of the platelet [8].

Acetaminophen is an analgesic and antipyretic but does not produce anti-inflammatory effects at clinical relevant doses [9,10]. The mechanisms of action of acetaminophen are still not well understood but recent research has shown that acetaminophen is a COX inhibitor in cells with low concentrations of arachidonic acid. Acetaminophen appears to be inhibiting the peroxidase portion of prostaglandin H_2 synthase (traditional NSAIDs inhibit the cyclo-oxygenase portion). There is also evidence that acetaminophen is a selective COX-2 inhibitor in selected tissues. Additionally, it appears to have an effect on a central COX-1 variant (previously called COX-3), inhibiting centrally mediated pain and pyrexia, especially in dogs [4,10–12]. Other proposed mechanisms of analgesia of acetaminophen include direct activation of serotonin receptors with serotonin-mediated stimulation of inhibitory pain pathways [4]. Readers are referred to Chapter 132 for further discussion on this topic.

Pharmacokinetics

Non-steroidal anti-inflammatory drugs have excellent bioavailability after parenteral and enteral administration but considerable species-specific differences exist in drug elimination [1]. Most NSAIDs are weak acids that are ionized at a physiologic pH while all NSAIDs are highly protein bound to albumin (98–99%), hence the volume of distribution (Vd) is very small. Only the unbound drug is pharmacologically active. Most NSAIDs are metabolized in the liver to inactive compounds via glucoronidation followed by renal and biliary excretion [1,4,13]. The high degree of protein binding limits renal excretion of the parent drug and restricts these drugs to the plasma compartment [1,4,13]. Once all albumin-binding sites are saturated, free drug concentrations increase quickly, leading to rapid efficacy of many NSAIDs while the kidney rapidly excretes free, unbound drug, preventing accumulation [13]. Elimination half-lives and enterohepatic recirculation vary considerably between drugs and species.

Aspirin is a weak acid that undergoes hepatic metabolism into salicylic acid; 70–90% of the drug is protein bound, mostly to albumin. Aspirin is minimally ionized and rapidly absorbed in the acidic environment of the stomach. Salicylic acid is eliminated via hepatic conjugation with glycine and glucoronidation followed by renal excretion [8].

Adverse Effects

From 2005 to 2010, the ASPCA Animal Poison Control Center reported 22 206 cases of dogs and cats exposed to different NSAIDs. Of these, 71% were dogs and 6% were cats [13]. A systematic review that evaluated prospective original studies on the safety of NSAID administration in dogs from 1990 to 2012 reported adverse effects in 55% of the studies [5]. Most common side-effects reported included vomiting, diarrhea, anorexia, lethargy, and melena. Less common clinical signs were fecal blood, bleeding, colitis, abdominal pain, aggressiveness or behavioral changes, hypersalivation, polydipsia, polyuria, adipsia, constipation, icterus, skin reactions, and weight loss. Two studies reported gastrointestinal perforations [5]. In general, the clinical effects of NSAID intoxication depend on the dose ingested. Lower toxic doses are likely to cause gastrointestinal signs while moderate doses can lead to gastrointestinal and renal injury and high doses can cause acute neurological signs (Table 133.1).

Gastrointestinal Toxicity

It is believed that NSAIDs cause gastrointestinal damage by direct and systemic effects. Direct effects are due to local irritation caused by NSAID-ion trapping. Systemic effects are mostly due to inhibition of COX-1-mediated endogenous PGE_2 but also PGI_2 production [1,13,14]. Gastrointestinal prostaglandins play an integral part in gastrointestinal cytoprotection by production of a protective, mucous gel layer, regulation of mucosal blood flow, cell turnover, and repair. Prostaglandin inhibition will diminish these protective effects. Aspirin may cause direct gastric irritation by disrupting surface phospholipids of the gastric mucosa [15]. Cats have limited ability to glucoronidate aspirin, which leads to prolonged excretion and half-life of aspirin and a higher incidence of gastrointestinal toxicity.

Renal Injury

Prostaglandin E_2 and PGI_2 play an important role in renal blood flow, and salt and water regulation. NSAIDs usually have little effect in healthy animals, but during episodes of decreased renal perfusion, they cause afferent arteriolar vasodilation and help to maintain renal blood flow. The kidneys become dependent on the vasodilatory effects of prostaglandins to maintain renal blood flow and glomerular filtration rate during episodes of dehydration, hemorrhage, anesthesia, heart failure and other conditions that would lead to decreased renal perfusion. Hence the use of NSAIDs during hemodynamic compromise is contraindicated. NSAID-induced renal injury includes papillary necrosis and interstitial nephritis [16].

Hepatic Injury

Hepatotoxicity induced by NSAIDs has been infrequently reported and is often idiosyncratic in origin. Clinical signs are often seen within the first 3 weeks of NSAID administration but can also occur after months to years of NSAID use. Idiosyncratic reactions are usually unpredictable and not dose related. Hepatocellular injury appears to be multifactorial in origin, including genetic variation in drug activation and detoxification and direct cellular effect leading to membrane dysfunction or cytotoxic T-cell response. It is unclear if pre-existing hepatic disease predisposes animals to hepatic injury due to NSAID administration [4,17,18]. Cats have limited ability to conjugate and glucoronidate aspirin as well as a relative deficiency in glutathione, all of which account for prolonged elimination, drug accumulation, and toxicity [15].

Coagulation and Hematological Issues

As COX inhibition can lead to inhibition of TXA_2 production by platelets, many NSAIDs can cause thrombocytopathy. Aspirin reduces platelet aggregation because it

Table 133.1 Pharmacokinetics and toxic doses of commonly administered NSAIDs in dogs and cats.

NSAID	Toxic dose	COX-1/COX-2 ratio*	Half-life (hr)†	V/D§ (L/kg)	Log P-value	Enterohepatic recirculation
Aspirin [4,32–36]	Dog: 25–50 mg/kg, BID-TID, gastric ulcerations, ≥450 mg/kg once, coma, hyperthermia, alkalosis, death. Cat: 25–100 mg/kg SID, gastric ulcerations, ≥100 mg/kg, lethal	0.3–0.39	7.5–12 (25 mg/kg); 22 (20 mg/kg)	0.17	1.19	No
Carprofen [4,29,35,37]	Dog: 5.3 mg/kg, vomiting, ≥50 mg/kg, renal damage. Cat: 3.9 mg/kg, vomiting, ≥8 mg/kg, renal damage	1.75–129	5–8.6; 19–20	0.12–0.22	4.13	Yes
Deracoxib [4,33,37]	Dog: ≥15 mg/kg, SID, vomiting, melena, ≥30 mg/kg renal injury. Cat: ≥4 mg/kg, gastrointestinal signs, ≥8 mg/kg, renal injury	1275	3; 8	1.5	–	Yes
Diclofenac [13,38,39]	Dog: 59–500 mg/kg LD$_{50}$	1–3.9	1.2–2	1.4 (human)	4.51	Yes
Etodolac [4,13,37,40]	Dog: 40 mg/kg/day, gastrointestinal ulcers, weight loss, emesis, 80 mg/kg/day, death, gastrointestinal and renal disease	0.52–7.92	8–12	>1	3.39	Yes
Firocoxib [33,37,40–42]	Dog: ≥25–50 mg/kg, gastrointestinal lesions in adult dogs, hepatic lesions, pancreatic edema. Duodenal ulcerations, death in 10–13-week-old dogs. Cat: not established	348	6–8	3–4.6	1.94	Yes
Flunixin [35,37,43,44]	Dog: ≥1.1 mg/kg, gastrointestinal lesions. Cat: not established	0.3 (horse)	3.7; 1–6 (1–2 mg/kg) (horse)	0.15 (horse)	–	Yes
Ketoprofen [35,37,38,45]	Dog: 0.44 mg/kg, gastrointestinal ulceration, 2000 mg/kg LD$_{50}$. Cat: 0.7–15 mg/kg renal toxicity	0.6	1.6; 0.5–1.5	0.22	3.12	Yes
Ibuprofen [3,4,13,46–48]	Dog: 8–16 mg/kg, SID for 30 days, gastric ulcerations, 100–125 mg/kg once, gastrointestinal problems, 175–300 mg/kg once, renal failure, >400 mg/kg, CNS effects, >600 mg/kg once, lethal. Cat: ~ twice as sensitive	0.6–15	3.9–5.3	0.05	3.97	Yes
Meloxicam [4,13,37]	Dog: not established. Cat: acute renal failure and death have been reported after repeat dosing	2.7–10	12–36; 15	0.3; 0.27	3.43	Yes
Naproxen [37,49,50]	Dog: >5 mg/kg, gastrointestinal signs, 10–25 mg/kg, renal damage, >50 mg/kg, CNS signs. Cat: not established	0.7	74	0.13	3.18	Yes
Phenylbutazone [4,35,37,38]	Dog: 332 mg/kg, LD$_{50}$. Cat: 44 mg/kg bone marrow suppression, gastrointestinal, renal and liver injury, death	0.6–9.7	2.5–6	0.14	3.16	Yes
Piroxicam [4,13,33,37]	Dog: 0.8 mg/kg, EOD for 10 days, gastric ulceration, hemorrhage, 1 mg/kg/day for 12–18 months, renal papillary necrosis, >700 mg/kg LD$_{50}$. Cat: not established	1.27–2	35–74; 12	0.3	3.06	Yes
Robenacoxib [37,51,52]	Dog: not established. Cat: 24 mg/kg/day for 21 days neurological signs, periportal hepatic necrosis, renal damage	32.2	1.2–1.7; 1.7	0.19	–	Yes

BID, twice a day (*bis in die*); CNS, central nervous system; COX, cyclo-oxygenase; EOD, every other day; NSAID, non-steroidal anti-inflammatory drug; SID, once a day (*semel in die*); TID, three times a day (*ter in die*); V/D, volume of distribution.

*In dog and human cell lines, based on 50% inhibitory concentration (IC$_{50}$), the higher the value above 1.0, the more specific the drug is for COX-2.

†Half-life for therapeutic dose unless indicated otherwise.

§Volume of distribution in dogs unless indicated otherwise.

irreversibly inhibits TXA_2 production. Consequently, as TXA_2 synthesis is inhibited for the lifespan of the platelet, new formation of TXA_2 requires the synthesis of new platelets [8]. The impact of other NSAIDs on platelet function is variable. Experimental research found decreased platelet aggregation in dogs that received aspirin and carprofen, increased clot strength in dogs that received deracoxib, and a minimal effect on clot strength with meloxicam administration [19]. In cats, experimental research showed that administration of aspirin and meloxicam had no effects on platelet aggregation, even though aspirin decreased TXA_2 significantly [20]. Unlike the effects of aspirin, the reversible inhibition of TXA_2 by other NSAIDs will allow platelet function to return to normal following metabolism of the drug.

Neurological Complications

Aseptic meningitis induced by NSAIDs has been reported in humans but not in veterinary medicine [21]. Salicylate-induced seizures in a dog have been reported [22]. Central nervous system (CNS) effects including seizures, ataxia, depression, and coma have been reported after ingestion of high doses of ibuprofen, naproxen, and robenacoxib (see Table 133.1).

Treatment of NSAID Intoxication

Animals that have ingested an accidental overdose of a NSAID should be treated promptly.

Decontamination should be performed immediately if the animal does not show clinical signs that prevent emesis (e.g. comatose, seizuring, tremoring, absent gag reflex) and if the ingestion was within the last 2 hours (see Chapter 127). Emesis can be induced with apomorphine (0.03–0.04 mg/kg IV once or a crushed tablet dissolved in 0.9% saline, administered in the conjunctival sac or intranasally). Alternatively, 3% hydrogen peroxide can be administered (2.2 mL/kg, PO to a maximum of 45 mL/dog), which can be repeated once if emesis did not occur [13,23]. In cats, emesis can be tried with xylazine (0.44 mg/kg, IM). Gastric lavage should be considered in animals that did not vomit and have recently ingested large, toxic doses as well as those in which neurological signs prevent the induction of emesis.

Activated charcoal (AC) (1–3 g/kg PO, q6–8h, 2–6 doses total) should be administered after induction of emesis. Repeated administration of AC is generally recommended as many NSAIDs undergo enterohepatic recirculation. The first dose of AC should contain a cathartic (e.g. sorbitol) to promote gastrointestinal transit time, followed by AC without a cathartic for consecutive dosing, to avoid dehydration and hypernatremia.

Recent research found that a single dose of AC is as effective as either multiple doses of AC or AC with sorbitol in reducing serum carprofen concentrations in moderately overdosed dogs [24]. This may mean that repeat doses of AC in NSAID intoxication are unnecessary, but until further research evaluating other NSAID drugs is performed, it would seem prudent to continue with repetitive AC dosing.

Fluid therapy with forced diuresis plays a key role in the intoxicated patient. Intravenous, balanced isotonic crystalloids (e.g. lactated Ringer's solution, Plasma-Lyte 148, Normosol-R) can be used at 1.5–2 times normal maintenance rates (see Chapter 167). This will aid in excretion of the drug, helps to vasodilate the renal vessels, which is particularly important in NSAID toxicosis, and prevents dehydration. Careful monitoring of packed cell volume, total protein, electrolyte abnormalities, and fluid balance during treatment is important.

Gastrointestinal support should be provided with H2 blockers such as famotidine, cimetidine or ranitidine as well as proton pump inhibitors such as omeprazole, esomeprazole or pantoprazole. Misoprostol (3 μg/kg PO q8–12h) is a synthetic PGE_1 analogue that was found to be beneficial in preventing gastrointestinal mucosal injury caused by aspirin [25] and might also be beneficial in NSAID intoxication to prevent injury. The use of metoclopramide should be avoided because it acts as a dopamine antagonist on a renal level and may decrease renal blood flow [26].

Intravenous lipid emulsions (ILE) have been used successfully in two recent case reports to treat intoxications with ibuprofen and naproxen in dogs [27,28] (see Chapter 128). The most commonly accepted mechanism of action of ILE is the "lipid sink" theory, where ILE sequesters lipophilic compounds into a newly created intravascular lipid compartment which results in decreased free drug concentrations. The lipophilicity of a drug is related to its log P value, which is a ratio of unionized solute concentrations dissolved in two solutions. Since most drugs are ionizable at a certain, adjusted pH, log P values may not always accurately predict the drug's lipophilicity. Drugs are considered lipophilic if their log P > 1.0; the higher the log P value, the more lipophilic the drug. The following dose recommendations are published in veterinary medicine for the administration of 20% ILE: initial bolus of 1.5–4 mL/kg (~0.3–0.8 g/kg), IV over 1 minute, followed by constant-rate infusion (CRI) of 0.25 mL/kg/min (0.05 g/kg/min) IV over 30–60 minutes. If the animal continues to be clinical, intermittent boluses at 1.5 mL/kg q4–6h might be necessary with an optional follow-up CRI of 0.5 mL/kg/h (0.1 g/kg/h) until clinical signs improve [29].

Extracorporeal therapy (ECT) recommendations are not well defined (see Chapter 129). The high protein-binding property and low volume of distribution of many NSAIDs favor the use of charcoal hemoperfusion followed by conventional hemodialysis if the animal has significant clinical signs or has ingested a large amount of the drug. Total plasma exchange followed by charcoal hemoperfusion has also been utilized for NSAIDs that are strongly protein bound [30,31].

References

1 Lees P, Landoni MF, Giraudel J, Toutain PL. Pharmacodynamics and pharmacokinetics of nonsteroidal anti-inflammatory drugs in species of veterinary interest. *J Vet Pharmacol Therap* 2004;27:479–490.

2 Simmons DL, Botting RM, Hla T. Cyclooxygenase osozymes: the biology of prostaglandin synthesis and inhibition. *Pharmacol Rev* 2004;56:387–437.

3 Ricciotti E, Fitzgerald GA. Prostaglandins and inflammation. *Arterioscler Thromb Vasc Biol* 2011;31(5):986–1000.

4 Papich MG. An update on nonsteroidal anti-inflammatory drugs (NSAIDS) in small animals. *Vet Clin Small Anim* 2008;38:1243–1266.

5 Monteiro-Steagall BP, Steagall PVM, Lascelles BDX. Systematic review of nonsteroidal anti-inflammatory drug-induced adverse effects in dogs. *J Vet Intern Med* 2013;27:1011–1019.

6 Wolfe MM, Lichtenstein DR, Singh G. Gastrointestinal toxicity of non-steroidal anti-inflammatory drugs. *N Engl J Med* 1999;340:1888–1899.

7 Matsui H, Shimokawa O, Kaneko T, et al. The pathophysiology of non-steroidal anti-inflammatory drug (NSAID)-induced mucosal injuries in stomach and small intestine. *J Clin Biochem Nutr* 2011;48(2):107–111.

8 Catella-Lawson F, Reilly MP, Kapoor SC, et al. Cyclooxygenase and the antiplatelet effects of aspirin. *N Engl J Med* 2001;345(25):1890–1817.

9 Mburu DN, Mbugua LA, Skoglund LA, Loekken P. Effects of paracetamol (acetaminophen) and acetylsalicylic acid on the post-operative course after experimental orthopaedic surgery in dogs. *J Vet Pharmacol Ther* 1988;11:163–171.

10 Graham GG, Davis MJ, Day RO, Mohamudally A, Scott KF. The modern pharmacology of paracetamol: therapeutic actions, mechanism of action, metabolism, toxicity and recent pharmacological findings. *Inflammopharmacology* 2013;21(3):201–232.

11 Aronoff DM, Oates JA, Boutaud O. New insights into the mechanism of action of acetaminophen: its clinical pharmacologic characteristics reflect its inhibition of two prostaglandin H2 synthases. *Clin Pharmacol Ther* 2005;79:9–19.

12 Chandrasekharan NV, Dai H, Roos KL, et al. COX-3, a cyclooxygenase-1 variant inhibited by acetaminophen and other analgesic/antipyretic drugs: cloning, structure, and expression. *Proc Natl Acad Sci USA* 2002;99(21):13926–13931.

13 Khan SA, McLean MK. Toxicology of frequently encountered nonsteroidal anti-inflammatory drugs an dogs and cats. *Vet Clin Small Anim* 2012;42:289–306.

14 Wilson JE, Chandrasekharan NV, Westover KD, Eager KB, Simmons DL. Determination of expression of cyclooxygenase-1 and -2 isozymes in canine tissues and their differential sensitivity to nonsteroidal anti-inflammatory drugs. *Am J Vet Res* 2004;65:810–818.

15 Davis LE. Clinical pharmacology of salicylates. *J Am Vet Med Assoc* 1980;176:65.

16 Musu M, Finco G, Antonucci R, et al. Acute nephrotoxicity of NSAIDS from the foetus to the adult. *Eur Rev Med Pharmacol Sci* 2011;15(12):1461–1472.

17 Lee WM. Drug-induced hepatotoxicity. *N Engl J Med* 2003;349:474–485.

18 Bessone F. Non steroidal anti-inflammatory drugs: what is the actual risk of liver damage? *World J Gastroenterol* 2010;16(45):5651–5661.

19 Brainard BM, Meredith CP, Callan MB, et al. Changes in platelet function, hemostasis, and prostaglandin expression after treatment with nonsteroidal anti-inflammatory drugs with various cyclooxygenase selectivities in dogs. *Am J Vet Res* 2007;68(3):251–257.

20 Cathcart CJ, Brainard BM, Reynolds LR, Al-Nadaf S, Budsberg SC. Lack of inhibitory effect of acetylsalicylic acid and meloxicam on whole blood platelet aggregation in cats. *J Vet Emerg Crit Care (San Antonio)* 2012;22(1):99–106.

21 Kepa L, Oczko-Grzesik B, Stolarz W, Sobala-Szczgiel B. Drug-induced aseptic meningitis in suspected central nervous system infections. *J Clin Neurosci* 2005;12:562–564.

22 Schubert TA. Salicylate-induced seizures in a dog. *J Am Vet Med Assoc.* 1984;185(9):1000–1001.

23 Khan SA, Mclean MK, Slater M, Hansen S, Zawistowski S. Effectiveness and adverse effects od the use of apomorphine and 3% hydrogen peroxide solution to induce emesis in dogs. *J Am Vet Med Assoc* 2012;241(9):1179–1184.

24 Koenigshoff AM, Beal MW, Poppenga RH, Jutkowitz LA. Effect of sorbitol, single and multidose activated charcoal administration on carprofen absorption following experimental overdose in dogs. *J Vet Emerg Crit Care (San Antonio)* 2015;25(5):606–610.

25 Ward DM, Leib MS, Johnston SA, Marini M. The effect of dosing interval on the efficacy of misoprostol in the prevention of aspirin-induced gastric injury. *J Vet Intern Med* 2003;17(3):282–290.

26 Smit AJ, Meijer S, Wesseling H, Donker AJ, Reitsma WD. Effect of metoclopramide on dopamine induced

changes in renal function in healthy controls and in patients with renal disease. *Clin Sci (Lond)* 1988;75(4):421–428.

27 Herring JM, McMichael MA, Corsi R, Wurlod V. Intravenous lipid emulsion therapy in three cases of canine naproxen overdose. *J Vet Emerg Crit Care (San Antonio)* 2015;25(5):672–678.

28 Bolfer L, McMichael MA, Ngwenyama TR, O'Brien M. Treatment of ibuprofen toxicosis in a dog with IV lipid emulsion. *J Am Anim Hosp Assoc* 2014;50:136–140.

29 Fernandez AL, Lee JA, Rahilly L, et al. The use of intravenous lipid emulsion as an antidote in veterinary toxicology. *J Vet Emer Crit Care (San Antonio)* 2011;21(4):309–320.

30 Palm CA, Kanakubo K. Blood purification for intoxications and drug overdose. In: *Small Animal Critical Care Medicine*, 2nd edn (eds Silverstein DC, Hopper K). Elsevier Saunders, Philadelphia, 2015.

31 Cowgill L, personal communication 2015.

32 Parton K, Balmer TV, Boyle J, Whittem T, MacHon R. The pharmacokinetics and effects of intravenously administered carprofen and salicylate on gastrointestinal mucosa and selected biochemical measurements in healthy cats. *J Vet Pharmacol Ther* 2000;23(2):73–79.

33 Talcott PA, Gwaltney-Brant SM. Nonsteroidal antiinflammatories. In: *Small Animal Toxicology*, 3rd edn (eds Peterson ME, Talcott PA). Elsevier Saunders, Philadelphia, 2012.

34 Dittert LW. Pharmacokinetic prediction of tissue residues. *J Toxicol Environ Health* 1977;2(4):735–756.

35 Lascelles BDX, Court MH, Hardie EM, Robertson SA. Nonsteroidal anti-inflammatory drugs in cats: a review. *Vet Anaesth Analg* 2007;34:228–250.

36 Brune K, Nuernberg B, Schneider HT. Biliary elimination of aspirin after oral and intravenous administration in patients. *Agents Actions Suppl* 1993;44:51–57.

37 Plumb DC. *Plumb's Veterinary Drug Handbook*, 8th edn. Wiley Blackwell, Hoboken, 2015.

38 Brideau C, van Staden C, Chan CC. In vitro effects of cyclooxygenase inhibitors in whole blood of horses, dogs and cats. *Am J Vet Res* 2001;62(11):1755–1760.

39 Committee for Veterinary Medicinal Products. Diclofenac. Summary Report. EMEA/MRL/885/03-FINAL. European Agency for the Evaluation of Medicinal Products, London, 2003, pp. 1–9.

40 Papich MG, Messenger K. Non-steroidal anti-inflammatory drugs. In: *Veterinary Anesthesia and Analgesia*, 5th edn (eds Grimm KA, Leigh AL). Wiley-Blackwell, Hoboken, 2015.

41 McCann ME, Rickes EL, Hora DF, et al. In vitro effects and in vivo efficacy of a novel cyclooxygenase-2 inhibitor in cats with lipopolysaccharide-induced pyrexia. *Am J Vet Res* 2005;66(7):1278–1284.

42 McCann ME, Andersen DR, Zhang D, et al. In vitro effects and in vivo efficacy of a novel cyclooxygenase-2 inhibitor in dogs with experimentally induced synovitis. *Am J Vet Res* 2004;65(4):503–512.

43 Stegelmayer BL, Bottoms GD, Denicola BD, Reed WM. Effects of flunixine meglumine in dogs following experimentally induced endotoxemia. *Cornell Vet* 1988;78(3):221–230.

44 Committee for Veterinary Medicinal Products. Flunixin. Summary Report. EMEA/MRL/661/99-FINAL. European Agency for the Evaluation of Medicinal Products, London, 1999.

45 Serrano-Rodriguez JM, Serrano JM, Rodriguez JM, et al. Pharmacokinetics of the individual enantiomer S-(+) ketoprofen after intravenous and oral administration in dogs at two dose levels. *Res Vet Sci* 2014;96(3):523–525.

46 Botting RM. Inhibitors of cyclooxygenases: mechanisms, selectivity and uses. *J Physiol Pharmacol* 2006;57(Suppl 5):113–124.

47 Scherkl R, Frey HH. Pharmacokinetics of ibuprofen in the dog. *J Vet Pharmacol Ther* 1987;10(3):261–265.

48 Au DS-L, Kuo TH, Lee CS, Mederski-Samoraj B. Disposition of ibuprofen in nephrectomized dogs. *J Pharmaco Sci* 1984;73(5):705–708.

49 Baigent C, Patrono C. Selective cyclooxygenase 2 inhibitors, aspirin, and cardiovascular disease: a reappraisal. *Arthritis Rheum* 2003;48(1):12–20.

50 Frey HH, Rieh B. Pharmacokinetics of naproxen in the dog. *Am J Vet Res* 1981;42(9):1615–1617.

51 Robenacoxib. Available at: www.fda.gov

52 Schmid VB, Seewald W, Lees P, King JN. In vitro and ex vivo inhibition of COX isoforms by robenacoxib in the cat: a comparative study. *J Vet Pharmacol Ther* 2010;33(5):444–452.

134

Grape, Raisin, and Lily Ingestion

J.D. Foster, VMD, DACVIM

Friendship Hospital for Animals, Washington, DC, USA

Grape, Raisin, and Currant Nephrotoxicity Pathogenesis

Grapes, raisins, and currants have been reported to cause acute kidney injury (AKI) in dogs. Affected dogs have been exposed to fresh grapes from grocery stores or vines in private yards, grape crushings, or fermented grapes from wineries [1]. Red seedless grapes were involved in most cases, but AKI has also been reported with golden seedless types. The raisins involved were mostly commercial sun-dried raisins of various brands, including both dark and golden seedless varieties. The estimated ingested amount of raisins causing toxicity ranges between 0.1 and 1.3 oz/kg (2.8–36.4 g/kg) and the estimated quantity of grapes causing toxicity ranges between 0.7 and 5.3 oz/kg (19.6–148.4 g/kg) [2].

The exact toxic substance within grapes, raisins, and currants is unknown. When tested, samples of grapes and raisins were found not to contain mycotoxin or ochratoxin A [2]. Dogs developing AKI were found to have moderate to severe renal tubular degeneration, mineralization of the tubular epithelium and basement membrane, and tubular obstruction caused by proteinaceous and cellular debris [2]. Another report showed similar findings, but the tubular basement membrane remained intact [3].

Presenting clinical complaints included vomiting (100% of dogs), lethargy, anorexia, diarrhea, ataxia, and weakness. Symptoms typically develop within 24 hours of exposure.

Lily Nephrotoxicity Pathogenesis

Acute kidney injury has been reported in cats following ingestion of *Lilium* and *Hemerocallis* species of lily plants (Box 134.1) [4–7]. There are numerous plants that are called "lily" but do not belong to these two species, such as the peace lily (genus *Spathiphyllum*). These other species of plants may result in additional toxic effects, such as oral and gastrointestinal irritation, vomiting, or cardiac effects, or may be non-toxic. Confusion arises in the identification of lily plants due to the existence of many hybrid species, as well as a lack of identification when flowers are received as gifts.

Owners should be directly questioned about possible lily exposure for any acutely azotemic cat. One study found that less than 30% of cat owners knew that lilies were toxic, so they may not willingly provide such important history [7]. All parts of the lily plant, including the petals, stamen, leaves, and pollen, are toxic to cats [5]. Just chewing on the petals or ingestion of a single flower has resulted in nephrotoxicity. The exact toxin is unknown, but has been demonstrated to be water soluble [5]. Easter lily flowers were shown to contain 16 different steroidal glycoalkaloids, which may be the nephrotoxic compounds, but this has not been confirmed *in vivo* [8]. Experimentally induced lily toxicity resulted in moderate to severe proximal tubular epithelial cell necrosis, edema, and tubular obstruction [5]. Pancreatitis has also been observed in some cats [6].

It should be noted that many cats (87% in one report) develop transient or no clinical signs following lily exposure [7]. Vomiting, lethargy, and hypersalivation are the

Box 134.1 Nephrotoxic lilies		
Asiatic lily	Japanese show lily	Tiger lily
Calla lily	Leopard lily	Trumpet lily
Daylily	Panther lily	White lily
Easter lily	Stargazer lily	Yellow lily

most common clinical signs, typically observed 1–5 days post exposure, with many cats showing these symptoms within 1–3 hours after ingestion [6]. Neurological abnormalities, including seizures and ataxia, have been reported in almost 40% of cats [9]. One report suggested that seizures often occurred following handling of cats, such as after physical examination [5].

Physical Examination

Physical examination may reveal abdominal pain, abnormal mentation, hypothermia, and dehydration. Abdominal pain was present in nearly 30% of dogs with grape and raisin toxicity. Renomegaly and renal pain may be present. It should be noted that many cats with lily nephrotoxicity have a normal examination and appear remarkably bright and asymptomatic despite severe uremia. It is important to note the size of the urinary bladder during initial examination.

Initial Diagnostics

Initial diagnostics should include complete blood count, serum chemistry with electrolytes, acid–base status, urinalysis (sample should be submitted for culture to rule out pyelonephritis), and blood pressure.

Grape and raisin toxicity commonly results in hyperphosphatemia (90%) and hypercalcemia (62%), as well as an increased $Ca \times P$ product (95% of dogs). Hypo- and hyperkalemia are frequently encountered. Thrombocytopenia (mean 50×10^3 PLT/µL) was found in nearly 30% of dogs. Isosthenuria, proteinuria, and glucosuria are found in the majority of dogs [2].

Common findings of lily nephrotoxicity include moderate to severe azotemia, isosthenuria, glucosuria, proteinuria, and often cylindruria. A common, but not pathognomonic, finding is a *more markedly elevated serum creatinine concentration compared to a more moderate blood urea nitrogen*. Cats may have serum creatinine concentrations of 15–30 mg/dL, whereas the BUN is typically < 250 mg/dL, resulting in a decreased BUN:Cr ratio. One study found that of cats presenting within 48 hours after lily exposure, only 20% had elevated BUN and 4.5% had elevated creatinine concentrations on initial labwork [10]. Metabolic acidosis resulting from uremic toxins and elevated serum lactate is often encountered. Hyperkalemia may be present and should prompt the clinician to inquire about urine output, as many cats with lily nephrotoxicity develop oligoanuria (see Chapter 95). Hypokalemia may be present in polyuric animals. Increased hematocrit and serum total protein may indicate dehydration.

Management of Non-Azotemic Animals Shortly After Exposure

Management recommendations vary depending on the degree of renal injury. Gastric decontamination through emesis, lavage, and activated charcoal is highly recommended for dogs following grape, raisin, or currant exposure (Box 134.2) (see Chapter 127). Induction of emesis more than 2 hours following ingestion may be warranted because *Vitis* fruits remain in the gastrointestinal tract for some time. It is unknown if activated charcoal binds to the nephrotoxic substances; in this case, repeated doses may be beneficial. Fluid therapy should be administered for a minimum of 48–72 hours and serum chemistry values monitored for at least 72 hours for indications of AKI [11].

For lily nephrotoxicity, asymptomatic cats and those with only mild azotemia within the first 48 hours following exposure should be managed with gastric decontamination and diuresis. Vomiting should be induced if exposure was recent (within 8–12 hours) to try to minimize the quantity of toxin absorbed. Alpha-2 adrenoceptor agonists or hydrogen peroxide can be used to induce emesis (see Chapter 127) [10]. Gastric lavage could be considered for cats ingesting a large amount of plant material, unless contraindicated. Oral activated charcoal may be considered to help reduce gastrointestinal absorption, but it is unknown if this is actually effective since the kinetics of the unknown nephrotoxin are still yet to be documented. Diuresis can be produced by administering normal saline intravenously at twice

---

Box 134.2 Initial gastric decontamination recommendations (see Chapter 127 for further details)

Inducing emesis
- Apomorphine (0.02–0.04 mg/kg IV or IM). It can also be administered by placing it directly behind the eyelid in the subconjunctival sac.
- Xylazine can be used in cats with limited effectiveness (0.44 mg/kg IM or SC).
- Dexmedetomidine 7–10 mcg/kg IM, SC

Charcoal
- Dosage varies with individual products.
- Powdered activated charcoal and water (2–5 g/kg of body weight (1 g activated charcoal in 5 mL water)). If sorbitol is added as a cathartic, it is given at a dose of 3 mg/kg and mixed with the activated charcoal. Repeat administration of activated charcoal every 4–6 hours for 2–3 days may be beneficial.

maintenance rates and continued for 48 hours (see Chapter 167).

Patients should be monitored very closely for lack of urine output, weight gain, and other signs of hypervolemia (serous nasal and ocular discharge, tachypnea, dyspnea, peripheral edema, etc.) as this may indicate the patient is oligoanuric. These patients are best managed as described below. The water solubility of the nephrotoxin suggests that it is amenable to removal via hemodialysis [12]. Although this may be considered as an adjunctive means of toxin removal, its efficacy is unknown, as is the intensity and duration of dialysis necessary to ensure sufficient toxin removal (see Chapter 129).

Managing Patients with Established Acute Kidney Injury

Dogs with grape/raisin nephrotoxicity may be polyuric or oligoanuric. Oligoanuric acute kidney injury is the most common result of significant lily nephrotoxicity. Affected cats may remain anuric for 1–2 weeks before starting to produce urine again. The return of urine production is often gradual and not typically associated with a massive polyuria phase, as observed with postobstruction diuresis and recovery from leptospirosis. Oligoanuric animals should be given intravenous fluids only if hypovolemic or dehydrated, with the volume of fluid administered being calculated to correct these abnormalities. Subsequent intravenous fluid therapy should be performed very cautiously, as patients are quite prone to iatrogenic hypervolemia when anuric. Hypervolemic patients should not receive intravenous fluids, and pharmacological conversion to polyuria may be attempted when extracorporeal renal replacement (ERRT) is not an option (see Chapter 129).

Hyperkalemia may be managed by administering intravenous insulin + dextrose, beta-2 agonists, sodium bicarbonate, and sodium polystyrene. Intravenous calcium is indicated for treating arrhythmias resulting from hyperkalemia, but the serum potassium concentration still needs to be corrected (see Chapter 109). Due to the severity of azotemia and prolonged duration of oligoanuria, extracorporeal renal replacement therapy or peritoneal dialysis should be considered. An esophagostomy tube can be used to provide enteral nutrition, medication delivery, and accessibility for enteral water. Jugular venepuncture or catheterization should be avoided in all candidates for ERRT. Hypertension should be managed with amlodipine (PO or rectal) to reach a target systolic blood pressure < 160 mmHg (see Chapter 63).

Nutritional support should be initiated as early as the patient will tolerate, with preference given to the enteral route. Parenteral nutrition can be considered in patients which have severe or protracted gastrointestinal symptoms, but vascular access may be difficult, particularly in patients that also require ERRT. Prescription renal diets are indicated, with the diet containing the lowest amount of potassium per 100 kcal likely being most helpful in the management of hyperkalemic patients. Due to the catabolic nature of AKI and ERRT, animals typically require more than their calculated metabolic energy requirements to prevent loss of fat and muscle mass. Phosphate binders can be administered with meals and antinausea medications and antacids given as needed.

Prognosis

Approximately 25–60% of dogs will remain asymptomatic following grape or raisin exposure [2,11]. Dogs which developed AKI reportedly had a 53% survival rate. The median time until resolution of azotemia in surviving dogs was 16 days for BUN and 30 days for creatinine, although some dogs took months until normalization occurred. Eighteen percent of surviving dogs failed to regain normal renal function [2]. ERRT was used to successfully manage a dog with currant nephrotoxicity, allowing management of uremia until return of renal function occurred [13].

The prognosis for cats which have been given supportive care shortly after exposure is good, up to 100% survival in one study [10]. Cats developing AKI have reportedly had a grave prognosis, 50–100% mortality in several studies [4,6,9,14]. Successful resolution of AKI has been reported following management with ERRT [15]. Survival rate for cats treated with dialysis is reportedly 50% [16].

References

1 Gwaltney-Brant S, Holding JK, Donaldson CW, Eubig PA, Khan SA. Renal failure associated with ingestion of grapes or raisins in dogs. *J Am Vet Med Assoc* 2001;218(10):1555–1556.

2 Eubig PA, Brady MS, Gwaltney-Brant SM, Khan SA, Mazzaferro EM, Morrow CMK. Acute renal failure in dogs after the ingestion of grapes or raisins: a retrospective evaluation of 43 dogs (1992–2002). *J Vet Intern Med* 2005;19(5):663–674.

3 Morrow CMK, Valli VE, Volmer PA, Eubig PA. Canine renal pathology associated with grape or raisin ingestion: 10 cases. *J Vet Diagn Invest* 2005;17(3):223–231.

4 Brady MA, Janovitz EB. Nephrotoxicosis in a cat following ingestion of Asiatic hybrid lily (Lilium sp). *J Vet Diagn Invest* 2000;12(6):566–568.

5 Rumbeiha WK, Francis JA, Fitzgerald SD, et al. A comprehensive study of Easter lily poisoning in cats. *J Vet Diagn Invest* 2004;16(6):527–541.

6 Langston CE. Acute renal failure caused by lily ingestion in six cats. *J Am Vet Med Assoc* 2002;220(1):49–52, 36.

7 Slater MR, Gwaltney-Brant S. Exposure circumstances and outcomes of 48 households with 57 cats exposed to toxic lily species. *J Am Anim Hosp Assoc* 2011;47(6):386–390.

8 Uhlig S, Hussain F, Wisløff H. Bioassay-guided fractionation of extracts from Easter lily (Lilium longiflorum) flowers reveals unprecedented structural variability of steroidal glycoalkaloids. *Toxicon* 2014;92:42–49.

9 Hadley RM, Richardson JA, Gwaltney-Brant SM. A retrospective study of daylily toxicosis in cats. *Vet Hum Toxicol* 2003;45(1):38–39.

10 Bennett AJ, Reineke EL. Outcome following gastrointestinal tract decontamination and intravenous fluid diuresis in cats with known lily ingestion: 25 cases (2001–2010). *J Am Vet Med Assoc* 2013;242(8):1110–1116.

11 Sutton NM, Bates N, Campbell A. Factors influencing outcome of Vitis vinifera (grapes, raisins, currants and sultanas) intoxication in dogs. *Vet Rec* 2009;164(14):430–431.

12 Monaghan KN, Acierno MJ. Extracorporeal removal of drugs and toxins. *Vet Clin North Am Small Anim Pract* 2011;41(1):227–238.

13 Stanley SW, Langston CE. Hemodialysis in a dog with acute renal failure from currant toxicity. *Can Vet J* 2008;49(1):63–66.

14 Worwag S, Langston CE. Acute intrinsic renal failure in cats: 32 cases (1997–2004). *J Am Vet Med Assoc* 2008;232(5):728–732.

15 Berg RIM, Francey T, Segev G. Resolution of acute kidney injury in a cat after lily (Lilium lancifolium) intoxication. *J Vet Intern Med* 2007;21(4):857–859.

16 Lippi I, Ross S, Masato F, Cowgill LD. Acute kidney injury secondary to lily intoxication in 30 cats. Presented at ACVIM Forum, Seattle, 2013.

135

Recreational Drug Intoxications
Melissa Bucknoff, DVM, DACVECC

School of Veterinary Medicine, Ross University, Bassetterre, St Kitts, West Indies

Cocaine

Cocaine is an illicit drug with profound sympathomimetic and psychostimulatory effects. Its use is prevalent, making it the second most problematic illicit drug after heroin [1]. Derived from the leaves of the alkaloid coca plant and processed into a powder, it can be insufflated (snorted), injected, or smoked in free-base form (crack). Solid white powder forms contain 12–16% cocaine salts that are cut with adulterants (lidocaine, benzoaine, caffeine, amphetamines) [2].

Despite its prevalent use in people, cocaine toxicity is uncommonly reported in dogs, and only one case report in a cat [3]. A recent retrospective study in dogs with presumptive cocaine intoxication found neurological abnormalities to be the most common presenting sign, followed by cardiovascular effects, and all dogs in the study survived to hospital discharge [1]. Due to the complex pharmacological properties of cocaine and its derivatives, it is still considered potentially life-threatening. Working police dogs may be at higher risk of exposure, and the use of a muzzle has been advocated to help minimize intoxications [4].

Mechanism and Toxicokinetics

Sympathomimetic effects are due to reuptake inhibition of norepinephrine (NE), serotonin, and dopamine. Stimulation of endogenous catecholamine release causes direct effects on the myocardium and CNS. Neuroendocrine system dysregulation occurs with effects on appetite, sleep, alertness, and body temperature.

Cocaine is rapidly acting and readily crosses the blood–brain barrier. Plasma concentrations peak within 15–20 minutes of exposure. Metabolism is through hydrolysis by plasma and hepatic esterases and 10–20% is excreted unchanged in the urine.

- Oral LD_{50} in dogs: 6–12 mg/kg and 3.5 mg/kg for IV/SC
- LD in cats: 7.5 mg/kg IV, 16 mg/kg SC

Clinical Signs

Hyperexcitability, hypervigilance, muscle tremors, ataxia, seizures, mydriasis, hypersalivation, tachycardia, tachyarrhythmias, hypertension, hyperthermia, and vomiting. Kidney injury may occur from rhabdomyolysis.

Differential Diagnoses

Stimulants such as amphetamines, methamphetamine, serotonergic drugs, and caffeine. Other causes of seizures and/or tremors include mycotoxins ("garbage gut"), strychnine, or metaldehyde. Additionally, pheochromocytomas may have similar clinical signs.

Diagnostics

Urine multidrug test kits for humans can be used as a point-of-care diagnostic tool, although they must be interpreted with caution (Table 135.1). Currently, there are no validated veterinary urine drug-screening tests. A positive test result is identified by the presence of a color change observed within each channel. The major limitation with these test kits is the possibility of false-negative results, which may occur in peracute cases or when drug concentrations are below the minimal detection limit. A positive test for cocaine may be seen for 2–3 days following exposure.

Minimum database is performed as a screening test. Urinalysis may reveal markers of acute kidney injury (myoglobinuria, granular casts, glucosuria, proteinuria) (see Chapter 94).

Treatment

No specific antidote exists and treatment is supportive (see Table 135.1). Decontamination through emesis is performed in cases when large quantities have been consumed, but must be avoided when neurological signs

Textbook of Small Animal Emergency Medicine, First Edition. Edited by Kenneth J. Drobatz, Kate Hopper, Elizabeth Rozanski and Deborah C. Silverstein.
© 2019 John Wiley & Sons, Inc. Published 2019 by John Wiley & Sons, Inc.
Companion Website: www.wiley.com/go/drobatz/textbook

Table 135.1 Treatment overview of recreational drug intoxication.

Treatment	Dosage and remarks
*Decontamination	Emesis: apomorphine 0.03 mg/kg IV
	Adsorption: activated charcoal
	Gastric lavage (intubation required)
Anxiolytics	Diazepam or midazolam 0.25–0.5 mg/kg IV
	Acepromazine 0.01–0.05 mg/kg IV, IM, SC, transmucosal
	Chlorpromazine 0.5–1 mg/kg IV
Anticonvulsants	Short-acting: diazepam or midazolam IV or intranasal
	Long-acting: phenobarbital 8–16 mg/kg IV loading dose or 2–4 mg/kg IV q12h; levetiracetam 20–40 mg/kg IV q8h
Antiarrhythmics	Lidocaine 2–8 mg/kg IV to effect in dogs; 0.25–0.5 mg/kg in cats (caution!)
	Propranolol 0.02 mg/kg IV slowly (maximum 1 mg/kg)
	Esmolol CRI
Reversal agents	Flumazenil 0.05 mg/kg IV
	Naloxone 0.01–0.04 mg/kg IV or IM
Antiemetics	Maropitant 1 mg/kg SC (off-label in cats)
	Ondansetron 0.1–0.2 mg/kg IV q8–12h

*Contraindicated with CNS depression.

CRI, constant-rate infusion; IM, intramuscular; IV, intravenous; SC, subcutaneous.

are present due to seizure potential and aspiration risk (see Chapter 127). Gastric lavage may be considered if the quantity ingested is potentially lethal. Activated charcoal with cathartic (sorbitol) can be given once, but repeated dosing is likely ineffective due to rapid absorption. Endoscopy or surgery can be considered to retrieve intact bags of cocaine, although caution must be taken to avoid their rupture.

Central nervous system (CNS) stimulation must be minimized to reduce mania and avoid seizure precipitation. A quiet, dim-lit room is ideal, but the patient must be in an area where ongoing monitoring is feasible. Monitor blood pressure and ECG and treat life-threatening arrhythmias as indicated (see Chapter 53). Hyperthermic patients should be actively cooled using water baths, ice packs, and fans (see Chapter 147). Take care to avoid overcooling (stop at 103–103.5 °F). IV fluids are used to promote renal excretion of the drug. Give antiemetics as needed.

Prognosis

Prognosis depends on quantity ingested and severity of signs. Outcome can be good with supportive care.

Multiple organ dysfunction may develop and cardiac arrest is possible (see Chapter 159).

Methamphetamine

Methamphetamine ("meth") is a highly addictive psychoactive stimulant. Its abuse as a recreational drug in people is widespread across the country. Crystal meth, the precipitated rock form, is used for smoking. Powdered meth can be insufflated, ingested, or injected IV. Effects are similar to cocaine, with much more potency [5].

Methamphetamine toxicity is almost certainly underreported due to the legal implications associated with its possession. Crude home laboratories are common sites for manufacturing methamphetamine from precursor drugs like ephedrine. Dogs may have unguarded access to such areas, creating exposure risk.

Mechanism and Toxicokinetics

Sympathomimetic stimulant effects are through inhibition of monoamine oxidase (MAO), increased catecholamine release, and direct dopamine and serotonin receptor agonism. Distribution is mainly to the kidneys, liver, and lung. Metabolism is via hepatic hydroxylation and deamination followed by renal excretion.

- Oral LD_{50} in dogs: 9–100 mg/kg [5]

Clinical Signs

Multisystemic effects include serotonin syndrome, hyperactivity, restlessness, hypersalivation, ataxia, tremors, seizures, altered mentation, and hyperthermia. Morbidity from cardiac arrhythmias, hypertension, and disseminated intravascular coagulation (DIC) may lead to death.

Diagnostics and Treatment

Urine can be tested for methamphetamine. Supportive treatment is indicated based on clinical signs. Urinary acidification increases rate of excretion.

Differential Diagnoses

Central nervous system stimulants, cocaine, Ma Huang (ephedra), MDMA, and other "designer drugs."

Prognosis

Respiratory, renal, and liver failure can cause death in severe cases.

Table 135.2 Sources of marijuana.

Preparation	THC source	Average THC concentration
Cigarette ("joint")	Crude plant material (dried)	3%
Seedless ("sinsemilla") Hashish	Resin from tops of flowering plant	≥10%
Hash oil		≥20%
Medical-grade butter	Extract from boiled plant	≥[THC] in plant
Synthetic cannabinoids	Synthetic herbal incenses	High potency

THC, delta-9-tetrahydrocannabinol.

Marijuana

Derived from the *Cannabis sativa* hemp plant, marijuana refers to tobacco-like dried preparations of leaves, flowers, seeds, and stems. Marijuana is the most common illicit drug in the United States and its availability has increased greatly over the past decade [6], now being legal for personal use in some states. Toxicity is due to the psychoactive compound delta-9-tetrahydrocannabinol (THC). "Hashish" refers to the highly concentrated resin from the flowering portion of the plant. Dogs are extremely susceptible to the effects of THC.

Marijuana has a wide safety margin. Toxic effects correlate with absorbed THC concentrations, which vary by preparation and cultivation technique. Medical-grade THC butter used in baked goods contains the most concentrated forms of the drug (Table 135.2).

Mechanism and Toxicokinetics

Intoxication is most commonly via oral exposure, but second-hand smoke inhalation is theoretically possible. THC absorption following ingestion is slower and more erratic than with smoking. Oral absorption can be increased with concurrent ingestion of fatty foods, such as brownies, or edibles infused with THC butter. Onset of clinical signs in dogs generally occurs within 1–2 hours following ingestion.

Delta-9-tetrahydrocannabinol is highly lipophilic with a large volume of distribution to the liver, brain, kidneys, and adipose tissue. Following ingestion, THC is converted in the liver and lung to 11-hydroxy-delta-9-THC, the primary metabolite. Excretion is 85% biliary via enterohepatic recirculation and 15% renal. Elimination half-life from adipose stores is approximately 30 hours [6].

Oral LD of THC in dogs is > 3 g/kg, approximately 1000 times the dose where behavioral or neurological effects are seen. An average joint contains 15–30 mg of THC [6]. Estimating toxic doses is challenging due to variable drug purities and lack of witnessed exposure in many cases.

The two major cannabinoid receptors are CB_1 and CB_2. The CB_1 receptor is located primarily within the CNS.he CB_2 receptor is found in peripheral tissues. CB_1 receptor activation inhibits multiple neurotransmitters (acetylcholine, glutamate, GABA, norepinephrine, dopamine, 5-HT). Both inhibit adenyl cyclase and increase potassium channel conductance [7]. All clinical effects of THC are thought to be due to activity at CB_1 receptors. CB_2 receptor effects are less well elucidated. Evidence suggests roles in inflammation, immune modulation, and analgesia, making it a therapeutic target for medically prescribed marijuana.

Clinical Signs

Delta-9-tetrahydrocannabinol can induce a wide range of non-specific clinical signs that vary in severity and duration, depending on the dose and route. The most common clinical signs in dogs are ataxia, depression, altered mentation, urinary incontinence, hypersalivation, mydriasis, vomiting, tremors, nystagmus, vocalizing, bradycardia, hypo- or hyperthermia, sensitivity to light and sound, and coma and death in severe cases. A recent retrospective study reported that nearly half the dogs presented with urinary incontinence, a finding that may be more common with exposure to medical-grade marijuana [8]. Additional effects include direct gastrointestinal irritation, particularly with large amounts of plant material. Patient factors, such as age, size, and co-morbidities, can influence severity of toxic effects. Signs can persist from 1–3 days in dogs (average 24 hours) [6].

In the event of concurrent chocolate ingestion, stimulatory effects from caffeine and theobromide may confound the classic clinical findings associated with marijuana. Dogs may be at risk for developing foreign body obstruction after consuming plastic bags full of marijuana [6].

Differential Diagnoses

Hallucinogenics, CNS stimulants or depressants, other recreational plants and drugs.

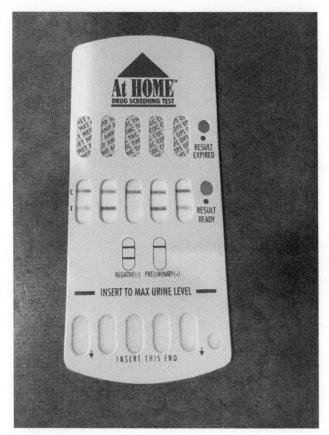

Figure 135.1 Example of a multichannel urine dipstick drug screening test with a positive result for THC.

Diagnostics

Urine can be tested for cannabinoids. However, dog urine may contain altered THC metabolites not detected via human drug-screening kits, making their use controversial [8] (Figure 135.1). Sample handling can also cause false-negative test results, as THC can bind to rubber stoppers and glass. While results of urine drug tests must be interpreted with caution, it is generally accepted that a positive test most likely indicates true THC toxicity and a negative test does not exclude the possibility of exposure [9].

Confirmatory testing through gas chromatography mass spectrometry is considered the gold standard for detection in people, but it is of questionable value in dogs. Stomach contents may be evaluated for cannabinoids. Consultation with a toxicology laboratory is recommended prior to specimen submission.

Treatment

There is no specific antidote for marijuana. Treatment objectives center around supportive care. As with other intoxicants, decontamination is the most effective way to minimize further drug absorption. Emesis induction may prove unrewarding due to the significant antiemetic effects of THC. Some dogs may vomit due to direct effects of the drug, resulting in autodecontamination.

Activated charcoal is an effective adsorption agent for a plethora of toxic compounds and may be given to reduce enterohepatic recirculation of THC. Case selection is paramount, as risks of treatment should never outweigh benefits. Aspiration of charcoal can result in severe morbidity or mortality. It is important to remember that the majority of marijuana toxicity cases are not fatal, even without specific gastrointestinal intervention.

Antianxiety medications are used to sedate acutely agitated patients. IV fluids can be given to treat volume deficits from significant vomiting. Patients may be debilitated in severe cases, requiring intensive nursing care, IV fluids, and airway management. Sternal positioning with elevation of the head may minimize risk of aspiration and atelectasis. Antiemetics may be indicated for ongoing vomiting or nausea.

Recently, the use of intravenous lipid therapy has been proposed for treatment of the highly lipophilic THC (see Chapter 128). The exact mechanism is unknown, but it likely works in several ways [10], although a full description is beyond this chapter's scope. Intralipid therapy is often well tolerated, but can be associated with adverse effects. While it cannot be advocated as part of routine treatment, it may be considered in severe cases of high-potency THC ingestion, such as medical-grade butter. Currently, there are no prospective studies evaluating its utility in dogs with THC toxicity.

Prognosis

Prognosis is very good in most cases, with full recovery made within 24–72 hours. Recovery may be prolonged in animals exposed to very large doses of THC. Two canine deaths have been reported following ingestion of medical-grade butter [8].

Conclusion

Exposure to recreational drugs is possible in dogs, and much less so in cats (Table 135.3). Thoughtful questioning as to possible exposure may result in a greater likelihood of gaining knowledge of possible exposure. In most accidental exposures, there are no legal ramifications, but it may be worthwhile to have a practice policy and consult with local officials.

Table 135.3 Summary of recreational drugs and their effects.

Generic name/street name	Mechanism of action	Clinical signs
MDMA (ecstasy, Molly)	SSRI; stimulates serotonin release	CNS stimulation, hallucinations
GHB (date rape drug)	Synthetic GABA derivative; modulates dopamine signaling	CNS depression
Flunitrazepam (Rohypnol)	Benzodiazepine; opens chloride channels on CNS GABA receptor	Muscle relaxation, sedation, disorientation, hallucinations
LSD (acid)	Serotonin receptor partial agonist; increases glutamate release; binds dopamine and alpha-adrenergic receptors	Hyperexcitability, hallucinations, vomiting, disorientation, mydriasis, tachycardia, depression, compulsive scratching in litter box, increased grooming (cats)
Lysergic acid amide substances (LSAs)	Hallucinogenic seeds from morning glory and Hawaiian baby rose plant; serotonergic	Similar to LSD
Ketamine (Special K)	Dissociative agent; antagonizes glutamate at NMDA receptor by blocking calcium influx	CNS stimulation, ataxia, hallucinations, nystagmus, aggression, cataplexy
PCP (angel dust)	Dissociative agent, similar to ketamine; prolonged effects	CNS stimulation or depression, tremors, tachycardia, arrhythmias, hypo- or hypertension, hyperthermia, rhabdomyolysis, renal failure
Opioids (opium, heroin, oxycodone, morphine, codeine, meperidine, hydromorphone, fentanyl)	Opioid receptor agonist/antagonist effects; varies with drug	CNS depression (dogs) and stimulation (cats), emesis, hypoventilation, ileus

CNS, central nervous system; GABA, gamma-aminobutyric acid; GHB, gamma-hydroxybutyric acid; LSD, lysergic acid diethylamide; MDMA, methylendioxymethamphetamine; PCP, phencyclidine; SSRI, selective serotonin reuptake inhibitor.

References

1 Thomas EK, Drobatz KJ, Mandell DC. Presumptive cocaine toxicosis in 19 dogs: 2004–2012. *J Vet Emerg Crit Care* 2014;24(2):201–207.
2 Bischoff K, Kang HG. Cocaine. In: *Small Animal Toxicology* (eds Osweiler GD, Hovda LR, Brutlag AG). Wiley-Blackwell, Ames, 2011, pp. 212–217.
3 Barfield DM, Pegrum SA, Snow D, et al. Pupillary dilation, tachycardia and abnormal behaviour in a young cat. Diagnosis: cocaine intoxication. *J Feline Med Surg* 2007;9(4):265–270.
4 Llera RM, Volmer PA. Toxicologic hazards for police dogs involved in drug detection. *J Am Vet Med Assoc* 2006;228(7):1028–1032.
5 Drotar TK. Methamphetamine. In: *Small Animal Toxicology* (eds Osweiler GD, Hovda LR, Brutlag AG). Wiley-Blackwell, Ames, 2011, pp. 230–236.
6 Fitzgerald KT, Bronstein AC, Newquist KL. Marijuana poisoning. *Topics Compan Anim Med* 2013;28:8–12.
7 McGuigon M. Cannabinoids. In: *Goldfrank's Toxicological Emergencies*, 8th edn (eds Goldfrank LR, Flomenabaum NE, Lewin NA). McGraw-Hill, New York, 2006, pp. 1212–1220.
8 Meola, SD, Tearney CC, Sharlee AH, et al. Evaluation of trends in marijuana toxicosis in dogs living in a state with legalized medical marijuana: 125 dogs (2005–2010). *J Vet Emerg Crit Care* 2012;22(6):690–696.
9 Teitler JB. Evaluation of a human on-site urine multidrug test for emergency use with dogs. *J Am Anim Hosp Assoc* 2009;45(2):59–66.
10 Gwaltney-Brant S, Meadows I. Use of intravenous lipid emulsions for treating certain poisoning cases in small animals. *Vet Clin Small Anim* 2012;42:251–262.

136

Household Toxins

Lindsey Nielsen, DVM, DACVECC

Veterinary Emergency and Specialty Centers of New Mexico, Albuquerque, NM, USA

Decontamination

One of the most effective ways to limit the clinical effects of toxins on patients is to perform decontamination processes as indicated. The type of toxin, time from exposure, and type of exposure can all influence which decontamination procedures are undertaken. Decontamination techniques are discussed in detail in Chapter 127.

Common Household Toxin Exposures

Foods

Xylitol

Xylitol is a sugar alcohol used as a sugar substitute or sweetener in sugar-free products. It is most commonly found in chewing gum, but can also be found in products like baked goods or even some peanut butters. Ingestion of over 0.1 g/kg of xylitol by dogs causes a massive increase in insulin secretion, leading to a subsequent hypoglycemia for 12–48 hours following ingestion [1]. In addition to hypoglycemia, ingestion of >0.5 g/kg of xylitol will cause subsequent hepatic necrosis and fulminant liver failure anywhere from 9 to 72 hours following ingestion [2].

Inducing emesis should be attempted for those cases presenting within a few hours of ingestion of the product, although most commonly the xylitol is rapidly absorbed within 30 minutes of ingestion (see Chapter 127) [3]. Following decontamination attempts, most dogs should be hospitalized for glucose monitoring with dextrose supplementation when indicated. For those exposed to >0.5 g/kg, administration of liver protectants (e.g. SaME, Denosyl) and antioxidants should be initiated. Xylitol toxicity has not been described in cats.

Chocolate

Chocolate is a very common toxin exposure frequently experienced by dogs, especially around holidays when chocolate is particularly common. Chocolate is among the top five toxicities seen in veterinary hospitals according to the Pet Poison Hotline [4]. The toxic components of chocolate are methylxanthines, with caffeine and theobromine causing the most clinical signs [5]. These components can cause a range of clinical signs, worsening with increasing amounts of chocolate ingested or type of chocolate. Baker's chocolate and dark chocolate have much higher concentrations of methylxanthines compared to milk chocolate, so it is important to confirm the type of chocolate ingested. Chocolate calculators are available to help determine toxicity. "White" chocolate is not chocolate at all, so is considered non-toxic.

Initially, gastrointestinal signs such as vomiting and diarrhea can occur, but this can progress to agitation, hyperactivity, ataxia, tremors, seizures, tachycardia, arrhythmias, hypertension, hyperthermia, and even death. Clinical signs typically begin within 6 hours of ingestion and can last for up to 72 hours. Pancreatitis is also possible following chocolate ingestion due to the high fat concentration of most chocolates.

Ideally, treatment should begin with decontamination if the patient is not neurologically affected (see Chapter 127) (Figure 136.1). This should be followed with repeated doses of activated charcoal, intravenous fluid management to enhance urinary excretion of the toxic metabolites, and close monitoring of the cardiac and neurological status of the patient. When abnormalities arise, most arrhythmias can be treated with beta-blockers, such as metoprolol if available, propranolol or esmolol. Propranolol may delay excretion of methylxanthines which is why metoprolol is preferred if available [6]. Most seizures can be controlled with diazepam, although

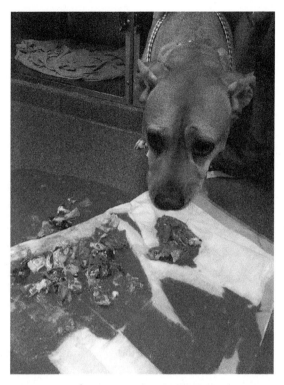

Figure 136.1 A dog being decontaminated after eating an entire bag of Halloween candy.

seizures are quite uncommon. Fortunately, most chocolate toxicity is limited to gastrointestinal signs and tachycardia, and most dogs recover uneventfully, with "death by chocolate" being very rare without co-morbidities or massive ingestion. Cats do not appear to like chocolate, so chocolate toxicity is unheard of in this species.

Onions and Garlic

Members of the *Allium* genus, such as onions, leeks, chives and garlic, have sulfur-containing compounds that when ingested in large amounts can cause red blood cell hemolysis, Heinz body formation, and methemoglobinemia [7]. Gastrointestinal signs such as vomiting and diarrhea are common, as are signs of weakness, tachypnea, and tachycardia from the anemia. Decontamination is recommended, followed by monitoring for development of anemia and symptomatic therapy for any gastrointestinal signs that develop, which may not occur for up to 5 days [8]. It should be noted that a large quantity of onions is required for clinical disease to develop. Transfusions may be required. Also, due to the differences between feline and canine hemoglobin, cats may be more sensitive to the toxic effects of *Allium* species than dogs [8]. Cat exposure has been particularly linked to human baby foods, which may have garlic or onion powder added. Dogs are most frequently exposed by ingestion of fried onions or onions mixed with meat products.

Bread Dough

Unrisen or raw bread dough can be perceived as a tasty treat by most dogs and even rarely by some cats, but when ingested, the yeast in the dough will begin to grow and ferment within the stomach. The rapid expansion of the yeast can cause abdominal distension and, more rarely, respiratory and vascular decompensation. Emesis induction is usually unsuccessful, and therefore decontamination is often achieved with gastric lavage. If the yeast ferments, ethanol will be produced and this can result in signs of alcohol intoxication, including ataxia and disorientation, with severe cases developing profound CNS depression that could require aggressive supportive care, including mechanical ventilation [9]. Recovery is usually uncomplicated and signs are resolved within 24 hours.

Outdoor Products

Many products people use in their yards for pest management can be toxic to animals. Rodenticides are a common culprit, and more information on their ingestion can be found in Chapter 130. Other common pest control products can pose a toxic threat to pets as well.

Metaldehyde

Metaldehyde is the active ingredient in snail and slug control products that can cause severe neurological derangements in animals. Most animals will develop severe muscle tremors and hyperesthesia as well as associated tachycardia and hyperthermia. Some patients may go on to develop depression, intractable seizures, respiratory failure, and death. Emesis can be attempted within 30 minutes following exposure, although the toxin is rapidly metabolized, and many patients are already showing clinical signs on presentation to the clinic [10]. Decontamination can be attempted via gastric lavage, followed by repeated doses of activated charcoal. Additional treatment is symptomatic, including diazepam for seizures, methocarbamol for tremors, and anesthesia with gas inhalants or propofol for those most severely affected until the metaldehyde is metabolized [11]. Full recovery in severely affected patients can take up to 3 days, though most patients are recovered within 24 hours.

Mulch and Fertilizer Products

Luckily, the majority of these products are not appetizing, but some can be and can contain components that can cause gastrointestinal upset and other problems. Many fertilizers contain nitrogen, phosphorus, and potassium, but some can also contain more harmful products like insecticides, cocoa, iron, or zinc [12]. Because of the wide variation in components of each product, having the client bring the packaging material or contacting poison control in each individual exposure may be helpful. Most will only cause mild gastrointestinal upset and ingestion can be treated symptomatically.

Strychnine

Strychnine is a poison historically found in various gopher baits and rodenticides used to kill ground squirrels. Its use is rare today, as it has been replaced by other pesticides. This is a highly potent poison and ingestion of only a few tablespoons can be lethal in both dogs and cats. Strychnine blocks the inhibitory actions of glycine in the central nervous system. This causes a disinhibition of motor neurons and interneurons, leading to exaggerated and overactive neuronal activity causing muscle spasms, hyperexcitability, seizures, hyperthermia, tetanus, and eventual death from respiratory paralysis [13]. The poison is rapidly absorbed and clinical signs can be seen within 15 minutes of exposure, making emesis induction difficult and often ineffective [14]. The remainder of treatments are geared towards supportive care and symptomatic treatment with diazepam, methocarbamol, and IV fluid therapy. For those severely affected, anesthesia and mechanical ventilation may be required until the toxin is cleared from the body, which can take up to 72 hours.

Cleaning Products

Most cleaning products are aversive and do not taste palatable, so ingestions are rare, but can be severe when they do occur. Additionally, exposure to the skin as well as eyes and mucosal surfaces can also pose threats to pets.

Soaps and Detergents

These products can be found in most of the hand soaps, body washes, and shampoos used by humans, as well as many cleaning products such as laundry or dishwashing detergents. When ingested, they can cause mild gastrointestinal signs including hypersalivation, vomiting, or diarrhea, or irritation of the skin or eyes [15]. Most of these signs are self-limiting but may require symptomatic therapy. If a patient has an ocular exposure, flushing the eye with sterile saline for 5 minutes is recommended (see Chapter 127).

Alcohols

Alcohols, including those found in beverages, medications, bread dough, windshield cleaner, and rubbing alcohol, are all rapidly absorbed through the gastrointestinal, inhalation, and dermal routes. The rapid absorption makes decontamination difficult, and supportive treatment of clinical signs that occur is often the treatment of choice. Patients can develop vomiting, ataxia, hypothermia, hypoglycemia, acidosis, respiratory depression, coma, and death [16]. Hemodialysis is an option to more rapidly eliminate the ethanol from those that have a severe toxicosis (Chapter 129) [17].

Acids

Many household cleaning products contain acids, which can be extremely toxic for pets both locally and systemically. The acids will cause local coagulative tissue necrosis and pain in those areas where exposed [14]. When exposed orally, this will cause pain, dysphagia, vomiting, and ulceration of the oral cavity and esophagus. Dermal exposure will cause irritation or ulceration. Ocular exposure can be severe, causing corneal ulceration or melting.

Acids are some of the few toxins where decontamination is not advocated due to the risk of worsening corrosive injury. Initially, administering water or milk to the patient may dilute the product and limit the effects of exposure. Following this, treatment is mostly symptomatic and geared towards pain management. For dermal or ocular exposures, flushing with copious amounts of water for over 15 minutes is recommended (see Chapter 127).

Alkalis

Alkalis are also found in many household cleaning products, including some cationic detergents, and many plumbing products. These agents will cause severe corrosive injury without associated pain, which is why clinical signs may not immediately be apparent. Clinical signs that do develop are often related to the underlying mucosal damage caused to the gastrointestinal tract, which can be severe enough to cause perforation [18]. Emesis should not be induced and charcoal is not effective in these patients. Supportive care and investigation for the extent of esophageal and gastrointestinal damage that has occurred should take place.

Foreign Objects

Many owners have experienced the stress that comes with a playful and inquisitive puppy ingesting a foreign object, which often poses more of a threat by potentially causing a gastrointestinal obstruction. However, some common household objects can also pose a toxic threat to the pets that ingest them.

Pennies

Pennies minted in the United States after 1982 are made primarily of zinc and coated with a thin layer of copper [19]. After a penny is ingested by an animal, the gastric juices will cause zinc to leach out of the coin and enter the systemic circulation, where it will cause zinc toxicity in the form of intravascular hemolysis [20]. Dogs with evidence of intravascular hemolysis should be radiographed to exclude penny ingestion.

Treatment includes removal of the penny so that the patient is no longer being exposed to zinc, which can be achieved by emesis induction, endoscopic removal or surgical removal. Following removal of the coin, treatment for the subsequent anemia with blood products and supportive care is advocated. Pancreatitis has been reported following zinc toxicity.

Batteries

Ingestion of batteries can pose several threats to pets. When chewed, they can release their contents, which are often alkaline in nature, causing alkali burns. When swallowed whole, they can cause foreign body obstructions that commonly require surgical intervention to remove.

Treatment of battery exposures often involves first treating for the possibility of alkali exposure by giving the patient water to delay the chance of internal corrosive damage to the gastrointestinal tract [21]. Feeding a bulky diet may help the battery pass through the intestinal tract without causing damage, but if there is any question or concern about the object not passing, surgical or endoscopic removal should be undertaken.

Magnets

In addition to potentially causing a foreign body obstruction, when multiple magnets are ingested by a pet they can attract each other from differing segments of bowel and can lead to pressure necrosis of the intestinal tract and subsequent septic peritonitis [22]. Magnet ingestion should be taken seriously, and if multiple magnets have been ingested, surgical intervention should be considered.

Conclusion

There are hundreds of potential toxic threats that a pet may be exposed to in the household. A basic understanding of decontamination and the results of exposure to the more commonly encountered household toxins can help the emergency clinician to provide the best care for the poisoned pet.

References

1 Dunayer EK, Gwaltney-Brand SM. Acute hepatic failure and coagulopathy associated with xylitol ingestion in eight dogs. *J Am Vet Med Assoc* 2006;229(7):1113–1117.

2 Dunayer EK. New findings on the effects of xylitol ingestion in dogs. *Vet Med* 2006;12:791–796.

3 Murphy LA, Coleman AE. Xylitol toxicosis in dogs. *Vet Clin Small Anim* 2012;42:307–312.

4 Pet Poison Helpline. Top 10 Dog Toxins of 2014. Available at: www.petpoisonhelpline.com/uncategorized/top-10-dog-toxins-of-2014/(accessed 7 February 2018).

5 Carson TL. Methylxanthines. In: *Small Animal Toxicology*, 2nd edn (eds Peterson ME, Talcott PA). Elsevier Saunders, St Louis, 2006, pp. 845–852.

6 Hooser SB, Beasley VR. Methylxanthine poisoning. In: *Current Veterinary Therapy: Small Animal Practice*, Volume IX (ed. Kirk RW). WB Saunders, Philadelphia, 1986, pp. 191–192.

7 Cope RB. Allium species poisoning in dogs and cats. *Vet Med* 2005;100(8):562–566.

8 Gugler K, Piscitelli CM, Denis J. Hidden dangers in the kitchen: common foods toxic to dogs and cats. *Compendium* 2013;35(7):E1–E6.

9 Means C. Bread dough toxicosis in dogs. *J Vet Emerg Crit Care* 2003;13(1):39–41.

10 Puschner B. Metaldehyde. In: *Small Animal Toxicology*, 2nd edn (eds Peterson ME, Talcott PA). Elsevier Saunders, St Louis, 2006, pp. 830–839.

11 Yas-Natan E, Segeve G, Aroch I. Clinical, neurological and clinicopathological signs, treatment, and outcome of metaldehyde intoxication in 18 dogs. *J Small Anim Pract* 2007;48(8):483–443.

12 Wismer T. Toxicology of common household hazards: the good, the bad, and the tasty. Proceedings of the Wild West Veterinary Conference, October 14–18 2009, Reno, NV.

13 Talcott PA. Strychnine. In: *Small Animal Toxicology*, 2nd edn (eds Peterson ME, Talcott PA). Elsevier Saunders, St Louis, 2006, pp. 1076–1082.

14 Wismer T. ABCDs of rodenticides. Proceedings of the Wild West Veterinary Conference, October 14–18 2009, Reno, NV.

15 Merck Manual for Pet Health. Household Hazards. Available at: www.merckvetmanual.com/pethealth/special_subjects/poisoning/household_hazards.html (accessed 7 February 2018).

16 Houston DM, Head LL. Acute alcohol intoxication in a dog. *Can Vet J* 1993;34:41–42.

17 Keno LA, Langston CE. Treatment of accidental ethanol intoxication with hemodialysis in a dog. *J Vet Emerg Crit Care* 2011;21(4):363–368.

18 Kore, AM, Nesselrodt A. Household cleaning products and disinfectants. *Vet Clin North Am Small Anim Pract* 1990;20(2):525–537.

19 United States Mint. The Composition of The Cent. www.usmint.gov/about_the_mint/fun_facts/?action=fun_facts2 (accessed 7 February 2018).

20 Torrance AG, Fulton RB. Zinc-induced hemolytic anemia in a dog. *J Am Vet Med Assoc* 1987;191(4): 443–444.

21 Tanaka J, Yamashita M, Yamashita M, et al. Effects of tap water on esophageal burns in dogs from button lithium batteries. *Vet Hum Toxicol* 1999;41(5):279–282.

22 Creedy N, Bates N. Ingestion of multiple magnets by a dog. *Vet Rec* 2011;169:504.

J. Skin and Soft Tissue Disease

137

Life-Threatening Dermatological Emergencies

Brian K. Roberts, DVM, DACVECC

Mountain Emergency Medical Center, Blue Ridge, GA, USA

Dermatological Emergencies

Dermatological disorders are a leading cause for pet owners to seek veterinary advice. While the incidence and prevalence of all dermatological diseases are unknown, recent surveys of dogs and cats indicate that clinical signs of alopecia, dermatitis, and otitis are in the top five reasons that prompt a visit to the veterinarian [1]. Dermatological disorders were the third most common problem at primary care practices in England, with a prevalence of 10.4% [2]. While many emergency veterinarians and specialists in emergency and critical care would not consider pruritus or alopecia as an emergency, some pet owners do. Pet owners may also visit the emergency service because of convenience which is common in human medicine [3,4]. Secondary pyoderma and dermatitis can cause systemic inflammatory response syndrome and associated organ dysfunction [5].

Methicillin-Resistant Staphylococcal Infections (MRSIs)

The rise of bacterial resistance has been a major issue in both human and veterinary medicine for decades [6,7]. Staphylococcal infections have become notorious for their resistance to multiple antibiotics (MRSA), cause of nosocomial infections, and zoonotic ability. MSRA can be caused by a variety of bacteria; most noted in humans is *Staphylococcus aureus*, while dogs and cats are typically associated with *Staphylococcus pseudointermedius* (MRSP) and *Staphylococcus schleiferi* (MRSS) [8,9]. MRSI sare found in the environment and on the surfaces of furniture, and are nasal cavity commensals in healthy persons (MRSA: 29–38%), healthy dogs (MRSP: 1.5–2%) and cats (MRSP: 4%) [10–12]. Humans are typically considered the source of a MRSA infection in pets and pets can serve as a reservoir for people [13].

Commensal MRSIs were noted in 14.5% of oral swabs of healthy, adult cats [14].

The antibiotic resistance of MRSIs is achieved through bacterial acquisition of the mecA gene which encodes a penicillin-binding protein (PBP2a) that has much lower binding affinity for beta-lactams. While most dogs and cats with MRSI pyodermas do not become systemically ill, the infections are difficult to treat since other classes of antibiotics are also rendered ineffective [15]. Methicillin-resistant *Staphylococcus pseudointermedius* growth was still present in 62% of cultures from dogs treated for pyoderma and 28.3% of dogs developed MRSP who were previously MRSP culture negative after treatment [16]. In emergency facilities, exposure to MRSIs may be more likely due to high caseload, increased numbers of patients with immunosuppression, and improper disinfection of the facility between cases.

Clinical signs of MRSIs include skin abscess, otitis externa, wounds, and pyoderma which are all common emergencies; 25% of bacterial dermatitis cultures were positive for MRSI in one study of 435 dogs [17]. Most cases of MRSI-associated dermatopathies consist of localized lesions characterized by papules, erosions, crusts, and exudates (Figure 137.1). However, there have been reports of necrotizing fasciitis with associated symptoms of sepsis (tachypnea, fever, depression), erythema multiforme (Figure 137.2), and non-healing abscesses in cats [18–20].

Differential diagnoses include superficial non-methicillin-resistant pyoderma, demodecosis, cutaneous fungal infection (*Malessezia*), cutaneous drug eruption, vasculitis, and pemphigus foliaceus. It is important to realize that MRSIs can look like almost anything which causes dermatitis.

Definitive diagnosis is based on culture and sensitivity. Since methicillin is no longer a commonly used antibiotic, oxacillin is used for sensitivity testing. Additional methods of diagnosis include PCR (gold standard) and

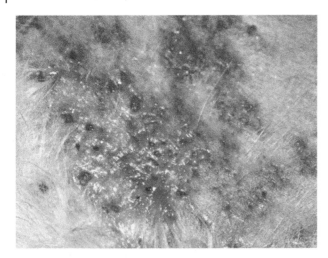

Figure 137.1 MRSA infection in a dog. Reproduced with permission of Kimberly Coyner.

latex agglutination testing to detect PBP2a. Disk diffusion combined with latex agglutination had the best specificity and sensitivity for MRSA [21]. If a *Staphylococcus* sp. is confirmed resistant to oxacillin, it is typically resistant to all beta-lactams. One should be suspicious of MRSI if a patient with a non-healing wound, folliculitis or abscess presents after completing a course of antibiotics, especially beta-lactams. Other risk factors of MRSI include use of fluoroquinolones, intravenous catheterization, having more than 10 veterinary staff employed, and postsurgery site infection [22,23].

Successful treatment of MRSI requires ruling out other causes of dermatitis and effective antimicrobial medication. The most commonly prescribed antibiotics for MRSP are chlormaphenicol and doxycycline. Other antibiotics which may be effective include aminoglycosides, minocycline, rifampin, and fluoroquinolones. The use of fluoroquinolones is not typically recommended for a number of reasons. Most importantly, these antimicrobials have the ability to create high-level MRSI mutants which are resistant to

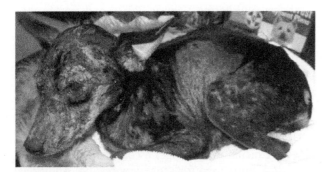

Figure 137.2 MRSA and secondary EM. Reproduced with permission of Kimberly Coyner.

many classes of antibiotics [24]. If fluoroquinolones are used, they should be limited to veterinary-labeled products because of their bioavailability and the fact that non-veterinary forms may not be well absorbed [25,26]. It is paramount that antibiotic selection is determined based on sensitivity testing. Parenteral antibiotics used in human medicine include the streptogramins (daptomycin, tigecycline, quinupristin, dalfopristin) which are administered intravenously. Use of these antimicrobials in veterinary medicine is not well documented [27].

Most infections will resolve within a month to 8 weeks of systemic antibiotic use. Like other chronic infections (i.e. fungal), antimicrobial treatment should extend for 2–3 weeks after clinical signs resolve. The time for the pyoderma to resolve is more likely to be due to the chronic nature of the dermatopathy, not the virulence of the MRSI [28].

Burns

Cutaneous thermal injuries or burns are not commonly reported in small animals [29]. The incidence and prevalence of burn injuries were not noted in the veterinary literature. Common causes of burns affecting dogs and cats include electric heating pads, open flames, mufflers of motor vehicles, hot water bottles, improperly grounded electrosurgical units, animal dryers, boiling liquids, sun exposure, and even garden hoses lying in the sun that contain residual water [30–33]. Other types of burns include chemical and radiation exposure which will not be discussed in this section. Due to haired skin, thermal injuries are sometimes overlooked. Heating pad and hot water bottle thermal injuries can take time to declare. Most importantly, other injuries to the respiratory system, cardiovascular system, kidneys, and neurological system may accompany thermal injuries, especially in cases of smoke exposure and carbon monoxide toxicity [34].

Cutaneous burns are classified based on surface area affected and depth of affected tissue. The "Rule of Nines" is a classification system used in human medicine, and sometimes in veterinary medicine, which describes percentage of total body surface area (TBSA) burned. In burned persons, the body is divided into affected zones with a corresponding percentage of surface area. Burns to the head, each forelimb and neck comprise 9% of TBSA. Burns affecting the dorsal trunk, ventral trunk and each hindlimb account for 18% of TBSA [35]. Local burns are those that injure < 20% of TBSA and typically do not cause SIRS. Severe burn injury affects > 20–30% of TBSA and usually leads to systemic derangements in homeostasis, causing SIRS (see Chapter 159).

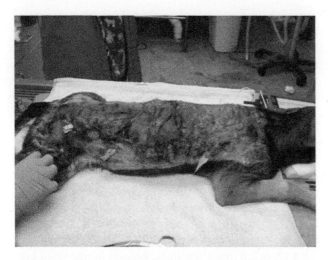

Figure 137.3 Five-day-old, third-degree burn injury post drain placement. Reproduced with permission of Kimberly Coyner.

Depth of burned tissue is classified as "degree" of injury. First-degree burns or superficial burns involve the epidermis, causing hyperemia and pain. Second-degree or partial-thickness burns affect the epidermis and upper portions of the dermis. These deeper burns are characterized by pain and blistering with the hair remaining intact. Third-degree or full-thickness burns encompass the epidermis and entire dermis (Figure 137.3). Fourth-degree burns have even deeper tissue injury, with not only the epidermis and dermis affected, but also extension to muscle, tendon and bone [36]. Neither method of burn classification has been validated in small animals, but they are generally accepted ways of characterizing burns.

Patients with severe burns to the muzzle, nose, and eyes may have smoke inhalation. Visualization of blisters in those areas, burn-induced alopecia, soot, black-tinged sputum, singed whiskers and erythema with blisters in the oropharynx are indicators of smoke inhalation. Confirmation using co-oximetry or comparison of pulse oximetry to arterial blood gas, and elevated central venous oxygen partial pressure can support the diagnosis.

Associated respiratory disorders include hypoventilation, bronchospasm, obstruction, and ARDS [37]. Cardiac arrhythmias and hypotension can result from carbon monoxide and cyanide toxicosis. Acute kidney injury may ensue from hypotension secondary to cardiovascular derangements and hypovolemia associated with cutaneous burns fluid loss (see Chapter 94). Hypoxia and cyanide will affect the neurological system, causing altered mentation such as stupor and coma, tremors, ataxia, and seizures [38].

The local response of the skin to thermal injury is characterized by cytokine activation by immunocytes, ischemia, and loss of cell membrane integrity. Increased cell membrane permeability, caused by cytoskeleton disruption and loss of hydrostatic forces, is the most important reason for tissue necrosis. Epidermal and deeper cells closest to the heat source undergo coagulation and vascular thrombosis, suffering the most damage. Surrounding tissues are affected by blood stasis and edema from capillary leak syndrome. These factors and hypoperfusion result in ischemia; however, these tissues may be salvageable [39].

Immediately after a severe burn injury, systemic inflammation develops and remains in place for months, causing ARDS, capillary leak, myocardial dysfunction, and poor perfusion (see Chapter 159). Edema from hypoalbuminemia and vasoactive substances such as thromboxane along with inducible nitric oxide (iNOS) worsen hypoxia. Cytokines and other inflammatory proteins produce marked hyperalgesia of the injury site. Levels of inflammatory mediators (interleukin-1 and -6, tumor necrosis factor alpha) are used as markers of burn severity in humans. High levels are associated with severe pain, hypermetabolism, and tissue catabolism [40]. Hyperglycemia and insulin resistance have been documented in human burn injury. Persistent, significant hyperglycemia is associated with bacterial and fungal sepsis with higher mortality rates in burned persons. Tight glycemic control with insulin can blunt the proinflammatory response but can also cause hypoglycemia and increased mortality [41,42].

Treatment of burn injuries is three-fold. First, life-threatening complications such as carbon monoxide poisoning, cyanide toxicity, ARDS, pain, and hypovolemia must be assessed for and treated with oxygen, mechanical ventilation (if indicated), analgesics, and judicious intravenous fluids (see Chapter 139). Monitoring of central venous pressure trends, especially in patients with ARDS, can assist in guiding fluid rates. Patients in shock and/or with SIRS need intravenous fluids (crystalloid 25 mL/kg over 15 min for dogs; 15 mL/kg over 15 min in cats then reassess vital signs and blood pressure) for optimized oxygen delivery (see Chapter 167) [43]. Severe burn patients will lose a significant amount of protein, water, and electrolytes from their wounds. These patients will have higher than maintenance (3–5 mL/kg/h) requirement of isotonic crystalloid [44]. Colloids (Vetstarch®, Hetastarch®) are alternatives to isotonic crystalloids for patients with hypoalbuminemia and capillary leak syndrome (see Chapter 168). However, colloids may also extravasate, worsening interstitial edema. Colloids have come under scrutiny for worsening and causing acute kidney in critically ill people but these complications have not been reported in small animals [45].

Oncotic pressure measurement can help guide dosage of intravenous colloids, which are generally provided at rates of 10–20 mL/kg/day [46]. Use of different isotonic crystalloids with different sodium content, correction of hypokalemia with added potassium chloride, and supplementation of magnesium (MgSO$_4$ 0.1–0.15 mEq/kg loading, 0.75–1 mEq/kg/day replacement) are based on serial monitoring of electrolytes (see Chapters 110 and 173) [47].

Monitoring of complications such as hypotension, hypoxia, and arrhythmias should be undertaken (see Chapter 53) [48]. Laboratory and cage-side testing of cell count, biochemical profile, acid–base balance, coagulation parameters, D-dimer or fibrin degradation products, lactate, ionized calcium, urine output, and central venous pressure should be performed. The burn itself should be immediately cooled with water or isotonic saline for at least 10 minutes. Ice water and ice packs must not be used as they will cause worsening vasoconstriction and necrosis [49]. Debridement of necrotic tissue and cleaning of the wound with adequate systemic and local analgesia is performed once vital signs are normalized and fluid therapy is under way (see Chapter 166).

Analgesia, both systemic and local, is important for adequate wound care and limiting the stress response (see Chapter 193). Opioids that are pure mu-agonists such as fentanyl (3–10 μg/kg/h), morphine (0.5–1 mg/kg SC q4h), and hydromorphone (0.025 mg/kg/min) are all good choices. Addition of lidocaine (1–3 mL/kg/h), ketamine (2–5 μg/kg/min), and gabapentin (7–10 mg/kg PO) to the opiate will provide neuroleptanalgesia, and decrease the "wind-up" phenomenon caused by NMDA stimulation.

Protecting the wound from infection, removal of necrotic tissue and providing adequate moisture are crucial for proper healing. Strict aseptic technique must be followed during debridement, cleaning, and bandaging of burns. Wounds should be assessed, cleaned, undergo debridement and bebandaged daily. Topical antiseptic solutions such as 0.25% chlorhexidine or dilute providone-iodine are used to clean the wound and flush away dead skin. After cleaning and debriding the wound, topical silver sulfadiazine or polysporin ointment is applied, followed by a three-layer bandage. Wound closure should not be attempted for a minimum of 3–7 days so that the full extent of the injury can be ascertained [48]. Systemic antibiotics are reserved for cases with documented wound infection, sepsis, pneumonia, and leukopenia or other immunosuppression. In general, potentiated pencillins (ampicillin 15–22 mg/kg IV q6–8h; amoxicillin-sulbactam 13.75–20 mg/kg IV q8–12h) and first-generation cephalosporins (cefazolin 22 mg/kg IV q6–8h) are used if one of the aforementioned conditions is complicating the burn-injured patient (see Chapter 200).

Dogs and cats with severe burns of high degree will likely need supplemental nutrition because of their hypermetabolic state and loss of protein. Enteral feeding using tubes placed in non-burned skin with high caloric diets such as Clinicare and critical care diets (A/D by Hills and Recovery by Royal Canin) are prescribed at resting energy rate $(70 \times [\text{body weight (kg)}]^{0.75} +/- \text{illness factor multiplier})$.

Frostbite

Frostbite is a term used to describe injury to tissues exposed to cold [50]. There are very few reports of cold-induced injuries affecting small animals and the incidence is likely much lower than burn injury. One brief description of chilblain syndrome (an acrally located eruption that occurs with exposure to cold) has been reported in service dogs, housed in unheated outdoor kennels, experiencing pain, erythema, and swelling of tail tips [51]. Most other references found were experimentally induced cold injury to animals or anecdotal reports on the Veterinary Information Network.

Dogs' extremities are well adapted to cold temperatures, characterized by arteriovenous anastomoses and vein-artery-vein triads which act as countercurrent heat exchangers [52]. Tissue injury is caused by formation of ice crystals, resulting in mild forms of erythema to full-thickness epidermal necrosis, similar to burns. Frostbite does have some important differences from burn injury, in that inflammation is less accentuated but persists longer and the extracellular matrix is rarely destroyed [53]. In humans, frostbite is separated into two major categories of superficial and deep, with four different degrees of severity. Superficial frostbite (types I and II) have a clinical appearance of redness, swelling, and numbness which progress to blisters, erosions, and loss of sensation. Deep frostbite (types III and IV) lesions are noted as hemorrhagic blisters, black/necrotic and edematous with no sensation to the affected areas [54].

During marked reduction in temperature, exposed tissues initially suffer vasoconstriction, with the most severe constriction occurring at 15 °C. If the temperature continues to drop and reaches 10 °C, the vasoconstriction is interrupted by vasodilation in an attempt to prevent complete loss of perfusion. This is known as the "hunting response." As the cold temperature persists, endothelial damage with formation of microthrombi follows. Edema formation, mediated by mast cell histamine release, further disrupts oxygenation of the tissues [55].

Similar to burns, small animals with frostbite should be assessed for concurrent injuries such as fractures and hemorrhage. If hypothermia (body temperature < 35 °C) is present, a number of systemic changes occur that can affect survival. Hypothermia results in catecholamine release which causes vasoconstriction, tachycardia, and hypertension (see Chapter 148). Severe hypothermia (body temperature < 30 °C) causes arrhythmias such as atrial fibrillation and refractory ventricular arrhythmias [56]. Additionally, delayed drug metabolism, impaired platelet function, immunosuppression, and sludging of blood occur [57].

Treatment depends on the severity of injury, degree of hypothermia, if present, and time point of the injury. Initially, the patient should be placed in a protected environment, not allowing re-exposure to cold. Alternation of freezing and thawing worsens the injury, causing severe thrombosis and ischemia. Rapid rewarming of an affected area is not recommended (unless the patient is hypothermic) due to reperfusion injury. Slow rewarming of the affected area should be performed using warm air current of 22–27 °C [58]. In cases of acute frostbite, affected areas may be bathed for 15–30 minutes in water at a temperature of 37–39 °C. Rapid rewarming for acute frostbite resulted in better clinical outcomes in dogs [59]. Wound management involves protecting deeper, exposed tissues from infection and removal of necrotic tissue. Analgesia, as discussed in the burn section, must be adequate and used judiciously.

Vasodilators, thromboprophylaxis, thrombolytics, hyperbaric oxygen, and NSAIDs have been studied experimentally with animal models and clinically in humans with frostbite. Vasodilators (prostaglandin E1) combined with slow rewarming of affected areas were noted to limit the degree of tissue damage in animal models [60]. Thrombolysis with tissue plasminogen activator within 24 hours of injury helped preserve tissue and lessened amputation rates in people (see Chapter 71) [61].

Drug Eruption

Dermal drug eruptions or cutaneous drug eruptions (CDE) are idiosyncratic reactions to any medication (topical, parenteral, or enteral). CDEs are a very important issue in human medicine, affecting 7% of the general population and 10–15% of hospitalized persons. Emergency room visits by persons affected by drug allergy made up 33.5% in one study [62]. Dermatopathies associated with drug reactions cost an estimated $136 billion annually [63].

In veterinary medicine, older reports noted an incidence range of 1.6% of all cats and 2% of all dogs presenting to a university hospital [64,65]. It is likely that the incidence is higher, since reporting of CDE is not mandatory. Compounding this is the fact that immune-mediated dermatopathies like toxic epidermal necrolysis, pemphigus foliaceus, and erythema multiforme can develop secondary to drug exposure [66]. Both immune-mediated hypersensitivity reactions of all types (I–IV) (Table 137.1) and non-immunological mechanisms such as altered arachidonic acid metabolism, complement activation and "danger" particles like cytokines and cell debris are attributed to the pathogenesis of CDE. Another means of immune activation is thought to occur through haptens and prohaptens

Table 137.1 Hypersensitivity reactions.

Hypersenstivity reaction	Common cutaneous lesions	Common lesion location	Immunoglobulin, cytokine and immunocyte activity	Pathophysiology	Associated systemic effects
Type I	Angioedema, urticaria, erythema	Trunk Muzzle Periocular	IgE-antigen complex binds to mast cells and basophils	Degranulation Release of histamine, leukotrienes, kinins, eosinophilic chemotactic factor	Anaphylactic shock Bronchoconstriction Upper airway obstruction
Type II	Vessicles, bullae, erosions, mucocutaneous ulcers	Extremities and mucocutaneous junction	IgM and IgG cytotoxicity	Antigen-antibody binding results in direct cytoxicity and complement activation	Immune-mediated anemia Immune-mediated thrombocytopenia
Type III	Urticaria, ulceration, alopecia, pitting or firm edema, hemorrhagic bullae, wheals, papules	Pinnae, footpads, mucocutaneous junction	IgG	Immune complexes deposit in endothelium of vessels	Systemic lupus erythematosus Glomerulonephritis
Type IV	Vesicles, bullae, papules, plaques and erythematous macules	Trunk, axilla, inguinal region, foot pads, pinnae	T-cell, interleukins, tumor necrosis factor-alpha	Antigens bound to T-cells resulting in tissue necrosis and activation of macrophages	

which are small drug molecules bound to proteins. These complexes invoke major histocompatibility complex to stimulate T-cell-mediated self-injury [66].

Many classes of drugs are known to cause CDE, with antibiotics representing a majority of reactions in dogs and cats. Sulfonamides, penicillins, cephalosporins, and topical antiparasitic agents are just a few of the many drugs associated with CDE. Table 137.2 lists the clinical findings and associated medications of cutaneous drug reactions and Figures 137.4, 137.5 and 137.6 are of a dog with CDE from cephalexin. Differential diagnoses include primary immune-mediated dermatopathies such as discoid lupus erythematosus, pemphigus complex (pemphigus foliaceus, pemphigus vulgaris, pemphigus erythematosus, bullous pemphigoid), vasculitis, demodecosis, panniculitis, and pyoderma. CDE can appear as almost any dermatopathy and other differential diagnoses are based on specifics of the lesions [67].

Cutaneous drug eruptions should be considered in dogs and cats with commonly described lesions

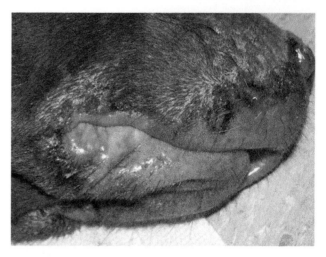

Figure 137.4 Cephalexin reaction 1. Reproduced with permission of Kimberly Coyner.

(mucocutaneous, erosive, ulcerative, vesicular, and necrotic), a history of medication use, vaccines given and topical treatments performed. Reactions to both

Table 137.2 Reactions, associated conditions and medications implicated in cutaneous drug reactions.

Reaction and associated conditions	Medications
Pruritus	Antibiotics
Facial excoriations	NSAIDs
	Opiates
	Methimazole
Sweet's syndrome: neutrophilic dermatitis	NSAIDs: carprofen, fircoxib
Erythematous plaques and nodules	
Systemic signs: pyrexia, thrombocytopenia, vasculitis, pain	
Lupus-like reactions	Sulfonamides
Erythema, depigmentation, crusts, erosions, ulcers	Hydralazine
Common locations: foot pads, pinnae, mucocutaneous junction	Vaccines
Pemphigus-like reactions	Trimethroprim-sulfamethoxypyridazine
Pemphigus foliaceus:	Cephalexin
Papules, crusts, alopecia,	Amoxicillin-clavulanic acid
Common locations: periocular, mucocutaneous, foot pads, muzzle and nose	Oxytetracycline
Pemphigus vulgaris:	Pencillin
Vesicles, bullae, erosions	Promeris (amitraz and metaflumizone)
Common locations: axilla, inguinal region, mucocutaneous, oral cavity	
Fixed drug eruption	Diethylcarbamazine
Erythema (well-circumscribed), edema, bullae, ulceration	5-Fluorocytosine
	Levothyroxine
	Cephalexin
	Amoxicillin-clavulanic acid

NSAID, non-steroidal anti-inflammatory drug.

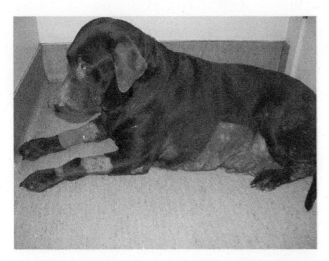

Figure 137.5 Cephalexin reaction 2. Reproduced with permission of Kimberly Coyner.

oral and topical medications can take days to months to develop so a thorough history of all medications must be recorded. Most cases will present 1–3 weeks after starting the medication or topical treatment. A strong suspicion of CDE is based on history and physical exam findings [67]. Additional diagnostic testing, especially in patients with systemic signs such as fever, tachycardia and tachypnea, should include complete cell count, minimum database, acid–base, lactate level, and urinalysis. Vasculitis, EM, and TEN are associated with SIRS and many secondary immune-mediated drug reactions can result in thrombocytopenia, anemia, nephritis, and hepatopathy.

Unfortunately, definitive diagnosis is only accomplished by rechallenge with the suspected medication; however, this can be dangerous and/or deadly [68]. Aspiration with cytology and biopsy with histopathology will provide diagnoses of erythema multiforme, toxic

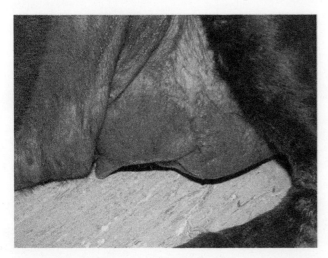

Figure 137.6 Cephalexin reaction 3. Reproduced with permission of Kimberly Coyner.

epidermal necrolysis, and pemphigus. In many cases, cytology and dermohistopathology are non-specific, but will assist in ruling out other differentials. Antibody testing to measure IgE reactions associated with type I immune hypersensitivity along with antidrug IgG and antitissue antibodies may be supportive of CDE.

Patients with systemic signs will need intensive monitoring and treatment. Intravenous fluid therapy to correct dehydration and support cardiac output should be instituted with isotonic crystalloids and/or colloids (see Chapters 167, 168, and 169). Colloids may be indicated for patients with hypoproteinemia and low colloidal oncotic pressure. Analgesia, nutritional support, vital sign monitoring, urine output, organ function, and cell counts should be provided and monitored as for any critically ill small animal. Criticalists should pay close attention to electrolyte, acid–base balance, and worsening lesions in patients suspected to have EM, TEN, and vasculitis. Protection against secondary infection and exposure should be accomplished by topical wound flushing (dilute chlorhexidine [14]) and bandage application. Soiled bandages or bandages with "strike-through" of wound effusion should be changed as necessary while providing adequate analgesia.

Definitive therapy is to discontinue the offending medication, cleanse any remaining topical product, and supportive care. Use of anti-inflammatory medications such as glucocorticoids is controversial [66]. Small animals with angioedema and pruritus may benefit from glucocorticoid administration, especially in the late phase of anaphylaxis. Long-term treatment of drug-induced pemphigus is often necessary. Different immunosuppressive agents such as cyclosporine and azathioprine are used in cases of EM and TEN whose dosages are mentioned in the respective sections of this chapter. Human IV immunoglobulins have been used in cases of drug-resistant pemphigus and CDE [69]. When using immunosuppressive medications, thoroughly monitor for nosocomial infection, MRSI, and sepsis.

Prognosis is good for most cases, except those with multiple organ dysfunction and extensive necrosis associated with TEN.

Vasculitis

Vasculitis is defined as inflammation of the blood vessels, caused by an abnormal immune response [70]. It is an uncommon disorder, noted in only 0.4% of cats seen for dermatopathies [3]. Vasculitis may be associated with infectious agents such as babesiosis, Rocky Mountain spotted fever, histoplasmosis, and feline infectious peritonitis, and with non-infectious disease such as lymphoma [71]. Vessel inflammation may be localized to an

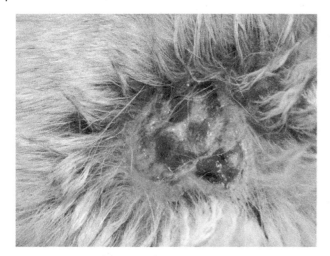

Figure 137.7 Vasculitis ulcerative lesion. Reproduced with permission of Kimberly Coyner.

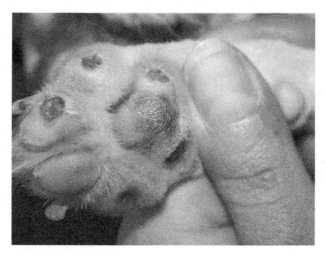

Figure 137.9 Vasculitis affecting foot pads. Reproduced with permission of Kimberly Coyner.

internal organ, disseminated systemically or only affect areas of the skin [72]. Most cases of cutaneous vasculitis in small animals are idiopathic (approximately 50%) and others have been associated with vaccination, food allergy, and medications. Implicated medications include those in Table 137.2 which can cause CDE. Vasculitis has been reported secondarily to human serum albumin, carbamizole, and fenbendazole [73,74].

Types I, II, and III hypersensitivity reactions are the pathogenic processes involved with vasculitis. Type I reactions are believed to be important initially, but are not likely to be the major pathogenic process [70]. Complement activation and neutrophil degranulation during type II reactions result in endothelial necrosis, interstitial edema, and altered blood flow. Immune-antibody complexes associated with type III reactions occlude blood vessels, attract activated leukocytes which release

cytokines that stimulate more inflammation and formation of reactive oxygen species. Vessel damage from any hypersensitivity process causes extravasation of fluid and blood, leading to tissue ischemia [75].

Clinical findings in small animals with cutaneous vasculitis may be isolated to the skin or be associated with systemic signs. Skin lesions include urticaria, ulcers, alopecia, edema that is pitting or firm, hemorrhagic bullae, wheals, and papules (Figures 137.7 and 137.8). Many lesions will be associated with pitting edema so palpation and testing for blanching with pressure are important during physical examination [70]. Ischemic changes of necrosis and ulcers commonly affect the extremities, pinna tips, nasal mucosa, footpads, and oral mucosa [67] (Figures 137.9 and 137.10). Dogs and cats with systemic signs of vasculitis are commonly painful. The pain is diffuse and most severe during the initial phase of the

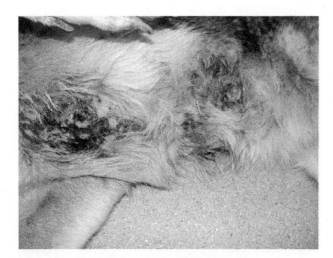

Figure 137.8 Vasculitis erosive and edematous lesions. Reproduced with permission of Kimberly Coyner.

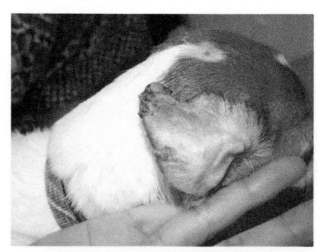

Figure 137.10 Vasculitis affecting pinna. Reproduced with permission of Kimberly Coyner.

disease. Fever, anorexia, neuropathy, polyarthropathy, gastroenteritis, polyuria, and lethargy are other systemic signs that can accompany the cutaneous signs [70]. History of oral medication use, vaccines, topical product application, food sensitivities, and ectoparasites such as ticks should be thoroughly investigated.

Diagnosis of vasculitis is accomplished by histopathological examination of biopsied tissue. Histological classification differentiates cutaneous vasculitis as leukocytoclastic, characterized by nuclear pyknosis and karyorrhexis, and non-leukocytoclastic. The dominant immunocytes are noted, with neutrophilic infiltrate being found in the majority of cases [76]. Differential diagnoses include diseases that can cause DIC such as neoplasia, sepsis, cold agglutinin disease, autoimmune disorders, infectious disease associated with vasculitis, neoplasia such as cutaneous lymphoma, EM, and TEN [77]. A complete blood count, biochemical profile, urinalysis, coagulation panel, serology or PCR for infectious diseases should be performed in cases where vasculitis is suspected. Dogs and cats with critical illness and extensive dermal lesions should also have vital signs, acid–base, ionized calcium, magnesium, and fluid balance (CVP, body weight, and urine output) monitored as needed.

Treatment entails a specific plan for the individual based on clinical findings, laboratory data, severity of disease, and underlying cause. Current medications associated with CDE and vasculitis should be stopped. Lesions should be clipped, gently cleaned with antiseptic solution and their extent marked to note any progression.

Immunomodulation is required in most cases of idiopathic vasculitis and even in some neoplastic, food-allergic and infectious cases. Glucocorticoids are used initially, especially in cases of disease progression, at lower doses of 0.5–1 mg/kg of prednisone. Lower dosages are less likely to have side-effects of delayed wound healing, infection, and sepsis [70]. Other immunomodulating drugs that can be considered, especially in patients that cannot tolerate glucocorticoids or those with treatment failure, include cyclosporine, azathioprine (1–2 mg/kg), and chlorambucil (0.1–0.2 mg/kg EOD). Doxycycline (5–10 mg/kg BID) and niacinamide (22 mg/kg q8–12h) are antibiotics which have immunomodulating effects of altering neutrophil and eosinophil chemotaxis [78]. Pentoxifylline (10–30 mg/kg PO q8–12h) is recommended for cutaneous vasculitis because of its hemorrheological properties which assist in tissue oxygenation. It requires long-term dosing and is rarely helpful as a single agent.

For patients that do not respond to immunomodulation using the aforementioned medications, sulfasalazine (25 mg/kg TID) should be considered in those cases without recent exposure to it.

Prognosis is dependent on the extent of the lesions, lesion progression, and degree of systemic involvement. Classification of vasculitis combining histological lesions and clinical presentation does not currently exist in veterinary medicine [70].

Erythema Multiforme

Erythema multiforme (EM) is a rare, immune-mediated dermatopathy. One retrospective study noted a 0.4% incidence of EM in dogs and 0.11% incidence in cats [79]. In humans, the majority of EM cases are triggered by herpesvirus and EM has five different variants, some self-limiting while others cause severe illness. Approximately 10% of human EM cases are thought to be drug induced [80].

The etiology of EM in small animals has been attributed to drug reactions in 19–59% of cases [81]. Drugs implicated include (1) antibiotics such as sulfonamides, penicillins, and cephalosporins, (2) levamisol, and (3) levothyroxine. Foods with beef and soy protein, neoplasia and infection with *Staphylococcus*, and parvovirus have been reported as triggers of EM. Approximately 23% of EM cases in small animals are idiopathic [79].

The pathogenesis of EM is not well known in small animals. In human EM, T-helper lymphocytes are involved in the immune response, mediated by cytokines such as interferon-alpha in cases of herpes viral EM and tumor necrosis factor-alpha in cases of drug reactions. One study of EM and graft-versus-host disease in dogs identified activated CD4 and T-lymphocytes but implicated cytokines remain unknown. Activated lymphocytes target keratinocytes, causing apoptotic cell death [82].

Lesions and disease of EM are classified as "EM minor" and "EM major." EM minor lesions affect one or less mucosal surfaces and less than 50% of TBSA. EM major lesions affect at least one or more mucosal surfaces (Figure 137.11). Both forms commonly affect the trunk, axillary, and inguinal regions. Pinnae and footpads can also be affected, similar to vasculitis. Most lesions have a similar appearance to cutaneous drug eruptions such as vesicles, bullae, papules, plaques, and erythematous macules [67] (Figure 137.12). Classic "target lesions" characterized by centrally clear necrosis with surrounding erythema are most frequently noted in cases of EM major. In a few instances, EM may have a more chronic form, causing thick crusts and plaques. Recurrence of EM lesions and chronic EM in dogs is most often noted affecting face and ears, mostly without target lesions [81].

Similar to cutaneous drug reactions, the differential diagnoses for EM include vasculitis, pemphigus, TEN, demodecosis, dermatophytosis, bacterial folliculitis,

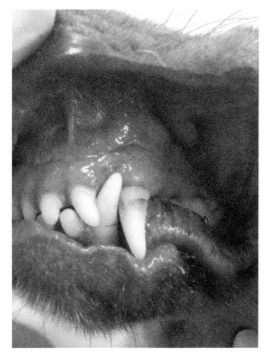

Figure 137.11 Erythema multiforme mucocutaneous lesion. Reproduced with permission of Kimberly Coyner.

and drug eruption. One of the most important aspects of diagnosis is to differentiate EM from urticaria. Small animals with edema and lesions that last less than 12 hours most likely have urticaria and not EM [82]. Target

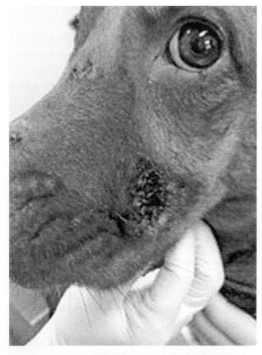

Figure 137.12 Erythema multiforme crusts and plaques. Reproduced with permission of Kimberly Coyner.

lesions, while not pathognomonic, are commonly noted in EM cases.

Diagnosis of EM is clinicopathological and confirmation can be obtained through histopathology. Patients with EM major are likely to have systemic signs of fever, lethargy, and anorexia. Organ dysfunction, DIC, and sepsis can occur also. Unfortunately, there are no clinical criteria to diagnose EM in small animals like the algorithms used for humans. Therefore, histopathology is commonly employed to obtain a definitive diagnosis; however, histopathological lesions of EM are very similar to TEN, making diagnosis difficult [81].

Erythema multiforme treatment entails first differentiating it from urticaria and removal of any inciting causes such as oral medications and bathing if a recent topical treatment is believed to be the culprit. Many cases of EM minor are self-limiting, especially if a causative agent is discontinued. Recurrent EM and idiopathic EM likely require immunosuppression using prednisone (1–2 mg/kg/day). Additional or alternative immunomodulators (Table 137.3) may be needed if a desired response is not obtained. Patients with SIRS, hypotension, and organ dysfunction may require intravenous crystalloids, colloids, and even plasma to replace fluid, albumin, and electrolyte losses from skin lesions (see Chapter 159).

Any small animal that is suspected of having EM should have a baseline minimal database. Patients with systemic signs, especially SIRS, should have additional clinicopathological diagnositics monitored routinely, including but not limited to venous blood gas, electrolytes, ionized calcium, magnesium, and lactate. Vital sign monitoring of heart rate, blood pressure, central

Table 137.3 Immunomodulators for life-threatening dermatopathies.

Immunomodulator	Dose	Dermatopathy
Prednisone	0.5–1 mg/kg/day	Vasculitis
Prednisone	1–2 mg/kg/day	Vasculitis, EM, TEN
Prednisone	2–4 mg/kg/day	Unresponsive EM, TEN
Cyclosporine	5–10 mg/kg/day	Vasculitis, EM, TEN
Azathioprine	1–2 mg/kg/day	Vasculitis, EM, TEN
Chlorambucil	0.1–0.2 mg/kg q48h	Vasculitis
Mycophenolate mofetil	20–40 mg/kg/day, divided TID	Vasculitis, EM major, TEN
Human intravenous gamma-globulin (hIVIG)	2 g/kg	TEN, EM major

EM, erythema multiforme; TEN, toxic epidermal necrolysis; TID, three times a day (*ter in die*).

venous pressure, and urine output should be considered in critically ill dogs and cats. Prognosis for EM minor cases is fair to good, with many small animals having lesion resolution in a matter of weeks. Persistent cases affecting senior dogs and those with EM major typically require life-long immunosuppression, with lesion relapses occurring commonly after medications are withdrawn. Dogs and cats that have extensive mucocutaneous lesions with systemic illness and associated complications of DIC and organ dysfunction carry a poor prognosis [67].

Toxic Epidermal Necrolysis and Stevens–Johnson Syndrome

Toxic epidermal necrolysis (TEN), which is similar to Stevens–Johnson syndrome (SJS), is another rare, immune-mediated skin disease that affects small animals and humans [83]. TEN/SJS was previously considered to be more severe variants of EM. TEN/SJS is now considered a separate disorder from EM and is commonly associated with various drugs such as sulfonamides, penicillins, cephalosporins, NSAIDs (-oxicams), and phenobarbital. Topical flea dips with D-limonene were noted to cause TEN in dogs and cats. There are also many isolated reports invoking rare triggers of TEN, including vaccines, commercial shampoos, and neoplasia. Very few cases of TEN/SJS are idiopathic [82].

The pathogenesis of TEN/SJS, similar to EM, is characterized by keratinocyte apoptosis. TEN/SJS has more extensive cell necrosis than EM and is caused by lymphocyte-mediated cytotoxicity. The major mediators of TEN/SJS are cytotoxic T-lymphocyte release of granulysin and natural killer (NK) cell activation [84]. In TEN/SJS, lesions progress from clusters of dying cells to full-thickness necrosis with less inflammation noted than in EM. Early TEN/SJS lesions have histological characteristics of burns [85]. The exact mechanism of how medications cause sensitization and resulting cell death is unknown. Experimentally, small moieties of certain drugs interacting with host peptides become antigenic and there is evidence of drug moieties directly interacting with T-cell receptors [86].

Lesions of TEN/SJS are acute and characterized by erythema and systemic signs of pain, pyrexia, and anorexia. As lesions develop, they progress from vesicles to bullae, developing ulcerations and erosions with the hallmark sign of epidermal detachment (positive pseudo-Nikolsky sign: pressure causes separation of erythematous skin versus normal skin) (Figures 137.13 and 137.14). Typical distribution involves the trunk, extremities, muzzle/face, and mucocutaneous junctions [67,82].

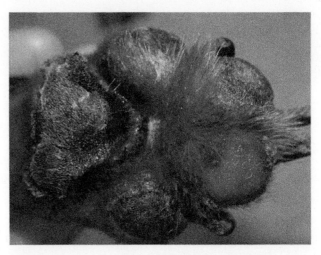

Figure 137.13 Toxic epidermal necrolysis food pad slough. Reproduced with permission of Kimberly Coyner.

Differential diagnoses for TEN/SJS include EM, burns, systemic lupus erythematosus, bullous autoimmune diseases (pemphigus), vasculitis, superficial suppurative dermatitis of miniature schnauzers, and epitheliotropic lymphoma. Histological examination of skin biopsies which describe full-thickness coagulation necrosis of the epidermis is the only method of obtaining a definitive diagnosis [67].

Toxic epidermal necrolysis and SJS are quickly progressive and require emergency intervention. Therapy is similar to EM and burns because the extensive dermal necrosis results in extensive fluid, protein, and electrolyte losses. Supportive care, as outlined in the burn section of this chapter, should be instituted immediately, including intravenous fluid resuscitation, support of colloidal pressure, provision of analgesia, wound care, and

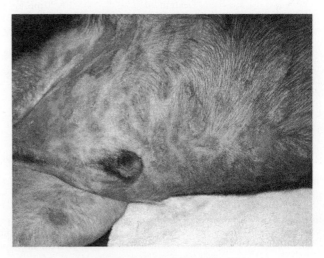

Figure 137.14 Toxic epidermal necrolysis target lesions. Reproduced with permission of Kimberly Coyner.

nutritional support. Any current medications that the animal is being given should be stopped.

Corticosteroids are the mainstay of therapy, but there is controversy regarding their use. It appears that they are most beneficial early on so a rapid clinical diagnosis is important [87]. Human intravenous immunoglobulin (hIVIG) was found to be effective in one cat and two dogs with TEN; however the expense and risks of using a potential human antigenic source must be considered. Additional therapies include plasmapheresis, N-acetyl-cysteine, pentoxifylline, and possibly TNF-alpha inhibitors (infliximab) but small animal research using these treatments is limited [82].

Unfortunately, the prognosis for TEN/SJS is poor. Mortality rates in humans approach 30–50% and are much higher in small animals, approaching 100% [66].

Table 137.4 Treatment and supportive care of selected dermatological emergencies in dogs and cats.

Therapy	Drug	Dosage*	Indication for use	Disease/condition
Immunosuppressants	Prednisone	1–2 mg/kg PO q24h[9]	Immunosuppression	EM, TEN, CV
	Cyclosporine**	5–10 mg/kg PO q12–24h	Reserved for idiopathic cases of EM/TEN	
	Azathioprine	2.2 mg/kg PO q24h[9] (d)		
	Dapsone	1 mg/kg PO q8h[19] (d)		
	Sulfasalazine	20–40 mg/kg PO q8h[19] (d)		
Antibiotics	Amoxicillin-clavulanic acid	13.75 mg/kg PO q12h	Prevent secondary infection/septicemia in patients with compromised epidermal barrier	EM, TEN, burns
	Ampicillin-sulbactam	22–30 mg/kg IV q8h		
	Cephalexin	22 mg/kg PO q12h[12]		
	Cefazolin	20 mg/kg IV q8h		
	Enrofloxacin	5 mg/kg PO, IV q24h		
Crystalloids	Plasmalyte	90 mL/kg/h: shock, dog	Hypovolemic/maldistributive shock	TEN, EM, burns
	0.9% NaCl	60 mL/kg/h: shock, cat		
	LRS	Weight (kg) × % estimated dehydration: replacement	Dehydration	
	Normosol		Maintain effective circulating volume	
		60–66 mL/kg/day: maintenance		
Colloids	Hetastarch	5–15 mL/kg: shock, dog	Hypovolemic/maldistributive shock	EM, TEN, burns
	Pentastarch	5–10 mL/kg: shock, cat		
	Dextran-70	10–20 mL/kg/d: maintenance	Hypoproteinemia, low colloidal oncotic pressure	
Opioids	Fentanyl	2–5 µg/kg/h IV or transdermal patch	Analgesia	EM, TEN, burns
	Hydromorphone	0.05–0.2 mg/kg IV q4–6h		
	Buprenorphine	0.005–0.02 mg/kg IV, buccal (c) q6–12h		
Nutrition	Enteral (nasoesophageal, nasogastric, esophageal)		Supportive care, promote wound healing	EM, TEN, burns
	Parenteral (PPN, TPN)			
Other	Pentoxifylline	10–15 mg/kg PO q8h[10,12]	Immunomodulation, anti-inflammatory, antithrombotic	CV
	Human IVIG	1 g/kg IV over 4h[11,12]		EM, TEN
			Immunomodulation	

c, cats only; CV, cutaneous vasculitis; d, dogs only; EM, erythema multiforme; IV, intravenous; IVIG, intravenous immunoglobulin; PO, by mouth (*per os*); PPN, partial parenteral nutrition; TEN, toxic epidermal necrolysis; TPN, total parenteral nutrition.

* Superscript numbers correspond to references cited in the text.

** Bioequivalent to Neoral.

References

1 Banfield Pet Hospital. State of Pet Health 2015 Report. Available at: www.banfield.com/state-of-pet-health (accessed 15 February 2018)

2 O'Neill DG, Church DB, McGreevy PD, Thomson PC, Brodbelt DC. Prevalence of disorders recorded in cats attending primary-care veterinary practices in England. *Vet J* 2014;202(2):286–291.

3 Turbitt E, Freed GL. Regular source of primary care and emergency department use of children in Victoria. *J Paediatr Child Health* 2016;52(3):303–307.

4 Chmiel C, Huber CA, Roseman T, et al. Walk-ins seeking treatment at an emergency department or general practitioner out-of-hours service: a cross-sectional comparison. *BMC Health Serv Res.* 2011;11:94.

5 Min S-H, Kang M-H, Sur JH, Park HM. Staphylococcus pseudintermedius infection associated with nodular skin lesions and systemic inflammatory response syndrome in a dog. *Can Vet J* 2014;55(5):480–483.

6 Pegram PS Jr. Staphylococcus aureus antibiotic resistance. *Am Fam Physician* 1981;24(3):165–170.

7 Dubel JR, Zink DL, Kelly LM, Naqi SA, Renshaw HW. Bacterial antibiotic resistance: frequency of gentamicin-resistant strains of Escherichia coli in the fecal microflora of commercial turkeys. *Am J Vet Res* 1982;43(010):1786–1789.

8 Carrell M, Perencevich EN, David MZ. USA300 Methicillin-resistant Staphylococcus aureus, United States, 2013. *Emerg Infect Dis* 2015;21(11):1973–1980.

9 Hanselman BA, Kruth SA, Rousseau J, Weese JS. Coagulase positive staphylococcal colonization of humans and their household pets. *Can Vet J* 2009;50(9):954–958.

10 Fritz SA, Hogan PG, Singh LN, et al. Contamination of environmental surfaces with Staphyloccocus aureus in households with children infected with methicillin-resistant S aureus. *JAMA Pediatr* 2014;168(1):1030–1038.

11 Kottler S, Middleton JR, Perry J, Weese JS, Cohn LA. Prevalence of Staphylococcus aureus and methicillin-resistant Staplyloccoccus aureus carriage in three populations. *J Vet Intern Med* 2010;24(1):132–139.

12 Griffeth GC, Traverse M, Abraham JL, Shofer FS, Rankin SC. Screening for skin carriage of methicillin-resistant coagulase-positive staphylococci and Staphylococcus schleiferi in dogs with healthy and inflamed skin. *Vet Dermatol* 2008;19(3):142–149.

13 Morris DO, Lautenbach E, Zaoutis T, et al. Potential for pet animals to harbor methicillin-resistant Staphylococcus aureus when residing with human MRSA patients. *Zoonoses Public Health* 2012;59(4):286–293.

14 Muniz IM, Penna B, Lilenbaum W. Methicillin-resistant commensal staphylococci in the oral cavity of healthy cats: a reservoir of methicillin resistance. *Vet Rec* 2013;173(20):502.

15 Bemis DA, Jones RD, Frank LA, Kania SA. Evaluation of susceptibility test breakpoints used to predict mecA-mediated resistance in Staphylococcus pseudointermidius isolated from dogs. *J Vet Diag Invest* 2009;21(1):53–58.

16 Beck KM, Waisglass SE, Dick HL, Weese JS. Prevalence of meticillin-resistant Staphylococcus pseudointermedius from skin and carriage sites of dogs after treatment of their meticillin-resistant or meticillin-sensitive staphylococcal pyoderma. *Vet Dermatol* 2012;23(4):369–375.

17 Hoet AE, Van-Balen J, Nava-Hoet RC, et al. Epidemiological profiling of methicillin-resistant Staphyloccous aureus-positive dogs arriving at a veterinary teaching hospital. *Vectorn Borne Zoonotic Dis* 2013;13(6):385–393.

18 Weese JS, Poma R, James F, et al. Staphylococcus pseudointermedius necrotizing fasciitis in a dog. *Can Vet J* 2009;50(6):655–656.

19 Coyner KS. The emergence and prevalence of MRSA, MRSP, and MRSS in pets and people. *Vet Med* 2012. Available at: http://veterinarymedicine.dvm360. com/emergence-and-prevalence-mrsa-mrsp-and-mrss-pets-and-people (accessed 15 February 2018).

20 Bender JB, Torres SMF, Gilbert SM, Olsen KE, LeDell KH. Isolation of methicillin-resistant Staphylococcus aureus from a non-healing abscess in a cat. *Vet Rec* 2005;157(13):388–389.

21 Alipour F, Ahmadi M, Javadi S. Evaluation of different methods to detect methicillin resistance in MRSA. *J Infect Public Health* 2014;7(3):186–191.

22 Vincze S, Brandenburg A, Espelage W, et al. Risk factors MRSA infection in companion animals: results from a case-control study within Germany. *Int J Microbiol* 2014;304(7):787–793.

23 Faires MC, Traverse M, Tatker KC, Pearl DL, Weese JS. Methicillin-resistant and -susceptible Staphylococcus aureus infections in dogs. *Emerg Infect Dis* 2010;16(1):69–75.

24 Dalhoff A, Schubert S. Dichotomous selection of high-level oxacillin resistance in Staphylococcus aureus by fluoroquinolones. *Int J Antimicrob Agents* 2010;36(3):216–221.

25 Papich MG, Riviere JE. Fluoroquinolone antimicrobial drugs. In: *Veterinary Pharmacology and Therapeutics*, 9th edn (eds Riviere JE, Papich MG). Wiley-Blackwell, Ames, 2009.

26 Papich MG. Ciprofloxacin pharmacokinetics and oral absorption of generic ciprofloxacin tablets in dogs. *Am J Vet Res* 2012;73(7):1085–1091.

27 Papich MG. Selection of antibiotics for methicillin-resistant Staphylococcus pseudintermedius: time to revisit some old drugs? *Vet Dermatol* 2012;23(4): 352–360.

28 Bryan J, Frank LA, Rohrbach BW, et al. Treatment outcome of dogs with methicillin-resistant

and methicillin-susceptible Staphylococcus pseudointermedius pyoderma. *Vet Dermatol* 2012;23(4):361–368, e65.

29 Gazotto CK. Thermal burn injury. In: *Small Animal Critical Care Medicine*, 2nd edn (eds Silverstein DC, Hopper K). Elsevier Saunders, St Louis, 2015, pp. 743–747.

30 Scott DW, Miller WH, Griffin CE. Envronmental skin disease: burns. In: *Muller and Kirk's Small Animal Dermatology*, 6th edn (eds Scott DW, Miller WH, Griffin CE). Elsevier Saunders, Phildelphia, 2001, pp. 1083–1087.

31 Papazoglou LG, Kazakos G. Thermal burns in two dogs associated with inadequate grounding of electrosurgical unit patient plates. *Aust Vet Pract* 2001;31(2):67–70.

32 Swaim SF, Lee AH, Hughes KS. Heating pads and thermal burns in small animals. *J Am Hosp Assoc* 1989;25(2):156–162.

33 Quist EM, Tanabe M, Mansell JE, Edwards JL. A case series of thermal scal injuries in dogs exposed to hot water from garden hoses (garden hose scalding syndrome). *Vet Dermatol* 2012;23(2):162–166, e33.

34 Vaughn L, Beckel N, Walters P. Severe burn injury, burn shock and smoke inhalation injury in animals. Part 2: diagnosis, therapy, complications and prognosis. *J Vet Emerg Crit Care* 2012;22(2):187–200.

35 Dupha N. Burn injury. In: *The Veterinary ICU Book* (eds Wingfield WE, Raffe M). Teton NewMedia, *Jackson Hole*, 2002, pp. 917–981.

36 Pavletic MM. Management of specific wounds: burns. In: *Atlas of Small Animal Wound Management and Reconstructive Surgery*, 3rd edn (ed. Pavletic MM). Wiley-Blackwell, Ames, 2010.

37 Fitzgerald J. Smoke inhalation. In: *Small Animal Toxicology*, 3rd edn (eds Peterson ME, Talcott MA). Elsevier Saunders, St Louis, 2013, p. 416.

38 Drobatz1 KJ, Walker, LM, Hendricks JC. Smoke exposure in dogs: 27 cases (1988–1997). *J Am Vet Med Assoc* 1999;215(9):1306–1311.

39 Orgill DP, Porter SA, Taylor HO. Heat injury to cells in perfused systems. *Ann NY Acad Sci* 2005;1066:106–118.

40 Gauglitz GG, Song J, Herndon DN, et al. Characterization of the inflammatory response during acute and post-acute phases after severe burn. *Shock* 2008;30(5):503–507.

41 Jeschke MG, Boehning DF, Finerty CC, Herndon DN. Effect of insulin on the inflammatory and acute phase response after burn injury. *Crit Care Med* 2007;35(Suppl 9):s519–s523.

42 Wiener RS, Wiener DC, Larson RJ. Benefits and risks of tight glucose control in critically ill adults: a meta-analysis. *JAMA* 2008;300(8):933–944.

43 Hopper K, Sliverstein D, et al. Shock syndromes. In: *Fluid, Electrolyte and Acid–Base Disorders in Small Animal Practice*, 4th edn (ed. DiBartola SP). Elsevier Saunders, St Louis, 2012, pp. 557–583.

44 Davis H, Jensen T, Johnson A, et al. AAHA/AAFP fluid therapy guidelines for dogs and cats. *J Am Anim Hosp Assoc* 2013;49(3):149–159.

45 Cazzolli D, Prittie J. The crystalloid-colloid debate: consequences of resuscitation fluid selection in veterinary critical care. *J Vet Emerg Crit Care* 2015;25(1):6–19.

46 Langston C. Managing fluid and electrolyte disorders in renal failure. In: *Fluid, Electrolyte and Acid–Base Disorders in Small Animal Practice*, 4th edn (ed. DiBartola SP). Elsevier Saunders, St Louis, 2012, pp. 544–556.

47 Bateman S. Disorders of magnesium: magnesium deficit and excess. In: *Fluid, Electrolyte and Acid–Base Disorders in Small Animal Practice*, 4th edn (ed. DiBartola SP). Elsevier Saunders, St Louis, 2012, pp. 212–229.

48 Frantz K, Byers CG. Thermal injury. *Compend Contin Educ Vet* 2011;33:E1.

49 Jutkowitz AL. Care of the burned patient. *Proceedings of IVECCS* 2005.

50 Frostbite. In: *Dorland's Medical Dictionary for Healthcare Consumers*. Available at: http://medical-dictionary.thefreedictionary.com/frostbite (accessed 15 February 2018).

51 Jepson PG. Chilblain syndrome in dogs. *Vet Rec* 1981;109(17):392.

52 Ninomiya H, Akiyama E, Simazaki K, et al. Functional anatomy of the footpad vasculature of dogs: scan electron microscopy of vascular corrosion casts. *Vet Dermatol* 2011;22(6):475–481.

53 Goertz O, Hirsch T, Buschhaus B, et al. Intravital pathophysiologic comparison of frostbite and burn injury in a murine model. *J Surg Res* 2011;167: e395–e401.

54 Imray C, Grieve A, Dhillon S, Caudwell Xtreme Everest Research Group. Cold damage to the extremeties: frostbite and non-freezing cold injuries. *Postgrad Med J* 2009;85:481–488.

55 Francis TJ, Golden FS. Non-freezing cold injury: the pathogenesis. *J R Nav Med Serv* 1985;71:3–8.

56 Greene S. *Veterinary Anesthesia and Pain Management Secrets*. Hanley & Belfus Inc, Philadelphia, 2002, pp. 139, 149–153.

57 Duffy T. Thermoregulation of the perioperative patient. Proceedings of the American College of Veterinary Surgeons, 2007, pp. 707–712.

58 Hallam MJ, Cubison T, Dheansa B, Imray C. Managing frostbite. *BMJ* 2010;341:c5864.

59 Entin MA, Baxter H. Influence of rapid warming on frostbite in experimental animals. *Plast Reconstr Surg* 1952;9:511–524.

60 Yeager RA, Campion TW, Kerr JC, Hobson RW 2nd, Lynch TG. Treatment of frostbite with intra-arterial prostaglandin E1. *Am Surg* 1983;49:665–667.

61 Bruen KJ, Ballard JR, Morris SE, et al. Reduction of the incidence of amputation in frostbite injury with thrombolytic therapy. *Arch Surg* 2007;142:546–551.

62 Bernard Y-H, Tan T. Epidemiology and risk factors for drug allergy. *Br J Clin Pharmacol* 2011;71(5):684–700.

63 Bigby M. Rates of cutaneous drug reactions to drugs. *Arch Dermatol* 2001;137:765–770.

64 Scott DW, Miller WH Jr. Idiosyncratic cutaneous adverse drug reactions in the cat: literature review and report of 14 cases (1990–1996). *Felin Pract* 1998;26(10):10–15.

65 Scott DW, Miller WH Jr. Idiosyncratic cutaneous adverse drug reactions in the dog: literature review and report of 101 cases (1990–1996). *Canine Pract* 1999;24:16–22.

66 Voie KL, Cambell, Lavergne SN. Drug hypersensitivity reactions targeting the skin in dogs and cats. *J Vet Intern Med* 2012;26:863–874.

67 Kersey KM, Rosales M, Roberts BK. Dermatologic emergencies: identification and treatment. *Compend Contin Educ Vet* 2013;35(1):E2.

68 Scott DW, Miller WH, Griffin CE. Immune-mediated disorders. In: *Muller and Kirk's Small Animal Dermatology*, 6th edn (eds Scott DW, Miller WH, Griffin CE). WB Saunders, Philadelphia, 2001, pp. 667–779.

69 Rahilly LJ, Keating JH, O'Toole TE. The use of intravenous human immunoglobulin the treatment of severe pemphigus foliaceus in a dog. *J Vet Intern Med* 2006;20:1483–1486.

70 Bloom PB. *Cutaneous vasculitis: what it is and how you treat it*. Proceedings of the 25th North American Dermatology Forum, Portland, April 14–17, 2010.

71 Tasaki Y, Miura N, Iyori K, et al. Generalized alopecia with vasculitis-like changes in a dog with babesiosis. *J Vet Med Sci* 2013;75(10):1367–1369.

72 Ridgway MD, Singh K. DIC and granulomatous vasculitis in a dog with disseminated histoplasmosis. *J Am Anim Hosp Assoc* 2011;47(3):e26–e30.

73 Jasani S, Boag AK, Smith KC. Systemic vasculitis with severe cutaneous manifestation as a suspected idiosyncratic hypersensitivity reaction to fenbendazole in a cat. *J Vet Intern Med* 2008;22(3):666–670.

74 Powell C, Thompson P, Murtaugh RJ. Type III hypersensitivity reaction with immune complex deposition in 2 critically ill dogs administered human serum albumin. *J Vet Emerg Crit Care* 2013;23(6):598–604.

75 Innera M. Cutaneous vasculitis in small animals. *Vet Clin North Am Small Anim Pract* 2013;43(1):113–134.

76 Gross TL, Ihrke PJ, Walder EJ, Affolter VK. *Skin Diseases of the Dog and Cat: Clinical and Histopathologic Diagnoses*, 2nd edn. Blackwell Science, Oxford, 2005, pp.238–247.

77 Nichols PR, Morris DO, Beale KM. A retrospective study of canine and feline cutaneous vasculitis. *Vet Dermatol* 2001;12(5):255–264.

78 White SD, Rosychuck RA, Reinke SI, Paradis M. Tetracycline and niacinamide for treatment of autoimmune skin disease in 31 dogs. *J Am Vet Med Assoc* 1992;200:1497–1500.

79 Scott DW, Miller W. Erythema multiforme in dogs and cats: literature review and case material from the Cornell University College of Veterinary medicine. *Vet Dermatol* 1999;10:297–309.

80 French LE, Prins C. Erythema multiforme, Stevens–Johnson syndrome and toxic epidermal necrolysis. In: *Dermatology*, vol. 1, 2nd edn (eds Bolongna JL, Jorizzo JL, Schaffer JV). Mosby Elsevier, Amsterdam, 2008, pp. 287–300.

81 Hinn AC, Olivry T, Luther PB. Erythema multiforme, Steven–Johnson syndrome, and toxic epidermal necrolysis in the dog: clinical classification, drug exposure and histopathologicical correlations. *J Vet Allergy Clin Immunol* 1998;6:14–20.

82 Yager JA. Erythema multiforme, Stevens–Johnson syndrome and toxic epidermal necrolysis: a comparative review. *Vet Dermatol* 2014;25(5); e406–e464.

83 Bastuji-Garin S, Rzany B, Stern RS, et al. Clinical classification of cases of toxic epidermal necrolysis, Stevens–Johnson syndrome and erythema multiforme. *Arch Dermatol* 1993;129:92–96.

84 Chung WH, Hung SI, Yang JY, et al. Granulysin is a key mediator for disseminated keratinocyte death in Stevens–Johnson syndrome and toxic epidermal necrolysis. *Nat Med* 2008;14:1343–1350.

85 Paquet P, Nikkels A, Arrese JE, Vanderkelen A, Pierard GE. Macrophages and TNF-α in toxic epidermal necrolysis. *Arch Dermatol* 1994;130:605–608.

86 Schwartz RA, McDonough PH, Lee BW. Toxic epidermal necrolysis: part 1. *J Am Acad Dermatol* 2013;69(173):e1–e13.

87 Schwartz RA, McDonough PH, Lee BW. Toxic epidermal necrolysis: part 2. *J Am Acad Dermatol* 2013;69(187):e1–e16.

138

Severe Soft Tissue Infections

Melissa Clark, DVM, PhD, DACVCP[1] and Yekaterina Buriko, DVM, DACVECC[2]

[1]*Animal Medical Center, New York, NY, USA*
[2]*Matthew J. Ryan Veterinary Hospital, University of Pennsylvania, Philadelphia, PA, USA*

Introduction

Infections of the skin and soft tissues are common in dogs and cats, and vary widely in their clinical severity. The phrase "severe soft tissue infections" (SSTIs) generally refers to those infections which involve deeper tissues (fascia, muscle) and have the potential to produce substantial tissue damage or systemic compromise if not aggressively treated. "Necrotizing" infections are SSTIs that exhibit clinical and/or histopathological features of necrosis [1]. The most well recognized of the necrotizing soft tissue infections (NSTIs), necrotizing fasciitis (NF), is a rapidly progressive infection that involves bacterial tracking along fascial planes, with local tissue destruction resulting from secretion of cellular and bacterial proteases. A variant of NF is Fournier's gangrene (FG), which involves the tissues of the perianal area [2,3]. NF and other SSTI can also be associated with toxic shock syndrome, in which massive cytokine release triggered by bacterial antigens leads to a systemic inflammatory response with multiple organ involvement. Early recognition and prompt intervention are essential components of limiting the sequelae of SSTIs/NSTIs [4].

Etiology

In humans, NSTIs are classified as type I (polymicrobial), type II (monomicrobial) or type III (caused by anaerobes such as *Clostridium*) [2,4]. Type I infections are most common and may include infection with methicillin-resistant *Staphylococcus aureus* (MRSA), although MRSA has also been reported as a cause of monomicrobial infections in recent years [2,4–6]. Type II infections are most often caused by group A streptococci, such as *Streptococcus pyogenes*, and can be associated with streptococcal toxic shock syndrome.

Polymicrobial, streptococcal, and anaerobic NSTIs have all been described in dogs and cats [7]. However, streptococcal necrotizing infections in small animals are usually caused by beta-hemolytic streptococci of Lancefield group G (e.g. *Streptococcus canis*) rather than by group A streptococci, as in humans [8,9]. In a retrospective study of 47 dogs with SSTIs, the most common bacterial species isolated in antemortem cultures were beta-hemolytic streptococci (monomicrobial in 9/13 cultures), *E. coli*, and staphylococci (including methicillin-resistant), with lower numbers of anaerobes (*Clostridium*, *Peptostreptococcus*) and a variety of other aerobes (*Pseudomonas*, *Serratia*, *Klebsiella*, *Enterococcus faecalis*, *Pasteurella*, *Enterobacter cloacae*).

In cats, *S. canis*, *Acinetobacter baumanni* (suspected nosocomial), and *Prevotella bivia* have been cultured in cases of NF, the former two associated with septic shock [10–12]. A polymicrobial infection with *Enterococcus faecium*, *Staphylococcus epidermidis*, and *E.coli* has been described in a cat with FG; the *S. epidermidis* was resistant to oxacillin and all other beta-lactams tested [13].

Pathophysiology

Streptococcus canis is a commensal organism, and many of the other organisms that cause SSTIs also arise from the patient's endogenous flora. In some cases, the development of established infection can be attributed to a loss of the skin barrier and/or altered systemic host defenses (i.e. a pre-existing chronic wound or immunosuppressive condition). However, an early observation in human medicine was that NSTIs could also develop following seemingly minor trauma ("trivial accidents") in otherwise healthy individuals [6].

In the above-mentioned study by Buriko et al. [7], 19% of dogs with NSTIs had a potentially immunomodulating condition (hyperadrenocorticism, hypothyroidism, IMPA, meningitis/vasculitis, IMHA, Evans' syndrome, neoplasia, or chronic UTI) at presentation; 13% were administered steroids and 17% were administered NSAIDs prior to the onset of clinical signs. Seventeen percent had a history of recent skin barrier compromise (injections, surgery at the affected site or a distant site, vehicular trauma with minor abrasions). Three other dogs had a history of blunt trauma, boarding with no obvious history of trauma, or grooming with razor burn [7]. An inciting factor was not identified in the remaining cases.

Other potential predisposing or inciting factors for NF described in dogs and cats include tooth extraction [14], minor dog bites or superficial pyoderma [9], and prior radiation therapy (with development of clinical signs after a small wound was noted in the irradiated area [15]). One cat developed NF emanating from a site of intravenous catheter replacement (suspected nosocomial infection) [12]. Additional cases following boarding with no witnessed trauma, or cases in which no inciting factor could be identified, have also been reported [9,16].

Because of the occurrence of some NSTIs without an obvious portal for inoculation, several recent investigations in human medicine have focused on molecular characterization of the processes by which necrotizing streptococcal infections are established and propagated. One hypothesis suggests that under certain circumstances, any disruption of normal musculoskeletal anatomy can lead to hematogenous seeding of the affected tissue by streptococcal organisms [17]. The intermediate filament vimentin, which can act as a tether for streptococci, has been found to be upregulated in injured skeletal muscle cells *in vitro* [18], and in mice, minor blunt trauma followed by intravenous delivery of group A streptococcal organisms led to homing of the streptococci to the injured area [17]. Subsequent bacterial proliferation in subcutaneous tissue and fascial planes results in elaboration of proteases, by both bacteria and host leukocytes; in addition, the antiphagocytic streptococcal M protein and other virulence factors activate local coagulation pathways and produce regional thrombosis and vasoconstriction. The result is widespread fascial digestion and ischemic and liquefactive necrosis of surrounding subcutaneous tissue, muscle, and skin [19].

Although the details of these processes have not been verified in dogs and cats, they are presumed to be similar based on similar clinical and histopathological findings. Group G streptococcal isolates have also been found to express some of the same bacterial superantigens as group A streptococci; these superantigens (pyrogenic exotoxins) bind to MHC II molecules on antigen-presenting cells and T-cell receptors, triggering generalized cytokine release and producing the signs of toxic shock syndrome [20].

Clinical Features (Table 138.1)

Physical examination findings in dogs and cats with SSTIs/NSTIs include heat, swelling, or erythema of the affected area, often with pain out of proportion to the apparent extent of tissue injury [8,9]. Bullous lesions (common in humans, uncommon in dogs) and skin sloughing may occur as the disease advances [8,16]. Dramatic progression may occur within 12–24 hours of initial presentation. Lesions may be found on the limbs (most common), ventral thorax and abdomen, flanks, dorsum, muzzle, or prepuce, or in the inguinal area (or perianal area in the case of FG) [7,9].

Other common initial physical examination findings in affected dogs include fever (63%), tachycardia (70%), and tachypnea (81%); hypotension or mental dullness may also be present, particularly in dogs with sepsis or toxic shock syndrome [7]. Initial laboratory assessment may reveal leukocytosis or leukopenia (with or without a left shift), mild thrombocytopenia, hypoalbuminemia, mild to moderate elevation of AST or ALP, mildly prolonged PTT, and elevated FDPs [7]. Additionally, hyperbilirubinemia and hypoglycemia (presumed associated with sepsis) have been reported in a dog with NF [16]. Similar physical examination and clinicopathological findings have been reported in cats with NF or FG [10–13].

Diagnosis (see Table 138.1)

The possibility of a severe or necrotizing soft tissue infection should be entertained for any skin or soft tissue lesion for which pain seems disproportionate to clinical appearance, as well as for lesions which progress very rapidly or those with potential signs of necrosis such as blistering, crepitus, discoloration, or tissue sloughing. Imaging may be helpful in increasing the index of suspicion or directing sample collection. In humans, MRI is the preferred imaging modality for differentiation of necrotizing from non-necrotizing infections; characteristic findings in NSTIs include hyperintensity of deep fascia and muscles on T2-weighted images. Computed tomography has been reported to be 80% sensitive based on detection of abscesses and fascial thickening [6]. However, advanced imaging is not commonly performed initially in dogs because of expense and the need for sedation.

Radiography and ultrasound findings have been described in 47 dogs with SSTIs/NSTIs; 23 of these dogs had radiographs performed of the affected area, and 16 had ultrasound examination. On radiographs, none of the dogs had bony involvement or gas visualized in the soft tissues (the latter is a specific but not sensitive sign

894 | *Textbook of Small Animal Emergency Medicine*

Table 138.1 Summary of recommendations for recognition, diagnosis, and treatment of severe and necrotizing soft tissue infections.

Suggestive historical and PE findings	Localized erythema, swelling, and warmth with pain out of proportion to clinical appearance
	Bullae, discoloration, or skin sloughing
	Rapidly progressive lesions
	History of recent trauma, injections, procedures, or immunosuppression
Diagnostic plan	Collect CBC, biochemistry, urinalysis, infectious disease testing as applicable to assess for:
	Evidence of SIRS/sepsis
	Concurrent conditions or organ dysfunction
	Imaging:
	Ultrasound of affected area
	Consider advanced imaging (CT/MRI)
	Radiographs may be performed but are likely to be low-yield.
	Collect microbiological samples.
	If open wound, obtain cytology and culture from leading edge (tissue swab or biopsy). If skin is intact, consider:
	Ultrasound-guided aspiration of affected tissue for cytology and culture
	Local anesthesia with skin incision, "finger test", and sample collection
Treatment plan	Appropriately support blood pressure and vital signs
	Opioids preferred for analgesia; avoid NSAIDs (controversial)
	Initiate parenteral antibiotic therapy
	Clindamycin + penicillin + either (1) an aminoglycoside, (2) a third-generation cephalosporin, or (3) meropenem
	Consider prior antibiotic therapy and potential adverse drug reactions
	Avoid fluoroquinolones as monotherapy
	Consider early surgical debridement
	Excision of all necrotic tissue, probing of wound pockets
	Repeated debridement or limb amputation if necessary
	Consider NPWT, skin grafts once infection is resolved
	Refractory cases of streptococcal toxic shock unstable for surgery: consider IVIG
	Continue supportive care (Rule of 20)

CBC, complete blood count; CT, computed tomography; IVIG, intravenous immunoglobulin; MRI, magnetic resonance imaging; NSAID, non-steroidal anti-inflammatory drug; NPWT, negative pressure wound therapy; PE, physical examination; SIRS, systemic inflammatory response syndrome.

of necrotizing infections in humans). Ultrasound identified a subcutaneous fluid pocket in 69% of dogs in which it was performed, and subcutaneous edema in all. Fine needle aspiration of the affected area was performed in 23 dogs (some under ultrasound guidance) and revealed evidence of subcutaneous bacterial infection in 62% [7]. Therefore, although ultrasound findings are neither sensitive nor specific for necrosis, imaging and aspirates may facilitate the assignment of a bacterial etiology to a rapidly progressive skin lesion and aid in acute management, and aspirates of affected tissue (preferably with ultrasound guidance to identify pockets) should be considered in all dogs with potential necrotizing infections.

The definitive diagnosis of NSTI is often made during surgical exploration of the diseased tissue. The "finger test" describes the ease with which tissues can be digitally separated along fascial planes; the characteristic lesions associated with necrotizing infections are a positive finger test, fascial edema, gray non-contracting muscle, and a thin, murky, foul-smelling "dishwater" discharge [6,8]. The finger test can be performed through a small incision with local anesthesia if a necrotizing infection is being considered and uncertainty exists regarding the need for surgical debridement [8].

Histopathologically, necrotizing infections are associated with polymorphonuclear cell infiltration, edema of the dermis and subcutaneous fat, and thrombosis of nutrient vessels to skin and muscle, in addition to liquefactive necrosis of fascia and tissues [6,8,21].

Treatment (see Table 138.1)

Treatment of SSTIs/NSTIs should include early initiation of broad-spectrum antibiotic therapy with activity against likely pathogens, source control (generally consisting of early, aggressive, and potentially repeated surgical debridement), and pathogen identification by culture, with appropriate tailoring of antimicrobial treatment [4] (see Chapter 200). Tissue cultures should be taken from the leading edge of a lesion if possible, as the central portion may contain contaminants [8]; blood cultures can also be considered if sepsis is suspected.

Once cultures are obtained, empirical antibiotic therapy directed against streptococci, other skin flora (including methicillin-resistant staphylococci), gram-negative organisms, and anaerobes should be initiated. In one recent human study, a combination of clindamycin, a penicillin, and gentamicin was adequate against the causative pathogen(s) in 95% of necrotizing infections, based on susceptibility testing [22]. Because protein synthesis inhibitors such as clindamycin may inhibit exotoxin synthesis by streptococci, and because a proportion of streptococci isolated in the study by Buriko et al. [7] were penicillin resistant, a similar regimen incorporating clindamycin might be appropriate as empirical therapy in dogs and cats. The risks of nephrotoxicity induced by aminoglycosides must be weighed against their potential benefits when using them in animals with possible sepsis-induced hypoperfusion or renal compromise. Alternatives to aminoglycosides in animals with known or potential renal compromise are third-generation cephalosporins or carbapenems (i.e. meropenem); it should be remembered that carbapenems, like other beta-lactams, are not effective against methicillin-resistant staphylococci.

Fluoroquinolones, although they provide good gram-negative coverage, may not be ideal as a first-line treatment for NSTIs. First, they have been shown to induce bacteriophage-mediated lysis of streptococci *in vitro*, with increased expression of superantigens [23], although the significance of this finding *in vivo* remains unknown. Second, in the study by Buriko et al. [7], over 50% of organisms isolated in antemortem culture were resistant to fluoroquinolones.

Surgical exploration and debridement should be considered early, as antibiotic access to necrotic tissues may be limited by thrombosis and poor local perfusion, and both reduction of bacterial load and exposure of tissues to oxygen may be beneficial in resolving infection [6,8] (see Chapter 166). Debridement should include removal of all questionable tissue and blunt probing of wound pockets in all directions [6,8]. Once debridement has been completed, the surgical site may be initially managed as an open wound, with antibacterial dressings and frequent bandage changes. Repeated debridement (every 24–48 hours) may be necessary, depending upon wound appearance and progression; in some cases, amputation of the affected limb has proved necessary to halt the spread of infection into adjacent tissues [6,8,16]. Negative pressure wound therapy (NPWT) has been shown to be beneficial in NSTIs in human medicine, and there are several reports of the use of NPWT to enhance healing after debridement in dogs and cats [24,25]. Skin grafts may also be considered once infection is resolved and a bed of healthy granulation tissue has formed [25]. Although surgery is indicated in most cases of SSTI, there have been three reports of successful treatment of FG in cats with conservative therapy [26].

Other aspects of patient care, including analgesia, correction of fluid, acid–base, and electrolyte abnormalities, nutrition, and recumbency care, are also integral components of treatment (see Sections 5 and 7). Animals with toxic shock syndrome and abnormal vascular responsiveness may require pressors to maintain appropriate perfusion. For analgesic therapy, opioids are an appropriate choice, with mu-agonists preferred because of the severe pain usually associated with SSTIs. The use of NSAIDs is controversial; they have been postulated to facilitate more rapid spread of NSTIs in humans because of interference with neutrophil chemotaxis,

and in mice, the NSAID ketorolac was associated with a marked increase in the number of group A streptococci in injured muscle when given 1 hour before injury [17]. However, more recent prospective human studies and a retrospective study in 47 dogs have not found an association between NSAID use prior to diagnosis and progression of disease and/or survival [7,27].

Other therapies that have been suggested to be beneficial in NSTIs include hyperbaric oxygen therapy (HBO) and intravenous immunoglobulin (IVIG). In humans, no prospective, randomized clinical trials have been conducted to evaluate the use of HBO, and delaying other treatment in favor of HBO is not advised [2,3]. However, there are reports of successful treatment of SSTIs using antibiotic therapy and IVIG in cases in which surgery was precluded by hemodynamic instability of the patient or extensive tissue involvement [28], and IVIG administration was associated with faster resolution of MODS in a small randomized study [29]. Proposed actions of IVIG in SSTIs include binding and neutralization of streptococcal or staphylococcal exotoxins and superantigens [6,28].

Hyperbaric oxygen therapy has been described in a dog with NF [16], but so far, as in human medicine, insufficient information exists in veterinary medicine to determine whether or not it has the capability to reduce morbidity and mortality associated with NSTIs. Administration of IVIG has not been formally described in dogs or cats with NSTIs, but could be considered in suspected streptococcal or staphylococcal SSTIs with toxic shock where surgical debridement must be delayed or is not possible.

Prognosis

In the study by Buriko et al. [7], the overall mortality rate for dogs with SSTIs (of which 85% were NSTIs) was 53%. The majority of deaths in this study were euthanasias, but a similarly guarded prognosis has been reported for SSTIs in human medicine (overall mortality of 25–30%, increasing to 70% in the presence of toxic shock syndrome [6]). Predictors of mortality in humans include white blood cell counts greater than 30000/μL, creatinine > 2 mg/dL, heart disease at hospital admission, and clostridial infection [30]. Delay in surgical debridement has also been identified as an independent negative prognostic factor in humans with NSTIs [31].

In dogs, although a number of clinicopathological variables, initial respiratory rate, and the proportion of patients undergoing initial surgical debridement have been found to differ between survivors and non-survivors of SSTIs, all of these findings were limited by the retrospective nature of the study and small sample size, and further studies are necessary to better characterize prognostic factors in dogs and cats with SSTIs/NSTIs [7].

References

1 Anaya DA, Dellinger EP. Necrotizing soft-tissue infection: diagnosis and management. *Clin Pract* 2007;44:705–710.

2 Phan HH, Cocanour CS. Necrotizing soft tissue infections in the intensive care unit. *Crit Care Med* 2010;38:S460–S468.

3 DeWaele JJ. Management of necrotizing skin and soft tissue infections. *Expert Rev Anti-Infect Ther* 2012;10:805–814.

4 Napolitano LM. Severe soft tissue infections. *Infect Dis Clin North Am* 2009;23:571–591.

5 Miller LG, Perdreau-Remington F, Rieg G, et al. Necrotizing fasciitis caused by community-acquired methicillin-resistant Staphylococcus aureus in Los Angeles. *N Engl J Med* 2005;352:1445–1453.

6 Lancerotto L, Tocco I, Salmoso R, et al. Necrotizing fasciitis: classification, diagnosis, and management. *J Trauma* 2012;72:560–565.

7 Buriko Y, van Winkle TJ, Drobatz KJ, et al. Severe soft tissue infections in dogs: 47 cases (1996–2006). *J Vet Emerg Crit Care* 2008;18:608–618.

8 Naidoo SL, Campbell DL, Miller LM, et al. Necrotizing fasciitis: a review. *J Am Anim Hosp Assoc* 2005;41: 104–109.

9 Prescott JF, Miller W, Mathews KA, et al. Update on canine streptococcal toxic shock syndrome and necrotizing fasciitis. *Can Vet J* 1997;38:241–242.

10 Mayer MN, Rubin JE. Necrotizing fasciitis caused by methicillin-resistant Staphylococcus pseudintermedius at a previously irradiated site in a dog. *Can Vet J* 2012;53:1207–1210.

11 Hess MO. Necrotising fasciitis due to Prevotella bivia in a cat. *J Small Anim Pract* 2009;50:558–560.

12 Sura R, Hinckley LS, Risatti GR, et al. Fatal necrotizing fasciitis and myositis in a cat. *Vet Rec* 2008;162:450–453.

13 Brachelente C, Wiener D, Malik Y, et al. A case of necrotizing fasciitis with septic shock in a cat caused by Acinetobacter baumannii. *Vet Dermatol* 2007;18: 432–438.

14 Berube DE, Whelan MF, Tater KC, et al. Fournier's gangrene in a cat. *J Vet Emerg Crit Care* 2010;20: 148–154.

15 Jenkins CM, Winkler K, Rudloff E, et al. Necrotizing fasciitis in a dog. *J Vet Emerg Crit Care* 2001;11: 299–305.

16 Plavec T, Zdovc I, Juntes P, et al. Necrotizing fasciitis caused by Serratia marcescens after tooth extraction in a Doberman Pinscher: a case report. *Vet Med* 2008;53:629–635.

17 Hamilton SM, Bayer CR, Stevens DL, et al. Muscle injury, vimentin expression, and nonsteroidal anti-inflammatory drugs predispose to cryptic group A streptococcal necrotizing infection. *J Infect Dis* 2008;198:1692–1698.

18 Bryant AE, Bayer CR, Huntington JD, et al. Group A streptococcal myonecrosis: increased vimentin expression after skeletal-muscle injury mediates the binding of streptococcus pyogenes. *J Infect Dis* 2006;193:1685–1692.

19 Olsen RJ, Musser JM. Molecular pathogenesis of necrotizing fasciitis. *Annu Rev Pathol Mechan Dis* 2010;5:1–31.

20 Igwe EI, Shewmaker PL, Facklam RR, et al. Identification of superantigen genes speM, ssa, and smeZ in invasive strains of beta-hemolytic group C and G streptococci recovered from humans. *FEMS Microbiol Lett* 2003;229:259–264.

21 Lamm CG, Ferguson AC, Lehenbauer TW, et al. Streptococcal infection in dogs: a retrospective study of 393 cases. *Vet Pathol* 2010;47:387–395.

22 Kulasegaran S, Cribb B, Vandal AC, et al. Necrotizing fasciitis: 11-year retrospective case review in South Auckland. *ANZ J Surg* 2016;86:826–830.

23 Ingrey KT, Ren J, Prescott JF. A fluoroquinolone induces a novel mitogen-encoding bacteriophage in Streptococcus canis. *Infect Immun* 2003;71: 3028–3033.

24 Maguire P, Azarara JM, Carb A, et al. The successful use of negative-pressure wound therapy in two cases of necrotizing fasciitis. *J Am Anim Hosp Assoc* 2015;51:43–48.

25 Nolfe MC, Meyer-Lindenberg A. Necrotising fasciitis in a domestic shorthair cat – negative pressure wound therapy assisted debridement and reconstruction. *J Small Anim Pract* 2014;56:281–284.

26 Vaske HH, Ragan IK, Harkin KR, et al. Successful conservative management of suspected Fournier's gangrene in cats: three cases. *J Feline Med Surg Open Rep* 2015;1–9.

27 Aronoff DM, Bloch KC. Assessing the relationship between the use of nonsteroidal anti-inflammatory drugs and necrotizing fasciitis caused by group A streptococcus. *Medicine* 2003;82:225–235.

28 Norrby-Teglund A, Muller MP, McGeer A, et al. Successful management of severe group A streptococcal soft tissue infections using an aggressive medical regimen including intravenous polyspecific immunoglobulin together with a conservative surgical approach. *Scand J Infect Dis* 2005;37:166–172.

29 Darenberg J, Ihendyane N, Sjolin J, et al., StreptIg Study Group. Intravenous immunoglobulin G therapy in streptococcal toxic shock syndrome: a European randomized, double-blind, placebo-controlled trial. *Clin Infect Dis* 2003;37:333–340.

30 Anaya DA, McMahon K, Nathens AB, et al. Predictors of mortality and limb loss in necrotizing soft tissue infections. *Arch Surg* 2005;140:151–157.

31 Wong C, Chan H, Pasupathy S, et al. Necrotizing fasciitis: clinical presentation, microbiology, and determinants of mortality. *J Bone Joint Surg* 2003; 85-A:1454–1460.

K. Environmental Emergencies

139

Smoke Inhalation Toxicity

Erin McGowan, VMD, DACVECC[1] and Kenneth J. Drobatz, DVM, MSCE, DACVIM (IM), DACVECC[2]

[1] *BluePearl Veterinary Specialty and Emergency Pet Hospital, Waltham, MA, USA*
[2] *University of Pennsylvania, Philadelphia, PA, USA*

Introduction

House and building fires are common occurrences in the United States, especially in large cities. Smoke inhalation in pets trapped within a house fire can have a multitude of different problems and presentations. Inhaled smoke and debris may contain respiratory irritants and toxins, and can cause heat damage to the skin, eyes, and the upper airway. In humans, inhalation injury is a greater contributor to overall mortality than the percentage of body surface area affected by burns [1]. Early recognition, intervention, and stabilization of smoke inhalation victims is necessary as these patients can rapidly progress to respiratory failure and life-threatening complications.

Pathophysiology of Smoke Inhalation

Smoke is a heterogenous mixture of chemicals and particulate matter in which the components are specific to each fire. The detrimental components of smoke include thermal heat, particulate matter, systemic toxins, and respiratory irritants [2,3]. The main clinical consequences of smoke inhalation include acute upper airway obstruction, bronchospasm, small airway occlusion, predisposition for pulmonary infection, and respiratory failure [2,3].

The thermal heat of smoke is damaging to the sensitive mucosa of the nose, oral cavity, and oropharynx. Thermal damage is commonly localized to the upper airway since the body is able to dissipate heat rapidly past the nasal pharynx. If the temperature of the smoke is hot enough to cause thermal injury to the lower airway, patients typically succumb to upper airway obstruction due to extensive edema prior to exhibiting clinical signs from the lower airway thermal burns [3].

The size of the particulate matter determines whether it is deposited in the upper or lower airway. The toxins associated with these particles may be water soluble and may dissolve within airway mucus and cause damage to the mucosa for 48 hours post inhalation [4]. The adherence of these toxins along with thermal injury predisposes the respiratory lining to acute inflammation, increased vascular permeability, and extensive edema. The damaged mucosal cells will produce large volumes of protein-rich exudate and inflammatory cells. Cytokines IL-1-alpha, IL-6, IL-8, and TNF-alpha are released and trigger neutrophilic migration to the airway lumen, furthering the inflammatory cycle and resulting in damage of the respiratory columnar cells and mucociliary apparatus. The combination of mucosal damage, loss of protective mechanisms, and reactive oxygen species results in distal migration of upper airway material and bacteria towards the lower airways, predisposing patients to bacterial pneumonia [2,3,5]. Obstruction of the bronchi, bronchioles, and terminal bronchioles with this debris can occur and further exacerbate respiratory distress. Damage to the upper airway, including the trachea and mainstem bronchi, can result in necrosis 3–5 days post exposure. The resulting pseudomembranous casts often slough and then obstruct the lower airways, resulting in surfactant disruption, lung lobe collapse, and further respiratory dysfunction [2,3,6].

One of the major complicating factors in patients with smoke inhalation is acute respiratory distress syndrome (ARDS). ARDS can develop as a response to smoke inhalation and can be further exacerbated and worsened by the damage to the upper respiratory tract and epithelial sloughing as previously described. The formation of nitric oxide (NO) synthase by the respiratory epithelial cells and alveolar macrophages resulting in formation of NO (a potent vasodilator) has been implicated in

Textbook of Small Animal Emergency Medicine, First Edition. Edited by Kenneth J. Drobatz, Kate Hopper, Elizabeth Rozanski and Deborah C. Silverstein.
© 2019 John Wiley & Sons, Inc. Published 2019 by John Wiley & Sons, Inc.
Companion Website: www.wiley.com/go/drobatz/textbook

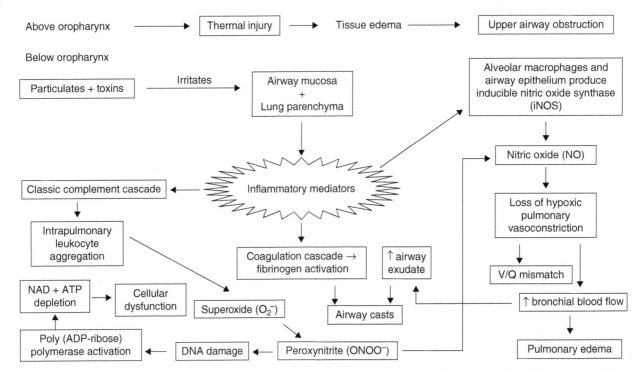

Figure 139.1 Pathophysiology of smoke inhalation induced-respiratory tract inflammation and pulmonary edema. Reproduced with permission of the College of Intensive Care Medicine of Australia and New Zealand.

increasing bronchial blood flow and decreasing hypoxic pulmonary vasoconstriction, resulting in V/Q mismatch. NO can also combine with the superoxide (O_2^-) produced by activated neutrophils to form peroxynitrite (ONOO$^-$). Peroxynitrite leads to DNA damage and subsequent activation of poly (ADP-ribose) polymerase which utilizes large amounts of ATP and NAD, resulting in energy depletion and cell death [3,7].

The pathophysiology of smoke inhalation is described in Figure 139.1. The combination of edema, increased blood flow, increased vascular permeability, vasodilation, and energy depletion can lead to ARDS and respiratory failure. The severity of lung damage and inflammation may predispose to pulmonary infection. Approximately 50% of human patients with smoke inhalation injury will develop a secondary infection [2,3,8].

Carbon Monoxide and Cyanide Exposure

Inhaled carbon monoxide (CM) and hydrogen cyanide (HC) can exacerbate respiratory and systemic collapse in smoke inhalation patients. The severity of intoxication from CM is dependent on the duration of exposure, concentration of inhaled CM, and underlying health status of the patient [2]. CM is rapidly absorbed across the alveolar membrane and has an affinity for hemoglobin that is 200–250 times greater than that of oxygen [2,3,6,9]. CM binds hemoglobin tightly to form carboxyhemoglobin (CO-Hgb), resulting in a functional anemia in which red blood cells are unable to facilitate oxygen carrying and release. This causes a left shift of the oxygen-hemoglobin dissociation curve and secondary cellular hypoxia. CM also competitively inhibits intracellular cytochrome oxidase enzyme systems, specifically cytochrome p450, which disrupts aerobic metabolism and cellular respiration. CM toxicity is associated with the induction of lipid peroxidation, direct cellular damage, reperfusion injury, and central nervous system demyelination [2,6,10].

While literature in the veterinary field is limited, a recent case series found that dogs with higher CO-Hgb concentrations had a significantly longer duration of hospitalization, altered mental status, abnormal respiratory sounds, increased respiratory effort, and hypothermia [11].

Carbon monoxide toxicity may result in both acute and delayed neurological abnormalities. Delayed neurological sequelae are more common in people that are more symptomatic at presentation. Delayed onset of neurological signs in these people manifests as memory loss, confusion, ataxia, and seizures 2–40 days post exposure [12]. Delayed neurological signs have been described in veterinary medicine [2,10,13,14].

One case report describes a dog that presented comatose secondary to CM toxicity from smoke inhalation with initial recovery, but re-presented 5 days later for progressive neurological signs including tetraparesis and mental dullness. This dog recovered completely with intensive supportive care and had no evidence of neurological abnormalities at a 34-month follow-up [10]. Another case series describes multiple animals from the same household hospitalized for CM toxicity from smoke inhalation. All but one animal recovered initially from CM toxicity. Two weeks after exposure, hearing deficits were found in all remaining animals, but resolved by 6 weeks post incident [14]. In a case series of three adult Chihuahuas hospitalized after smoke inhalation, the patients showed initial improvement but later developed seizures. Despite intensive hospitalization and supportive care, all three dogs died and multiple intracranial lesions were found on histopathological examination that were consistent with CM exposure [13]. Another case series describes 21 dogs caught in a kennel fire; those with neurological signs had significantly increased CO-Hgb levels and all five of the dogs that presented with neurological deficits had CO-Hgb levels >24% [11].

Thermal combustion of nitrogen-containing polymers produces HC. HC is rapidly absorbed upon inhalation and inhibits cellular use of oxygen. Once absorbed, cyanide combines with Fe^{3+} in the mitochondrial cytochrome a3 complex and inhibits electron transport and cellular respiration [15]. The inhalation of CM and HC results in synergistic effects that rapidly inhibit the body's ability to utilize oxygen. This leads to tissue hypoxia, acidosis, and a decrease in cerebral oxygen consumption [16–18].

Physical Examination Findings

A clinical diagnosis of smoke inhalation should be based on the patient's history and physical examination. Indications of smoke inhalation include singed nasal vibrissae, oropharyngeal blistering, facial burns, a smoke smell to the fur, and dark, soot-filled sputum [6,9,19]. Patients should be immediately assessed for respiratory difficulty (both upper and lower airway). Lung auscultation may reveal increased breath sounds, wheezes secondary to bronchoconstriction, or crackles. The patient should be evaluated for hypoventilation secondary to either poor pulmonary or chest wall compliance. Patients may present initially with only mild clinical signs that may worsen over 24–36 hours.

Smoke inhalation and associated CM toxicity can result in significant cardiovascular abnormalities such as hypotension, cardiac arrhythmias, and dehydration. Neurological assessment should evaluate for signs of head trauma as well as evidence of neurotoxicity.

Agitation, confusion, ataxia, decreased mentation, loss of consciousness, and seizures are highly suggestive of CM or cyanide toxicity [6,19–21]. Intracranial signs are supportive of hypoxic events to the brain which can lead to intracranial edema, swelling, and an increase in intracranial pressure.

A thorough eye exam should be performed as exposure keratopathy and corneal ulceration are common secondary to smoke exposure. A patient with suspected smoke exposure should have their eyes liberally irrigated to minimize continued topical exposure of toxicants and irritants. Significant burn injury is a rare finding in smoke inhalation patients. In two retrospective studies, only one of 27 dogs and one of 22 cats had a major burn injury. The most common dermatological abnormalities seen in animals that presented to the emergency department following smoke inhalation were minor injuries such as singed fur and skin lacerations [22,23]. It is possible that patients with more severe burns and inhalation injury died at the scene.

Diagnostics

Patients with respiratory difficulty should have diagnostics such as pulse oximetry and arterial blood gas analysis performed, but results should be interpreted carefully if CM or cyanide toxicity is suspected. A standard two-wavelength pulse oximeter will provide a falsely elevated peripheral saturation of oxygen (SpO_2) reading due to the inability to differentiate between oxyhemoglobin and CO-Hgb [8,10,19,21,24]. An arterial blood gas (PaO_2) only reflects the dissolved oxygen which should be unchanged in CM or cyanide toxicity. To evaluate the amount of CO-Hgb in patients with CM toxicity, a CO-oximeter is required. The blood of normal cats and dogs should have <1% CO-Hgb [25,26]. Elevations of this value, along with clinical presentation and history, should be used to make a diagnosis of CM toxicity. If the CO-Hgb is normal but a patient presents with neurological signs, metabolic acidosis, high lactate concentration despite adequate perfusion parameters, and a reduction in the arterial-venous oxygen gradient, then cyanide toxicity should be considered.

Thoracic radiographs may be performed, but often parenchymal abnormalities will be absent initially, but may appear over the first 24 hours following smoke inhalation. Radiographic abnormalities associated with smoke inhalation include a diffuse interstitial pattern, focal alveolar pattern, and lung lobe collapse secondary to obstruction of the main stem bronchi with debris [22,23].

Laryngoscopy is often useful to evaluate the upper airway and determine the extent of edema and damage. In human patients, bronchoscopy is a standard diagnostic tool and patients are graded to determine the extent of injury and prognosis [16]. Bronchial lavage is also useful to obtain a sample for culture and susceptibility testing, and to remove excessive debris.

Bronchoscopy is of limited use in veterinary medicine due to the need for general anesthesia if a tracheostomy tube is not in place.

Treatment

Immediate treatment with supplemental oxygen is imperative for supporting arterial oxygen content and increasing the elimination of CM (see Chapter 181). Rapid clinical improvement is common with the addition of supplemental oxygen, and it is becoming increasingly common for first responders to administer oxygen as soon as possible. At 21% inspired oxygen, the half-life of CM is 5 hours. The half-life decreases to 1 hour at 100% oxygen and 20 minutes with 100% hyperbaric oxygen therapy at 2.5–3 times atmospheric pressure [9,12,19]. The use of hyperbaric oxygen therapy has theoretical benefits, but the results of a Cochrane review evaluating seven randomized controlled trials failed to show sufficient evidence to justify its use in the treatment of CM toxicity [27]. While the use of hyperbaric oxygen therapy is rare in veterinary medicine, oxygen supplementation given via mask, oxygen cage, endotracheal intubation, or other methods is adequate in most cases.

Ensuring an adequate airway is a priority after the administration of supplemental oxygen. Severe edema may be seen initially, but can also develop rapidly. Ensuring a functional and open airway is vital. If there is concern, either intubation with positive pressure ventilation or a tracheostomy tube should be considered (see Chapter 180).

Mechanical ventilation may be indicated for both persistent hypoxia despite supplemental oxygen or hypoventilation due to poor pulmonary compliance and chest wall injuries. Low tidal volume mechanical ventilation with associated permissive hypercapnia has been shown to reduce ventilator-induced lung injury [3,28]. Positive pressure ventilation along with positive end-expiratory pressure (PEEP) helps decrease atelectasis and maintain adequate oxygenation and increase compliance of damaged lungs (see Chapter 188).

Intravenous fluid resuscitation with a balanced isotonic crystalloid should be instituted, if indicated, to support the cardiovascular system and maintain hydration (see Chapter 167). While smoke inhalation patients typically need only maintenance rates of fluids, if dermal burns are present the patient's fluid requirements may be significantly increased [19]. See Section 5 for further details.

If HC is highly suspected and the patient has not improved significantly with supportive care, then antidotes such as amyl nitrate and sodium thiosulfate may prove beneficial. These antidotes oxidize hemoglobin to methemoglobin, which preferentially binds cyanide to create cyanomethemoglobin and allows free cyanide to be converted to thiocyanate by the liver and metabolized [7]. Since treatment of cyanide requires the formation of methemoglobinemia, the use of this antidote is controversial as it may worsen hypoxemia. Hydroxocobalamin (vitamin B12a) administration may also be considered since it binds cyanide to form cyanocobalamin which is excreted via the urine [3].

Supportive treatments include the use of beta-2 agonists to reduce bronchoconstriction-induced airflow resistance and improve dynamic compliance. Beta-2 agonists such as terbutaline (0.01 mg/kg IV, SC, IM, PO) or inhaled albuterol decrease histamine release, leukotriene levels, and TNF-alpha concentrations, thereby conferring an anti-inflammatory effect. There is also evidence that beta-2 agonists may improve fluid clearance within the respiratory tract and promote mucosal repair [3,29–31].

Even though it is reported that 50% of humans treated for smoke inhalation develop bacterial pneumonia, preventive antibiotics are not recommended (see Chapter 200) [8,19]. If a patient develops clinical signs of pneumonia and culture and susceptibility tests are not available, empirical antimicrobial therapy covering the most common isolates, *Staphylococcus aureus* (cefazolin 15 mg/kg IV q12h) and *Pseudomonas* (ceftazidime 30 mg/kg IV q6h or amikacin 15 mg/kg IV q24h), should be instituted (see Chapter 37) [6,19].

Nebulization of epinephrine and corticosteroids is reported to help minimize edema of the upper airway. Use of systemic steroids has resulted in higher infection and mortality rates in clinical animal studies [6,32,33]. In children, a significant decrease in the incidence of reintubation for pulmonary failure, decreased atelectasis, and decreased mortality was shown following nebulization with heparin and N-acetylcycsteine [34]. Future treatments attempting to target nitric oxide synthase and inflammation in an attempt to restore hypoxic vasoconstriction in the lungs may prove beneficial, in addition to the use of nebulized antioxidants such as gamma-tocopherol (vitamin E) [3,35–37]. A recent study in dogs looked at high-volume lung lavage to reduce toxin exposure and minimize inflammatory mediators and found an improved short-term outcome [38].

Prognosis

In humans, the mortality rate of patients admitted for smoke inhalation without concurrent dermal burn injury is <10% [39]. The overall survival rate of dogs and cats suffering from smoke inhalation without accompanying severe dermal burns has been variable. In a case series looking at dogs presenting to an urban veterinary hospital for smoke inhalation, 11/27 cases were deemed more complicated, and of those, 8/11 either died or were euthanized [22]. In a case series looking at cats presenting to that same institution, only 5/22 were deemed complicated, and there was a survival rate of 20/22 [23]. The majority of the cats and dogs that did well had significant improvement within 24 hours of admission [22,23]. These studies may provide an overly optimistic prognosis as the only patients that were included were ones that made it to the hospital for treatment.

After treatment for smoke inhalation, the potential for delayed complications continues. Delayed neurological signs have been discussed already and chronic respiratory conditions, such as bronchitis, bronchiectasis, pulmonary fibrosis, and atelectasis, are possible. However, long-term studies have not been performed in veterinary patients. As the exact outcome of patients with smoke inhalation is unknown, it is important to have appropriate client communication as well as long-term follow-up, if indicated.

References

1 Shirani KZ, Pruitt BA Jr, Mason AD Jr. The influence of inhalation injury and pneumonia on burn mortality. *Ann Surg* 1987;205:82–87.

2 Vaughn L, Beckel N. Severe burn injury, burn shock, and smoke inhalation injury in small animals. Part 1: burn classification and pathophysiology. *J Vet Emerg Crit Care* 2012;22:179–186.

3 Toon MH, Maybauer MO, Greenwood JE, Maybauer DM, Fraser JF. Management of acute smoke inhalation injury. *Crit Care Resusc* 2010;12:53–61.

4 Nugen N, Herndon DN. Diagnosis and treatment of inhalation injury. In: *Total Burn Care*, 2nd edn (ed. Herndon DN). WB Saunders, London, 2001, pp. 262–270.

5 Cox RA, Burke AS, Jacob S, et al. Activated nuclear factor kappa and airway inflammation after smoke inhalation and burn injury in sheep. *J Burn Care Resusc* 2009;30:489–498.

6 Fitzgerald KT, Flood AA. Smoke inhalation. *Clin Tech Small Anim Pract* 2006;21(4):205–214.

7 Murakami K, Traber DL. Pathophysiological basis of smoke inhalation injury. *News Physiol Sci* 2003;18: 125–129.

8 Sheridan RL. Burns. In: *Textbook of Critical Care*, 5th edn (eds Fink MP, Abraham E, Vincent JL, Kochanek PM). Elsevier Saunders, Philadelphia, 2005, pp. 2065–2075.

9 Duffy BJ, McLaughlin PM, Eichelberger MR. Assessment, triage, and early management of burns in children. *Clin Pediatr Emerg Med* 2006;7:82–93.

10 Mariani CL. Full recovery following delayed neurologic signs after smoke inhalation in a dog. *J Vet Emerg Crit Care* 2003;13:235–239.

11 Ashbaugh EA, Mazzaferro EM, McKiernan BC, et al. The association of physical examination abnormalities and carboxyhemoglobin concentrations in 21 dogs trapped in a kennel fire. *J Vet Emerg Crit Care* 2012;22:361–367.

12 Kao LW, Nanagas KA. CM poisoning. *Med Clin North Am* 2005;89:1161–1194.

13 Kent M, Creevy KE, Delahunta A. Clinical and neuropathological findings of acute CM toxicity in Chihuahuas following smoke inhalation. *J Am Anim Hosp Assoc* 2010;46:259–264.

14 Berent AC, Todd J, Sergeeff J, Powell LL. CM toxicity: a case series. *J Vet Emerg Crit Care* 2005;15:128–135.

15 Prien T, Traber D. Toxic smoke compounds and inhalation injury – a review. *Burns* 1988;14:451–460.

16 Dries DJ, Endorf FW. Inhalation injury: epidemiology, pathology, treatment strategies. *Scand J Trauma Resusc Emerg Med* 2013;21:31.

17 McCall JE, Cahill TJ. Respiratory care of the burn patient. *J Burn Care Rehabil* 2005;26:200–206.

18 Moore SJ, Ho IK, Hume AS. Severe hypoxia produced by concomitant intoxication with sublethal doses of CM and cyanide. *Toxicol Appl Pharmacol* 1991;109:412–420.

19 Vaughn L, Beckel N, Walters P. Severe burn injury, burn shock, and smoke inhalation injury in small animals. Part 2: diagnosis, therapy, complications, and prognosis. *J Vet Emerg Crit Care* 2012;22:187–200.

20 Jackson DL, Menges H. Accidental CM poisoning. *J Am Med Assoc* 1980;243:772–774.

21 Prockop LD, Chichkova RI. CM intoxication: an updated review. *J Neurol Sci* 2007;262:122–130.

22 Drobatz KJ, Walker LM, Hendricks JC. Smoke exposure in dogs: 27 cases (1988–1997). *J Am Vet Med Assoc* 1999;207:1306–1311.

23 Drobatz KJ, Walker LM, Hendricks JC. Smoke exposure in cats: 22 cases (1986–1997). *J Am Vet Med Assoc* 1999;207:1312–1316.

24 Desanti LB. Pathophysiology and current management of burn injury. *Adv Skin Wound Care* 2005;18:323–332.

25 Wray JD. Methaemoglobinaemia caused by hydroxycarbamide (hydroxyurea) ingestion in a dog. *J Small Anim Sci* 2008;49:211–215.

26 Ayres DA. Pulse oximetry and CO-oximetry. In: *Advanced Monitoring and Procedures for Small Animal Emergency and Critical Care* (eds Creedon JMB, Davis H). Wiley-Blackwell, Chichester, 2012, pp. 274–285.

27 Buckley NA, Juurlink DN, Isbister G, Bennett MH, Lavonas EJ. Hyperbaric oxygen for CM poisoning. *Cochrane Database Syst Rev* 2011;4:CD002041.

28 Acute Respiratory Distress Syndrome Network, Brower RG, Matthay MA, et al. Ventilation with lower tidal volumes for acute lung injury and the acute respiratory distress syndrome. *N Engl J Med* 2000;342:1301–1308.

29 Morina P, Herrera M, Venegas J, et al. Effects of nebulized salbutamol on respiratory mechanics in adult respiratory distress syndrome. *Intensive Care Med* 1997;23:58–64.

30 Zhang H, Kim YK, Govindarajan A, et al. Effect of adrenoreceptors on endotoxin induced cytokines and lipid peroxidation in lung explants. *Am J Respir Crit Care Med* 1999;160:1703–1710.

31 Mcauley DF, Frank JA, Fang X, Matthay MA. Clinically relevant concentrations of beta2-adrenergic agonists stimulate maximal cyclic adenosine monophosphate-dependent airspace fluid clearance and decrease pulmonary edema in experimental acid-induced lung injury. *Crit Care Med* 2004;32:1470–1476.

32 McFadden ER. Therapy of acute asthma. *J Allergy Clin Immunol* 1989;84(2):151–158.

33 Nieman GF, Clark WR, Hakim T. Methylprednisolone does not protect the lung from inhalation injury. *Burns* 1991;17:384–390.

34 Desai MH, Mlcak R, Richardson J, et al. Reduction in mortality in pediatric patients with inhalation injury with aerolized heparin/N-acetylcysteine therapy. *J Burn Care Rehabil* 1998;19:210–212.

35 Enkhbaatar P, Connelly R, Wang J, et al. Inhibition of neuronal nitric oxide synthase in ovine model of acute lung injury. *Crit Care Med* 2009;37:208–214.

36 Westphal M, Enkhbaatar P, Schmalstieg FC, et al. Neuronal nitric oxide synthase inhibition attenuates cardiopulmonary dysfunctions after combined burn and smoke inhalation injury in sheep. *Crit Care Med* 2008;36:1196–1204.

37 Enkhbaatar P, Murakami K, Shimoda K, et al. The inducible nitric oxide synthase inhibitor BBS-2 prevents acute lung injury in sheep after burn and smoke inhalation injury. *Am J Respir Crit Care Med* 2003;167:1021–1026.

38 Nie F, Su D, Shi Y, et al. Early high volume lung lavage for acute severe smoke inhalation injury in dogs. *Mol Med Rep* 2014;9:863–871.

39 Clark WR. Smoke inhalation: diagnosis and treatment. *World J Surg* 1999;16:24.

140

Porcupine Quilling
Elizabeth Rozanski, DVM, DACVIM (SAIM), DACVECC

Cummings School of Veterinary Medicine, Tufts University, North Grafton, MA, USA

Introduction

Porcupines are rodents indigenous to much of the north-ern parts of the United States and throughout Canada [1]. They are the second largest rodent in the US, second only to the beaver. They live in wooded areas and dens, where they eat leaves, twigs, berries, and other vegetation. Porcupines are strong tree climbers. They are nocturnal, near-sighted, and non-aggressive, and have evolved to use their modified hairs (quills) as protection against predators. Quills are hollow and barbed, and range in length from less than 1 cm to 8–9 cm. Shed quills are replaced, and quills in newborn porcupines (porcupettes) harden within a few days. The quill itself is an engineering marvel, with small barbs that help the quill to slide into the tissue of the attacker, but prevent easy withdrawal [2]. This characteristic has recently been exploited to create a suture, aptly named Quill™ [3].

Importantly, the quills are not actively thrown at an attacker, but when the porcupine is threatened, the quills will stand up and will be more easily dislodged. Thus, the porcupine is never the aggressor, but rather the victim in dog:porcupine interactions [4]. Interestingly, porcupine quills have antimicrobial properties, as self-quilling in falls is not uncommon in porcupines [5]. Free-roaming large-breed dogs often encounter and attack porcupines [4] (Figure 140.1). Cats are rarely, if ever, quilled. Keeping a dog leashed will prevent porcupine quillings, but this may be harder to do in more rural areas.

Prehospital Care

Owners of dogs that have been quilled should be advised to bring them to the veterinarian for removal. Quill removal is painful and, in all but the most minor quillings, should be performed under sedation or general anesthesia. If immediate removal is not possible, dogs should be prevented from rubbing at the quills as

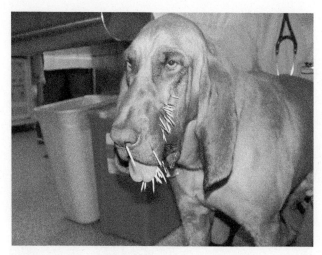

Figure 140.1 A bloodhound with a minor quilling after a porcupine encounter.

this will push them in deeper and make them harder to remove, as well as more likely to migrate.

Quill Removal

After sedation or anesthesia, quill removal is performed by gently grasping the quill at its base with a hemostat and pulling it out. Intubation may be challenging or impossible with severe quillings as the quills may be lodged in the larynx (Figure 140.2). The hemostat may be rinsed in a bowl of water, which serves to contain the quills as well for easier clean-up (Figure 140.3). Removed quills are still sharp. After all visible quills have been removed, the head, neck, chest, and front limbs should be carefully palpated for migrating quills. Small incisions may be required to retrieve these quills.

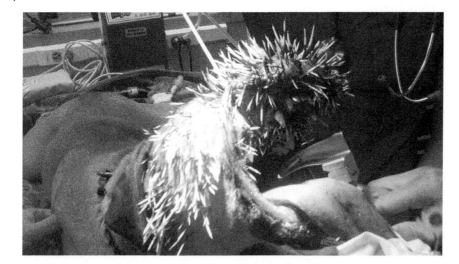

Figure 140.2 A pit bull terrier type dog with a severe quilling, including quills in the larynx. Note the quill through the tongue, as well as the catheter in the saphenous vein. It may be easier to restrain a severely quilled dog for a hindlimb catheter in order to prevent the restrainer from being injured by the quills.

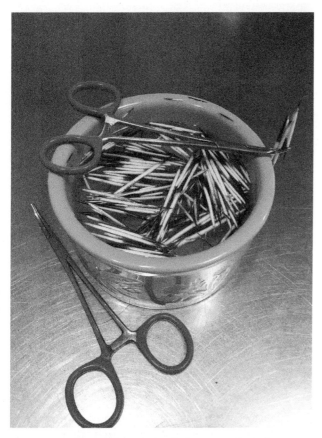

Figure 140.3 Hemostats and a bowl of water used to help remove quills.

Discharge Instructions

Dogs may be discharged as soon as recovered. Analgesics, such as NSAIDs, are often prescribed. Due to the antimicrobial nature of quills, infection is rare but a short course of antimicrobials may be prescribed if removal is accompanied by multiple incisions (see Chapter 200).

Owners should be advised that dogs will not avoid porcupine encounters in the future and additionally, that some quills might remain.

Rabies has not been reported after a quilling. One study identified that raccoons found with quills imbedded were more likely to be rabid, but this appears to reflect rabies infection in the raccoon, as rabies encephalitis caused the raccoons to attack porcupines, rather than the other way around [6]. A rabies booster vaccine is therefore not necessary after a dog attacks a porcupine, unless there is some other reason for considering rabies infection, such as a true porcupine attack during daylight hours. In the most recent report on rabies surveillance, there were no reported rabies infection in porcupines [7].

Complicated Quillings

Complicated quillings are defined as the presence of migrating quills that cause significant morbidity or even mortality [8–12]. Complicated quillings should be suspected in dogs that show signs of lameness, altered mentation, difficulty breathing, or swellings within a few days to several weeks after the quilling. Quills have been reported in the eyes, central nervous system, joints, and thorax [8–12]. Intrathoracic quills are associated with pneumothorax in some cases, usually within days of the initial quilling.

Treatment of quill-associated pneumothorax is surgical exploration and removal of the quill and any damaged lung parenchyma. Quills have also been found and removed from the heart and pericardium. Quills are hard to find with diagnostic imaging, although experienced and patient radiologists may be able to localize some migrating quills, particularly with ultrasound [9] (Figure 140.4). Complicated quillings are more common with severe quillings and those quillings that are not promptly addressed.

Figure 140.4 Ultrasound image of a quill in the front leg of a German short-haired pointer. This dog was non-weight-bearing lame 2 weeks after a severe quilling. Image courtesy of Dr. Heather Spain.

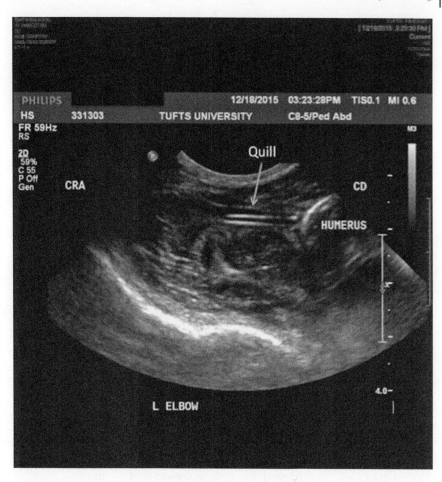

Conclusion

Most quillings are uncomplicated, and treated successfully in emergency rooms. Severe or complicated quillings may be much more challenging and require careful evaluation and planning.

References

1 https://en.wikipedia.org/wiki/Porcupine (accessed 7 February 2018).

2 Cho WK, Ankrum JA, Guo D, et al. Microstructured barbs on the North American porcupine quill enable easy tissue penetration and difficult removal. *Proc Natl Acad Sci USA* 2012;109(52):21289–21294.

3 Ruff GL. The history of barbed sutures. *Aesthet Surg J* 2013;33(3 Suppl):12S–16S.

4 Johnson MD, Magnusson KD, Shmon CL, et al. Porcupine quill injuries in dogs: a retrospective of 296 cases (1998–2002). *Can Vet J* 2006;47(7):677–682.

5 Roze U, Locke DC, Vatakis N. Antibiotic properties of porcupine quills. *J Chem Ecol* 1990;16(3):725–734.

6 Rosatte R, Wandeler A, Muldoon F, et al. Porcupine quills in raccoons as an indicator of rabies, distemper, or both diseases: disease management implications. *Can Vet J* 2007;48(3):299–300.

7 Monroe BP, Yager P, Blanton J, et al. Rabies surveillance in the United States during 2014. *J Am Vet Med Assoc* 2016;248(7):777–788.

8 Sauvé CP, Sereda NC, Sereda CW. Identification of an intra-cranial intra-axial porcupine quill foreign body with computed tomography in a canine patient. *Can Vet J* 2012;53(2):187–189.

9 Brisson BA, Bersenas A, Etue SM. Ultrasonographic diagnosis of septic arthritis secondary to porcupine quill migration in a dog. *J Am Vet Med Assoc* 2004;224(9):1453–1454, 1467–1470.

10 Nucci DJ, Liptak J. The Diagnosis and surgical management of intracardiac quill foreign body in a dog. *J Am Anim Hosp Assoc* 2016;52(1):73–76.

11 Guevara JL, Holmes ES, Reetz J, Holt DE. Porcupine quill migration in the thoracic cavity of a German shorthaired pointer. *J Am Anim Hosp Assoc* 2015;51(2):101–106.

12 Schneider AR, Chen AV, Tucker RL. Imaging diagnosis – vertebral canal porcupine quill with presumptive secondary arachnoid diverticulum. *Vet Radiol Ultrasound* 2010;51(2):152–154.

141

Crotalinae Snake Envenomation

Raegan J. Wells, DVM, MS, DACVECC

Phoenix Veterinary Emergency and Referral, Phoenix, AZ, USA

Introduction

Snake envenomation is a clinically significant cause of presentation to veterinary hospitals for small animal patients. Approximately 162 snake taxa are native to the United States, about 27 of which are front-fanged venomous taxa, with the majority of these belonging to the family Viperidae, subfamily Crotalinae. Pit vipers (Crotalinae), including rattlesnakes (*Crotalus* spp), copperheads and water moccasins (*Agkistrodon* spp), and pygmy rattlesnakes and massasaugas (*Sistrurus* spp), are responsible for approximately 99% of the venomous bites sustained in the US [1]. Crotalinae envenomation in the United States will be discussed, but general concepts of treatment and disease can be applied to victims in any region. Practicing veterinarians should orient themselves to the venomous snakes indigenous to the region in which their patients may have exposure.

A good deal of dogma surrounds snake behavior, characteristics of envenomation, and resultant clinical signs in victims. A common misconception is that young pit vipers cannot control the amount of venom injected with a bite, therefore resulting in a larger dose of venom. All pit vipers control the amount of venom injected during a bite, with the volume injected dependent upon the size of the snake's venom glands and the nature of the bite. Studies evaluating the flow and volume of venom injected with various types of bites (predatory or defensive) have confirmed that there is a percentage of bites without measureable venom delivery, and there may be a trend toward lower volumes injected with defensive bites [2].

While the mechanics of pit viper venom delivery is fascinating, the clinical reality is that most veterinary patients will present with clinical signs of envenomation. The decision to treat these symptoms will be directed by the severity of clinical signs and available resources.

Snake envenomation can occur at any time of year, depending upon the activity of the snakes and exposure of veterinary patients. In very warm climates, such as the Sonoran Desert, crotalinae envenomation occurs year round [3].

Crotalinae Envenomation

There is relatively more information available on Crotalinae envenomation in dogs compared to cats. The published mortality rates for Crotalinae envenomation are low, ranging from 1.8% to 24% in dogs and 6% to 18% in cats [3–14]. Non-survivors typically suffer envenomations to the head, including the eye and tongue, which may provide a more direct route to the central nervous system or predispose to asphyxiation. Dogs that have suffered distal limb envenomations and acutely died are suspected to have experienced intra-arterial envenomation. Envenomations to the trunk may lead to profound clinical signs, including hemoperitoneum and acute respiratory muscle paralysis [6,15]. Relatively speaking, cats appear more susceptible to profound muscle weakness [6,14]. Dogs with advanced age and increased time from envenomation to treatment are risk factors for death [3]. It is well accepted that Crotalinae envenomation has an overall low mortality rate, but patient suffering and morbidity may be profound, requiring significant and costly therapies. Nearly any body system may be affected following envenomation.

Crotalinae venom is a complex mixture of water, proteins, and peptides. Most of the proteins are enzymatic, while the peptides exert organ toxicity [4,5,16]. The classically described enzymes include hyaluronidase, which facilitates rapid spread of the venom by breakdown of the connective tissues; phospholipase A2, which leads to cytotoxicity, including the characteristic echinocytosis and spherocytosis observed as well as anticoagulation via anti-Xa activity; thromboxane, which is at least partially responsible for the thrombocytopenia often observed; as well as snake venom metalloproteinases (SMVPs) which contribute to platelet dysfunction, leading to clinical hemorrhage [16–18].

Crotalinae venoms can cause profound and complicated alterations in the coagulation system, leading to both thrombosis and hemorrhage. These proteins can be broadly classified as FV and FX activators, activators of prothrombin, thrombin-like enzymes, anticoagulant factor IX/X binding proteins, activators of protein C, thrombin inhibitors, fibrinolytic enzymes as well as plasminogen activator (see Chapter 70) [19]. Some venoms contain potent neurotoxins, such as the Mojave venom that causes presynaptic inhibition and may lead to progressive paralysis. These toxins have been identified in the venoms of the Mojave rattlesnake (*C. scutulatus*), western diamondback (*C. atrox*), prairie rattlesnake (*C. viridis*) and southern pacific rattlesnake (*C. helleri*) and pose a significant risk of life-threatening neurological complications associated with envenomation [6]. Myotoxins have been identified in a number of venoms, placing patients at risk for widespread myonecrosis and profound neuromuscular weakness. The most salient point is that nearly any body system may be affected.

Clinical Signs of Envenomation

The classic clinical signs of Crotalinae envenomation involve pain, swelling, regional ecchymosis, and one to two small puncture wounds. It is reported that the Mojave rattlesnake may have pure neurotoxins, therefore making identification of a wound difficult.

Most animals presenting for evaluation following envenomation will exhibit local disease at the bite site, in addition to systemic clinical signs. Dogs often suffer bites to their muzzle, with extremity as the next most common site. Cats will often suffer bites to multiple regions of their body. These patients may present anywhere along the spectrum of compensatory to decompensatory shock (see Chapter 152). Bites to the tongue or mouth may swell rapidly, leading to upper airway obstruction. Hyperglycemia and hypokalemia may be appreciated as a consequence of catecholamine surge. Cardiac arrhythmias are common and should be monitored for (see Chapter 53). Pigmenturia may occur due to hemolysis, rhabdomyolysis or both (see Chapter 66). Anemia may occur due to hemorrhage, hemolysis or both. Thrombocytopenia may be observed, with or without prolonged bedside coagulation times (PT, aPTT) (see Chapter 67). Hyperlactatemia is common,

and likely due to both tissue damage and hypoperfusion. Widespread hemorrhage may occur, leading to hematemesis, hematuria, melena, epistaxis, pulmonary infiltrates or any combination thereof. Neurotoxicity may lead to seizures, nystagmus, or paralysis. Hypoventilation is a risk factor for patients with profound weakness and/or central nervous system involvement. Patients may exhibit any combination or degree of severity of these clinical signs.

Patient Evaluation and Stabilization

An extensive human snake bite severity score has been proposed for use in applying objective assessment to veterinary envenomations [20]. Computation of this score requires measurement of coagulation times and platelet count, so it may not be a practical tool for widespread application in veterinary medicine.

A practical approach to assessment of envenomation is to complete a thorough physical examination. Further measurements may be directed based upon abnormalities noted during physical examination. Additional monitoring to consider includes measurement of systolic blood pressure, electrocardiogram, venous blood gas and electrolytes, a complete blood count with blood smear for evaluation of manual platelet count, echinocyte and spherocyte assessment, chemistry panel to assess renal and hepatic function, urinalysis to assess for pigmenturia, and coagulation times. If client or hospital resources are limited, then an abbreviated laboratory evaluation may consist of a blood smear to evaluate for red blood cell abnormalities and platelet count, venous blood gas and electrolytes, packed cell volume and total protein, measurement of blood urea nitrogen and/or creatinine, and a urine specific gravity with visual inspection for pigmenturia. Cystocentesis is contraindicated due to risk of hemorrhage. Circumferential measurement of the bite site is painful and unlikely to confer any significant advantage to the patient, and is not routinely performed by the author.

Patients should receive a triage assessment immediately upon arrival to the hospital (see Chapter 2). If clinical signs of pain, any form of shock or any other abnormalities are noted, rapid venous access should be obtained while the remaining baseline evaluation of perfusion parameters is assessed. Hypovolemic shock should be treated with isotonic balanced electrolyte fluids, in titrated aliquots of blood volume (see Chapter 153). Analgesia should be provided, ideally with a reversible opioid agonist such as hydromorphone or fentanyl (see Chapter 193). Opioid administration is safe and should not be withheld for fear of exacerbating neurological symptoms.

Finally, neutralization of the circulating venom with antivenom is the ideal treatment for patients with clinical signs of Crotalinae snake envenomation. Advances in antivenom manufacturing have occurred in recent years, providing the clinician with safer and more effective options. Veterinarians must familiarize themselves with the venoms in their region, evaluate their patient's clinical signs and then decide if antivenom administration is necessary. It is important, however, to remember that neutralization of circulating venom is the most direct method to reverse or halt progression of clinical signs and minimize patient suffering.

Antivenoms

There are currently two Crotalinae antivenoms approved by the United States Department of Agriculture (USDA) for use in veterinary medicine: Antivenin (Crotalidae) Polyvalent (ACP) and Venom Vet™. Other antivenoms that have been demonstrated safe and effective in the peer review literature include CroFab™ and an F(ab')2 polyvalent Crotalinae antivenom produced by Veteria Labs, in Mexico (Table 141.1) [3,10,11,14,21].

One antivenom product has predominated veterinary medicine for years: Antivenin (Crotalidae) Polyvalent (ACP), an equine origin antivenom comprised of whole immunoglobulin G (IgG) molecules. Newer antivenoms have been developed from enzymatic digestion of the whole IgG to cleave off the antigen (venom) binding region, termed fragment antigen binding (Fab) region, from the fragment crystallizable (Fc) portion. The creation of a smaller product lacking the Fc portion is believed to increase the volume of distribution and possibly result in a less antigenic product [22–25] These Fab-based antivenoms include Crotalinae Polyvalent Immune Fab (Crofab™), an ovine origin single Fab-based molecule antivenom, and Fab dimer (F(ab')2) equine origin antibody-derived antivenoms (Table 141.1). The Fab-based antivenoms tend to have a relatively short half-life and move outside of the intravascular compartment faster than other antivenoms and may necessitate re-administration if re-envenomation occurs. Compared to the Fab monomer, F(ab')2 antivenoms have a longer half-life and remain in the vascular compartment longer. They also have 2 antigen binding sites per molecule, compared to 1 antigen-binding site on the Fab monomer.

Table 141.1 Commonly available Crotalinae antivenom formulations.

Immunoglobulin type	Formulation	Supplied as	Venoms used in production	Approval status as of March 2018
IgG – equine Longest $T_{1/2}$ 150 kDa 2 venom-binding sites	Antivenom Crotalidae Polyvalent (ACP) Distributed by Boehringer Ingelheim Vetmedica	Lyophilized powder Slow reconstitution Room temperature storage	*Crotalus atrox,* *C. adamanteus,* *C. terrificus,* *Bothrops asper*	USDA approved for use in veterinary medicine
Fab – ovine Shortest $T_{1/2}$ 50 kDa 1 venom-binding site	CroFab® Distributed by Protherics	Lyophilized powder Fast reconstitution Room temperature storage	*Crotalus atrox,* *C. adamanteus,* *C. scutulatus,* *Agkistrodon piscovorus*	FDA approved for use in human medicine Off-label use in veterinary medicine
F(ab')2 – equine Longer $T_{1/2}$ than Fab, shorter than IgG 110 kDa 2 venom-binding sites	Venom Vet™ Produced by Instituto Biologico, Argentino S.A.I.C.	Liquid No reconstitution necessary Refrigeration necessary	*C. durissus, C. simus,* *Lachesis muta,* *Bothrops asper,* *B. alternatus, B. diporus*	USDA approved for use in dogs
F(ab')2 – equine Longer $T_{1/2}$ than Fab, shorter than IgG 110 kDa 2 venom-binding sites	Antivenom – *Bothrops asper* and *Crotalus durissus* Produced by Veteria Labs, S.A. de C.V.	Lyophilized powder Slow reconstitution Room temperature storage	*C. durissus,* *C. oreganus, C. o. helleri,* *C. adamanteus,* *C. scutulatus,* *C. atrox, C. horridus,* *Agkistrodon contortix,* *A. piscivorus,* *Bothrops asper*	Pending USDA approval for use in veterinary medicine Import permits required for experimental use

There is one USDA approved F(ab')2 antivenom available at the time of writing, Venom Vet™. This product is labeled to neutralize the venom of all North American Crotalinae snakes, and is a collection of purified pooled immunoglobulins from healthy horses immunized against multiple species (Table 141.1). There are no peer-review publications describing the clinical efficacy or use of this antivenom. Another widely used F(ab')2 antivenom is Antivenom Bothrops asper & Crotalus durissus, imported from Mexico and distributed by Veteria Labs. This antivenom has been described in multiple peer review publications, and appears to be safe and effective [3,6,9,10,13,14]. The author finds this antivenom to be effective at clinical improvement with neurotoxins and myotoxins. One vial has been shown to be sufficient to neutralize clinical signs of rattlesnake envenomation in most dogs. Dogs with lower body weight and increased time from bite to presentation require more antivenom [3]. A safety study reported that up to 6 vials could be administered intravenously within one hour safely to healthy dogs [21].

A definitive dose of antivenom has not been established. Each batch of antivenom may have different antigen-binding abilities. It is reasonable to consider starting with two vials of F(ab')2 antivenom in very small dogs or patients presenting with severe clinical signs such as cardiovascular collapse. Once it has been determined that antivenom is indicated, timely neutralization of venom should be prioritized, so the infusion should be administered as rapidly as possible. Intitial infusion rates of 0.25–0.5 mL/kg/h are recommended while monitoring for signs of reaction. If no reaction is appreciated, the rate can be increased to administer the entire dose within 30–60 minutes. Cats may be more likely to experience a reaction to antivenom infusion, so close monitoring and slower infusion rates may be warranted in this species [14].

Some patients experience severe and protracted signs of envenomation, requiring multiple repeat boluses of antivenom. In these instances, it is sometimes advised to administer the antivenom as a constant-rate infusion (CRI). The dosing is empirical, and based upon human CRI protocols for bleeding diathesis [26]. Consider 1–2 vials over 6 hours continuously. Examples include patients with ongoing severe clinical signs such as neuromuscular collapse, profound hemolysis and/or rhabdomyolysis. It is not necessary to perform intradermal testing prior to antivenom administration, nor is it necessary to administer prophylactic diphenhydramine or glucocorticoids [1,3,11].

Endpoints to consider include optimization of perfusion parameters (heart rate, blood lactate, systolic blood pressure, electrocardiogram), resolution of coagulopathy as demonstrated by normalized coagulation times and/or platelet count, sustained resolution or significant improvement in echinocytosis and spherocytosis if noted at baseline, lack of pigmenturia and/or progressive hemolysis, control of pain, and lack of progressive swelling or tissue damage.

Additional Therapies

There is an equine plasma protein product, RTLR™ (MG Biologics), marketed as snake bite protein support for dogs. This is from horses that have been vaccinated against the Mojave, eastern diamondback, western diamondback, and prairie rattlesnake. The manufacturer recommends administration at about 4 mL/kg. Each bag contains 100 mL of unpurified equine plasma. Peer review literature evaluating safety or efficacy does not exist at this time. The author cautions against offering this therapy to canine and feline patients in lieu of purified antivenom products. Potential complications include volume overload due to relatively larger dose of colloid product compared to antivenom, and risk of acute and delayed hypersensitivity reactions.

Antibiotic prophylaxis has been a controversial topic in the treatment of Crotalinae envenomation. The consensus in human medicine is that antibiotics are not indicated unless evidence of an infection develops [27,28]. Recent veterinary literature evaluating dogs with rattlesnake envenomation does not support routine antibiotic prophylaxis [3,9]. Some wounds will require treatment, likely due to secondary compartment syndrome and opportunistic infections (see Chapter 166). When indicated, single agent with the narrowest spectrum and shortest treatment duration possible, guided by bacterial culture and susceptibility, is recommended.

Routine administration of glucocorticoids is not recommended. No morbidity or mortality benefit has been documented with use of glucocorticoids in dogs envenomated by Crotalinae spp, and potential risks of use outweigh the potential benefit.

Local wound treatment with laser therapy has been promoted by some veterinarians. Peer review evidence of this therapy is lacking. It is a reasonable therapy to offer, should only be used by individuals with proper training, and should not be applied more than every 8 hours. This is an adjunctive therapy and should not be offered in lieu of standard treatments such as neutralizing antivenom, fluid therapy, and analgesia. Non-steroidal anti-inflammatory medications are not recommended, as these patients are at risk for kidney injury due to hypoperfusion, coagulopathy, nephrotoxins in the venom, and pigmenturia. Additionally, gastrointestinal ulceration is possible secondary to hypoperfusion and coagulopathy.

Some patients may require transfusion of red blood cells to treat secondary anemia due to blood loss, hemolysis or both (see Chapter 176). Hemolysis with spherocytosis may be observed, sometimes as late as 72 hours following initial envenomation. It is most likely that these patients are experiencing ongoing envenomation, and treatment with antivenom should be prioritized over immune suppression. In patients experiencing hemorrhagic complications of envenomation, treatment with fresh frozen plasma is not indicated. The mechanism of coagulopathy in most cases is not due to factor deficiency, but rather a complex syndrome of factor inhibition, activation, platelet inhibition, and endothelial dysfunction. As such, neutralization of circulating venom with antivenom is the treatment of choice.

The only reliable means of envenomation prevention is avoidance. Common attempts at envenomation prophylaxis include aversion training and use of a rattlesnake vaccine, *Crotalus atrox* toxoid manufactured by Hygieia Biological Laboratories and distributed by Red Rock Biologics. This vaccine claims efficacy against *C. atrox* venom, and the manufacturer also notes possible protection against venoms of many other Crotalinae snakes. Canine challenge studies evaluating postvaccine antibody titers in dogs or support of clinical efficacy are lacking. A retrospective evaluation of dogs suffering rattlesnake envenomation reported no measurable benefit of vaccination [3]. There is no peer review evidence supporting prophylaxis of snake bite by using avoidance training, behavioral modification, or prophylactic vaccination.

References

1 Peterson ME. Snake bite: pit vipers. *Clin Tech Small Anim Pract* 2006;21(4):174–182.

2 Young BA, Zahn K. Venom flow in rattlesnakes: mechanics and metering. *J Experiment Biol* 2001;204:4345-4351.

3 Witsil AJ, Wells, RJ, Woods C. 272 cases of rattlesnake envenomation in dogs: demographics and treatment including safety of F(ab')2 antivenom use in 236 patients. *Toxicon* 2015;105:19–26.

4 Julius T, Kaelble M, Leech E, et al. Retrospective evaluation of neurotoxic rattlesnake envenomation in dogs and cats: 34 cases (2005–2010). *J Vet Emerg Crit Care* 2012;22(4):460–469.

5 McCown J, Cooke K, Hanel R, et al. Effect of antivenin dose on outcome from crotalid envenomations: 218 dogs (1988–2006). *J Vet Emerg Crit Care* 2009;19(6):603–610.

6 Willey JR, Schaer M. Eastern diamondback (Crotalus adamanteus) envenomation of dogs: 31 cases (1982–2002). *J Am Anim Hosp Assoc* 2005;41:22–33.

7 Carr A, Schultz J. Prospective evaluation of the incidence of wound infection in rattlesnake envenomation in dogs. *J Vet Emerg Crit Care* 2015;25(4):546–551.

8 Katzenbach J, Foy D. Retrospective evaluation of the effect of antivenom administration on hospitalization duration and treatment cost for dogs envenomated by Crotalus viridis: 113 dogs (2004–2012). *J Vet Emerg Crit Care* 2015;25(5):655–659.

9 Peterson M, Matz M, Seibold K, et al. A randomized multicenter trial of Crotalidae polyvalent immune Fab antivenom for the treatment of rattlesnake envenomation in dogs. *J Vet Emerg Crit Care* 2011;21(4):335–345.

10 Hackett TB, Wingfield WE, Mazzaferro EM, et al. Clinical findings associated with prairie rattlesnake bites in dogs: 100 cases (1989–1998). *J Am Vet Med Assoc* 2002;220(11):1675–1680.

11 Hoose J, Carr A. Retrospective analysis of clinical findings and outcome of cats with suspected rattlesnake envenomation in Southern California: 18 cases (2007–2010). *J Vet Emerg Crit Care* 2013;23(3):314–320.

12 Pashmakova M, Bishop M, Black D, et al. Multicenter evaluation of the administration of crotalid antivenom in cats: 115 cases (2000–2011). *J Am Vet Med Assoc* 2013;243:520–525.

13 Istvan S, Walker J, Hansen B, et al. Presumptive intraperitoneal envenomation resulting in hemoperitoneum and acute abdominal pain in a dog. *J Vet Emerg Crit Care* 2015;25(6):770–777.

14 Gopalakrishnakone P, Hawgood BJ, Holbrooke SE, et al. Sites of action of Mojave toxin isolated from the venom of the Mojave rattlesnake. *Br J Pharmacol* 1980;69:421–437.

15 Powell RS, Lieb CS, Rael ED. Identification of a neurotoxic venom component in the tiger rattlesnake Crotalus tigris. *J Herpetol* 2004;38(1):149–152.

16 Gold BS, Dart RC, Barish RA. Bites of venomous snakes. *N Engl J Med* 2002;347(5):347–356.

17 Kini RM. Structure-function relationships and mechanism of anticoagulant phospholipase A2 enzymes from snake venoms. *Toxicon* 2005;45:1147–1161.

18 Kamiguti AS. Platelets as targets of snake venom metalloproteinases. *Toxicon* 2005;45:1041–1049.

19 Lu Q, Clemetson JM, Clemetson KJ. Snake venoms and hemostasis. *J Thromb Haemost* 2005;3:1791–1799.

20 Dart RC, Hurlbut KM, Garcia R. Validation of a severity score for the assessment of crotalid snakebite. *Ann Emerg Med* 1996;27(3):321–326.

21 Woods C, Young D. Clinical safety evaluation of F(ab)2 antivenom (Crotalus durissus-Bothrops asper) administration in dogs. *J Vet Emerg Crit Care* 2011;21(5):565–569.

22 Gutierrez JM, Leon G, Lomonte B. Pharmacologic-pharmacodynamic relationships of immunoglobulin therapy for envenomation. *Clin Pharmacokinet* 2003;42(8):721–741.

23 Lavonas EJ. Antivenoms for snakebite: design, function, and controversies. *Curr Pharm Biotechnol* 2012;13:1980–1986.

24 Morais VM, Massaldi H. Snake antivenoms: adverse reactions and production technology. *J Venom Anim Toxins* 2009;15(1):2–18.

25 Seifert SA, Boyer LV. Recurrence phenomena after immunoglobulin therapy for snake envenomations: part 1. *Pharmacokinetics and pharmacodynamics of immunoglobulin antivenoms and related antibodies. Ann Emerg Med* 2001;37(2):189–195.

26 Bush SP, Seifert SA, Oakes J. Continuous IV Crotalidae polyvalent immune Fab (Ovine) (FabAV) for selected North American Rattlesnake bite patients. *Toxicon* 2013;69:29–37.

27 Clark RF, Selden BS, Furbee B. The incidence of wound infection following crotalid envenomation. *J Emerg Med* 1993;11:583–586.

28 LoVecchio F, Klemens J, Welch S, Rodriguez R. Antibiotics after rattle-snake envenomation. *J Emerg Med* 2002;23(4):327–328.

142

Elapid Snake Envenomation: North American Coral Snakes and Australian Elapids (Tiger Snakes, Brown Snakes, Taipans, Death Adders, and Black Snakes)

Katrin Swindells, BVSc, MANZCVS, DACVECC[1] and Michael Schaer, DVM, DACVIM (SAIM), DACVECC[2]

[1] *Western Australian Veterinary Emergency and Specialty, Perth, WA, Australia*
[2] *College of Veterinary Medicine, University of Florida, Gainesville, FL, USA*

Introduction

Elapids are venomous front-fanged snakes found in Australia, North America, South and Central America, Asia, Africa, India, and the Middle East. Fangs are often small, resulting in minimally traumatic bites. Therefore, failure to identify a bite site does not rule out envenomation. Elapid snakes may also give a 'dry bite' without injection of venom into the patient. The authors recommend that antivenom is used when there is clinical evidence of Australian elapid envenomation in dogs and cats. Because of the potential for anaphylactic reactions to equine immunoglobulins, antivenom should not be used in the absence of definitive signs of envenomation, and epinephrine should always be available when antivenom

is going to be used. In America, prompt treatment with antivenom is recommended for dogs found in close contact with a recently found dead or mutilated coral snake.

This chapter primarily discusses elapid envenomations in Australia and North America. The basic principles of treatment of envenomation may be helpful to guide treatment decisions for elapid envenomations in other countries, with the proviso that the correct antivenom needs to be administered (Table 142.1). Worldwide veterinary-specific information about elapids is often limited; a useful source of information about the human envenomation syndromes for individual species of snakes worldwide and recommended antivenoms can be found at the following website: www.toxinology.com

Table 142.1 Australian and North American elapid snakes, toxins, and recommended antivenoms.

Genus	Species	Venom toxins	Potential clinical effects	Recommended antivenom type and starting dose
North America elapids				
Coral snakes (*Micruroides; Micrurus*)	Western coral snake or Arizona coral snake (*Micruroides euryxanthus*)	Neurotoxin (dogs, cats) Hemolysin (dogs)	Paralysis (severe) Hemolysis (mild, uncommon)	Suero Antiofidico Anticoral – Liquido- Solucion injectable-Instituto Clodomiro Picado, Universidad de Cosa Rica
	North American coral snake or Eastern coral snake or harlequin coral snake (*Micrurus fulvius*)			Coralmyn, Polivalent Anticoral Fabotherapic, Instituto Bioclon SA de CV, Mexico Both require special permission to import
	Texas coral snake (*Micrurus tener*)			1–2 vials. Increase dose to 5 vials if severe signs such as paralysis and hypoventilation, if the owners can afford

Genus	Species	Venom toxins	Potential clinical effects	Recommended antivenom type and starting dose
Australian elapids				
	There are over 100 different species of elapids within Australia; only those commonly associated with envenomation in animals are discussed below			Australian polyvalent snake antivenom 40 000 units (CSL) can be used to treat envenomation by all Australian elapid species. It is extremely expensive compared to monovalent antivenoms listed below
Brown snakes (*Pseudonaja*)	Dugite (*Pseudonaja affinis*) Eastern brown snake (*Pseudonaja textilis*) Western brown snake or Gwardar (*Pseudonaja nuchalis*) Speckled brown snake (*Pseudonaja guttata*)	Procoagulant Neurotoxin	Coagulopathy (severe) Paralysis (severe)	Brown snake antivenom 1000 units. If requires intubation and ventilation, 3000 units
Black snakes (*Pseudechis*)	Red-bellied black snake (*Pseudechis porphyriacus*)	Procoagulant (mild?) Hemolysin Myotoxin Neurotoxin	Hemolysis (severe) Anemia (severe) Rhabdomyolysis (severe) Paralysis (minimal to severe)	Tiger snake antivenom 3000 units (black snake antivenom 18 000 units can be used but is more expensive)
	Mulga snake or king brown snake (*Pseudechis australis*)	Hemolysin Myotoxin Neurotoxins Anticoagulant	Hemolysis (mild to severe) Anemia Rhabdomyolysis (severe) Paralysis (mild to severe)	Black snake antivenom 18 000 units
Copperheads (*Austrelaps*)	Common copperhead or lowlands copperhead (*Austrelaps superbus*)	Neurotoxins Myotoxins Hemolysins Anticoagulant	Paralysis (mild to severe) Rhabdomyolysis (severe) Hemolysis (severe) Anemia (severe)	Tiger snake antivenom 3000 units
Death adders (*Acanthophis*)	Common death adder (*Acanthophis antarcticus*)	Neurotoxins Anticoagulant	Paralysis (severe)	Death adder antivenom 6000 units
Taipan (*Oxyuranus*)	Coastal taipan or common taipan (*Oxyuranus scutellatus*)	Neurotoxins Myotoxin Procoagulants Hemolysins	Paralysis (severe) Rhabdomyolysis (severe) Coagulopathy (severe) Hemolysis (mild)	Taipan antivenom 12 000 units
Tiger snake (*Notechis*)	Mainland tiger snake, Western tiger snake, island tiger snake (*Notechis scutatus*)	Procoagulant toxins Neurotoxins Myotoxin	Coagulopathy (severe) Paralysis (severe) Rhabdomyolysis (severe) Hemolysis (rare, mild)	Tiger snake antivenom 3000 units. If requires intubation and ventilation, 9000 units

Elapid Species Identification

North America

The venomous Eastern coral snake can be easily identified as having a black snout, and yellow, black, and red bands encircling the body. The red and black rings are wider than the interposed yellow rings (Figure 142.1). Care should be taken not to become confused with the harmless scarlet king snake in which the yellow and red rings are separated by black rings ("Red on yellow kill a fellow, red on black, venom lack"). The other species of coral snakes in the Americas and Mexico will have color pattern variations specific to the species in a particular geographic location.

Australia

Snake coloration or relying on the public's description is notoriously inaccurate for identifying snake species within Australia, with the majority of snakes being brown in colour even if they are a member of the Black (*Pseudechis*), Taipan (*Oxyuranus*), Copperhead (*Austrelaps*) or Brown (*Pseudonaja*) snake family or one of the many mildly venomous species of snakes. The following methods are recommended to help determine which type of antivenom should be administered.

- Identification of the snake by an experienced herpetologist. Veterinarians can attempt to identify dead snakes using a snake identification key for their local area which identifies snakes according to scale counts, body shape, and color. Catching, attempting to kill or examination of live elapid snakes by inexperienced

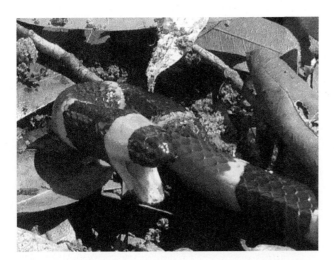

Figure 142.1 The Eastern coral snake, *Micrurus fulvius fulvius*, is a venomous elapid snake characterized by the red and yellow colors lying adjacent to one another. It is geographically distributed in the south-eastern part of the United States.

snake handlers should be strongly discouraged due to the significant risk of life-threatening human envenomation.
- Use of the Commonwealth Serum Laboratory (CSL) snake venom detection kit (SVDK) on the bite site, urine or blood. This kit determines the most appropriate antivenom to administer. The SDVK is not suitable for use outside Australia and Papua New Guinea.
- Knowledge of elapid snakes within the specific locality together with clinical signs can help determine the most appropriate antivenom to use [1]. See Table 142.1 for clinical signs of the major venomous elapid species. However, failure to respond appropriately to antivenom should always raise concerns that the wrong antivenom has been administered.

Pathophysiology of Elapid Venoms

Elapid snake venoms are a complex combination of toxins, with the venom of many species containing multiple neurotoxins, peptides, and enzymatically active and non-active compounds [2]. Despite the prodigious amount of research into elapid venom toxins, their mechanisms of action and treatment efficacy *in vitro* and recent studies of antivenom efficacy in human envenomations, there is limited research into the clinical syndrome of envenomation in dogs and cats. Additionally, there are many mild to moderately venomous elapids whose venom has not been researched.

There appear to be significant clinical differences in the envenomation syndromes of humans and other species, with humans being less susceptible to the neurotoxin effects of envenomation in comparison to dogs and cats [3]. It is also possible that the high incidence of severe paralysis in dog and cat envenomation is due to higher amounts of venom being injected by the snake, potentially due to the unrelenting attacking behavior of dogs and cats when hunting snakes.

Neurotoxins

Neurotoxins are classed as either presynaptic or postsynaptic and exert their effects at the neuromuscular junction, causing a rapid onset of lower motor neuron (LMN) paralysis. Many venoms contain both presynaptic and postsynaptic neurotoxins. Presynaptic neurotoxins belong to the phospholipase A_2 group of toxins and cause structural changes to the nerve terminal, preventing release of acetylcholine. *In vitro* studies have shown that presynaptic neurotoxins can become irreversibly bound and unresponsive to antivenom. Postsynaptic neurotoxins (as found in the western hemisphere elapids and some Australian elapids) act as antagonists at acetylcholine receptors, and *in vitro* studies do not support irreversible binding, so theoretically there should be a rapid response to administration of appropriate antivenom.

Clinical experience in dogs and cats with Australian brown (*Pseudonaja*) and tiger (*Notechis*) snake envenomations which contain presynaptic neurotoxins indicates that severe acute paralysis can rapidly reverse with high doses of antivenom, and irreversible binding is likely to take longer than 24 hours and potentially several days [4]. Conversely, reports of envenomations when postsynaptic neurotoxins are present in both dogs and humans (in Australasia) have revealed cases in which improvement of paralysis has been delayed post antivenom [5,6].

Higher doses of neurotoxic venom have been associated with a more rapid onset of paralysis in dogs envenomated with tiger snake venom and the same is thought to occur in other elapid envenomations [7]. Dogs and cats which are active post envenomation tend to have a faster onset of clinical signs, probably due to muscular activity increasing lymphatic flow and absorption of the venom from the bite site. Paralysis is non-painful and humans have been reported to progress to severe paralysis while sleeping in a hospital bed.

Procoagulant Toxins

Prothrombin activators which are present in some Australian elapid venoms are either classed as group C prothrombin activators (*Oxyuranus* and *Pseudonaja* venoms), similar to factor XaVa prothombinase complex, or group D prothrombin activators (*Notechis* venom) which is similar to factor Xa and requires the presence of the patient's factor Va for the procoagulant effects to be manifested. Procoagulant toxins cause diffuse intravascular thrombosis, consuming clotting factors and then resulting in venom-induced consumptive coagulopathy (VICC) with depletion of fibrinogen, factor V and factor VIII. Coagulation testing reveals prolongation of PT and aPTT commonly beyond the limits of test detection [4,8]. VICC and cerebral haemorrhage are the most common causes of human death in Australian snake bite. Acute renal failure occasionally occurs in patients with VICC and is potentially due to renal ischemia secondary to intrarenal microthrombosis.

Normalization of the patient's clotting times post antivenom administration takes a significant period of time due to the requirement for hepatic synthesis of replacement clotting factors, commonly at least 12 hours in dogs and cats after antivenom and 24–36 hours in humans [4,8]. Current human guidelines and clinical experience with animals indicate that one vial of antivenom should be sufficient to neutralize procoagulant toxins. Clinical signs of hemorrhage are infrequent, and fresh frozen plasma is rarely indicated and should never be given before antivenom as it may worsen thrombosis formation [9]. Because of the severe coagulopathy and the potential for life-threatening bleeding, strict confined rest is recommended until clotting times normalize [10].

Anticoagulant Toxins

Several phospholipase A_2 toxins in Australian elapids have an anticoagulant effect on blood, causing prolongation of aPTT and potentially PT. Spontaneous hemorrhage does not occur and the prolonged bleeding times improve rapidly after antivenom administration [11,12].

Myotoxins

Various phospholipase A_2 toxins in Australian elapids can cause severe rhabdomyolysis. Increases in creatinine kinase (CK) are generally delayed for at least 3–6 hours post bite, and minimizing patient muscular activity and early administration of antivenom prevent the development of rhabdomyolysis; delayed administration of antivenom is still worthwhile as it potentially prevents the worsening of rhabdomyolysis. CK can be severely elevated >5000 U/L, and in some patients massive elevations >500 000 U/L can occur. Elevations in CK do not immediately resolve post administration of antivenom; instead, CK plateaus and then gradually decreases [11,13]. Myoglobinuria is common and severe myoglobinuria may cause acute kidney injury (AKI) to develop [7,13,14]. Megaoesophagus secondary to myotoxins has been reported as a complication of Australian tiger snake envenomation in dogs, with reports of resolution taking up to 5 weeks [15].

Hemolytic Toxins

Some phospholipase toxins in North American and Australian elapids cause lysis of red cells, resulting in severe anemia, hemoglobinemia and hematuria, and potentially AKI [16]. Echinocytes or burr cells and evidence of red cell damage may be visualized on blood smear examination (see Chapter 66). The risk of development of anemia from exposure to hemolytic toxins appears to be species specific, with dogs having an increased susceptibility compared to humans and cats [11,13,16]. Rare cases of immune-mediated delayed hemolytic anemia in dogs have also been reported [17]. In envenomations due to Australian tiger snake bites and US coral snake bites, hemolysis may occur without significant anemia developing. Severe hemolytic anemia can develop in bites from Australian black snakes, copperheads, and taipans.

Local-Acting Cytotoxins

Localized tissue reactions or injury around the bite site are not a significant component of North American or Australian elapid envenomations and in most cases the bite is difficult to identify in dogs and cats. Mild local tissue swelling may occur associated with envenomating bites from Australian black snakes, taipans, and copperheads. Severe local tissue injury can occur to secondary to African and Asian cobra bites, which are also members of the elapid family [18].

Clinical Signs of Envenomation

Any of the following clinical signs are an indication for antivenom administration.

Preparalytic Signs

Preparalytic signs most commonly occur within 30 minutes or less of the bite, and can include one or more of vomiting, salivation, inappropriate urination or defecation, trembling, tachypnea or collapse and then a period of apparent recovery. In dogs, preparalytic signs have been associated with an LD_{50} dose or higher of *Notechis* venom or progression to clinical signs of envenomation [4,7].

Paralysis

Elapid venoms are primarily neurotoxic, resulting in paralysis, and in severe cases death from ventilatory failure. Any signs of LMN paralysis, even if mild, are an indication for antivenom if there is known contact with an elapid. Elapid snake envenomation should be considered as a differential diagnosis for any animal which develops rapidly progressive LMN paralysis in endemic areas.

Australia
Classically, clinical signs start with a decreased gag, weak or absent palpebral reflex, then weakness of the limbs and a mildly ataxic gait, followed by recumbency, inability to hold the head up, difficulties swallowing and ptyalism due to pharyngeal paralysis, loss of all withdrawal reflexes and complete LMN paralysis with signs of respiratory distress, hypoventilation, and then finally respiratory arrest. Mydriasis is a relatively late clinical sign. Brachycephalic breeds can develop respiratory distress as an early sign when envenomated. Because of the potential for irreversible binding of neurotoxins and requirement for prolonged periods of hospitalization or ventilation, sufficient antivenom should be administered early in the course of envenomation. The onset

and speed of progression of paralysis is highly variable. Dogs occasionally require ventilation within 30 minutes of being bitten or can take 6–12 hours to develop signs with rare reports of longer time periods. Therefore, the patient must never be left unobserved when monitoring for potential snake bite.

Cats occasionally have a more delayed presentation and may be presented with signs of severe paralysis after their owners notice that the cat hasn't moved off the same piece of furniture for 12–24 hours.

Complications of paralysis include aspiration pneumonia, corneal ulcers, and detrusor atony. If ventilation is required then multiple vials of antivenom are associated with a more rapid improvement in tiger and brown snake envenomations [4].

North America
Coral snake envenomations have a similar progression of paralysis as above and also have a variable time course for onset of clinical signs of paralysis, varying from immediately post bite to 36 hours later, with the majority showing clinical signs within 2–4 hours of being bitten. Any sign of weakness or illness after close contact with a coral snake is an indication for antivenom, especially if the venous PCO_2 is increasing toward 65 mmHg.

Coagulopathy

Coagulopathy can occur with Australian elapid envenomations and is an indication for administration of antivenom (see Chapter 70). VICC is associated with severe prolongations of PT, aPTT, and ACT test beyond the limits of test detection. Clinical bleeding occurs infrequently in dogs and cats and can include bleeding from oral wounds, hematuria, hyphema, gastrointestinal hemorrhage and, very rarely in small animals, internal bleeding or central nervous system hemorrhage [4,17]. Large hematomas can occur associated with venepuncture, cystocentesis, and oral wounds; therefore jugular venepuncture should be avoided if possible and pressure bandages placed over sites of venepuncture. Occasionally, dogs and cats will not develop coagulopathy despite other clinical signs of envenomation from a species of snake known to have procoagulant toxins. Anticoagulant toxins may just cause a mild prolongation of APTT which does not progress to a severe coagulopathy.

Rhabdomyolysis

Rhabdomyolysis commonly occurs with Australian elapid envenomations at least 3–6 hours post bite and is primarily detected by recognition of myoglobinuria or elevated CK on testing. Myoglobinuria can be severe, with urine dark brown to black in color. Humans often report significant muscle pain secondary to venom-induced rhabdomyolysis although this is more difficult to appreciate in dogs and cats. Regurgitation secondary to megaesophagus may occur in dogs and take weeks to resolve.

Hemolysis and Anemia

Severe hemolysis and anemia can develop in bites from Australian black snakes, copperheads and taipans; antivenom is indicated and blood transfusions may be required.

In envenomations due to Australian tiger snake and US coral snake bites, hemolysis may occur without significant anemia developing. Hemolysis only occurs in approximately 50% of the dogs that are bitten by North American coral snakes. The hemolysis is usually not life-threatening but pigmenturia should be treated with intravenous crystalloid solutions and is an indication for antivenom (see Chapter 167).

First Aid Advice for Owners

Because of the potential for rapid onset of clinical signs of paralysis, any owner who phones to say that their pet has been bitten or may have been in close contact with a snake should be advised to minimize activity and present their pet for immediate veterinary examination. If owners describe an already collapsed patient, provide instructions on how to perform mouth-to-nose ventilation if required en route, as the most common cause of acute death in dogs and cats is hypoxemia secondary to respiratory paralysis. A firm crepe pressure bandage can be applied to a bitten limb and has been shown to slow venom absorption; however, in dogs and cats, most bites are found on the head, neck, and thorax and in these locations pressure bandages are contraindicated.

Treatment of Envenomation in Dogs and Cats

Patients should be under constant observation because of the significant risk of rapid onset of paralysis. Dogs occasionally progress from walking to respiratory arrest within 15–30 minutes.

Asymptomatic Patients

An IV catheter should be placed (avoid the jugular vein) and blood collected to evaluate PT, aPTT or ACT, PCV, TP, hemolysis, and CK (where geographically indicated). Urine should be collected to assess for pigmenturia. In Australia, a SVDK is recommended if signs of envenomation are present and there is an uncertainty regarding which antivenom to administer. Cystocentesis should be avoided, if coagulopathic. Neurological assessment is performed to assess for evidence of paralysis. The presence of paralysis, coagulopathy, hemolysis or anemia and known contact with an elapid snake are indications for antivenom.

When a severely envenomated patient presents, the first steps in treatment follow the ABC approach (see Chapter 2). Assess if the patient has a patent airway (suction/swab any saliva present), intubate if the patient is apneic or severely paralyzed and unable to breathe and start manual or machine ventilation with 100% oxygen if apneic or hypoventilating (ETCO$_2$ >60 mmHg) (see Chapter 188). Most severely envenomated dogs and cats will respond well to oxygen support and assisted ventilation, allowing time to perform diagnostics and start appropriate treatment. Bradycardia is common during severe envenomations, is not associated with hypotension and normally resolves with improvement in oxygenation. Hypotension can occur but normally resolves with appropriate correction of hypoxemia or a conservative fluid bolus.

Antivenom is administered diluted at least 1:1 in Hartmann's/lactated Ringer's or 0.9% NaCl and administered over 20–30 minutes with close monitoring for evidence of anaphylaxis occurring, unless cardiac arrest has occurred in which case it is administered as a bolus. Epinephrine should always be readily available. If anaphylaxis is suspected 0.01 mg/kg epinephrine is administered IM, and it may be necessary to repeat it in 15–20 minutes if the vital signs do not stabilize. Intravenous adrenaline should be avoided except in the situation of cardiac arrest because of the potential for cardiac arrhythmias and intracranial hemorrhage if VICC is present.

There is significant variation between the purity and potential risk of anaphylaxis between antivenoms from different countries. If dexamethasone and antihistamines are recommended by the manufacturer prior to administration, this recommendation should be followed. In Australia, antivenom is highly purified and the incidence of anaphylactic reactions in dogs and cats is 10%; when they do occur, reactions are rarely severe [4].

The patient's neurological status should be reassessed immediately after administration of antivenom. If there is deterioration in neurological status, further antivenom should be administered.

In Florida, cost restrictions usually limit the administered dose to 1–2 vials of coral snake antivenom [19]. The Costa Rican product used is purified and requires no preventative hypersensitivity treatment. In Australia, if VICC or anticoagulant coagulopathy is present, a single dose of antivenom should be sufficient to neutralize the effects of the procoagulant or anticoagulant toxins. With VICC, the coagulopathy normally improves within 12 hours in dogs and cats although normalization of clotting times may take up to 24 hours post antivenom. Fresh frozen plasma is only recommended if it has been at least 6 hours post bite and only if life-threatening hemorrhage is suspected and antivenom has already been administered [9]. Strict confined rest is recommended until the patient's clotting times have normalized.

If myolysins are present and CK continues to rise significantly 6 hours after antivenom, and there is severe myoglobinuria, further antivenom should be administered

and intravenous crystalloid should be infused at an approximate twice maintenance dose of 120 ml/kg/day until the pigmenturia clears. The urine output should be closely monitored because of the risk of AKI developing. Pigmenturia secondary to myoglobinuria often improves rapidly once sufficient antivenom has been administered. Humans report significant muscle pain associated with myotoxins and opiate analgesia should be administered to dogs and cats (see Chapter 191).

Dogs and cats should remain under close observation until all signs of envenomation have resolved. Strict confined rest for 1–2 weeks is recommended after discharge.

References

1 Shea GM. The distribution and identification of dangerously venomous Australian terrestrial snakes. *Aust Vet J* 1999;77:791–798.
2 Fry BG. Structure-function properties of venom components from Australian elapids. *Toxicon* 1999;37:11–32.
3 Barber CM, Isbister GK, Hodgson WC. Solving the 'Brown snake paradox': in vitro characterisation of Australasian snake presynaptic neurotoxin activity. *Toxicol Lett* 2012;210:318–323.
4 Swindells KL, Sor J. Unpublished study data. Retrospective study of 178 confirmed brown snake bites in dogs and cats at Murdoch University. Presented at Australian and New Zealand College of Veterinary Scientists – College Science Week Conference 2011.
5 Johnston CI, O'Leary MA, Brown SGA, et al. Death Adder envenoming causes neurotoxicity not reversed by antivenom – Australian Snakebite Project (ASP-16). *PLoS Negl Trop Dis* 2012;6(9):e1841.
6 Swindells KL, Russell NJ, Angles JM, et al. Four cases of snake envenomation responsive to death adder antivenom. *Aust Vet J* 2006;84:22–29.
7 Lewis PF. Common tiger snake envenomation in dogs and mice – relationship between the amount of venom injected and the onset of clinical signs. *Aust Vet J* 1994;71:130–132.
8 Isbister GK, Scorgie FE, O'Leary MA, et al. Factor deficiencies in venom-induced consumption coagulopathy resulting from Australian elapid envenomation: Australian Snakebite Project (ASP-10). *J Thromb Haemost* 2010;8(11):2504–2513.
9 Isbister GK, Buckley NA, Page CA, et al. A randomized controlled trial of fresh frozen plasma for treating venom-induced consumption coagulopathy in cases of Australian snakebite (ASP-18). *J Thromb Haemost* 2013;11:1310–1318.
10 Ong RKC, Lenard ZM, Swindells KL, Raisis AL. Extradural haematoma secondary to brown snake (*Pseudonaja species*) envenomation. *Aust Vet J* 2009;87:152–156.
11 Churchman A, O'Leary MA, Buckley NA, et al. Clinical effects of red-bellied black snake (*Pseudechis porphyriacus*) envenoming and correlation with venom concentrations: Australian Snakebite Project (ASP-11). *Med J Aust* 2010;193:696–700.
12 Johnston CI, Brown SGA, O'Leary MA, et al. Mulga snake (*Pseudechis australis*) envenoming: a spectrum of myotoxicity, anticoagulant coagulopathy, haemolysis and the role of early antivenom therapy – Australian Snakebite Project (ASP-19). *Clin Toxicol* 2013;51:417–424.
13 Heller J, Bosward KL, Hodgson DR, et al. Anuric renal failure in a dog after Red-bellied Black snake (*Pseudechis porphyriacus*) envenomation. *Aust Vet J* 2006;84:158–162.
14 Lewis PF. Myotoxicity and nephrotoxicity of common tiger snake (*Notechis scutatus*) venom in the dog. *Aust Vet J* 1994;71:136–139.
15 Hopper K, Beck C, Slocombe RF. Megaoesophagus in adult dogs secondary to Australian tiger snake envenomation. *Aust Vet J* 2001;79:652–675.
16 Heller J, Mellor DJ, Hodgson JL, et al. Elapid snake envenomation in dogs in New South Wales: a review. *Aust Vet J* 2007;85:469–479.
17 Ong HM, Witham A, Kelers K, et al. Presumed secondary immune-mediated haemolytic anaemia following elapid snake envenomation and its treatment in four dogs. *Aust Vet J* 2015;93;319–326.
18 White J. Snake venoms and coagulopathy. *Toxicon* 2005;45;951–967.
19 Perez ML, Fox K, Schaer M. A retrospective review of coral snake envenomation in the dog and cat: 20 cases 1996 to 2011. *J Vet Emerg Crit Care* 2012;22(6):682–689.

143

Spider and Scorpion Envenomation

Kate Hopper, BVSc, PhD, DACVECC

School of Veterinary Medicine, University of California, Davis, CA, USA

Spider Envenomation

There are more than 41 000 species of spiders in the world and although almost all of them are technically venomous, only a few of them are considered medically important. The two most important clinical syndromes associated with spider bite worldwide are loxoscelism and latrodectism. There are other venomous spiders of significant medical importance but they are confined to relatively small geographical regions and will not be addressed here. Spiders of the family Theraphosidae will be briefly discussed as they can cause significant envenomation of dogs and cats.

The actual incidence of spider bites is very difficult to determine, especially in veterinary patients where it is unlikely that a spider bite can be verified. The risk of spider bites as perceived by clinicians and the lay public far exceeds the actual risk and leads to frequent misdiagnoses [1].

Loxoscelism

Loxoscelism describes the bite of spiders from the genus *Loxosceles*, commonly known as recluse, fiddle-back or brown spiders. There are alleged cases of necrotic arachnidism due to non-*Loxosceles* spiders, but these have not been definitively diagnosed. There are more than 100 species of *Loxosceles* spider and most are found in South America. They are endemic in the central and southern United States but are not found in the states on the east or west coasts or along the Canadian border.

The classic abnormality associated with loxoscelism is dermonecrosis. The exact pathogenesis of *Loxosceles* venom is not fully understood. Key components of the venom include phospholipases and hyaluronidase [2]. The venom can trigger an intense inflammatory response and has direct hemolytic effects. The bite itself is not painful and human patients are often unaware that they have been bitten. This makes a definitive diagnosis challenging. It is believed that most bites by *Loxosceles* spiders cause minor erythema and edema and are self-limiting. Cutaneous loxoscelism describes the development of skin necrosis and ulceration at the bite site. Skin necrosis in human patients takes 72 hours or more to become evident. A dry necrotic eschar forms and detaches after 2–3 weeks, leaving an ulcerated lesion that can take weeks or months to heal.

Cutaneous loxoscelism is associated with non-specific systemic signs in many cases such as fever and vomiting. In contrast, systemic loxoscelism is very uncommon and is associated with intravascular hemolytic anemia developing over 7–14 days. Acute kidney injury in systemic loxoscelism is rare and has been associated with a poorer outcome in human cases [1,2].

The diagnosis is generally based on the presence of a cutaneous lesion with non-specific systemic signs in a patient with an appropriate epidemiological history. This means the patient must have been in a geographical area known to have *Loxosceles* spiders for the diagnosis to even be considered. In reality, loxoscelism is exceedingly rare. These spiders hide in dry dark places and are not aggressive; most human bites occur when the spider is trapped against the person. The likelihood of them biting animals is considered very low.

There are numerous other diseases that can cause necrotic skin lesions that may be misdiagnosed as a brown recluse spider bite. These include severe soft tissue infection (streptococcal or staphylococcal infections), pyoderma, neoplasia, toxic epidermal necrolysis, erythema multiforme, purpura fulminans, and localized vasculitis (see Chapter 137). All possible diagnoses should be investigated before considering necrotic arachnidism as a likely cause.

Textbook of Small Animal Emergency Medicine, First Edition. Edited by Kenneth J. Drobatz, Kate Hopper, Elizabeth Rozanski and Deborah C. Silverstein.
© 2019 John Wiley & Sons, Inc. Published 2019 by John Wiley & Sons, Inc.
Companion Website: www.wiley.com/go/drobatz/textbook

There are no confirmed cases of loxoscelism published in the veterinary literature. There is a case report from Brazil of a dog with necrotic skin lesions "probably" due to a *Loxosceles* spider. This lesion was treated symptomatically and the lesions took 2 months to heal [3]. There are innumerable anecdotal cases of skin lesions attributed to a spider bite in veterinary medicine; many are from geographical regions that do not have loxoscele spiders. It is likely that most of these cases are a misdiagnosis and unfortunately there is no way to determine the true incidence or nature of spider envenomation in our patients at this time. Readers are directed to Isbister and Whyte for a suggested diagnostic approach to patients with necrotic, ulcerative skin lesions [4].

Recommended first aid for a brown recluse spider bite includes elevation and immobilization of the affected limb, ice packing of the bite site, and local wound care. Supportive care is provided as indicated. Other adjunctive therapies have been suggested but none has been proven to be of benefit. Most loxoscele spider bites are self-resolving without medical intervention. Cases of severe necrosis may require surgical management but this is very uncommon and is rarely life threatening (see Chapter 166). There are conflicting reports regarding the possible benefits of glucocorticoid therapy. No detrimental effects of glucocorticoid therapy have been reported and they are commonly given to human cases of spider bite. There is no loxosceles antivenom available in the United States, although *L. lateum* antivenom is available in Mexico and South America and may be of benefit if administered within 8 hours of the bite.

The prognosis for recovery from a brown recluse spider bite is excellent; severe necrosis may lead to subsequent scarring but this is a rare occurrence [1,2].

Lactrodectism

The widow spider group is the most medically important group of spiders in the world, causing the greatest number of human deaths. These spiders are from the genus *Lactrodectus* and are found worldwide. The venom of these spiders contains numerous toxins; the most clinically relevant toxin in mammalian envenomation is the alpha-latrotoxin. It has a unique selective effect on nerve endings, causing initial activation followed by depletion of neurotransmitters and subsequent flaccid paralysis. The female spider has fangs long enough to envenomate animals or people [2,5].

People often report little or no pain at the time of the bite but in 5–60 minutes local pain develops with increasing intensity. There may be local swelling or visible puncture marks but the major clinical sign is pain. About a third of human widow bite cases will have systemic signs, as outlined in Table 143.1. Pain is still the dominant sign; acute abdominal pain, muscle cramps, and/or spasms are all reported. Weakness, malaise, blepharoconjunctivitis, rhinitis, and photophobia are the more common systemic signs reported in people suffering lactrodectism in North America. Infants commonly present screaming in pain and often appear to have an acute abdomen and rigidity without pyrexia. Death is rare in human medicine and usually occurs in young, old or infirm patients [2].

There is considerable species variability in susceptibility to black widow envenomation. Guinea pigs and horses are highly susceptible, cats are moderately susceptible, and dogs are relatively resistant to the effects of the venom [6,7]. The single well-described case of feline black widow spider envenomation in the literature reports acute distress with muscle stiffness and pain of the abdomen and pelvic limbs. These signs progressed to muscle weakness, flaccid paralysis, and respiratory difficulties. There was significant elevation in creatine kinase and aspartate aminotransferase. The cat was treated with a vial of antivenom and slowly improved over 5–6 days [8]. There are many anecdotal reports of black widow spider bites in dogs and cats. Most of the cases are unsubstantiated but the general clinical presentation is one of acute pain and cats tend to be more severely affected than dogs.

There is little first aid indicated for a widow spider bite; application of an ice pack may help relieve the local pain. The majority of widow spider bites in people do not require medical therapy. In more severe

Table 143.1 Systemic signs reported in human patients with lactrodectism.

Organ system	Abnormality
Cardiovascular	Bradycardia, tachycardia, arrhythmias, hypertension
Respiratory	Bronchial secretions, bronchoconstriction, pulmonary edema
Central nervous system	Psychoses, amnesia, confusion, insomnia, hallucinations, delirium
Peripheral nervous system	Pain, lacrimation, salivation, rhinitis, priapism, mydriasis, miosis
Skeletal and smooth muscle	Hypertonia, clonic contractions, fasciculations
Gastrointestinal	Nausea, vomiting, heartburn, hypersalivation, acute abdomen
Renal	Urine retention due to sphincter tone Nephritis
Hematology	Leukocytosis, neutrophilia, lymphopenia, eosinophilia, monocytosis, hemoconcentration

envenomations, supportive care should be provided, including parenteral opioid analgesia, as indicated. Antivenom therapy has been commonly recommended for patients with systemic signs, although antivenom administration is controversial as strong evidence for its efficacy is currently lacking. A randomized placebo-controlled study of widow spider envenomation in Australia found no improvement associated with antivenom therapy [5,9]. Muscle relaxant therapy with methocarbamol or diazepam has been used to treat muscle spasms.

Other therapies suggested for latrodectism include corticosteroids, magnesium, and calcium administration. Evidence for the efficacy of these therapies is scarce and they are not currently recommended in human medicine [2].

Theraphosidae Spiders

Spiders from the family Theraphosidae are commonly known as tarantulas, bird-eating, spiders or whistling spiders. Envenomation by these spiders has minor effects in humans but can have fatal effects in animals, including cats, dogs, rats, mice, and birds. There are several cases of Theraphosidae envenomation reported in dogs in Australia. All nine cases reported died, including two dogs that were 40–50 kg in size. Many of the dogs died within 1–2 hours of being bitten [10,11]. There is limited information on the venom of Theraphosidae. As there are no reports of pets suffering tarantula bites from North or South America that the author is aware of, it is possible that members of this spider family from Australia are more venomous than other regions of the world. But given the increasing popularity of keeping Theraphosidae spiders as pets where dogs and cats may be exposed, it is important to be aware of the possible risks.

There are no specific treatment recommendations currently for Theraphosidae envenomation other than symptomatic and supportive care.

Scorpion Envenomation

Scorpions, like spiders, are members of the class Arachnida. They have eight legs, grasping appendages at the head known as pedipalps, and a long, segmented tail. The terminal segment of the tail is a venomous stinger known as a telson. There are over 1700 species of scorpions, although only a small number of them are considered capable of causing clinically significant envenomation. Scorpions live in tropical and temperate regions of the world and pose a significant human health issue in many areas. Some of the important genera are *Centruroides*

in North America, Central America, and parts of South America, *Tityus* in South America, *Androctonus* and *Buthus* in North Africa, *Buthotus* and *Leiurus* in the Middle East, and *Mesobuthus tamulus* in India. In the United States and Mexico, stings of *Centruroides sculpturatus* (bark scorpion) are potentially fatal to small children [12]. There is very little published information regarding scorpion envenomation of dogs or cats and our understanding is largely based on the human literature.

Pathophysiology of Envenomation

Scorpion venom is a complex mixture of numerous toxic substances and there is substantial variation in composition between species. The venom can contain acetylcholinesterases, serotonin, histamine, protease inhibitors, phospholipase, hyaluronidase, and neurotoxins [7,12]. The toxins with the greatest medical importance are neurotoxins that bind to sodium, potassium, and calcium channels. Scorpion alpha-toxins bind to mammalian voltage-gated sodium channels causing membrane hyperexcitability and repetitive, uncontrolled axonal firing. The result is autonomic dysfunction and neuromuscular activity. In addition, there can be massive endogenous release of catecholamines and other vasoactive peptides, including neuropeptide Y and endothelin-1.

Clinical Effects of Scorpion Envenomation in People

Scorpion envenomation varies in severity and clinical signs, but overall the clinical consequences are a manifestation of neurotoxic excitation syndromes leading to primarily cardiovascular and neurological abnormalities.

Pain, paresthesiae, and numbness are commonly reported in the region of the scorpion sting, soon after envenomation. Most stings only have local signs but it is possible to see systemic signs with stings of the more venomous scorpions.

Stimulation of the sympathetic nervous system can result in tachycardia, hypertension, mydriasis, restlessness, and seizures. If cholinergic stimulation is significant, it can lead to bradycardia, vasodilation, miosis, salivation, lacrimation, vomiting, and priapism. Abnormal sympathetic and/or parasympathetic tone can cause cardiac arrhythmias, including atrial tachycardia, ventricular premature contractions, ST segment changes and, less commonly, bundle branch block (see Chapter 53) [13]. Generally, the more severe envenomations are associated with predominantly sympathetic signs. Myocardial ischemia and myocarditis can occur following some species of scorpion envenomation found in Africa, the Middle East, and Asia. Neuromuscular excitation in people can be manifested as visual disturbances, abnormal ocular movements, fasciculations, paralysis, and unco-ordinated muscular activity.

A simple grading system for evaluation of scorpion stings in human patients was recently published. A slightly abbreviated version of this grading system and general treatment recommendations is shown in Table 143.2 [13].

Treatment of Scorpion Envenomation in People

The treatment approach to scorpion envenomation varies with the severity of the sting and a summary is provided in Table 143.2. It has been recommended that patients who present with grade 1 or 2 envenomation remain under observation for 4 hours in case of progression to a higher grade of severity. Antivenom therapy is controversial and results of studies to date have been variable. In North America, scorpion antivenom is considered beneficial but not cost-effective for routine use and it has been suggested that it should be reserved for severe envenomations [14]. In addition, the benefit of antivenom is questionable once severe systemic envenomation has been established. Benzodiazepines are

Table 143.2 Classification and treatment of scorpion stings for human patients [13].

Clinical Grade	Clinical Effects	Potential Treatment
Grade 1	Local manifestations only	
	Pain	Analgesia
	Paresthesia	Local anesthesia
	Numbness	
Grade 2	Autonomic excitation	Antivenom
	Hypertension	Prazosin
	Agitation and anxiety	Oral benzodiazepines
Grade 3		Antivenom
	Pulmonary edema	Oxygen therapy +/− mechanical ventilation, vasodilators (e.g. prazosin)
	Hypotension & cardiogenic shock	Dobutamine, other inotropes
	Severe neuromuscular excitation	Benzodiazepine infusion
Grade 4	Multiorgan failure including coma, seizures and end organ damage due to hypotension	Antivenom
		Mechanical ventilation
		Inotropes
		Benzodiazepine infusion
		Supportive care

used in human patients to control the neuromuscular hyperactivity and opioids are commonly indicated for analgesia. Atropine administration is often avoided as, although it can alleviate many of the cholinergic signs, it may worsen the adrenergic effects. Alpha-adrenergic receptor antagonists such as prazosin and doxazosin may be of benefit to reduce some of the cardiovascular abnormalities and prevent pulmonary edema [15].

Scorpion Envenomation in Dogs and Cats

There are numerous anecdotal reports of scorpion envenomation in dogs and some suspected cases in cats. In 2008 the Veterinary Pet Insurance company reported that scorpion stings were the fifth most common animal-induced injury to pets reported for claims.

The only published case report the author could find described scorpion envenomation (*Tityus bahiensis*) in a dog from Brazil. The presenting signs included intermittent drowsiness with bouts of vocalization and aggressiveness, tachypnea, tachycardia, and a painful region of the right thoracic limb. The animal was managed with supportive care, including a local anesthetic block around the area of the sting, and was asymptomatic by 24 hours [16].

Anecdotal reports of scorpion stings in dogs in the US are commonly described as having local signs with pain at the site of the sting but very little swelling. The *Centruroides sculpturatus* scorpion may also cause coughing. Potential reasons for scorpion envenomation to cause a cough include paresthesia of the mouth and oropharynx, as well as pulmonary edema.

Anecdotal reports of treatment of scorpion stings in dogs in the US commonly describe the use of antihistamines and glucocorticoids. There is no mention of antihistamine therapy in the treatment of human patients with scorpion stings. Given the commonly reported clinical signs of scorpion envenomation in dogs, it seems unlikely that antihistamines would be of benefit. Similarly, glucocorticoids are not used in routine therapy for scorpion envenomations in people. Studies evaluating the role of hydrocortisone in treating scorpion stings in adults and children found no benefit [17,18]. Unless there is a specific indication for their use, routine administration of glucocorticoids to treat scorpion envenomation cannot be recommended.

Analgesia is an important part of management of these cases (see Chapter 193). If severe systemic signs are present, supportive care as outlined for human patients is indicated. If severe adrenergic signs such as hypertension and tachyarrhythmias are evident, there may be a role for alpha-adrenergic receptor antagonist drugs such as prazosin (see Chapter 63). Scorpion antivenom may be beneficial in severe envenomations, but may not be feasible in veterinary patients given the costs associated with this product.

To the author's knowledge, there are no published reports of scorpion envenomation in cats. It has been sug-gested that cats may be more resistant to scorpion venom than dogs but there is no evidence to support this claim. It is possible that cats are more careful and agile than dogs so may not be as likely to be exposed to scorpion stings.

References

1 Swanson DL, Vetter RS. Bites of brown recluse spiders and suspected necrotic arachnidism. *N Engl J Med* 2005;352(7):700–707.
2 Isbister GK, Fan HW. Spider biter. *Lancet* 2011;378:2039–2047.
3 Machado L, Antunes M, Mazini A, et al. Necrotic skin lesion in a dog attributed to Loxosceles (brown spider) bite: a case report. *J Venom Anim Toxins Trop Dis* 2009;15(3):572–581.
4 Isbister GK, Whyte IM. Suspected white-tail spider bite and necrotic ulcers. *Intern Med J* 2004;34:38–44.
5 Da Silva PH, da Silveira R, Appel M, et al. Brown spiders and loxoscelism. *Toxicon* 2004;44:693–709.
6 Brown RA. Red back spider envenomation in dogs. Control and Therapy #989. Post Grad Committee in Veterinary Science, University of Sydney, 1980.
7 Meier J, White J (eds). *Handbook of Clinical Toxicology of Animal Venoms and Poisons.* CRC Press, Boca Raton, 1995.
8 Twedt DC, Cuddon PA, Horn TW. Black widow spider envenomation in a cat. *J Vet Intern Med* 1999;13: 613–616.
9 Isbister GK, White J. Clinical consequences of spider bites: recent advances in our understanding. *Toxicon* 2004;43:477–492.
10 O'Hagan BJ, Raven RJ, McCormick KM. Death of two pups from spider envenomation. *Aust Vet J* 2006;84(8):291.

11 Isbister GK, Page CB, Buckley NA, et al. Randomized controlled trial of intravenous antivenom versus placebo for latrodectism: the second Redback Antivenom Evaluation (RAVE-II) study. *Ann Emerg Med* 2014;64(6):620–628.
12 Skolnik AB, Ewald MB. Pediatric scorpion envenomation in the United States: morbidity, mortality, and therapeutic innovations. *Pediatr Emerg Care* 2013;29(1):98–103.
13 Isbister GK, Bawaskar HS. Scorpion envenomation. *N Engl J Med* 2014;371(5):457–463.
14 Armstrong EP, Bakall M, Skrepnek GH, Boyer LV. Is scorpion antivenom cost-effective as marketed in the United States? *Toxicon* 2013;76:394–398.
15 Bawaskar HS, Bawaskar PH. Prazosin therapy and scorpion envenomation. *J Assoc Physicians India* 2000;48(12):1175–1180.
16 Cardoso MJL, Sakate M, Ciampolini P, et al. Envenomation by scorpion in dog – case report. *J Venom Anim Toxins Trop Dis* 2004;10:98–105.
17 Bahloul M, Chaari A, Dammak H, et al. Impact of hydrocortisone hemisuccinate use on outcome of severe scorpion-envenomed adult patients. *Am J Ther* 2014;21(6):e181–188.
18 Bahloul M, Chaari A, Ammar R, et al. Severe scorpion envenomation among children: does hydrocortisone improve outcome? A case-control study. *Trans R Soc Trop Med Hyg* 2013;107(6):349–355.

144

Bufo Toad Toxicosis

Leo Londoño, DVM, DACVECC and Gareth Buckley, MA, VetMB, MRCVS, DACVECC, DECVECC

University of Florida, College of Veterinary Medicine, Gainesville, FL, USA

Introduction

The cane or giant toad, previously classified as *Bufo marinus*, now classified as *Rhinella marina*, is a large terrestrial toad native to Central and South America. While hundreds of species belonging to the *Bufo* genus are distributed throughout the tropical and temperate regions of the world, the classic toxicity is seen with the cane or giant toad; these are widely distributed through Central and South America, parts of the US such as southern Florida and Texas, and northern Australia. Other species of *Bufo* toads are more widely spread but are associated with less severe clinical signs.

The cane toad was first introduced to the states of Florida and Hawaii in North America, and Queensland, Australia, in the early 1900s as a biological pest control measure in sugar cane and other plantations. They owe their colonizing success to the lack of predators, their ability to eat other animals, including native frogs and toads, their adaptability to agricultural and urban settings, and their high fecundity. Shortly after introduction to different regions of the world, the cane toad became a significant threat to local species and companion animals.

Bufo toads can measure 10–23 cm and females can weigh up to 1.5 kg [1], hence they are often referred to as "giant toads." These stout and short-legged amphibians vary in color from tan to dark brown with spotted patterns; the source of their venom is two large parotid, warty-like glands located behind each eye extending from the temporal region past their shoulder area (Figure 144.1). These glands secrete a milky venomous fluid, which serves to deter predators, helping this species to survive in difficult environments.

As with many venomous animals, the composition of this venom is very complex. The venom's main two components are biogenic amines and steroid derivatives (Table 144.1) but the composition of the venom varies significantly, depending on the species of the toad and geographical differences [2,3]. The components of the venom have significant effects on the victim's neurological, cardiovascular and gastrointestinal systems, leading to the signs of toxicosis observed in both humans and companion animals.

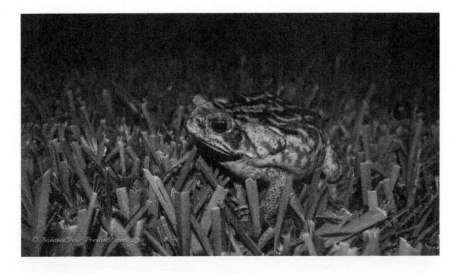

Figure 144.1 Adult cane toad on a residential lawn in North Palm Beach, Florida. Reproduced with permission of Michael West.

Table 144.1 Components of *Bufo* venom and associated systemic effects.

	Components	Effects
Biogenic amines	Epinephrine, norepinephrine	Tachycardia, hypertension, hyperthermia, visceral vasoconstriction, bronchodilation
	Bufotenin, bufotionin, dihidrobufotenin	Hallucinogenic effects
	Serotonin, 5-hydroxytryptophan	Hallucinogenic effects, seizures, tremors, ptyalism, abdominal pain
Steroid derivatives	Ergosterol, cholesterol, gamma-sistosterol	No effects
	Bufagins and bufadienolids (e.g. arenobufagin, bufotalin, cinobufagin, marinobufagin)	Cardiac effects with digitalis-like action

Incidence

Because of the curious nature of dogs and cats, *Bufo* toads are a highly attractive, venomous threat to companion animals. According to a survey among general practice and emergency veterinarians from the United States, Canada, Australia, and the UK, 51% of the respondents chose animal envenomation as the most common toxin exposure in dogs and 9% of these cases were associated with toad toxicosis [4]. On the other hand, 40% of respondents to the survey chose animal envenomation as the most common exposure in cats, and only 1% of these cases were related to toads. *Bufo* toxicosis in dogs is most commonly reported during the warm months of the year in south Florida (March–November) with no events reported during the month of December [5]. The seasonal distribution of *Bufo* toxicosis follows a similar pattern in Australia, where the incidence of toad toxicosis drops between the months of June and September, when the temperature and rainfall averages are lowest [6]. Seasonal increases in cases of envenomation during the summer and heavy-rainfall months are correlated to the time of peak breeding activity of the giant toads, while the drop in case reports during the winter months is likely due to hibernation behavior.

Signalment

Cats are not commonly envenomated by *Bufo* toads compared to dogs, and reports of *Bufo* toxicosis in cats are not found in the veterinary literature. The reason for the apparent low incidence of *Bufo* toxicosis in cats is likely multifactorial but it may be due to the fact that outdoor cats are less likely to receive veterinary attention when exposed to a toxin, or in this case shortly after exposure to a venomous animal, and are less likely to bite or ingest relatively large animals.

Toad envenomation can affect dogs of all breeds and ages. Small breeds represent the vast majority of dogs affected by toad toxicosis. Terriers appear to be the breed most commonly affected with *Bufo* toxicosis. In one retrospective study, 76% of dogs in Australia intoxicated by cane toads were small breed and from this group of dogs, 73.5% were considered pure- or mixed-breed terriers [6]. These findings were also observed in a previous study in south Florida, where the most common breeds affected by this toxicity included Yorkshire terriers, Jack Russell terriers, West Highland white terriers, dachshunds, and toy poodles [5]. No sex predilection was identified in these studies. Younger dogs, less than 4 years old, appeared to be more frequently affected in one study [6].

Clinical Signs of Envenomation

Absorption of the *Bufo* toxins is through the oral mucosa and upper gastrointestinal mucosa, or cutaneous wounds. Dogs and cats are exposed to the toxin after mouthing or ingesting the toad. The hallmark clinical sign of *Bufo* toxicosis is hyperemic "brick-red" mucous membranes (Figure 144.2). Hyperemic gums were recorded in 51% and 63% of dogs with suspected *Bufo* toxicosis in two retrospective studies [5,6]. Among the clinical signs of dogs affected with cane toad toxicosis in south Florida, neurological abnormalities were most frequently observed,

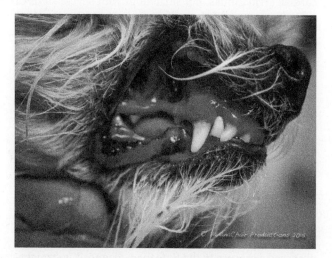

Figure 144.2 An 11-year-old, neutered male West Highland white terrier with signs of *Bufo* toxicosis; note the hyperemic mucous membranes. Reproduced with permission of Michael West.

followed by hyperemic mucous membranes, ptyalism, collapse, tachypnea, and vomiting [5]. Another retrospective study of dogs in Australia found that increased salivation was the most common clinical sign observed followed by hyperemic mucous membranes, seizures, weakness/ataxia, cardiac arrhythmias, muscle tremors, and vomiting [6]. Dogs with mild envenomation or envenomation with other, less toxic species of *Bufo* toads are likely to present with signs of hypersalivation and red mucous membranes. Moderate to severely envenomated dogs most commonly present in status epilepticus or during the postictal phase after having seizures at home or on their way to the hospital.

In humans, *Bufo* toxicosis is associated with gastrointestinal signs and cardiotoxicity due to the resemblance of the bufogenic toxins to cardiac glycosides and digoxin toxicity [3,7]. There are reports of envenomation in people after ingesting aphrodisiacs or Asian herbal supplements containing bufogenic toxins, as well as ingestion of *Bufo* toad eggs, leading to life-threatening cardiac arrhythmias [7–9]. In one of these case reports, a 40-year-old man had positive digoxin serum concentrations after ingesting aphrodisiac pills, despite never taking digoxin [8]. Successful treatment with digoxin Fab fragments for toad envenomation has been reported in two men and in mice [10,11].

Dogs receiving lethal doses of bufogenic toxins were reported to develop ventricular fibrillation leading to 100% mortality in all untreated dogs [12]. In dogs with natural exposure to bufogenic toxins, the incidence of cardiac arrhythmias is less prevalent, approximately 21% in one study [6], and bradycardia with heart rates less than 50 beats per minute was the indication for treatment with IV atropine in another study [5] (see Chapter 53). In the authors' experience, dogs infrequently present with cardiac arrhythmias, but small dogs with severe signs of toxicity are more likely to show these signs. Smaller dogs are also more likely to be hospitalized than larger dogs according to one study [5], suggesting that a higher ratio of toxin to body weight may cause more severe clinical signs, although the correlation between body weight and development of cardiac arrhythmias has not been formally investigated. No studies have been performed looking at digoxin serum concentrations in dogs with *Bufo* toxicosis.

Diagnosis

The diagnosis of *Bufo* toad toxicosis is made purely based on history and clinical exam findings. In cases of observed exposure to the *Bufo* toad, diagnosis is straightforward. At this time there are no biochemical, hematological or biomarkers that can aid the clinician in the diagnosis of *Bufo* toxicosis. Veterinarians practicing in areas where *Bufo* toads are endemic should be aware of the clinical signs associated with toad toxicosis in order to promptly recognize and treat the affected animal.

History taking plays a major role in the diagnosis of *Bufo* toxicosis. Dogs with cane toad envenomation have no previous history of seizures or other neurological disorders [6]; they may have had previous environmental exposure to these toads [5] and develop acute onset of clinical signs consistent with a toxicity. In one study, 18% of dogs had a history of previous exposure to *Bufo* toads ranging from one to eight encounters in the past [5]. Dogs do not appear to learn precautionary behaviors towards these venomous toads, despite previous encounters and development of toxicosis.

Treatment and Monitoring

Initial treatment of dogs and cats with *Bufo* toxicosis should be tailored towards oral decontamination and treatment of seizure activity. The owner can be instructed to start decontamination techniques at home as long as the animal is not actively seizing in order to prevent injuries to the owners. At-home decontamination should be performed with a damp towel or damp clean rag used to wipe the oral mucous membranes and prevent further absorption of the toxins. A common mistake made by veterinarians is to recommend owners to lavage the animal's mouth with a hose or running tap water, increasing the risk of aspiration pneumonia. Several dogs that have died in hospital while being treated for *Bufo* toxicity died due to aspiration pneumonia caused by owners attempting to lavage the mouth with water or by administration of products such as milk or olive oil believed to decrease toxin absorption.

If the animal is observed ingesting the toad or parts of the toad, emesis can be induced if the animal is neurologically stable. Orogastric lavage can also be attempted in the animal with neurological signs once seizure activity has been controlled. The use of activated charcoal in *Bufo* toxicosis has not been evaluated or reported in retrospective studies. Currently, charcoal or charcoal with cathartics in cases of severe envenomation is not used routinely due to the risk of aspiration pneumonia.

Treatment of seizures is described in further detail in Chapter 21. In cases *of Bufo* toad envenomation, standard doses of benzodiazepines are used to control seizures or to help control neurological signs of muscle rigidity. If boluses of benzodiazepines are not enough to control seizure activity, continuous-rate infusions of benzodiazepines or propofol can be administered. Other anticonvulsants such as phenobarbital or levetiracetam can also be administered in refractory cases. Treatment of cardiac arrhythmias should be based on electrocardiogram findings (see Chapter 53). Atropine is the treatment of choice for bradyarrhythmias as recommended in previous studies [5,6]. In cases of tachyarrhythmias, propranolol was used in two dogs due to prolonged (>30 min) sinus tachycardia in one study [5]; the use of other drugs such as esmolol, lidocaine, amiodarone, and verapamil has also been suggested [6,13]. Treatment of *Bufo*-envenomated dogs with digoxin Fab fragments has not been reported.

Intravenous fluid therapy is commonly administered to hospitalized animals with signs of *Bufo* toxicosis (see Chapter 167). There is a lack of information regarding blood pressure, lactate levels, and other hemodynamic parameters in envenomated dogs, but clinical experience indicates that true cardiovascular shock is rare in *Bufo* toxicity, and so routine use of aggressive fluid resuscitation is not typically required. Maintenance fluid therapy at conventional rates is therefore recommended in addition to replacement of any ongoing losses. In cases of tachyarrhythmia, ECG monitoring should be performed before and during patient assessment and treatment, and those with persistent tachyarrhythmia may require treatment with antiarrhythmic agents, depending on its severity. Typically, short-acting beta-blockers are the drug of choice for the treatment of these arrhythmias (see Chapter 53). Indiscriminate fluid therapy may lead to fluid overload in debilitated animals and worsen lung pathology in cases of aspiration pneumonia.

Animals with mild signs of *Bufo* envenomation (hypersalivation and hyperemic mucous membranes) can be treated as outpatients after oral decontamination and owners should continue monitoring at home for development of neurological signs. For moderately to severely affected animals, hospitalization with supportive care and monitoring for seizure activity should be recommended. In the two retrospective studies mentioned earlier, 55–61% of the dogs were admitted to hospital and monitored for periods ranging between 11 and 48 hours [5,6]. Long-term monitoring is not required once the animal is discharged from hospital after recovery from envenomation.

Prognosis

Prognosis is excellent for dogs with *Bufo* toxicosis and prompt appropriate treatment. The prognosis in cats is unknown. Mortality in dogs with *Bufo* toad envenomation has been reported to be 4% [5,6]. The incidence of short-term complications such as aspiration pneumonia or long-term complications such as neurological deficits has not been reported.

Acknowledgments

The authors would like to thank Dr Michael West, associate ER veterinarian at Pet Emergency and Referral Center of Palm Beach Gardens, for the photographs and clinical input provided.

References

1 Somma LA. *Rhinella marina*. USGS Nonindigenous Aquatic Species Database. Available at: http://nas.er.usgs.gov/queries/FactSheet.aspx?speciesID=48 (accessed 8 February 2018).

2 Sakate M, Lucas de Oliveira PC. Toad envenoming in dogs: effects and treatment. *J Venom Anim Toxins* 2000;6:52–62.

3 Eubig PA. Bufo species toxicosis: big toad, big problem. *Vet Med* 2001;96:594–599.

4 Hall K. Toxin exposures and treatments: a survey of practicing veterinarians. In: *Kirk's Current Veterinary Therapy*, 14th edn (eds Bonagura JD, Twedt DC). Saunders-Elsevier, St Louis, 2009, pp. 95–99.

5 Roberts BK, Aronsohn MG, Moses BL, et al. *Bufo marinus* intoxication in dogs: 94 cases (1997–1998). *J Am Vet Med Assoc* 2000; 216:1941–1944.

6 Reeves MP. A retrospective report of 90 dogs with suspected cane toad (*Bufo marinus*) toxicity. *Aust Vet J* 2004;82:608–611.

7 Yei CC, Deng JF. Toad or toad cake intoxication in Taiwan: report of four cases. *J Formos Med Assoc* 1993;92:S135–139.

8 Gowda RM, Cohen RA, Khan IA. Toad venom poisoning: resemblance to digoxin toxicity and therapeutic implications. *Heart* 2003;89:e14.

9 Kuo HY, Hsu CW, Chen JH, et al. Life-threatening episode after ingestion of toad eggs: a case report with literature review. *Emerg Med J* 2007;24(3):215–216.

10 Brubacher JR, Ravikumar PR, Bania T, et al. Treatment of toad venom poisoning with digoxin-specific Fab fragments. *Chest* 1996;110:1282–1288.

11 Brubacher JR, Lachmanen D, Ravikumar PR, et al. Efficacy of digoxin specific Fab fragments (Digibind) in the treatment of toad venom poisoning. *Toxicon* 1999;37:931–942.

12 Palumbo NE, Perry SF, Read G. Experimental induction and treatment of toad poisoning in the dogs. *J Am Vet Med Assoc* 1975;167:1000–1005.

13 Sakate M, Lucas de Oliveira PC. Use of lidocaine, propranolol, amiodarone, and verapamil in toad envenoming (Genus *Bufo*) in dogs. *J Venom Anim Tox* 2001;7:240–259.

145

Hymenoptera Envenomation

Rebecca Flores, DVM and Vincent Thawley, VMD, DACVECC

Matthew J. Ryan Veterinary Hospital, University of Pennsylvania, Philadelphia, PA, USA

Apoidea

The family Apoidea includes the social honey bees, bumble bees, and solitary bees. These insects are social and herbivorous, feeding off flower pollen and nectar. They build their nests (hives) in hollow trees or other cavities. Nests of bumble bees contain 100–200 insects and are typically not involved in mass envenomations whereas honey bee (*Apis mellifera*) hives often contain thousands of workers, with 40 000 workers in some managed colonies [1].

Africanized honey bees (AHB) are a tropical variety of honey bee that was imported from Africa to Brazil in 1956 to improve honey production [2]. This variety of bee, known for its aggressive temperament leading to mass envenomation, escaped and replaced the local honey bee variety in Brazil, reaching the United States by 1990 [3]. As of 2011, AHBs have spread to 10 US states although attacks have not been noted in all of these states [4]. AHBs are quicker to attack and will chase their victims up to 0.6 miles, as compared to European honey bees which will follow for up to 500 yards. AHBs also tend to establish a larger number of colonies in less protected locations within a particular geographic area, making them more easily disturbed [5].

Bees can only sting once, as their barbed stinger remains in the victim's skin following envenomation. After a sting, the stinger and venom sac are pulled out of the bee's abdomen, resulting in the insect's death shortly thereafter [6,7].

Vespoidea

The family Vespoidea includes the wasps, hornets, and yellowjackets. These insects are predacious carnivores, feeding on other insects and sweet substances such as sap and nectar, that frequently forage near open food containers and garbage. Stings typically occur via a single vespid and most commonly occur in the late summer and early fall when hungry yellowjackets are attracted to the smell of human food prepared outdoors [6]. Mass envenomation may occur when a colony is disturbed. Hornets and wasps typically inhabit trees and shrubs, while yellowjackets are frequently ground dwellers. Compared to the Apoidea, vespids tend to be more aggressive and possess smooth stingers which allow them to deliver multiple stings [7,8].

Formicidea

The family Formicidea contains the ants. Those medically relevant include the black and red imported fire ant (*Solenopsis invicta* and *S. richteria*). Both are native to South America and entered the United States in the 1900s [9], where they formed hybrids with native species. The black imported fire ants are mostly confined to Alabama and Mississippi but the red imported fire ants and hybrids are highly adaptive and have spread to 12 southern states. Red fire ant hybrids appear to be cold resistant and can overwinter, allowing for northward migration into areas with a cooler climate [10].

Fire ants form mounds which can interfere with farming. They may attack livestock and other native species and increasingly are reported to attack pets and debilitated humans [11]. Imported fire ants are omnivorous, stinging and killing invertebrates as their primary food source. Fire ants can quickly swarm a victim, using pheromone cues to sting simultaneously. The fire ant initially bites its prey with its prominent mandibles and, once anchored, tucks its abdomen to sting with a non-barbed stinger. The ant then remains attached by its mandibles, removes its stinger, rotates its body, and stings again.

This is repeated 6–7 times in a circular pattern, with venom slowly injected over 20–30 seconds. This results in a slower onset and less painful sting than those delivered by bees or vespids [12,13].

Venom

Bee venom is a complex mixture of proteins and biologically active peptides. Mellitin, the major component and the main cause of pain following a sting, is a detergent, which alters cell membrane integrity. Mellitin works synergistically with the primary allergen of venom, phospholipase A2, to cause red blood cell, platelet, leukocyte, and vascular endothelial cell lysis [1,14], and is suspected to cause myelinolysis of the spinal cord [13,15]. Other venom components include mast cell degranulating factor, which causes histamine and vasoactive amine release from mast cells, and hyaluronidase, which disrupts collagen, allowing venom to spread to adjacent tissues. Bee venom also contains vasoactive amines such as histamine, dopamine, and norepinephrine, and apamin, a neurotoxin that acts on the spinal cord [13].

Wasp venoms are more heterogeneous but most contain three major allergenic peptides as well as vasoactive amines (serotonin, histamine, tyramine, catecholamines), wasp kinins, and acetylcholine. The vasoactive substances are responsible for the intense pain of wasp stings. Antigen 5 is the most allergenic component but its activity is poorly understood. Other venom components include phospholipase A and B, which cleave lipid bilayers, and hyaluronidase. Vespid venom does not contain mellitin [16].

Unlike the venom of other Hymenoptera, which are composed primarily of proteins in an aqueous solution, fire ant venom is composed of 95% water-insoluble alkaloids. These alkaloids are primarily piperidines which have cytotoxic, hemolytic, antibacterial, and insecticidal properties [13]. They do not produce an IgE-mediated reaction, but instead produce sterile pustules secondary to tissue inflammation which are almost pathognomonic for fire ant stings [17].

Lethal Dose

Stinging insects are not able to meter their venoms like some venomous snakes and deliver a relatively standard volume of venom per sting. The European honey bee is thought to inject 147 μg of venom per sting, with most wasps injecting about 17 μg of venom per sting [17]. Africanized honey bees likely inject a slightly smaller volume of venom per sting than their European counterparts. The lethal dose for bee, wasp

or hornet envenomation is approximately 500 stings per adult human [1,8,18] and is estimated to be 20 stings/kg in most mammals [1,19]. Each fire ant sting can deliver 0.11 μL of venom, with up to 20 consecutive stings being delivered before venom stores are depleted. Severe systemic reactions have been reported following 50–100 fire ant stings in humans. While fatal envenomation can occur in animals, the lethal dose is unknown [20].

Clinical Manifestations of Envenomation

Hymenoptera envenomation may result in local tissue reactions, immune-mediated responses or, rarely, venom systemic toxic effects. A local reaction, characterized by edema, erythema, and pain at the site of envenomation, occurs following all Hymenoptera envenomation as a result of the vasoactive properties of the venom. This is typically self-limiting and generally resolves within 24 hours [13].

Immune-Mediated Response

Immune-mediated response to envenomation can be divided into three subtypes: regional reaction, systemic anaphylaxis, and delayed hypersensitivity reaction. Regional reactions are thought to be IgE mediated and involve the area immediately surrounding the site of the sting. Regional reactions can be extensive and may lead to erythema and edema encompassing an entire extremity. This may not be apparent for up to 24 hours following a sting and will typically peak in severity within 48 hours, although signs may not resolve for several days and may be confused with cellulitis [13,21].

Systemic anaphylaxis, though rare, is the most life-threatening reaction to Hymenoptera envenomation (see Chapter 146). It is mediated by IgE and is characterized by all or a combination of clinical signs related to cardiovascular collapse, respiratory difficulty, or cutaneous or gastrointestinal signs. Clinical signs are due to massive release of a variety of chemical mediators, primarily histamine, from mast cells and basophils. Cutaneous signs include urticaria, erythema, angioedema, and pruritus. Respiratory signs include dyspnea, bronchospasm, stridor, and cough as a result of laryngeal and pharyngeal edema, increased mucus production, and bronchoconstriction. Circulatory compromise is characterized by hypotension and signs of poor tissue perfusion (pale mucous membranes, prolonged capillary refill time, poor pulse quality, and dull mentation) due to vasodilation and increased vascular permeability. Tachycardia or, less commonly, vagally mediated bradycardia may be seen. Arrhythmias, myocardial ischemia, and cardiac arrest may also occur. Gastrointestinal signs may include nausea, vomiting, and diarrhea or hematochezia. Other clinical signs which may occur include weakness, syncope, lacrimation, conjunctival hyperemia, and seizures.

Clinical signs of anaphylaxis typically occur within 15 minutes of the insult and are unlikely to occur if no signs are noted within 30 minutes. The time to onset of signs is directly proportional to the severity of the signs. Depending on the severity and manifestation of anaphylaxis, death can occur within minutes [22].

Delayed hypersensitivity reactions are uncommon but can occur within days to weeks of envenomation, resulting from tissue deposition of antigen-antibody complexes. The resultant inflammatory cascade leads to complement binding and subsequent formation of anaphylatoxin, causing mast cell degranulation and histamine release which results in damage to the basement membrane. This may result in vasculitis, polyarthritis, glomerulonephritis, and myocardial lesions [13,22].

Systemic Toxic Reactions

Systemic toxic reactions occur due to the direct effects of venom and are related to the total volume of venom injected. Clinical signs can include fever, depression, ataxia, seizures, pigmenturia, hypotension, and melena or hematochezia [23]. Secondary immune-mediated hemolytic anemia and thrombocytopenia have been reported in dogs following massive bee and vespid envenomation [24–31] (see Chapter 66). Mellitin and phospholipase A2 may cause rhabdomyolysis, leading to myoglobinemia, myoglobinuria and potentially a pigment nephropathy. Ataxia, transient facial nerve paralysis, seizure, and other neurological dysfunction secondary to the effects of mellitin and apamin have been reported in dogs [13,25]. Acute respiratory distress syndrome (ARDS) may occur following massive envenomation [24,26,32]. One case report describes a dog which was mechanically ventilated for suspected ARDS secondary to massive bee envenomation; this dog ultimately recovered to discharge [33]. Coagulopathy and disseminated intravascular coagulation are also commonly reported, likely due to hepatocellular injury and release of tissue thromboplastin and endothelial cell disruption [26,34] (see Chapter 70).

Only one published case report describes massive envenomation of two dogs by fire ants in Australia. Both dogs developed acute kidney injury (see Chapter 94). One dog died, and necropsy revealed evidence of mesenteric and myocardial hemorrhage as well as renal tubular necrosis [35].

Diagnosis

Definitive diagnosis may be challenging if the incident was not witnessed, but the circumstances may raise a clinical suspicion for Hymenoptera envenomation. Depending on the type of reaction, there may be few biochemical or radiographic changes noted. Local and regional reactions are diagnosed on physical examination. Anaphylaxis is often a clinical diagnosis, but elevations in ALT and ultrasound evidence of gall bladder wall edema have been associated with anaphylaxis in dogs [36–38]. Animals presenting with delayed or toxic reactions may show evidence of hepatopathy (elevated ALT, AST, ALP, GGT, bilirubin), azotemia secondary to acute kidney injury, urinary casts, evidence of rhadomyolysis (elevated CK, myoglobinemia, myoglobinuria), evidence of immune-mediated hemolytic anemia or thrombocytopenia (spherocytosis, anemia, thrombocytopenia, hemoglobinemia, hemoglobinuria), or coagulopathy (prolonged PT/PTT, thrombocytopenia, and elevated D-dimers). Complete blood count may also reveal an inflammatory leukogram [13].

Treatment

Local or mild regional reactions often do not require treatment but application of ice or cool compresses, and oral or injectable antihistamines (1–2 mg/kg diphenhydramine IM, PO) may be helpful [14]. Sarna lotion (camphor and menthol) can be applied topically for fire ant stings. Topical use of meat tenderizer (papain) or aluminum sulfate has not been demonstrated to be effective. Animals with multiple stings or with severe regional reactions should be hospitalized to monitor for the development of systemic toxic reactions. Human recommendations are to hospitalize patients for 24 hours following massive envenomation of >50 stings [39].

Hypotension should be treated aggressively with intravenous fluid therapy see (Chapter 167). Maintenance of normotension and adequate tissue perfusion is of utmost importance. Appropriate analgesia (see Chapter 193) should be provided and while broad-spectrum antibiotics are not typically required, they should be administered if secondary infection develops [13,22,24].

Treatment of Systemic Anaphylaxis

Anaphylaxis is a medical emergency and survival is dependent on immediate patient assessment and stabilization (see Chapter 146). Immediate administration of epinephrine (Table 145.1) given as an IV bolus is indicated, followed by CRI of epinephrine titrated to

Table 145.1 Treatment of systemic anaphylaxis [22].

Medication	Dog dosage	Cat dosage
Epinephrine	0.01 mg/kg (1 mg/mL solution) IM/IV q5–15 min	0.01 mg/kg (1 mg/mL solution) IM/IV q5–15 min
	Max dose: 0.3 mg < 40 kg, 0.5 mg > 50 kg	CRI: 0.05 μg/kg/min if shock is present
	CRI: 0.05 μg/kg/min if shock is present	
Isotonic crystalloid	90 mL/kg (in aliquots, to effect)	60 mL/kg (in aliquots, to effect)
Colloids (Hetastarch)	5 mL/kg bolus, up to 20 mL/kg	5 mL/kg bolus, up to 20 mL/kg
Methylprednisolone sodium succinate	30 mg/kg IV	30 mg/kg IV
Dexamethasone sodium phosphate	1–4 mg/kg IV	1–4 mg/kg IV
Prednisone sodium succinate	10–25 mg/kg IV	10–25 mg/kg IV
Diphenhydramine	1–4 mg/kg IM or PO q8–12h	0.5–2 mg/kg IM or PO q8–12h
	0.5–1 mg/kg IV slowly (not >50 mg total)	
Ranitidine	0.5–2 mg/kg IV, PO or SC	0.5–2 mg/kg IV, PO or SC
	Give IV slowly over 10 min	Give IV slowly over 10 min
Albuterol	0.5 mL of 0.5% solution in 4 mL isotonic saline by nebulizer q6h,	0.5 mL of 0.5% solution in 4 mL isotonic saline by nebulizer q6h,
	90 μg/actuation (1–2 puffs) by metered dose q15min for 3 doses	90 μg/actuation (1–2 puffs) by metered dose q15min for 3 doses
Aminophylline	5–10 mg/kg IM or slowly IV	5–10 mg/kg IM or slowly IV
Vasopressin	CRI: 0.5–1.25 mU/kg/min	CRI: 0.5–1.25 mU/kg/min
Norepinephrine	CRI: 0.1–1 μg/kg/min	CRI: 0.1–1 μg/kg/min
Dopamine	CRI: 2.5–10 μg/kg/min	CRI: 2.5–10 μg/kg/min
Glucagon	1–2 mg/kg followed by	1–2 mg/kg followed by
	CRI: 5–15 mg/min	CRI: 5–15 mg/min
Atropine	0.02–0.04 mg/kg IV	0.02–0.04 mg/kg IV
Ipratropium	18 μg/actuation, via inhalation	18 μg/actuation, via inhalation

CRI, constant-rate infusion; IM, intramuscular; IV, intravenous; PO, by mouth (*per os*); SC, subcutaneous.

clinical response if shock is present. The airway should be secured and the patient intubated if necessary, and supplemental oxygen should be provided.

Aggressive fluid resuscitation is recommended in hypotensive patients. Bolus IV infusion of an isotonic crystalloid solution should be administered at resuscitative volumes (90 mL/kg in dogs and 60 mL/kg in cats, given in aliquots to effect). Colloids may be beneficial in providing a more sustained hemodynamic response and can be administered in bolus form.

Glucocorticoid use is controversial and a Cochrane review showed no benefit of administration during systemic anaphylaxis [40]; however, glucocorticoid use may reduce the severity of inflammation in late stages of anaphylaxis. Antihistamines (H1 and H2 antagonists) may be administered to relieve symptoms, particularly urticaria and pruritus, and they may decrease gastric acid secretion.

Bronchodilators may be another useful adjunctive therapy. Albuterol acts to relieve bronchospasm by relaxing bronchial smooth muscle [41]. Aminophylline, in addition to smooth muscle relaxation, also increases endogenous epinephrine release and decreases histamine release via phosphodiesterase inhibition [42].

Refractory hypotension may require treatment with vasopressors such as norepinephrine, vasopressin or dopamine. Refractory bronchospasm can be treated with glucagon or inhaled ipratropium. Persistent bradycardia or previous administration of beta-blockers may necessitate treatment with an anticholinergic [22].

Treatment of Toxic and Delayed Reactions

Massive envenomation requires aggressive, rapid stabilization with IV fluids to improve perfusion as well as provision of analgesia. Depending on the clinical manifestation, ancillary therapies may include antihistamine and corticosteroid administration to reduce upper airway edema and pruritus, plasma transfusion to treat DIC or coagulopathy, hemodialysis for severe or oligoanuric acute kidney injury (see Chapter 94), and oxygen support or mechanical ventilation for acute lung injury/acute respiratory distress syndrome (see Chapter 181). Epinephrine should be considered if there is suspicion of an anaphylactic component to the reaction. Broad-spectrum antibiotic therapy should be considered, particularly for fire ant massive envenomation [13] (see Chapter 200).

References

1 Vetter RS, Camazine S. Mass envenomation by honey bees and wasps. *West J Med* 1999;170(4):223–227.

2 Gonsalves LS. The introduction of the African Bees (Apis mellifera adasonii) into Brazil and some comments on their spread in South America. *Am Bee J* 1974;114:414–419.

3 Rowell MS, Bradley L, Cole C. The range expansion of the Africanized honey bee in Texas. *Am Bee J* 1993;133:84–85.

4 United States Department of Agriculture. Agriculture Research Service: Spread of Africanized Honey Bees by Year, updated March, 2011. www.ars.usda.gov/Research/docs.htm?docid=11059&page=6 (accessed 8 February 2018).

5 Kim KT, Oguro J. Update on the status of Africanized honey bees in the Western States. *West J Med* 1999;170:220–222.

6 Goddard J. *Physicians Guide to Arthropods of Medical Importance*, 3rd edn. WB Saunders, Philadelphia, 2000.

7 Winston ML. Form and function: honey bee anatomy. In: *The Biology of the Honey Bee*. Harvard University Press, Cambridge, 1987, pp. 13–45.

8 Smallheer BA. Bee and wasp stings: reactions and anaphylaxis. *Crit Care Nurs Care Clin North Am* 2013;25(2):151–164.

9 Logren CS, Banks WS, Glancey BM. Biology and control of imported fire ants. *Ann Rev Entomol* 1975;20:1–30.

10 Kemp SF, deShazo RD, Mofitt JE, et al. Expanding habitat of the imported fire ant (Solensis invicta): a public health concern. *J Allergy Immunol* 2000;105:683–691.

11 deShazo RD, Kemp SF, deShazo MD, Goddard J. Fire ant attacks on patients in nursing homes: an increasing problem. *Am J Med* 2004;116(12):843–846.

12 Stafford CT. Hypersensitivity to fire ant venom. *Ann Allergy Asthma Immunol* 1996;77:87–95.

13 Fitzgerald KT, Flood AA. Hymenoptera stings. *Clin Techn Small Anim Pract* 2006;21(4):194–204.

14 Peters LJ, Kovacic JP. Histamine: metabolism, physiology, and pathophysiology with applications in veterinary medicine. *J Vet Emerg Crit Care* 2009;19(4):311–328.

15 Schmidt JO, Blum MS, Overal WL. Comparative enzymology of venoms from stinging Hymenoptera. *Toxicon* 1986;24(9):907–921.

16 Bachman DS, Paulson MD, Jerry R, Mendell MD. Acute inflammatory polyradiculoneuropathy following Hymenoptera stings. *JAMA* 1982;247(10):1443–1445.

17 Nakajima T. Pharmacological biochemistry of vespid venoms. In: *Venoms of the Hymenoptera: Biochemical, Pharmacological and Behavioral Aspects* (ed. Piek T). Academic Press, Orlando, 1986, pp. 309–327.

18 Vetter RS, Visscher PK. Bites and stings of medically important venomous arthropods. *Int J Dermatol* 1998;37:481–496.

19 Franca FO, Benvenuti LA, Fan HW, et al. Severe and fatal mass attacks by "killer bees" in Brazil: clinicopathological studies with measurement of serum venom concentrations. *QJ Med* 1994;87:269–282.

20 Brand JM, Blum MS, Fales HM, et al. Fire ant venoms: comparative analysis of alkaloidal components. *Toxicon* 1972;10:259–271.

21 Reisman RE. Current concepts: insect stings. *N Engl J Med* 1994;331(8):523–527.

22 Shmuel DL, Cortes Y. Anaphylaxis in dogs and cats. *J Vet Emerg Crit Care* 2013;23(4):377–394.

23 Riches KJ, Gillis D, James RA. An autopsy approach to bee sting related deaths. *Pathology* 2002;34:257–262.

24 Cowell AK, Cowell RL. Management of bee and other Hymenoptera stings. In: *Kirk's Current Veterinary Therapy XII* (ed. Bonagura JD). WB Saunders, Philadelphia, 1995, pp. 226–228.

25 Waddell LS, Drobatz KJ. Massive envenomation by Vespula spp. *in two dogs. J Vet Emerg Crit Care* 1999;9(2):67–71.

26 Wysoke JM, van den Berg PB, Marshall C. Bee sting-induced haemolysis, spherocytosis and neural dysfunction in three dogs. *J S Afr Vet Assoc* 1990;61(1):29–32.

27 Cowell AK, Cowell RL, Tyler RD, et al. Severe systemic reactions to Hymenoptera stings in three dogs. *J Am Vet Med Assoc* 1991;198(6):1014–1016.

28 Noble SJ, Armstrong PJ. Bee sting resulting in secondary immune-mediated hemolytic anemia in two dogs. *J Am Vet Med Assoc* 1999;214(7):1026–1027.

29 Nakamura RK, Fenty RK, Biancio D. Presumptive immune-mediated thrombocytopenia secondary to massive Africanized bee envenomation in a dog. *J Vet Emerg Crit Care* 2013;23(6):652–656.

30 Grisotto LSD, Mendes E, Castro I, et al. Mechanisms of bee venom-induced acute renal failure. *Toxicon* 2006;48:44–54.

31 Oliveira EC, Pedroso PMO, Meirelles AE, et al. Pathologic findings in dogs after multiple Africanized bee stings. *Toxicon* 2007;49:1214–1218.

32 Mughal MN, Abbas G, Saqib M, Muhammad G. Massive attack by honeybees in a German Shepherd dog: description of a fatal case and review of the literature. *J Venom Anim Toxins Trop Dis* 2014;20:55.

33 Walker W, Tidwell AS, Rozanski EA, et al. Imaging diagnosis: acute lung injury following massive bee envenomation in a dog. *Vet Radiol* 2005;46(4): 300–303.

34 Fighera RA, Mello de Souza T, Lombardo de Barros CS. Bee sting as a cause of death in dogs. *Ciência Rural* 2007;37(2):590–593.

35 Abraham LA, Hinkley CJ, Tatarczuch L, et al. Acute renal failure following Bull Ant mass envenomation in two dogs. *Aust Vet J* 2004;82(1,2):43–47.

36 Peters GA, Karnes WE, Bastron JA. Near-fatal and fatal anaphylactic reactions to insect sting. *Ann Allergy* 1978;41:268–273.

37 Quantz JE, Miles MS, Reed AL, et al. Elevation of alanine transaminase and gallbladder wall abnormalities as biomarkers of anaphylaxis in canine hypersensitivity patients. *J Vet Emerg Crit Care* 2009;19(6):536–544.

38 Thomas E, Mandell DC, Wadell LS. Survival after anaphylaxis induced by a bumblebee sting in a dog. *J Am Anim Hosp Assoc* 2013;49(3):210–215.

39 Kolecki PK. Delayed toxic reaction following massive bee envenomation. *Ann Emerg Med* 1999;33(1):114–116.

40 Choo KJ, Simmons FE, Sheikh A. Glucocorticosteroids for the treatment of anaphylaxis: Cochrane systematic review. *Allergy* 2010;65(10):1205–1211.

41 Simons FE. Anaphylaxis. *J Allergy Clin Immunol* 2010;125(2 suppl 2):S161–181.

42 Plumb DC. *Plumb's Veterinary Drug Handbook*, 6th edn. Blackwell Publishing, Ames, 2008.

146

Hypersensitivity and Anaphylaxis

Sabrina N. Hoehne, DVM, DACVECC and Kate Hopper, BVSc, PhD, DACVECC

University of California Davis, Davis, CA, USA

Incidence and Definitions

In the United States, 1% of all human emergency department visits are allergy related. The majority of visits are composed of acute allergic and hypersensitivity reactions, with only 1% considered anaphylactic reactions [1]. The prevalence of acute allergic and anaphylactic reactions in veterinary medicine remains unknown, but is assumed to be increasing due to the growing exposure of small animals to antigenic substances [1–3].

Hypersensitivity reactions are defined as "objectively reproducible symptoms or signs initiated by exposure to a defined stimulus at a dose tolerated by normal persons" while an *allergy* or *allergic reaction* is a hypersensitivity reaction initiated by a specific immunological mechanism such as IgE-mediated allergies (see below) [4].

Atopy is an individual or familial tendency to become sensitized and produce IgE antibodies in response to ordinary exposure to antigens that can lead to the typical symptoms of allergies [4].

Definitions of *anaphylaxis* commonly include acute, serious, generalized or systemic allergic or hypersensitivity reactions that are rapid in onset, can be life threatening or fatal, and occur suddenly after contact with an allergy-causing substance [4–7]. The World Allergy Organization proposes a brief definition of anaphylaxis as "a serious, life-threatening, generalized or systemic hypersensitivity reaction" [8].

Classification and Pathophysiology of Hypersensitivity Reactions and Anaphylaxis

Acute allergic reactions can clinically be divided into localized and systemic hypersensitivity reactions. *Local* hypersensitivity reactions are restricted to cutaneous abnormalities such as erythema, pruritus, urticaria, or angioedema (Figure 146.1) whereas *systemic or generalized* hypersensitivity reactions lead to signs of systemic inflammatory mediator release [9,10].

In people, *mild generalized* hypersensitivity reactions are defined as causing cutaneous reaction only, such as generalized erythema, urticaria, and angioedema [9]. *Moderate generalized* hypersensitivity reactions comprise manifestations of severe illness with respiratory, cardiovascular, and gastrointestinal involvement [9]. Symptoms can include nausea, vomiting, and dizziness, along with processes known to lead to hypotension or hypoxemia such as dyspnea and stridorous respiration [9]. *Severe generalized* hypersensitivity reactions are defined by documented hypotension (systolic blood pressure <90 mmHg) or hypoxemia (SpO2 <92%), as well as clinical signs of neurological compromise resulting from hypotension or hypoxia, such as collapse and altered mental status [9]. Moderate and severe generalized hypersensitivity reactions are defined by features associated with hypoxemia and hypotension and therefore can be classified as *anaphylactic reactions* [9].

Immunologically, hypersensitivity as well as anaphylactic reactions are immediate (type 1) hypersensitivity reactions. Mast cells and basophils express Fc-epsilon-RI receptors on their cell surface that have a high affinity for the Fc portion of immunoglobulin E (IgE) antibodies [11]. Initial exposure to an antigen leads to increased production of IgE antibodies, which are subsequently bound to mast cell Fc-epsilon-RI receptors in sensitized individuals. After re-exposure to the same antigen, the antigen induces cross-linking of two adjacent surface IgE antibodies, leading to mast cell degranulation [11,12]. Multiple vasoactive mediators are released during mast cell degranulation, including histamine, tryptase, heparin, and cytokines [13]. Histamine effects are exerted via histamine receptors and receptor stimulation

Textbook of Small Animal Emergency Medicine, First Edition. Edited by Kenneth J. Drobatz, Kate Hopper, Elizabeth Rozanski and Deborah C. Silverstein.
© 2019 John Wiley & Sons, Inc. Published 2019 by John Wiley & Sons, Inc.
Companion Website: www.wiley.com/go/drobatz/textbook

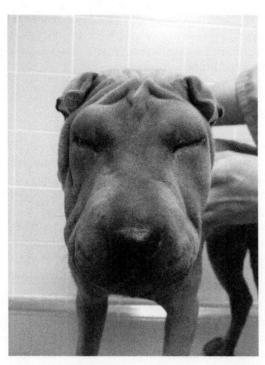

Figure 146.1 Localized hypersensitivity reaction in a Shar-Pei following Hymenoptera sting to the paw with facial urticaria, erythema, and pruritus.

can lead to pruritus, urticaria, angioedema, conjunctivitis, and rhinitis in allergic reactions as well as the vasodilation and increased vascular permeability responsible for cardiovascular collapse in anaphylactic reactions [3,13,14]. Platelet-activating factor (PAF) has also been shown to play a major role in anaphylactic reactions. PAF is a potent bronchoconstrictor, increases vascular permeability, and enhances platelet aggregation, histamine release, and vasodilation [11].

Apart from the classic IgE-mediated immunological pathway, a second pathway of systemic anaphylaxis was recently identified in murine models of anaphylaxis. This alternative pathway is mediated by immunoglobulin G (IgG) production and binding to the low-affinity IgG receptor Fc-gamma-RIII on macrophages. Re-exposure to an antigen induces anaphylaxis by formation of IgG antigen complexes. Complexes bind to Fc-gamma-RIII and cross-linkage of the receptor causes release of PAF from macrophages. In the alternative pathway, PAF rather than histamine is primarily responsible for development of hemodynamic alterations [12]. The significance of an alternative pathway of anaphylaxis in dogs and cats is yet to be determined.

Immunological mechanisms of hypersensitivity all require initial exposure to an antigen to stimulate the antibody response, also known as sensitization. Hypersensitivity responses only occur upon re-exposure to the antigen [11].

Lastly, in addition to the immunological; forms of anaphylaxis described above, non-immunological triggers for anaphylaxis have also been described when physical factors such as heat, cold, or pharmaceuticals cause degranulation of mast cells and basophils without participation of immunoglobulins [3,13]. This mechanism does not require sensitization, so hypersensitivity or anaphylaxis can occur upon the first exposure to an antigen.

The term *anaphylactic reaction* traditionally refers to IgE-mediated events, while *anaphylactoid reactions* are mediated by IgE-independent immunological or non-immunological events. Clinically, the two entities are not distinguishable and the World Allergy Organization suggests that the term *anaphylaxis* be used in preference to anaphylactoid reaction, regardless of the pathophysiology [7].

Etiologies and Clinical Manifestations

Hypersensitivity reactions and anaphylaxis occur as a dynamic continuum and any antigen capable of activating mast cells can trigger a reaction. The most common substances reported in veterinary medicine include vaccine proteins, insect and reptile venoms and their antivenoms, blood products, antimicrobial agents, non-steroidal anti-inflammatory agents, opioids, radiographic contrast agents, food, and physical factors such as heat or cold [15–24]. Single cases of fatal anaphylaxis associated with a dexamethasone suppression test and an intraoperative anaphylactic reaction to accidental dissection of an adult heartworm during lung lobectomy have also been reported in dogs [25,26].

After initial exposure to the antigenic stimulus, hypersensitivity and anaphylactic reactions occur within minutes of contact [6,12,13]. The time to onset of clinical signs and the severity of systemic anaphylactic reactions correlate, and as a general rule, the more rapidly the symptoms manifest, the more severe a reaction will be and the more likely it is to progress to being life threatening [13]. Manifestations of hypersensitivity and anaphylactic reactions can include cutaneous, cardiovascular, respiratory, gastrointestinal, and neurological symptoms [9]. The clinical presentation and course are dictated by the organ systems primarily affected by the reaction and directly relate to the distribution of the largest mast cell population, which varies between species [10,13].

In dogs with hypersensitivity reactions, cutaneous and gastrointestinal signs predominate. Specifically, in vaccine-associated adverse events, dermal signs including facial edema, pruritus, erythema, and urticaria are the most common clinical manifestations in 68% of patients, followed by gastrointestinal signs such as vomiting, diarrhea, and anorexia in 45% of patients [19]. Young adult small-breed dogs were found to be at greater risk for vaccine-associated adverse events and the risk has been shown to significantly increase with an increasing number of vaccines administered per visit [27]. Anaphylactic reactions following vaccine administration are less commonly observed and appear to rarely be fatal [19]. It is important to note that the clinical signs of hypersensitivity and anaphylaxis can vary with the antigen responsible.

In anaphylactic reactions, the liver and gastrointestinal tract are most commonly affected in the dog. Histamine released from the gastrointestinal tract leads to significant sinusoidal and hepatic venous congestion, which in some cases may progress to hepatic hemorrhage and hepatocellular necrosis [10,28]. This can lead to distributive shock (see Chapter 155). Increased vascular permeability can contribute to cardiovascular collapse and massive fluid shifts of up to 35% of the intravascular volume to the interstitial space can occur [3,29]. Rapid hemodynamic compromise can occur without preceding cutaneous signs. A study of canine hypersensitivity reactions reported that only 57% of dogs showed cutaneous signs during anaphylactic reactions, and that their manifestations were more subtle than in milder allergic reactions [10]. Respiratory manifestations of anaphylaxis in the dog are rare but can consist of pulmonary congestion or hemorrhage clinically manifesting as tachypnea and increased respiratory effort [28].

The most common clinical signs with vaccine-associated allergic reactions in cats include lethargy with or without fever, localized vaccination site reactions such as soreness or inflammation, vomiting, facial edema, or generalized pruritus [30]. Cats with anaphylactic reactions more commonly exhibit pulmonary and gastrointestinal signs such as open mouth breathing, tachypnea, respiratory distress, salivation, vomiting, and diarrhea [3,18]. Respiratory signs are thought to result from bronchoconstriction, laryngeal edema, and increased mucus production [31]. The risk for vaccine-associated adverse reactions in cats also increases with the number of vaccines administered per visit, but severe hypersensitivity reactions are rare [30]. Anaphylactic reactions have also been reported in cats following administration of ophthalmic medications, the most commonly reported signs being respiratory and gastrointestinal in nature [18]. Less commonly, dermatological signs such as angioedema, pruritus, urticaria, chemosis and conjunctival hyperemia, and neurological signs including ataxia have been described in cats suffering from anaphylactic events [18].

The most severe anaphylactic reactions, such as cardiovascular collapse and respiratory compromise, are most commonly observed after parenteral administration of antigen [28,29]. Oral ingestion of antigens can cause gastrointestinal symptoms as well as dermal reactions, and topically applied antigen can cause cutaneous and ocular signs, as well as systemic signs of anaphylaxis [18,31]. Lastly, antigen inhalation commonly causes local signs of rhinitis and bronchoconstriction [31].

Diagnosis

The diagnosis of hypersensitivity reactions and anaphylaxis is clinical and based on history and recognition of classic clinical signs on physical examination. A detailed history that investigates recent exposure to potential triggers such as vaccinations, new medications, insect bites and stings can help raise the suspicion for an allergic reaction. As discussed previously, cutaneous, gastrointestinal, respiratory, cardiovascular, neurological, and ocular signs can be encountered in patients suffering from hypersensitivity and anaphylactic reactions.

Clinical criteria for the diagnosis of anaphylaxis have been formulated in people, but to date universal criteria have not been established for veterinary species. Based on the criteria reported in people and previous reports of hypersensitivity in small animals, suggested clinical criteria that make hypersensitivity and anaphylactic reactions likely in dogs and cats are summarized in Box 146.1 [6].

One study found both increased ALT and changes in gall bladder wall appearance to be significantly associated with anaphylaxis in canine patients [10]. Gall bladder wall changes found in patients with anaphylaxis include increased wall thickness >3 mm and striated

---

Box 146.1 Suggested diagnostic criteria for hypersensitivity and anaphylaxis in dogs and cats

Known recent exposure to antigen greatly increases the diagnostic likelihood

Hypersensitivity in dogs
One or both of the following:
- Acute cutaneous signs
- Gastrointestinal signs

Hypersensitivity in cats
Any one or more of the following:
- Gastrointestinal signs
- Respiratory signs
- Cutaneous signs

Anaphylaxis in dogs and cats
Life-threatening abnormality with one or more of the following:
- Cutaneous signs
- Gastrointestinal signs
- Respiratory signs
- Cardiovascular signs

gall bladder wall (halo or double rim effect) suggestive of subserosal edema [10]. More than 100 biomarkers for mast cell and basophil activation, such as plasma histamine and tryptase concentrations, have been described, none of which are readily available in clinical veterinary medicine [32].

Treatment

The treatment for hypersensitivity reactions is largely symptomatic and dictated by the severity of the reaction. Anaphylaxis is a medical emergency and initial patient assessment should focus on circulation, airway, and breathing (see Chapter 2). Life-threatening signs of anaphylactic reactions to Hymenoptera stings (bees, wasps) in dogs are usually apparent within 10–15 minutes of venom exposure and in a small number of susceptible animals can rapidly progress to death (see Chapter 145). This is likely the case for anaphylactic reactions to a variety of antigens [15]. In veterinary medicine, no randomized controlled trials have been performed to evaluate the medications most commonly used in the treatment of anaphylaxis and the choice of treatment therefore remains controversial. Treatment recommendations are summarized in Table 146.1.

Antihistamines

Antihistamines are commonly used in veterinary medicine to treat hypersensitivity reactions. While H1 antihistamines have been shown to reduce pruritus associated

Table 146.1 Suggested drugs and dosages for treatment of hypersensitivity and anaphylactic reactions in dogs and cats.

Drug	Dose and route
Diphenhydramine	Dogs: 1–4 mg/kg PO or IM
	Cats: 0.5–2 mg/kg PO or IM
Dexamethasone sodium phosphate	0.1 mg/kg IV
Epinephrine	0.01–0.025 mg/kg IV
	0.05 µg/kg/min IV as CRI
Albuterol	0.5 mL of 0.5% solution in 4 mL of isotonic saline by nebulizer
	1–2 puffs (90 µg/actuation)
Terbutaline	0.01 mg/kg IM or IV
	0.625–1.25 mg PO
Aminophylline	5–10 mg/kg IM or IV

CRI, constant-rate infusion; IM, intramuscular; IV, intravenous; PO, by mouth (*per os*).

with antigen exposure in allergic reactions, treatment with antihistamines has not been proven effective in alleviating cardiovascular signs of anaphylaxis [33,34]. In a Cochrane review on the role of H1 antihistamines for the treatment of human anaphylaxis, no strong evidence was found for or against their use and no recommendations for clinical practice could be formulated [35]. Antihistamines should therefore only be considered in the treatment of mild to moderate hypersensitivity reactions or as an ancillary treatment in anaphylactic shock to relieve cutaneous, ocular, and nasal signs.

Recommended dosages for diphenhydramine, an H1 antihistamine, are 1–4 mg/kg PO or IM, in dogs and 0.5–2 mg/kg IM or PO in cats [36]. Some evidence exists that concurrent administration of H2 with H1 antihistamines can alleviate flushing, headache, and other symptoms in people [8]. It is possible that H2 receptor antagonists lead to similar relief in animals, but this has yet to be shown. Similar to H1, H2 antihistamines should be considered ancillary treatment of anaphylaxis only.

Glucocorticoids

Glucocorticoids are another drug class frequently used in the treatment of all hypersensitivity reactions. Similar to H1 antihistamines, a Cochrane review was unable to find evidence to justify the use of steroids in the emergency management of anaphylaxis, and currently their use can neither be supported nor refuted [37]. When using glucocorticoid drugs, it is important to remember that the onset of effects of this drug class takes several hours and it therefore does not relieve acute signs associated with hypersensitivity reactions [8].

The dose for oral administration of prednisone for mild hypersensitivity reactions is recommended to be 1 mg/kg and equivalent doses of parenterally administered glucocorticoids are appropriate (e.g. dexamethasone sodium phosphate at 0.1 mg/kg IV) [6].

Epinephrine

The World Health Organization and several published anaphylaxis treatment guidelines consider epinephrine to be an essential medication and recommended first-line treatment in human anaphylaxis [6–8]. The predominant clinical signs in human patients are respiratory failure, laryngeal edema, and cardiovascular collapse [38–40]. The beneficial effects of epinephrine in human anaphylaxis are believed to be due to both alpha- and beta-adrenergic effects [41]. Alpha-1 adrenergic stimulation is responsible for potent vasoconstriction of the small arterioles, which can have life-saving cardiovascular effects [41]. Furthermore, the vasoconstriction decreases mucosal edema and helps relieve upper airway obstruction [41]. Beta-2 effects further alleviate respiratory signs by increased bronchodilation and decreased histamine release, while beta-1 adrenergic effects increase cardiac contractility [41].

In contrast to these findings in human medicine, distributive shock in canine anaphylaxis may be due to pooling of venous blood in the hepatic circulation and the use of epinephrine as a first-line treatment is controversial [28]. In experimental models of canine anaphylactic shock, low-rate constant-rate infusions of epinephrine were considered more effective than a single bolus dose [42–44]. Subcutaneous administration is not recommended due to potent vasoconstriction and unpredictable absorption in states of anaphylactic shock [44].

Epinephrine is supplied as either a 1:1000 (1 mg/mL) or 1:10000 (0.1 mg/mL) solution. Epinephrine autoinjector (EpiPen) use is not recommended by the authors due to several concerns. Injectors are most commonly available in two fixed doses of 0.15 and 0.3 mg and therefore cannot be safely administered to patients weighing less than 15 kg. Furthermore, the needle size is limited and might preclude the intramuscular administration of the drug in obese animals. At-home administration of first aid drugs could additionally delay appropriate presentation of an at-risk animal to a veterinarian within the critical time period.

Bronchodilators

Beta-2 agonists such as albuterol and terbutaline, as well as xanthine derivates, can be beneficial as an additional treatment for respiratory manifestation of anaphylaxis.

Intravenous Fluids and Other Ancillary Treatments

Due to the potential of rapid extravasation of significant amounts of plasma volume and distributive shock due to venous pooling, intravenous fluid resuscitation is recommended for anaphylactic patients (see Chapter 153). Patients with refractory clinical hypoperfusion or hypotension might also require vasopressor administration (see Chapter 155).

Prognosis

The prognosis of hypersensitivity reactions is variable and depends on the allergenic trigger, severity, and progression of the reaction. Once a diagnosis of allergic or anaphylactic reaction is suspected, a detailed history should be taken and recommendations made to avoid exposure to the suspected trigger.

References

1 Gaeta TJ, Clark S, Pelletier AJ, Camargo CA. National study of US emergency department visits for acute allergic reactions, 1993 to 2004. *Ann Allergy Asthma Immunol* 2007;98(4):360–365.

2 Armitage-Chan E. Anaphylaxis and anaesthesia. *Vet Anaesth Analg* 2010;37(4):306–310.

3 Shmuel DL, Cortes Y. Anaphylaxis in dogs and cats. *J Vet Emerg Crit Care* 2013;23(4):377–394.

4 Johansson SG, Bieber T, Dahl R, et al. Revised nomenclature for allergy for global use: Report of the Nomenclature Review Committee of the World Allergy Organization, October 2003. *J Allergy Clin Immunol* 2004;113(5):832–836.

5 Johansson SGO, Hourihane JO'B, Bousquet J, et al. A revised nomenclature for allergy: an EAACI position statement from the EAACI nomenclature task force. *Allergy* 2001;56(9):813–824.

6 Sampson HA, Muñoz-Furlong A, Campbell RL, et al. Second Symposium on the Definition and Management of Anaphylaxis: Summary Report – Second National Institute of Allergy and Infectious Disease/ Food Allergy and Anaphylaxis Network Symposium. *Ann Emerg Med* 2006;47(4):373–380.

7 Simons FER, Ardusso LR, Bilò M, et al. International consensus on (ICON) anaphylaxis. *World Allergy Organ J* 2014;7(1):9.

8 Simons FER, Ardusso LRF, Bilò MB, et al. World Allergy Organization guidelines for the assessment and management of anaphylaxis. *World Allergy Organ J* 2011;4(2):13–36.

9 Brown SG. Clinical features and severity grading of anaphylaxis. *J Allergy Clin Immunol* 2004;114(2): 371–376.

10 Quantz JE, Miles MS, Reed AL, White GA. Elevation of alanine transaminase and gallbladder wall abnormalities as biomarkers of anaphylaxis in canine hypersensitivity patients: anaphylaxis biomarkers in canine hypersensitivity. *J Vet Emerg Crit Care* 2009;19(6):536–544.

11 Robbins SL, Kumar V, Cotran RS (eds). *Robbins and Cotran Pathologic Basis of Disease*, 8th edn. Elsevier Saunders, Philadelphia, 2009.

12 Finkelman F. Anaphylaxis: lessons from mouse models. *J Allergy Clin Immunol* 2007;120(3):506–515.

13 Khan BQ, Kemp SF. Pathophysiology of anaphylaxis: *Curr Opin Allergy Clin Immunol* 2011;11(4):319–325.

14 Limsuwan T, Demoly P. Acute symptoms of drug hypersensitivity (urticaria, angioedema, anaphylaxis, anaphylactic shock). *Med Clin North Am* 2010;94(4):691–710.

15 Fitzgerald KT, Flood AA. Hymenoptera stings. *Clin Tech Small Anim Pract* 2006;21(4):194–204.

16 Girard NM, Leece EA. Suspected anaphylactoid reaction following intravenous administration of a gadolinium-based contrast agent in three dogs undergoing magnetic resonance imaging: anaphylactoid reaction to MRI contrast agent in dogs. *Vet Anaesth Analg* 2010;37(4):352–356.

17 Heller J, Mellor D, Hodgson J, et al. Elapid snake envenomation in dogs in New South Wales: a review. *Aust Vet J* 2007;85(11):469–479.

18 Hume-Smith KM, Groth AD, Rishniw M, et al. Anaphylactic events observed within 4 h of ocular application of an antibiotic-containing ophthalmic preparation: 61 cats (1993–2010). *J Feline Med Surg* 2011;13(10):744–751.

19 Miyaji K, Suzuki A, Shimakura H, et al. Large-scale survey of adverse reactions to canine non-rabies combined vaccines in Japan. *Vet Immunol Immunopathol* 2012;145(1-2):447–452.

20 Moore GE, HogenEsch H. Adverse vaccinal events in dogs and cats. *Vet Clin North Am Small Anim Pract* 2010;40(3):393–407.

21 Niza MMR, Félix N, Vilela CL, Peleteiro MC, Ferreira AJ. Cutaneous and ocular adverse reactions in a dog following meloxicam administration. *Vet Dermatol* 2007;18(1):45–49.

22 Ohmori K, Masuda K, Maeda S, et al. IgE reactivity to vaccine components in dogs that developed immediate-type allergic reactions after vaccination. *Vet Immunol Immunopathol* 2005;104(3-4):249–256.

23 Tocci LJ. Transfusion medicine in small animal practice. *Vet Clin North Am Small Anim Pract* 2010;40(3):485–494.

24 Walker T, Tidwell AS, Rozanski EA, de Laforcade A, Hoffman AM. Imaging diagnosis: acute lung injury following massive bee envenomation in a dog. *Vet Radiol Ultrasound* 2005;46(4):300–303.

25 Carter JE, Chanoit G, Kata C. Anaphylactoid reaction in a heartworm-infected dog undergoing lung lobectomy. *J Am Vet Med Assoc* 2011;238(10): 1301–1304.

26 Schaer M, Ginn PE, Hanel RM. A case of fatal anaphylaxis in a dog associated with a dexamethasone suppression test: a case of fatal anaphylaxis. *J Vet Emerg Crit Care* 2005;15(3):213–216.

27 Moore GE, Guptill LF, Ward MP, et al. Adverse events diagnosed within three days of vaccine administration in dogs. *J Am Vet Med Assoc* 2005;227(7):1102–1108.

28 Dean HR, Webb RA. The morbid anatomy and histology of anaphylaxis in the dog. *J Pathol Bacteriol* 1924;27(1):51–64.

29 Kitoh K, Watoh K, Chaya K, Kitagawa H, Sasaki Y. Clinical, hematologic, and biochemical findings in dogs after induction of shock by injection of heartworm extract. *Am J Vet Res* 1994;55(11):1535–1541.

30 Moore GE, DeSantis-Kerr AC, Guptill LF, et al. Adverse events after vaccine administration in cats: 2,560 cases (2002–2005). *J Am Vet Med Assoc* 2007;231(1):94–100.

31 Dowling LL. Anaphylaxis. In: *Small Animal Critical Care Medicine* (eds Silverstein DC, Hopper K). Elsevier Saunders, Philadelphia, 2015.

32 Simons FER. Anaphylaxis: recent advances in assessment and treatment. *J Allergy Clin Immunol* 2009;124(4):625–636.

33 Rhoades R. Suppression of histamine-induced pruritus by three antihistaminic drugs*1. *J Allergy Clin Immunol* 1975;55(3):180–185.

34 Silverman HJ, Taylor WR, Smith PL, et al. Effects of antihistamines on the cardiopulmonary changes due to canine anaphylaxis. *J Appl Physiol* 1988;64(1):210–217.

35 Sheikh A, ten Broek VM, Brown SG, Simons FER. H1-antihistamines for the treatment of anaphylaxis with and without shock. *Cochrane Database Syst Rev* 2007;1:CD006160.

36 Plumb DC. Plumb's Veterinary Drug Handbook: *Desk*, 7th edn. Wiley-Blackwell, Ames, 2011.

37 Choo KJL, Simons E, Sheikh A. Glucocorticoids for the treatment of anaphylaxis: Cochrane systematic review. *Allergy* 2010;65(10):1205–1211.

38 Kemp SF, Lockey RF. Anaphylaxis: a review of causes and mechanisms. *J Allergy Clin Immunol* 2002;110(3):341–348.

39 Marone G, Bova M, Detoraki A, et al. The human heart as a shock organ in anaphylaxis. In: *Anaphylaxis (Novartis Foundation Symposium)*. John Wiley and Sons, Chichester, 2004.

40 Triggiani M, Patella V, Staiano RI, Granata F, Marone G. Allergy and the cardiovascular system. *Clin Exp Immunol* 2008;153:7–11.

41 Simons KJ, Simons FER. Epinephrine and its use in anaphylaxis: current issues: *Curr Opin Allergy Clin Immunol* 2010;10(4):354–361.

42 Bautista E, Simons FER, Simons KJ, et al. Epinephrine fails to hasten hemodynamic recovery in fully developed canine anaphylactic shock. *Int Arch Allergy Immunol* 2002;128(2):151–164.

43 Mink S. Effect of bolus epinephrine on systemic hemodynamics in canine anaphylactic shock. *Cardiovasc Res* 1998;40(3):546–556.

44 Mink SN, Simons FER, Simons KJ, Becker AB, Duke K. Constant infusion of epinephrine, but not bolus treatment, improves haemodynamic recovery in anaphylactic shock in dogs. *Clin Exp Allergy* 2004;34(11):1776–1783.

147

Canine Heat Stroke

Yaron Bruchim, DVM, IVIMS, DACVECC, DECVECC[1] and Efrat Kelmer, DVM, DACVECC, DECVECC[2]

[1]*The Hebrew University of Jerusalem, Jerusalem, Israel*
[2]*The Hebrew University Veterinary Teaching Hospital, Koret School of Veterinary Medicine, Israel*

Pathophysiology

Elevation of body temperatures above the normal hypothalamic set point can be due to pyrogenic or non-pyrogenic causes. Non-pyrogenic hyperthermia occurs when heat-dissipating mechanisms cannot adequately compensate for heat production, or when these mechanisms are impaired [1]. In dogs, under normal environmental conditions, more than 70% of total body heat is dissipated through radiation and convection from body surfaces. As environmental temperatures increase and approach body temperature, evaporation, primarily through panting, becomes more important for maintaining normothermia. The nasal turbinates provide a large surface area for water loss from the moist mucous membranes, and play an important role in heat dissipation. Hypersalivation increases the evaporative efficiency, although high environmental temperatures and increased humidity (>35%) will decrease its effectiveness; when humidity is >80%, this cooling measure will be negated [2,3].

Heat stroke is caused by the inability to dissipate accumulated heat. In dogs, it is characterized by core temperatures above 41 °C (105.8 °F) with central nervous system (CNS) dysfunction [3,4]. It results from exposure to a hot and humid environment (classic heat stroke), from voluntary strenuous physical exercise (exertional heat stroke) or severe, uncontrolled tremors or seizures [1,5].

In the initial stages of heat stress, cardiac output increases due to peripheral vasodilation and decreased vascular resistance. As hyperthermia progresses, cutaneous and splanchnic blood pooling combines with dehydration, which results in decreasing circulating blood volume – hypotension. Consequently, cardiac output declines due to decreased circulating blood volume, leading to failure of heat loss through the mechanisms of radiation and convection, causing an elevation in body temperature that may progress to heat stroke.

Accumulation of blood in these organs is a major contributor to the shock and consequent intestinal ischemia, hypoxia, and endothelial hyperpermeability that many heat stroke patients develop. Cytokine production, reactive oxygen and nitrogen species generation, endotoxemia, and endothelial injury are all contributors to increased vascular permeability and subsequent interstitial edema [6–8]. Activation of inflammatory and hemostatic pathways initiates a systemic inflammatory response syndrome (SIRS) which often progresses to multiorgan dysfunction syndrome (MODS) [7,9] (see Chapter 159).

Serious complications of heat stroke include rhabdomyolysis, acute kidney injury (AKI) (see Chapter 94), acute respiratory distress syndrome (ARDS), and disseminated intravascular coagulation (DIC) [10–12] (see Chapter 70). Consequently, despite appropriate cooling and supportive treatments, mortality rates above 50% have been reported in humans and canines suffering from heat stroke because no specific treatment is available to ameliorate the activated inflammatory and hemostatic pathways [13–16]. It seems that the main causes of death from heat stroke in canines are systemic hemodynamic deterioration and pulmonary lesions, as determined from postmortem studies of 11 dogs that suffered naturally occurring heat stroke [12].

Risk Factors for Developing Heat Stroke

Several factors are associated with the risk of developing heat stroke. These include prior occurrence of heat stroke or heat stress, obesity, breed (brachiocephalic, golden and Labrador Retrievers), body weight (>15 kg), high environmental temperature and humidity, and lack of acclimation and fitness [14,17,18]. Prior heat stroke may affect the thermoregulatory center in the preoptic zone which is responsible for heat sensation and dissipation. Excess body fat increases the body's natural thermal isolation and impairs normal heat dissipation mechanisms in obese people and animals [3,19]. Large-breed dogs are significantly more at risk of developing heat stroke, particularly exertional heat stroke, suggesting that the ratio between body size and surface area is an important factor in heat dissipation during heat stress. The median body weight of 54 dogs with naturally occurring heat stroke was 31 kg, also supporting this theory [14].

Two endogenous adaptive mechanisms are directly invoked to combat heat stress: heat acclimation and the rapid heat shock response. Heat acclimation induces adaptive physiological and behavioral changes that improve the individual's ability to cope with extreme environmental heat. Acclimation is a time-dependent process leading to a dynamic expansion of the body temperature regulatory range due to left and right shifts in the temperature threshold for heat dissipation and thermal injury, respectively.

The heat shock response is a rapid molecular cytoprotective mechanism that involves production of heat shock proteins (HSP). When subjected to sublethal heat stress, the body enhances HSP transcription and synthesis to increase HSP72 cellular reserves, thus providing cytoprotection [20]. In a recent prospective study, the correlation between HSP 72, heat acclimation, and physical performance in military working dogs was evaluated. During the study, three consecutive physical performance tests were performed over a 2-year training period. Serum HSP72 concentrations and lymphocyte HSP72 and its corresponding mRNA levels were analyzed before and after the physical endurance test. Results showed that together with the profound enhancement of aerobic power and physical performance, HSP72 mRNA was induced and progressively increased, and there was also a significant rise in basal and peak serum HSP72 concentrations after physical exercise [17].

Clinical Signs and Diagnosis

The most common clinical signs of canine heat stroke include collapse, shock, tachypnea, spontaneous bleeding (e.g. petechiae, hematemesis, and hematochezia), disorientation/stupor, coma, and seizures. Although the definition of heat stroke is based on hyperthermia causing shock and hypotension, it is important to remember that patients can be hyper-, normo- or hypothermic on presentation, particularly if cooling measures were initiated by the owners prior to presentation. Furthermore, in a retrospective study of canine heat-related illness, hypothermia upon admission was a poor prognostic indicator [15]. Therefore, heat stroke should not be disregarded in

a patient with normal or low core temperature if the history reveals recent exercise or confinement in a hot and humid environment, recent cooling by the owner and clinical and/or clinicopathological findings compatible with heat-related illness.

Acute collapse, abnormal mentation, hypoglycemia, and hyperemic mucous membranes are common in dogs with heat-induced illness. Nonetheless, the median systolic and diastolic blood pressure upon admission to medical treatment in a prospective study of 30 dogs with naturally occurring heat stroke were in the normal range (>90 mmHg and >60 mmHg, respectively and HR of 160 bpm), except for one dog [21]. This is in contrast to the hypotension documented in both experimental models and human clinical reports [22]. The lack of hypotension suggests that the dogs were in a state of compensatory shock at the time of admission to the hospital (after cooling by their owners and/or by the referring veterinarian). The neurohormonal compensatory response of blood pressure is likely to be faster than the recovery/disruption of biochemical parameters.

Hematological Disorders and Biochemical Abnormalities

The most common hematological findings in canines with heat stroke are thrombocytopenia and increased packed cell volume (PCV) and hemoglobin concentrations. In a retrospective study of 54 dogs with heat stroke, 83% had thrombocytopenia upon admission and during hospitalization, although it was not found to be a significant risk factor for death (Table 147.1) [23]. In that study, only 50% of the dogs suffered from DIC, so thrombocytopenia is most likely caused by a combination of vasculitis, splenic sequestration with blood pooling, gastrointestinal bleeding, and hyperthermia-induced platelet aggregation [23].

Nucleated red blood cells (nRBCs) on peripheral blood smear are abundant in dogs with heat stroke (10–120%) and represent a significant risk factor for mortality. They most likely occur secondary to heat-induced damage to the bone marrow. Dogs presenting with >18 nRBC/100 WBC on peripheral blood smear were significantly more likely to die, have renal complications, and develop DIC. The maximum level of nRBC was detected upon admission with a gradual decline over the first 36 hours from the insult in all the dogs [10]. This phenomenon can be attributed to thermal lesions within the bone marrow, leading to blood–bone marrow barrier injury and subsequent release of nRBCs to the peripheral circulation. An alternative hypothesis might be that bone marrow release of nRBCs to the peripheral circulation in canine heat stroke is mediated via the actions of cytokines.

Table 147.1 Risk factors for mortality in 54 dogs with naturally occurring heat stroke.

Variable	RF present		RF not present		RR	Exact CI 95%	P
	n	Number of deaths (%)	n	Number of deaths(%)			
Timelag >90 min	34	21 (62)	15	4 (27)	2.32	1.08–5.90	0.032
Cooling by owners before admission	26	10 (39)	28	17 (61)	0.63	0.35–1.12	0.173
Obesity	11	9 (82)	36	15 (42)	1.96	1.11–3.21	0.040
Coma/semicoma upon admission	22	15 (68)	20	8 (41)	1.71	0.95–3.32	0.060
Seizures during illness	19	14 (74)	35	13 (37)	2.00	1.17–3.37	0.020
Prothrombin time >18 sec upon admission	8	7 (88)	39	18 (46)	1.90	1.05–2.94	0.050
aPTT >30 sec upon admission	14	13 (93)	33	12 (36)	2.55	1.57–4.28	<0.001
Thrombocytopenia* during illness	42	19 (45)	8	3 (37)	0.83	0.28–1.80	1.000
Creatinine >1.5 mg/dL at 24h from admission	20	15 (75)	17	4 (24)	3.19	1.41–8.39	0.003
Glucose <47 mg/dL upon admission	12	10 (83)	12	5 (42)	2.00	1.01–5.27	0.03
Presence of DIC	28	19 (68)	26	8 (31)	2.21	1.22–4.31	0.013
Presence of AKI	18	14 (78)	36	13 (36)	2.15	1.28–3.64	0.008
Presence of DIC + AKI	12	11 (92)	21	6 (29)	3.21	1.63–7.01	0.001
Presence of environmental heat stroke	20	10 (50)	34	17 (50)	1.00	0.55–1.72	1.000
Presence of exertional heat stroke	34	17 (50)	20	10 (50)	1.00	0.58–1.82	1.000

*Platelet count $150 \times 10^3/mm^3$.

AKI, acute kidney injury; aPTT, activated partial thromboplastin time; CI, confidence interval; DIC, disseminated intravascular coagulation; RF, risk factor; RR, relative risk.

Rhabdomyolysis is a prominent feature of heat stroke during and following the heat insult, and is exacerbated during the first 24 hours of hospitalization due to muscular hypoperfusion resulting from distributive shock and DIC. The degree of increase in serum muscle enzyme activities reflects the extent of cellular damage and direct thermal injury to myocardial and skeletal muscle myocytes [24]. Liver damage and acute liver failure have been described in humans and animals with heat stroke [25–28]. Therefore, the most commonly observed serum biochemistry abnormalities in canine heat stroke include increased serum activities of creatine kinase, alanine aminotransferase (ALT), aspartate aminotransferase (AST), alkaline phosphatase (ALP), gamma-glutamyl transpeptidase (GGT), and hypoglycemia [10,14]. In 46 dogs with heat stroke, CK was reported to be elevated in 97% at presentation, with a median of 11 000 U/L (range 107–345 000 U/L), AST and ALT in 80% (median 750, range 40–14 500 and median 225, range 44–3200 U/L), and ALP and GGT only in 25% of the dogs (median 135, range 24–586 U/L, median 5.5, range 1–38 U/L) (Bruchim et al. 2016, unpublished data). Interestingly, only ALP and GGT were significantly higher among non-survivors, perhaps indicating the role of sepsis-induced cholestasis and hepatic failure, as described in human heat stroke victims and animal models [26,27].

In a retrospective study of 54 dogs with heat stroke, hypoglycemia was evident in 62% of the dogs upon admission, and was found to be a significant risk factor of mortality. Hypoglycemia can result from increased utilization or decreased production of glucose, or be due to hepatic failure or sepsis, as seen in some dogs with persistent hypoglycemia despite initial stabilization of serum glucose levels (see Table 147.1) [14].

Coagulation Disorders and Disseminated Intravascular Coagulation

Thermal endothelial cell injury leads to diffuse vascular damage and initiation of coagulation and subsequent microvascular thrombosis. In addition, multiorgan cellular necrosis further stimulates the coagulation system and results in DIC, an important factor in the morbidity and mortality of heat stroke patients [29] (see Chapter 62). The injured endothelium releases thromboplastin and factor XII, which activate coagulation and the complement cascade, inducing SIRS and widespread DIC. Hepatic injury and failure due to hypoperfusion, microembolism, and direct hyperthermic damage may exacerbate the hemostatic disorders [29].

In vitro studies have shown that high temperatures (>42 °C) lead to platelet aggregation, activation of the coagulation cascade, and enhanced fibrinolysis [1,7,11,30,31]. Normalization of body temperatures inhibits fibrinolysis but not the coagulation cascade or platelet aggregation [30]. In a retrospective study of 54 dogs with naturally occurring heat stroke, 50% were diagnosed with DIC [14]. In 11 such dogs, severe bleeding and widespread microthrombosis, characteristic of hemorrhagic diathesis, were invariably noted at necropsy [12]. As DIC may appear hours to days after the initial hyperthermic insult, dogs with heat stroke should be monitored closely for coagulation abnormalities and clinical signs of DIC for at least 24 hours after the insult.

In a recent study in which serial monitoring of coagulation parameters was followed during the first 36 hours of hospitalization in 30 dogs with heat stroke, hemostatic analytes at presentation were not associated with mortality. However, prolonged PT and aPTT at 12–24 hours, lower total protein C activity at 12 hours, and hyperfibrinogenemia at 24 hours post presentation were significantly associated with mortality. Increased D-dimer concentration and low antithrombin activity were common at all time-points, but were not associated with mortality (Figure 147.1) [32]. Interestingly, in that study, which was performed 10 years following the first one at the same institution, DIC was not associated with mortality, the median number of fresh frozen plasma units administered increased from 2 to 4 units per dog, and mortality decreased from 50% to 40%.

Other Complications: Acute Kidney Injury, Central Nervous System Dysfunction, ARDS, Cardiac Arrhythmias, and Gastrointestinal Bacterial Translocation

Acute Kidney Injury

Azotemia is a common finding in patients with heat stroke (see Chapter 94). It results from prerenal and renal mechanisms, such as severe hypovolemia and direct renal tissue damage leading to tubular necrosis, a frequent finding at necropsy of dogs with heat stroke [12]. This probably occurs as a result of direct renal thermal injury, hypovolemia, hypoxia, and endotoxemia, release of cytokines and vasoactive mediators and microthrombosis associated with DIC [1,33]. The presence of AKI during hospitalization and serum creatinine levels >1.5 mg/dL at 12 and 24 hours after presentation were found to be independent risk factors for death in dogs with heat stroke (see Table 147.1) [14,21,34]. Therefore, careful monitoring of renal function and early intervention are warranted.

Central Nervous System Dysfunction

Severe hyperthermia may lead to cerebral hypoperfusion, neuronal necrosis, direct vascular damage, cerebral edema, hemorrhage, and multifocal vascular thrombosis with tissue infarction that may lead to CNS dysfunction and death. The canine brain is considered more resistant to thermal injury than the human brain and other physiological factors, such as respiratory alkalosis, shock and hypoglycemia, may play a more significant role in the observed CNS clinical signs in canine heat stroke [35].

Acute Respiratory Distress Syndrome

Thermal and biochemical injury to the pulmonary endothelium may lead to non-cardiogenic pulmonary edema, also known as ARDS (see Chapters 39 and 159). Histopathological lung lesions in dogs suffering from heat stroke include pulmonary infarcts, marked alveolar hemorrhage, and edema [12].

Cardiac Arrhythmias

A few extracardiac mechanisms were proposed as contributing to the development of cardiac arrhythmias: myocardial hypoperfusion, lactic acidosis and electrolyte imbalance, and possibly direct thermal injury. Postmortem findings in 11 dogs with heat stroke showed mild to severe subendocardial, myocardial and epicardial hemorrhages and hyperemia in all dogs [12]. These findings suggest that DIC has a pivotal role in the pathogenesis of the reported cardiac arrhythmias. Antiarrhythmic therapy should be considered, however, only if the patient has related clinical signs (see Chapter 53).

Gastrointestinal Bacterial Translocation

In humans and experimental studies, marked increases in core temperatures are associated with blood flow redistribution, which is characterized by cutaneous vasodilation that occurs at the expense of decreased intestinal blood flow [4,6]. This splanchnic vasoconstriction may cause ischemia and limit local vascular heat exchange, thereby promoting bowel tissue hyperthermia. Both intestinal ischemia and hyperthermia may promote oxidative stress that stimulates cytoskeletal relaxation, thus contributing to the opening of tight junctions and/or injuries to the epithelium [6,36]. These morphological and functional changes enhance intestinal permeability, thus facilitating the translocation of bacteria and endotoxins that are normally contained within the intestinal lumen, and subsequently worsening a systemic inflammatory response syndrome that may culminate in multiorgan system failure and death [6,37].

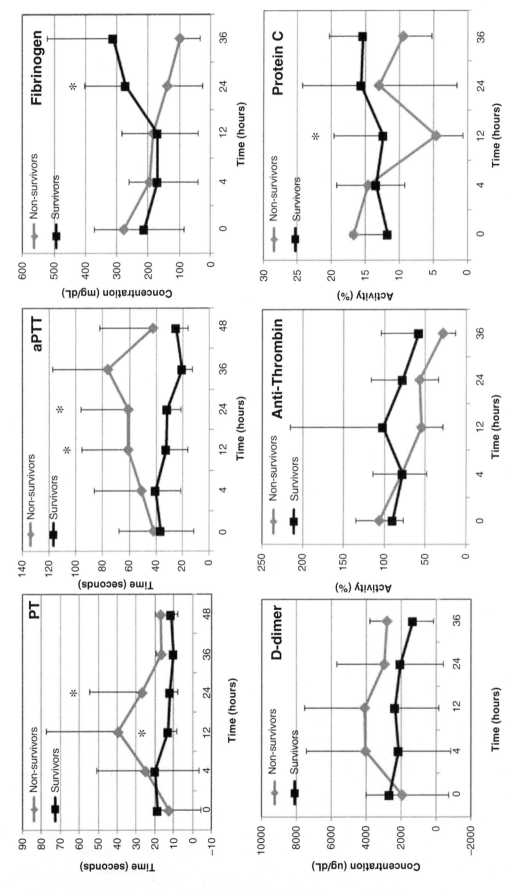

Figure 147.1 Trends in hemostatic parameters throughout hospitalization in 30 dogs with naturally occurring heat stroke. Mean values of survivors (n = 18, *black squares*) and non-survivors (n = 12, *gray diamonds*) are depicted. Whiskers represent the SD. * depicts significant difference between survivors and non-survivors. aPTT, activated partial thromboplastin time; PT, prothrombin time.

Gastrointestinal bacterial translocation has not been specifically documented in dogs with naturally occurring heat stroke but given the massive hemorrhagic diarrhea and hematemesis that rapidly ensue in dogs with severe heat stroke, it is reasonable to assume that it is a major contributing factor to SIRS, sepsis, and MODS that may occur in severe cases (see Chapter 159).

In summary, clinicopathological findings in canine heat stroke are mainly related to the primary thermal insult; however, secondary deterioration occurs due to dehydration, shock, and a poor perfusion to the tissues. Thus, early diagnosis and intervention are crucial to prevent further multiorgan dysfunction and exacerbation of coagulation abnormalities. Time lag from insult to admission (>1.5 h) was a crucial factor for survival in canines suffering from heat stroke [14].

Treatment Options

Whole-body cooling prior to admission is highly recommended. The literature suggests different cooling methods (e.g. cold enema, gastric lavage, ice baths); however, other successful and perhaps more practical methods use evaporative cooling via whole-body irrigation with tap water and placement of a fan facing the animal. Animals with thick undercoats may benefit from shaving prior to wetting. A cool environment with low humidity is also beneficial. Cooling with ice directly on body surfaces and/or peripheral blood vessels should be avoided as it may result in cutaneous vasoconstriction and decrease heat loss ability. During cooling, the patient's temperature should be monitored every 5–15 minutes to avoid hypothermia. Cooling should be terminated when body temperature has reached 39.5 °C (103 °F). Cooling does not result in suppression of the inflammatory response, but will prevent further cellular destruction.

Most canine heat stroke victims suffer from distributive shock, as described above. Although the absolute intravascular volume has not changed significantly, vasodilation and venous pooling of blood lead to a relative hypovolemia (see Chapters 153 and 155). As the animal is cooled, the vasomotor tone will return to normal. Therefore, judicious fluid therapy is warranted. An initial crystalloid dose of 10–20 mL/kg should be administered and perfusion parameters (HR, MM, CRT, pulse quality, blood pressure, mentation, urine output) continuously reassessed to help guide additional fluid therapy (see Chapter 167). When perfusion cannot be restored with crystalloids alone, synthetic colloids (hydroxyethyl starch solutions), vasopressor agents (dopamine, vasopressin, norepinephrine) and positive inotropes (dobutamine) should be considered (see Chapters 159 and 168).

Dextrose should be administered to hypoglycemic dogs as a single bolus (1 mL/kg of diluted 50% dextrose not to exceed a maximum of 10 mL) followed by a 2.5–5% dextrose CRI, with close monitoring of the glucose concentrations (see Chapter 111).

All dogs with heat stroke should be given oxygen therapy during triage (see Chapter 181). Animals with severe dyspnea or laryngeal edema should be intubated, although this can decrease self-cooling mechanisms inherent with panting. In the most severe cases, general anesthesia with 100% oxygen or positive pressure ventilation may be required.

Mannitol therapy may be beneficial in animals with cerebral edema causing intracranial hypertension, although it can also worsen cerebral hemorrhage, if present. Mannitol administration has beneficial effects on the kidney and will help restore urine output and flush tubular casts out in animals with AKI. A suggested treatment regime might be 0.5–1 g/kg of mannitol over 10–20 minutes after the initial fluid resuscitation, followed by 1–2 additional boluses over the ensuing 12 hours.

Benzodiazepines (diazepam, midazolam) are administered as a bolus followed by a CRI if the animal seizures (about 33% of the cases). Other causes for seizures such as hypoglycemia or metabolic and electrolyte imbalances should be ruled out (see Chapter 21).

Antimicrobial treatment is not warranted in mild to moderate cases. In severe cases, broad-spectrum antibiotics are indicated to treat sepsis due to presumed gastrointestinal bacterial translocation (see Chapter 200). A combination of antimicrobials effective against gram-positive, gram-negative, and anaerobic bacteria is recommended in severe cases, utilizing the "escalation–de-escalation" method. A combination of a potentiated penicillin and a fluoroquinolone or third-generation cephalosporin could be considered.

Gastric protectants such as H2 blockers (e.g. famotidine) or proton pump inhibitors (pantoprazole) should be administered to prevent further gastric damage (see Chapter 77). Antiemetics and promotility agents are essential for prevention of vomiting and consequent aspiration pneumonia.

If urine output remains insufficient despite adequate fluid replacement and mean arterial blood pressure is >60 mmHg, medical therapy with furosemide and/or mannitol should be considered (see Chapter 95). Overrhydration must be avoided in anuric/oliguric patients and fluid therapy adjusted based on urine output and intravascular volume status of the patient. Hemodialysis may be indicated in dogs with oligoanuria despite medical therapy, as well as those patients with severe overhydration, uremia or electrolyte derangements.

Treatment of the hemostatic abnormalities due to DIC is based on stabilization of the coagulation system with fresh frozen plasma and concurrent prevention of thrombosis with anticoagulants (see Chapters 62 and 71).

Hemofiltration has been suggested as an effective treatment modality in an experimental model of severe canine heat stroke, causing early clearance of accumulated serum cytokines, creatinine, and BUN [38]. Clinical data are unavailable at this time.

Monitoring

Serial monitoring of the patient's clinical and clinico-pathological parameters is essential for early identification of complications and appropriate intervention. Continuous monitoring of vital signs is warranted, including temperature, femoral pulse rate and quality and capillary refill time to assess perfusion, hydration and shock status. In addition, PCV/TS, serum glucose, coagulation profile (including TEG or ROTEM when available), CBC, lactate, blood gas (arterial or venous), arterial blood pressure, and urine output should be monitored. The mental status of the patient should be evaluated frequently and continuous ECG monitoring is recommended as arrhythmias may develop during the first 24 hours after the heat stroke occurs.

Prognosis

Mortality rates in dogs suffering from severe heat stroke are reportedly 40–50% [14,21,34,39]. Animals with heat-induced illness have a reportedly lower mortality rate (35%) [15]. At the authors' institution, mortality rates decreased to 40% and 43% in two recent studies [21,34] compared to 50% 10 years earlier [14]. However, larger scale studies are needed to determine if this trend is real.

Conclusion

In conclusion, heat stroke in dogs is a life-threatening condition, resulting in serious secondary complications such as DIC, AKI, and ARDS, and a high mortality rate despite appropriate treatment. Early admission and treatment along with whole-body cooling by the owners and caregivers are important for survival. The diagnosis of canine heat stroke should not rely exclusively on hyperthermia or the presence of neurological abnormalities upon admission, but should be based on the combination of the history, clinical signs, and laboratory results. Treatment and monitoring should be intensive and prolonged since complications can have a delayed onset and present serious risk factors for mortality (see Table 147.1).

References

1 Leon LR, Bouchama A. Heat stroke. *Compr Physiol* 2015;5(2):611–647.

2 Hemmelgarn C, Gannon K. Heat stroke: clinical signs, diagnosis, treatment, and prognosis. *Compend Contin Educ Vet* 2013;35(7):E3.

3 Hemmelgarn C, Gannon K. Heat stroke: thermoregulation, pathophysiology, and predisposing factors. *Compend Contin Educ Vet* 2013;35(7):E4.

4 Bouchama A, Knochel JP. Heat stroke. *N Engl J Med* 2002;346(25):1978–1988.

5 Epstein Y, Roberts WO. The pathopysiology of heat stroke: an integrative view of the final common pathway. *Scand J Med Sci Sports* 2011;21(6):742–748.

6 Hall DM, Buettner GR, Oberley LW, et al. Mechanisms of circulatory and intestinal barrier dysfunction during whole body hyperthermia. *Am J Physiol Heart Circ Physiol* 2001;280(2):H509–H521.

7 Leon LR, Helwig BG. Heat stroke: role of the systemic inflammatory response. *J Appl Physiol (1985)* 2010a;109(6):1980–1988.

8 Russell, JA. Management of sepsis. *N Engl J Med* 2006;355(16):1699–1713.

9 Leon LR, Helwig BG. Role of endotoxin and cytokines in the systemic inflammatory response to heat injury. *Front Biosci (Schol Ed)* 2010b;2:916–938.

10 Aroch I, Segev G, Loeb E, Bruchim Y. Peripheral nucleated red blood cells as a prognostic indicator in heat stroke in dogs. *J Vet Intern Med* 2009;23(3): 544–551.

11 Bouchama A, Roberts G, Al Mohanna F, et al. Inflammatory, hemostatic, and clinical changes in a baboon experimental model for heat stroke. *J Appl Physiol* 2005;98(2):697–705.

12 Bruchim Y, Loeb E, Saragusty J, Aroch I. Pathological findings in dogs with fatal heat stroke. *J Comp Pathol* 2009;140(2-3):97–104.

13 Argaud L, Ferry T, Le Q, et al. Short- and long-term outcomes of heat stroke following the 2003 heat wave in Lyon, France. *Arch Intern Med* 2007;167(20):2177–2183.

14 Bruchim Y, Klement E, Saragusty J, et al. Heat stroke in dogs: A retrospective study of 54 cases (1999–2004) and analysis of risk factors for death. *J Vet Intern Med* 2006;20(1):38–46.

15 Drobatz KJ, Macintire DK. Heat-induced illness in dogs: 42 cases (1976–1993). *J Am Vet Med Assoc* 1996;209(11):1894–1899.

16 Misset B, De Jonghe B, Bastuji-Garin S, et al. Mortality of patients with heat stroke admitted to intensive care units during the 2003 heat wave in France: a national

multiple-center risk-factor study. *Crit Care Med* 2006;34(4):1087–1092.

17 Bruchim Y, Aroch I, Eliav A, et al. Two years of combined high-intensity physical training and heat acclimatization affect lymphocyte and serum HSP70 in purebred military working dogs. *J Appl Physiol (1985)* 2014;117(2):112–118.

18 Horowitz M. Heat acclimation: Heat acclimation: phenotypic plasticity and cues to the underlaying molecular mechanism. *J Therm Biol* 2001;26:357–363.

19 Chung NK, Pin CH. Obesity and the occurrence of heat disorders. *Mil Med* 1996;161(12):739–742.

20 Horowitz M. From molecular and cellular to integrative heat defense during exposure to chronic heat. *Comp Biochem Physiol A Mol Integr Physiol* 2002;131(3): 475–483.

21 Bruchim Y, Segev G, Kelmer E, et al. Hospitalized dogs recovery from naturally occurring heat stroke; does serum heat shock protein 72 can provide prognostic biomarker? *Cell Stress Chaperones* 2016;21(1):123–130.

22 Dehbi M, Baturcam E, Eldali A, et al. Hsp-72, a candidate prognostic indicator of heat stroke. *Cell Stress Chaperones* 2010;15(5):593–603.

23 Mohanty D, Gomez J, Mustafa KY, Khogali M, Das KC. Pathophysiology of bleeding in heat stress: an experimental study in sheep. *Exp Hematol* 1997;25(7):615–619.

24 Alzeer AH, el-Hazmi MA, Warsy AS, Ansari ZA, Yrkendi MS. Serum enzymes in heat stroke: prognostic implication. *Clin Chem* 1997;43(7):1182–1187.

25 Borregaard L, Lyngsoe BK, Fenger-Eriksen C, Gronbaek H, Brandsborg B. [Acute liver failure following heat stroke after participating in a running event.] *Ugeskr Laeger* 2014;176(28):VO1130075.

26 Geng Y, Ma Q, Liu YN, et al. Heat stroke Induces liver injury via IL-1beta and HMGB1-induced pyroptosis. *J Hepatol* 2015;63(3):622–633.

27 Hadad E, Ben-Ari Z, Heled Y, et al. Liver transplantation in exertional heat stroke: a medical dilemma. *Intensive Care Med* 2004;30(7):1474–1478.

28 Kurowski J, Lin HC, Mohammad S, Krug S, Alonso EM. Exertional heat stroke in a young athlete resulting in acute liver failure. *J Pediatr Gastroenterol Nutr* 2016;63(4):e75–e76.

29 Krau SD. Heat-related illness: a hot topic in critical care. *Crit Care Nurs Clin North Am* 2013;25(2): 251–262.

30 Bouchama A, Bridey F, Hammami MM, et al. Activation of coagulation and fibrinolysis in heat stroke. *Thromb Haemost* 1996;76(6):909–915.

31 Diehl KA, Crawford E, Shinko PD, Tallman RD Jr, Oglesbee MJ. Alterations in hemostasis associated with hyperthermia in a canine model. *Am J Hematol* 2000;64(4): 262–270.

32 Bruchim Y, Kelmer E, Cohen A, Codner C, Segev G, Aroch I. Hemostatic abnormalities in dogs with naturally occurring heatstroke. *J Vet Emerg Crit Care* 2017;27(3):315–324.

33 Lin YF, Wang JY, Chou TC, Lin SH. Vasoactive mediators and renal haemodynamics in exertional heat stroke complicated by acute renal failure. *QJM* 2003;96(3):193–201.

34 Segev G, Daminet S, Meyer E, et al. Characterization of kidney damage using several renal biomarkers in dogs with naturally occurring heat stroke. *Vet J* 2015;206(2):231–235.

35 Oglesbee MJ, Alldinger S, Vasconcelos D, et al. Intrinsic thermal resistance of the canine brain. *Neuroscience* 2002;113(1):55–64.

36 Shapiro Y, Alkan M, Epstein Y, Newman F, Magazanik A. Increase in rat intestinal permeability to endotoxin during hyperthermia. *Eur J Appl Physiol Occup Physiol* 1986;55(4):410–412.

37 Soares AD, Costa KA, Wanner SP, et al. Dietary glutamine prevents the loss of intestinal barrier function and attenuates the increase in core body temperature induced by acute heat exposure. *Br J Nutr* 2014;112(10):1601–1610.

38 Chen GM, Lan YY, Wang CF, et al. Clearance of serum solutes by hemofiltration in dogs with severe heat stroke. *Scand J Trauma Resusc Emerg Med* 2014;22:49.

39 Teichmann S, Turkovic V, Dorfelt R. [Heat stroke in dogs in southern Germany. A retrospective study over a 5.5-year period]. *Tierarztl Prax Ausg K Kleintiere Heimtiere* 2014;42(4):213–222.

148

Cold Exposure

Karol A. Mathews, DVM, DVSc, DACVECC

Ontario Veterinary College, University of Guelph, Guelph, ON, Canada

Introduction

Cold exposure may result in accidental hypothermia, defined as an unintentional decrease in core temperature without preoptic and anterior hypothalamic nuclei disease [1,2]. The normal range for core temperature in dogs and cats is 37.5–39.5 °C (99.5–102.5 °F). Hypothermia is defined as a core body temperature 2 °C below normal in humans (35 °C) (95 °F) [3] which would correlate with a temperature below 36.0 °C (97 °F) in cats and dogs. Of importance is that, in the clinical setting, the rectal temperature is the initial mode of temperature assessment. Digital thermometers register to 32 °C (89.8 °F), making an accurate determination of degree of hypothermia difficult. In addition, the poor depth of measurement gives a lower reading compared to esophageal monitoring. This may continue through rewarming for up to an hour, during which time the rectal temperature may even drop by several degrees while the heart and esophageal temperatures are rising [4]. The electronic thermometers with probes approximately 10 Fr and 1 metre long (Sonatemp 400–700 Thermometer, Sheridan, Argyle, NY) record temperatures below 21 °C (69.8 °F) and can be placed intranasally into the esophagus or into the colon per rectum. It is recommended to cautiously place the rectal probe in at least 15 cm (10 http); however, this is patient size dependent. Infrared otic thermometers have inherent inconsistencies.

In addition to exposure to low environmental temperatures, other factors exacerbating the effects of cold exposure resulting in hypothermia are immersion in water [5], trauma, and exhaustion. Freezing injuries (frostbite) of the extremities are common injuries associated with cold exposure. Underlying conditions such as hypothyroidism, very young or very old age, cardiac disease or malnutrition may predispose animals to accidental hypothermia at a temperature higher than would occur in a healthy animal. Recreational drugs, ethylene glycol, and phenothiazines, as examples, can disrupt normal heat production and conservation by impairing perception of changes in ambient temperature, depressing mental status, and inhibiting the shivering response. These etiologies should be considered in any unexplained case of hypothermia.

Pathophysiology of Effects of Cold Exposure [1–3,6–10]

At temperatures 1–2 °C below normal, thermogenesis, through shivering and hypermetabolism, attempts to compensate for heat loss. Intense vasoconstriction in peripheral tissues results in acrocyanosis and cool extremities due to shunting of blood away from the cold body surface to help sustain core body temperature. With prolonged exposure, thermoregulation fails as heat production is unable to offset the rate of heat loss from the body surface; further reduction in core temperature then occurs, leading to progressive multiorgan dysfunction. The increased circulating catecholamines result in increased respiratory rate, minute ventilation and oxygen consumption, increased heart rate, cardiac output and mean arterial pressure and elevated levels of serum cortisol, lactate, glycerol, ketones, and glucose.

Respiratory compromise occurs via various mechanisms. After the initial tachypnea, central respiratory depression occurs at 2–5 °C below normal, leading to decreased respiratory rate and tidal volume. As core temperature approaches 25 °C (85 °F) or less, bronchiolar mucous plugs and atelectasis occur, increasing the risk of bronchitis and bronchopneumonia (see Chapter 37). Immersion injury/near drowning frequently results in pneumonia (see Chapter 40). Increased intracranial pressure may result in non-cardiogenic pulmonary edema. The compromised pulmonary gas exchange coupled with decreased perfusion to the tissues results in lactic acidosis, the significance of which increases with

Textbook of Small Animal Emergency Medicine, First Edition. Edited by Kenneth J. Drobatz, Kate Hopper, Elizabeth Rozanski and Deborah C. Silverstein.
© 2019 John Wiley & Sons, Inc. Published 2019 by John Wiley & Sons, Inc.
Companion Website: www.wiley.com/go/drobatz/textbook

decreasing temperature. Also, oxygen affinity for hemoglobin increases with low temperatures which further reduces oxygen delivery to the tissues.

Cardiovascular function decreases after the initial increase in arterial blood pressure and heart rate. Progressive hypothermia reduces cardiac output and mean arterial blood pressure as bradycardia, hypovolemia, and decreased ejection fraction occur.

Electrocardiogram changes related to body temperature can be seen. At approximately 32 °C (90 °F), the Osborn J wave may appear. The J waves are usually upright in aVL, aVF, in leads II and V6, at the junction of the QRS complex and ST segment. The size of these waves increases with temperature depression, but is unrelated to arterial pH. The waves are diagnostic but not prognostic or pathognomonic of hypothermia, as they are also associated with central nervous system lesions, focal cardiac ischemia, and sepsis. Atrial fibrillation may occur. Ventricular fibrillation (VF) and asystole may follow with core temperatures below 28 °C (83 °F) and 20 °C (68 ° F) respectively. ECG changes accompanying mild hypothermia include prolongation of the P-R, Q-T and QRS intervals, atrial ectopy, and T-wave inversion. Ventricular fibrillation may be triggered by mechanical irritation, such as placing central lines, but mere handling of the patient can precipitate VF. In general, caution is warranted when handling these patients and extremely gentle care is required when drying the wet patient.

Neurological abnormalities, both central and peripheral, are frequently present. Cerebral blood flow is reduced at temperatures 2–5 °C below normal, and patients may be uncoordinated, stuporous and eventually comatose as the temperature drops below 30 °C (86 °F). An increase in intracranial pressure may occur secondary to "cold edema," an osmotic gradient associated with changing serum glucose levels, ischemic injury, or head injury. In humans, hyperreflexia predominates from 35 °C (95 ° F) to 32.2 °C (90 ° F), and is followed by hyporeflexia. The plantar response remains flexor until 26 °C, when areflexia develops. The patellar reflex is usually the last reflex to disappear, and is the first to reappear during rewarming. From 30 °C (86 °F) to 26 °C (78.8 °F), both the contraction and relaxation phases of the reflexes are equally prolonged. Various traumatic injuries may also result in neurological abnormalities and true injury (spinal) cannot be assessed until the patient is rewarmed, unless obvious lesions are present.

Urinary output ranges from polyuria to anuria (see Chapter 95). Glomerular filtration rate (GFR) is enhanced as core temperature decreases below normal by 2–3 ° C, due to peripheral vasoconstriction, shunting of blood centrally, and increase in central blood volume. The resultant increase in GFR promotes withdrawal of antidiuretic hormone (ADH), leading to "cold diuresis." Cold-related impairment of renal enzymatic activity inhibits tubular

reabsorption of glucose, sodium, and water with loss of extremely dilute urine contributing further to dehydration. As hypothermia progresses, cardiac output drops despite activation of the RAAS. The resultant afferent and efferent renal arteriolar vasoconstriction reduces glomerular plasma flow and peritubular capillary pressure. Renal blood flow is depressed by 50% at 27–30 °C (80.6–86 °F) which decreases glomerular filtration rate.

Acute kidney injury, secondary to depressed renal blood flow and defective tubular activity, often develops in patients who have prolonged and profound hypothermia (see Chapter 94). Acute tubular necrosis may be observed prior to azotemia. Blood urea nitrogen (BUN) and creatinine are often elevated because of decreased nitrogenous waste clearance by the cold diuresis. Prior renal disease is a possibility. The BUN is a poor indicator of volume status because of ongoing fluid shifts. The SDMA (IDEXX), an assessment of GFR, is more accurate.

Testicular torsion may occur due to cremasteric contractions (see Chapter 126).

Splanchnic blood flow and gastrointestinal motility diminish as the core temperature approaches 34 °C (93 °F). Ileus develops when the temperature drops below 30 °C (86 °F). Gastric dilation in pediatrics, abdominal distension or rigidity, obstipation, and poor rectal tone are frequently present in humans. As vasoactive amines histamine and serotonin are released in response to vascular compromise, punctate erosions of the stomach, duodenum, ileum and colon, and pancreatitis have been reported to occur in humans and animals (Mathews, personal observations) (see Chapter 86). Severe hypothermia often induces a hemorrhagic pancreatitis as a consequence of depressed pancreatic perfusion. The liver is relatively resistant to the effects of cold injury but depletion of glycogen stores occurs early in hypothermia and a general decrease in metabolic function leads to decreased detoxification and conjugation activity and diminished lactate metabolism. This is an important point to consider when administering various medications and lactate-containing fluids.

Hematological, biochemical, and coagulation parameters are altered as hypothermia progresses. Initially, hypokalemia may be present but K^+ increases as temperature decreases. Hyperkalemia (>12 mmol/L) is a potential index of irreversibility (see Chapter 109). High lactic acid levels may predict a bad outcome. Alkalosis appears protective. In canine deep hypothermia studies, puppies and dogs with arterial pH reduced to, and maintained at, 7.4 had decreased cardiac performance and myocardial damage when compared to the control group, left uncorrected (alkalemic) pH >7.4. The control group had increased cerebral blood flow, normal cardiac indices and improved electrical stability of the heart [11]. The fibrillation threshold of dogs markedly decreased when arterial pH was held at 7.4 [11]. Isotonic dehydration increases the hematocrit and hemoglobin concentrations and total plasma solids. White blood cells and platelets may sequester within the spleen and perivascular tissue, causing leukopenia and thrombocytopenia. Disseminated intravascular coagulation may occur after prolonged hypothermia and hypoperfusion as a result of microvascular disruption, hemoconcentration, and activation of the clotting cascades (see Chapter 70).

Although coagulopathies occur in hypothermia, the clotting factor levels are normal. In a reported study of human trauma patients who developed lethal coagulopathies, the average temperature was 31.2 °C. High CPK levels may indicate rhabdomyolysis.

Gluconeogenesis occurs with depression of insulin release and an increased peripheral receptor resistance to insulin due to the stress-induced catecholamine release. Hyperglycemia that persists during rewarming signals the potential for diabetic ketoacidosis or hemorrhagic pancreatitis (see Chapter 112). Insulin is ineffective until well above 30 °C(86 °F), and should be withheld to avoid iatrogenic hypoglycemia after rewarming

Aspiration of gastric contents may occur after immersion/near drowning hypothermia or due to hypothermia itself [5]. Therefore, dyspnea may be present or develop upon rewarming.

Management [1–3,7–10]

Carefully place the patient on a warm surface. Noting all the above sequelae of hypothermia, management of hypothermic animals should include monitoring of all possible events.

Initially, establish the ABCs of resuscitation (see Chapter 2). Should cardiac arrest be suspected, ensure that the patient is arrested prior to commencing cardiopulmonary resuscitation as chest compression frequently causes VF. Due to severe vasoconstriction, it is often difficult to feel a pulse and weak myocardial contractions are barely, if at all, audible. Confirm myocardial wall motion with tFAST (see Chapter 182) [12]. A "flat ECG" may be due to asystole or just bad electrical conductance through cold skin or problems of adhesion of ECG electrodes. Sterile hypodermic needles should be placed through the gel portion of the electrodes which will improve adhesion and conduction, or place a 23–25 gauge hypodermic needle through the skin and attach the alligator clip to the needle. ECG monitoring may be difficult due to shivering (may look like VF). Oxygen administration may reduce the risk of VF during resuscitation (see Chapter 181). Should VF be diagnosed, note that the cold myocardium is relatively insensitive to DC shock defibrillation; however, administer three immediately and if no response,

administer a further three shocks after the patient has been rewarmed to 28–30 °C (83–86 °F) (see Chapter 150). The hypothermic heart is unresponsive to pacing and cardioactive drugs.

Medication to treat arrhythmias should not be given until body temperature is 30–32 °C (86–90.3 °F) as drugs are ineffective at temperatures below this. Atropine is ineffective for bradyarrhythmias at low temperatures. Rewarming alone will usually correct this rhythm and, frequently, atrial fibrillation [1,13]. Also, the heart generally cannot sustain rhythmic electrical function until this temperature is reached. Basic cardiopulmonary resuscitation should be performed, if cardiac arrest diagnosed, until the temperature is ≥32 °C (90.3 °F) when advanced cardiac life support (the use of medication) can be added if required. Administration of normal doses, and repeat doses of any medication, will lead to accumulation and be toxic to the patient when rewarmed. Patients may appear "dead" if the temperature is <28 °C (83 °F) but resuscitation should be attempted as occasional success has been recorded in individuals with temperatures <14 °C (57.2 °F). The American Heart Association recommendations are to rewarm patients to at least 35 °C (95 °F) before declaring futility and withdrawing support [14]. The saying "you're not dead until you're warm and dead" should be remembered.

Secondly, assess the cause and duration of hypothermia and institute appropriate therapy for the cause. Injuries associated with trauma, possible abusive elicit drug or alcohol administration, drowning or medical problems predisposing to exposure hypothermia should be identified. Following this, restoration of normothermia is the main objective.

Rewarming techniques depend on the degree of hypothermia, duration, and predisposing events. Blood should be collected for packed cell volume (PCV), total plasma solids (TS), blood urea nitrogen (BUN) or urea, creatinine, electrolytes, blood gases, glucose and ALT, prior to fluid administration. As even mild hypothermia causes a cold diuresis, all hypothermic animals should receive warmed intravascular fluid support; an alkalinizing solution, Plasma-lyte A, 148 or Normosol R, is recommended. Lactated Ringer's should be avoided in severe hypothermia as the liver may be unable to metabolize the lactate.

Fluids should be warmed to 50 °C (120 °F) when hung with a standard intravenous delivery set or to 42 °C (107.5 °F) when using 60 mL syringes, short tubing, and a syringe pump. The temperature of the fluid drops rapidly due to ambient room temperature, even when warmed, therefore slow delivery will reach room temperature at the IV catheter [15]. Placing the intravenous delivery line under a warm water bottle or heating blanket will maintain warm fluid temperature. Ensure the directly administered temperature is not higher than 42 °C (107.6 °F).

Hydration status should be assessed and fluid requirements calculated. It is advisable to administer fluids cautiously initially due to possible depressed cardiac function and intense peripheral vasoconstriction. Blood pressure measurements should be attempted. Where indicated, after rewarming, a urinary catheter should be placed to measure urine output. Constant assessment is required as the core temperature increases; fluid therapy can be altered based on blood pressure, urine production, PCV, TS, mentation, and tolerance of fluids delivered.

External rewarming is usually adequate for temperatures >32 °C (90.3 °F). This can be in an active or passive form. If the patient is wet, dry them gently with a towel to remove as much water as possible.

Passive rewarming is usually adequate for the mildly hypothermic animal ~ 34 °C (93.5 °F). Shivering is usually present at temperatures ≥35 °C (95 °F), but may be absent below this. Holding a small patient, covered with a blanket, close to your body is an efficient means of rewarming. For the larger patient, place them in a warm room wrapped in a blanket, where the animal can rewarm themselves via shivering and heat conservation. The head should also be covered. Ensure good coverage of the body and not just the limbs. With this method, the temperature can increase by 0.4–2 °C/h. A degree of peripheral vasoconstriction is maintained which minimizes the risk of both hypotension and the temperature afterdrop. Afterdrop refers to a drop in the core temperature as a result of sudden peripheral rewarming and vasodilation where the cold acidemic blood is returned to the core. Hypotension and potentially fatal dysrhythmias can result (especially notable in spinal cord transection where peripheral thermoregulation fails).

Active rewarming is required for patients with moderate to severe hypothermia and core temperatures below 34 °C (93.5 °F); this may include those which are hypoglycemic, hypothyroid, adrenal insufficient or have other disorders that limit endogenous thermogenesis, and patients with diabetic ketoacidosis or an unstable cardiovascular system. Active rewarming must be performed in any patient, whatever the degree of hypothermia, if initial passive rewarming methods fail to elevate body temperature. Warm water bottles (avoid contact to avoid thermal burns), heated blankets (Hot Dog warming blanket; Augustine Medical Incorporated, MN) or a warmed incubator for small animals can accomplish active external rewarming. Warming the ambient air and cage with hot water bottles will reduce heat loss. Fans should not be used as stationary air is less conducive to heat losses by radiation. However, forced air enclosed around the patient, has proved effective in core rewarming. Temperatures of 28.8 ± 2.5 °C increased by 2.4 ± 1.0 °C/h using the forced air system of disposable plastic and paper covers

and a heat source that directs warm air across the skin (Bair Hugger; Augustine Medical Incorporated, MN) in humans and dogs (Mathews, personal observation) who recovered rapidly and uneventfully. *Caution*: cutaneous burns may occur due to inability to move and the initial vasoconstriction blocks dissipation of heat from surface tissues. The temperature of external heat sources therefore should not exceed 45 °C (113 °F).

Afterdrop may develop with these heat sources, which may predispose to worsening of cardiac arrhythmias. Also, vasodilation associated with warming of the limbs may precipitate further hypotension. While it is recommended to limit the application of external heat to the trunk to minimize the afterdrop effect, where the limbs/feet are affected by frostbite, this and body rewarming is managed simultaneously [16]. Frostbite can result in severe injury/amputation which will frequently result in euthanasia, so frostbite must be treated immediately (see Frostbite below) (see Chapter 137). The warmed blood traversing the extensive AV network in the feet can be transferred into the body through the dilated AV shunt network, reducing afterdrop [17]. A soft padded bandage will reduce peripheral edema of the limbs.

The risk of circulatory collapse is determined primarily by the patient's degree of tolerance of intravenous fluids, the extent of hypothermia, and intensity of rewarming. If intolerance to fluids or colloids is demonstrated and ventricular function is impaired, a slow titration of dobutamine, starting at 1 µg/kg/min slowly increasing to effect and a maximum of 5 µg/kg/min until rewarmed, then a further increase, has been suggested.

Invasive internal rewarming is recommended for animals that have cardiac-arrested hypothermia, core temperatures <30 °C (<86 °F) or higher if cardiovascular function is unstable and where other forms of rewarming are unsuccessful. Core rewarming minimizes afterdrop and potential deterioration, and hastens normalization of body temperature. In addition to using warm intravenous fluids, peritoneal dialysis with 10–20 mL/kg of 43 °C (109.5 °F) 0.9% saline or 1.5% dextrose dialysis fluid (similar to lactated Ringer's) is suggested [18]. Administer fluid with caution so as not to jeopardize ventilation. Do not use Plasma-lyte or Normosol as these appear painful when placed into the abdomen. An exchange every 30 minutes is recommended. The dialysate must be kept at ~43 °C (109.4 °F) or core rewarming may not occur or a temperature drop may be encountered. Avoid dialysis in patients with suspected abdominal trauma and/or where surgery was recently performed.

The author has used warm (43 °C, 109.5 °F) saline irrigation of the urinary bladder via a urinary catheter and found this to be very effective and less invasive than lavage of the peritoneal cavities. Gastric or colonic lavage with 43 °C (109.4 °F) 0.9% saline has also been suggested but there is a potential for regurgitation/aspiration, alterations in electrolytes, and inability to obtain accurate rectal or esophageal temperature.

Heating inspiratory oxygen is also recommended in warming the patient. This may be accomplished by applying a heat and moisture exchange device (Intersurgical Inc., Liverpool, NY) between the oxygen tubing and the endotracheal tube or face mask.

There is no definitive recommendation on the rate of rewarming. Some recommend that the rate should not exceed 1.5–2 °C/h to avoid development of pulmonary/cerebral edema. However, a more rapid technique may be desirable to facilitate treatment of associated medical problems. Quickly increasing the temperature to 30 °C (86 °F) may reduce the risk of VF and cardiovascular collapse, improve myocardial performance, and minimize acidosis and hypoxia associated with slower methods. Unless severe, do not correct the acidosis until after corrective fluid administration as this tends to normalize with fluid administration. Frequent measurement is required to monitor the trend. Acidosis causes a shift of the oxyhemoglobin dissociation curve to the right which will counter the shift to the left produced by hypothermia. However, if pH remains <7.3 after appropriate fluid administration, judicious correction is advised. Canine studies indicate that a pH >7.4 was cardioprotective during rewarming of extreme hypothermia [11]. It is recommended not to temperature correct for blood gas measurements [1,19].

Pain must be managed in patients whose temperature was <34 °C (93 °F). Human patients frequently complain of total body muscle aches, which can be quite severe for several days. This, in part, accounts for the depression observed post resuscitation. In both cats and dogs, slowly titrate fentanyl 3–5 µg/kg IV to effect, to avoid overdose, then continue the effective dose/hour, or titrate methadone or morphine 0.2–0.5 mg/kg to effect and continue the effective dose over 4 hours, or use hydromorphone 0.03–0.3 mg/kg administered in a similar way as methadone or morphine, once rewarmed.

Opioids may prevent the shivering reflex but where pain is evident, opioid analgesia is warranted during the active external rewarming process [6]. Avoid non-steroidal anti-inflammatory analgesics (NSAIAs) initially.

Continuous monitoring is essential as the rewarmed patient is at risk for developing multiple complications, including those associated with reduced splanchnic perfusion. Frostbite of peripheral tissues (ears, tail, distal limbs) may also be noted as rewarming progresses.

While the above are guidelines, not all hypothermic animals will present as described nor will they necessarily require the rewarming technique described. How-ever, initial presentation and trending will dictate the appropriate therapeutic modality to pursue.

Frostbite

Pathophysiology [1,2,16,20]

Frostbite is the freezing, or effect of freezing, of a part of the body, the extent of which is dependent on time of exposure and degree of hypothermia. Intracellular water crystallization, temperature-induced protein changes, and membrane damage result in cellular injury.

Extracellular water crystallizes, decreasing the interstitial water in the liquid phase with subsequent increased osmolarity. In response, water moves out of cells, affecting intracellular electrolyte concentrations and modifying cellular protein structure. In addition, diversion of oxygen and nutrients away from the periphery due to vasoconstriction and hypoperfusion predisposes to cell death. The associated vasculitis, exacerbated by hemoconcentration, hyperviscosity, platelet sequestration/dysfunction and cold-induced inhibition of coagulation cascade enzymes, predisposes to thromboembolism [20]. This may also cause bleeding, which becomes evident on thawing of the tissues. As tissues thaw, marked edema occurs because of melting of water crystals, cellular damage, loss of endothelial integrity, and thrombosis.

Over a few days, the degree of necrosis +/- gangrene will be established. Local production of prostaglandins and thromboxanes enhances the degree of injury. In addition to limbs and feet, dogs and cats may also have frostbite of ears and nose. Dogs may also acquire freezing injury due to contact of parts of the body (penis, tongue) to ice or frozen metal which will accelerate the freezing process. Coccygeal muscle injury (limber tail) has been reported in working dogs when exposed to cold weather. The tail carriage is affected to a varying degree, and the tail appears flaccid (see Chapter 202) [21].

Superficial frostbite results when the epidermis and dermis are affected; deep frostbite occurs when the underlying structures freeze. After initial therapy, a further assessment is made. A first degree manifests as erythema after warming; second degree leads to blistering; third degree is skin necrosis and fourth degree devitalization of the whole part (gangrene). Third- and fourth-degree injuries are susceptible to infection and tissue loss. However, the severity of the injury cannot be fully assessed for several days. Superficial frostbite in people has been described as white, without blanching or evidence of capillary filling after mild pressure and feels somewhat soft or rubbery to palpation. Deep frostbite, which involves all tissues including bone, produces a hard or wooden-like extremity.

Management

Frostbitten tissues should be rapidly warmed. Immerse the affected part in water at 40–42 °C (104–108 °F) for at least 20 minutes or until thawing is complete. Dry heat should not be used. Never rub or massage the tissues. For mild injury, application of soft, dry bandages to the injured part is required to protect the area from self-inflicted, or other, trauma and reduce edema. Cage rest is required to reduce injury. Analgesics *must* be given as this injury is extremely painful. Where there are no contraindications in a fluid-resuscitated patient, a COX-2 selective/preferential NSAIA may be administered and could be therapeutic due to the anti-inflammatory and antithromboxane effect.

In third- and fourth-degree frostbite, it is recommended that blisters containing clear or milky fluid should be aspirated/debrided and covered in aloe vera q8h, which also has an antiprostaglandin, antithromboxane effect.

Padding should be put between the patient's digits, if affected; the limbs/feet should be wrapped in a loose, protective dressing, then splinted and elevated to reduce reperfusion edema. Hemorrhagic blisters should be left intact to prevent desiccation of the underlying tissue; however, aspiration, leaving the skin intact, is recommended if reduction is necessary due to location. Topical antiseptics may help prevent infection of necrotic tissue or ruptured blisters.

Prophylactic antibiotics are not recommended. Culture of an infected wound and antibiogram should be performed to select the appropriate antibiotic, when indicated. A superficial infection will respond to topical administration of raw honey with daily rinsing and bandaging until cleared (usually 3 days) [22]. Surgical management should be delayed until spontaneous amputation of necrotic tissue has occurred and is complete. Definitive surgical management is based on the individual injury. Heparin or low-molecular weight dextrans have not proven beneficial.

References

1 Danzl DF, Pozos R, Hamlet M. Accidental hypothermia. In: *Management of Wilderness and Environmental Emergencies*, 2nd edn (eds Auerbach P, Geehr E). Mosby, St Louis, 1989, pp. 35–76.

2 Danzl DF, Pozos RS. Accidental hypothermia. *N Engl J Med* 1994;331:1756–1760.

3 Kerpainen RR, Brunette DD. The evaluation and management of accidental hypothermia. *Respir Care* 2004;49(2):192–205.

4 Giesbrecht GG. Cold stress, near drowning and accidental hypothermia: a review. *Aviat Space Environ Med* 2000;71:733–752.

5 Hooper AJ, Hockings LE. Drowning and immersion injury. *Anesth Intens Care Med* 2011; 12:399–402.

6 Hanania NA, Zimmerman JL. Accidental hypothermia. *Crit Care Clin* 1999;15(2):235–249.

7 Dhupa N. Hypothermia in dogs and cats. *Comp Contin Educ Pract Vet* 1995;7:265–271.

8 Todd JM. Hypothermia. In: *Small Animal Critical Care Medicine*, 2nd edn (eds Silverstein DC, Hopper K. Elsevier, St Louis, 2015, pp. 789–795.

9 Ahn AH. Approach to the hypothermic patient. In: *Kirk's Current Veterinary Therapy XII* (ed. Bonagura J). Saunders, Philadelphia, 1995, pp. 157–161.

10 http://crashingpatient.com/

11 Becker H, Vinten-Johansen, Buckberg GD, et al. Myocardial damage caused by keeping pH 7.40 during systemic deep hypothermia. *Thorac Cardiovasc Surg* 1981;82:810–820.

12 Boysen SR, Lisciandro GR. The use of ultrasound for dogs and cats in the emergency room: AFAST and TFAST. *Vet Clin North Am Small Anim Pract* 2013;43(4):773–797.

13 Campbell SA, Day TK. Spontaneous resolution of hypothermia-induced atrial fibrillation in a dog. *J Vet Emerg Critical Care* 2004;14(4):293–298.

14 Emergency Cardiac Care Committee and Subcommittees, American Heart Association. Guidelines for cardiopulmonary resuscitation and emergency cardiac care. *Part IV. Special resuscitation situations. JAMA* 1992;268:2242–2250.

15 Handrigan MT, Wright RO, Becker BM, Linakis JG, Jay GD. Factors and methodology in achieving ideal delivery temperatures for intravenous and lavage fluid in hypothermia. *Am J Emerg Med* 1997;15: 350–353.

16 Biem J, Koehncke N, Classen D, et al. Out of the cold: management of hypothermia and frostbite. *Can Med Assoc J* 2003;168(3):305–311.

17 Cabell LW, Perkowski SZ, Gregor T, Smith GK. The effects of active peripheral skin warming on perioperative hypothermia in dogs. *Vet Surg* 1997;26:79–85.

18 Bersenas AMEB. A clinical review of peritoneal dialysis. *J Vet Emerg and Crit Care* 2011;21(6):605–617.

19 http://crashingpatient.com/intensive-care/alpha-stat-vs-ph-stat.htm/

20 Rohrer MJ, Natale AM. Effect of hypothermia on the coagulation cascade. *Crit Care Med* 1992;20: 1402–1405.

21 Steiss J, Braund K, Wright J. Coccygeal muscle injury in English pointers (limber tail). *J Vet Intern Med* 1999;13:540–548.

22 Mathews KA, Binnington AG. Management of wounds using honey. *Compend Cont Educ Pract Vet* 2002;24(1):53–60.

149

Electrical and Lightning Injuries

F.A. (Tony) Mann, DVM, MS, DACVS, DACVECC

University of Missouri, Columbia, MO, USA

Introduction

Electrocution may occur by contact with high-voltage or low-voltage electrical sources or by a lightning strike. It is generally accepted that chewing through household electrical cords is the most common cause of electrocution in dogs and cats. From 1968 through 2014, a database compiling patient encounter data from several veterinary institutions recorded that 318 dogs and 98 cats sustained electrical injuries. (The Veterinary Medical Databases (VMDB) are currently housed at the University of Missouri, Columbia, Missouri (https://vmdb.org). The VMDB does not make any implicit or implied opinion on the subject of this chapter.) Of these, 54 dogs and 26 cats had chewed electrical cords, and four dogs and no cats had been struck by lightning. It is likely that many of the unspecified electrocutions were low-voltage injuries from chewing household electrical cords.

Electrical Injury

Mechanisms of Electrical Injury

The mechanisms of electrical injury are related to the direct effects of the electrical current and the transformation of electrical energy to heat. The electrical current may disrupt electrophysiological activity, leading to muscle spasms, cardiac arrhythmias, loss of consciousness, and respiratory arrest [1–3]. Direct cellular injury may occur through the process of electroporation, which is the development of momentary holes in cellular membranes induced by electrical shock. The holes allow passage of macromolecules across membranes, which causes osmotic damage to cells [4].

As electrical current is transformed into heat, intracellular and extracellular fluids may become superheated, which results in coagulation of tissue proteins,

thrombosis of small vessels, and degenerative changes in small arterial walls [1,2,4]. Ultimately, the result is necrosis of the superheated tissues, as well as tissues that become ischemic from the vascular consequences. Direct thermal injury may also occur from arcing of a current that leaves the electrical source, crosses an air gap, and strikes tissue [1].

The severity of electrical injury varies depending on the electrical resistance of the part of the body that is struck, the nature of the current (alternating versus direct), and the intensity of the current (amperage) [1,4]. Less energy will be transferred to areas of the body that have high resistance to electrical flow. Dry skin has high resistance so less energy will be transferred in dry skin than in wet skin. Wet skin and moist mucous membranes have low electrical resistance so one can expect high flow of electricity in these tissues and a propensity for maximal tissue damage.

Alternating current (AC) tends to cause more severe injury than direct current (DC) at the same amperage. Higher exposure may occur with AC than with DC because the former elicits muscular contractions that prevent the victim from releasing the power source. For this reason, the exposure time is typically longer with AC than with DC. Direct current electricity does not usually cause muscular tetany.

Given the same resistance, high-voltage electricity can be expected to cause more damage than low-voltage electricity. One might expect more injury from 240 volt outlets used for large household appliances than from standard 120 volt wall outlets. However, current (measured in amperes) is a function of voltage divided by resistance (Ohm's Law; $I = V/R$) so the magnitude of the current depends on the affected tissue as discussed previously [1,4].

Predisposition to Electrical Injury

Young dogs and cats are the most common victims of electrical injury because they are more likely to chew

Textbook of Small Animal Emergency Medicine, First Edition. Edited by Kenneth J. Drobatz, Kate Hopper, Elizabeth Rozanski and Deborah C. Silverstein.
© 2019 John Wiley & Sons, Inc. Published 2019 by John Wiley & Sons, Inc.
Companion Website: www.wiley.com/go/drobatz/textbook

on electrical cords than are older animals. The average age of dogs with electrical injury has been reported as 3.5 months (range, 5 weeks to 1.5 years; n = 29); the range of ages of seven cats with electrical injury was reported to be 2 months to 2 years [1]. A database compiled from several veterinary institutions revealed that, from 1968 through 2014, the most common age range for electrical injuries was 2–12 months; 213 (67%) of 318 dogs and 48 (49%) of 98 cats that had electrical injuries and 38 (70%) of 54 dogs and 12 (46%) of 26 cats that sustained electrical injury from chewing electrical cords were 2–12 months old. A seasonal predisposition is generally accepted, but there is some difference of opinion as to what time of year most injuries are seen. Holiday seasons characterized by use of decorative lights (Halloween, Christmas) certainly pose electrical risks [4], but one study reported that 79% of canine cases occurred during the 6 months from March through August [1].

Clinical Findings

Surface burns may be noted at the point of contact with the electrical source. The thermal injury may be superficial, characterized by mild hyperemia, or may manifest as a severe full-thickness burn. Burns from chewing electrical cords have been noted on the lips, gums, tongue (Figure 149.1) and palate [1–6]. Some oral cavity electrical shocks produce enough trauma to cause dental fractures and oronasal fistulae [6].

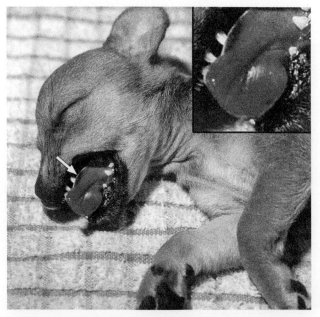

Figure 149.1 Puppy brought in dead on arrival after chewing an electrical cord. Note the burn evident on the left lateral tongue margin (*arrow*). Reproduced with permission of Elsevier.

Cardiac arrhythmias may be present, the severity of which depends on the intensity of the electrical current. Sudden death from electrical shock is likely due to ventricular fibrillation caused by low-voltage current, as with most household exposures [4–7]. High-voltage exposure may cause asystole [4]. Animals that survive the shock may experience ventricular arrhythmias, but ventricular tachycardia progressing to ventricular fibrillation is unlikely in survivors of the initial electrocution event [8] (see Chapter 53).

Respiratory distress is a common clinical feature noted in the form of tachypnea, cyanosis, orthopnea, coughing, or apnea (see Chapter 39). Respiratory arrest from tetanic contractions of respiratory muscles occurs during contact with the electrical source, but breathing typically resumes when the victim is separated from the source of electricity [9].

Causes of respiratory distress include facial or nasopharyngeal edema, diaphragmatic tetany, and neurogenic pulmonary edema. Non-cardiogenic pulmonary edema is typically considered to be a result of increased capillary permeability [10,11]. However, neurogenic pulmonary edema is a form of non-cardiogenic pulmonary edema with multiple possible etiologies, including both hydrostatic and permeability edema secondary to massive sympathetic outflow (see Chapter 39). The typical radiographic pattern is alveolar infiltration of the caudo-dorsal quadrants (Figure 149.2).

Respiratory distress is less severe with pulmonary edema induced by electrical cord shock than with other causes of non-cardiogenic pulmonary edema. Likewise, there is less radiographic involvement than with other causes of non-cardiogenic pulmonary edema [10], and there is often radiographic evidence of resolving pulmonary infiltrates within 18–24 hours (Figures 149.2 and 149.3) [1].

Neurological injury as a result of direct CNS stimulation may be noted immediately upon electrical contact. Stiffening of the animal has been noted by people who have witnessed a dog or cat biting an electrical cord [3]. The victim usually loses consciousness [3]. There may be focal muscle tremors or seizures, sometimes accompanied by defecation or vomiting [3,4]. Extensor rigidity and death may occur rather rapidly. Tetanic limb contraction has been noted after survival of high-voltage electrical shock [12]. Non-ambulatory tetraparesis due to focal cervical myelopathy has been reported in a dog immediately after chewing an electrical cord [13]. The acute neurological manifestations of electrocution are thought to be due to electrically induced neural activity rather than electroporation and resultant tissue hypoxia, although hypoxia from excess energy consumption could play a role [14]. Delayed neurological manifestations are thought to result from electroporation and free radical mechanisms [15].

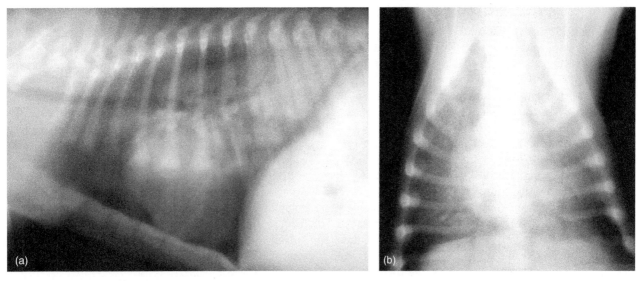

Figure 149.2 Lateral (a) and ventrodorsal (b) thoracic radiographs of a puppy that experienced severe electrical injury by chewing on an electrical cord. Note the prominent infiltration of the caudodorsal lung fields. Reproduced with permission of Elsevier.

Gastrointestinal (GI) abnormalities may result from electrical interference with motility. Abdominal radiographs or ultrasonography may show GI gas patterns characteristic of ileus [4].

Ocular manifestations of electrical injury (cataracts) are usually later findings, noted several months after the episode. Cataracts are commonly seen in human beings following near-fatal electrical injury and lightning strike and have been reported in a dog that was electrocuted by chewing an electrical cord [16].

Secondary Effects of Electrical Injury

Although complete blood count and serum chemistry results are usually within normal limits, tissue hypoxia from electrically induced ischemia and pulmonary edema may lead to necrosis of the affected tissues and subsequent hematological changes and additional organ damage. Tissue necrosis may lead to hyperkalemia, myoglobinemia, myoglobinuria, hemoglobinemia, and hemoglobinuria [4]. Hyperkalemia may also result from

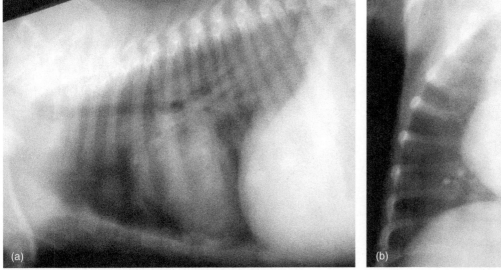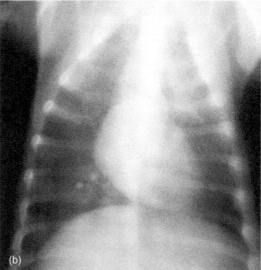

Figure 149.3 Lateral (a) and ventrodorsal (b) thoracic radiographs of the puppy in Figure 149.2 taken approximately 24 hours after the radiographs in Figure 149.2. Note the significant progress in resolution of the pulmonary infiltration. Reproduced with permission of Elsevier.

excessive muscular activity during electrical shock; this muscular activity also contributes to acidemia and hyperlactatemia [17]. Hypoproteinemia may ensue in patients with severe burns [4].

Treatment of Electrical Injury

Initial treatment at the scene of the exposure includes precautions to prevent inadvertent injury to rescuers. The source of electricity should be turned off before the victim is touched. Preferably, the electricity should be turned off at the electrical panel but alternatively, the offending electrical cord may be unplugged carefully from the outlet. Once the victim is removed from the electrical source, immediate medical attention should be sought regardless of the victim's apparent condition. Victims in cardiopulmonary arrest require cardiopulmonary resuscitation (see Chapter 150). Better results might be expected in a hospital environment, but life-saving techniques on the scene may be required if there is to be any hope of success.

Treatment of animals that survive the initial electrical insult is tailored to the clinical effects. Animals in shock are treated with intravenous fluids to expand intravascular volume because the mechanism of shock is likely a relative hypovolemia (see Chapters 39 and 152). However, because there may be a cardiogenic component to the shock from arrhythmias and subsequent decreased stroke volume, and because neurogenic pulmonary edema may develop quickly, judicious fluid therapy is indicated. Fluids that typically are given in low volumes (e.g. hypertonic saline, synthetic colloids) may be beneficial (see Chapters 167 and 168).

Respiratory distress requires prompt attention. Airway obstruction from edematous oropharyngeal tissues may require temporary tracheostomy tube placement. Partial obstructions may be managed conservatively with sedation and, if not contraindicated, anti-inflammatory drugs and diuretics. Supplemental oxygen is recommended (see Chapter 181), but if the respiratory distress is due entirely to obstruction, relief of the obstruction should return oxygenation to normal.

Oxygen supplementation should continue until it is ascertained that neurogenic pulmonary edema has not developed or has resolved (see Chapter 181). Positive pressure ventilation may be required if the patient is hypoxic and does not respond appropriately to supplemental oxygen (see Chapter 188).

Burned tissues are treated conservatively using standard wound treatment principles (see Chapter 166). Reconstructive surgery, if indicated, is performed after recovery from the electrical shock when it is determined that the patient is a stable anesthetic candidate and the tissues are healthy enough to expect good surgical results.

Ventricular arrhythmias are managed by administering antiarrhythmic agents and by reversing the underlying pathophysiological derangements (see Chapter 53). Seizures are controlled with anticonvulsant therapy (see Chapter 21). Gastrointestinal abnormalities are best managed with early nutritional support, via an appropriate feeding tube if necessary.

Pain management is necessary because burn wounds are painful and because there is likely muscle soreness from excessive activity during the electrical stimulation (see Chapter 190). Initially, opioids are preferred, but non-steroidal anti-inflammatory drugs may be used when GI integrity and renal and hepatic function are presumed to be normal.

Prognosis

The prognosis for victims that survive the initial shock episode is generally good, as long as the clinical effects are reversible. Respiratory abnormalities are the sequela most likely to alter prognosis. Most cases of electrically induced non-cardiogenic pulmonary edema resolve quickly, but one study reported a fatality rate of 38.5% [1]. Some animals will require follow-up surgery to treat residual effects of burns. Recovering victims should be monitored for potential long-term effects. Owners should be instructed to observe for cataract development, which could occur several months after recovery.

Delayed consequences of electrical injury in people (pain, peripheral neurological manifestations, neuropsychological disturbances, and cataract formation) have reportedly taken up to 5 years or longer to surface in some cases [18]. Incidence of late-onset consequences in veterinary species is unknown.

Lightning Injury

Lightning injury is more likely to occur in large animal species [19–22] than in dogs and cats because of their greater outdoor exposure. However, companion animals, especially dogs, share outdoor activities with human beings and, therefore, may occasionally be exposed. A carefully studied lightning strike at a scene where two adults and 26 girls were camping also affected seven dogs [23]. Fatal injuries occurred in four of the girls and four of the dogs.

Of the surviving dogs, the smallest one, a Maltese-poodle mix, escaped injury. One of the remaining surviving dogs sustained burns and the other suffered damage to an eye that subsequently became opaque. Because the deceased dogs were farther from the struck tent pole than surviving people, it was speculated that dogs might be more susceptible to the effects of lightning injury than are human beings [23]. It is possible that small dogs, as in the camping site incident, are less susceptible to lightning injury than larger dogs [23]. Among cattle, adults are more likely to be struck by lightning than are calves [20]. Electrical injury from lightning strike has been reported to cause visual impairment in cattle as a result of cerebrocortical necrosis [24] and renal failure in people due to myoglobinuria from muscle damage [25]. These consequences have not been reported in dogs and cats, but are nonetheless possible.

The pathophysiology of lightning injury is similar to that of other electrical injuries, except for the mechanism by which the electricity reaches the victim and the potential for injury from mechanical energy. There are five possible mechanisms by which lightning can deliver electrical energy to a victim: direct lightning strike, direct strike of an object that the victim is touching (referred to as contact injury), side flash (splash) from a struck object, step voltages (ground potential) produced by current flowing through the soil beneath, and an upward streamer that does not connect or complete a full lightning strike [26–30]. With the latter mechanism, injury is caused by the upward streamer of charge that is induced from an object on the ground as a lightning leader of flash approaches the ground from a thundercloud [23,26–30].

In addition to electrical and thermal injury, a sixth method of lightning-induced injury, barotrauma, may occur [30]. In this mechanism, internal injury is caused by the massive pressure differential created by the blast. The blast effect occurs when rapid air movement results from superheated air that is then cooled. The resultant mechanical energy imparted to the lightning victim can result in various forms of physical injury. People are often thrown to the ground and report muscle pain. Lumbosacral fracture with resultant spinal cord injury was the only lesion identified in three pigs in an outdoor pen that was struck by lightning [21]. Spinal fracture due to lightning strike has also been noted in pond fish [31], and the blast effect of lightning strike has been reported to cause vestibular injury in horses and human beings [32]. Although such injuries have not been reported in dogs and cats, the occurrence of mechanical energy effects similar to those reported in other species should not be surprising.

References

1 Kolata RJ, Burrows CF. The clinical features of injury by chewing electrical cords in dogs and cats. *J Am Anim Hosp Assoc* 1981;17:219–222.

2 Marks SL. Electrocution. *Proc North Am Vet Conf* 2004;18:176–177.

3 Morgan RV. Environmental injuries. In: *Veterinary Pediatrics: Dogs and Cats from Birth to Six Months of Age* (ed. Hoskins J). Saunders, Philadelphia, 1990, pp. 505–516.

4 Presley RH, Macintire DK. Electrocution and electrical cord injury. *Stand Care Emerg Crit Care Med* 2005;7(9):7–11.

5 Decosne-Junot C, Junot S. Electrocuted cats and dogs: diagnosis and treatment. *A Hora Veterinária* 2004;24:65–68.

6 Legendre LFJ. Management and long term effects of electrocution in a cat's mouth. *J Vet Dent* 1993;10:6–8.

7 Geddes LA, Bourland JD, Ford G. The mechanism underlying sudden death from electric shock. *Med Instrum* 1986;20(6):303–315.

8 Kroll MW, Fish RM, Lakkireddy D, et al. Essentials of low-power electrocution: established and speculated mechanisms. Presented at the Annual International Conference of the IEEE Engineering in Medicine and Biology Society, 2012, pp. 5734–5740.

9 Bradford A, O'Regan RG. The effects of low-voltage electric shock on respiration in the anaesthetized cat. *J Exp Physiol* 1985;70:115–127.

10 Drobatz KJ, Saunders M, Pugh CR, Hendricks JC. Noncardiogenic pulmonary edema in dogs and cats: 26 cases (1987–1993). *J Am Vet Med Assoc* 1995;206(11):1732–1736.

11 Haldane S, Marks SL, Raffe M. Noncardiogenic pulmonary edema. *Stand Care Emerg Crit Care Med* 2003;5(7):1–5.

12 Ridgway RL. High-voltage electric shock in a cat. *Vet Med Small Anim Clin* 1975;70(3):31.

13 Ros C, de la Fuente C, Pumarola M, Anor S. Spinal cord injury secondary to electrocution in a dog. *J Small Anim Pract* 2015; doi 10.1111/jsap.12325: 1–3.

14 McCreery DB, Agnew WF, Bullara LA, Yuen TGH. Partial pressure of oxygen in brain and peripheral nerve during damaging electrical stimulation. *J Biomed Eng* 1990;12:309–315.

15 Reisner AD. Possible mechanisms for delayed neurological damage in lightning and electrical injury. *Brain Injury* 2013;27:565–569.

16 Brightman AH, Brogdon JD, Helper LC, Everds N. Electric cataracts in the canine: a case report. *J Am Anim Hosp Assoc* 1984;20:895–898.

17 Bradford A, O'Regan RG. Acidaemia and hyperkalemia following low-voltage electric shock in the anaesthetized cat. *Q J Exp Physiol* 1985;70:101–113.

18 Wesner ML, Hickie J. Long-term sequelae of electrical injury. *Can Fam Physician* 2013;59:935–939.

19 Williams MA. Lightning strike in horses. *Compend Contin Educ Pract Vet* 2000;22(9):860–867.

20 Tartera P, Schelcher F. Lightning strike in cattle. *Point Vétérinaire* 2001;32:48–51.

21 Van Alstine WG, Widmer WR. Lightning injury in an outdoor swine herd. *J Vet Diagn Invest* 2003;15: 289–291.

22 Vanneste E, Weyens P, Poelman DR, et al. Lightning related fatalities in livestock: veterinary expertise and the added value of lightning location data. *Vet J* 2015;203:103–108.

23 Carte AE, Anderson RB, Cooper MA. A large group of children struck by lightning. *Ann Emerg Med* 2002;39:665–670.

24 Boevé MH, Huijben R, Grinwis G, Djajadiningrat-Laanen SC. Visual impairment after suspected lightning strike in a herd of Holstein-Friesian cattle. *Vet Rec* 2004;154(13):402–404.

25 Okafur UV. Lightning injuries and acute renal failure: a review. *Ren Fail* 2005;27(2):129–134.

26 Anderson RB. Does a fifth mechanism exist for explain lightning injuries? *IEEE Eng Med Biol Mag* 2001;20:105–113.

27 Cooper MA. A fifth mechanism of lightning injury. *Acad Emerg Med* 2002;9(2):172–174.

28 Cooper MA, Holle RL, Andrews C. Distribution of lightning injury mechanisms. Proceedings of the 20th International Lightning Detection Conference and 2nd International Lightning Meteorology Conference, Tucson, Arizona, April 24, 2008, pp. 1–4.

29 Gomes C. Lightning safety of animals. *Int J Biometeorol* 2012;56(6):1011–1023.

30 Thomson EM, Howard TM. Lightning injuries in sports and recreation. *Curr Sports Med Rep* 2013;12(2): 120–124.

31 Barlow AM. "Broken backs" in koi carp (Cyprinus carpio) following lightning strike. *Vet Rec* 1993;133(20):503.

32 Bedenice D, Hoffman AM, Parrott B, McDonnel J. Vestibular signs associated with suspected lightning strike in two horses. *Vet Rec* 2001;149(17):519–522.

Section 4

Trauma and Resuscitation

A. Cardiopulmonary Resuscitation

150

Cardiopulmonary Resuscitation in the Emergency Room

Daniel J. Fletcher, PhD, DVM, DACVECC[1] and Manuel Boller, DMV, MTR, DACVECC[2]

[1] *Cornell University College of Veterinary Medicine, Ithaca, NY, USA*
[2] *Melbourne Veterinary School, University of Melbourne, Werribee, Victoria, Australia*

Recognition of Cardiopulmonary Arrest

Cardiopulmonary arrest (CPA) should be ruled out in any unresponsive patient presenting on emergency or being found collapsed while being treated in the emergency room. The Reassessment Campaign on Veterinary Resuscitation (RECOVER) guidelines recommend the use of the rapid airway-breathing (AB) assessment, which should be completed in no more than 10–15 seconds on triage examination [1–7].

Airway Assessment

The airway is visually inspected by opening the mouth and pulling out the tongue to examine the entire oral cavity for evidence of foreign objects or pathology causing airway obstruction. Suction or careful manual extraction is used to remove any fluid or foreign objects present in the upper airway. If the patient responds during the manipulation, the exam should be halted immediately, as CPA has been ruled out and the clinician should move on to a primary survey (see Chapter 2).

Breathing Assessment

The breathing assessment is focused on identifying apnea and hence a diagnosis of CPA. Breathing may be assessed by identification of a chest rise or feeling for air movement through the nares.

Diagnosis of CPA

Due to evidence of a high rate of false-positive assessments of the presence of a pulse, evaluation of the circulation is no longer recommended [8,9]. Unresponsive, apneic patients should be presumed to be in CPA and cardiopulmonary resuscitation (CPR) should be initiated immediately. Figure 150.1 shows the RECOVER

CPR algorithm, which summarizes the approach to the two aspects of CPR: Basic Life Support (BLS in blue) and Advanced Life Support (ALS in green).

Basic Life Support

Basic Life Support aims to restore oxygenation, ventilation, and blood flow to tissues using chest compressions and positive pressure ventilation. Numerous studies have documented that delays and prolonged pauses in BLS lead to lower rates of return of spontaneous circulation (ROSC) and decreased survival to discharge [10,11].

Chest Compressions

Once CPA is diagnosed, chest compressions must be started immediately. They can be done most effectively with the patient in right or left lateral recumbency in most cases [12]. Deep compressions, one-third to one-half the chest width, are delivered at a rate of 100–120 per minute, and full elastic recoil is allowed between compressions. Uninterrupted 2-minute compression cycles should be done because it takes 1 minute of continuous compressions to reach a stable arterial blood pressure [13]. After each cycle, a new compressor rotates in to reduce fatigue and maintain compression quality.

Larger breed dogs with chests that are approximately as wide as they are deep (round-chested conformations) likely benefit most from compressions over the highest point on the thorax with the patient in lateral recumbency, which will maximally employ the thoracic pump approach, dependent on increasing overall intrathoracic pressure (Figure 150.2a). In large dogs with chests that are deeper than wide (keel-chested dogs), the cardiac pump theory should be employed, with chest compressions delivered directly over the ventricles (the third–fifth

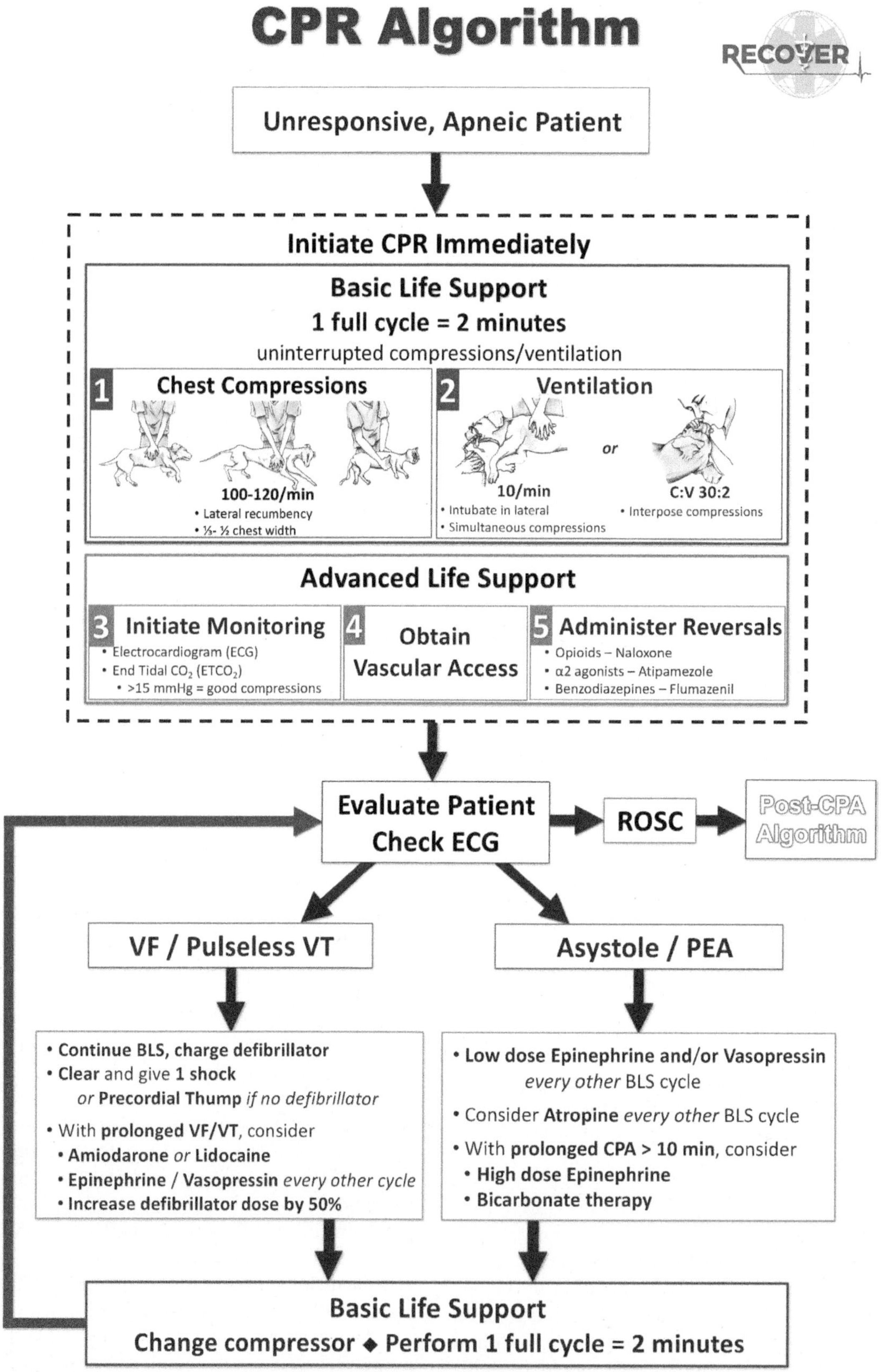

CPR Algorithm

RECOVER

Unresponsive, Apneic Patient

Initiate CPR Immediately

Basic Life Support
1 full cycle = 2 minutes
uninterrupted compressions/ventilation

1 Chest Compressions

100-120/min
- Lateral recumbency
- ⅓- ½ chest width

2 Ventilation

or

10/min
- Intubate in lateral
- Simultaneous compressions

C:V 30:2
- Interpose compressions

Advanced Life Support

3 Initiate Monitoring
- Electrocardiogram (ECG)
- End Tidal CO₂ (ETCO₂)
  - >15 mmHg = good compressions

4 Obtain Vascular Access

5 Administer Reversals
- Opioids – Naloxone
- α2 agonists – Atipamezole
- Benzodiazepines – Flumazenil

Evaluate Patient Check ECG → **ROSC** → *Post-CPA Algorithm*

VF / Pulseless VT

- **Continue BLS, charge defibrillator**
- **Clear** and give **1 shock**
  or **Precordial Thump** *if no defibrillator*
- With **prolonged VF/VT**, consider
  - **Amiodarone** or **Lidocaine**
  - **Epinephrine / Vasopressin** *every other cycle*
  - **Increase defibrillator dose by 50%**

Asystole / PEA

- **Low dose Epinephrine and/or Vasopressin**
  every other BLS cycle
- Consider **Atropine** *every other* BLS cycle
- With **prolonged CPA > 10 min**, consider
  - **High dose Epinephrine**
  - **Bicarbonate therapy**

Basic Life Support
Change compressor ◆ Perform 1 full cycle = 2 minutes

Figure 150.1 RECOVER CPR algorithm. Reprinted with permission from Fletcher et al. [7]. Reproduced with permission of John Wiley & Sons, Ltd.

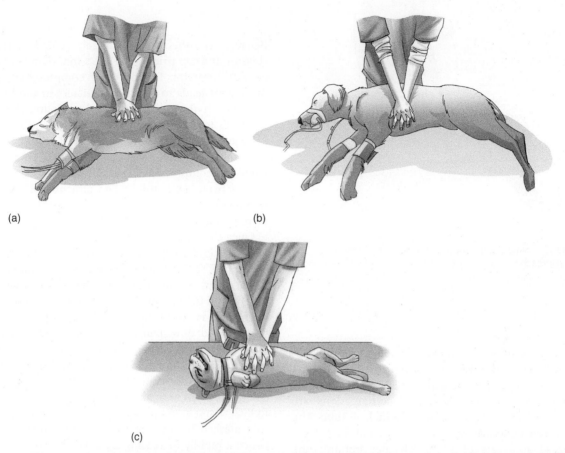

(a)

(b)

(c)

Figure 150.2 The approach to chest compressions in medium- to large-breed dogs. (a) The thoracic pump approach in round-chested dogs. (b) The cardiac pump approach in keel-chested dogs. (c) Sternal compressions in dorsal recumbency in flat-chested dogs.

intercostal space) (Figure 150.2b). In dogs with chests that are wider than they are deep (flat-chested dogs such as English bulldogs), compressions directly over the sternum with the dog in dorsal recumbency may be optimal (Figure 150.2c). Regardless of the chest shape of larger dogs, it is important to lock the elbows and interlace the fingers of both hands, with one hand on top of the other and the shoulders directly above the hands at all times. This compression posture maximally employs the core abdominal muscles rather than the arms, reducing rescuer fatigue (Figure 150.3).

For small patients with narrow chests, a one-handed technique with the thumb on one side of the chest directly over the heart and the other fingers on the opposite side may help reduce the potential to overcompress the heart to greater than one-half its width (Figure 150.4).

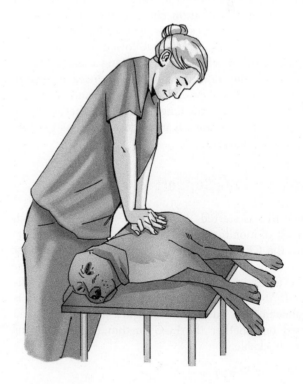

Figure 150.3 Rescuer posture for chest compressions in large and medium-sized dogs, with shoulders directly above hands, elbows locked, and compressions achieved by bending at the waist and engaging the core muscles.

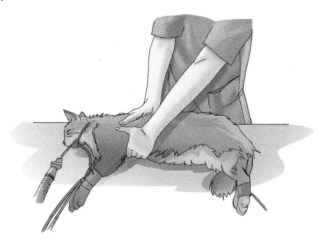

Figure 150.4 Single-handed compressions using the cardiac pump approach in cats and small dogs.

Ventilation

Ventilation should be started as soon as possible in dogs and cats with CPA. Whenever possible, patients should be intubated immediately in lateral recumbency (or dorsal recumbency if sternal compressions are being delivered) with a cuffed endotracheal tube. The tube is secured to prevent dislodgment and the patient ventilated at a rate of 10 breaths per minute (one breath every 6 seconds). If intubation equipment is not immediately available, mouth-to-snout ventilation can be used until intubation supplies are available. For non-intubated ventilation, chest compressions must be paused while breaths are delivered, so BLS should consist of 30 chest compressions followed by a brief pause to deliver two quick breaths by making a seal over both nares with the mouth, extending the neck to ensure that the snout is aligned with the spine and observing the chest to ensure the lungs inflate. Another round of 30 chest compressions is initiated as soon as the two breaths are delivered.

Advanced Life Support

Once BLS is started, ALS therapies can begin, which consist of monitoring and drug and defibrillation therapy. The CPR algorithm in Figure 150.1 lists the first three steps of ALS: initiating monitoring, obtaining vascular access, and administering reversal agents if indicated. At the end of the first cycle of BLS, the ECG is evaluated, and additional therapies are administered based on whether the ECG rhythm is shockable or non-shockable.

Initiating ALS

Because ALS therapies are largely guided by the ECG rhythm, the top priority for ALS initiation is attaching an ECG monitor. During chest compressions, patient movement leads to electrical artifacts in the ECG that preclude rhythm identification, so it is imperative that the ECG leads be attached before the end of the first 2-minute cycle of BLS to ensure that the ECG can be analyzed during the brief pause in chest compressions while the compressors are rotating. Only non-flammable electrode gel is used when attaching ECG leads to minimize the risk of fire should electrical defibrillation be required.

Once the ECG leads are attached, the next priority is end-tidal carbon dioxide ($ETCO_2$) monitoring. Unlike the ECG, $ETCO_2$ monitors are highly resistant to motion artifact, and because the CO_2 exhaled with each breath is delivered to the lungs by blood from the tissues, when ventilation is consistent, the $ETCO_2$ is proportional to tissue blood flow. During CPR, an $ETCO_2$ of at least 15 mmHg suggests adequate tissue blood flow to limit tissue ischemia, and an $ETCO_2$ above this target during CPR has been associated with increased survival to discharge in small animal patients [14]. In addition, upon ROSC, tissue blood flow increases dramatically, leading to a marked increase in CO_2 delivery to the lung and hence a rapidly increasing $ETCO_2$. Therefore, a sudden dramatic increase in $ETCO_2$ during CPR (often to values in excess of 45–50 mmHg) is a sign of ROSC, and corroboration of this finding via pulse palpation or auscultation of the heart is indicated.

Once monitoring devices have been attached to the patient, the next ALS priority is securing vascular access. If an intravenous catheter is already in place, its patency is tested with a saline flush. If vascular access has not yet been secured, a peripheral catheter as close to the heart as possible (most commonly a cephalic catheter) should be placed as quickly as possible. Because of poor venous return during CPR, veins are often difficult to see even if occluded, and if a vein is not obvious on visual inspection, a cutdown procedure should be used to obtain vascular access. A large incision may be made parallel to or directly over the location of the vessel after tenting the skin above it to prevent laceration, and the vein isolated from the subcutaneous tissues using blunt dissection with a hemostat. After placing tension on the vessel using the hemostat, a catheter is introduced into the vein and secured with suture. In puppies and kittens, intraosseous (IO) catheterization with an 18 or 20 gauge needle can often be done quickly. If a spinal needle is available, it will be less likely to become plugged with bone than a regular needle. The authors prefer the use of the femur for this procedure during CPR because it is most easily accessible without interfering with chest compressions. IO drill devices also facilitate very rapid vascular access in adult small animal patients.

Finally, in any patients that have received sedative drugs prior to CPA, reversal agents are administered as soon as possible. Because of slow drug metabolism in patients with poor perfusion, these drugs should be administered even if it has been several hours since the sedative was given. Figure 150.5 is the RECOVER drug and dosing chart, which lists the doses for the common reversal agents used in small animal medicine as well as dosing regimens for other ALS drugs. Naloxone may be used to reverse opioids, flumazenil for benzodiazepines, and atipamezole (or yohimbine) for alpha-2 agonists.

Interpreting the ECG

At the end of each 2-minute cycle of BLS, chest compressions are paused briefly as a new compressor rotates in. During this pause, every member of the team should look at the ECG monitor and assess the rhythm. The team leader should call out the rhythm diagnosis and ask all team members to weigh in on the diagnosis. If there is disagreement about the rhythm diagnosis, chest compressions are resumed and the team members in disagreement should discuss their perspectives on the diagnosis. Ultimately, based on input from the team, the team leader will make a final decision on the rhythm diagnosis. ECG interpretation is important during CPR because it determines the best ALS therapies.

CPR Emergency Drugs and Doses

Weight (kg)		2.5	5	10	15	20	25	30	35	40	45	50
Weight (lb)		5	10	20	30	40	50	60	70	80	90	100
DRUG	DOSE	ml	ml	ml	ml	ml	ml	ml	ml	ml	ml	ml
Epi Low (1:1000; 1mg/ml) every other BLS cycle x3	0.01 mg/kg	0.03	0.05	0.1	0.15	0.2	0.25	0.3	0.35	0.4	0.45	0.5
Epi High (1:1000; 1 mg/ml) for prolonged CPR	0.1 mg/kg	0.25	0.5	1	1.5	2	2.5	3	3.5	4	4.5	5
Vasopressin (20 U/ml)	0.8 U/kg	0.1	0.2	0.4	0.6	0.8	1	1.2	1.4	1.6	1.8	2
Atropine (0.54 mg/ml)	0.04 mg/kg	0.2	0.4	0.8	1.1	1.5	1.9	2.2	2.6	3	3.3	3.7
Amiodarone (50 mg/ml)	5 mg/kg	0.25	0.5	1	1.5	2	2.5	3	3.5	4	4.5	5
Lidocaine (20 mg/ml)	2 mg/kg	0.25	0.5	1	1.5	2	2.5	3	3.5	4	4.5	5
Naloxone (0.4 mg/ml)	0.04 mg/kg	0.25	0.5	1	1.5	2	2.5	3	3.5	4	4.5	5
Flumazenil (0.1 mg/ml)	0.01 mg/kg	0.25	0.5	1	1.5	2	2.5	3	3.5	4	4.5	5
Atipamezole (5 mg/ml)	100 µg/kg	0.06	0.1	0.2	0.3	0.4	0.5	0.6	0.7	0.8	0.9	1
External Defib (J)	4-6 J/kg	10	20	40	60	80	100	120	140	160	180	200
Internal Defib (J)	0.5-1 J/kg	2	3	5	8	10	15	15	20	20	20	25
External Defib (J)	2-4 J/kg	5	10	20	30	40	50	60	70	80	90	100
Internal Defib (J)	0.2-0.4 J/kg	1	2	2	3	4	5	6	7	8	9	10

Row categories (left margin): Arrest (Epi Low through Atropine); Anti-Arrhyth (Amiodarone, Lidocaine); Reversal (Naloxone, Flumazenil, Atipamezole); Defib Monophasic (first External/Internal Defib); Defib Biphasic (second External/Internal Defib).

Figure 150.5 CPR drug and dosing chart.

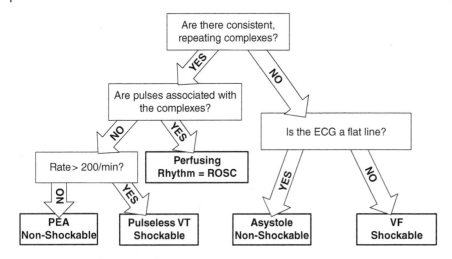

Figure 150.6 ECG algorithm for differentiating shockable, non-shockable, and perfusing rhythms during CPR.

After each cycle of BLS, the ECG rhythm is characterized as one of the following: ROSC, a non-shockable rhythm (the most common arrest rhythms in small animals), or a shockable rhythm. Figure 150.6 demonstrates a simple algorithm for characterizing the ECG rhythm during CPR. First, determine if the ECG contains consistent, repeating complexes. If it does not, determine if the ECG is a flat line, which would indicate asystole, a non-shockable rhythm. If it instead consists of apparently random activity on the baseline, this is most likely ventricular fibrillation (VF), a shockable rhythm. If the ECG does contain consistent, repeating complexes, feel for pulses. If some complexes are associated with pulses, the patient has achieved ROSC. If there are no pulses, the rate is evaluated. If it is less than 200 per minute, the most likely diagnosis is pulseless electrical activity (PEA), a non-shockable rhythm. If the rate is greater than 200 per minute, this is most likely pulseless ventricular tachycardia (pulseless VT), a shockable arrest rhythm.

Non-Shockable Arrest Rhythms

Figure 150.1 summarizes ALS therapies recommended for non-shockable arrest rhythms (asystole and PEA). Because cardiac output during external CPR is approximately 30% of normal, maintenance of adequate perfusion to the core organs is critical. Therefore, therapy targeted at peripheral vasoconstriction and redirection of blood flow to the core organs is recommended. Options include low-dose epinephrine (0.01 mg/kg) and vasopressin (0.8 U/kg). These drugs may be administered IV, IO, or intratracheally (IT) if vascular access has not yet been secured. Vagolytic therapy (atropine 0.04 mg/kg IV, IO or IT) may also be considered for routine use, and may confer additional benefit in patients arresting due to high vagal tone (e.g. bradyarrhythmias due to gastrointestinal, respiratory, and ocular disease). Both

vasopressor and vagolytic drugs are repeated every other cycle of BLS (i.e. every 4 minutes) during CPR.

High-dose epinephrine (0.1 mg/kg) should only be used in cases of prolonged CPA (greater than 10 minutes) where the rescuers are considering stopping CPR because of a lack of response. Although it has been associated with a higher rate of ROSC than low-dose epinephrine, it leads to a decreased rate of survival to discharge [15]. For patients with acute, reversible causes of CPA, further delay beyond 10 minutes before considering high-dose epinephrine is likely warranted. Sodium bicarbonate therapy (1 mEq/kg IV or IO, but not IT) may also be considered for patients with prolonged CPA, but ideally should only be administered after confirming the presence of severe metabolic acidosis on blood gas analysis.

Shockable Arrest Rhythms

The only effective therapy for shockable rhythms is electrical defibrillation. Dosing depends on the type of defibrillator (summarized in Figure 150.5). All personnel should be trained in the safe use of the electrical defibrillator.

The defibrillator paddles are placed on opposite sides of the chest directly over the heart with the patient in dorsal recumbency. The person delivering the shock should shout a warning to all other personnel and ensure that no one is touching the patient or the table before discharging the defibrillator. The goal is to stop the uncoordinated electrical activity of the ventricular myocardial cells, allowing the normal pacemakers in the sinus node to take over. Non-shockable arrest rhythms should never be shocked, as this will only lead to myocardial injury and reduced likelihood of achieving ROSC.

If an electrical defibrillator is not available, a precordial thump (a firm blow with the heel of the hand delivered directly over the heart) may be attempted. Unfortunately, this has extremely low efficacy, and should never be used if electrical defibrillation is available [16].

Defibrillation is repeated after each 2-minute cycle of BLS until a non-shockable rhythm or ROSC is achieved. Defibrillator doses may be increased by approximately 50% after each shock up to a maximum dose of 10 J/kg.

For patients with prolonged CPA (greater than 10 minutes) due to a shockable rhythm, antiarrhythmic medications (amiodarone 5 mg/kg or lidocaine 2 mg/kg slow IV or IO) may be considered as adjunctive therapy to defibrillation. Studies using monophasic defibrillators demonstrated potential deleterious effects of lidocaine on electrical defibrillation efficacy, but this phenomenon has not been observed with biphasic defibrillators [17]. In addition, vasopressors as described for non-shockable rhythms may be considered for patients with prolonged CPA due to shockable rhythms.

Prognosis

Dogs and cats with perianesthetic CPA had greater survival to discharge (approaching 50%) than the overall CPA patient population (6–7%) [14]. When considering initiating CPR, it is important to differentiate patients with CPA due to acute reversible conditions, who likely have a fair prognosis, from those with progressive, irreversible diseases leading to death. By applying the evidence-based guidelines summarized in this chapter, it is likely that many patients with acute, reversible conditions can survive to discharge if the CPA is identified rapidly and CPR is initiated immediately.

References

1 Boller M, Fletcher DJ. RECOVER evidence and knowledge gap analysis on veterinary CPR. Part 1: Evidence analysis and consensus process: collaborative path toward small animal CPR guidelines. *J Vet Emerg Crit Care* 2012;22 Suppl 1:S4–S12.

2 McMichael M, Herring J, Fletcher DJ, Boller M. RECOVER evidence and knowledge gap analysis on veterinary CPR. Part 2: Preparedness and prevention. *J Vet Emerg Crit Care* 2012;22 Suppl 1:S13–S25.

3 Hopper K, Epstein SE, Fletcher DJ, Boller M. RECOVER evidence and knowledge gap analysis on veterinary CPR. Part 3: Basic life support. *J Vet Emerg Crit Care* 2012;22 Suppl 1:S26–S43.

4 Rozanski E, Rush JE, Buckley GJ, et al. RECOVER evidence and knowledge gap analysis on veterinary CPR. Part 4: Advanced life support. *J Vet Emerg Crit Care* 2012;22 Suppl 1:S44–S64.

5 Brainard BM, Boller M, Fletcher DJ. RECOVER evidence and knowledge gap analysis on veterinary CPR. Part 5: Monitoring. *J Vet Emerg Crit Care* 2012;22 Suppl 1:S65–S84.

6 Smarick SD, Haskins SC, Boller M, Fletcher DJ. RECOVER evidence and knowledge gap analysis on veterinary CPR. Part 6: Post-cardiac arrest care. *J Vet Emerg Crit Care* 2012;22 Suppl 1:S85–S101.

7 Fletcher DJ, Boller M, Brainard BM, et al. RECOVER evidence and knowledge gap analysis on veterinary CPR. Part 7: Clinical guidelines. *J Vet Emerg Crit Care* 2012;22 Suppl 1:S102–S131.

8 Eberle B, Dick WF, Schneider T, et al. Checking the carotid pulse check: diagnostic accuracy of first responders in patients with and without a pulse. *Resuscitation* 1996;33(2):107–116.

9 Dick WF, Eberle B, Wisser G, Schneider T. The carotid pulse check revisited: what if there is no pulse? *Crit Care Med* 2000;28(11 Suppl):N183–N185.

10 Christenson J, Andrusiek D, Everson-Stewart S, et al. Chest compression fraction determines survival in patients with out-of-hospital ventricular fibrillation. *Circulation* 2009;120(13):1241–1247.

11 Kitamura T, Iwami T, Kawamura T, et al. Time-dependent effectiveness of chest compression-only and conventional cardiopulmonary resuscitation for out-of-hospital cardiac arrest of cardiac origin. *Resuscitation* 2011;82(1):3–9.

12 Maier GW, Tyson GS, Olsen CO, et al. The physiology of external cardiac massage: high-impulse cardiopulmonary resuscitation. *Circulation* 1984;70(1):86–101.

13 Kern KB, Hilwig RW, Berg R, Ewy G. Efficacy of chest compression-only BLS CPR in the presence of an occluded airway. *Resuscitation* 1998;39(3):179–188.

14 Hofmeister EH, Brainard BM, Egger CM, Kang S. Prognostic indicators for dogs and cats with cardiopulmonary arrest treated by cardiopulmonary cerebral resuscitation at a university teaching hospital. *J Am Vet Med Assoc* 2009;235(1):50–57.

15 Vandycke C, Martens P. High dose versus standard dose epinephrine in cardiac arrest – a meta-analysis. *Resuscitation* 2000;45(3):161–166.

16 Nehme Z, Andrew E, Bernard S, Smith K. Treatment of monitored out-of-hospital ventricular fibrillation and pulseless ventricular tachycardia utilising the precordial thump. *Resuscitation* 2013;84(12):1691–1696.

17 Sims JJ, Miller AW, Ujhelyi MR. Lidocaine increases the proarrhythmic effects of monophasic but not biphasic shocks. *J Cardiovasc Electrophysiol* 2001;12(12):1363–1368.

151

Small Animal Cardiopulmonary Resuscitation Initiatives

Manuel Boller, DMV, MTR, DACVECC[1] and Daniel J. Fletcher, PhD, DVM, DACVECC[2]

[1]*Melbourne Veterinary School, University of Melbourne, Werribee, Victoria, Australia*
[2]*Cornell University College of Veterinary Medicine, Ithaca, NY, USA*

Strategically Advancing the Field of Veterinary CPR

Cardiopulmonary arrest (CPA) in dogs and cats is a highly lethal process and constitutes a significant problem in small animal practice across all clinical settings. Proficiency in conducting CPR is considered an important skill for veterinarians and especially emergency and critical care clinicians, but CPR is a source of stress and anxiety for resuscitation team members [1,2]. A perception of futility may prevail when considering the more recently published survival-discharge rates of 6% percent in dogs and 3–6% percent in cats [3,4]. However, evidence suggests that survival rates are not just dependent on patient factors, but can be improved through systems changes such as improving CPA treatment recommendations and CPR training programs. A recent Japanese study indicates that a marked increase in rates of return of spontaneous circulation (ROSC) and survival to discharge can occur after implementing staff training according to RECOVER CPR guidelines [5]. In human medicine, training initiatives and improved CPR guidelines were associated with increased survival rates of sudden cardiac arrest victims [6,7]. The survival rates of sudden cardiac arrest patients with ventricular fibrillation also varied substantially with the geographic region of arrest, and ranged from 7.7% (Alabama) to 39.9% (Seattle) [8].

Taken together, these data indicate that the survival rate can be significantly improved by preparedness initiatives. The Reassessment Campaign on Veterinary Resuscitation (RECOVER) set out to implement a systematic review of knowledge to generate treatment recommendations for dogs and cats with CPA in 2011, and published the first evidence-based small animal CPR guidelines in 2012 [9].

RECOVER, founded by the American College of Veterinary Emergency and Critical Care (ACVECC) and the Veterinary Emergency and Critical Care Society (VECCS), is evolving into an international organization with the intent to encourage and facilitate veterinary resuscitation research around the globe. An important milestone to that end is recently published consensus guidelines on standardized reporting of small animal CPR, as they present fundamental instruments to conduct collaborative CPR research and establish CPR registries [10]. A strategy that consists of:

- continuing reassessment of knowledge relevant to veterinary CPR
- development and dissemination of evidence-based guidelines
- identification of knowledge gaps
- conducting studies to address these gaps, and
- measuring shifts in the epidemiology of CPR in response to treatment recommendations and training programs

may lead to sustained progress in survival rates in veterinary patients (Figure 151.1).

Evidence-Based Consensus Small Animal CPR Guidelines

RECOVER brought together almost 100 collaborators, predominantly specialists in veterinary ECC and anesthesia, who volunteered to systematically review the literature relevant to small animal CPR and to devise treatment guidelines [9,11]. RECOVER partnered with the International Liaison Committee on Resuscitation (ILCOR), which conducts evidence analysis and provides CPR treatment recommendations in people [12]. Consequently, RECOVER utilized a process similar to ILCOR

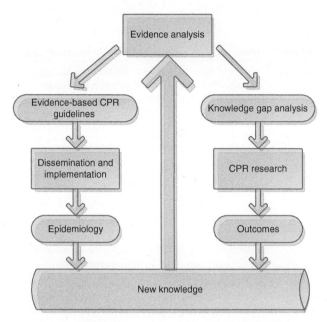

Figure 151.1 Veterinary resuscitation science strategy. Evidence analysis leads to CPR practice guidelines and a knowledge gap analysis. Through passive (publications) and active (training initiatives) dissemination steps, a change in the CPR practice in veterinary hospitals is evoked with an effect on the epidemiology of CPA (i.e. ROSC, survival). This will provide important new knowledge on the effect of the applied guidelines and of different implementation strategies and training initiatives. Knowledge gaps will be addressed by conducting specific observational studies, interventional trials, and/or by analysis of registry data. The outcomes that result from these studies will provide new understanding on how to better treat CPA in dogs and cats. This new evidence will in turn influence revised guidelines and change the list of knowledge gaps.

to systematically review the literature and to summarize findings in a process aimed at minimizing reviewer bias [11].

This process was initiated by identifying key clinical questions in five domains of CPR: preparedness/prevention, Basic Life Support (BLS), Advanced Life Support (ALS), monitoring, and post-cardiac arrest (PCA) care. Each question was posed in PICO format (Patient – Intervention – Comparator – Outcome). The results of all studies relevant to a specific question were categorized in an evidence grid according to level of evidence, study quality, and direction of the effect (e.g. benefit or harm). Based on the number and quality of studies and the risk:benefit ratio of the examined interventions, each treatment recommendation was assigned a level (Level A: High-quality evidence; Level C: Consensus/expert opinion) and class (Class I: Benefit >>> risk; Class III: Risk > benefit) designation. This approach allowed clear recommendations to be made while explicitly stating the strength of the evidence.

RECOVER led to 101 treatment recommendations (see Chapter 150) that were published open-access and have been widely disseminated with translations into several languages [9,13]. Revised versions of the RECOVER guidelines will be published as new relevant knowledge emerges. In addition, future guidelines will target additional issues that could not be addressed during the RECOVER 2012 process due to a lack of reviewers.

Knowledge Gaps

The RECOVER evidence analysis process exposed a large list of knowledge gaps, which lowered the level of recommendation for many of the guidelines (Table 151.1). The identified knowledge gaps serve as a list of prioritized research objectives that should be addressed by the veterinary resuscitation science community. More clinical veterinary CPR studies are needed to improve the quality of evidence available. While RECOVER guidelines are based on the best available evidence, the vast majority of this evidence consisted of research conducted in species other than dogs and cats. To the authors' knowledge, there was only one clinical veterinary randomized controlled trial published in the English literature by March 2018 [14].

Clinical veterinary CPR research is challenging. The unforeseen nature of CPA makes enrollment of cases difficult and the immediacy of CPR renders acquisition of informed consent impossible. The high mortality rate makes investigation of the most relevant outcomes, such as survival to hospital discharge and functional recovery, exceedingly challenging. The general lack of funding available for veterinary research leads to underpowered studies. Lack of technology to measure quality of CPR in dogs and cats further limits high-quality studies. Finally, a common nomenclature and consistent definitions of key data elements of veterinary CPR are necessary for multicenter studies and meta-analyses across studies.

Some of the above roadblocks are not readily overcome in the short term. Others, such as the development of a uniform set of terms surrounding veterinary CPR, are easier to address.

Glossary and Guidelines For Standardized Reporting

A common CPR terminology is of central importance for clear communication and collaborative studies. Unambiguous operational definitions for terminology used in CPR research studies and registries are a prerequisite for valid data collection.

Table 151.1 Select knowledge gaps across all five domains of CPR.

Preparedness and prevention	Basic Life Support	Advanced Life Support	Monitoring	Post-cardiac arrest care
Influence of cause of CPA on outcome in dogs and cats	CPR-related injuries in dogs and cats	Dose of epinephrine in dogs and cats	Utility of pulse palpation and apex beat for diagnosis of CPA in dogs and cats	Evidence on the utility of a hemodynamic optimization strategy on outcome in dogs and cats
CPA risk factors in anesthetized patients in dogs and cats	Efficacy of non-invasive ventilation in dogs and cats	Epinephrine versus vasopressin in dogs and cats	The utility of bedside echocardiography during CPR in dogs and cats	Evidence on the utility of a respiratory optimization strategy on outcome in dogs and cats
Effectiveness of CPR training programs and simulation in dogs and cats	Optimal ventilation parameters in dogs and cats	Efficacy of atropine in small animal CPR or subset of CPA populations	The utility of $ETCO_2$ values at initiation and over the course of CPR in dogs and cats	PCA hemodynamic performance and influence on outcome in dogs and cats
Influence of leadership training on CPR team performance	Optimal compression depth in dogs and cats	The effect of amiodarone for refractory VF in dogs and cats	The utility of $ETCO_2$ to confirm endotracheal intubation during CPR in dogs and cats	PCA blood gas, electrolyte, and acid–base abnormalities and influence on outcome in dogs and cats
Influence of team size on CPR team performance	Optimal compression location in dogs with various chest conformations	The effect of buffer administration during CPR in dogs and cats	Prognostic value of $ETCO_2$ during CPR in dogs and cats	Feasibility of TTM in dogs and cats
Influence on debriefing on CPR team performance/patient outcomes	Optimal compression rate in dogs and cats	Timing and effect of open-chest CPR on outcome in dogs and cats	Blood gas, electrolyte and acid–base abnormalities during CPR in dogs and cats	Temperature goals of TTM in dogs and cats
Influence of posttraining assessment on knowledge/skill retention	Timing of rescuer fatigue during veterinary CPR, and in relation to animal size/species	Effect of impedance threshold device in dogs	Frequencies of heart rhythms and association with outcome in dogs and cats	PCA rewarming rates of hypothermic dogs and cats
	Extent of no-compression fraction in dogs and cats	Evidence toward development of stopping recommendations in dogs and cats	Development and utility of feedback technology to guide CPR performance	Effects of PCA neuroprotective and metabolic drugs on outcome in dogs and cats
			Development and utility of physiological feedback technology to guide CPR effectiveness	Impact of referral to critical care department for PCA care on outcome of dogs and cats

CPA, cardiopulmonary arrest; CPR, cardiopulmonary resuscitation; $ETCO_2$, end-tidal carbon dioxide; PCA, post-cardiac arrest; TTM, targeted temperature management.

Standardized reporting of data in the field of resuscitation science is commonly referred to as the "Utstein style." Utstein Abbey was the location of a meeting on the Norwegian island of Mosteroy where a group of resuscitation experts convened in 1990 to develop consensus guidelines for standardized reporting of CPR in people [15]. In 2013, the RECOVER initiative formed an international group of veterinary emergency and critical care experts, representatives of veterinary critical care organizations and ILCOR, to develop Utstein-style guidelines for uniform reporting of small animal CPR events. The finalized consensus guidelines were published in 2016 and provide an important tool to veterinary researchers to conduct clinical studies [10]. The document contains a veterinary CPR glossary and also suggests key data elements to be reported in clinical veterinary CPR studies and included in research reports.

It is the hope of the RECOVER initiative that the veterinary Utstein-style reporting guidelines will increase the quality of small CPR research, facilitate data comparison across studies, and encourage multicenter studies.

CPR Registry

A registry is a health-related database that contains clinical and demographic information about individuals and serves a specific health-related purpose [16]. While observational research projects focus on short-term data collection, medical registries are used for long-term data gathering.

The RECOVER initiative developed a CPR registry with the principal objective of collecting epidemiological information of CPR in dogs and cats. Such epidemiological data are currently only reported in observational studies conducted in single academic centers [3,4,17,18]. Because the veterinary CPA population is heterogeneous, large sample sizes are needed to examine the effects of specific variables (e.g. co-morbidities) on outcome. A more accurate description of the CPA population may allow a more appropriate focus of future CPR guidelines.

Although study designs such as randomized controlled trials are required to prove cause and effect of a specific therapeutic intervention, this registry will be able to address many significant knowledge gaps. As an example, the characteristics of CPA cases that are associated with a favorable outcome can be more fully elucidated. In addition, determining ROSC and survival rates after CPR

of various durations would be of great value. What is the association between the duration of CPR and the length of recovery? How are survival rates of animals changing over the years and with the advent of new guidelines? A registry is an indispensable tool to create new knowledge on small animal CPR. The RECOVER initiative CPR registry utilizes the Utstein-style reporting guidelines as a data collection framework. These provide clear operational definitions for all data elements included and identify data elements that absolutely require reporting (i.e. core variables), and those that cannot always be reliably collected or are of hypothesis-generating value (i.e. supplemental variables). The registry is implemented in an electronic, secure data capture system that can be accessed internationally via the internet.

Conclusion

The RECOVER evidence-based clinical guidelines serve as an important foundation in our attempts to improve CPR outcomes, but future progress in veterinary resuscitation science will depend upon addressing the identified knowledge gaps and actively observing the effects of new training programs and broader acceptance of these clinical approaches. While still lagging behind the dramatic progress in human resuscitation over the last 20 years, these strategies for advancing veterinary resuscitation science through systematic evidence evaluation, training programs to improve guideline adoption, uniform reporting of small animal CPR in an international registry, and research focused on identified knowledge gaps have the potential to improve outcomes in dogs and cats with CPA.

References

1 Boller M, Kellett-Gregory L, Shofer FS, et al. The clinical practice of CPCR in small animals: an internet-based survey. *J Vet Emerg Crit Care* 2010;20:558–570.

2 Hofmeister EH, Thompson BF, Brainard BM, et al. Survey of academic veterinarians' attitudes toward provision of cardiopulmonary-cerebral resuscitation and discussion of resuscitation with clientele. *J Vet Emerg Crit Care* 2008;18:133–141.

3 Hofmeister EH, Brainard BM, Egger CM, et al. Prognostic indicators for dogs and cats with cardiopulmonary arrest treated by cardiopulmonary cerebral resuscitation at a university teaching hospital. *J Am Vet Med Assoc* 2009;235:50–57.

4 McIntyre RL, Hopper K, Epstein SE. Assessment of cardiopulmonary resuscitation in 121 dogs and 30 cats at a university teaching hospital (2009–2012). *J Vet Emerg Crit Care* 2014;24:693–704.

5 Kawase K, Ujiie H, Takaki M, et al. Clinical outcome of canine cardiopulmonary resuscitation following RECOVER clinical guidelines at a Japanese nighttime animal hospital. *J Vet Med Sci* 2018;80:518–525.

6 Olasveengen TM, Vik E, Kuzovlev A, Sunde K. Effect of implementation of new resuscitation guidelines on quality of cardiopulmonary resuscitation and survival. *Resuscitation* 2009;80:407–411.

7 Lick CJ, Aufderheide TP, Niskanen RA, et al. Take Heart America: a comprehensive, community-wide, systems-based approach to the treatment of cardiac arrest. *Crit Care Med* 2011;39:26–33.

8 Nichol G, Thomas E, Callaway CW, et al. Regional variation in out-of-hospital cardiac arrest incidence and outcome. *JAMA* 2008;300:1423–1431.

9 Fletcher DJ, Boller M, Brainard BM, et al. RECOVER evidence and knowledge gap analysis on veterinary

CPR. Part 7: Clinical guidelines. *J Vet Emerg Crit Care* 2012;22 Suppl:S102–131.

10 Boller M, Fletcher DJ, Brainard BM, et al. Utstein-style guidelines on uniform reporting of in-hospital cardiopulmonary resuscitation in dogs and cats. A RECOVER statement. *J Vet Emerg Crit Care* 2016;26:11–34.

11 Boller M, Fletcher DJ. RECOVER evidence and knowledge gap analysis on veterinary CPR. Part 1: Evidence analysis and consensus process: collaborative path toward small animal CPR guidelines. *J Vet Emerg Crit Care* 2012;22 Suppl:S4–S12.

12 Hazinski MF, Nolan JP, Aickin R, et al. Part 1: Executive Summary: 2015 International Consensus on Cardiopulmonary Resuscitation and Emergency Cardiovascular Care Science With Treatment Recommendations. *Circulation* 2015;132(16 suppl 1):S2–S39.

13 VECCS. RECOVER – Spanish: Veterinary Emergency and Critical Care Society. Available at: http://veccs .org/recover-cpr/recover-spanish/

14 Buckley GJ, Rozanski EA, Rush JE. Randomized, blinded comparison of epinephrine and vasopressin for treatment of naturally occurring cardiopulmonary arrest in dogs. *J Vet Intern Med* 2011;25:1334–1340.

15 Cummins RO, Chamberlain DA, Abramson NS, et al. Recommended guidelines for uniform reporting of data from out-of-hospital cardiac arrest: the Utstein style. A statement for health professionals from a task force of the American Heart Association, the European Resuscitation Council, and Heart and Stroke Foundation of Canada, and the Australian Resuscitation Council. *Circulation* 1991;84:960–975.

16 Solomon DJ, Henry RC, Hogan JG, et al. Evaluation and implementation of public health registries. *Public Health Rep* 1991;106:142–150.

17 Wingfield WE, van Pelt DR. Respiratory and cardiopulmonary arrest in dogs and cats: 265 cases (1986–1991). *J Am Vet Med Assoc* 1992;200:1993–1996.

18 Kass PH, Haskins SC. Survival following cardiopulmonary resuscitation in dogs and cats. *J Vet Emerg Crit Care* 1992;2:57–65.

B. Circulatory Shock

152

Pathophysiology of Shock

Edward Cooper, VMD, MS, DACVECC

Veterinary Medical Center, Ohio State University, Columbus, OH, USA

Introduction

Shock can be defined in a number of ways. Classically, shock has been considered to be any situation which results in insufficient perfusion (blood flow) to tissues, resulting in cellular oxygen debt. Categorical examples of perfusion-related shock include hypovolemic, obstructive, maldistributive, and cardiogenic. However, situations may arise in which perfusion is adequate but oxygen delivery is still compromised (such as with severe anemia and hypoxemia). These potential causes of shock and their underlying mechanisms can be elucidated by consideration of the major "players" in cardiovascular hemostasis and oxygen delivery – as represented by the so-called "tree of life" (Figure 152.1). And while

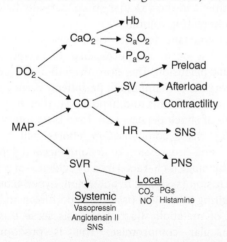

Figure 152.1 Schematic representation of the "tree of life" – factors that determine perfusion pressure and oxygen delivery. CaO_2, blood oxygen content; CO, cardiac output; CO_2, carbon dioxide; DO_2, oxygen delivery; Hb, hemoglobin; HR, heart rate; MAP, mean arterial pressure; NO, nitric oxide; PaO_2, arterial partial pressure of oxygen; PGs, prostaglandins; PNS, parasympathetic nervous system; SaO_2, arterial oxygen saturation; SNS, sympathetic nervous system; SV, stroke volume; SVR, systemic vascular resistance.

disruption of these factors encompasses many types of shock, it does not take into account the possibility of impaired cellular oxygen utilization and/or energy production, despite adequate delivery (such as severe hypoglycemia or mitochondrial dysfunction). And so in the broadest sense, shock is the result of any condition in which the metabolic demand for oxygen exceeds uptake and utilization, resulting in a cellular energy debt and a measurable change in organ function.

Specific causes, clinical manifestations, and potential management of shock will be covered in greater detail in subsequent chapters (see Chapters 153, 154, and 155). What follows is a description of the pathophysiological impact of a shock state, the ensuing compensatory efforts, and (if left untreated) progression to cardiovascular collapse. In addition, there will be consideration of the subsequent systemic impact of tissue ischemia, necrosis, and reperfusion injury which can occur even if shock reversal is successful.

Cellular Impact

Regardless of underlying cause, shock is characterized by an imbalance between oxygen and nutrient delivery to tissues, cellular consumption, and the removal of cellular metabolic end-products. Delivery of oxygen to tissues (DO_2) is a function of cardiac output (CO) and the oxygen-carrying capacity of the blood (CaO_2) (see Figure 152.1). The major determinants of CO are heart rate and stroke volume. CaO_2 is dictated predominantly by hemoglobin content (Hb) and percent saturation (SO_2), with dissolved oxygen (PaO_2) contributing only a small amount ($CaO_2 = 1.34 \times Hb \times SO_2 + 0.003\, PaO_2$). Normally the delivery of oxygen is well in excess of what is needed for cellular metabolism. This redundancy provides a buffer so that a significant decrease in delivery will not have a major impact on cellular oxygen consumption

Textbook of Small Animal Emergency Medicine, First Edition. Edited by Kenneth J. Drobatz, Kate Hopper, Elizabeth Rozanski and Deborah C. Silverstein.
© 2019 John Wiley & Sons, Inc. Published 2019 by John Wiley & Sons, Inc.
Companion Website: www.wiley.com/go/drobatz/textbook

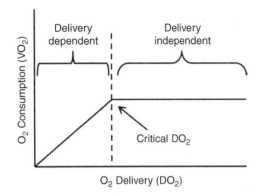

Figure 152.2 Schematic representation of the relationship between oxygen delivery (DO_2) and cellular oxygen consumption (VO_2).

(VO_2), also known as "delivery independent" (Figure 152.2).

Tissues can further offset a decrease in oxygen delivery by increasing oxygen extraction. Under normal circumstances, approximately 25% of oxygen is removed as arterial blood moves across the capillary and in times of need this can potentially increase to 70–80% or more [1]. However, eventually the reduction in DO_2 will reach a threshold (or critical DO_2) and O_2 consumption will necessarily diminish ("delivery dependent"). At this stage demand outweighs supply, resulting tissue ischemia and cellular hypoxia [2].

As such, the initial impacts of shock occur at the cellular level. Mitochondria function at the lowest oxygen tension in the body but consume almost all of the available oxygen in order to provide more than 95% of aerobic chemical energy for cellular metabolism [3]. Decreased oxygen delivery and cellular uptake (especially in muscle and splanchnic organs) impairs the ability of mitochondria to perform oxidative phosphorylation and produce adequate amounts of adenosine triphosphate (ATP). In response, cells will try to decrease metabolic activity of "non-essential" functions to reduce energy (and oxygen) consumption [4]. Eventually, even this capacity is exceeded, resulting in a switch to anaerobic metabolism and lactic acid production.

Intracellular acidosis can lead to denaturing of proteins, diminished enzyme function, and disruption of transport mechanisms. In addition, without the oxygen-dependent ability to produce adequate cellular energy, multiple intracellular systems, including membrane-associated ion transport pumps, begin to fail [5]. Cells are no longer able to maintain membrane integrity and an intracellular shift of fluid results in cellular edema and further dysfunction.

If injury is severe enough, cellular necrosis or apoptosis will be triggered. Sufficient loss of cells will result in loss of tissue function and ultimately organ failure. Insufficient availability of ATP, largely related to mitochondrial dysfunction, results in cellular acidosis, oxygen free radical formation, and loss of adenine nucleotides from the cell, all further contributing to tissue injury [2].

Systemic Impact

On a global scale, the systemic impact of shock can be characterized in three phases. The initial phase involves the body's attempt to maintain/restore core tissue perfusion and oxygenation. This primarily involves activation of the sympathetic nervous system mediated through baroreceptors (sensing decreased vessel wall distension) and chemoreceptors (sensing hypoxia, hypercapnia, and/or acidemia) [6]. The ensuing release of catecholamines promotes peripheral vasoconstriction, tachycardia, and increased cardiac contractility (and also creates most of the outward clinical signs of shock). The associated increase in cardiac output and systemic vascular resistance helps to restore mean arterial (perfusing) pressure [7]. In addition, activation of the renin-angiotensin-aldosterone system and increased release of vasopressin (antidiuretic hormone) serve to promote further vasoconstriction and diminished urinary water losses [7]. In patients with hypovolemia (whether absolute or relative), the associated decrease in hydrostatic pressure will naturally cause a shift of fluid from the interstitial compartment to the vascular space, partially helping to restore circulating volume.

It is important to note that these compensatory changes may occur at the expense of peripheral and splanchnic perfusion. Therefore, even though blood flow to vital organs is maintained, peripheral tissues may be experiencing ischemia and hypoxia. Further, if the inciting cause of shock persists and there is no intervention, eventually these compensatory efforts will be overwhelmed and progression to decompensated shock will occur. This stage is characterized by evidence of impaired core perfusion (systemic hypotension, hyperlactatemia). The resulting prolonged tissue hypoperfusion and development of metabolic (lactic) acidosis serve to worsen cardiovascular compromise. This is predominantly mediated by progressive catecholamine insensitivity and eventual exhaustion of compensatory mediators, leading to vasodilation and bradycardia [7]. Loss of vasomotor tone is especially prominent in skeletal muscle, leading to a reduction of blood flow to "non-essential" organs, with further impairment of venous return and cardiac output [8]. This terminal stage of shock is irreversible, ultimately progressing to complete cardiovascular collapse and death.

Secondary Systemic Sequelae

Given the potentially progressive and fatal impact of shock itself, early recognition and intervention are key. Clinical signs should reflect the presence of a shock state, whereas history and diagnostic evaluation serve to reveal the specific (or at least categorical) cause to help guide resuscitation. Therapy is then aimed at rapidly restoring tissue perfusion/oxygen delivery as well as addressing the underlying cause (see Chapters 153–155 for specific aspects of shock diagnosis and treatment). However, it is important to remember that significant tissue injury may have occurred even if initial resuscitation is successful. Depending on the cause, extent, and duration of shock, multiple systemic implications can arise in the postresuscitation period. As such, awareness, recognition, and management of these sequelae can be just as important as management of shock itself.

Systemic Inflammatory Response

Systemic inflammatory response syndrome (SIRS) occurs secondary to the widespread tissue ischemia and/or reperfusion injury that can be associated with shock. It is covered in greater detail elsewhere (see Chapter 159), so a brief overview is provided here in the context of shock sequelae.

Cellular damage or death triggers a complex cascade of events that ultimately results in further tissue destruction and potentially organ failure [9]. One of the initial steps in this process involves upregulation and release of inflammatory cytokines such as interleukin-6 (IL-6) and granulocyte colony stimulating factor (G-CSF) that serve as chemotactic factors for enhanced infiltration of neutrophils into affected tissues [10]. Increased rolling and sticking of neutrophils to the endothelium can lead to capillary plugging and obstruction of microcirculatory blood flow and transcapillary exchange [11]. Once diapedesis occurs, neutrophils release reactive oxygen and nitrogen species as well as proteolytic enzymes (elastases, metalloproteinases, etc.), leading to vasodilation, increased capillary permeability, and destruction of the extracellular matrix [9]. This results in leakage of protein and fluid into the interstitium and associated tissue edema. Ultimately, this can lead to disturbance of oxygen and metabolite exchange and cellular swelling and dysfunction [9].

Activation of the complement system also plays a major role in the pathogenesis of systemic inflammation secondary to shock [12]. Tissue injury leads to the release of split-products, including C3a and C5a, the anaphylatoxins. These mediators can increase vascular permeability, stimulate histamine and arachidonic acid product release, induce cytokine production and release, and promote adherence and aggregation of granulocytes to the vascular endothelium [13–15].

Hypoxic cellular injury also leads to an increased activity of phospholipases A_2 and C, which stimulate production of prostaglandins and leukotrienes [9]. These mediators exert a variety of effects, including further recruitment of inflammatory cells, alterations in vascular permeability and vasomotor tone, and enhanced platelet activity and aggregation [9]. The intestinal tract serves as another portal for systemic inflammation when reduced intestinal perfusion associated with shock results in increased permeability and intestinal barrier dysfunction (so-called "shock gut") [16]. These changes allow for translocation of bacteria and other mediators from the intestinal lumen, leading to infectious complications (sepsis) and thereby further upregulation of the inflammatory cascade.

Yet another major contributing factor is the liberation of toxic metabolites and reactive oxygen species after reperfusion occurs. Accumulation of hypoxanthine (a breakdown product of ATP) during ischemia leads to the formation of potent free radicals once oxygen is reintroduced [9]. These reactive oxygen species are then responsible for lipid peroxidation, disruption of cell membranes, and DNA damage, resulting in cellular apoptosis or necrosis (see Chapter 158 for additional information) [9].

Coagulopathy

Inflammation-induced activation of the coagulation pathway can lead to microvascular thrombosis, exacerbation of ischemic injury and eventually disseminated intravascular coagulopathy (DIC). Most of the proinflammatory cytokines (such as IL-1, IL-6, TNF-alpha, and arachidonic acid metabolites) are also procoagulant, leading to platelet and clotting factor activation [17]. One of the major contributing steps is an increased expression of tissue factor on endothelium and monocytes which, in conjunction with factor VII, initiates the coagulation cascade [9]. The resulting increased generation of thrombin is then a multifactorial catalyst for driving platelet aggregation and fibrin formation. Further contributing to excessive clot formation is the consumption and downregulation of natural anticoagulants, such as antithrombin and protein C [18]. Finally, increased activity of plasminogen activator inhibitor (PAI-1), as well as thrombin-activatable fibrinolysis inhibitor (TAFI), impairs clot degradation and worsens thrombosis [18].

The excessive clot formation associated with this hypercoagulable state promotes the formation of microthrombi throughout the vasculature. On the arterial side, these thrombi will cause occlusion of flow and result in downstream ischemic injury (and further tissue damage, inflammatory response, etc.). Venous thrombosis can cause obstruction in venous return, resulting in tissue edema, decreased right ventricular preload, and/or hypoxemia (with pulmonary thromboembolism). Eventually consumption of platelets and clotting factors will cause a switch to a hypocoagulable state and bleeding tendency. The associated potential hypovolemia and anemia can then worsen global perfusion and oxygen delivery.

Mitochondrial Dysfunction

As previously indicated, diminished mitochondrial energy production plays a major role in the pathogenesis of shock and cellular hypoxia. However, even when oxygen delivery is restored, there is evidence to suggest that mitochondrial function can still be impaired. This is related to the effects of various inflammatory mediators, such as tumor necrosis factor alpha (TNF-alpha), leading to uncoupling of oxidative phosphorylation and increased mitochondrial permeability and apoptosis [19].

Increased production of reactive oxygen and nitrogen species is another major contributor to mitochondrial injury. Reactive species are produced through normal cellular metabolism and removed by natural antioxidant systems. However, in the face of cellular injury and inflammation, the ability to scavenge free radicals is significantly reduced [20]. The formation of various reactive species is further increased in the face of ischemia and reperfusion (as previously mentioned). The membrane-bound nature of mitochondria is particularly susceptible to lipid peroxidation and free radical injury, as are the various proteins associated with electron transport [20]. As such, the resulting structural and functional damage to the mitochondria can lead to persistent dysfunction even after resuscitation.

Microcirculatory Dysfunction

In a shock state, decreased microvascular perfusion can certainly be expected (secondary to hypovolemia, hypotension, vasoconstriction, etc.). However, microvascular derangements can persist or develop even after resuscitation. One potential contributor to impaired flow through the microcirculation is endothelial edema secondary to ischemic injury, increased permeability, and influence of inflammatory mediators [21]. Given their normal diameter (<10 μm), even small increases in capillary wall thickness can have a significant impact on flow. In addition, inflammation-induced endothelial activation and increased leukocyte adhesion can result in capillary plugging, as can less deformable red blood cells [21]. The development of arterial microthrombi (associated with SIRS and DIC) can also severely impair blood flow to downstream microcirculatory units.

Finally, tissue ischemia, necrosis, reperfusion, and inflammation can all result in disruption of metabolic flow coupling that normally plays a major role in local regulation of microvascular flow [21].

Multiple Organ Dysfunction Syndrome

The widespread tissue damage that occurs with severe shock, in conjunction with the ensuing systemic inflammatory response (and other mechanisms described above), can ultimately lead to multiple organ dysfunction syndrome (MODS). The gastrointestinal tract is believed to be one of the earliest organ systems to be affected in this process as both victim and perpetrator. As previously mentioned, prolonged hypotension with shock can lead to epithelial injury and loss of mucosal barrier function with subsequent translocation [16]. In addition, recovery from shock is associated with decreased gut motility, resulting in gastrointestinal atony and functional ileus [17]. The lungs are also highly susceptible to systemic inflammatory injury, leading to acute respiratory distress syndrome (ARDS). The pathogenesis of ARDS involves inflammation-induced diffuse alveolar-capillary injury and subsequent severe accumulation of proteinaceous edema in the pulmonary interstitium and alveoli [17].

The kidneys can be very sensitive to microcirculatory disorders (thrombosis, hypoperfusion) with renal ischemia leading to tubular necrosis [17]. The resulting acute kidney injury is typically characterized by an increase in serum creatinine and blood urea nitrogen along with an onset of oliguria (urine production < 0.5 mL/kg/h) or anuria (see Chapters 94 and 95). During a shock state, there can be primary ischemic injury to the highly metabolically active hepatocytes. In addition, inflammatory mediators can cause hepatocytes to undergo significant alterations in synthetic activity, biliary transport, bile flow, and glucose metabolism [22]. Kupffer cells, macrophages found within the hepatic parenchyma, release chemokines that attract neutrophils into the liver and activate them [22]. After migrating into the parenchyma, activated neutrophils produce oxygen-derived radicals and proteases that cause further injury to hepatocytes and ultimately lead to organ failure (see Chapter 90) [22].

Conclusion

The conditions that occur during shock can be fatal if not sufficiently addressed. In addition, a shock state can initiate a self-perpetuating cycle of tissue injury, inflammation, coagulation, microvascular dysfunction, and organ failure, even after successful resuscitation. Therefore, early recognition and intervention are essential to limit the extent of tissue damage and minimize the ensuing systemic impacts.

References

1 Leach RM, Treacher DF. Oxygen delivery and consumption in the critically ill. *Thorax* 2002;57(2):170–177.

2 Guitierrez G, Reines HD, Wulf-Guitierrez ME. Clinical review: hemorrhagic shock. *Crit Care* 2004;8:373–381.

3 Garrioch MA. The body's response to blood loss. *Vox Sang* 2004;87(S1):S74–S76.

4 Duran-Bedolla J, Montes de Oca-Sandoval MA, Saldana-Navor V, et al. Sepsis, mitochondrial failure and multiple organ dysfunction. *Clin Invest Med* 2014;37(2):E58–E69.

5 Boutilier RD. Mechanisms of cell survival in hypoxia and hypothermia. *J Exp Biol* 2001;204: 3171–3181.

6 Guyton A. Nervous regulation of the circulation, and rapid control of arterial pressure. In: *Textbook of Medical Physiology*, 12th edn (ed. Hall J). Elsevier, Philadelphia, 2011, pp. 201–211.

7 Peitzman AB, Billiar TR, Harbrecht BG, et al. Hemorrhagic shock. *Curr Probs Surg* 1995;32(11): 929–1002.

8 Cryer HM, Gosche J, Harbrecht J, et al. The effect of hypertonic saline resuscitation on response to severe hemorrhagic shock by the skeletal muscle, intestinal, and renal microcirculation systems: seeing is believing. *Am J Surg* 2005;190(2):305–313.

9 Keel M, Trentz O. Pathophysiology of polytrauma. *Injury* 2005;36:691–709.

10 Hierkolzer C, Billiar TR. Molecular mechanisms in the early phase of hemorrhagic shock. *Langenbeck's Arch Surg* 2001;386:302–308.

11 Ambrosio G, Weisman HF, Mannisi JA, et al. Progressive impairment of regional myocardial perfusion after initial restoration of postischemic blood flow. *Circulation* 1989;80:1846–1861.

12 Yao YM, Redl H, Bahrami S, et al. The inflammatory basis of trauma/shock-associated multiple organ failure. *Inflamm Res* 1998;47:201–210.

13 Schlag G, Redl H. Mediators of injury and inflammation. *World J Surg* 1996;20:406–410.

14 Gallinaro R, Cheadle WG, Applegate K, et al. The role of the complement system in trauma and infection. *Surg Gynecol Obstet* 1992;174:430–440.

15 Cavaillon JM, Fitting C, Haeffner Cavaillon N. Recombinant C5a enhances interleukin 1 and tumor necrosis factor release by lipopolysaccharide-stimulated monocytes and macrophages. *Eur J Immunol* 1990;20:253–257.

16 Wattenasirichaigoon S, Menconi MJ, Delude RL, et al. Effect of mesenteric ischemia and reperfusion or hemorrhagic shock on intestinal mucosal permeability and ATP content in rats. *Shock* 1999;112:127–133.

17 Osterbur K, Mann FA, Kuroki K, et al. Multiple organ dysfunction syndrome in humans and animals. *J Vet Intern Med* 2014;28:1141–1151.

18 Hopper K, Bateman S. Updated view of hemostasis: mechanisms of hemostatic dysfunction associated with sepsis. *J Vet Emerg Crit Care* 2005;15(2):83–91.

19 Crouser ED. Mitochondrial dysfunction in septic shock and multiple organ dysfunction syndrome. *Mitochondrion* 2004;4:729–741.

20 Duran-Bedolla J, Montes de Oca-Sandoval MA, Saldana-Navor V, et al. Sepsis, mitochondrial failure and multiple organ dysfunction. *Clin Invest Med* 2014;37(2):E58–E69.

21 Moore JP, Dyson A, Singer M, et al. Microcirculatory dysfunction and resuscitation: why, when and how. *Br J Anaesth* 2015;115(3):366–375.

22 Tsiotou AG, Sakorafas GH, Anagnostopoulos G, et al. Septic shock: current pathogenic concepts from a clinical perspective. *Med Sci Monit* 2005;11:RA76–85

153

Hypovolemic Shock

Corrin Boyd, BVMS (Hons), MVetClinStud, DACVECC and Lisa Smart, BVSc (Hons), DACVECC

School of Veterinary and Life Sciences, Murdoch University, Murdoch, WA, Australia

Pathophysiology of Hypovolemic Shock

Hypovolemia may be caused by loss of crystalloid-like fluid, plasma-like fluid or whole blood. Physiological compensation for loss of volume is fairly similar across the different types of volume loss, although fluid shifts across the endothelium may be different depending on oncotic pressure balance.

Loss of blood volume, whether it is due to plasma fluid loss or hemorrhage, causes a cascade of physiological responses [1–3], starting with a decrease in venous return and cardiac output (Box 153.1). Decreased cardiac output leads to a decrease in wall stretch of the aortic arch and carotid arteries, which is detected by baroreceptors in these areas. Subsequently, several neural pathways are stimulated that cause an overall increase in sympathetic tone, including increased inotropy, chronotropy, and lusitropy due to direct cardiac innervation, and peripheral arteriole constriction due to circulating catecholamines and increased transmural pressure. Epinephrine and norepinephrine are released from the adrenal medulla in proportion to the degree of shock and explain the typical physical examination signs of arterial vasoconstriction, including tachycardia, pale mucous membranes, prolongation of capillary refill time (CRT), small pulse wave amplitude, and cool limbs. Venoconstriction, as well as splenic contraction in some species, also provides an increase to central circulating blood volume, although these changes are not as visible on physical examination. This compensation for hypovolemic shock can normalize and maintain arterial blood pressure. In contrast to the periphery, the cerebral and coronary arterioles dilate during the sympathetic response in response to beta-2 adrenergic receptor stimulation.

When oxygen delivery decreases below the level needed for oxygen consumption of the cell, cellular oxygen demand is no longer being met and oxygen consumption becomes dependent on delivery. Below this point, termed the critical oxygen delivery point, anaerobic metabolism predominates and cellular lactate and hydrogen ion production increases. Due to intracellular buffering of hydrogen ions, carbon dioxide (CO_2) also increases. These changes cause hyperlactatemia, metabolic acidosis, and increased venous partial pressure of CO_2 (PCO_2). Increased venous and tissue PCO_2 can be utilized by various monitoring techniques to detect decreased tissue perfusion (see Diagnosis of Hypovolemic Shock). Peripheral chemoreceptors detect decreased pH and enhance local vasoconstriction, as well as stimulating ventilatory drive in order to excrete more CO_2. This may be detected clinically by tachypnea and hyperventilation.

As renal perfusion decreases, the renin-angiotensin-aldosterone system is stimulated due to decreased stretch in the afferent arteriole and decreased chloride delivery to the macula densa. Angiotensin II also causes peripheral vasoconstriction and maintains glomerular filtration rate by constriction of the efferent arteriole. Aldosterone release from the adrenal gland causes sodium reabsorption in the cortical collecting tubule. Antidiuretic hormone (ADH) is released from the pituitary due to decreased stretch in the cardiac atria and the stimulation of angiotensin II. In addition to stimulating peripheral vasoconstriction, ADH also increases water reabsorption in the collecting tubule. In this way, sodium and water reabsorption together help to increase circulating blood volume.

Starling's forces also help to restore blood volume by favoring fluid movement from the interstitium to the intravascular space, which is one reason why packed cell volume (PCV) starts to fall during mild prolonged hemorrhage. This decrease in interstitial volume is not usually detectable by assessing dehydration parameters in the acute phase but may become more obvious if the animal has a slow blood loss over a number of hours to days. There is also some degree of interstitial osmotic drive

Textbook of Small Animal Emergency Medicine, First Edition. Edited by Kenneth J. Drobatz, Kate Hopper, Elizabeth Rozanski and Deborah C. Silverstein.
© 2019 John Wiley & Sons, Inc. Published 2019 by John Wiley & Sons, Inc.
Companion Website: www.wiley.com/go/drobatz/textbook

Box 153.1 Physiological responses to hypovolemic shock.

Compensated
- Decreased venous return
  - Decreased stroke volume
  - Decreased aortic and carotid arterial wall stretch
- Increased sympathetic nervous system tone
  - Increased cardiac inotropy, chronotropy, lusitropy
  - Release of catecholamines from adrenal medulla
  - Peripheral arteriolar vasoconstriction
  - Cerebral and coronary arteriolar vasodilation
  - Venoconstriction
  - Splenic contraction
- Supply-dependent oxygen consumption
  - Hyperlactatemia
  - Increased cellular hydrogen ion production
  - Peripheral chemoreceptor stimulation
  - Local arteriolar vasoconstriction
  - Increased ventilatory drive
- Stimulation of renin-angiotensin-aldosterone system
  - Increased angiotensin II
  - Peripheral vasoconstriction
  - Maintenance of glomerular filtration rate
  - Increased aldosterone
  - Increased renal sodium reabsorption
- Increased antidiuretic hormone
  - Peripheral vasoconstriction
  - Increased renal water reabsorption
  - Increased thirst
- Decreased intravascular hydrostatic pressure
  - Fluid movement from interstitial space

Decompensated
- Decreased sensitivity of adrenergic receptors
- Exhaustion of antidiuretic hormone stores
- Local release of vasodilatory mediators
- Progressive intracellular acidosis
- Progressive bradycardia and hypotension

Post-resuscitation after severe shock
- Ischemia and reperfusion injury
- Intestinal villous sloughing
- Systemic inflammation
- Microthrombosis
- Coagulopathy
  - Initial hypercoagulability
  - Subsequent hypocoagulability

that favors some water movement from the intracellular space. It is theorized that ischemic tissues release products from proteolysis and lipolysis, therefore increasing osmolality in the extracellular fluid space. Lastly, hypovolemia also stimulates thirst, via ADH, and increased sodium "appetite," which helps to restore blood volume.

Decompensation

The vasoconstrictive response eventually wanes due to decreased sensitivity of adrenergic receptors to catecholamines and exhaustion of ADH stores. Ischemic tissues also release chemicals that cause local vasodilation. Progressive intracellular acidosis in the myocardium reduces calcium concentration and decreases contractility, and progressive myocardial necrosis leads to ultimate failure. Acidosis also interferes with pump mechanisms in the cell membrane, disturbing the cardiac conduction system. The result of these effects on the patient is progressive hypotension, bradycardia, and death. This degree of shock may be irreversible; the patient may die despite subsequent blood volume expansion.

If the patient responds to blood volume expansion during severe shock, consequences of ischemia and reperfusion injury can still cause complications (see Chapter 158). Cellular necrosis, interstitial edema, and microthrombi in vital organ systems can lead to organ failure, similar to the pathophysiology of septic shock. Sloughing of intestinal villi and increased intestinal permeability, especially in dogs, lead to further losses due to intestinal hemorrhage, endotoxin release, and bacterial translocation. Hypercoagulability due to the initial response of the hypoxic endothelium soon turns to hypocoagulability and bleeding complications can further impair organ function. Intensive support and monitoring are often required for patients that have suffered from severe shock and develop multiple organ dysfunction (see Chapter 159).

Diagnosis of Hypovolemic Shock

Physical Examination

Physical examination is central to the diagnosis of hypovolemic shock and can be rapidly performed during the initial evaluation. Hypovolemic shock alters six key physical examination parameters, termed the *perfusion parameters*: mentation, heart rate, pulse quality, mucous membrane color, CRT, and extremity temperature (Table 153.1). Changes in these parameters reflect both the effects of decreased perfusion and the sympathetic compensatory response. Tachycardia is a consistent feature of compensated shock in dogs whereas cats often present with bradycardia, even with mild to moderate shock. It is often the first parameter to change. Thorough evaluation of perfusion parameters should include palpation of both the femoral and distal limb pulse, as changes in pulse amplitude typically occur distally first. With progression of shock, the number of abnormal variables increases, as well as the severity of these changes.

Table 153.1 Changes in the six perfusion parameters that are expected with hypovolemic shock of increasing severity.

Perfusion parameters	Severity of shock		
	Mild	Moderate	Severe
Mentation	Mildly obtunded	Obtunded	Stuporous to comatose
Heart rate	Increased	Increased (may be decreased in cats)	Increased or decreased
Pulse quality	Fair to good	Poor	Non-palpable
Mucous membranes	Pink to mildly pale	Pale pink	White/gray
Capillary refill time	2 seconds	2–3 seconds	>3 seconds
Extremity temperature	Normal	Cool	Cold

Tachypnea and increased respiratory effort also typically accompany shock, although they are not consistent indicators of decreased perfusion.

Similar alterations in perfusion parameters will also occur with cardiogenic or obstructive forms of shock (see Chapters 154 and 155). Differentiation of these types of shock can be challenging at times, but the presence of jugular vein distension should increase the suspicion for cardiogenic or a form of obstructive shock, rather than hypovolemic shock.

Blood Pressure

Blood pressure is often maintained in mild to moderate hypovolemic shock as a result of the compensatory response, but it will be reduced as shock progresses. In the circumstance of severe shock, physical examination parameters should be obviously abnormal and measurement of blood pressure should not delay diagnosis or treatment of shock. Direct arterial blood pressure measurement is usually not available in the emergency setting and non-invasive techniques may be inaccurate [4], so the measurement of blood pressure is not prioritized until treatment of hypovolemic shock has been implemented.

The shock index is a triage tool employed by some emergency clinicians to simplify detection of shock. It is calculated from the heart rate divided by the systolic blood pressure and may assist in the detection of mild shock states where neither parameter alone is abnormal. Although this parameter has not been validated against a criterion standard diagnosis of shock, its clinical use has been reported in dogs [5,6], with a shock index of greater than 0.9–1.0 being generally consistent with a clinical diagnosis of shock. However, further research is required before it can be recommended in the routine evaluation for hypovolemic shock in an individual patient.

Pulse pressure, or pulse amplitude, variation with the respiratory cycle may also assist with diagnosis of hypovolemia, especially in a patient receiving positive pressure ventilation (PPV). There is a normal variation in pulse pressure during the respiratory cycle generated by PPV due to several factors, primarily increased right atrial pressure and subsequent decreased venous return during inspiration [7]. This difference is increased in hypovolemia, due to the greater collapsibility of the vena cava, greater right atrial compliance, and greater sensitivity of the ventricles to preload changes when operating on the steep portion of the Frank–Starling curve [7]. A pulse pressure variation greater than 10–15% is consistent with hypovolemia [7–9]. In patients without an arterial catheter, it may be possible to estimate pulse pressure variation from the pulse oximeter plethysmograph [10]. Frequency domain analysis of the plethysmograph can improve the utility of this technique [11]. Pulse pressure variation has not yet been clinically evaluated in small animals presenting as emergencies and may be of limited value in spontaneously breathing patients.

Electrocardiogram

Electrocardiogram R-wave amplitude may decrease during hypovolemia, with one dog model showing amplitude reduction in all leads during hemorrhagic shock [12]. In humans, ECG changes are less sensitive than pulse pressure variation in detecting hypovolemia [13]. Lack of R-R interval variation is also an indicator of increased sympathetic tone and may be an early sign of hypovolemia [14]. Calculation is complicated and not standardized, and there is currently limited evidence of clinical utility [15,16].

Laboratory Tests

Several point-of-care laboratory tests can serve as an adjunct to the assessment of hypovolemic shock, including blood lactate concentration and arteriovenous blood gas differences. These tests should be used in conjunction with clinical assessment of the patient, as the cause of changes in these parameters may be multifactorial.

Blood lactate concentration increases in moderate to severe shock due to inadequate oxygen delivery, but this is not a specific finding as lactate will increase with severe tissue hypoxia of any cause [17]. Lactate will also increase in some non-hypoxic scenarios such as diseases that affect tissue oxygen utilization or lactate metabolism [17]. Infusion of lactate-containing fluids such as lactated Ringer's solution may transiently increase blood lactate concentration [18]. Elevated lactate has been associated with worse outcomes in traumatized dogs [19] and humans [20], and has been associated with more severely abnormal perfusion parameters in cats [21]. Base excess has been used as a surrogate marker for lactate [22] but it is important to remember that this will be confounded by other metabolic acid–base disturbances (see Chapter 107). Lactate can be serially monitored during resuscitation (see Chapter 156). While it is not specific for shock, a persistently elevated lactate should prompt careful evaluation for ongoing shock.

Several blood gas parameters may also be altered in hypovolemic shock. These parameters should only be interpreted from mixed venous blood samples, which may not be possible to attain in the emergency room, or from central venous blood as a surrogate [23]. Peripheral venous samples may not reflect systemic oxygen utilization, as the peripheral tissues are affected by the compensatory response, including arteriovenous shunting of blood. In all types of shock, the mixed or central venous oxygen saturation of hemoglobin ($S_{mv}O_2$ or $S_{cv}O_2$) will decrease due to increased tissue oxygen extraction. An $S_{cv}O_2$ of < 70% is considered consistent with shock [23]. This parameter is unlikely to be a sensitive measure of shock when an animal is heavily sedated or under general anesthesia due to decreased oxygen utilization.

The arteriovenous partial pressure of carbon dioxide difference ($P_{v-a}CO_2$) is an indicator of the adequacy of cardiac output, with increased levels seen due to increased tissue CO_2 production [24]. Once again, this is not specific for hypovolemia. Dividing the $P_{v-a}CO_2$ by the arteriovenous oxygen content difference ($C_{a-v}O_2$) provides an assessment of the degree of anaerobic metabolism occurring in the tissues, which will also be elevated in shock [24].

Diagnostic Imaging

Bedside ultrasound is a rapid and relatively easy modality to use for detecting hypovolemic shock, without delaying other assessment or treatments. A short-axis view of the ventricles can be assessed subjectively for diastolic filling and contractility using the standard thoracic focused assessment with sonography for triage

(TFAST) pericardial chest site view (see Chapter 182) [25–27]. Caudal vena cava size can be estimated using the diaphragmaticohepatic view of the TFAST, where the vena cava crosses the diaphragm. Decreased vena cava diameter and dynamic collapse of the vena cava during inspiration are supportive of hypovolemia [27]. Other echocardiographic parameters supporting hypovolemia in dogs include decreased left ventricular end-diastolic volume, cardiac index, and mitral valve E-wave velocity [28]. In cats, hypovolemia causes a decrease in the left atrial to aortic root diameter ratio and an increased wall thickness in diastole [29].

Changes detected on thoracic radiography that occur during hypovolemia include reduction in the size of the heart, caudal vena cava, and pulmonary vasculature. Due to the time and restraint required, thoracic radiographs should not be used as a primary means of diagnosing hypovolemic shock, but may be supportive in conjunction with other clinical data.

Response to Treatment

Response to treatment is a useful tool in supporting a diagnosis of hypovolemic shock. This takes the form of a *fluid challenge* [30,31]. An intravenous fluid bolus, for example 10–20 mL/kg of an isotonic crystalloid for a dog (see below), is rapidly administered (see Chapter 167). Perfusion parameters, especially heart rate, should be constantly monitored during the fluid bolus. Improvement, even if transient, in perfusion parameters or adjunctive tests is supportive of a diagnosis of hypovolemic shock. If central venous pressure measurement is available, large increases (increase > 3–5 mmHg or final reading > 15 mmHg) should prompt ceasing the fluid challenge [31]. For most animals, there is low risk in administering a fluid challenge. A lack of response to the fluid challenge should prompt investigation of other causes, such as septic shock. Fluid challenges should be performed with caution in animals with pulmonary disease, cardiac disease, and anuria. Also, the approach should be more conservative in cats due to the risk of adverse effects of fluid overload; therefore, 5–10 mL/kg of an isotonic crystalloid fluid is recommended for a fluid challenge in cats.

Emerging Diagnostic Techniques

Near infra-red spectroscopy (NIRS) measures oxygenated and deoxygenated hemoglobin and myoglobin in tissues, reflecting the balance of tissue oxygen delivery and consumption [11]. It can predict the need for blood transfusion in traumatized humans that otherwise appear hemodynamically stable [32]. This technology has not been clinically evaluated in small animals.

Transthoracic bioimpedance is a non-invasive technology that can be used to estimate cardiac output [11]. It can discriminate between normovolemia and hypovolemia in humans [33] but has not been clinically evaluated in small animals.

Treatment of Hypovolemic Shock

Treatment of hypovolemic shock requires rapid replacement of circulating blood volume with intravenous (or intraosseous) fluid boluses. Several different fluid types are available for this purpose, including isotonic crystalloids, hypertonic crystalloids, synthetic or natural colloids, and blood products (see Chapters 167–170 and 176). The fluid chosen will depend on the type of hypovolemia: loss of crystalloid-like fluid, loss of plasma-like fluid, or loss of whole blood.

Loss of crystalloid-like fluid is treated with isotonic crystalloids. Doses are often expressed as a percentage of blood volume (approximately 80–90 mL/kg in a dog and 50–60 mL/kg in a cat). As a rough guide, mild hypovolemia will require approximately 25% of blood volume, and moderate to severe hypovolemia approximately 50–100% of blood volume. Only approximately 25% of the administered dose remains in the intravascular space within 1 hour [34], with the remainder redistributing to the interstitial space. These patients are usually also interstitially dehydrated, and the fluid redistribution will assist in rehydration. This should be taken into account in the subsequent formulation of a rehydration plan (see Chapter 171). If available, serum electrolyte concentrations can also guide the choice of an appropriate isotonic crystalloid. The isotonic crystalloid of choice is usually lactated Ringer's solution (LRS). Plasmalyte-148 and Normosol-R contain acetate, which may cause vasodilation when rapidly administered [35]. Large-volume administration of 0.9% sodium chloride can cause a hyperchloremic metabolic acidosis [36].

Loss of plasma-like fluid is also often treated with isotonic crystalloids, which are certainly the initial fluid of choice. This may lead to hypoproteinemia and, consequently, decreased colloid osmotic pressure, favoring fluid movement into the interstitial space. In a normally hydrated patient, this can rapidly lead to interstitial edema. Synthetic colloids may be considered as an alternative in order to maintain colloid osmotic pressure and avoid excessive tissue edema, but adverse effects of synthetic colloids, including coagulopathy and acute kidney injury (see Chapters 168 and 169), need to be weighed against the possible benefit of maintaining colloid osmotic pressure (COP).

The ideal treatment of blood loss is transfusion of fresh whole blood, but availability is often limited. Blood component therapy with packed red blood cells and fresh frozen plasma is often used instead (see Chapter 176). These should generally be administered after the initial resuscitative period with isotonic crystalloids, to avoid the need for rapid administration. However, speed of administration will be guided by the current state of active bleeding. Management of hemorrhagic shock is further covered in Chapter 170.

Resuscitation Endpoints

Whilst fluid doses can be estimated based on the severity of shock, treatment of an individual patient should continue until appropriate resuscitation endpoints are reached. These endpoints are parameters that indicate that shock has resolved and tissue oxygen delivery is adequate. They may include normalization of perfusion parameters, blood pressure, blood lactate concentration, and subjective assessment of volume on bedside echocardiogram.

In situations where there is ongoing hemorrhage, resuscitation may be performed to subnormal endpoints until there is definitive control of hemorrhage. *Hypotensive resuscitation* refers to fluid resuscitation to a blood pressure that is subnormal but still supports major organ function, such as systolic blood pressure of 90 mmHg or mean arterial pressure of 60 mmHg. *Delayed resuscitation* involves not administering any fluid therapy until after definitive control of hemorrhage. See Chapter 170 for further detail.

Complications of Hypovolemic Shock

Several detrimental complications may occur following the treatment of hypovolemic shock. These complications are more likely to occur if treatment is delayed, inadequate or excessive. This emphasizes the need for prompt recognition of hypovolemic shock and close monitoring during treatment towards appropriate endpoints.

Reperfusion injury may occur when tissue oxygen delivery is restored following a period of tissue hypoxia. This may result in a systemic inflammatory response and multiple organ dysfunction (see Chapter 158).

Large volumes of crystalloid, colloid or packed red blood cells can result in a dilutional coagulopathy and thrombocytopenia (see Chapter 70). In turn, this may result in further hemorrhage and perpetuation of hypovolemia. When large volumes of fluid resuscitation are needed, it is prudent to monitor coagulation tests and treat appropriately if these tests are abnormal and there is ongoing hemorrhage (see Chapter 176).

Administration of high volumes of intravenous fluids can result in interstitial edema, especially in the lung, with subsequent impairment of organ function. The endothelial glycocalyx can also be damaged by hypervolemia, leading to multiple adverse effects including increased vascular permeability, hypercoagulability, and a proinflammatory response [37,38]. Patients should be closely monitored during treatment of hypovolemic shock. Fluid therapy should be stopped if resuscitation endpoints are reached before the entire empiric dose has been given.

References

1 Haddy F, Scott J, Molnar J. Mechanism of volume replacement and vascular constriction following hemorrhage. *Am J Physiol* 1965;208:169–181.

2 Szczepanska-Sadowska E, Oppermann CS, Simon E, Gray DA, Pleschka K, Szczypaczewska M. Central ANP administration in conscious dogs responding to dehydration and hypovolemia. *Am J Physiol Reg I* 1992;262:R746–R753.

3 Haddy F, Scott J. Metabolically linked vasoactive chemicals in local regulation of flow rates. *Am J Physiol* 1958;195:97–110.

4 Shih A, Robertson S, Vigani A, da Cunha A, Pablo L, Bandt C. Evaluation of an indirect oscillometric blood pressure monitor in normotensive and hypotensive anesthetized dogs. *J Vet Emerg Crit Care* 2010;20:313–318.

5 Peterson KL, Hardy BT, Hall K. Assessment of shock index in healthy dogs and dogs in hemorrhagic shock. *J Vet Emerg Crit Care* 2013;23:545–550.

6 Porter AE, Rozanski EA, Sharp CR, Dixon KL, Price LL, Shaw SP. Evaluation of the shock index in dogs presenting as emergencies. *J Vet Emerg Crit Care* 2013;23:538–544.

7 Michard F. Changes in arterial pressure during mechanical ventilation. *Anesthesiology* 2005;103:419–428.

8 Berkenstadt H. Pulse pressure and stroke volume variations during severe haemorrhage in ventilated dogs. *Br J Anaesth* 2005;94:721–726.

9 Montenij LJ, de Waal EEC, Buhre WF. Arterial waveform analysis in anesthesia and critical care. *Curr Opin Anaesthesiol* 2011;24:551–556.

10 Cannesson M, Besnard C, Durand PG, Bohé J, Jacques D. Relation between respiratory variations in pulse oximetry plethysmographic waveform amplitude and arterial pulse pressure in ventilated patients. *Crit Care* 2005;9:R562–R568.

11 Middleton P, Davies S. Noninvasive hemodynamic monitoring in the emergency department. *Curr Opin Crit Care* 2011;17:342–350.

12 Torre PD, Zaki S, Govendir M, Church D, Malik R. Effect of acute haemorrhage on QRS amplitude of the lead II canine electrocardiogram. *Aust Vet J* 1999;77:298–300.

13 Soltner C, Dantec R, Lebreton F, Huntzinger J, Beydon L. Changes in R-wave amplitude in DII lead is less sensitive than pulse pressure variation to detect changes in stroke volume after fluid challenge in ICU patients postoperatively to cardiac surgery. *J Clin Monit Comput* 2010;24:133–139.

14 Ryan ML, Thorson CM, Otero CA, Vu T, Proctor KG. Clinical applications of heart rate variability in the triage and assessment of traumatically injured patients. *Anesthesiol Res Pract* 2011; Article ID 416590.

15 Edla S, Reisner AT, Liu J, Convertino VA, Carter R, Reifman J. Is heart rate variability better than routine vital signs for prehospital identification of major hemorrhage? *Am J Emerg Med* 2015;33:254–261.

16 Elstad M, Walløe L. Heart rate variability and stroke volume variability to detect central hypovolemia during spontaneous breathing and supported ventilation in young, healthy volunteers. *Physiol Meas* 2015;36:671–681.

17 Allen SE, Holm JL. Lactate: physiology and clinical utility. *J Vet Emerg Crit Care* 2008;18:123–132.

18 Vail DM, Ogilvie GK, Fettman MJ, Wheeler SL. Exacerbation of hyperlactatemia by infusion of lactated Ringer's solution in dogs with lymphoma. *J Vet Intern Med* 1990;4:228–232.

19 Hall KE, Holowaychuk MK, Sharp CR, Reineke E. Multicenter prospective evaluation of dogs with trauma. *J Am Vet Med Assoc* 2014;244:300–308.

20 Lefering R, Zielske D, Bouillon B, Hauser C, Levy H. Lactic acidosis is associated with multiple organ failure and need for ventilator support in patients with severe hemorrhage from trauma. *Eur J Trauma Emerg Surg* 2013;39:487–493.

21 Reineke EL, Rees C, Drobatz KJ. Association of blood lactate concentration with physical perfusion variables, blood pressure, and outcome for cats treated at an emergency service. *J Am Vet Med Assoc* 2015;247:79–84.

22 Stillion JR, Fletcher DJ. Admission base excess as a predictor of transfusion requirement and mortality in dogs with blunt trauma: 52 cases (2007–2009). *J Vet Emerg Crit Care* 2012;22:588–594.

23 Walley KR. Use of central venous oxygen saturation to guide therapy. *Am J Respir Crit Care Med* 2011;184:514–520.

24 Lamia B, Monnet X, Teboul J. Meaning of arterio-venous PCO2 difference in circulatory shock. *Minerva Anestesiol* 2006;72:597–604.

25 Carr BG, Dean AJ, Everett WW, et al. Intensivist bedside ultrasound (INBU) for volume assessment in the intensive care unit: a pilot study. *J Trauma Acute Care Surg* 2007;63:495–502.

26 Lisciandro GR, Lagutchik MS, Mann KA, et al. Evaluation of a thoracic focused assessment with sonography for trauma (TFAST) protocol to detect pneumothorax and concurrent thoracic injury

in 145 traumatized dogs. *J Vet Emerg Crit Care* 2008;18:258–269.

27 Zengin S, Al B, Genc S, Yildirim C, Ercan S, Dogan M, Altunbas G. Role of inferior vena cava and right ventricular diameter in assessment of volume status: a comparative study: ultrasound and hypovolemia. *Am J Emerg Med* 2013;31:763–767.

28 Fine D, Durham H Jr, Rossi N, Spier A, Selting K, Rubin L. Echocardiographic assessment of hemodynamic changes produced by two methods of inducing fluid deficit in dogs. *J Vet Intern Med* 2010;24:348–353.

29 Campbell F, Kittleson M. The effect of hydration status on the echocardiographic measurements of normal cats. *J Vet Intern Med* 2007;21:1008–1015.

30 Cecconi M, Singer B, Rhodes A. The fluid challenge. In: *Annual Update in Intensive Care and Emergency Medicine* (ed. Vincent JL). Springer, Amsterdam, 2011, pp. 332–339.

31 Vincent JL, Weil MH. Fluid challenge revisited. *Crit Care Med* 2006;34:1333–1337.

32 Beekley AC, Martin MJ, Nelson T, et al. Continuous noninvasive tissue oximetry in the early evaluation of the combat casualty: a prospective study. *J Trauma Acute Care Surg* 2010;69:S14–S25.

33 Reisner A, Xu D, Ryan K, Convertino V, Rickards C, Mukkamala R. Monitoring non-invasive cardiac output and stroke volume during experimental human hypovolaemia and resuscitation. *Br J Anaesth* 2011;106:23–30.

34 Silverstein DC, Aldrich J, Haskins SC, Drobatz KJ, Cowgill LD. Assessment of changes in blood volume in response to resuscitative fluid administration in dogs. *J Vet Emerg Crit Care* 2005;15:185–192.

35 Saragoça MA, Mulinari R, Bessa A, et al. Comparison of the hemodynamic effects of sodium acetate in euvolemic dogs and in dogs submitted to hemorrhagic shock. *Braz J Med Biol Res* 1985;19:455–458.

36 Cazzolli D, Prittie J. The crystalloid-colloid debate: consequences of resuscitation fluid selection in veterinary critical care. *J Vet Emerg Crit Care* 2015;25:6–19.

37 Chappell D, Jacob M, Hofmann-Kiefer K, Conzen P, Rehm M. A rational approach to perioperative fluid management. *Anesthesiology* 2008;109:723–740.

38 Woodcock T, Woodcock TM. Revised Starling equation and the glycocalyx model of transvascular fluid exchange: an improved paradigm for prescribing intravenous fluid therapy *Br J Anaesth* 2012;108:384–394.

154

Cardiogenic Shock

Luiz Bolfer, DVM, Dipl. BCVECC and Meg M. Sleeper, VMD, DACVIM

University of Florida, Gainesville, FL, USA

Introduction

The definition of cardiogenic shock is decreased cardiac output and evidence of tissue hypoxia in the presence of adequate intravascular volume. The clinical definition, originating from studies of a cardiogenic shock model in dogs, is persistent hypotension (systolic blood pressure < 90 mmHg or mean arterial pressure < 65 mmHg) with severe reduction in cardiac index ($<1.8\,\text{L/min/m}^2$ without support or < 2.0 to 2.2 L/min/m^2 with support) and left ventricular end-diastolic pressure (LVEDP) > 18 mmHg [1]. These parameters are obtained with pulmonary artery (PA) catheterization, which is not routinely performed in veterinary medicine. However, Doppler echocardiography may be used to estimate elevations of the ventricular filling pressure [2]. Cardiogenic shock may develop secondary to an acute and rapidly progressive cardiac disorder or may be the end stage of a previously diagnosed cardiac disease. In either situation, the fatality rate may be high.

Essentially, cardiogenic shock may occur with any disease that causes myocardial damage or otherwise inhibits the cardiac contractile mechanism [3].

Pathophysiology (see Chapter 152)

Shock is identified in most patients based on findings of hypotension and inadequate organ perfusion and cellular energy production. This condition may be caused by either low cardiac output or low systemic vascular resistance (SVR). Circulatory shock can be subdivided into four distinct classes: hypovolemic, cardiogenic, obstructive, and distributive.

Cardiogenic shock is characterized by primary myocardial dysfunction resulting in inability of the heart to maintain cardiac output despite adequate intravascular volume (forward flow failure). Cardiac output (CO) is a product of stroke volume (SV) and heart rate (HR).

$$\text{CO (L min}^{-1}) = (\text{SV}) \times (\text{HR})$$

A state of shock develops when the decrease in cardiac output is severe enough to cause inadequate tissue perfusion. A vicious cycle is initiated when the deficient cardiac output decreases coronary perfusion, causing global metabolic derangements to the myocardium (Figure 154.1). These patients demonstrate clinical signs of hypotension, cool extremities, poor capillary refill time, tachycardia, low urine output, and altered mentation.

Tachycardia is a normal physiological response triggered by baroreceptor-mediated sympathetic stimulation to preserve blood pressure and tissue perfusion. In most cases, sinus tachycardia is an appropriate reflex and best addressed by treating the underlying cause such as hypotension, hypoxia, and/or acid–base disorders. As contractility worsens, although hypotension results in decreased afterload and augments cardiac output to an extent, cardiac output worsens. The degree to which the left ventricular end-systolic volume increases is a powerful hemodynamic predictor of mortality in people with systolic dysfunction and an echocardiographic parameter for the diagnosis of systolic dysfunction in both human and veterinary medicine [4–7].

In the face of systolic dysfunction (decreased contractility) and systemic hypotension (decreased afterload), neurohormonal mechanisms to increase preload (i.e. renin-angiotensin-aldosterone system) are activated to increase diastolic filling and augment cardiac output. However, ultimately, the elevated left ventricular diastolic filling pressures increase myocardial oxygen demand and can lead to pulmonary edema and congestive heart failure. Arterial oxygen desaturation ensues from the increased tissue oxygen extraction, which is due

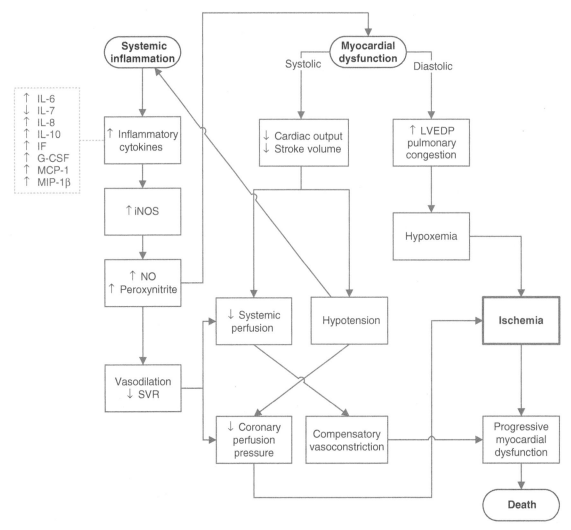

Figure 154.1 Systolic and/or diastolic myocardial dysfunction lead to a decrease in cardiac output with derangements to the systemic perfusion and arterial blood pressure resulting in a cascade of events that further exacerbates myocardium function, leading to myocardial ischemia and ultimately death.

to the low cardiac output, combined with intrapulmonary shunting [8].

The reduction in cardiac output triggers the release of catecholamines that result in peripheral vasoconstriction and help maintain perfusion to vital organs. Vasopressin and angiotensin II levels increase, which leads to improvement in coronary and peripheral perfusion at the cost of increased afterload. The increased afterload further impairs myocardial function, and decreased perfusion to the myocardium, coupled with systemic hypotension, can lead to systemic inflammatory response syndrome (SIRS) (see Chapter 159). SIRS can result in impaired perfusion of the intestinal tract, enabling transmigration of bacteria and sepsis [9]. Cytokine levels rise over the 24–72 hours after the development of cardiogenic shock. Tumor necrosis factor-alpha and interleukin-6 have myocardial depressant action and in

combination with other factors (e.g. complement, procalcitonin, neopterin, C-reactive protein) have been reported to contribute to SIRS and vasodilation during cardiogenic shock (see Figure 154.1) [10,11]. Microcirculatory abnormalities are present in addition to the global hemodynamic derangement [12,13].

Incidence and Etiology

There are no data available regarding the true incidence of cardiogenic shock in the veterinary patient. In humans, the American Heart Association (AHA) estimates that cardiogenic shock occurs in approximately 10% of patients with acute myocardial infarction [14]. Regardless of the underlying condition, cardiogenic shock is typically the result of severe left ventricular contractile failure (systolic dysfunction). Other types of cardiac dysfunction leading to cardiogenic shock have been reported in animals, including diastolic dysfunction (e.g. cardiac tamponade, hypertrophic cardiomyopathy (HCM), valvular dysfunction (e.g. degenerative mitral valve disease (DMVD)), and cardiac arrhythmias (tachyarrhythmias or bradyarrhythmias) [15] (Box 154.1). When an underlying cardiac disease is present, cardiogenic shock usually is the result of an acute exacerbation of the disease. Patients with decompensated heart failure and concomitant diseases (e.g. hypertension, diabetes mellitus, neoplasia, pneumonia, kidney disease) may be at higher risk of developing cardiogenic shock.

Studies in human patients with myocardial ischemia complicated by cardiogenic shock demonstrated that approximately three-fourths develop shock after hospital presentation and initiation of therapy [16]. The use of beta-blockers, angiotensin converting enzyme inhibitors, morphine, and diuretics translated into a substantial number of cardiogenic shock events [17,18]. There are no studies evaluating the effects of common cardiac drugs and the development of iatrogenic cardiogenic shock in animals.

Sepsis-induced cardiomyopathy (SICM) is characterized by left ventricular dilation and a depressed ejection fraction [19]. Several studies exist in dogs reporting that left ventricular dysfunction followed sepsis and neoplasia [20–22]. Theoretically, sepsis, or severe illness, induces chemical mediators (e.g. endotoxins, cytokines, and nitric oxide), resulting in depressed cardiac contractility and subsequent cardiogenic shock.

Diagnosis

Cardiogenic shock affects various organs and may be present with a large array of symptoms. When suspecting cardiogenic shock in people, the diagnosis is often made with a combination of invasive techniques (e.g. PA catheterization) to obtain hemodynamic parameters as well as non-invasive techniques such as echocardiography. A patient with cardiogenic shock is expected to have low cardiac output and an increase in the preload parameters of central venous pressure and pulmonary arterial pressure. In veterinary critical patients, the diagnosis is usually suspected by findings noted during history, physical exam, thoracic radiographs, electrocardiography, indirect blood pressure, and echocardiography.

Physical Examination

The physical examination findings vary according to the underlying disease as well as the degree of hypoperfusion/hypotension. The presence of altered mentation,

Box 154.1 Examples of cardiac dysfunction that can result in cardiogenic shock.

Left ventricular failure
Systolic dysfunction
 Ischemia/myocardial infarction
 Global hypoxemia
 Valvular disease
 Myocardial depressant drugs (e.g. beta-blockers, calcium channel blockers)
 Myocardial contusion
 Respiratory acidosis
 Metabolic derangements (e.g. acidosis, hypophosphatemia, hypocalcemia)
 Myocarditis
 Cardiomyopathy
 Cardiotoxic drugs (e.g. doxorubicin)
Diastolic dysfunction
 Ischemia
 Ventricular hypertrophy
 Restrictive cardiomyopathy
 Prolonged hypovolemic or septic shock
 External compression by pericardial tamponade
Increased afterload
 Aortic stenosis
 Hypertrophic cardiomyopathy
 Dynamic aortic outflow tract obstruction
 Coarctation of the aorta
 Systemic hypertension
Valvular and structural abnormalities
 Mitral stenosis and/or regurgitation
 Endocarditis
 Obstruction due to cardiac neoplasia or thrombus
 Chordae tendinea rupture
 Tamponade

Right ventricular failure
Increased afterload
 Pulmonary thromboembolism
 Pulmonary vascular disease
 Hypoxic pulmonary vasoconstriction
 High alveolar pressure
 Acute respiratory distress syndrome
 Pulmonary fibrosis
 Chronic obstructive pulmonary disease
Valvular and structural abnormalities
 Tricuspid valve dysplasia
 Tricuspid regurgitation
 Pulmonic stenosis

disorientation, poor responsiveness, or unconsciousness is indicative of poor central nervous system perfusion. Poor perfusion is usually apparent from cool extremities and pale mucous membranes; the pulse strength may be weak or absent as a result of poor cardiac output. Pulses may also be irregular if arrhythmias are present. Animals with right-sided congestive heart failure often exhibit peripheral venous distension and jugular pulses. The respiratory system may be affected by the development of lactic acidosis and secondary tachypnea or pulmonary edema if left heart failure is present. Cardiac auscultation may reveal muffled sound in patients with pericardial effusion. Tachycardia is the most common heart rate observed unless severe bradyarrhythmia (e.g. third-degree AV block) is the cause of the cardiogenic shock. Pulse deficits may be noted with some arrhythmias (premature ectopic beats and atrial fibrillation). A heart murmur should be present in dogs with DMVD and may or may not be present in dogs with dilated cardiomyopathy (DCM). Cats with HCM may develop a gallop sound associated with increased left ventricular filling pressure.

Electrocardiogram (ECG)

Multiple types of arrhythmias might be present in a patient in a state of shock. ECG monitoring should always be performed when cardiogenic shock is suspected. The most common arrhythmias are sinus tachycardia/bradycardia, atrial fibrillation, and ventricular tachycardia, but the presence of an arrhythmia does not imply that the patient has cardiogenic shock. Patients with other types of shock may also develop arrhythmias (see Chapter 53).

Thoracic Radiography

The decision to obtain thoracic radiographs should be exercised with caution in a very fragile patient. It is highly recommended to postpone radiographs in favor of emergency treatment and patient stabilization. Common changes noted on thoracic radiographs of patients with underlying cardiac disease include an enlarged cardiac silhouette, pulmonary venous and caudal vena cava engorgement. Patients with congestive heart failure will have changes consistent with a pulmonary infiltrate or pleural effusion. Pericardial effusion results in a globoid cardiac silhouette and loss of the normal contour of the cardiac silhouette (see Chapter 54).

Laboratory Exam findings, Lactate, Biomarkers, and Arterial Blood Pressure

The hemogram is often normal in these patients unless there is evidence of generalized inflammation or infection. A chemistry profile may reveal azotemia and elevated liver enzymes reflective of poor perfusion to the kidney and liver. Venous or arterial blood is helpful to evaluate the patient's acid–base status as well as oxygenation capacity. Patients with cardiogenic shock are often acidotic due to the combination of inadequate

cellular oxygenation leading to anaerobic metabolism and metabolic acidosis. Hyperlactatemia, a prominent feature of cardiogenic shock, can be attributed to increased tissue production or impaired utilization of lactate caused by dysoxia or tissue underperfusion, respectively.

In humans, biomarkers may be helpful to diagnose and monitor patients with cardiogenic shock. In veterinary patients, BNP and cardiac troponin-I can be used to help distinguish between heart and lung disease as well as to identify patients with myocardial injury [23]. Increased levels of NT-pro-BNP and cTnI were associated with worse prognosis in dogs with DCM and cardiogenic shock [24].

Arterial blood pressure (ABP) monitoring is recommended with Doppler ultrasound and sphygmomanometry in a continuous manner to help titrate therapeutic efforts. Placement of an arterial catheter, commonly in the dorsal pedal artery, allows direct measurement and continuous monitoring of arterial blood pressure. This method provides the most accurate measurement of blood pressure but is more invasive, and placement of arterial catheters can be challenging, especially in small patients or those with severe hypoperfusion.

Echocardiography

Echocardiography is important for definitively diagnosing the form of underlying heart disease (if present) and monitoring therapy in patients with cardiogenic shock. Based on echocardiography, a diagnosis of cardiogenic shock can be made if there is evidence of systolic dysfunction in the presence of adequate end-diastolic volume.

Sublingual Microcirculation

Because cardiogenic shock affects the microcirculation and may exacerbate hypotension and increase the risk of developing sepsis, a more direct assessment of the microcirculation can be performed using handheld video microscopy for observation of the sublingual microcirculation [25].

Treatment and Monitoring

Cardiogenic shock results in temporary or permanent derangement of the entire circulatory system, much of which is partially or completely reversible with appropriate treatment. Since cardiogenic shock has multiple etiologies, treatment should be directed to correct the underlying disease when possible (e.g. relief of cardiac tamponade with pericardiocentesis, addressing sepsis, etc.). Unfortunately, these conditions make up only a small proportion of cases of cardiogenic shock. In the absence of an intervention that can reverse the underlying pathology, treatment of cardiogenic shock in animals aims to acutely improve hemodynamics with the goal that chronic medical management may result in clinical compensation [15].

The hallmark of cardiogenic shock in the veterinary patient is the combination of hypotension and heart failure, which offers a therapeutic challenge because the treatment of either abnormality can worsen the other (Figure 154.2). If systolic dysfunction is present, the use of inotropes such as dobutamine is warranted. If the animal is stable enough for oral medications, pimobendan may be considered. Although pimobendan is considered an inodilator, it rarely causes a reduction in systemic blood pressure. Glucagon may have a role as an adjunctive

therapy in patients with cardiogenic shock unresponsive to initial therapy. Exogenously administered glucagon has a positive inotropic effect on the heart that results in increased cardiac output and blood pressure [26]. Pulmonary edema is treated with diuretics (furosemide) and oxygen support. The use of vasodilators for managing pulmonary edema is contraindicated in the presence of hypotension.

Vasopressors are used with caution in patients with cardiac dysfunction because the increased afterload negatively affects cardiac output. While the use of inotropic agents and vasopressors may temporarily improve cardiac output and peripheral perfusion, these agents increase myocardial oxygen demand and ATP consumption, predisposing to the development of arrhythmias. There are no studies in veterinary patients to draw any recommendations for the use of one inotropic/vasopressor agent

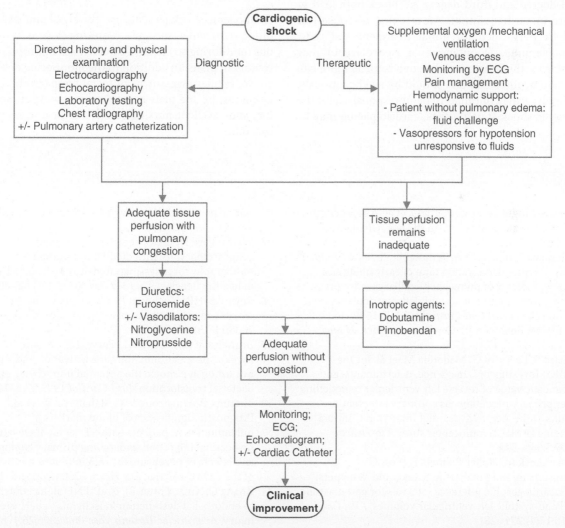

Figure 154.2 Treatment of patients with poor tissue perfusion and congestion is always challenging. If systolic dysfunction is present, the use of inotropes such as dobutamine is warranted. Pulmonary edema is treated with diuretics (normally furosemide). The goal is to eliminate congestion while re-establishing good tissue perfusion.

versus another, but higher doses of vasopressors were associated with poorer prognosis and survival in people with cardiogenic shock [27]. Dopamine has been shown to increase arrhythmias and likely mortality and for that reason, it is no longer recommended in the management of cardiogenic shock [28]. In patients with cardiogenic shock without an underlying cardiac disease (e.g. sepsis-induced cardiomyopathy), there is widespread agreement that standard treatment should focus on optimization of hemodynamic parameters by fluid resuscitation and vasopressor therapy as well as infection control in the case of sepsis [29].

Some arrhythmias may predispose the heart to inadequate ventricular filling and decreased venous return (see Chapter 53). Therapy of tachyarrhythmias includes vagal maneuvers, calcium channel blockers, and beta-blockers. However, if systolic dysfunction is suspected, beta-blockers should be avoided. High-grade second-degree and third-degree AV block both lead to decrease in cardiac output. An atropine response test should be performed for initial treatment and therapeutic planning. Dobutamine or isoproterenol may help increase the heart rate, although isoproterenol can exacerbate hypotension and should be used cautiously. If the bradycardia continues to be unresponsive and the cardiogenic shock state persists, cardiac pacing may be indicated.

Pulmonary artery catheterization and the resultant hemodynamic data, particularly cardiac power and stroke work index, have been shown to be useful for diagnosis and monitoring of humans with cardiogenic shock [30]. However, there has been a decline in PA catheterization in human medicine after the publication of a prospective observational study that suggested that PA catheters were associated with poor outcome [31]. PA catheterization is rarely used in the management of critical veterinary patients due to patient size, cost, special equipment requirements, etc. Contractile function can be assessed with echocardiography or left ventricle angiography. If available, an indwelling PA catheter allows ongoing evaluation of CO in response to changes in therapy and volume status. Diastolic function is more difficult to assess.

Conclusion

Cardiogenic shock patients are gravely ill and their condition is extremely unstable, requiring close and continuous monitoring so changes can be made appropriately to treatment plans. In addition to the monitoring described above, regular assessment of rectal temperature, coagulation testing and platelet counts, urine output monitoring, and excellent nursing care are critical to successful outcome.

References

1 Lluch S, Moguilevsky C, Pietra G, et al. A reproductive model of cardiogenic shock in the dog. *Circulation* 1969;39:205–218.
2 Giannuzzi P, Imparato A, Temporelli PL, et al. Doppler-derived mitral deceleration time of early filling as a strong predictor of pulmonary capillary wedge pressure in post-infarction patients with left ventricular systolic dysfunction. *J Am Coll Cardiol* 1994;23:1630–1637.
3 Califf RM, Bengtson JR. Cardiogenic shock. *N Engl J Med* 1994;330:1724–1730.
4 Funaro S, La Torre G, Madonna M, et al, for the AMICI Investigators. Incidence, determinants, and prognostic value of reverse left ventricular remodelling after primary percutaneous coronary intervention: results of the Acute Myocardial Infarction Contrast Imaging (AMICI) multicenter study. *Eur Heart J* 2009;5:566–575.
5 Seckerdieck M, Holler P, Smets P, Wess G. Simpson's method of discs in Salukis and Whippets: echocardiographic reference intervals for end-diastolic and end-systolic left ventricular volumes. *J Vet Cardiol* 2015;17(4):271–281.
6 Kim JH, Lee MS, Lee SY, et al. Contrast echocardiography to assess left ventricular volume and function in Beagle dogs: comparison with 3-Tesla dual

source parallel cardiac magnetic resonance imaging. *Vet J* 2013;198(2):450–456.
7 Lee M, Park N, Lee S, et al. Comparison of echocardiography with dual-source computed tomography for assessment of left ventricular volume in healthy Beagles. *Am J Vet Res* 2013;74(1):62–69.
8 Reynolds HR, Hochman JS. Cardiogenic shock: current concepts and improving outcomes. *Circulation* 2008;117(5):686–697.
9 Brunkhorst FM, Clark AL, Forycki ZF, Anker SD. Pyrexia, procalcitonin, immune activation and survival in cardiogenic shock: the potential importance of bacterial translocation. *Int J Cardiol* 1999;72:3–10.
10 Theroux P, Armstrong PW, Mahaffey KW, et al. Prognostic significance of blood markers of inflammation in patients with ST-segment elevation myocardial infarction undergoing primary angioplasty and effects of pexelizumab, a C5 inhibitor: a substudy of the COMMA trial. *Eur Heart J* 2005;26:1964–1970.
11 Zhang C, Xu X, Potter BJ, et al. TNF-alpha contributes to endothelial dysfunction in ischemia/reperfusion injury. *Arterioscler Thromb Vasc Biol* 2006;26:475–480.
12 Donati A, Tibboel D, Ince C. Towards integrative physiological monitoring of the critically ill: from cardiovascular to microcirculatory and cellular

function monitoring at the bedside. *Crit Care* 2013;17:5–11.

13 Jung C, Fritzenwanger M, Lauten A, et al. Evaluation of microcirculation in cardiogenic shock: current diagnostic and therapeutic aspects. *Dtsch Med Wochenschr* 2010;135:80–83.

14 Antman EM. ST-elevation myocardial infarction: management. In: *Braunwald's Heart Disease. A Textbook of Cardiovascular Medicine*, 7th edn (eds Zipes DP, Libby P, Bonow RO, Braunwald E). Elsevier Saunders, Philadelphia, 2005, pp. 1167–1226.

15 Côté E. Cardiogenic shock and cardiac arrest. *Vet Clin North Am* 2001;31(6):1129–1145.

16 Babaev A, Frederick PD, Pasta DJ, Every N, Sichrovsky T, Hochman JS. Trends in management and outcomes of patients with acute myocardial infarction complicated by cardiogenic shock. *JAMA* 2005;294:448–454.

17 ISIS-4 (Fourth International Study of Infarct Survival) Collaborative Group. ISIS-4: a randomized factorial trial assessing early oral captopril, oral mononitrate, and intravenous magnesium sulphate in 58,050 patients with suspected acute myocardial infarction. *Lancet* 1995;345:669–685.

18 ACE Inhibitor Myocardial Infarction Collaborative Group. Indications for ACE inhibitors in the early treatment of acute myocardial infarction: systematic overview of individual data from 100,000 patients in randomized trials. *Circulation* 1998;97:2202–2212.

19 Parker MM, Shelhamer JH, Bacharach SL, et al. Profound but reversible myocardial depression in patients with septic shock. *Ann Intern Med* 1984;100(4):483–490.

20 Dickinson AE, Rozanski EA, Rush JE. Reversible myocardial depression associated with sepsis in a dog. *J Vet Intern Med* 2007;21(5):1117–1120.

21 Nelson OL, Thompson PA. Cardiovascular dysfunction in dogs associated with critical illnesses. *J Am Anim Hosp Assoc* 2006;42(5):344–349.

22 Kenney EM, Rozanski EA, Rush JE, et al. Association between outcome and organ system dysfunction in dogs with sepsis: 114 cases (2003–2007). *J Am Vet Med Assoc* 2010;236(1):83–87.

23 Langhorn R, Willesen JL. Cardiac troponins in dogs and cats. *J Vet Intern Med* 2016;30:36–50.

24 Noszczyk-Nowak A. NT-pro-BNP and troponin I as predictors of mortality in dogs with heart failure. *Pol J Vet Sci* 2011;14(4):551–556.

25 Sherman H, Klausner S, Cook WA. Incident dark-field illumination: a new method for microcirculatory study. *Angiology* 1971;22:295–303.

26 White CM. A review of potential cardiovascular uses of intravenous glucagon administration. *J Clin Pharmacol* 1999;39:442–447.

27 Valente S, Lazzeri C, Vecchio S, et al. Predictors of in-hospital mortality after percutaneous coronary intervention for cardiogenic shock. *Int J Cardiol* 2007;114:176–182.

28 De Backer P, Biston J, Devriendt C, et al. Comparison of dopamine and norepinephrine in the treatment of shock. *N Engl J Med* 2010;362(9):779–789.

29 Sato R, Nasu M. A review of sepsis-induced cardiomyopathy. *J Intens Care* 2015;3:48.

30 Fincke R, Hochman JS, Lowe AM, et al. Cardiac power is the strongest hemodynamic correlate of mortality in cardiogenic shock: a report from the SHOCK trial registry. *J Am Coll Cardiol* 2004;44:340–348.

31 Connors AF Jr, Speroff T, Dawson NV, et al., for the SUPPORT Investigators. The effectiveness of right heart catheterization in the initial care of critically ill patients. *JAMA* 1996;276:889–897.

155

Additional Mechanisms of Shock

Sean Smarick, VMD, DACVECC and Iain Keir, BVMS, DACVECC, DECVECC

Avets, Monroeville, PA, USA

Introduction

Shock as proposed by Cox and Hinshaw in 1972 was classified as hypovolemic, cardiogenic, distributive, or obstructive [1]. Despite the popularity and persistence of this classification system, its utility is limited in that it only addresses causes of circulatory compromise leading to tissue ischemia. Other mechanisms beyond ischemia can be responsible for the shock state. Regardless of the classification, shock results in cellular dysfunction through a lack of energy (ATP) production by the mitochondria (see Chapter 152).

A recent veterinary reference has approached shock utilizing an expanded functional system beyond the classic model to include hypovolemic, cardiogenic, distributive, metabolic, and hypoxemic shock. Hypoxemic refers to not only decreased oxygen tension (partial pressure), but also hemoglobin and oxygen content in the arterial blood. Metabolic refers to hypoglycemia and aberrations in cellular respiration. This paradigm deviates from the classic model by including cardiac tamponade under cardiogenic shock and obstructive causes under distributive [2].

Conditions such as sepsis can have multiple contributors to the decrease in cellular energy production and do not fit neatly into one classification. Despite any inconsistencies in such classifications and artificial delineation as applied to clinical patients, the clinician should adopt a paradigm that will provide a comprehensive approach to the etiology of shock in the emergent patient. Hypovolemic and cardiogenic shock have been addressed in Chapters 153 and 154 but other causes should also be considered upon presentation, especially if initial efforts to resuscitate the patient are unsuccessful. See Box 155.1 for additional rule-outs for shock.

Box 155.1 Shock beyond hypovolemic and cardiogenic causes.

Distributive
SIRS/sepsis
Anaphylaxis/anaphylactoid
Hypoadrenocorticism
Neurogenic

Obstructive
Cardiac tamponade
Pleural space disease
    Pleural effusion
    Pneumothorax
    Diaphragmatic hernia
Pulmonary thromboemboli
GDV

Decreased arterial blood oxygen content
Decreased arterial oxygen tension in blood
    Decreased PiO_2
    Hypoventilation
    V/Q mismatching
    Diffusion barrier
    Anatomical shunting
Decreased oxygen-carrying capability
    Anemia
    Dyshemoglobinemias

Metabolic
Hypoglycemia
Mitochondrial dysfunction
    Intoxications
    Disease related

GDV, gastric dilation-volvulus; PiO_2, partial pressure of inspired oxygen = $FiO_2 \times$ (barometric pressure – saturated vapor pressure of H_2O); SIRS, systemic inflammatory response syndrome; V/Q, ventilation/perfusion.

Textbook of Small Animal Emergency Medicine, First Edition. Edited by Kenneth J. Drobatz, Kate Hopper, Elizabeth Rozanski and Deborah C. Silverstein.
Companion Website: www.wiley.com/go/drobatz/textbook

Distributive Shock

When there is a maldistribution of blood flow due to a marked decrease in systemic vascular resistance, shock results from inadequate perfusion. Vascular volume and cardiac function may be normal but clinically, there are conditions in which an aspect of hypovolemia and cardiac compromise also contributes to the shock state. While increasing the vascular volume or cardiac output may provide a degree of compensation, distributive shock often requires pharmacological intervention to reverse the decrease in systemic vascular resistance along with therapies aimed at the inciting cause [3]. Distributive shock may also result from a marked increase in systemic vascular resistance from an overdosage of, for example, epinephrine, cocaine, amphetamines, phenylpropanolamine, pseudoephedrine, etc. (see Chapter 135) or in animals with a functional pheochromocytoma. Treatment typically involves addressing the underlying cause and the use of alpha-adrenergic antagonists.

SIRS and Sepsis

Distributive shock is the predominant mechanism of shock in the patient with systemic inflammatory response syndrome (SIRS) and sepsis (SIRS secondary to an infection; see Chapter 159). Distributive shock is commonly associated with SIRS or sepsis due to inappropriate vasodilation induced by release of inflammatory cytokines, resulting in a relative hypovolemia, so that the blood volume remains constant but the total vascular capacity increases, resulting in a drop in blood pressure [4].

This also causes leakage of fluid from the vascular compartment. The release of inflammatory cytokines into the peripheral circulation will cause a breakdown in the normally non-porous endothelial glycocalyx and fluid extravasation into the interstitial space, resulting in a degree of hypovolemic shock. The component of hypovolemic shock may be exacerbated by continued loss of fluid into the peritoneal or pleural space, as seen with septic peritonitis and pyothorax, respectively. To complicate the management of the patient with SIRS/sepsis further, the presence of cytokines in the systemic circulation can also directly cause cellular metabolic dysfunction through reduced energy production (ATP) by the mitochondria; this can occur in the presence of increased or decreased blood flow to the tissue.

The patient with distributive shock caused by SIRS/sepsis can have one of two distinct clinical characteristics, "warm shock" or "cold shock," depending upon cardiac function. In a patient with warm shock, there is a compensatory increase in cardiac output caused by an increase in cardiac contractility, in response to the vasodilation (see Chapter 159). Examination of this patient will reveal hyperdynamic pulses, hyperemic mucous membranes with a rapid capillary refill time, warm extremities, and increased rectal temperature. The increased cardiac output results in normal or even increased blood flow to organs and tissue beds. However, despite this increased blood flow, these patients remain at risk for the development of organ dysfunction.

The patient with cold shock will have the same vasodilation but there is an associated reduction in cardiac output caused by decreased cardiac contractility. The cause of this decrease in cardiac contractility is multifactorial but includes cytokine-induced mitochondrial dysfunction, altered cellular substrate provision, and desensitization of beta-adrenergic receptors of the myocardium; these changes are reversed once the patient recovers (see Chapter 154). Upon examination, the patient in cold shock will have reduced pulse quality, pale mucous membranes with a prolonged capillary refill time, cold extremities, and hypothermia. The decrease in cardiac output (cardiogenic shock) will result in reduced perfusion of organs and tissue beds, putting these patients at risk of developing organ dysfunction induced by ischemic and sepsis [5] (see Chapter 154).

Anaphylaxis

Anaphylaxis is an acquired immune reaction mediated by immunoglobulin E (IgE) from a previous sensitization while anaphylactoid reactions do not require previous exposure and are not IgE mediated (see Chapter 146). Coronary artery vasoconstriction plays a role in the pathogenesis. History may yield exposure to antigens commonly associated with allergic reactions (e.g. vitamin K1, envenomation, etc.). Acute cardiovascular collapse often ensues with or without signs attributable to upper airway swelling, bronchial constriction, and gastric acid production. Epinephrine is the mainstay of treatment in addition to IV fluid support, corticosteroids and histamine antagonists (see Chapter 146) [6].

Hypoadrenocorticism

Hypoadrenocorticism is a lack of or decrease in the hormones produced by the adrenal medulla resulting in corticosteroid and mineralocorticoid deficiencies. Hypovolemia and electrolyte abnormalities ensue, in addition to a decrease in vascular tone, possibly due to an overproduction of nitric oxide (NO). History and physical exam can range from classic presentations of weakness, vomiting, diarrhea and electrolyte abnormalities to those that are more subtle. If hypoadrenocorticism is suspected, in addition to supportive care with replacement IV fluids, for example, corticosteroid therapy is instituted. Dexamethasone should be used if the patient is undergoing cortisol testing as it does not cross-react with cortisol measurements (see Chapter 115) [7–9]. Critical illness-related corticosteroid insufficiency has also been described in patients with sepsis and results in hypotension resistant to fluid support and vasopressor therapy [10].

Neurogenic Shock

A neurogenic component of shock was proposed and demonstrated in dogs in 1942 [11]. Clinically, disruption of sympathetic pathways (e.g. a spinal cord injury, SCI) can lead to both cardiogenic shock in the form of brad-yarrhythmias and distributive shock with loss of sympathetic input to the distal vasculature. A central nervous system (CNS) lesion, such as a SCI, would be supported by history, physical examination, and advanced imaging. Maintaining appropriate blood pressure with IV fluids and vasopressors, along with anticholinergics to address bradyarrhythmias, is appropriate to maintain perfusion, especially to the CNS which may have lost autoregulation since further ischemia may worsen the insult [12].

Obstructive Shock

Physical impedance to blood flow resulting in decreased perfusion is referred to as obstructive shock [3].

Cardiac Tamponade

If pericardial effusion accumulates within the pericardium, it will eventually distend the sack and transmit the increase in pericardial pressure to the external heart wall, decreasing ventricular filling and therefore cardiac output [13]. Although air is compressible, when confined within the pericardium, it may result in enough pressure to cause cardiac tamponade [14]. History may include progressive exercise intolerance or lethargy, vomiting, or acute collapse. In addition to signs of circulatory shock, physical exam findings may include distended jugular veins, pulsus paradoxus, and muffled heart sounds. Electrical alternans may be seen on ECG. Pericardiocentesis should offer immediate relief [15] (see Chapter 54, Pericardial Effusion).

Pleural Space Disease

Fluid, air, or tissue within the pleural space often leads to hypoxemia due to compression of lung lobes. Additionally, pressure on the heart or great vessels limits venous return and therefore cardiac output, exacerbating the shock state. History usually includes some symptom attributable to respiratory embarrassment. Trauma

raises a high index of suspicion for pneumothorax, hemothorax or diaphragmatic hernia, but many other conditions, ranging from spontaneous pneumothorax to neoplasia, can lead to pleural space disease. Physical examination can include abnormal respiratory rates and effort to include paradoxical breathing along with dull breath sounds, distended jugular veins, and pulsus paradoxus [16]. Imaging such as radiographs, ultrasound, and laboratory analysis of the fluid will help delineate the cause. Thoracocentesis should be viewed as an emergent *diagnostic* tool as well as a therapeutic procedure in the case of air or fluid [17] (see Chapters 44–49 and 183).

Pulmonary Thromboembolism (see Chapters 42 and 62)

The presence of a pulmonary embolism (PE) causes obstruction on the pulmonary vascular bed, with the severity of obstructive shock dependent upon the size of the obstruction (see Chapter 42). Causes of pulmonary embolism include fat, metastatic neoplasia, parasites, and blood clots. Pulmonary thromboembolism is the result of blood clots forming at a distant site, dislodging and traveling to the pulmonary vasculature, clots forming in the right side of the heart and migrating to the pulmonary vasculature, or they can form *in situ* associated with other pulmonary artery pathology, such as pulmonary hypertension or heartworm disease.

The initial approach to a patient with suspected PE is focused on stabilizing the patient while clinical evaluation and diagnostic testing are carried out. The majority of patients with a PE will be hemodynamically stable and therefore the clinician should instigate general supportive measures including intravenous fluids, oxygen supplementation, and empiric anticoagulation (see Chapter 71). In the subset of patients that are hemodynamically unstable, significant hypotension will be present and the initial treatment focus is on restoring perfusion with intravenous fluid resuscitation and vasopressor support, in addition to oxygen support which may require intubation and mechanical ventilation (see Chapter 188) [18].

Gastric Dilation-Volvulus

In gastric dilation-volvulus (GDV) syndrome, the stomach is distended with gas (see Chapter 82). The distended stomach places pressure on the low pressure vena cava, decreasing or occluding venous return, leading to a decrease in cardiac output. The stomach may undergo ischemia directly from increased transmural pressure within the gastric wall or due to a torsion of the stomach (and associated vasculature). Beyond obstructive mechanisms, SIRS, cardiogenic compromise, and hypoventilation add to the shock state [19]. The classic presentation is a large- to giant-breed dog that is retching unproductively with a distended abdomen and clinical signs of shock; however, any dog presenting in shock, especially with signalments associated with the disease, should have GDV ruled out with radiographs. In addition to intravascular volume expansion, decompression of the stomach and surgical derotation and exploration are warranted.

Non-Circulatory Shock

The arterial circulation delivers oxygen and fuel to the cells. While cardiogenic, hypovolemic, distributive, and obstructive mechanisms lead to circulatory shock, the lack of oxygen, its utilization at the cellular (mitochondrial) level or lack of energy substrate also lead to or contribute to the shock state.

Decreased Oxygen Content

Oxygen is carried in the blood, with over 98% normally bound to hemoglobin in the red blood cell and < 2% dissolved in the plasma. Hypoxemia usually refers to low arterial oxygen tension or partial pressure of oxygen dissolved in the blood and is caused by decreased inspired oxygen, hypoventilation, ventilation-perfusion mismatching, alveolar diffusion impairment, and anatomical shunting of venous blood into the arterial system. However, due to the oxygen hemoglobin dissociation curve, low oxygen tensions result in low saturation of hemoglobin and therefore decreased *content* of oxygen [20]. However, even with normal or high oxygen tensions, that is, partial pressure of oxygen, the content may be low if there is a lack of hemoglobin, for example due to anemia (see Chapter 10) or the hemoglobin's ability to carry oxygen is compromised, as with carboxyhemoglobin (HbCO) [21] or methemoglobin (HbMet) [22].

Respiratory embarrassment would be indicated by history and physical examination. Pale mucous membranes may indicate anemia and decreased hemoglobin concentration; packed cell volume and hematocrit can also help in assessing adequate red cells numbers. History of intoxications, such as acetaminophen in cats that can lead to HbMet (see Chapter 132), or smoke or other combustion inhalation (see Chapter 139) that can lead to HbCO should raise the index of suspicion for dyshemoglobinemia. Pulse oximetry can screen for hypoxemia, although blue mucous membranes make this an academic exercise; however, the converse is not true – the presence of pink mucous membranes does not indicate the absence of hypoxemia. Brown and bright red mucous membranes upon physical examination support HbMet and HbCO, respectively, and co-oximetry can confirm their presence. Pulse oximetry, unless equipped to assess HbMet or HbCO, is misleading in patients with dyshemoglobinemias [23,24]. Oxygen therapy (see Chapter 181) is initially administered and transfusions (see Chapters 176 and 177) are given as needed.

Metabolic Aspects

In the face of adequate circulation and arterial oxygen content, shock can occur if there is not an energy substrate, as in hypoglycemia, or the energy-generating capability of the cell, such as in the mitochondria, is compromised.

Hypoglycemia can be ruled out in patients with obtundation, seizures or hypothermia with simple point-of-care testing and treated with intravenous administration of dextrose (see Chapter 111).

Mitochondrial dysfunction is seen in certain intoxications, such as bromethalin [25,26] (see Chapter 130), and is known to occur in a number of metabolic derangements, including sepsis [27]. In the emergent patient with altered mentation, and in the absence of supporting history, such dysfunction becomes a diagnosis of exclusion after ruling out the other causes of shock.

References

1 Hinshaw L. *The Fundamental Mechanisms of Shock.* Plenum Publishing, New York, 1972.
2 de Laforcade A. *Small Animal Critical Care Medicine.* Elsevier, St Louis, 2015, pp. 26–30.
3 Vincent JL, de Backer D. Circulatory shock. *N Engl J Med* 2013;369(18):1726–1734.
4 Angus DC, van der Poll T. Severe sepsis and septic shock. *N Engl J Med* 2013;369(21):2062–2063.
5 Rudiger A, Singer M. Mechanisms of sepsis-induced cardiac dysfunction. *Crit Care Med* 2007;35(6):1599–1608.
6 Shmuel DL, Cortes Y. Anaphylaxis in dogs and cats. *J Vet Emerg Crit Care* 2013;23(4):377–394.
7 Orbach P, Wood CE, Keller-Wood M. Nitric oxide reduces pressor responsiveness during ovine hypoadrenocorticism. *Clin Exp Pharmacol Physiol* 2001;28(5–6):459–462.
8 Klein SC, Peterson ME. Canine hypoadrenocorticism: part I. *Can Vet J* 2010;51(1):63–69.
9 Klein SC, Peterson ME. Canine hypoadrenocorticism: part II. *Can Vet J* 2010;51(2):179–184.
10 Burkitt JM, Haskins SC, Nelson RW, Kass PH. Relative adrenal insufficiency in dogs with sepsis. *J Vet Intern Med* 2007;21(2):226–231.
11 Phemister DB, Schachter RJ. Neurogenic shock: I. the effects of prolonged lowering of blood pressure by

continuous stimulation of the carotid sinus in dogs. *Ann Surg* 1942;116(4):610–622.

12 Smith PM, Jeffery ND. Spinal shock – comparative aspects and clinical relevance. *J Vet Intern Med* 2005;19(6):788–793.

13 Shaw SP, Rush JE. Canine pericardial effusion: pathophysiology and cause. *Compend Contin Educ Vet* 2007;29(7):400–403; quiz 404.

14 Agut A, Costa-Teixeira MA, Cardoso L, Zarelli M, Soler M. What is your diagnosis? Pneumopericardium. *J Am Vet Med Assoc* 2010;237(4):363–364.

15 Shaw SP, Rush JE. Canine pericardial effusion: diagnosis, treatment, and prognosis. *Compend Contin Educ Vet* 2007;29(7):405–411.

16 Le Boedec K, Arnaud C, Chetboul V, et al. Relationship between paradoxical breathing and pleural diseases in dyspneic dogs and cats: 389 cases (2001–2009). *J Am Vet Med Assoc* 2012;240(9):1095–1099.

17 Padrid P. Canine and feline pleural disease. *Vet Clin North Am Small Anim Pract* 2000;30(6):1295–1307, vii.

18 Goggs R, Benigni L, Fuentes VL, Chan DL. Pulmonary thromboembolism. *J Vet Emerg Crit Care* 2009;19(1): 30–52.

19 Miller TL, Schwartz DS, Nakayama T, Hamlin RL. Effects of acute gastric distention and recovery on tendency for ventricular arrhythmia in dogs. *J Vet Intern Med* 2000;14(4):436–444.

20 Scott NE, Haskins SC, Aldrich J, Rezende M, Gallagher RM, Henderson MM. Comparison of measured oxyhemoglobin saturation and oxygen content with analyzer-calculated values and hand-calculated values obtained in unsedated healthy dogs. *Am J Vet Res* 2005;66(7):1273–1277.

21 Ashbaugh EA, Mazzaferro EM, McKiernan BC, Drobatz KJ. The association of physical examination abnormalities and carboxyhemoglobin concentrations in 21 dogs trapped in a kennel fire. *J Vet Emerg Crit Care* 2012;22(3):361–367.

22 McKenna JA, Sacco J, Son TT, et al. Congenital methemoglobinemia in a dog with a promoter deletion and a nonsynonymous coding variant in the gene encoding cytochrome b_5. *J Vet Intern Med* 2014;28(5):1626–1631.

23 Love L, Singer M. Anesthesia Case of the Month. *J Am Vet Med Assoc* 2013;242:753–756.

24 Feiner JR, Rollins MD, Sall JW, Eilers H, Au P, Bickler PE. Accuracy of carboxyhemoglobin detection by pulse CO-oximetry during hypoxemia. *Anesth Analg* 2013;117(4):847–858.

25 Coppock R. Advisory: Bromethalin rodenticide – no known antidote. *Can Vet J* 2013;54(6):557–578.

26 Bates MC, Roady P, Lehner AF, Buchweitz JP, Heggem-Perry B, Lezmi S. Atypical bromethalin intoxication in a dog: pathologic features and identification of an isomeric breakdown product. *BMC Vet Res* 2015;11:244.

27 Lee I, Hüttemann M. Energy crisis: the role of oxidative phosphorylation in acute inflammation and sepsis. *Biochim Biophys Acta* 2014;1842(9): 1579–1586.

156

Lactate Monitoring

Casey Kohen, DVM, DACVECC[1] and Kate Hopper, BVSc, PhD, DACVECC[2]

[1]*MarQueen Veterinary Emergency and Specialty Group, Roseville, CA, USA*
[2]*School of Veterinary Medicine, University of California, Davis, CA, USA*

Introduction

Lactate was first measured in patients in the early 1900s, and it was found that the accumulation of lactic acid accounted for the metabolic acidosis observed in patients with decreased blood flow and shock [1]. Later, Huckabee described populations of hospitalized patients with marked accumulation of lactate and acid–base disturbances [2]. Based on categorization of these patients on the presence or absence of an acidosis and clinical hypoperfusion or hypoxia, marked differences in mortality were noted, suggesting the use of lactate as a monitoring and prognostic tool. Following this seminal work, decades of research have been dedicated to the utilization of lactate monitoring in both human and veterinary patients.

Lactate Physiology

Lactate is a negatively charged molecule that is almost completely dissociated at physiological pH. It exists in two isoforms, D-lactate and L-lactate, but most clinical analyzers will only measure the L-lactate isoform. D-lactate is produced by some forms of bacteria, whereas L-lactate is produced by mammalian cells. Under normal aerobic conditions, glucose enters glycolysis, resulting in the production of pyruvate and a net of 2 moles of adenosine triphosphate (ATP) per mole of glucose. Pyruvate then enters the mitochondria and undergoes further metabolism to produce 36 moles of ATP per mole of glucose. Using this pathway, only a small amount of pyruvate is converted to lactate via the cytosolic enzyme lactate dehydrogenase [3].

Causes of Hyperlactatemia

Hyperlactatemia has traditionally been thought to arise due to inadequate oxygen delivery, and as such has been considered a marker of anaerobic metabolism. However, hyperlactatemia can also occur in the presence of aerobic metabolism. In his seminal papers discussing elevations in plasma lactate, Huckabee described three categories of patients with increased plasma lactate: patients with hyperlactatemia with no change in serum pH (type 1 hyperlactatemia) versus patients with hyperlactatemia and concurrent acidemia (type 2 hyperlactatemia). He further divided type 2 hyperlactatemia into type A lactic acidosis (2A) and type B lactic acidosis (2B). Type 2A describes lactic acidosis due to inadequate oxygen delivery to meet cellular demand, while type 2B includes all causes of lactic acidosis that occur despite adequate oxygen delivery [4]. Causes of hyperlactatemia are shown in Box 156.1 [2,4].

Type 1 Hyperlactatemia without Acidosis

Although commonly associated with an acidosis, hyperlactatemia can occur without a decrease in plasma pH (acidemia). This may be due to the presence of a concurrent metabolic alkalosis or as a result of the underlying mechanism for lactate production. Detecting the presence of a concurrent alkalotic process may require advanced acid–base analytical techniques such as the semi-quantitative approach [5]. There are also causes of increased lactate production that are not associated with a concomitant accumulation of hydrogen ions.

When lactic acidosis develops, the production of lactate occurs through a different cellular pathway from that of hydrogen ion accumulation (discussed further below). If accelerated glycolysis occurs in the face of normal mitochondrial function, increases in pyruvate production lead to increased lactate due to a mass effect. Hydrogen ions do not accumulate in the extracellular space in these circumstances, as they can enter the functional mitochondria for use in oxidative phosphorylation [6].

Box 156.1 Classification and etiology of lactic acidosis [3,6,7].

Type A – inadequate oxygen delivery for cellular demands
- Shock (cardiogenic, septic, hypovolemic, hypoxic)
- Regional hypoperfusion (splanchnic)
- Severe hypoxemia ($PaO_2 < 40\,mmHg$)
- Severe, acute anemia (hematocrit < 15%)
- Carbon monoxide toxicity
- Muscle activity: seizures, trembling, shivering, exercise, excessive restraint

Type B – no clinical evidence of inadequate oxygen delivery
- 1B– associated with underlying disease
  - Diabetes mellitus
  - Liver disease
  - Neoplasia
  - Sepsis
  - Pheochromocytoma
  - Thiamine deficiency
- 2B – caused by drugs or toxins
  - Ethanol
  - Methanol
  - Ethylene glycol
  - Sorbitol
  - Xylitol
  - Salicylates
  - Acetaminophen
  - Epinephrine
  - Terbutaline
  - Cyanide
  - Propylene glycol
- 3B – due to inborn errors of metabolism
  - Glycogen storage diseases
  - Pyruvate dehydrogenase phosphatase-1 deficiency
  - Mitochondrial oxidative phosphorylation disorders

Type 2A Lactic Acidosis

In states of inadequate oxygen supply, the rate of glycolysis outstrips that of mitochondrial metabolism. This results in the accumulation of both pyruvate and nicotinamide adenine dinucleotide (NADH), altering the cellular NADH to NAD ratio (cellular redox state). In this state, ongoing glycolysis may become the main source of cellular energy production. In order to provide adequate substrate for glycolysis to continue, pyruvate is converted to lactate, producing oxidized nicotinamide adenine dinucleotide (NAD) (Figure 156.1). Lactate dehydrogenase activity significantly increases due to the redox state present in anaerobic conditions, increasing

the lactate to pyruvate ratio [7]. The process of lactate generation from pyruvate consumes hydrogen ions, providing protection from intracellular acidosis. Lactic acidosis occurs as a result of concomitant accumulation of lactate and hydrogen ions through two separate cellular pathways. The hydrogen ions responsible for the acidosis are the product of hydrolysis of ATP. In the healthy state, these hydrogen ions diffuse into the mitochondria. In anaerobic conditions, hydrogen ions accumulate and are transported out of the cell via various mechanisms. This adaptive strategy prevents worsening of a cellular acidosis. This results in the commonly observed acidosis associated with hyperlactatemia.

Once oxygen delivery or supply is restored, lactate is converted back to pyruvate, with conversion rates in humans of up to 320 mmol/L/h, far exceeding normal rates of production [7].

Type 2B Lactic Acidosis

Type 2B lactic acidosis occurs in patients without clinical evidence of decreased oxygen delivery such as hypoperfusion, anemia or hypoxemia. When lactic acidosis is recognized in the emergency room patient, every effort should be made to ensure that oxygen delivery to tissues is adequate. Evaluation of perfusion parameters, blood pressure, packed cell volume, and blood oxygenation status are all recommended. If lactic acidosis persists without any evidence of inadequate oxygen delivery, a type B lactic acidosis should be suspected. Causes of type B lactic acidosis are shown in Box 156.1. Treatment is based on resolution of the primary disease [6,7].

Lactate Measurement

Various devices are available for lactate monitoring, including handheld point-of-care (POC) analyzers and large benchtop blood gas and acid–base analyzers. Lactate can be measured in plasma or whole blood.

The most common technique for lactate analysis is amperometry, where a lactate-sensitive electrode is coated with lactate oxidase, converting lactate to pyruvate and hydrogen peroxide. Hydrogen peroxide is then measured amperometrically [8]. Although there is some difference between arterial, venous, and capillary blood lactate values, several studies have concluded that this variation is unlikely to be clinically significant [8,9]. It is important to note that the majority of lactate analyzers only measure the L-lactate isoform. Analysis for the D-lactate isoform is available from specialty laboratories.

A few studies have evaluated the agreement of point-of-care analyzers with benchtop machines. Based on these studies, POC analyzers may result in slight

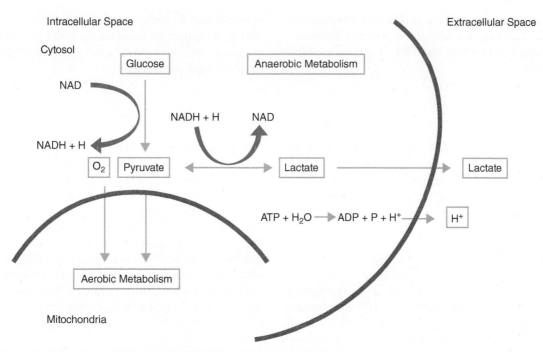

Figure 156.1 Overview of cellular lactate production. Glucose is converted to pyruvate through glycolysis. This is an anaerobic pathway occurring in the cytosol. Pyruvate can be converted back to glucose through the Cori cycle or can move into the mitochondria for further metabolism. Mitochondrial metabolism of pyruvate requires the presence of oxygen. When pyruvate cannot be metabolized by the mitochondria, such as in anaerobic states, pyruvate will be reduced to lactate and transported out of the cell. The hydrogen ions responsible for a lactic acidosis are not produced through the same pathway as lactate. Instead they are the result of hydrolysis of adenosine triphosphate (ATP) in the cytosol. NAD +, oxidized nicotinamide adenine dinucleotide; NADH, reduced nicotinamide adenine dinucleotide.

underestimation and larger disagreement noted at higher lactate levels [10,11]. In general, disagreements between POC and benchtop analyzers were less than what would be clinically significant, but the reader is encouraged to review the various studies assessing specific analyzers for more information.

Since hyperlactatemia can exist with or without concurrent acid–base derangements, accompanying acid–base parameters will likely provide valuable information regarding the significance and etiology of hyperlactatemia. For this reason, lactate is ideally analyzed in conjunction with a complete acid–base and electrolyte panel. Finally, some analyzers using lactate oxidase methodology will report erroneously elevated lactate levels in patients with ethylene glycol toxicity [12]. Markedly elevated lactate values measured in patients without an obvious cause should be interpreted with caution if exposure to ethylene glycol is possible.

Sample Handling

In many circumstances, blood lactate is measured in ill or injured animals with POC or rapid turnround diagnostic analyzers. Therefore, prolonged storage time prior to

analysis is unlikely to occur. A delay in measuring whole-blood lactate may cause as much as a 70% increase in lactate due to ongoing glycolysis, especially in the presence of leukocytosis or polycythemia [8]. Samples that cannot be analyzed immediately should be placed on ice, in the appropriate sample tube for the analyzer, and analyzed preferably no more than 60 minutes post sampling [13]. As some, if not all of the sodium lactate within lactate-containing fluids such as lactated Ringer's or Hartmann's is L-lactate, it will be measured by lactate analyzers causing falsely elevated levels. Special attention to appropriate scavenging technique is important if blood samples are collected from catheters through which lactate-containing fluids are running [14].

Patient Selection

Lactate monitoring is indicated in many animals presenting to the emergency room. It should be considered in any patient with perfusion abnormalities or evidence of significant systemic disease. Lactic acidosis is a common cause of an elevated anion gap metabolic acidosis and should be measured whenever this acid–base abnormality is identified. It is important to note that the presence of a normal anion gap does not exclude hyperlactatemia, as many emergency and critically ill patients have concurrent hypoalbuminemia, leading to a decreased anion gap [15,16].

Normal Lactate Concentration

Normal resting plasma lactate levels have been reported to be less than 2.5 mmol/L in people and dogs [17]. There has been variability in the reported lactate concentration of healthy cats; this likely reflects the impact of struggling and muscle activity on lactate levels [18,19].

Assessment of Hyperlactatemia

When hyperlactatemia is identified in an emergency room patient, it should prompt an immediate evaluation for potential life-threatening abnormalities. This should include assessment of perfusion parameters, blood pressure, and hematocrit. Any significant abnormalities should be addressed as indicated. Muscle activity can rapidly increase blood lactate concentration so hyperlactatemia identified in the post-seizure patient or the patient with tremors or difficulties with restraint should be interpreted with caution. The patient with hyperlactatemia that has no evidence of decreased oxygen delivery or other obvious cause identified should have a further diagnostic work-up. This may or may not be necessary on an emergency basis, depending on the overall severity of illness of the animal. Concurrent acid–base analysis can be of diagnostic benefit. Consideration of diseases that can cause type B lactic acidosis or hyperlactatemia without acidosis (see Box 156.1) will aid in guiding the diagnostic approach.

In addition to its diagnostic role, blood lactate measurement can be an excellent tool for monitoring response to therapy. Following identification of hyperlactatemia due to inadequate oxygen delivery, serial monitoring of blood lactate is recommended. Ideally, monitoring should be continued until the blood lactate concentration has returned to normal. Changes in blood lactate over time not only help guide therapy but have been shown to have prognostic significance in many patient populations and are generally considered superior over a single admission value of lactate for prognosis [20–23].

Administration of a large quantity (180 mL/kg in an hour) of lactate-containing fluids to healthy dogs has been shown to cause a small but significant increase in blood lactate concentration [24]. Studies in experimental animals suggest that resuscitation of animals in hemorrhagic shock with lactate-containing fluids can be associated with persistence of hyperlactatemia despite improvement in cardiovascular performance [25]. Caution is advised when interpreting blood lactate concentration in patients following volume resuscitation with lactate-containing fluids.

Prognostic Implications

Elevations in serum lactate have been evaluated in several small animal veterinary populations. In general, an increase in lactate has been associated with an increased mortality or other negative outcomes in the following diseases or conditions in dogs: IMHA [21], gastric dilation-volvulus (GDV) [22], hypotension in ICU [26], SIRS [27], severe soft tissue infections [28], *Babesia* [29], and heartworm-associated caval syndrome [30]; and in cats with hypertrophic cardiomyopathy [31] or septic peritonitis [32,33]. Additionally, lactate has been incorporated into a veterinary illness severity scoring system for both dogs and cats, and is one of the most significant variables included [34,35].

In addition to its possible prognostic utility in certain veterinary patient populations, lactate was also found to be an independent predictor of mortality in a large population of dogs and cats presenting to an emergency room [36]. Interestingly, in this study, mortality in dogs with hyperlactatemia and normal acid–base parameters was not different than in dogs with a normal lactate. This underscores the importance of concurrent acid–base analysis along with lactate. In a separate study in cats presenting to the emergency room, increased lactate concentration was associated with decreased systolic blood pressure and worsening physically assessed perfusion variables. Interestingly, in this study, there was no statistically significant difference in lactate between survivors and non-survivors [37].

The prognostic value of blood lactate concentration has been extensively studied in dogs with GDV. The initial blood lactate value has been evaluated for its association with both gastric necrosis and mortality. In these studies, the median lactate in dogs with gastric necrosis was between 6.35 and 6.95 mmol/L whereas lactate in dogs without gastric necrosis was between 3.3 and 4.5 mmol/L. Dogs that survived had median lactates between 3.4 and 6.2 mmol/L and those that died had a median lactate between 6.8 and 10.3 mmol/L [22,38,39]. It is important to note that no single lactate value resulted in 100% sensitivity and specificity for gastric necrosis or mortality, and as a result, lactate values obtained from patients with GDV should be interpreted similarly to any other patient with injury or illness.

Although hyperlactatemia and lactic acidosis have prognostic implications, they should not be used solely to determine whether or not treatment for the primary disease process should be attempted. Rather, they should be used to document patients that may have severe, unexplained or occult perfusion or oxygen delivery deficits, where attentive monitoring and appropriate therapy are paramount to a successful outcome. Lactate monitoring is not a substitute for a thorough physical examination and must be interpreted in concert with the entire clinical picture.

Lactate Measurement in Other Body Fluids

Due to the difficulty in consistently documenting bacterial peritonitis, and the significant difference in management strategies, there has been interest in utilizing abdominal effusion lactate concentration to increase sensitivity and specificity in diagnosing septic peritonitis (see Chapter 87). It was shown that in dogs, an abdominal fluid lactate value of 2 mmol/L higher than

a peripheral lactate had 100% sensitivity and specificity in detecting bacterial peritonitis [40]. It should be noted that this study only had peritoneal lactate concentrations for seven dogs, therefore peritoneal lactate concentration should not overshadow other clinically important findings.

A separate study reported that all dogs with septic peritonitis had peritoneal effusion lactates greater than 2.5 mmol/L, and a peritoneal effusion lactate concentration higher than blood lactate [41]. It is also important to note that these studies evaluated dogs on presentation prior to any other surgical procedure. It has been reported that the presence of a closed suction drain may alter lactate concentrations in abdominal fluid, therefore the utility of abdominal fluid lactate concentration is questionable in the postoperative patient [42].

Based on previous studies, it does not appear that peritoneal lactate concentration is useful in detecting septic peritoneal effusion in cats [40,41].

References

1 Fuller BM, Dellinger RP. Lactate as a hemodynamic marker in the critically ill. *Curr Opin Crit Care* 2012;18(3):267–272.

2 Huckabee WE. Abnormal resting blood lactate: I. The significance of hyperlactatemia in hospitalized patients. *Am J Med* 1961;30(6):833–839.

3 Levy B. Lactate and shock state: the metabolic view. *Curr Opin Crit Care* 2006;12(4):315–321.

4 Huckabee WE. Abnormal resting blood lactate: II. Lactic acidosis. *Am J Med* 1961;30(6):840–848.

5 Tuhay G, Pein MC, Masevicius FD, et al. Severe hyperlactatemia with normal base excess: a quantitative analysis using conventional and Stewart approaches. *Crit Care* 2008;12(3):R66.

6 Fall PJ, Szerlip HM. Lactic acidosis: from sour milk to septic shock. *J Intensive Care Med* 2005;20(5):255–271.

7 Kraut JA, Madias NE. Lactic acidosis. *N Engl J Med* 2014;371(24):2309–2319.

8 Fine-Goulden MR, Durward A. How to use lactate. *Arch Dis Child Educ Pract* 2014;99(1):17–22.

9 Jansen TC, van Bommel J, Bakker J. Blood lactate monitoring in critically ill patients: a systematic health technology assessment. *Crit Care Med* 2009;37(10):2827–2839.

10 Thorneloe C, Bédard C, Boysen S. Evaluation of a hand-held lactate analyzer in dogs. *Can Vet J* 2007;48(3):283–288.

11 Acierno MJ, Mitchell MA. Evaluation of four point-of-care meters for rapid determination of blood lactate concentrations in dogs. *J Am Vet Med Assoc* 2007;230(9):1315–1318.

12 Hopper K, Epstein SE. Falsely increased plasma lactate concentration due to ethylene glycol

poisoning in 2 dogs. *J Vet Emerg Crit Care* 2013;23(1):63–67.

13 Noordally O, Vincent JL. Evaluation of a new, rapid lactate analyzer in critical care. *Intensive Care Med* 1999;25(5):508–513.

14 Jackson EV, Wiese J, Sigal B, et al. Effects of crystalloid solutions on circulating lactate concentrations: Part 1. *Implications for the proper handling of blood specimens obtained from critically ill patients. Crit Care Med* 1997;25(11):1840–1846.

15 Chawla LS, Jagasia D, Abell LM, et al. Anion gap, anion gap corrected for albumin, and base deficit fail to accurately diagnose clinically significant hyperlactatemia in critically ill patients. *J Intensive Care Med* 2008;23(2):122–127.

16 Iberti TJ, Leibowitz AB, Papadakos PJ, et al. Low sensitivity of the anion gap as a screen to detect hyperlactatemia in critically ill patients. *Crit Care Med* 1990;18(3):275–277.

17 Hughes D, Rozanski ER, Shofer FS, et al. Effect of sampling site, repeated sampling, pH, and PCO2 on plasma lactate concentration in healthy dogs. *Am J Vet Res* 1999;60(4):521–524.

18 Tynan B, Kerl ME, Jackson ML, et al. Plasma lactate concentrations and comparison of two point-of-care lactate analyzers to a laboratory analyzer in a population of healthy cats. *J Vet Emerg Crit Care* 2015;25(4):521–527.

19 Redavid LA, Sharp CR, Mitchell MA, et al. Plasma lactate measurements in healthy cats. *J Vet Emerg Crit Care* 2012;22(5):580–587.

20 Cortellini S, Seth M, Kellett-Gregory LM. Plasma lactate concentrations in septic peritonitis: a

retrospective study of 83 dogs (2007–2012). *J Vet Emerg Crit Care* 2015;25(3):388–395.

21 Holahan ML, Brown AJ, Drobatz KJ. The association of blood lactate concentration with outcome in dogs with idiopathic immune-mediated hemolytic anemia: 173 cases (2003–2006). *J Vet Emerg Crit Care* 2010;20(4):413–420.

22 Mooney E, Raw C, Hughes D. Plasma lactate concentration as a prognostic biomarker in dogs with gastric dilation and volvulus. *Top Compan Anim Med* 2014;29(3):71–76.

23 Stevenson CK, Kidney BA, Duke T, et al. Serial blood lactate concentrations in systemically ill dogs. *Vet Clin Pathol* 2007;36(3):234–239.

24 Boysen SR, Dorval P. Effects of rapid intravenous 100% L-isomer lactated Ringer's administration on plasma lactate concentrations in healthy dogs. *J Vet Emerg Crit Care* 2014;24(5):571–577.

25 Aarnes TK, Bednarski RM, Bednarski RM, et al. Effect of intravenous administration of lactated Ringer's solution or hetastarch for the treatment of isoflurane-induced hypotension in dogs. *J Am Vet Med Assoc* 2009;70(11):1345–1353.

26 Ateca LB, Dombrowski SC, Silverstein DC. Survival analysis of critically ill dogs with hypotension with or without hyperlactatemia: 67 cases (2006–2011). *J Am Vet Med Assoc* 2015;246(1):100–104.

27 Butler AL, Campbell VL, Wagner AE, et al. Lithium dilution cardiac output and oxygen delivery in conscious dogs with systemic inflammatory response syndrome. *J Vet Emerg Crit Care* 2008;18(3):246–257.

28 Buriko Y, van Winkle TJ, Drobatz KJ, et al. Severe soft tissue infections in dogs: 47 cases (1996–2006). *J Vet Emerg Crit Care* 2008;18(6):608–618.

29 Nel M, Lobetti RG, Keller N, et al. Prognostic value of blood lactate, blood glucose, and hematocrit in canine babesiosis. *J Vet Intern Med* 2004;18(4):471–476.

30 Kitagawa H, Yasuda K, Kitoh K, et al. Blood gas analysis in dogs with heartworm caval syndrome. *J Vet Med Sci* 1994;56(5):861–867.

31 Bright JM, Golden AL, Gompf RE. Evaluation of the calcium channel-blocking agents diltiazem and verapamil for treatment of feline hypertrophic cardiomyopathy. *J Vet Intern Med* 1991;5(5):272–282.

32 Costello MF, Drobatz KJ, Aronson LR, et al. Underlying cause, pathophysiologic abnormalities, and response to treatment in cats with septic peritonitis: 51 cases (1990–2001). *J Am Vet Med Assoc* 2004;225(6):897–902.

33 Parsons KJ, Owen LJ, Lee K, et al. A retrospective study of surgically treated cases of septic peritonitis in the cat (2000–2007). *J Small Anim Pract* 2009;50(10):518–524.

34 Hayes G, Mathews K, Doig G, et al. The Feline Acute Patient Physiologic and Laboratory Evaluation (Feline APPLE) Score: a severity of illness stratification system for hospitalized cats. *J Vet Intern Med* 2011;25(1):26–38.

35 Hayes G, Mathews K, Doig G, et al. The acute patient physiologic and laboratory evaluation (APPLE) score: a severity of illness stratification system for hospitalized dogs. *J Vet Intern Med* 2010;24(5):1034–1047.

36 Kohen CJ, Hopper K, Kass PH, Epstein SE. Retrospective evaluation of the prognostic utility of lactate, base deficit, pH, and anion gap in canine and feline emergency patients. *J Vet Emerg Crit Care* 2018;28:54–61.

37 Reineke EL, Rees C, Drobatz KJ. Association of blood lactate concentration with physical perfusion variables, blood pressure, and outcome for cats treated at an emergency service. *J Am Vet Med Assoc* 2015;247(1):79–84.

38 Beer KAS, Syring RS, Drobatz KJ. Evaluation of plasma lactate concentration and base excess at the time of hospital admission as predictors of gastric necrosis and outcome and correlation between those variables in dogs with gastric dilatation-volvulus: 78 cases (2004–2009). *J Am Vet Med Assoc* 2013;242(1):54–58.

39 de Papp E, Drobatz KJ, Hughes D. Plasma lactate concentration as a predictor of gastric necrosis and survival among dogs with gastric dilatation-volvulus: 102 cases (1995–1998). *J Am Vet Med Assoc* 1999;215(1):49–52.

40 Bonczynski JJ, Ludwig LL, Barton LJ, et al. Comparison of peritoneal fluid and peripheral blood ph, bicarbonate, glucose, and lactate concentration as a diagnostic tool for septic peritonitis in dogs and cats. *Vet Surg* 2003;32(2):161–166.

41 Levin GM, Bonczynski JJ, Ludwig LL, et al. Lactate as a diagnostic test for septic peritoneal effusions in dogs and cats. *J Am Anim Hosp Assoc* 2004;40(5):364–371.

42 Szabo SD, Jermyn K, Neel J, Mathews KG. Evaluation of postceliotomy peritoneal drain fluid volume, cytology, and blood-to-peritoneal fluid lactate and glucose differences in normal dogs. *Vet Surg* 2011;40(4):444–449.

157

Emerging Monitoring Techniques

Rodrigo C. Rabelo, DVM, EMT, MSc, PhD, DBVECC

Intensivet Veterinary Consulting, Brazil

Introduction

Animals with hemodynamic compromise often require intensive and continuous monitoring to assess the response to treatment as well as to rapidly identify deterioration in clinical status. There are numerous potential tools for hemodynamic monitoring and this chapter will review some of the newer monitoring techniques available.

Venous Oxygen Monitoring

Venous hemoglobin oxygen saturation (SvO_2) has been utilized as an effective resuscitation endpoint. SvO_2 is an indirect measure of tissue oxygenation. There are three main determinants of SvO_2: cardiac output, hemoglobin concentration, and arterial oxygen content (CaO_2). An uncompensated rise in VO_2 (such as fever or seizure activity) or a decrease in DO_2 will reduce SvO_2. On the other hand, an improvement of oxygen supply, as well as reductions in VO_2, can increase the SvO_2[1,2].

Venous hemoglobin oxygen saturation can be measured continuously by an indwelling oximetry catheter, or intermittently evaluated via blood gas analysis or co-oximetry. Most blood gas machines measure PvO_2 and use a human algorithm for the oxygen-hemoglobin dissociation curve to calculate the corresponding SvO_2. Some blood gas machines contain a co-oximeter and assess hemoglobin saturation directly. It is important to note that all commercial blood gas machines designed for human blood and can impair their accuracy for assessment of SvO_2 in animals.

Venous hemoglobin oxygen saturation measured via a pulmonary artery catheter has been considered ideal for hemodynamic assessment but as mixed venous blood samples are unlikely to be available in the emergency room patient, central venous SvO_2 ($ScvO_2$) is most commonly used for monitoring purposes. Central venous SvO_2 values of $\geq 70\%$ are recommended as a resuscitation endpoint [3,4]. The SvO_2 of peripheral venous blood may not reflect central venous values in the hemodynamically unstable patient and are not recommended for use as a resuscitation endpoint. Central venous blood samples can be obtained by intermittent jugular venepuncture or more ideally an indwelling jugular catheter.

A reduction in SvO_2 may be an early indicator that the patient's clinical condition is deteriorating, even when blood pressure or heart rate are normal after resuscitation in dogs [5,6]. When SvO_2 is less than 65%, it indicates increased oxygen extraction due to decreased oxygen supply. This oxygen supply may drop with inadequate cardiac output, anemia, hypoxemia or even with a rise in oxygen demand. On the other hand, an SvO_2 higher than 75% may suggest an underlying defect in oxygen extraction, as can occur with mitochondrial dysfunction with sepsis or cytotoxic tissue hypoxia (cyanide poisoning for example) (see Chapter 159) [2].

The $ScvO_2$ was used as a gold standard parameter for resuscitation of human septic patients and as a guide by the Global Sepsis Alliance and the Surviving Sepsis Campaign until 2015. Although some studies on early goal-directed therapy in patients with severe sepsis and septic shock showed that maintenance of a continuously measured $ScvO_2$ above 70% resulted in a reduction in mortality compared with the same treatment without $ScvO_2$ monitoring, new evidence has shown that its interpretation should be carefully assessed in conjunction with a complete clinical examination and lactate clearance, preferably with the circulatory system sonographic assessment [4,7–10].

One study in dogs with severe sepsis and/or septic shock evaluated changes in tissue perfusion parameters in response to goal-directed hemodynamic resuscitation. In this study, resuscitation was aimed at restoring parameters related to tissue perfusion, including capillary refill time, central venous pressure, blood pressure, lactate, base deficit, and $ScvO_2$. A higher $ScvO_2$ was associated with a lower risk of death [5].

Given the current evidence, $ScvO_2$ appears to be an effective endpoint to guide resuscitation but integration with other parameters such as lactate concentration and physical examination is important (see Chapter 156).

Peripheral Hemodynamic Parameters

Being very well defined as "acute circulatory failure" by Weil in 1979, when the cardiovascular system fails to provide cells with adequate oxygen flow to maintain physiology, shock is a very complex syndrome that continues to challenge many emergency doctors [11,12].

Clinically, arterial hypotension represents as a cardinal sign of classic shock, but it is not always present with occult or cryptic shock [11,13]. Therefore, the diagnosis of peripheral vasoconstriction (peripheral hypothermia, pale mucous membrane, delayed capillary refil time, oliguria, decrease of bowel sounds or loss of sensitivity to detect a pulse curve by pulse oximeter) is an essential part of emergency patient evaluation. When vasoconstriction is caused by activation of the sympathetic nervous system, it can prevent the fall in blood pressure [14–19]. Parameters such as peripheral temperature, sublingual capnometry, and tissue oximetry may allow identification of patients with hemodynamic instability despite the absence of hypotension.

Temperature Gradient Monitoring

In most species (dogs, cats, and humans, for example), the physiological response in the face of low tissue perfusion consists of raising the sympathetic tone while reducing the vagal efferent activity (parasympathetic). This reflex will induce tachycardia and vasoconstriction reflex, mainly in the skin, skeletal muscle, kidneys, gastrointestinal tract, and splanchnic vascular bed, thereby enabling it to divert blood to the central circulation. This will maintain the activity of essential components for immediate survival, including the heart, central nervous system (CNS), and lungs [18,20–22].

Temperature gradient monitoring is based on the concept that skin vasoconstriction is an early sign of hypoperfusion [15,19]. The technique is performed by checking the temperature of the interdigital space or the plantar pad of the posterior limb of dogs and cats. A double laser infra-red thermometer with emissivity adjusted to 0.98E is directed to the interdigital membrane (metatarsal if possible) or the plantar pad (if smooth and absent of hyperkeratosis), as shown in Figure 157.1. The peripheral temperature is compared to the core temperature measured simultaneously. It is critical to measure the peripheral temperature at other points (tip of the nose, axillary and inguinal areas) to evaluate whether there is heterogeneity of peripheral flow, common in severe sepsis and septic shock, indicative of poor prognosis [22–27].

In a worldwide multicenter study performed by the author and colleagues, with 523 patients treated in emergency services in Spain, Portugal, and Brazil, the vast majority of emergency patients had a normal level of consciousness and heart rate, systemic blood pressure, and rectal temperature, all within physiological limits. These parameters, when analyzed separately, generate a false sense of safety, since they are considered the gold standard in assessing systemic perfusion, when in fact they reflect the status of the central circulatory bed, with low sensitivity in the evaluation of the peripheral hemodynamic segment [28,29]. Many of these same patients demonstrated peripheral hypothermia and hyperlactatemia (occult or cryptic shock), often with concurrent low urinary output and no bowel sounds. This supports the concept that the central circulation is maintained thanks to this flow deviation from the peripheral bed [28,30–33].

The temperature gradient between the core and the periphery (delta Tcp) should be <6.5 °C in dogs and ≤7.5 °C in cats. If delta Tcp is increased but core temperature is still within the normal range, this suggests that peripheral vasoconstriction is compensating effectively. If delta Tcp is reduced and core temperature is low, the animal is more seriously hemodynamically compromised [31,32,34]. Figure 157.2 describes the Line of Life counted from the hemodynamic evolution of the critically ill patient.

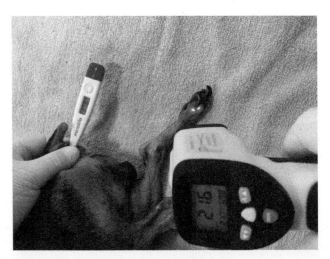

Figure 157.1 Peripheral and rectal temperatures are measured for calculating the delta Tcp.

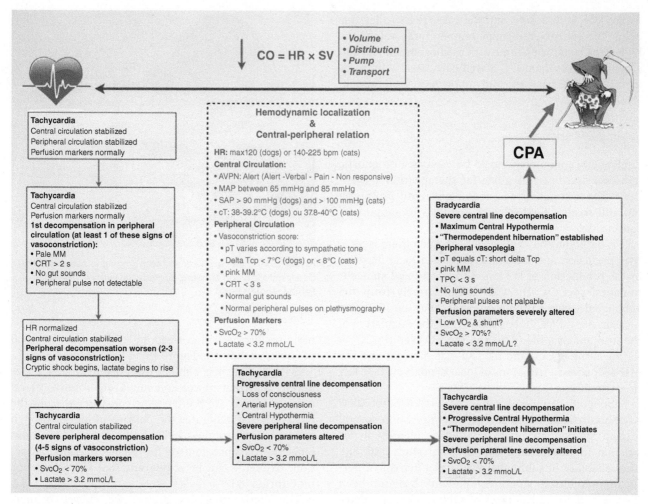

Figure 157.2 The Line of Life describes the hemodynamic evolution and the organic response to low cardiac output of the critically ill patient.

It is also important to stress that the values of 6.5 °C and 7.5 °C are alert indicators, based on the studies of Joly and Weil (1969), Kaplan (2001), and Lima and colleagues (2009) in human patients, and in our recent studies with populations of normal dogs and cats (unpublished data) [21,26,33]. More studies are in progress to improve the sensitivity and specificity of this parameter.

It is necessary to be attentive to the following information when assessing delta Tcp.

- The higher the peripheral vasoconstriction, the higher the core–peripheral temperature gradient.
- There is grave concern when the gradient is greater than 10 °C or when the delta Tcp persists above the normal range for more than 24 hours.
- The peripheral sensor needs to be placed where there is production of heat and minimal movement (interdigital space of the left hindlimb is the standard).
- The presence of central hypothermia, an ambient temperature lower than 20 °C and/or vasodilatory

shock tends to limit the use of this central–peripheral gradient.
- In cases of severe vasoplegia, the gradient tends to be shorter with an associated central hypothermia.

Evaluation of other temperature gradients can also be extremely useful for monitoring the peripheral circulatory state in the severely ill patient.

Delta Tskin-diff is the gradient obtained when the temperature sensor is directed to the interdigital space of the left forelimb compared to the medial aspect of the same limb in the region of the midradius. This technique is more suitable for environments where the temperature may vary (mainly the operating room, OR). Values of delta Tskin-diff greater than 4 °C indicate severe vasoconstriction in anesthetized patients, and the normal would be a delta Tskin-diff close to 0 °C [15,19].

When the gradient between the patient's skin (measured at the same point as described for delta Tcp) and the room temperature reaches a value lower than 4–6 °C over 12 hours of hospitalization, there is a correlation with a poor survival rate. The smaller this delta Tpr (peripheral–room temperature) value, the higher the lactate in people with cardiogenic shock, and a delta Tpr less than 5 °C is well correlated with lower cardiac indexes (the same did not occur in septic shock) [15,19,35].

Sublingual Capnometry

Sublingual capnometry should be used as a prognostic indicator and not as a guide for therapeutic interventions. The technique is recent and apparently promising but still require further clinical studies to support its routine use.

It is based on the knowledge that when there is local hypoperfusion and ischemia, there is a local increase in the production of H+ions and lactate and an accumulation of CO_2. The CO_2 diffuses freely from the sublingual tissue to the tonometer, allowing its direct measurement ($PgCO_2$ or $PsICO_2$) and the calculation of the intramucosal pH (pHi) and the CO_2 gap ($PgCO_2$ – $PaCO_2$). The $PgCO_2$ and the CO_2 gap increase and the pHi decreases in situations of local hypoxia such as low flow conditions.

Sublingual capnometry has been shown to identify hemorrhagic shock and predict survival in several human studies, although it failed to identify hypovolemia in one human experimental study [36–38]. The reliability of sublingual PCO_2 as a marker of perfusion in clinical veterinary patients has not been determined. The advantages of sublingual capnometry include it being non-invasive, simple, easy to operate and with good correlation with gastrointestinal tonometry, serum lactate levels, and SvO_2. Its disadvantages include its newness, high cost, paucity of clinical experience with the method, a risk of infection (contamination of the solution with thecapnoprobe) and it does not evaluate oxygenation. The $PsICO_2$ can only be correctly interpreted as an indicator of hypoperfusion in the light of $PaCO_2$ [39].

Hemodynamic Component of Pulse Oximetry

In addition to analyzing the respiratory component of pulse oximetry, the waveform generated by the pulse oximeter, the plethysmograph, permits the verification of some hemodynamic parameters especially relevant to the management of critical patients [40–42].

Even the systolic blood pressure can be measured with the aid of the oximeter. The system can be attached to a sphygmomanometer, and whenever the cuff is compressed, the plethysmographic curve will disappear. To deflate the cuff slowly, the first curve to appear on the

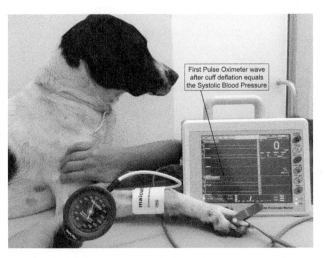

Figure 157.3 Pulse oximeter and sphygmomanometer used to check systolic blood pressure. Reproduced with permission of Pablo Ezequiel Otero.

monitor display will correspond to the systolic blood pressure, as shown in Figure 157.3.

Even though it is similar, the pulse oximeter curve is only a virtual image and not a quantitative blood pressure curve. As the curve is constructed from the pulsation that generates the passage of blood through the tissue, it produces information about tissue flow. Since flow is a prerequisite for normal metabolic function, oximetry can be a relevant tool for emergency monitoring [43].

The plethysmograph draws two curves primarily. The pulse wave is a high-frequency curve that responds to pressure variations, becoming a specular image of the blood pressure curve. The low-frequency curve, which reflects the respiratory changes, the product of cyclical fluctuations promoted by the variations that experience the systolic discharge. Figure 157.4 identifies the two curves and describes the components of the plethysmograph's dynamics. The amplitude and the design of the curve (with its ascendant lift, the baseline and the area under the curve, AUC) will enable the correct interpretation of the whole system [43].

Plethysmogram Monitoring (Delta P_{pleth})

The changes in intrathoracic pressure that occur with the respiratory cycle are registered in a plethysmograph, by moving the baseline and modifying the amplitude of each wave. These variations are a reflection of the alterations of the central venous system during the respiratory cycle, directly affecting right atrial filling, which then affects the next volume to be

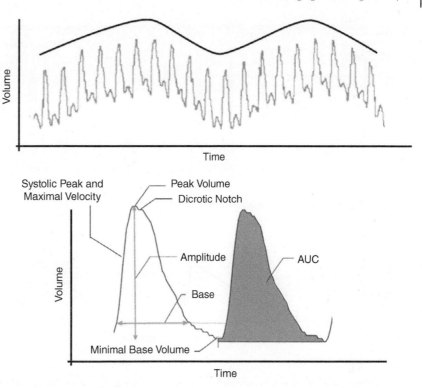

Figure 157.4 Components of the plethysmograph's dynamics. The amplitude and the design of the curve will enable the correct interpretation of the whole system. AUC, area under the curve.

ejected by the left ventricle, and reflected in time by the arterial pulse [44].

In spontaneous ventilation, during the inspiratory phase, the subatmospheric pressure produced in the thoracic cavity during inspiration draws both air and blood into the lungs. The blood is guided from the vena cava to the right circuit of the heart and then to the pulmonary vascular bed when a slight decline of peripheral venous pressure is registered. Simultaneously, the left ventricle decreases systolic ejection by 1–2 beats due to the retention of blood in the pulmonary circuit. In the expiratory phase, the positive pressure that occurs during expiration increases the systolic ejection, peripheral flow, amplitude, and peripheral venous pressure. Even if these changes are minimal, they can all be observed as a wave of lower frequency in the plethysmograph in association with inspiration [43,45–47].

During ventilation with positive pressure, changes recorded in the plethysmograph are exactly opposite to those observed during spontaneous ventilation.

The delta P_{pleth} is determined by analyzing the plethysmographic curve obtained from the pulse oximetry during the respiratory cycle, under controlled mechanical ventilation, using the same principle of arterial pulse contour analysis [45,46]. As the plethysmographic curve is obtained, the variation is calculated as a percentage of baseline amplitude obtained during apnea (without positive intrathoracic pressure):

Delta P_{pleth} Formula:

$$\Delta P_{pleth} (\%) = 100 \times (Ppleth_{max} - Ppleth_{min}) / [(Ppleth_{max} + Ppleth_{min}) / 2]$$

The delta P_{pleth} should be 9–15% in normovolemic patients, and Figure 157.5 shows the relationship between the plethysmographic curve and breathing during mechanical ventilation [43,48].

In general, no dynamic indicator employed to identify which patients are responsive to fluid therapy should be considered reliable in patients with cardiac arrhythmias, as well as significant changes in the chest wall or pulmonary distensibility. Also, as previously mentioned, this type of measurement have been validated in human patients under mechanical ventilation and using the contour of the blood pressure curve as a guide, and will probably not be fully trusted in patients with spontaneous ventilation in the emergency setting. This technique should be used in association with all other available methods of hemodynamic monitoring [44,47,49].

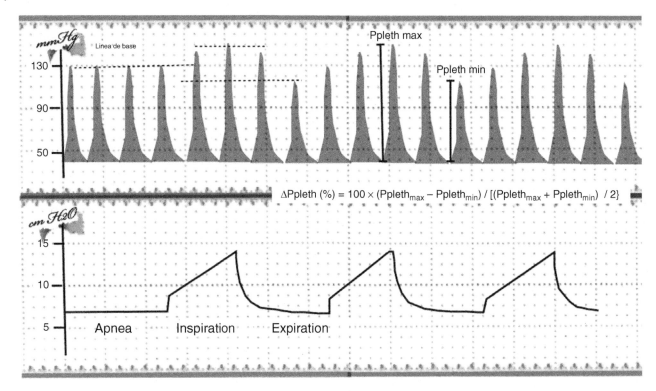

$$\Delta Ppleth\ (\%) = 100 \times (Ppleth_{max} - Ppleth_{min}) / [(Ppleth_{max} + Ppleth_{min}) / 2]$$

Figure 157.5 Relationship between the plethysmographic curve and breathing during a controlled ventilador cycle.

References

1 de Laforcade A, Silverstein D. Shock. In: *Small Animal Critical Care Medicine*, 2nd edn (eds Silverstein D, Hopper K). Elsevier Saunders, Philadelphia, 2015, pp. 26–29.

2 Hayes MA, Timmis AC, Yau EH, et al. Elevation of systemic oxygen delivery in the treatment of critically ill patients. *N Engl J Med* 1994;330(24):1717–1722.

3 Rivers EP, Yataco AC, Jaehne AK, Gill J, Disselkamp M. Oxygen extraction and perfusion markers in severe sepsis and septic shock: diagnostic, therapeutic and outcome implications. *Curr Opin Crit Care* 2015;21:381–387.

4 Rivers EP, Nguyen B, Havstad S, et al. Early goal-directed therapy in the treatment of severe sepsis and septic shock. *N Engl J Med* 2001;345:1368–1377.

5 Conti-Patara A, de Araujo Caldeira J, de Mattos-Junior E, et al. Changes in tissue perfusion parameters in dogs with severe sepsis/septic shock in response to goal-directed hemodynamic optimization at admission to ICU and the relation to outcome. *J Vet Emerg Crit Care* 2012; 22(4):409–418.

6 Young BC, Prittie JE, Fox P et al. Decreased central venous oxygen saturation despite normalization of heart rate and blood pressure post shock resuscitation in sick dogs. *J Vet Emerg Crit Care* 2014;24(2):154–161.

7 ProCESS Investigators, Yealy DM, Kellum JA, et al. A randomized trial of protocol-based care for early septic shock. *N Engl J Med* 2014;370(18):1683–1693.

8 ARISE Investigators, ANZICS Clinical Trials Groups, Peake SL, et al. Goal-directed resuscitation for patients with early septic shock. *N Engl J Med* 2014;371(16):1496–1506.

9 Mouncey PR, Osborn TM, Power GS, et al. Trial of early, goal-directed resuscitation for septic shock. *N Engl J Med* 2015;372:1301–1311.

10 Gattinoni L, Brazzi L, Pelosi P, et al. A trial of goal-oriented hemodynamic therapy in critically ill patients. *N Engl J Med* 1995;333(16):1025–1032.

11 Weil MH, Henning RJ. New concepts in the diagnosis and fluid treatment of circulatory shock. *Anesth Analg* 1979;58:124–132.

12 Levy MM, Dellinger RP, Townsend SR, et al. The Surviving Sepsis Campaign: results of an international guideline-based performance improvement program targeting severe sepsis. *Crit Care Med* 2010;38(2):367–374.

13 Chien LC, Lu KJ, Wo CC, et al. Hemodynamic patterns preceding circulatory deterioration and death after trauma. *J Trauma* 2007;62:928–932.

14 Holcomb JB, Salinas J, Mc Manus JM, et al. Manual vital signs reliably predict need for life-saving

interventions in trauma patients. *J Trauma* 2005;59:821–829.

15 Lima A, Bakker J. Noninvasive monitoring of peripheral perfusion. *Intensive Care Med* 2005;31:1316–1326.

16 Evans JA, May J, Ansong D, et al. Capillary refill time as an independent prognostic indicator in severe and complicated malaria. *J Pediatr* 2006;149:676–681.

17 Schriger DL, Baraff L. Capillary refill: is it a useful predictor of hypovolemic states? *Ann Emerg Med* 1991;20:601–605.

18 Lima AP, Beelen P, Bakker J. Use of a peripheral perfusion index derived from the pulse oximetry signal as a noninvasive indicator of perfusion. *Crit Care Med* 2002;30:1201–1213.

19 Lima A, Bakker J. Clinical monitoring of peripheral perfusion: there is more to learn. *Crit Care Med* 2014;18:113.

20 Miyagatani Y, Yukioka T, Ohta S, et al. Vascular tone in patients with hemorrhagic shock. *J Trauma* 1999;47:282–287.

21 Lima A, Jansen TC, Van Bommel J, et al. The prognostic value of the subjective assessment of peripheral perfusion in critically ill patients. *Crit Care Med* 2009;37(3): 934–938.

22 Mansel JC, Shaw DJ, Strachan FA, Gray A, Clutton RE. Comparison of peripheral and core temperatures in anesthetized hypovolaemic sheep. *Vet Anaesth Analg* 2008;35:45–51.

23 Tomasic M, Nann LE. Comparison of peripheral and core temperatures in anesthetized horses. *Am J Vet Res* 1999;60:648–651.

24 Burton AC. Temperature of skin: measurement and use as index of peripheral blood flow. *Meth Med Res* 1948;1:146–166.

25 Felder D, Russ E, Montgomery H, Horwitz O. Relationship in the toe of skin surface temperature to mean blood flow measured with a plethysmograph. *Clin Sci* 1954;13:251–257.

26 Kaplan LJ, McPartland K, Santora TA, et al. Start with a subjective assessment of skin temperature to identify hypoperfusion in intensive care unit patients. *J Trauma* 2001;50:620–627.

27 Sessler DI. Skin-temperature gradients are a validated measure of fingertip perfusion. *Eur J Appl Physiol* 2003;89:401–402.

28 Rabelo RC. Estudio y valor pronóstico de los parámetros relacionados con supervivencia en clínica de urgencias de pequeños animales: estudio multicéntrico. Doctoral thesis, *Universidade Complutense de Madrid*, 2008.

29 Rabelo RC, Arnold CF, Alsua SC. RICO Score – classificação rápida de sobrevida em cuidados intensivos. Variáveis inter-relacionadas em cães. *Clín Vet* 2009;78:28–38.

30 Isola JGMP. Parâmetros clínicos e laboratoriais, relacionados ao prognóstico, em cães hospitalizados com gastroenterite. Doutorado em Cirurgia Veterinária – FCAV UNESP, Jaboticabal, 2014.

Available at: https://repositorio.unesp.br/ handle/11449/122009 (accessed 19 February 2018).

31 Isola JGM, Santana AE, Moraes PC, Rabelo RC. Incidência da vasoconstrição e da parvovirose relacionadas com a sobrevivência em cães com gastroenterite. *J Latin Am Vet Emerg Crit Care Soc* 2014;6:120–126.

32 Isola JGM, Santana AE, Moraes PC, Rabelo RC. Relação da vasoconstrição, alterações neurológicas, e o nível de consciência em cães atendidos com gastroenterite. *J Latin Am Vet Emerg Crit Care Soc* 2014;6:127–133.

33 Joly HR, Weil MH. Temperature of the great toe as an indication of the severity of shock. *Circulation* 1969;39;131–138.

34 Isola, JGM, Santana AE, Pereira-Neto GB, Rabelo RC. Severe sepsis and septic shock survival in a clinical canine model. *Crit Care* 2013;17 Suppl 4:105.

35 Vincent JL, Moraine JJ, van der Linden P. Toe temperature versus transcutaneous oxygen tension monitoring during acute circulatory failure. *Intensive Care Med* 1988;14:64–68.

36 Baron BJ, Dutton RP, Zehtabchi S, et al. Sublingual capnometry for rapid determination of the severity of hemorrhagic shock. *J Trauma* 2007;62(1): 120–124.

37 Cammarata GA, Weil MH, Castillo CJ, et al. Buccal capnometry for quantitating the severity of hemorrhagic shock. *Shock* 2009;31(2):207–211.

38 Chung KK, Ryan KL, Rickards CA, et al. Progressive reduction in central blood volume is not detected by sublingual capnography. *Shock* 2012;37(6):586–591.

39 Weil MH, Nakagawa Y, Tang W, et al. Sublingual capnometry: a new noninvasive measurement for diagnosis and quantitation of severity of circulatory shock. *Crit Care Med* 1999;27(7):1225–1229.

40 Renner J, Broch O, Gruenewald M, et al. Non-invasive prediction of fluid responsiveness in infants using pleth variability index. *Anaesthesia* 2011;66(7):582–589.

41 Westphal GA, Silva E, Gonçalves AR, et al. Pulse oximetry wave variation as a noninvasive tool to assess volume status in cardiac surgery. *Clinics* 2009;64(4):337–343.

42 Murray WB, Foster PA. The peripheral pulse wave: information overlooked. *J Clin Monit* 1996;12:365–377.

43 Otero P, Portela D. Oximetria de pulso. In: *Emergências de Pequenos Animais* (ed. Rabelo RC). Elsevier, São Paulo, 2013, pp. 163–170.

44 Bartels K, Thiele RH. Advances in photoplethysmography: beyond arterial oxygen saturation. *Can J Anaesthesiol* 2015;62(12):1313–1328.

45 Zimmermann M, Feibicke T, Keyl C, et al. Accuracy of stroke volume variation compared with pleth variability index to predict fluid responsiveness in mechanically ventilated patients undergoing major surgery. *Eur J Anaesthesiol* 2010;27(6):555–561.

46 Díaz F, Erranz B, Donoso A, et al. Influence of tidal volume on pulse pressure variation and stroke volume

variation during experimental intra-abdominal hypertension. *BMC Anesthesiol* 2015;15:127.

47 Liu Y, Wei LQ, Li GQ, et al. Pulse pressure variation adjusted by respiratory changes in pleural pressure, rather than by tidal volume, reliably predicts fluid responsiveness in patients with acute respiratory distress syndrome. *Crit Care Med* 2016;44(2):342–351.

48 Mallat J, Meddour M, Durville E, et al. Decrease in pulse pressure and stroke volume variations after mini-fluid challenge accurately predicts fluid responsiveness. *Br J Anaesth* 2015;115(3):449–456.

49 Hamzaoui O, Monnet X, Teboul JL. Evolving concepts of hemodynamic monitoring for critically ill patients. *Indian J Crit Care Med* 2015;19(4):220–226.

158

Ischemia-Reperfusion Injury

Josh Smith, DVM, DACVECC[1] and Robert Goggs, BVSc, DACVECC, DECVECC, PhD, MRCVS[2]

[1] *Veterinary Emergency Service, Middleton, MI, USA*
[2] *College of Veterinary Medicine, Cornell University, Ithaca, NY, USA*

Pathophysiology

Ischemia-reperfusion injury (IRI) occurs secondary to an initial restriction or cessation of blood flow to an organ followed by a return of perfusion and oxygen delivery [1]. Ischemia reduces oxygen delivery resulting in tissue hypoxia, and initiates a series of events that prime cells for dysfunction and necrosis upon reintroduction of blood flow. During ischemia, anaerobic metabolism leads to accumulation of hydrogen ions, resulting in intracellular acidosis and subsequent enzyme dysfunction and damage to regulatory and membrane channel proteins. Failure of ATP generation and subsequent ATPase pump dysfunction result in potassium efflux and influx of sodium, chloride, and calcium [2]. Increased intracellular sodium concentrations induce water influx by diffusion, resulting in cellular swelling [3]. Cytoplasmic calcium concentrations increase through release from organelles and influx from extracellular fluid, facilitating reactive oxygen species (ROS) generation and initiating both apoptosis and necrosis [4].

During ischemia, available ATP is progressively degraded to adenosine, followed by inosine and then hypoxanthine (Figure 158.1). In health, hypoxanthine is metabolized to urate by xanthine dehydrogenase (XD). In ischemic tissue, increased intracellular calcium concentrations activate calpain, which converts XD into xanthine oxidase (XO). Oxygen is required for XO-catalyzed metabolism of hypoxanthine. Thus in ischemic tissues, hypoxanthine cannot be metabolized normally and as hypoxia persists, both hypoxanthine and XO accumulate [2].

Reperfusion is necessary to restore oxygen delivery to ischemic tissues and increase ATP production, but it paradoxically worsens cellular injury and organ dysfunction. When oxygen is reintroduced, it enables XO to catalyze the conversion of water and hypoxanthine into urate and superoxide (Figure 158.2). A burst of ROS formation is seen within seconds of the onset of reperfusion wherein approximately 70% of the oxygen provided to the tissue is oxidized to superoxide by XO [3]. Xanthine oxidase is present in much higher amounts in dogs and rats compared to humans and rabbits, suggesting that it is a major player in canine reperfusion injury [2]. The superoxide formed can combine with nitric oxide to form peroxynitrite or be converted into hydrogen peroxide by superoxide dismutase (SOD). Catalase can then convert this hydrogen peroxide to water and oxygen, but hydrogen

Figure 158.1 During ischemia, ATP is sequentially hydrolyzed to hypoxanthine. The resultant reduction in available ATP leads to potassium efflux and movement of sodium, chloride, and calcium ions into cells. Increased intracellular calcium concentrations enable calpain activation which converts xanthine dehydrogenase to xanthine oxidase. These events cause cell dysfunction and swelling and set the stage for the damage that occurs following reintroduction of perfusion and an increased availability of oxygen and glucose. Reproduced with permission of John Wiley and Sons.

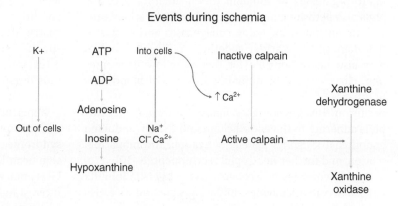

Textbook of Small Animal Emergency Medicine, First Edition. Edited by Kenneth J. Drobatz, Kate Hopper, Elizabeth Rozanski and Deborah C. Silverstein.
© 2019 John Wiley & Sons, Inc. Published 2019 by John Wiley & Sons, Inc.
Companion Website: www.wiley.com/go/drobatz/textbook

Events during reperfusion

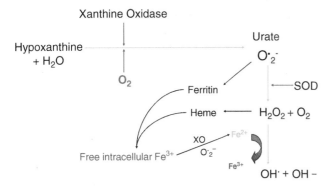

Figure 158.2 When oxygen availability increases following restoration of blood flow, the accumulated hypoxanthine is converted to urate and the superoxide radical by the action of xanthine oxidase. The superoxide radical can be converted into hydrogen peroxide by superoxide dismutase (SOD) or it can interact with ferritin to liberate intracellular ferric iron (Fe^{3+}). The hydrogen peroxide produced by SOD is also able to liberate intracellular ferric iron from hemoglobin. This reduced iron species can be oxidized to ferrous iron (Fe^{2+}). In turn, the ferrous iron enables the conversion of hydrogen peroxide into highly reactive hydroxyl radicals through a process that results in the regeneration of ferric iron that can continue to perpetuate the generation of further reactive oxygen species. Reproduced with permission of John Wiley and Sons.

peroxide can also combine with transition metals (usually free iron) to form the hydroxyl radical. Peroxynitrite and hydroxyl radicals are responsible for lipid peroxidation of cell membranes, oxidative damage to DNA, loss of membrane selective permeability, and degradation of structural proteins [2,5].

Neutrophils may mediate the majority of mucosal and microvascular injury with ischemia-reperfusion [1,6]. Neutrophils are attracted to ischemic tissue by XO and ROS and their infiltration is mediated by enhanced adhesion molecule expression. Activated neutrophils contribute to tissue injury in IRI through synthesis of additional ROS during the respiratory burst, with a 50–100-fold increase in oxidant production following exposure to micro-organisms or inflammatory mediators. Neutrophils also activate complement and release various proteolytic enzymes, including collagenases and elastases, that damage the vascular endothelium [7]. Neutrophils may also be responsible for the no-reflow phenomenon, characterized by diminished or absent blood flow in an area of tissue despite relief of prolonged vascular occlusion. This phenomenon may occur through neutrophils adhering to the endothelium and thereby inducing endothelial swelling, platelet activation, thrombus formation, and further neutrophil recruitment [8–10].

During episodes of ischemia, tissue hypoxia inhibits oxygen-sensitive enzymes, initiating signaling cascades

that control the transcription factor nuclear factor-kappa B (NF-kappa-B) [1]. Activation of NF-kappa-B leads to increases in inflammatory mediators and augmented expression of adhesion molecules, specifically intracellular adhesion molecule-1 and E-selectin [1,2]. During tissue ischemia-reperfusion, cyclo-oxygenase-2 (COX-2) is activated, leading to the formation of proinflammatory prostaglandins and ROS from arachidonic acid and the subsequent activation of phospholipase A_2. The cell death that accompanies IRI activates both the innate and adaptive immune systems via stimulation of the toll-like pattern recognition receptors (TLRs). During IRI, the TLRs are activated by interactions with damage-associated molecular pattern molecules including cfDNA, histones and high mobility group box 1 that are released from dying cells [1,11]. Activation of the TLRs results in production of inflammatory mediators, perpetuating tissue injury.

Tissues are protected from oxidative injury by antioxidant molecules, including proteins such as haptoglobin, ferritin, and ceruloplasmin [12], water-soluble compounds such as ascorbic acid (vitamin C) and glutathione [13], and fat-soluble molecules such as alpha-tocopherol (vitamin E), beta-carotene (vitamin A), and ubiquinol-10 [14]. Ultimately during IRI, however, the generation of ROS through the above mechanisms exceeds the capacity of the host antioxidant defenses. Lipid peroxidation, cell death, and accelerated inflammation result [15].

Disorders Associated with Ischemia-Reperfusion Injury

Ischemia-reperfusion injury likely contributes to the pathogenesis of a number of important emergent conditions of small animals (Table 158.1). A common cause is gastric dilation-volvulus (GDV) syndrome [16]. In animals with GDV syndrome, dilation and rotation of the stomach result in increased intragastric pressures and decreased venous return. This causes relative hypovolemia and obstructive shock as well as decreased gastric perfusion. Treatment of the condition involves restoration of intravascular volume, gastric decompression, and surgical correction. Irrespective of how these procedures are performed, reperfusion and hence IRI may result and can affect various organs including the stomach, intestines, spleen, liver, heart, and brain [17].

Reperfusion injury typically manifests within 3 hours of decompression [18]. In experimentally induced GDV syndrome, ATP concentrations in the fundus were not significantly different from baseline after 120 minutes of GDV, but were significantly reduced after 210 minutes. Interestingly, jejunal ATP concentrations were reduced

Table 158.1 Diseases in small animal emergency medicine associated with ischemia-reperfusion injury.

Disease process	Species affected	References
Arterial (aortic) thromboembolism	Cats > dogs	[21,22,24,26,88–97]
Cardiopulmonary arrest	Dogs, cats	[27,97]
Cardiopulmonary bypass	Dogs > cats	[98–106]
Crush injury	Dogs, cats	[33,107]
Diaphragmatic rupture with herniation	Cats > dogs	[108–111]
Gastric dilation-volvulus syndrome	Dogs	[17,81,112,113]
Intestinal incarceration/ strangulation	Dogs, cats	[114,115]
Mesenteric volvulus	Dogs > cats	[116–118]
Myocardial infarction	Dogs, cats	[119,120]
Organ transplantation	Cats	[121–125]
Spinal cord injury	Dogs > cats	[126–129]
Traumatic brain injury	Dogs, cats	[130–133]

within 120 minutes of GDV syndrome induction, concomitant with more severe mucosal injury, suggesting that the intestine may be compromised at least as quickly as the stomach with GDV syndrome [19]. Biomarkers of oxidative stress and antioxidant status have been assessed clinically in patients with GDV syndrome [20]. Consistent with IRI occurring in these patients, there were significant reductions in concentrations of key antioxidants including tocopherol and ascorbate during hospitalization.

Arterial thromboembolism (ATE) is a debilitating and potentially fatal complication of critical illness. Typically with ATE, thrombosis or embolization interrupts blood flow to the iliac arteries, although other vascular beds can be affected. ATE occurs most commonly secondary to feline cardiomyopathy [21], although low plasma arginine concentrations have also been associated with ATE [22]. This is potentially significant, because low arginine levels may contribute to increased platelet aggregation and potentiate IRI [23]. Thrombolytic therapy has been attempted in feline patients with ATE, but the complication rate is high. Reported adverse effects include hyperkalemia, azotemia, neurological signs, arrhythmias, acidosis, and sudden death (see Chapter 62) [24–26].

Reperfusion injury contributes significantly to the challenges faced after return of spontaneous circulation (ROSC) following cardiopulmonary arrest (CPA) [27]. During CPA, blood flow ceases and widespread ischemia occurs. After ROSC is achieved, oxygenated blood returns to ischemic, vasodilated tissues. In this setting, normoxic reperfusion in CPA is less damaging than hyperoxic reperfusion [28].

Myocardial infarction (MI) is an uncommon condition in dogs compared to humans [29], although dogs have been commonly used as models for MI in people. Myocardial ischemia causes the release of chemotactic factors with subsequent neutrophil migration, lipid peroxidation, and antioxidant depletion [30]. The invading neutrophils generate ROS and result in further injury to the vessels of the heart. Experimental studies in canine models have shown that administration of superoxide dismutase plus catalase reduced infarct size if given up to 75 minutes after occlusion [30]. A follow-up study showed that SOD had an equivalent effect to the combination, suggesting that IRI with MI is mediated principally by superoxide [31].

Although infrequent, crush injuries can result in IRI from reperfusion of skeletal muscles after removal of the crushing force [32]. Given the potential for crush injury with bite trauma, it is possible that IRI may also contribute to the pathogenesis of bite injuries. Crushed, ischemic tissue is markedly inflammatory such that following reperfusion, neutrophils invade in large numbers. The inflammation generated by the crush injury activates these neutrophils, leading to generation of high ROS concentrations that result in myocyte lipid peroxidation, myoglobin release, and subsequent myoglobinuria [33].

Ischemia-reperfusion injury likely contributes to the pathogenesis of spinal cord injury (SCI), myelomalacia, and ischemic myelopathy [34]. Previous landmark clinical trials in people evaluated the use of high-dose methylprednisolone sodium succinate (MPSS) to mitigate lipid peroxidation in SCI [35]. Although these data remain controversial, MPSS had no meaningful beneficial impact on outcomes in SCI and is not currently recommended [36].

Traumatic brain injury (see Chapter 19) can cause IRI due to ischemia that results from primary brain injury or develops secondary to excitotoxic or vasogenic edema formation and subsequent alterations in cerebral perfusion [36]. Given the very high brain lipid content and the limitations of neuronal repair and regeneration, cerebral IRI can have profound consequences. During cerebral IRI, alterations of endothelial cell reactivity, coagulation system activation, and granulocyte–endothelial cell interactions have been shown to affect the microvascular of the brain [37].

Identification of Ischemia-Reperfusion Injury

While the detrimental downstream effects of IRI on organ function may be readily apparent [38], specific identification of IRI is challenging. Various methods have been reported including measurement of reaction products, markers of oxidative stress, endogenous antioxidants, or markers of inflammation [39]. Few are widely available, straightforward to use, or well validated [40]. Although ROS can be measured directly [41], their high reactivity results in a fleeting existence that precludes easy quantification. Therefore, most methods focus on the downstream effects of IRI and ROS generation.

Measurement of reaction products involves measurement of malondialdehyde (MDA) or isoprostanes. Malondialdehyde forms when endoperoxides combine with unsaturated fatty acids and free iron and indicates that lipid peroxidation (although not necessarily IRI) has occurred. Measurement of MDA can be performed with the thiobarbituric acid reactive substances test or by ELISA and has been used to evaluate oxidative stress in dogs with hemolytic anemia, heart failure, nephrotoxicity, and parvoviral enteritis [42–45]. Measurement of MDA as a marker of IRI is confounded by generation of the compound *ex vivo* and as a result of thromboxane synthesis [40].

Isoprostanes are prostaglandin-like compounds formed when ROS oxidize cell membrane arachidonic acid. Isoprostanes, particularly F_2 forms, are considered a more reliable measurement of lipid peroxidation *in vivo* than MDA [46]. Isoprostane measurement has been used to identify lipid peroxidation in dogs with spinal cord injury [47,48], lymphoma [49], and critical illness [50]. However, they are best measured by mass spectrometry [51], which limits their clinical utility.

Detection of low levels of endogenous antioxidants offers an alternative means to assess a patient's oxidative stress. Glutathione occurs in the body in two forms: a reduced form (GSH) and an oxidized form (GSSG). In IRI, more glutathione will exist as the oxidized form, such that the ratio of the two forms can be used to determine the level of oxidative stress occurring [52]. This method is susceptible to spontaneous oxidation *ex vivo*, which artifactually increases the concentrations of GSSG. Measurements of glutathione have been used to identify oxidative stress in patients with GDV syndrome [20], critical illness [53], and various infectious and parasitic diseases [54–57]. Measurements of blood tocopherol concentrations also provide insight into IRI-induced oxidative stress. Abnormally low tocopherol concentrations have been identified in dogs with lymphoma [49], mast cell tumor [58], anesthesia [59], and in dogs enduring intense exercise [60]. In racing sled dogs, supplementing vitamin E prior to exercise can increase antioxidant levels post race [61], although the clinical relevance of this is unclear.

Numerous additional biomarkers have been evaluated for assessment of IRI, including tumor necrosis factor-alpha, interleukin (IL)-1, IL-6, IL-8, transforming growth factor-beta and cell-free DNA (cfDNA) [62,63]. Concentrations of these biomarkers can vary greatly during the course of illness, however. Many of these substances are labile and for some, their measurement is time-consuming and expensive [64]. Point-of-care tests for cfDNA hold promise for assessing patients with traumatic brain injury, sepsis, and cardiopulmonary arrest [65–67], although more work remains to be done validating cfDNA in IRI patients before it can be considered an alternative to standard testing [68]. As with many complex processes, maximum diagnostic accuracy may be obtained through the measurement of a panel of assays including peroxidation reaction products, antioxidants, and inflammatory markers. Such in-depth analyses are expensive and time-consuming and currently remain predominantly in the research realm.

Management of Ischemia-Reperfusion Injury

Numerous drugs and therapies have been evaluated for the prevention and treatment of IRI (Table 158.2) [69].

Table 158.2 Proposed therapies for IRI.

Proposed therapy	Disease or model studied	References
N-acetylcysteine	Canine myocardial dysfunction post CPA	[74]
Allopurinol	Feline intestinal ischemia, canine GDV syndrome	[84,112]
Deferoxamine	Canine experimentally induced GDV syndrome	[81]
DMSO	Canine GDV syndrome, renal ischemia	[81]
Hypothermia	Canine myocardial ischemia	[134]
Ischemic preconditioning	Canine myocardial ischemia	[135]
Ketamine	Canine cerebral ischemia	[136]
Lazaroids	Canine stroke, subarachnoid hemorrhage, sepsis	[137–140]
Lidocaine	Canine GDV syndrome	[71,72]
Nicardipine	Canine cerebral ischemia	[141]
Vitamin C	Canine renal transplant	[142]
Vitamin E	Canine ischemic stroke	[143]

CPA, cardiopulmonary arrest; DMSO, dimethyl sulfoxide; GDV, gastric dilation-volvulus.

Many have demonstrated promise in preclinical evaluations that use model systems, but most have failed once applied to real-world situations in human and veterinary clinical trials. In some cases, the therapy is effective only if given before the IRI injury occurs – a scenario that is rarely possible in clinical medicine. Here we discuss the therapies for which there is some evidence of benefit or where more work appears warranted.

Lidocaine

Lidocaine is an attractive therapy for the treatment of IRI because of its multimodal effects [70]. Lidocaine is a use-dependent fast sodium channel antagonist used as a local anesthetic and a class Ib antiarrhythmic agent. Additionally, it is an antagonist of ATP-sensitive potassium channels, a scavenger of superoxide and hydroxyl radicals, an inflammatory modulator, and an inhibitor of granulocytes [70].

There is moderate evidence for the prophylactic use of lidocaine in patients with GDV syndrome. Two studies have been performed. The first, a retrospective study, evaluated IV lidocaine administered after medical treatment and decompression, but before surgery [71]. That study showed no difference in complication rate or mortality between treated and untreated groups. The second study was a prospective trial that implemented lidocaine prior to fluid therapy and gastric decompression [72]. When administered prior to decompression and hence before the likely peak of reperfusion injury, lidocaine treatment significantly decreased the incidence of kidney injury, cardiac arrhythmias and coagulation disorders and shortened hospitalization. There was no significant effect on mortality, although the study was not powered to detect such a benefit [71,72].

N-Acetylcysteine

N-acetylcysteine (NAC) is a glutathione precursor that penetrates into cells and acts to replenish intracellular glutathione concentrations. Such increases in glutathione availability may result in improved cellular antioxidant capabilities. In experimental models, NAC reduces cardiopulmonary bypass-induced lung injury, preserves systolic function, and reduces myocardial edema in cardiopulmonary arrest [73,74]. Administration of NAC to critically ill dogs significantly increased glutathione availability but did not affect illness severity or outcome, although the study was likely underpowered to detect such differences [50]. Although dogs with spinal cord injury have demonstrable oxidative stress, administration of NAC intravenously before hemilaminectomy has no effect on urinary isoprostane excretion or neurological outcome [75].

Currently, the evidence for safety of NAC is excellent, but the evidence for efficacy of clinically meaningful endpoints is equivocal. Until further studies are conducted, the use of NAC is a reasonable pragmatic choice.

Ischemic Preconditioning

Ischemic preconditioning is a process by which short, controlled episodes of ischemia and reperfusion prime tissues in an effort to protect them from subsequent damage during IRI [76]. Preconditioning has most frequently been studied in myocardial ischemia models, with promising early results. In dogs, preconditioned hearts appear to have improved antioxidant capacity with less severe IRI following subsequent ischemia [77]. At this time, preconditioning has not been clinically studied in veterinary medicine, but two recent human clinical trials suggest the benefits may not translate from bench to bedside [78,79]. The reason is unclear, but may relate to patient heterogeneity, intercurrent disease or the limited benefit attainable from any one novel intervention [80].

Deferoxamine

During ischemia, intracellular iron bound to ferritin is released. Superoxide and hydrogen peroxide generated during reperfusion also mobilize iron from ferritin and heme, respectively, resulting in large amounts of free iron following reperfusion. Ferric iron (Fe^{3+}) is required for the Haber–Weiss reaction that results in formation of the hydroxyl radical, a potent oxidizing agent principally responsible for lipid peroxidation [2,40]. Deferoxamine, an iron chelator, has been evaluated experimentally in the treatment of IRI associated with GDV syndrome and was shown to decrease mortality, but the safety and clinical efficacy of this treatment have not been assessed [81].

Allopurinol

Allopurinol is a potent XO inhibitor that has been shown to attenuate the IRI in canine liver [82] and myocardium [83], and feline intestine [84]. The evidence to date, however, suggests that allopurinol may only be efficacious when used as a pretreatment. Clinical studies in which allopurinol is administered after or during IRI are lacking, and hence there is currently little to support its use in veterinary patients.

Cyclosporine

Cyclosporine is a calcineurin inhibitor that decreases activity of lymphocytes, especially T-cells. Calcineurin mediates calcium-triggered apoptosis in cells deprived of growth factors and is likely to be involved in the initiation of calcium-triggered apoptosis in IRI [4]. As such, there has been considerable interest in the potential use of calcineurin inhibitors to reduce IRI. Cyclosporine is also hypothesized to inhibit the opening of mitochondrial permeability-transition pores, and attenuate lethal myocardial injury associated with reperfusion in patients with myocardial infarction [29].

An initial small-scale prospective trial in people assessed the use of cyclosporine at the time of percutaneous coronary intervention, and demonstrated a reduction in the infarct size in the treatment group [85]. A larger follow-up study was unable to confirm this potential benefit, however [86]. The drug is widely used as an immunosuppressive in veterinary medicine and there are some experimental data suggesting efficacy in canine IRI model systems [82], but there are currently no studies investigating its use as an agent for IRI in veterinary patients.

Remifentanil

Remifentanil is a short-acting mu-agonist opioid that is degraded by plasma and tissue esterases. It has been investigated in mouse models as a preconditioning agent for IR injury with intestinal ischemia. Initiation of remifentanil prior to reperfusion of mouse intestines

was associated with decreased destruction of villi and IR injury [87]. This therapy has not yet been investigated clinically in veterinary or human medicine.

Conclusions and Clinical Recommendations

In IRI, tissue injury results from both diminished blood flow (ischemia) and subsequent reperfusion. Ischemia damages cells and primes tissue for injury following restoration of blood flow wherein generation of reactive oxygen species and activation of the innate immune system occur. Commonly associated conditions include GDV syndrome, feline arterial thromboembolism, and brain and spinal cord injury. Reperfusion injury can be difficult to identify, and the necessary biochemical testing is rarely conducted in a clinical setting. It is reasonable to assume that IRI has occurred or will occur during the management of patients with associated conditions and hence therapy may be initiated on an empiric basis. Evidence of efficacy is lacking for the majority of available therapies. Evidence exists supporting the use of lidocaine in dogs with GDV syndrome and may support the use of N-acetylcysteine in GDV syndrome and in other disease processes associated with IRI.

References

1 Eltzschig HK, Eckle T. Ischemia and reperfusion – from mechanism to translation. *Nat Med* 2011;17(11):1391–1401.

2 McMichael M, Moore RM. Ischemia-reperfusion injury pathophysiology, part I. *J Vet Emerg Crit Care* 2004;14(4):231–241.

3 Yapca OE, Borekci B, Suleyman H. Ischemia-reperfusion damage. *Eurasian J Med* 2013;45(2):126–127.

4 Shibasaki F, McKeon F. Calcineurin functions in Ca(2+)-activated cell death in mammalian cells. *J Cell Biol* 1995;131(3):735–743.

5 Radi R, Beckman JS, Bush KM, Freeman BA. Peroxynitrite-induced membrane lipid peroxidation: the cytotoxic potential of superoxide and nitric oxide. *Arch Biochem Biophys* 1991;288(2):481–487.

6 Schofield ZV, Woodruff TM, Halai R, et al. Neutrophils – a key component of ischemia-reperfusion injury. *Shock* 2013;40(6):463–470.

7 Korthuis RJ, Granger DN. Reactive oxygen metabolites, neutrophils, and the pathogenesis of ischemic-tissue/reperfusion. *Clin Cardiol* 1993;16(4 Suppl 1):I19–I26.

8 Barroso-Aranda J, Schmid-Schonbein GW, Zweifach BW, Engler RL. Granulocytes and no-reflow phenomenon in irreversible hemorrhagic shock. *Circ Res* 1988;63(2):437–447.

9 Kuijper PH, Gallardo Torres HI, Lammers JW, et al. Platelet and fibrin deposition at the damaged vessel wall: cooperative substrates for neutrophil adhesion under flow conditions. *Blood* 1997;89(1): 166–175.

10 Weber C, Springer TA. Neutrophil accumulation on activated, surface-adherent platelets in flow is mediated by interaction of Mac-1 with fibrinogen bound to alphaIIbbeta3 and stimulated by platelet-activating factor. *J Clin Invest* 1997;100(8):2085–2093.

11 Yu Y, Tang D, Kang R. Oxidative stress-mediated HMGB1 biology. *Front Physiol* 2015;6:93.

12 Halliwell B. Antioxidant defence mechanisms: from the beginning to the end (of the beginning). *Free Radic Res* 1999;31(4):261–272.

13 Jomova K, Valko M. Advances in metal-induced oxidative stress and human disease. *Toxicology* 2011;283(2-3):65–87.

14 Esterbauer H, Puhl H, Dieber-Rotheneder M, et al. Effect of antioxidants on oxidative modification of LDL. *Ann Med* 1991;23(5):573–581.

15 Jaeschke H. Reactive oxygen and mechanisms of inflammatory liver injury: present concepts. *J Gastroenterol Hepatol* 2011;26 Suppl 1:173–179.

16 Sharp CR. Gastric dilatation-volvulus. In: *Small Animal Critical Care Medicine*, 2nd edn (eds

Silverstein DC, Hopper D). Elsevier Saunders, Philadelphia, 2015, pp. 649–653.

17 Bruchim Y, Kelmer E. Postoperative management of dogs with gastric dilatation and volvulus. *Top Compan Anim Med* 2014;29(3):81–85.

18 Vajdovich P. Free radicals and antioxidants in inflammatory processes and ischemia-reperfusion injury. *Vet Clin North Am Small Anim Pract* 2008;38(1):31–123.

19 Peycke LE, Hosgood G, Davidson JR, et al. The effect of experimental gastric dilatation-volvulus on adenosine triphosphate content and conductance of the canine gastric and jejunal mucosa. *Can J Vet Res* 2005;69(3):170–179.

20 Walker TG, Chan DL, Freeman LM, et al. Serial determination of biomarkers of oxidative stress and antioxidant status in dogs with naturally occurring gastric dilatation-volvulus. *J Vet Emerg Crit Care* 2007;17(3):250–256.

21 Luis Fuentes V. Arterial thromboembolism: risks, realities and a rational first-line approach. *J Feline Med Surg* 2012;14(7):459–470.

22 McMichael MA, Freeman LM, Selhub J, et al. Plasma homocysteine, B vitamins, and amino acid concentrations in cats with cardiomyopathy and arterial thromboembolism. *J Vet Intern Med* 2000;14(5):507–512.

23 Johnson G 3rd, Tsao PS, Lefer AM. Cardioprotective effects of authentic nitric oxide in myocardial ischemia with reperfusion. *Crit Care Med* 1991;19(2):244–252.

24 Koyama H, Matsumoto H, Fukushima RU, Hirose H. Local intra-arterial administration of urokinase in the treatment of a feline distal aortic thromboembolism. *J Vet Med Sci* 2010;72(9):1209–1211.

25 Welch KM, Rozanski EA, Freeman LM, Rush JE. Prospective evaluation of tissue plasminogen activator in 11 cats with arterial thromboembolism. *J Feline Med Surg* 2010;12(2):122–128.

26 Pion PD. Feline aortic thromboemboli and the potential utility of thrombolytic therapy with tissue plasminogen activator. *Vet Clin North Am Small Anim Pract* 1988;18(1):79–86.

27 Smarick SD, Haskins SC, Boller M, Fletcher DJ. RECOVER evidence and knowledge gap analysis on veterinary CPR. Part 6: post-cardiac arrest care. *J Vet Emerg Crit Care* 2012;22 Suppl 1:S85–S101.

28 Marsala J, Marsala M, Vanicky I, et al. Post cardiac arrest hyperoxic resuscitation enhances neuronal vulnerability of the respiratory rhythm generator and some brainstem and spinal cord neuronal pools in the dog. *Neurosci Lett* 1992;146(2):121–124.

29 Yellon DM, Hausenloy DJ. Myocardial reperfusion injury. *N Engl J Med* 2007;357(11):1121–1135.

30 Werns SW, Shea MJ, Lucchesi BR. Free radicals in ischemic myocardial injury. *J Free Radic Biol Med* 1985;1(2):103–110.

31 Werns SW, Shea MJ, Driscoll EM, et al. The independent effects of oxygen radical scavengers on canine infarct size. Reduction by superoxide dismutase but not catalase. *Circ Res* 1985;56(6):895–898.

32 Malinoski DJ, Slater MS, Mullins RJ. Crush injury and rhabdomyolysis. *Crit Care Clin* 2004;20(1):171–192.

33 Thompson WW, Campbell GS. Studies on myoglobin and hemoglobin in experimental crush syndrome in dogs. *Ann Surg* 1959;149(2):235–242.

34 Okada M, Kitagawa M, Ito D, et al. Magnetic resonance imaging features and clinical signs associated with presumptive and confirmed progressive myelomalacia in dogs: 12 cases (1997–2008). *J Am Vet Med Assoc* 2010;237(10):1160–1165.

35 Bracken MB, Shepard MJ, Collins WF, et al. A randomized, controlled trial of methylprednisolone or naloxone in the treatment of acute spinal-cord injury. Results of the Second National Acute Spinal Cord Injury Study. *N Engl J Med* 1990;322(20):1405–1411.

36 DiFazio J, Fletcher DJ. Updates in the management of the small animal patient with neurologic trauma. *Vet Clin North Am Small Anim Pract* 2013;43(4):915–940.

37 del Zoppo GJ, Mabuchi T. Cerebral microvessel responses to focal ischemia. *J Cereb Blood Flow Metab* 2003;23(8):879–894.

38 Barie PS, Hydo LJ, Pieracci FM, et al. Multiple organ dysfunction syndrome in critical surgical illness. *Surg Infect* 2009;10(5):369–377.

39 McMichael MA. Oxidative stress, antioxidants, and assessment of oxidative stress in dogs and cats. *J Am Vet Med Assoc* 2007;231(5):714–720.

40 McMichael M. Ischemia-reperfusion injury: assessment and treatment, part II. *J Vet Emerg Crit Care* 2004;14(4):242–252.

41 Brisson BA, Miller CW, Chen G, et al. Detection of free radicals in ischemic and reperfused canine gracilis muscle flaps by use of spin-trapping electron paramagnetic resonance spectroscopy. *Am J Vet Res* 2001;62(3):384–388.

42 Pesillo SA, Freeman LM, Rush JE. Assessment of lipid peroxidation and serum vitamin E concentration in dogs with immune-mediated hemolytic anemia. *Am J Vet Res* 2004;65(12):1621–1624.

43 Freeman LM, Rush JE, Milbury PE, Blumberg JB. Antioxidant status and biomarkers of oxidative stress in dogs with congestive heart failure. *J Vet Intern Med* 2005;19(4):537–541.

44 Varzi HN, Esmailzadeh S, Morovvati H, et al. Effect of silymarin and vitamin E on gentamicin-induced nephrotoxicity in dogs. *J Vet Pharmacol Ther* 2007;30(5):477–481.

45 Panda D, Patra RC, Nandi S, Swarup D. Oxidative stress indices in gastroenteritis in dogs with canine parvoviral infection. *Res Vet Sci* 2009;86(1):36–42.

46 Morrow JD, Roberts LJ. The isoprostanes: unique bioactive products of lipid peroxidation. *Prog Lipid Res* 1997;36(1):1–21.

47 McMichael MA, Ruaux CG, Baltzer WI, et al. Concentrations of 15F2t isoprostane in urine of dogs with intervertebral disk disease. *Am J Vet Res* 2006;67(7):1226–1231.

48 Marquis A, Packer RA, Borgens RB, Duerstock BS. Increase in oxidative stress biomarkers in dogs with ascending-descending myelomalacia following spinal cord injury. *J Neurol Sci* 2015;353(1–2):63–69.

49 Winter JL, Barber LG, Freeman L, et al. Antioxidant status and biomarkers of oxidative stress in dogs with lymphoma. *J Vet Intern Med* 2009;23(2):311–316.

50 Viviano KR, VanderWielen B. Effect of N-acetylcysteine supplementation on intracellular glutathione, urine isoprostanes, clinical score, and survival in hospitalized ill dogs. *J Vet Intern Med* 2013;27(2):250–258.

51 Soffler C, Campbell VL, Hassel DM. Measurement of urinary F2-isoprostanes as markers of in vivo lipid peroxidation: a comparison of enzyme immunoassays with gas chromatography-mass spectrometry in domestic animal species. *J Vet Diagn Invest* 2010;22(2):200–209.

52 Center SA, Warner KL, Erb HN. Liver glutathione concentrations in dogs and cats with naturally occurring liver disease. *Am J Vet Res* 2002;63(8):1187–1197.

53 Viviano KR, Lavergne SN, Goodman L, et al. Glutathione, cysteine, and ascorbate concentrations in clinically ill dogs and cats. *J Vet Intern Med* 2009;23(2):250–257.

54 Kiral F, Karagenc T, Pasa S, et al. Dogs with Hepatozoon canis respond to the oxidative stress by increased production of glutathione and nitric oxide. *Vet Parasitol* 2005;131(1–2):15–21.

55 Almeida BF, Narciso LG, Melo LM, et al. Leishmaniasis causes oxidative stress and alteration of oxidative metabolism and viability of neutrophils in dogs. *Vet J* 2013;198(3):599–605.

56 Da Silva AS, Munhoz TD, Faria JL, et al. Increase nitric oxide and oxidative stress in dogs experimentally infected by Ehrlichia canis: effect on the pathogenesis of the disease. *Vet Microbiol* 2013;164(3–4):366–369.

57 Dimri U, Singh SK, Sharma MC, et al. Oxidant/antioxidant balance, minerals status and apoptosis in peripheral blood of dogs naturally infected with Dirofilaria immitis. *Res Vet Sci* 2012;93(1):296–299.

58 Finotello R, Pasquini A, Meucci V, et al. Redox status evaluation in dogs affected by mast cell tumour. *Vet Comp Oncol* 2014;12(2):120–129.

59 Lee JY. Oxidative stress due to anesthesia and surgical trauma and comparison of the effects of propofol and thiopental in dogs. *J Vet Med Sci* 2012;74(5):663–665.

60 Hinchcliff KW, Reinhart GA, DiSilvestro R, et al. Oxidant stress in sled dogs subjected to repetitive endurance exercise. *Am J Vet Res* 2000;61(5):512–517.

61 Baskin CR, Hinchcliff KW, DiSilvestro RA, et al. Effects of dietary antioxidant supplementation on oxidative damage and resistance to oxidative damage during prolonged exercise in sled dogs. *Am J Vet Res* 2000;61(8):886–891.

62 Arnalich F, Maldifassi MC, Ciria E, et al. Association of cell-free plasma DNA with perioperative mortality in patients with suspected acute mesenteric ischemia. *Clin Chim Acta* 2010;411(17-18):1269–1274.

63 Saini HK, Xu YJ, Zhang M, et al. Role of tumour necrosis factor-alpha and other cytokines in ischemia-reperfusion-induced injury in the heart. *Exp Clin Cardiol* 2005;10(4):213–222.

64 Kjelgaard-Hansen M, Goggs R, Wiinberg B, Chan DL. Use of serum concentrations of interleukin-18 and monocyte chemoattractant protein-1 as prognostic indicators in primary immune-mediated hemolytic anemia in dogs. *J Vet Intern Med* 2011;25(1):76–82.

65 Rodrigues Filho EM, Simon D, Ikuta N, et al. Elevated cell-free plasma DNA level as an independent predictor of mortality in patients with severe traumatic brain injury. *J Neurotrauma* 2014;31(19):1639–1646.

66 Garnacho-Montero J, Huici-Moreno MJ, Gutierrez-Pizarraya A, et al. Prognostic and diagnostic value of eosinopenia, C-reactive protein, procalcitonin, and circulating cell-free DNA in critically ill patients admitted with suspicion of sepsis. *Crit Care* 2014;18(3):R116.

67 Gornik I, Wagner J, Gasparovic V, et al. Prognostic value of cell-free DNA in plasma of out-of-hospital cardiac arrest survivors at ICU admission and 24 h post-admission. *Resuscitation* 2014;85(2):233–237.

68 Lippi G, Sanchis-Gomar F, Cervellin G. Cell-free DNA for diagnosing myocardial infarction: not ready for prime time. *Clin Chem Lab Med* 2015;53(12):1895–1901.

69 Verma S, Fedak PW, Weisel RD, et al. Fundamentals of reperfusion injury for the clinical cardiologist. *Circulation* 2002;105(20):2332–2336.

70 Cassutto BH, Gfeller RW. Use of intravenous lidocaine to prevent reperfusion injury and subsequent multiple organ dysfunction syndrome. *J Vet Emerg Crit Care* 2003;13(3):137–148.

71 Bruchim Y, Itay S, Shira BH, et al. Evaluation of lidocaine treatment on frequency of cardiac arrhythmias, acute kidney injury, and hospitalization time in dogs with gastric dilatation volvulus. *J Vet Emerg Crit Care* 2012;22(4):419–427.

72 Buber T, Saragusty J, Ranen E, et al. Evaluation of lidocaine treatment and risk factors for death associated with gastric dilatation and volvulus in dogs: 112 cases (1997–2005). *J Am Vet Med Assoc* 2007;230(9):1334–1339.

73 Qu X, Li Q, Wang X, et al. N-acetylcysteine attenuates cardiopulmonary bypass-induced lung injury in dogs. *J Cardiothorac Surg* 2013;8:107.

74 Fischer UM, Cox CS Jr, Allen SJ, et al. The antioxidant N-acetylcysteine preserves myocardial function and diminishes oxidative stress after cardioplegic arrest. *J Thorac Cardiovasc Surg* 2003;126(5):1483–1488.

75 Baltzer WI, McMichael MA, Hosgood GL, et al. Randomized, blinded, placebo-controlled clinical trial of N-acetylcysteine in dogs with spinal cord trauma from acute intervertebral disc disease. *Spine* 2008;33(13):1397–1402.

76 Lutz J, Thurmel K, Heemann U. Anti-inflammatory treatment strategies for ischemia/reperfusion injury in transplantation. *J Inflamm* 2010;7:27.

77 Murry CE, Jennings RB, Reimer KA. Preconditioning with ischemia: a delay of lethal cell injury in ischemic myocardium. *Circulation* 1986;74(5):1124–1136.

78 Meybohm P, Bein B, Brosteanu O, et al. A multicenter trial of remote ischemic preconditioning for heart surgery. *N Engl J Med* 2015;373(15):1397–1407.

79 Hausenloy DJ, Candilio L, Evans R, et al. Remote ischemic preconditioning and outcomes of cardiac surgery. *N Engl J Med* 2015;373(15):1408–1417.

80 Zaugg M, Lucchinetti E. Remote ischemic preconditioning in cardiac surgery – ineffective and risky? *N Engl J Med* 2015;373(15):1470–1472.

81 Lantz GC, Badylak SF, Hiles MC, Arkin TE. Treatment of reperfusion injury in dogs with experimentally induced gastric dilatation-volvulus. *Am J Vet Res* 1992;53(9):1594–1598.

82 Yamanoi A, Nagasue N, Kohno H, et al. Attenuation of ischemia-reperfusion injury of the liver in dogs by cyclosporine. A comparative study with allopurinol and methylprednisolone. *Transplantation* 1991;52(1):27–30.

83 Konya L, Bencsath P, Szenasi G, Feher J. Lack of effect of antioxidant therapy during renal ischemia and reperfusion in dogs. *Experientia* 1993;49(3):235–237.

84 Granger DN, McCord JM, Parks DA, Hollwarth ME. Xanthine oxidase inhibitors attenuate ischemia-induced vascular permeability changes in the cat intestine. *Gastroenterology* 1986;90(1):80–84.

85 Piot C, Croisille P, Staat P, et al. Effect of cyclosporine on reperfusion injury in acute myocardial infarction. *N Engl J Med* 2008;359(5):473–481.

86 Cung TT, Morel O, Cayla G, et al. Cyclosporine before PCI in patients with acute myocardial infarction. *N Engl J Med* 2015;373(11):1021–1031.

87 Cho SS, Rudloff I, Berger PJ, et al. Remifentanil ameliorates intestinal ischemia-reperfusion injury. *BMC Gastroenterol* 2013;13:69.

88 Killingsworth CR, Eyster GE, Adams T, et al. Streptokinase treatment of cats with experimentally induced aortic thrombosis. *Am J Vet Res* 1986;47(6):1351–1359.

89 Laste NJ, Harpster NK. A retrospective study of 100 cases of feline distal aortic thromboembolism: 1977–1993. *J Am Anim Hosp Assoc* 1995;31(6):492–500.

90 Pion PD. Feline aortic thromboemboli: t-PA thrombolysis followed by aspirin therapy and rethrombosis. *Vet Clin North Am Small Anim Pract* 1988;18(1):262–263.

91 Pion PD. Feline aortic thromboemboli. *Vet Clin North Am Small Anim Pract* 1988;18(1):260–262.

92 Reimer SB, Kittleson MD, Kyles AE. Use of rheolytic thrombectomy in the treatment of feline distal aortic thromboembolism. *J Vet Intern Med* 2006;20(2):290–296.

93 Schoeman JP. Feline distal aortic thromboembolism: a review of 44 cases (1990–1998). *J Feline Med Surg* 1999;1(4):221–231.

94 Boswood A, Lamb CR, White RN. Aortic and iliac thrombosis in six dogs. *J Small Anim Pract* 2000;41(3):109–114.

95 Lake-Bakaar GA, Johnson EG, Griffiths LG. Aortic thrombosis in dogs: 31 cases (2000–2010). *J Am Vet Med Assoc* 2012;241(7):910–915.

96 Winter RL, Sedacca CD, Adams A, Orton EC. Aortic thrombosis in dogs: presentation, therapy, and outcome in 26 cases. *J Vet Cardiol* 2012;14(2):333–342.

97 Fletcher DJ, Boller M, Brainard BM, et al. RECOVER evidence and knowledge gap analysis on veterinary CPR. Part 7: clinical guidelines. *J Vet Emerg Crit Care* 2012;22 Suppl 1:S102–S131.

98 Fujiwara M, Harada K, Mizuno T, et al. Surgical treatment of severe pulmonic stenosis under cardiopulmonary bypass in small dogs. *J Small Anim Pract* 2012;53(2):89–94.

99 Mizuno T, Kamiyama H, Mizuno M, et al. Plasma cytokine levels in dogs undergoing cardiopulmonary bypass. *Res Vet Sci* 2015;101:99–105.

100 Mizuno T, Mizukoshi T, Uechi M. Long-term outcome in dogs undergoing mitral valve repair with suture annuloplasty and chordae tendinae replacement. *J Small Anim Pract* 2013;54(2):104–107.

101 Uechi M, Harada K, Mizukoshi T, et al. Surgical closure of an atrial septal defect using cardiopulmonary bypass in a cat. *Vet Surg* 2011;40(4):413–417.

102 Uechi M, Mizukoshi T, Mizuno T, et al. Mitral valve repair under cardiopulmonary bypass in small-breed dogs: 48 cases (2006–2009). *J Am Vet Med Assoc* 2012;240(10):1194–1201.

103 Arai S, Griffiths LG, Mama K, et al. Bioprosthesis valve replacement in dogs with congenital tricuspid valve dysplasia: technique and outcome. *J Vet Cardiol* 2011;13(2):91–99.

104 Griffiths LG, Orton EC, Boon JA. Evaluation of techniques and outcomes of mitral valve repair in dogs. *J Am Vet Med Assoc* 2004;224(12):1941–1945.

105 Orton EC, Hackett TB, Mama K, Boon JA. Technique and outcome of mitral valve replacement in dogs. *J Am Vet Med Assoc* 2005;226(9):1500, 1508–1511.

106 Orton EC, Herndon GD, Boon JA, et al. Influence of open surgical correction on intermediate-term outcome in dogs with subvalvular aortic stenosis: 44 cases (1991–1998). *J Am Vet Med Assoc* 2000;216(3):364–367.

107 Song J, Ding H, Fan HJ, et al. Canine model of crush syndrome established by a digital crush injury device platform. *Int J Clin Exp Pathol* 2015;8(6):6117–6125.

108 Gibson TW, Brisson BA, Sears W. Perioperative survival rates after surgery for diaphragmatic hernia in dogs and cats: 92 cases (1990–2002). *J Am Vet Med Assoc* 2005;227(1):105–109.

109 Hambrook LE, Kudnig ST. Lung lobe torsion in association with a chronic diaphragmatic hernia and haemorrhagic pleural effusion in a cat. *J Feline Med Surg* 2012;14(3):219–223.

110 Minihan AC, Berg J, Evans KL. Chronic diaphragmatic hernia in 34 dogs and 16 cats. *J Am Anim Hosp Assoc* 2004;40(1):51–63.

111 Peterson NW, Buote NJ, Barr JW. The impact of surgical timing and intervention on outcome in traumatized dogs and cats. *J Vet Emerg Crit Care* 2015;25(1):63–75.

112 Badylak SF, Lantz GC, Jeffries M. Prevention of reperfusion injury in surgically induced gastric dilatation-volvulus in dogs. *Am J Vet Res* 1990;51(2):294–299.

113 Sharp CR, Rozanski EA. Cardiovascular and systemic effects of gastric dilatation and volvulus in dogs. *Top Compan Anim Med* 2014;29(3):67–70.

114 Di Cicco MF, Bennett RA, Ragetly C, Sippel KM. Segmental jejunal entrapment, volvulus, and strangulation secondary to intra-abdominal adhesions in a dog. *J Am Anim Hosp Assoc* 2011;47(3):e31–e35.

115 Hassinger KA. Intestinal entrapment and strangulation caused by rupture of the duodenocolic ligament in four dogs. *Vet Surg* 1997;26(4):275–280.

116 Junius G, Appeldoorn AM, Schrauwen E. Mesenteric volvulus in the dog: a retrospective study of 12 cases. *J Small Anim Pract* 2004;45(2):104–107.

117 Knell SC, Andreoni AA, Dennler M, Venzin CM. Successful treatment of small intestinal volvulus in two cats. *J Feline Med Surg* 2010;12(11):874–877.

118 Matushek KJ, Cockshutt JR. Mesenteric and gastric volvulus in a dog. *J Am Vet Med Assoc* 1987;191(3):327–328.

119 Hsu K, Snead E, Davies J, Carr A. Iatrogenic hyperadrenocorticism, calcinosis cutis, and myocardial infarction in a dog treated for IMT. *J Am Anim Hosp Assoc* 2012;48(3):209–215.

120 Mete A, McDonough SP. Epicardial coronary artery fibromuscular dysplasia, myocardial infarction and sudden death in a dog. *J Comp Pathol* 2011;144(1): 78–81.

121 Mehl ML, Kyles AE, Reimer SB, et al. Evaluation of the effects of ischemic injury and ureteral obstruction on delayed graft function in cats after renal autotransplantation. *Vet Surg* 2006;35(4): 341–346.

122 Schmiedt CW, Holzman G, Schwarz T, McAnulty JF. Survival, complications, and analysis of risk factors after renal transplantation in cats. *Vet Surg* 2008;37(7):683–695.

123 Schmiedt CW, Mercurio A, Vandenplas M, et al. Effects of renal autograft ischemic storage and reperfusion on intraoperative hemodynamic patterns and plasma renin concentrations in clinically normal cats undergoing renal autotransplantation and contralateral nephrectomy. *Am J Vet Res* 2010;71(10):1220–1227.

124 Schmiedt CW, Mercurio AD, Glassman MM, et al. Effects of renal autograft ischemia and reperfusion associated with renal transplantation on arterial blood pressure variables in clinically normal cats. *Am J Vet Res* 2009;70(11):1426–1432.

125 Snell W, Aronson L, Phillips H, et al. Influence of anesthetic variables on short-term and overall survival rates in cats undergoing renal transplantation surgery. *J Am Vet Med Assoc* 2015;247(3):267–277.

126 Olby N. The pathogenesis and treatment of acute spinal cord injuries in dogs. *Vet Clin North Am Small Anim Pract* 2010;40(5):791–807.

127 De Risio L, Adams V, Dennis R, et al. Magnetic resonance imaging findings and clinical associations in 52 dogs with suspected ischemic myelopathy. *J Vet Intern Med* 2007;21(6):1290–1298.

128 De Risio L, Adams V, Dennis R, et al. Association of clinical and magnetic resonance imaging findings with outcome in dogs suspected to have ischemic myelopathy: 50 cases (2000–2006). *J Am Vet Med Assoc* 2008;233(1):129–135.

129 Nakamoto Y, Ozawa T, Mashita T, et al. Clinical outcomes of suspected ischemic myelopathy in cats. *J Vet Med Sci* 2010;72(12):1657–1660.

130 Balbino M, Capone Neto A, Prist R, et al. Fluid resuscitation with isotonic or hypertonic saline solution avoids intraneural calcium influx after traumatic brain injury associated with hemorrhagic shock. *J Trauma* 2010;68(4):859–864.

131 Beltran E, Platt SR, McConnell JF, et al. Prognostic value of early magnetic resonance imaging in dogs after traumatic brain injury: 50 cases. *J Vet Intern Med* 2014;28(4):1256–1262.

132 Sande A, West C. Traumatic brain injury: a review of pathophysiology and management. *J Vet Emerg Crit Care* 2010;20(2):177–190.

133 Sharma D, Holowaychuk MK. Retrospective evaluation of prognostic indicators in dogs with head trauma: 72 cases (January–March 2011). *J Vet Emerg Crit Care* 2015;25(5):631–639.

134 Piktel JS, Rosenbaum DS, Wilson LD. Mild hypothermia decreases arrhythmia susceptibility in a canine model of global myocardial ischemia. *Crit Care Med* 2012;40(11):2954–2959.

135 Chen CL, Zheng H, Xuan Y, et al. The cardioprotective effect of hypoxic and ischemic preconditioning in dogs with myocardial ischemia-reperfusion injury using a double-bypass model. *Life Sci* 2015;141:25–31.

136 Werner C, Reeker W, Engelhard K, et al. [Ketamine racemate and S-(+)-ketamine. Cerebrovascular effects and neuroprotection following focal ischemia]. *Anaesthesist* 1997;46 Suppl 1:S55–S60.

137 Perkins WJ, Milde LN, Milde JH, Michenfelder JD. Pretreatment with U74006F improves neurologic outcome following complete cerebral ischemia in dogs. *Stroke* 1991;22(7):902–909.

138 Zoerle T, Ilodigwe DC, Wan H, et al. Pharmacologic reduction of angiographic vasospasm in experimental subarachnoid hemorrhage: systematic review and meta-analysis. *J Cereb Blood Flow Metab* 2012;32(9):1645–1658.

139 Maruki Y, Koehler RC, Kirsch JR, et al. Effect of the 21-aminosteroid tirilazad on cerebral pH and somatosensory evoked potentials after incomplete ischemia. *Stroke* 1993;24(5):724–730.

140 Johnson D, Hurst T, Prasad K, et al. Lazaroid pretreatment preserves gas exchange in endotoxin-treated dogs. *J Crit Care* 1994;9(4): 213–222.

141 Iwatsuki N, Ono K, Takahashi M, Tajima T. The effects of nicardipine given after 10-minutes complete global cerebral ischemia on neurologic recovery in dogs. *J Anesth* 1990;4(4):337–342.

142 Lee JI, Son HY, Kim MC. Attenuation of ischemia-reperfusion injury by ascorbic acid in the canine renal transplantation. *J Vet Sci* 2006;7(4): 375–379.

143 Rink C, Christoforidis G, Khanna S, et al. Tocotrienol vitamin E protects against preclinical canine ischemic stroke by inducing arteriogenesis. *J Cereb Blood Flow Metab* 2011;31(11):2218–2230.

159

Systemic Inflammatory Response Syndrome, Sepsis, and Multiple Organ Dysfunction Syndrome

Claire R. Sharp, BSc, BVMS (Hons), MS, DACVECC

School of Veterinary and Life Sciences Murdoch University, Murdoch, WA, Australia

Introduction

The systemic inflammatory response syndrome (SIRS) and sepsis are surprisingly common and associated with high morbidity and mortality in dogs and cats [1,2]. Dogs and cats commonly present to veterinary emergency rooms (ERs) with evidence of SIRS and it is vital for the emergency veterinarian to take an aggressive diagnostic and treatment approach to these patients in order to maximize the likelihood of a successful outcome. Identifying the underlying cause of SIRS and, specifically, differentiating infectious from non-infectious causes of SIRS, as well as recognizing organ dysfunction(s), are vital to guide appropriate and timely treatment.

Definitions

The current definitions for SIRS and sepsis used in veterinary medicine are derived from those originally published in human medicine [3,4]. Of note, revised definitions of sepsis and septic shock were recently introduced in human medicine (Sepsis-3) [5], so it is likely that the current veterinary definitions, used below, will ultimately be reconsidered.

Systemic inflammatory response syndrome is a clinical diagnosis, made on the basis of abnormalities in vital signs and white blood cell count. While specific criteria are published [6–10], there is no consensus in veterinary medicine; what denotes SIRS varies between species and publications (Table 159.1). Essentially, SIRS is considered present if the animal fulfills two (dogs) or three (cats) out of the four following SIRS criteria: (1) abnormal temperature, (2) abnormal heart rate, (3) tachypnea; and/or (4) a change in the leukon [6–10]. Sick cats with SIRS and sepsis are more likely to be hypothermic and bradycardic than dogs [9]. Since the primary aim of

having SIRS criteria is to flag patients that are systemically unwell and require prompt attention, the exact cutoff points for these parameters are less important than the overall assessment of the patient in light of their signalment, history, and physical examination findings.

Sepsis is the systemic inflammatory response to infection. Diagnosis of sepsis requires identification (or a high index of suspicion) of infection and fulfillment of SIRS criteria.

Severe sepsis is the presence of sepsis with decreased perfusion to the tissues and/or organ dysfunction(s). While there is no consensus definition for what denotes organ dysfunctions in veterinary medicine, various parameters have been suggested by different authors [1,5,11] (see Table 159.1).

Septic shock is said to occur in patients with sepsis and persistent arterial hypotension that is non-responsive to intravascular volume expansion; by definition, patients with septic shock are vasopressor dependent.

Multiple organ dysfunction syndrome (MODS) is defined as two or more dysfunctional organs in patients with SIRS or sepsis (Table 159.2) [1,5,11].

The changes in the Sepsis-3 definitions in human medicine occurred so as to remove an excessive focus on inflammation as the pathological process in sepsis, and move away from the misleading model that sepsis follows a continuum from sepsis, through severe sepsis, to septic shock, amongst other reasons [12].

As part of the new consensus definitions, sepsis is defined as life-threatening organ dysfunction caused by a dysregulated host response to infection. With this change, the term *severe sepsis* becomes superfluous. Sepsis-3 also includes a lay definition of sepsis as a life-threatening condition that arises when the body's response to an infection injures its own tissues and organs. In the new definition, organ dysfunction is identified as any acute change in total Sequential Organ

Textbook of Small Animal Emergency Medicine, First Edition. Edited by Kenneth J. Drobatz, Kate Hopper, Elizabeth Rozanski and Deborah C. Silverstein.
© 2019 John Wiley & Sons, Inc. Published 2019 by John Wiley & Sons, Inc.
Companion Website: www.wiley.com/go/drobatz/textbook

Table 159.1 Criteria for the systemic inflammatory response syndrome (SIRS) used in dogs and cats by various authors.

Criteria	Dogs (2/4 criteria)			Cats (3/4 criteria)	
	Hauptman et al. 1997 [13]	de Laforcade et al. 2003 [14]	Okano et al. 2002 [15]	Brady et al. 2000 [16]	DeClue et al. 2011 [17]
Temperature (°F/°C)					
• Fever	>102.2 °F (>39 °C)	>103 °F (>39.4 °C)	>103.5 °F (>39.7 °C)	>103.5 °F (>39.7 °C)	≥103.5 °F (>39.7 °C)
• Hypothermia	<100.4 °F (<38 °C)	<100 °F (<37.8 °C)	<100 °F (<37.8 °C)	<100 °F (<37.8 °C)	≤100 °F (<37.8 °C)
Heart rate (beats/min)	>120	>140	>160	>225	≥225
• Tachycardia					
• Bradycardia				<140	≤140
Respiratory rate (breaths/min)	>20	>20	>40	>40	≥40
• Tachypnea					
White blood cell count (cells/μL)	>16 000	>16 000	>12 000	>19 500	≥19 500
• Leukocytosis	<6000	<6000	<4000	<5000	≤5000
• Leukopenia					
• Band neutrophils (% bands)	>3%	>3%	>10%	>5%	≥5%

Table 159.2 Specific treatment considerations for organ dysfunctions that can occur in patients with SIRS and sepsis.

Organ dysfunction	Possible manifestations of organ dysfunction requiring treatment	Objective characterization of dysfunction	Treatment considerations
Cardiovascular dysfunction	Septic shock	MAP < 65 mmHg despite IV fluid resuscitation	Vasopressor agents
		Vasopressor dependence	
	Decreased myocardial contractility/myocardial dysfunction	Decreased fractional shortening, ejection fraction	Positive inotropes
		Biventricular dilation	
		Increased cTnI	
	Malignant cardiac arrhythmias	Recognized on ECG	Antiarrhythmics
Coagulation dysfunction (DIC)	Hypercoagulable state • Thromboembolic events possible	Hypercoagulable trace on viscoelastic testing	Antithrombotics (e.g. heparin, clopidogrel, aspirin)
		Decreased endogenous anticoagulants (AT, aPC)	
		Increased D-dimers	
	Hypocoagulable state/ consumptive coagulopathy • Bleeding possible	Prolonged clotting times (PT, aPTT)	Blood product transfusion if hypocoagulable and bleeding or prior to an invasive procedure
		Thrombocytopenia (Plt count ≤100,000/μL)	
		Hypocoagulable trace on viscoelastic testing	
Endocrine dysfunction	Hypoglycemia	BG < 60 mg/dL (3.3 mmol/L)	IV glucose supplementation
	Hyperglycemia	BG > 180 mg/dL (10 mmol/L)	Insulin therapy
	Critical illness-related corticosteroid insufficiency (CIRCI)	Low delta cortisol on ACTH stimulation test	Physiological hydrocortisone therapy

(Continued)

Table 159.2 (*Continued*)

Organ dysfunction	Possible manifestations of organ dysfunction requiring treatment	Objective characterization of dysfunction	Treatment considerations
Gastrointestinal dysfunction	Vomiting	Increased gastric residual volumes	Antiemetics (e.g. maropitant, ondansetron, dolasetron)
	Regurgitation, functional ileus, intolerance of enteral nutrition		Prokinetics (e.g. metoclopramide, erythromycin)
	Gastrointestinal ulcers		Antacids (e.g. PPIs, H_2 RAs)
			Sucralfate
	Diarrhea		Generally no specific therapy indicated
	Constipation		Laxatives, enemas
Hepatobiliary dysfunction	Icterus	Hyperbilirubinemia (TBili>0.5 mg/dL)	No clear role for specific therapy
	Increased hepatic transaminases (esp. ALT)		
	Impaired synthetic function		
Neurological	Seizures		Antiepileptic drugs
	Encephalopathy/impaired level of consciousness		
	Delirium		
Pulmonary dysfunction	Acute lung injury (ALI) and acute respiratory distress syndrome (ARDS)	A-a gradient>10 mmHg	Oxygen supplementation
		SpO_2<95% (FiO_2 0.21)	Lung protective mechanical ventilation
		P/F ratio<300 mmHg	
Kidney dysfunction	Acute kidney injury (AKI)	Oliguria, anuria	Consider diuretic therapy (e.g. furosemide, fenoldopam)
		Rise in [Creatinine]>0.3–0.5 mg/dL, in the absence of prerenal or postrenal causes	Continuous renal replacement therapy or intermittent hemodialysis
Vascular/ endothelial dysfunction	Endothelial glycocalyx damage, vascular leak		No specific therapy at this time

ACTH, adrenocorticotropic hormone; ALT, alanine aminotransferase; aPTT, activated partial thromboplastin time; BG, blood glucose; Cr, creatinine; cTnI, cardiac troponin I; H_2 RAs, H_2 receptor antagonists; MAP, mean arterial pressure; PPI, proton pump inhibitor; PT, prothrombin time; TBili, total bilirubin; UOP = urine output.

Failure Assessment (SOFA) score≥2 points as a result of the infection. And finally, septic shock is a subset of sepsis in which underlying circulatory and cellular/metabolic abnormalities are profound enough to substantially increase mortality. Based on the new definitions, patients with septic shock can be identified with a clinical construct of sepsis with persisting hypotension requiring vasopressors to maintain MAP≥65 mmHg and having a serum lactate>2 mmol/L (18 mg/dL) despite adequate volume resuscitation. In addition, hospitalized patients can be screened for sepsis using a quick SOFA (qSOFA) consisting of an abnormal Glascow Coma Scale Score, increased respiratory rate, and decreased blood pressure.

Pathophysiology

The SIRS, sepsis, and MODS share common pathogenic processes, although the clinical spectrum of disease is extremely varied. When inflammation in response to an insult has systemic effects, rather than remaining localized to the site of the insult, the resultant clinical manifestations are characterized as SIRS. Explained most simply, SIRS refers to a systemic proinflammatory state, inadequately controlled by endogenous anti-inflammatory responses. Although localized inflammation is a protective response to tissue injury, systemic inflammation is often deleterious. Sustained systemic inflammation can result in organ dysfunctions, and it is generally MODS that causes mortality in these patients.

Systemic inflammatory response syndrome can be the result of a non-infectious or an infectious insult (sepsis). Table 159.3 displays common causes of SIRS and sepsis in dogs and cats. Non-infectious SIRS and sepsis can be challenging to differentiate clinically because their pathophysiology is almost identical, with the exception only of the initial insult [13]. In patients with sepsis, pathogen-associated molecular patterns (PAMPs), expressed by the pathogen, stimulate pattern recognition receptors (PRRs), such as the toll-like receptors (TLRs), in the host. PAMPs include motifs such as lipopolysaccharide on gram-negative bacteria. Although most clinicians commonly think of bacterial causes of sepsis, viruses, fungal organisms, and parasites also have PAMPs that

Table 159.3 Commonly recognized causes of non-infectious SIRS and sepsis in dogs and cats. Some of these disorders are also covered in other chapters.

Non-infectious SIRS	Sepsis
Trauma • Blunt trauma (e.g. motor vehicle accident) • Penetrating trauma (e.g. gunshot wounds) • Surgical/iatrogenic trauma	Peritonitis/abdominal sepsis • Gastrointestinal perforation • Septic bile peritonitis when an infected biliary tract ruptures • Rupture of infected urogenital tract
Neoplasia	Pneumonia
Pancreatitis	Pyothorax
Immune-mediated diseases	Pyometra
Submersion injury	Prostatitis/prostatic abscess
Electrocution	Pyelonephritis
Burn injury	Lower urinary tract infection
Heatstroke	Hepatic abscess
Ischemic diseases • Gastric dilation-volvulus (GDV) • Splenic torsion • Mesenteric volvulus • Colonic torsion • Thromboembolic disease	Skin and soft tissue infections, including necrotizing fasciitis
Transfusion reactions	Rickettsial diseases • Babesiosis, ehrlichiosis, and others
Toxicoses and adverse drug reactions	Systemic mycoses
Anaphylaxis	Systemic viral infections
Envenomation	Systemic protozoal and parasitic infections

stimulate receptors of the host's innate immune system and can trigger SIRS. Stimulation of PRRs drives an intracellular signaling cascade that ultimately results in the upregulation of nuclear transcription of a variety of inflammatory mediators.

The inflammatory mediators of SIRS include cytokines, chemokines, vasoactive substances, and mediators of coagulation. Prototypical proinflammatory cytokines include tumor necrosis factor and interleukins-1 and 6; these cytokines contribute to the development of fever, leukocyte production and activation, cardiovascular instability, increased vascular permeability, and acute-phase protein synthesis. Chemokines induce neutrophil chemotaxis to sites of inflammation. Vasoactive substances released include inducible nitric oxide (NO), a potent vasodilator. Stimulation of inflammation also activates coagulation [14].

In non-infectious SIRS, tissue damage results in the expression or release of damage-associated molecular patterns (DAMPs) on/from host cells. DAMPS include cellular components such as heat shock proteins, high mobility group box 1 protein, ATP, and DNA. DAMPs also stimulate PRRs, initiating the same intracellular signaling cascades as PAMPs to produce SIRS.

Multiple organ dysfunction syndrome is a multifactorial phenomenon that occurs secondary to both non-infectious SIRS and sepsis. MODS refers to the presence of two or more dysfunctional organs in an acutely ill patient such that homeostasis cannot be maintained without intervention [3]. Organ dysfunctions result from inflammation, decreased tissue oxygen delivery (DO_2), energetic failure (impaired mitochondrial function), heterogenous microvascular flow, apoptosis, and microthrombosis.

Coagulation dysfunction and disseminated intravascular coagulation (DIC) in patients with systemic inflammation are due to the concurrent activation of coagulation, with an initial prothrombotic phase, followed by a consumptive coagulopathy (see Chapter 70) [14]. Endothelial activation also likely contributes to a hypercoagulable state *in vivo*. Microvascular thromboses and hemorrhage in turn can contribute to other organ dysfunctions (see Chapter 62). Cardiovascular dysfunction and septic shock are at least in part explained by the actions of NO. Additionally, critical illness-related corticosteroid insufficiency (CIRCI) causes vascular hyporeactivity [15,16]. Respiratory dysfunction is explained by leukocyte infiltration and fluid leak into alveoli, as well as impaired blood flow in the pulmonary circulation associated with thrombosis, leading to diffusion impairment and ventilation/perfusion mismatch (see Chapter 42) [17,18]. Other organ dysfunctions such as acute kidney injury (AKI) (see Chapter 94), and acute hepatic dysfunction are less well understood (see Chapter 90) [19].

Diagnostic Approach to SIRS and Sepsis

The history and clinical signs of dogs and cats that present with SIRS and sepsis are often non-specific and vary depending on the underlying disease process. The presenting complaint of the animal may be quite vague, including symptoms such as lethargy, depression, and inappetence. Vomiting and diarrhea may be due to gastrointestinal tract disease or secondary to the systemic disease (i.e. extragastrointestinal in origin). As with any case presenting on an emergency basis, identifying clinical signs that localize the primary problem to a body system is invaluable, if possible, to guide the diagnostic process.

Physical examination of patients with SIRS and sepsis reflects the systemic inflammatory state with possible derangements in temperature, heart rate, and respiratory rate as discussed. Dehydration and/or evidence of shock are also common. Assessing perfusion parameters (level of consciousness, heart rate, pulse quality, oral mucous membrane color, and capillary refill time (CRT)) should be a priority of the initial physical examination, since treatment of shock should be initiated immediately (see Section 4B, Circulatory Shock). Dogs present most commonly in the early decompensatory phase of shock, with pale mucous membranes, prolonged CRT, and weak pulses. That being said, a hyperdynamic state of shock or vasodilatory shock can also be present in dogs with SIRS and sepsis, resulting in hyperemic mucous membranes, a rapid CRT (<1 sec), and strong or bounding pulses. Concurrent dehydration (if present) will manifest as abnormalities such as dry mucous membranes, increased skin tenting, dehydrated abdominal contents and sunken eyes, and should be addressed following resuscitation from shock (see Chapter 171).

Point-of-care diagnostic tests such as measurement of blood pressure, blood lactate (see Chapter 156), and venous blood gases are often performed concurrent with the initial physical examination and patient stabilization. Hypotension and/or hyperlactatemia may be present in patients with compromised perfusion, and should prompt an aggressive approach to improve DO_2. Pulse oximetry and arterial blood gas analyses are usually performed in animals with evidence of respiratory compromise.

Screening diagnostic tests, including a complete blood count, blood smear, biochemistry profile, urinalysis, and coagulation tests, are also part of the initial diagnostic approach to a systemically unwell patient. Screening diagnostics are performed to assess for the presence of underlying disease, identify abnormalities requiring treatment, and assess for the presence of organ dysfunctions. Hematological and biochemical abnormalities typically reflect the underlying disease process and derangements in organ dysfunction secondary to SIRS. Hematological abnormalities may include abnormalities in the leukon (see Table 159.3) and toxic changes in leukocytes. Hemoconcentration consistent with hypovolemia and splenic contraction (dogs) may be present, while anemia may reflect chronic underlying disease, blood loss or hemolysis. Thrombocytopenia is common.

Biochemical abnormalities may include hypoalbuminemia, dysglycemia, ionized hypocalcemia, and hyperbilirubinemia. Hypoalbuminemia is generally multifactorial but thought to be associated with albumin's status as a negative acute-phase protein (i.e. decreased hepatic synthesis), and increased loss (e.g. gastrointestinal, urinary or into body cavity effusions). Hypoglycemia tends to be a terminal finding in dogs and cats with SIRS and sepsis, reflecting increased consumption and/or decreased hepatic synthesis. Hyperglycemia is more common and may reflect decreased insulin sensitivity, and the effects of high circulating concentrations of cortisol and catecholamines (i.e. stress hyperglycemia). Ionized hypocalcemia is thought to be predominantly due to hypovitaminosis D [20]. Hyperbilirubinemia may be secondary to intrahepatic cholestasis or hemolysis [9,21]. Azotemia with isosthenuria may reflect underlying chronic kidney disease or AKI. Kidney injury may be direct and primary (e.g. pyelonephritis) or an organ dysfunction secondary to SIRS. Urine sediment evaluation should be performed and urine collected by cystocentesis should be submitted for culture and susceptibility testing to screen for a urinary tract infection.

Coagulation testing is also commonly performed in veterinary patients with SIRS and sepsis (see Chapter 70). The hypercoagulable phase of DIC may be detected by hypercoagulable tracings on viscoelastic tests. Increased D-dimers suggest the formation and subsequent degradation of fibrin clots. Reduced circulating concentrations of endogenous anticoagulants, such as activated protein C (aPC) and antithrombin, also suggest a hypercoagulable state [7]. A hypocoagulable state can also be documented using viscoelastic tests, but is more commonly characterized by prolongations in prothrombin time and activated partial thromboplastin time.

Identification of the SIRS criteria in a patient should prompt a search for the underlying cause, either non-infectious or infectious. In order to diagnose sepsis, a patient must fulfill SIRS criteria and have a confirmed (or highly suspected) infection. Definitive diagnosis of bacterial infection requires identification of bacteria by cytology, histopathology or culture, while definitive diagnosis of infections with other types of pathogens may involve ancillary diagnostics such as identification of pathogen antigen, DNA or RNA in the host, or an antibody response suggestive of acute infection. In some cases, the underlying cause of systemic inflammation is immediately obvious, while in others it is not and exhaustive diagnostics are required. The preliminary search for infection may include point-of-care infectious disease testing, screening ultrasound, thoracic radiographs, abdominal ultrasound, and urine sediment examination.

Further testing based on these initial diagnostics may include additional infectious disease testing, spinal radiographs, and echocardiogram.

Point-of-care infectious disease testing in an animal with SIRS should include testing for feline immunodeficiency virus and feline leukemia virus in cats, and tick-borne pathogens (*Borrelia burgdorferi*, *Anaplasma phagocytophilum*, and *Ehrlichia canis*) in dogs in endemic areas. Send-out testing for other rickettsial diseases, fungal, viral and other pathogens may also be indicated. Fecal diagnostics can be used to screen for pathogens in-house and are particularly indicated in patients with SIRS and diarrhea as a prominent clinical sign. Fecal immunoassays are available for canine parvovirus (which cross-reacts with feline panleukopenia virus), and *Giardia*. Routine fecal diagnostics such as fecal floatation, fecal cytology, and wet-prep may also be useful.

Ultrasound examinations can be used in the ER (see Chapter 182) to evaluate for cavitary effusion or other obvious abnormalities. Standard approaches to using ultrasound in the veterinary ER are described for the thorax (thoracic focused assessment with sonography for trauma, tFAST), abdomen (aFAST), and pulmonary parenchyma (Veterinary Bedside Lung Ultrasound Examination; VetBLUE) [22,23].

Three-view thoracic radiographs or thoracic computed tomography (CT) should be obtained, particularly in animals with respiratory abnormalities. Thoracic imaging may reveal evidence of pneumonia, pleural effusion (although this is usually detected on tFAST first), or primary or secondary neoplasia. Abdominal ultrasound or CT by a specialist radiologist can also be invaluable in the search for an underlying cause, particularly in a patient with clinical signs or laboratory abnormalities suggestive of intra-abdominal disease. Imaging findings can be used to guide surgical exploration of effusions, for example in patients with abdominal sepsis or pyothorax.

Any abnormal fluid accumulations identified during physical examination or diagnostic imaging should be sampled for cytology, culture, and susceptibility. This may include peritoneal effusion (see Chapter 87), pleural effusion or joint fluid. Biochemical tests on cavitary effusions may also be helpful [24–26]. Other specific fluid samples that may be obtained as part of the diagnostic process for a patient with SIRS or sepsis include blood, lower airway fluid (collected by endotracheal wash, transtracheal wash or bronchoalveolar lavage), cerebrospinal fluid, urine, joint fluid, and organ aspirates.

Obtaining samples for culture and susceptibility testing should be performed as promptly as possible. Ideally, samples are obtained before, but should not delay the administration of, antimicrobials in a septic patient [27]. Current recommendations for blood cultures are to obtain two samples 30 minutes apart from different vessels, generally one central (jugular vein) and one peripheral, in an aseptic fashion. Generally, both aerobic and anaerobic cultures are submitted, perhaps with the exception of lower airway fluid culture where an anaerobic culture is less likely to be needed unless there is evidence of pulmonary abscessation.

Other diagnostic tests are based on signalment, history, clinical signs, and diagnostic findings in an individual patient.

Treatment Approach to SIRS and Sepsis

Treating Shock

The first and foremost consideration when stabilizing a patient with SIRS or sepsis is to ensure adequate DO_2. Animals with SIRS and sepsis may have decreased stroke volume due to hypovolemia, maldistribution, obstructive shock, cardiogenic shock or a combination of these. Identifying the contributors to shock in a particular patient with SIRS or sepsis is important to ensure appropriate treatment. Septic patients with shock generally have hypovolemic and/or distributive shock (see Section 4B, Circulatory Shock).

Restoring adequate DO_2 is achieved by sequentially considering and normalizing each contributor to DO_2. This is essentially the foundation of the early goal-directed therapy (EGDT) approach for the management of patients with severe sepsis and septic shock [27]. Although strict adherence to the published EGDT protocol has been questioned in human medicine, the principles of shock resuscitation that it embodies remain the same. Preload is addressed first, and the surviving sepsis guidelines suggest that boluses of isotonic crystalloids administered to predetermined endpoints should be the fluid of choice for restoration of intravascular volume [27]. Perfusion parameters and point-of-care tests are used to guide resuscitation to endpoints. Ideally, if the clinician uses resuscitation endpoints (e.g. mean arterial pressure ≥65 mmHg), the minimum amount of fluid needed to restore acceptable perfusion parameters will be administered. The use of synthetic colloids for increasing preload is no longer recommended in septic humans due to the risk of AKI and coagulation derangements, but there is some evidence of a beneficial effect of albumin [27].

The role of synthetic colloids and albumin for shock resuscitation in veterinary medicine is unclear (see Chapter 168). Packed red blood cell transfusions are indicated in those patients whose anemia is of sufficient severity to contribute to decreased DO_2 (see Chapter 176).

Treating Cardiovascular Dysfunction

In patients with septic shock, increasing preload alone is inadequate to restore DO_2 due to inappropriate peripheral vasodilation and distributive shock. As such, vasopressor administration is often beneficial. Norepinephrine is the first-line agent in human medicine [27]. Vasopressin, epinephrine, and dopamine may also be used. Myocardial depression may require specific therapy with positive inotropes, such as dobutamine, levosimendan or pimobendan. In patients with vasopressor-dependent hypotension, physiological hydrocortisone therapy is recommended due to the likelihood of CIRCI.

Antimicrobial Therapy (see Chapter 200)

In addition to fluid resuscitation from shock, the mainstays of sepsis treatment are antimicrobial therapy, source control, and aggressive supportive care. Early appropriate use of IV antimicrobials is perhaps the single most important factor in stabilizing the septic patient. Evidence in people with severe sepsis and septic shock suggests that every hour delay in administration of appropriate antimicrobials increases mortality [28,29]. In veterinary medicine, there is good evidence that implementation of a sepsis protocol improved the time to first administration of an antimicrobial in dogs with abdominal sepsis [30], although currently there is no evidence that this affects outcome [31].

Giving an appropriate antimicrobial requires an understanding of the origin of sepsis, the likely pathogens involved, and local resistance patterns. Generally, the goal is to start with broad-spectrum antimicrobial coverage and later de-escalate based on the results of culture and susceptibility testing. For example, community-acquired, secondary abdominal sepsis of gastrointestinal origin may be treated with amoxicillin + sulbactam for gram-positive aerobic and anaerobic coverage, and enrofloxacin for gram-negative aerobic coverage. In animals with recent exposure to antimicrobials or a high local burden of fluoroquinolone-resistant *E. coli*, amikacin (if normal renal function) or cefotaxime (if azotemic) would be more appropriate empiric antimicrobials for treatment of gram-negative aerobes. For animals that develop hospital-acquired sepsis, empiric antimicrobial choices are usually based on the assumption of multidrug-resistant (MDR) organisms.

Source Control

Following identification of the septic patient, sample collection, administration of IV antimicrobials, and resuscitation from shock, the next step of management is source control. Without effective source control measures, there is less chance of success, especially if infection is confined within a closed space (e.g. septic peritonitis, septic arthritis, pyothorax). Source control must be pursued as soon as is reasonably possible following initial patient stabilization. This often means emergency surgery. Provision of analgesia also becomes an important part of management when surgical source control is needed.

Supportive Care and Managing Organ Dysfunctions

The remainder of the therapeutic approach to dogs and cats with SIRS and sepsis focuses on treating the underlying disease, good supportive care, and managing organ dysfunctions (see Table 159.2). Close monitoring is also imperative. Parameters requiring serial monitoring include perfusion parameters, hydration parameters, heart rate, respiratory rate and effort, temperature, blood pressure, urine output, and electrolytes.

Prognosis for SIRS, Sepsis, and MODS

The prognosis for animals with SIRS, sepsis, and MODS varies markedly depending on the severity of illness and the specific nature of the underlying disease. It may not always be possible to provide pet owners with an accurate prognosis for a specific patient with SIRS or sepsis at the time of presentation to the ER; rather, daily reassessment, to assess response to treatment, is helpful for prognostication.

Some studies suggest that the more SIRS criteria an animal meets, the worse their prognosis [8], although this does not always hold true. There is also good evidence in dogs with septic peritonitis that the greater the number of organ dysfunctions, the worse the prognosis [1]. Septic shock carries a particularly grave prognosis. Nonetheless, given the confounding influence of euthanasia in veterinary studies assessing outcome, all efforts should be made for patient treatment when owners have intent to treat.

References

1 Kenney EM, Rozanski EA, Rush JE, et al. Association between outcome and organ system dysfunction in dogs with sepsis: 114 cases (2003–2007). *J Am Vet Med Assoc* 2010;236(1):83–87.
2 Babyak JM, Sharp CR. Epidemiology of systemic inflammatory response syndrome and sepsis in cats in a veterinary teaching hospital. *J Am Vet Med Assoc* 2016;249(1):65–71.
3 Bone RC, Balk RA, Cerra FB, et al. Definitions for sepsis and organ failure and guidelines for the use of innovative therapies in sepsis. The ACCP/SCCM Consensus Conference Committee. American College of Chest Physicians/Society of Critical Care Medicine. *Chest* 1992;101(6):1644–1655.
4 Levy MM, Fink MP, Marshall JC, et al. 2001 SCCM/ESICM/ACCP/ATS/SIS International

Sepsis Definitions Conference. *Crit Care Med* 2003;31(4):1250–1256.

5 Silverstein DC. Systemic inflammatory response syndrome and sepsis. Part 1: Recognition and diagnosis. *Today's Vet Pract* 2015;5(1).

6 Hauptman JG, Walshaw R, Olivier NB. Evaluation of the sensitivity and specificity of diagnostic criteria for sepsis in dogs. *Vet Surg* 1997;26(5):393–397.

7 de Laforcade AM, Freeman LM, Shaw SP, Brooks MB, Rozanski EA, Rush JE. Hemostatic changes in dogs with naturally occurring sepsis. *J Vet Intern Med* 2003;17(5):674–679.

8 Okano S, Yoshida M, Fukushima U, Higuchi S, Takase K, Hagio M. Usefulness of systemic inflammatory response syndrome criteria as an index for prognosis judgement. *Vet Rec* 2002;150(8):245–246.

9 Brady CA, Otto CM, van Winkle TJ, King LG. Severe sepsis in cats: 29 cases (1986–1998). *J Am Vet Med Assoc* 2000;217(4):531–535.

10 Declue AE, Delgado C, Chang CH, Sharp CR. Clinical and immunologic assessment of sepsis and the systemic inflammatory response syndrome in cats. *J Am Vet Med Assoc* 2011;238(7):890–897.

11 Ateca LB, Drobatz KJ, King LG. Organ dysfunction and mortality risk factors in severe canine bite wound trauma. *J Vet Emerg Crit Care* 2014;24(6):705–714.

12 Singer M, Deutschman CS, Seymour CW, et al. The Third International Consensus Definitions for Sepsis and Septic Shock (Sepsis-3). *JAMA* 2016;315(8):801–810.

13 Lewis DH, Chan DL, Pinheiro D, Armitage-Chan E, Garden OA. The immunopathology of sepsis: pathogen recognition, systemic inflammation, the compensatory anti-inflammatory response, and regulatory T cells. *J Vet Intern Med* 2012;26(3):457–482.

14 Hopper K, Bateman S. An updated view of hemostasis: mechanisms of hemostatic dysfunction associated with sepsis. *J Vet Emerg Crit Care* 2005;15(2):83–91.

15 Burkitt JM, Haskins SC, Nelson RW, Kass PH. Relative adrenal insufficiency in dogs with sepsis. *J Vet Intern Med* 2007;21(2):226–231.

16 Martin LG, Groman RP, Fletcher DJ, et al. Pituitary-adrenal function in dogs with acute critical illness. *J Am Vet Med Assoc* 2008;233(1):87–95.

17 Ware LB, Matthay MA. The acute respiratory distress syndrome. *N Engl J Med* 2000;342(18):1334–1349.

18 Declue AE, Cohn LA. Acute respiratory distress syndrome in dogs and cats: a review of clinical findings and pathophysiology. *J Vet Emerg Crit Care* 2007;17(4):340–347.

19 Keir I, Kellum JA. Acute kidney injury in severe sepsis: pathophysiology, diagnosis, and treatment recommendations. *J Vet Emerg Crit Care* 2015;25(2):200–209.

20 Holowaychuk MK, Birkenheuer AJ, Li J, Marr H, Boll A, Nordone SK. Hypocalcemia and hypovitaminosis D in dogs with induced endotoxemia. *J Vet Intern Med* 2012;26(2):244–251.

21 Taboada J, Meyer DJ. Cholestasis associated with extrahepatic bacterial infection in five dogs. *J Vet Intern Med* 1989;3(4):216–221.

22 Lisciandro GR. Abdominal and thoracic focused assessment with sonography for trauma, triage, and monitoring in small animals. *J Vet Emerg Crit Care* 2011;21(2):104–122.

23 Lisciandro GR, Fosgate GT, Fulton RM. Frequency and number of ultrasound lung rockets (B-lines) using a regionally based lung ultrasound examination named VetBLUE (veterinary bedside lung ultrasound exam) in dogs with radiographically normal lung findings. *Vet Radiol Ultrasound* 2014;55(3):315–322.

24 Bonczynski JJ, Ludwig LL, Barton LJ, Loar A, Peterson ME. Comparison of peritoneal fluid and peripheral blood pH, bicarbonate, glucose, and lactate concentration as a diagnostic tool for septic peritonitis in dogs and cats. *Vet Surg* 2003;32(2):161–166.

25 Levin GM, Bonczynski JJ, Ludwig LL, Barton LJ, Loar AS. Lactate as a diagnostic test for septic peritoneal effusions in dogs and cats. *J Am Anim Hosp Assoc* 2004;40(5):364–371.

26 Stafford JR, Bartges JW. A clinical review of pathophysiology, diagnosis, and treatment of uroabdomen in the dog and cat. *J Vet Emerg Crit Care* 2013;23(2):216–229.

27 Dellinger RP, Levy MM, Rhodes A, et al. Surviving Sepsis Campaign: international guidelines for management of severe sepsis and septic shock: 2012. *Crit Care Med* 2013;41(2):580–637.

28 Kumar A, Roberts D, Wood KE, et al. Duration of hypotension before initiation of effective antimicrobial therapy is the critical determinant of survival in human septic shock. *Crit Care Med* 2006;34(6):1589–1596.

29 Paul M, Shani V, Muchtar E, Kariv G, Robenshtok E, Leibovici L. Systematic review and meta-analysis of the efficacy of appropriate empiric antibiotic therapy for sepsis. *Antimicrob Agents Chemother* 2010;54(11):4851–4863.

30 Abelson AL, Buckley GJ, Rozanski EA. Positive impact of an emergency department protocol on time to antimicrobial administration in dogs with septic peritonitis. *J Vet Emerg Crit Care* 2013;23(5):551–556.

31 Keir I, Dickinson AE. The role of antimicrobials in the treatment of sepsis and critical illness-related bacterial infections: examination of the evidence. *J Vet Emerg Crit Care* 2015;25(1):55–62.

C. Trauma

160

Trauma Overview

Erica L. Reineke, VMD, DACVECC

School of Veterinary Medicine, University of Pennsylvania, Philadelphia, PA, USA

Introduction

Trauma is defined as any tissue injury that occurs more or less suddenly as a result of an external force [1]. Injury to tissues may be classified by the type of forces applied to the body, such as blunt and penetrating, and can occur secondary to motor vehicle accidents, animal abuse, falls, gunshot wounds, and animal–animal interactions. Traumatic injuries may be minor, such as lacerations or single bite wounds that are easily addressed and fixed. However, trauma can be severe and life threatening with injuries to multiple body systems. These severely injured patients may die acutely due to overwhelming injury typically associated with severe blood loss, hypoxemia, or traumatic brain injury. Other severely injured patients may survive initially but subsequently die due to complications such as delayed hemorrhage, infection, or multiple organ dysfunction. Finally, other severely injured patients may be treated and survive to hospital discharge.

It is important for the veterinarian to understand the epidemiology of small animal trauma in order to rapidly evaluate for common life-threatening injuries. Rapid and accurate recognition of life-threatening injuries is key in the initial triage evaluation to institute life-saving therapy and improve the animal's chances of survival. Trauma scoring systems help to identify the more severely injured patients, evaluate hospital patient outcomes, and aid patient enrollment in clinical trials.

Overview of the Pathophysiology of Trauma

In polytrauma patients, hemorrhage, hypoxemia, and tissue injury may either directly or indirectly contribute to decreases in tissue perfusion and oxygen delivery. An accumulating oxygen debt and systemic release of inflammatory mediators are responsible for triggering the systemic inflammatory response syndrome (SIRS) and multiple organ dysfunction syndrome (MODS), ultimately contributing to the death of the patient (see Chapter 159). Both SIRS and MODS have been identified in veterinary patients as a complication of both blunt and penetrating trauma and, similar to people, they are associated with non-survival [2,3].

In hemorrhagic shock, a decrease in cardiac output and mean arterial pressure is a key element leading to initial tissue hypoperfusion. Tissue hypoperfusion results in activation of the neuroendocrine stress response characterized by enhanced release of pituitary hormones, increased sympathoadrenal activity, pancreatic hypersecretion, and activation of inflammation [4]. When tissues and cells become deprived of oxygen, anaerobic metabolism is initiated, leading to increases in blood lactate and overproduction of oxygen radicals and other toxic metabolites [5]. Re-establishing effective circulation during resuscitation causes a steep increase in the levels of these toxic compounds, overwhelming tissue free radical scavengers and resulting in significant cellular injury (see Chapter 158). If oxygen delivery is not restored quickly, cell membrane pumps fail irreversibly and cell death occurs. The ischemic cell takes up interstitial fluid and swells, reducing perfusion to its neighbors [6,7]. Uncontrolled hemorrhage can lead to fatal shock characterized by a lack of contractile power of the heart and great vessels, inappropriate vasodilation, lack of response to catecholamines, and eventually brain death [6,7].

The systemic response to severe injury is characterized by a complex interaction across the hemostatic, inflammatory, endocrine, and neurological systems which may exacerbate the initial damage caused by hypoperfusion and reperfusion [8]. Following tissue injury, extracellular release of damage-associated molecular patterns (DAMPs) or alarmins from activated neutrophils or necrotic cells activates cells of the innate immune system (neutrophils and monocytes) and complement (C3a and C5a) [9–13]. Complement and inflammatory

Textbook of Small Animal Emergency Medicine, First Edition. Edited by Kenneth J. Drobatz, Kate Hopper, Elizabeth Rozanski and Deborah C. Silverstein.
© 2019 John Wiley & Sons, Inc. Published 2019 by John Wiley & Sons, Inc.
Companion Website: www.wiley.com/go/drobatz/textbook

cell activation triggers the production and release of inflammatory mediators such as interleukins (i.e. IL-6 and IL-8), generating the systemic response seen in SIRS [14]. Platelets activated by trauma and coagulation can also contribute to release of proinflammatory mediators and further promote SIRS [15]. Activated neutrophils migrate across the damaged vascular endothelium and become sequestered in "bystander" organs, leading to organ dysfunction [16]. Simultaneously, a compensatory anti-inflammatory response occurs characterized by increases in anti-inflammatory cytokines (IL-10 and TGF-beta) and cytokine antagonists (IL-1Ra) [17].

Depending on the balance of proinflammatory and anti-inflammatory factors, these responses may return to baseline or progress to persistent inflammation, immunosuppression, and increased risk for multiple organ dysfunction and sepsis [18].

Epidemiology of Small Animal Trauma

Trauma is common in small animal patients, accounting for 11–13% of emergency visits at Urban Teaching Hospitals [19,20]. In a large epidemiological study of approximately 75 000 North American dogs over a 20-year time period, trauma was the second leading cause of death in both juvenile and adult dogs [21]. To the author's knowledge, a similar epidemiological study has not been done in cats.

A large retrospective study and one multi-institutional prospective study describe trauma patterns in dogs. These studies found that trauma is most common in young male dogs, with blunt trauma occurring in approximately 50% of dogs, followed by penetrating trauma (34%), unknown trauma (11%), and crush injury (~2.5%) [19,22]. Polytrauma secondary to blunt injury is common, occurring in up to 72% of dogs [2]. The prognosis following trauma is excellent in dogs, with survival to hospital discharge reported to be around 90% [22].

There are two large studies describing trauma patterns in cats [19,23]. In these studies, male cats were most commonly injured and the majority were indoor-outdoor cats. The causes of trauma were similar in both studies, with unknown trauma the most common cause (34–39.5%), followed by blunt trauma (16.3–17%), multiple bite wounds (~14%), crush injury (13–14%), non-bite penetrating wounds (4–10%), and falls (8.6–14%). The survival to hospital discharge rate in the most recent study in cats was 76% [23]. Present-day information regarding trauma patterns in both dogs and cats will soon be available as a result of data being collected from veterinary trauma centers through an international veterinary trauma registry overseen by the American

College of Veterinary Emergency and Critical Care (see Chapter 161).

Animals suffering from blunt trauma may sustain injuries to multiple parts of the body, including the chest, abdomen, head, soft tissues, and extremities, as a consequence of widespread energy transfer to the body. Table 160.1 outlines the type and incidence of blunt traumatic injuries that have been described in the veterinary literature. Factors in several studies identified with non-survival included recumbency at admission, development of hematochezia, cardiac arrhythmias, hemoperitoneum, body wall hernias, severe soft tissue injury, vertebral fractures, pneumonia, disseminated intravascular coagulation, acute respiratory distress syndrome, MODs, requirement for mechanical ventilation, use of vasopressors. and cardiopulmonary arrest [2,24].

A recent veterinary study evaluated injuries sustained in dogs and cats secondary to animal abuse [25]. In this study, cats were more likely to suffer from non-accidental injuries compared to dogs and both dogs and cats were significantly younger than a cohort of animals with blunt trauma secondary to motor vehicle accidents. Injuries significantly associated with non-accidental trauma

Table 160.1 Types and frequency of injuries sustained in blunt trauma in dogs.

Type of injury	Frequency reported
Thoracic injury	
Pulmonary contusions	44–83% [1–3]
Pneumothorax	7–47% [1–3]
Hemothorax	3–18% [1,2]
Rib fractures	9–14% [1–3]
Diaphragmatic hernia	2–6% [1–3]
Flail chest	2% [1]
Pulmonary bullae	2% [1]
Abdominal injury	
Hemoperitoneum	23–38% [1,3]
Abdominal hernias	5% [1]
Urinary tract rupture	2–3% [1–3]
Head trauma	25% [1,2]
Fractures	
Pelvic and sacral fractures/luxations	21–39% [1–3]
Other hindlimb appendicular fractures	17–36% [1,2]
Forelimb appendicular fractures	12–15% [1,2]
Spinal fractures	9–10% [1,2]
Skull fractures	5–11% [1,2]
Soft tissue injuries (lacerations, abrasions, degloving wounds)	81–90% [1,3]

included scleral hemorrhage, damage to the claws, skull fractures, vertebral fractures, and rib fractures (usually on one side of the chest). Older fractures are also often identified [25].

Penetrating wounds may result from animal–animal interactions or foreign objects such as gunshot wounds or impalements. In penetrating injuries, shearing, compressive, and tensile forces combine to damage soft tissue, bone, and viscera [26]. Often, the degree of skin damage in these cases does not predict the underlying tissue damage. Penetrating abdominal injuries from bite wounds, gunshot wounds, and impalements can result in significant internal organ injury and surgical exploration is typically recommended following patient stabilization. Bite wounds appear to occur more commonly in male dogs compared to female dogs, with small dogs more likely to suffer multiple injuries [27]. A majority of studies report that *Pasteurella* spp, *Staphylococcus* spp, and *Streptococcus* spp were the bacteria commonly cultured from bite wounds, but mixed infections with both aerobic and anerobic bacteria are also reported [28–32].

In a recent study evaluating severe extensive bite wounds in 94 dogs requiring ICU admission, the majority were small-breed dogs (<10 kg) attacked by larger dogs (i.e. big dog–little dog interactions) and all dogs had surgical intervention [3]. Many dogs had evidence of SIRS, disseminated intravascular coagulation, and MODs and all were independently and significantly associated with mortality [3]. The most common organ dysfunction in this study was the respiratory system. Additionally, dogs with postoperative cardiovascular dysfunction (defined as a systolic arterial blood pressure <60 mmHg or requirement for vasopressors) or coagulation dysfunction were 29 times and 16 times respectively more likely to die [3].

Gunshot wounds can occur in both civilian and military working dogs. In two retrospective veterinary studies describing civilian gunshot wounds, injuries to the appendicular skeleton were most common, followed by the thorax (22%), head or neck (14%), and abdomen (14%) [33,34]. In a single paper describing gunshot wounds in 29 deployed military working dogs, the thorax was the most common site of injury (50%), followed by extremity wounds (46%) [35].

Trauma Scoring Systems

The Animal Trauma Triage Score (ATT) was developed for use in dogs to aid in identification of severely injured animals and for survival prediction [36]. In this scoring system, animals are scored on a 0–3 scale (0 = slight injury or no injury with 3 = severe injury) in six different

categories based on the initial physical examination: perfusion, cardiac, respiratory, eye/muscle/integument, skeletal, and neurological [36]. The ATT score assigned can range from 0 (an animal with only no or only slight injury in all categories) to 18 (an animal with severe injuries in all categories). In the initial prospective validation study, the survivors of trauma were found to have significantly higher mean ATT scores than non-survivors [36].

The utility of the ATT for predicting both severity of injury and outcome has been validated in several additional studies [22,24,35], with the most recent prospective study in traumatically injured dogs finding that an ATT >5 was 83% sensitive and 91% specific for predicting survival [22]. Although other variables have been evaluated for survival prediction, such as age, preexisting disease, type of trauma, and number of injuries, the ATT score appears to be the best outcome predictor available to date [22,24].

The Modified Glasgow Coma Scale (MGCS) is another scoring system used for outcome prediction in animals with head trauma [37]. In this system, animals with head trauma are scored on a scale from 1 to 6 in three different categories: motor activity, brainstem reflexes, and level of consciousness. The MGCS can range from 18, an animal with normal or only slight evidence of head injury, to 3, an animal with the highest score in all categories. Similar to the ATT score, the MGCS has been evaluated in both retrospective and prospective studies [22,37,38]. In these studies, lower scores have been found to be associated with more severe injury and non-survival. In the most recent retrospective study evaluating prognostic indictors in dogs with head trauma, a MGCS of <11 was 84% sensitive and 73% specific for predicting non-survival [38].

It is important to note that although these scoring systems can be useful to identify animals that may require more aggressive intervention, to evaluate specific hospital trauma patient outcomes or for patient enrollment in clinical trials, they should be used very cautiously in the individual patient and should not be used solely to advise a pet owner on whether to pursue treatment for their pet.

General Approach to the Polytrauma Patient

Animals with significant trauma often have injuries to multiple body systems and a thorough physical examination should be performed. As stated previously, in traumatically injured patients an accumulating tissue oxygen debt, due to either decreased tissue perfusion and/or hypoxemia, can trigger processes that lead to SIRS and MODS. Therefore, the initial approach to the emergency stabilization and resuscitation of traumatically injured patients should be aimed at improving and restoring tissue perfusion and oxygenation.

Initial assessment of cardiac output and circulating blood volume to evaluate for evidence of shock includes an evaluation of the patient's mucous membrane color, capillary refill time, heart rate, peripheral pulse quality, and rectal and extremity temperature (see Chapter 2). Pale mucous membranes, prolonged capillary refill time (>2 sec), tachycardia (or bradycardia in a cat), weak peripheral pulses, and hypotension indicate inadequate tissue perfusion. In the trauma patient, shock is typically the result of hemorrhage, but hypoxic, cardiogenic or septic shock may also occur [39]. Clinically significant hemorrhage secondary to trauma typically occurs in the thoracic cavity, peritoneum, retroperitoneal space, tissue compartments of the thigh (i.e. femoral fractures) and outside the body. These spaces should be investigated for the source of bleeding both during the physical exam and with diagnostic imaging (see below on abdominal FAST and thoracic FAST). External bleeding should be managed by application of direct pressure and ligation of exposed vessels. Generally, bleeding from the low-pressure pulmonary circuit resulting in a hemothorax will resolve spontaneously unless a major vessel has been injured or in cases of diaphragmatic hernia where hemorrhage originates from a displaced organ such as the liver.

In hemorrhagic shock, when only small volumes of blood are lost (10–12 mL/kg of blood or <15% of blood volume), there may only be mild changes in tissue perfusion parameters, such as a mild tachycardia, and arterial blood pressure may be normal or even elevated due to activation of compensatory mechanisms. These animals are at risk for ongoing hemorrhage and decompensation. As increasing amounts of blood are lost (>15% of blood volume), clinical signs of shock become more apparent. Absent pedal pulses is a very specific physical examination finding in hypotensive dogs and cats; the pedal pulses are no longer palpable when the blood pressure is less than 55 mmHg in dogs [40] and 70 mmHg in cats [41]. Arterial blood pressure should always be measured as many animals with hypoperfusion will have palpable peripheral pulses. This can be performed either directly through the placement of an arterial catheter or indirectly by Doppler or oscillometric techniques. Recently, the utility of the shock index (SI), which is the ratio of heart rate to systolic blood pressure, has been evaluated in dogs with hemorrhage. In this study, an SI>1.0 was found to be 79% sensitive and 69% specific for diagnosing blood loss [42].

An electrocardiogram should be performed to assess heart rate and evaluate for the presence of sustained cardiac arrhythmias that may affect cardiac output. Arrhythmias may result from shock, myocardial contusions or autonomic imbalance. Ventricular tachycardia and ventricular premature contractions (VPCs) are the most common cardiac arrhythmias in traumatically injured dogs, occurring in approximately 20% of cases [2,43,44]. Ventricular tachycardia may warrant therapy if sustained rates develop (see Chapter 53).

Injuries to the thorax may result in hypoxemia and decreased tissue oxygen delivery. In the veterinary literature, the incidence of blunt thoracic trauma is reported to be approximately 39–72% [2,45–48] (see Chapter 49). In one study of appendicular fractures in dogs, 25% were found to have concurrent hypoxemia [48]. Pulmonary contusions and pneumothorax are the most common thoracic injuries but other injuries that can occur include hemothorax, rib fractures, flail chest, and diaphragmatic hernia (see Table 160.1). Therefore, both the triage and serial physical examinations should include an evaluation of the animal's respiratory rate, respiratory effort, and a thorough thoracic auscultation.

Patients that are not breathing should be intubated and positive pressure ventilation initiated. Oxygen supplementation should be provided by mask or flow-by during the initial patient assessment (see Chapter 181). A pulse oximetry reading and/or arterial blood gas analysis can also be done to assess for hypoxemia. Dull lung sounds or an inverse or asynchronous breathing pattern should alert the clinician to the possibility of pleural space disease secondary to a pneumothorax, hemothorax, or diaphragmatic hernia [49] (see Chapters 44, 45, and 47). Moist lung sounds or fine pulmonary crackles, coughing, and/or blood in the mouth without evidence of oral or facial trauma may be seen in animals with pulmonary contusions.

In dyspneic patients in which pleural space disease is suspected, a needle thoracocentesis can be a life-saving intervention. A thoracic focused assessment with sonography for trauma (tFAST) examination could be done prior to needle thoracocentesis to confirm the presence of pleural space disease as indicated by an absent glide sign in patients with pneumothorax or the presence of echogenic effusion in animals with a hemothorax (see below and Chapter 180). For animals with suspected hemothorax, a needle thoracocentesis should only be done to relieve dyspnea as blood in the thoracic cavity will be reabsorbed by the lymphatic circulation, with 65% of red blood cells re-entering the systemic circulation within 2 days [50] (see Chapter 183).

In animals with abnormalities in thoracic auscultation or with penetrating thoracic injuries, thoracic radiography and/or computed tomography (CT) should be done to assess for intrathoracic injury. However, these diagnostic tests should be delayed until the patient has been stabilized. Of note, thoracic radiographs may be initially normal in dogs with pulmonary contusions, especially if radiographs are taken immediately after the traumatic event [51,52]. In general, pulmonary lesions develop within the first 4 hours following the traumatic event but it can take up to 24 hours for radiographic changes to occur [51,52].

Following evaluation of the cardiovascular and respiratory systems, an evaluation of the neurological system should be performed to evaluate for evidence of traumatic brain injury or spinal cord injury (see Chapters 19 and 24). A full neurological examination should be delayed until life-threatening conditions of the respiratory and cardiovascular systems have been addressed. Animals with injuries to the neurological system, including animals with traumatic brain injury, may have an abnormal level of consciousness, brainstem reflexes, and motor responses. Non-ambulatory patients should be evaluated for both spinal cord injury and pelvic fractures. Movement of these animals should be restricted until injury to the spinal cord can be excluded.

Evaluation of traumatic injury to the urinary system should include an admission and serial evaluation of blood urea nitrogen (BUN) and creatinine to assess renal function and monitoring of urine output. A normal urine output should be at least 1–2 mL/kg/h in a normotensive, euhydrated patient. Urinary ultrasound, urinary contrast studies, and/or CT can be performed to evaluate for integrity of the urinary tract if urinary tract rupture is suspected.

Finally, the patient should be assessed for fractures and wounds. Pelvic fractures are extremely common in dogs suffering from blunt trauma and may be identified during a rectal examination. Long bone fractures should be immobilized with a soft padded bandage initially and wounds should be clipped of hair, copiously flushed to remove debris, aseptically prepared and covered with a sterile dressing until further evaluation or definitive treatment can be performed.

During the triage evaluation, an intravenous catheter should be placed immediately in any animal with significant trauma, including animals with cardiovascular or respiratory instability or if there is evidence of traumatic brain injury. The intravenous catheter can be used for administration of intravenous fluid therapy for intravascular resuscitation and/or for administration of medications such as analgesia. Blood should be drawn at the time of intravenous catheter placement for packed cell volume (PCV), total protein (TP), lactate, blood gas analysis, blood electrolytes, blood urea nitrogen, and creatinine. In animals with significant hemorrhage, coagulation testing (PT, PTT, and/or thromboelastography) should be performed to evaluate for acute traumatic coagulopathy (see Chapter 163). In dogs with acute hemorrhage, the PCV may be initially normal due to release of red blood cells from splenic stores, and therefore a low TP should raise suspicion for hemorrhage.

A recent study investigating transfusion practices in dogs following trauma found that PCV of 39% and total solids of 4.5 g/dL were specific (92% and 89%), but insensitive (43% and 55%) predictors of the need for blood transfusion [53]. In a different study of 52 dogs with blunt trauma, admission base excess of −6.6 was 88% sensitive and 73% specific for predicting the need for a blood transfusion [54].

Animals with cardiovascular or respiratory instability should have both an initial and serial abdominal and thoracic FAST ultrasound examinations to evaluate for peritoneal, retroperitoneal, and thoracic effusions, diaphragmatic hernia, pneumothorax, and the presence of a urinary and gall bladder (see Chapter 182). During the thoracic FAST examination, an evaluation for pericardial effusion, cardiac chamber size, and contractility should also be done. These minimally invasive examinations can be done at the cage side and immediately following the triage physical examination (see Chapter 182). Serial FAST ultrasound examinations should be done especially in an animal with signs of shock in which fluid is not initially identified or in animals with unresponsive or recurrent shock following intravenous fluid resuscitation. In one study of dogs with blunt trauma, 17% of dogs were found to have an increasing volume of abdominal effusion on serial aFAST examinations [55].

If abdominal fluid is identified, an abdominocentesis should be performed to obtain a sample of fluid for analysis. For hemorrhagic effusions, a PCV and TP should be performed on the effusion. In acute hemorrhage, the PCV and TP of the effusion should reflect the patient's venous PCV and TP. In non-hemorrhagic or serohemorrhagic effusions, a creatinine and potassium of the effusion should be compared to a venous creatinine and potassium. An effusion-to-serum creatinine concentration >2.0 and an effusion-to-serum potassium >1.9 in cats and >1.4 in dogs are diagnostic for uroabdomen (see Chapter 103) [56,57]. Uroabdomen as a complication of trauma has been reported to occur in approximately 1.6–3% of dogs [2,24,58,59]. Bile peritonitis, although a rare condition, results from rupture of the gall bladder or bile ducts from either penetrating or blunt trauma [60,61]. Bile pleuritis has also been reported occurring secondary to a biopleural fistula, diaphragmatic hernia, or movement of peritoneal fluid across the intact diaphragm [62,63] (see Chapter 87). Both conditions can be diagnosed by an effusion bilirubin that is at least twice the serum bilirubin and/or the presence of bile pigments on microscopic evaluation of the effusion [60].

While both biliary rupture and uroperitoneum require surgical intervention, it is rare that surgery is indicated in fluid-responsive patients with traumatic hemoperitoneum caused by blunt trauma. In one study, only three of 53 dogs (6%) with hemoperitoneum secondary to blunt trauma required surgical intervention [2]. In most of these animals, hemorrhage is likely originating from the liver or spleen and the intact abdominal wall and the limited space within the peritoneum allow for compression limiting ongoing hemorrhage. However, indications for surgical intervention in blunt traumatic hemoperitoneum include animals that are unresponsive to intravenous fluid resuscitation (i.e. uncontrolled hemorrhage) or that have recurrence of bleeding and increased requirements for blood products. Animals with penetrating abdominal and thoracic injury secondary to bite wounds and impalements should be managed surgically once the patient has been hemodynamically stabilized. Surgical intervention is also indicated for abdominal gunshot wounds due to a high rate of peritonitis but thoracic gunshot wounds can often be managed conservatively with intermittent needle thoracocentesis or a tube thoracostomy to evacuate air and fluid [33].

Considerations for Intravenous Fluid Resuscitation in Trauma

The goal of intravenous fluid resuscitation in the traumatically injured patient is to restore tissue perfusion and oxygen delivery, thereby preventing organ failure. Intravascular volume replacement with crystalloids, colloids, hypertonic saline or blood products is the mainstay of treatment in hemorrhagic shock until hemorrhage ceases or is controlled. However, despite significant research in this field in both experimental animal studies and traumatically injured people, the optimal fluid resuscitation strategy in trauma remains elusive. In several randomized controlled trials comparing the safety and efficacy of different fluid therapy strategies in people with trauma, no clear benefit of one type of fluid therapy was found [64–66] (see Chapters 167–170).

Crystalloid fluid therapy with a balanced electrolyte solution such as Normosol-R or Plasmalyte is generally recommended as the first-line treatment in hemorrhagic shock (see Chapters 167 and 170). Intravenous boluses of 10–30 mL/kg of a balanced electrolyte solution given over 20–30 minutes should be administered until endpoints of resuscitation have been met (i.e. normalized tissue perfusion parameters, urine output, lactate clearance). The potential deleterious effects of aggressive crystalloid administration include the development of tissue edema, coagulopathy, and diluting the oxygen-carrying capacity of the blood. Tissue edema results from the redistribution of crystalloids into the extravascular space within minutes following administration, with only about 10–25% or less of the volume infused

remaining in the circulation after 1 hour [67]. Vascular endothelial injury as a result of the trauma can lead to increased permeability, and dilution of plasma proteins with crystalloids can aggravate the SIRS and interstitial edema [68]. Additionally, hemodilution of clotting proteins and platelets may impair coagulation.

Synthetic colloids, such as hydroxyethyl starch, are another intravascular volume replacement option and remain in the intravascular space for longer compared with crystalloids (see Chapters 168 and 169). Boluses of 5–10 mL/kg over 15–30 minutes are generally used and it is not recommended to exceed the maximum daily dose of 20 mL/kg. In a study that compared the use of crystalloids to hydroxyethyl starch (HES 130/0.4) in severely injured people with penetrating trauma who had already received 2 liters of crystalloids, those who received hetastarch had a faster resuscitation and lactate clearance without evidence of renal injury than people who received additional crystalloids [69] (see Chapter 169). However, synthetic colloids can impair coagulation and their use has been associated with acute kidney failure in people with sepsis [64]. High molecular weight hetastarch reduces factor VIII and von Willebrand's factor and will cause a coagulopathy [70,71]. The nephrotoxic effects of colloids are believed to be secondary to osmotic nephrosis, a condition in which the renal proximal tubular epithelial cells take up colloids, ultimately causing swelling and cellular dysfunction.

In the veterinary literature, there are few studies evaluating whether the administration of colloids is associated with acute kidney injury. In a recent retrospective study of critically ill dogs, the majority of which had septic peritonitis, neoplasia and gastrointestinal tract disease, the use of 6% tetrastarch (hydroxyethyl starch 130/0.4) was not associated with an increase in acute kidney injury as indicated by an increase in creatinine [72]. In people, a recent Cochrane systemic review of 78 randomized controlled trials comparing crystalloids to colloids in critically ill people concluded that there is no evidence to suggest that colloids reduce the mortality risk compared with crystalloids in patients with trauma or burns or following surgery [64]. Although colloids likely still have a role in trauma resuscitation in animals, consideration should be given to the increased cost and possible detrimental effects prior to their administration.

Hypertonic saline (7.2–7.5%) causes a marked osmotic fluid shift from the intracellular space to the extracellular space, leading to an increase in intravascular volume many times the volume infused [67,73]. An infusion of hypertonic saline causes an increase in heart rate and contractility, and a reduction in peripheral vascular resistance, and may improve microcirculatory hemodynamics [74]. Additionally, hypertonic saline may exert an anti-inflammatory effect by reducing proinflammatory cytokines and increasing anti-inflammatory interleukins in hemorrhagic shock, which may limit SIRS [75]. The addition of a colloid to hypertonic saline will extend its intravascular persistence. Studies in people and experimental animal studies have shown that similar to both crystalloids and colloids, the use of hypertonic saline can lead to impaired hemostasis [76–80]. Proposed mechanisms include a dilutional coagulopathy, platelet dysfunction, diminished clot propagation, and clot strength as well as impaired fibrin formation [76–80].

Administration of 3–5 mL/kg of hypertonic saline +/− a colloid intravenously may be particularly useful in animals with severe cardiovascular collapse, either before or during a crystalloid bolus. Additionally, hypertonic saline may be the preferred initial fluid resuscitation choice in hypotensive animals with traumatic brain injury due to its simultaneous effects of expanding intravascular volume and reducing intracranial pressure (see Chapter 19).

In people without traumatic brain injury, different fluid resuscitation strategies for shock have been evaluated due to concerns that aggressive crystalloid resuscitation strategy in uncontrolled hemorrhage results in increased intra-abdominal bleeding and worse outcomes. These strategies include "hypotensive," "controlled", and "limited volume" resuscitation, almost all of which refer to strategies in which the blood pressure is allowed to remain lower than normal during resuscitation compared with conventional resuscitation. Generally, when employing these types of strategies, smaller amounts of balanced isotonic crystalloids, colloids, hypertonic saline, and/or vasopressors are administered to a lower target blood pressure (i.e. 70–100 mmHg). The goal is to avoid artificially elevating the blood pressure and displacing tenuous blood clots after bleeding stops or diminishes in the hypotensive trauma patient.

Evidence from both experimental animal studies and human clinical studies has shown that an aggressive fluid resuscitation strategy results in increased intra-abdominal bleeding and a worse outcome compared to a hypotensive resuscitation strategy. In experimental animal studies, aggressive fluid resuscitation in hemorrhagic shock associated with penetration injuries led to hydraulic disruption of the thrombus, dilution of coagulation factors, and lowering of blood viscosity which was associated with a risk of rebleeding [81–83]. In a landmark study, Bickell et al. demonstrated that in people with penetrating torso injuries, prehospital aggressive fluid administration was associated with lower survival and higher complication rates compared with fluid therapy that was delayed and initiated at the time of surgery [84]. It should be noted that the time to surgical treatment in this study was <30 minutes, a time frame that is generally not achievable in most veterinary practices and therefore limits the applicability of this approach in veterinary

medicine. However, in another clinical trial evaluating different in-hospital fluid resuscitation strategies in traumatically injured people, there was no difference in mortality in people who received conventional fluid therapy compared to a hypotensive resuscitation strategy [85].

To date, the use of a hypotensive fluid resuscitation strategy and blood pressure targets has not been investigated in veterinary trauma patients with hemorrhage. To the author's knowledge, there is only one veterinary study investigating the use of a limited volume fluid strategy protocol compared to conventional resuscitation with large volumes of crystalloids in dogs with hemorrhage secondary to spontaneous hemoperitoneum. In this study [86], dogs in the limited volume fluid resuscitation group were given up to 8 mL/kg of hypertonic saline and 10 mL/kg of hydroxyethyl starch until endpoints of resuscitation were met (HR <120 bpm, RR <40 bpm, and SAP >90 mmHg). Dogs in the conventional resuscitation group received up to 80 mL/kg of crystalloids with the same resuscitation goals. Dogs in the limited volume group reached resuscitation goal endpoints significantly sooner than dogs in the conventional group. However, there was no difference in survival nor a significant difference in red blood cell transfusion requirements, although the study did not have the power to detect a difference in transfusion requirements between the two groups of dogs [86].

In this author's opinion, a limited volume resuscitation strategy may be useful in hemorrhagic shock secondary to trauma but to date, it has not been definitively shown to have a benefit over conventional resuscitation with crystalloids in animals with trauma. A fluid resuscitation strategy that targets a lower than normal blood pressure should be used cautiously (if at all) and only in animals without evidence of traumatic brain injury and in which surgical control of hemorrhage is being emergently pursued.

Administration of blood products (whole blood, packed red blood cells, fresh frozen plasma) may be used as part of the resuscitation strategy of a traumatically injured patient with hemorrhage (see Chapter 176). The benefits of packed red blood cells (pRBCs) and fresh frozen plasma transfusions include intravascular volume expansion while concurrently increasing oxygen carrying capacity and reversing coagulopathy. Accumulating evidence in the human trauma literature suggests that a cumulative ratio of fresh frozen plasma to pRBCs of at least 1:2 is associated with improved survival in people with massive hemorrhage, with some authors recommending a 1:1 ratio until hemorrhage has been controlled [7,87]. However, blood products are expensive, generally in short supply, and can lead to transfusion reactions. Therefore, the administration of blood products is generally reserved for animals with severe hemorrhage unresponsive to conventional fluid resuscitation or those that initially respond to fluid resuscitation but have recurrence of bleeding and shock. Dogs with penetrating trauma may be more likely to require transfusion and approximately 15–36% of dogs will require a pRBC transfusion [2,53,54].

Finally, the syndrome of acute traumatic coagulopathy may contribute to ongoing hemorrhage and need for blood transfusion. This condition is not simply a dilutional or consumptive coagulopathy as a result of intravascular fluid resuscitation and initial hemorrhage, but is thought to also occur secondary to an imbalance of the equilibrium between procoagulant factors, anticoagulant factors, platelets, endothelium, and fibrinolysis. In people, this syndrome may be characterized by factor V inhibition, dysfibrinogenemia, systemic anticoagulation, impaired platelet function, and hyperfibrinolysis [88,89]. Therefore, the early use of antifibrinolytics, such as tranexamic acid or ε-aminocaproic acid, to prevent clot dissolution and additional hemorrhage in trauma patients is intriguing given the limited availability and cost associated with blood transfusions in veterinary medicine (see Chapter 68). This interest stems from the results of the CRASH-2 trial that found that the administration of tranexamic acid to traumatically injured people who were bleeding or at risk of bleeding within 8 hours of injury reduced the risk of death from hemorrhage and decreased overall mortality as compared to placebo [90]. Interestingly, there was no difference in blood transfusions or the number of blood products transfused between the two groups, calling into question the mechanism of the beneficial effect of tranexamic acid [90].

Both tranexamic acid and epsilon-aminocaproic acid (EACA) are lysine derivatives that block the lysine site on plasminogen, thus preventing binding of tPA and preventing fibrinolysis. In veterinary medicine, there have been two clinical studies evaluating EACA in greyhounds undergoing either ovariohysterectomy or limb amputation, both of which demonstrated significant reductions in postoperative bleeding compared to a control group [91,92]. There have also been two recent veterinary retrospective studies describing the use of EACA and tranexamic acid in dogs [93,94]. It is difficult to reach conclusions regarding whether these medications reduce hemorrhage as there was no control group in the EACA study and in the tranexamic study, there were very few dogs with traumatic hemorrhage. However, based on the current data, these medications appear to be safe although tranexamic acid can cause vomiting.

References

1 Muir W. Trauma: physiology, pathophysiology, and clinical implications. *J Vet Emerg Crit Care* 2006;16:253–263.

2 Simpson SA, Syring R, Otto CM. Severe blunt trauma in dogs: 235 cases (1995–2003). *J Vet Emerg Crit Care* 2009;19(6):588–602.

3 Ateca LB, Drobatz K, King LG. Organ dysfunction and mortality risk factors in severe canine bite wound trauma. *J Vet Emerg Crit Care* 2014;24(6):705–714.

4 Neligan PJ, Barnov D. Trauma and aggressive homeostasis management. *Anesthesiol Clin* 2013;31(1):21–39.

5 Dunham CM, Siegel JH, Weireter L, et al. Oxygen debt and metabolic acidaemia as quantitative predictors of mortality and the severity of the ischemic insult in hemorrhagic shock. *Crit Care Med* 1991;19:231–243.

6 Duchesne JC, McSwain NE, Cotton BA, et al. Damage control resuscitation: the new face of damage control. *J Trauma* 2010;69(4):976–990.

7 Dutton RP. Fluid management for trauma: where are we now? *Contin Educ Anesth Crit Care Pain* 2006;6(4):144–147.

8 Lord JM, Midwinter MJ, Chen YF, et al. The systemic immune response to trauma: an overview of pathophysiology and treatment. *Lancet* 2014;384(9952):1455–1465.

9 Zhang Q, Raoof M, Chen Y, et al. Circulating mitochondrial DAMPS cause inflammatory responses to injury. *Nature* 2010;464:104–107.

10 Manson J, Theimermann C, Brohi K. Trauma alarmins as activators of damage induced inflammation. *Br J Surg* 2012;99 Suppl 1:12–20.

11 Burk AM, Martin M, Fleirl MA, et al. Early complementopathy after multiple injuries in humans. *Shock* 2012;37:348–354.

12 Neher MD, Weckbach S, Flierl MA, et al. Molecular mechanisms of inflammation and tissue injury after major trauma – is complement the "bad guy"? *J Biomed Sci* 2011;18:90.

13 Huber-Lang M, Kovtun A, Ignatius A. The role of complement in trauma and fracture healing. *Semin Immunol* 2013;25:73–78.

14 Ward PA. The dark side of C5a in sepsis. *Nat Rev Immunol* 2004;4:133–142.

15 Jenne CN, Urrutia R. Kubes P. Platelets: bridging hemostasis, inflammation, and immunity. *Int J Lab Hematol* 2013;35:254–261.

16 Reino DC, Palange D. Feketeova E, et al. Activation of toll-like receptor 4 is necessary for trauma hemorrhagic shock-induced gut injury and polymorphonuclear neutrophil priming. *Shock* 2012;38:107–114.

17 Xiao W, Mindrinos MN, Seok J, et al. The inflammation and host reponse to injury large-scale collaborative

research program. A genomic storm in critically injured humans. *J Exp Med* 2011;208:2581–2590.

18 Gentile LF, Cuenca AG, Efron PA, et al. Persistent inflammation and immunosuppression: a common syndrome and new horizon for surgical intensive care. *J Trauma Acute Care Surg* 2012;72:1491–1501.

19 Kolata RJ, Kraut NH, Johnston DE. Patterns of trauma in urban dogs and cats: a study of 1000 cases. *J Am Vet Med Assoc* 1974;164:499–502.

20 Hayes G, Matthews K, Doig G, et al. The acute patient physiologic and laboratory evaluation (APPLE) score: a severity of illness stratification system for hospitalized dogs. *J Vet Intern Med* 2010;24:1034–1047.

21 Fleming JM, Creevy KE, Promisolw DEL. Mortality in North American dogs from 1984 to 2004: an investigation into age-, size-, and breed-related causes of death. *J Vet Intern Med* 2011;25(2):187–198.

22 Hall KE, Holowaychuk MK, Sharp CR, Reineke E. Multicenter prospective evaluation of dogs with trauma. *J Am Vet Med Assoc* 2014;244(3):300–308.

23 Hall K, Sharp C, Reineke E, et al. A multicenter prospective cohort study of feline patients sustaining trauma: interim analysis. *J Vet Emerg Crit Care* 2013;23(S1):S7.

24 Streeter EM, Rozanski EA, de Laforcade-Buress A, et al. Evaluation of vehicular trauma in dogs: 239 cases (January–December 2001). *J Am Vet Med Assoc* 2009;235(4):405–408.

25 Intarapanich NP, McCobb EC, Reisman RW, et al. Characterization and comparison of injuries caused by accidental and non-accidental blunt force trauma in dogs and cats. *J Forensic Sci* 2016;61(4):993–999.

26 Mehler SJ, Otto CM. Penetration injury in the dog and cat. In: *Small Animal Surgical Emergencies* (ed. Aronson LR). John Wiley & Sons, Ames, pp. 456–464.

27 Shamir MH, Leisner S, Klement E, et al. Dog bite wounds in dogs and cats: a retrospective study of 196 cases. *J Vet Med A Physiol Pathol Clin Med* 2002;49(2):107–112.

28 Griffin GM, Holt DE. Dog-bite wounds: bacteriology and treatment outcome in 37 cases. *J Am Anim Hosp Assoc* 2001;37(5):453–460.

29 Meyers B, Schoeman JP, Goddard A. The bacteriology and antimicrobial susceptibility of infected and non-infected dog bite wounds: fifty cases. *Vet Microbiol* 2008;127(3–4):360–369.

30 Black DM, Rankin SC, King LG. Antimicrobial therapy and aerobic bacteriologic culture patterns in canine intensive unit patients: 74 dogs (January–June 2006). *J Vet Emerg Crit Care* 2009;19(5):489–495.

31 Abrahamian FM, Goldstein EC. Microbiology of animal bite wound infections. *Clin Microbiol Rev* 2011;24(2):231–246.

32 Mouro S, Vilela CL, Niza M. Clinical and bacteriological assessment of dog-to-dog bite wounds. *Vet Microbiol* 2010;144(1-2):127–132.

33 Fullington RJ, Otto CM. Characteristics and management of gunshot wounds in dogs and cats: 84 cases (1986–1995). *J Am Vet Med Assoc* 1997;5:658–662.

34 Olsen LE, Streeter EM, DeCook RR. Review of gunshot injuries in cats and dogs and the utility of a triage scoring system to predict short term outcome: 37 cases (2003–2008). *J Am Vet Med Assoc* 2014;245(8):923–929.

35 Baker JL, Havas KA, Miller LA, et al. Gunshot wounds in military working dogs in Operation Enduring Freedom and Operation Iraqi Freedom: 29 cases (2003–2009). *J Vet Emerg Crit Care* 2013;23(1):47–52.

36 Rockar RA, Drobatz KS. Development of a scoring system for the veterinary trauma patient. *J Vet Emerg Crit Care* 1994;4(2):77–82.

37 Platt SR, Radaelli T, McDonnell JJ. The prognostic value of the modified Glasgow coma scale in head trauma in dogs. *J Vet Intern Med* 2001;15:581–584.

38 Sharma D, Holowaychuk MK. Retrospective evaluatuion of prognostic indicators in dogs with head trauma: 72 cases (January–March 2011). *J Vet Emerg Crit Care* 2015;25(5):631–639.

39 Driessen B, Brainard B. Fluid therapy for the traumatized patient. *J Vet Emerg Crit Care* 2005;16(4):276–299.

40 Ateca LB, Reineke EL, Drobatz KJ. Relationship between metatarsal pulse palpation and systolic Doppler blood pressure in dogs presenting to an emergency service. *J Vet Emerg Crit Care* 2014;24(S1):S4.

41 Reineke EL, Rees C, Drobatz KJ. Prediction of systolic blood pressure using peripheral pulse palpation in cats. *J Vet Emerg Crit Care* 2016;26(1):52–57.

42 Peterson KL, Hardy BT, Hall K. Assessment of shock index in healthy dogs and dogs in hemorrhagic shock. *J Vet Emerg Crit Care* 2013;23(5):545–550.

43 Macintire DK, Snider TG. Cardiac arrhythmias associated with multiple trauma in dogs. *J Am Vet Med Assoc* 1984;184:541–545.

44 Buttrick ML, Riedesel DH, Selcer BA, et al. Hypoexemia in the acutely traumatized canine patient. *J Vet Emerg Crit Care* 1992;2(2):73–79.

45 Spackman CJ, Caywood DD. Feeney DA, et al. Thoracic wall and pulmonary trauma in dogs sustaining fractures as a result of motor vehicle accidents. *J Am Vet Med Assoc* 1984;185(9):975–977.

46 Tamas PM, Paddleford RR, Krahwinkel DJ. Thoracic trauma in dogs and cats presented for limb fractures. *J Am Anim Hosp Assoc* 1984;21(2):161–166.

47 Selcer BA. The incidence of thoracic trauma in dogs with skeletal injury. *J Small Anim Pract* 1987;28:21.

48 Cook JL. Cook CR, Tomlinson JL, et al. Scapular fractures in dogs: epidemiology, classification, and concurrent injuries in 105 cases (1988–1994). *J Am Anim Hosp Assoc* 1997;33(6):528–532.

49 Sigrist NE. Adamik KN, Doherr MG, Spreng DE. Evaluation of respiratory parameters at presentation as clinical indicators of the respiratory localization in dogs and cats with respiratory distress. *J Vet Emerg Crit Care* 2001;21(1):13–23.

50 Clark CH, Woodley CH. The absorption of red blood cells after parenteral injection at various sites. *Am J Vet Res* 1959;20:1062–1066.

51 Nichols RT, Pearce HU, Greenfield LJ. Effects of experimental pulmonary contusion on respiratory exchange and lung mechanics. *Arch Surg* 1968;96:723–730.

52 Erickson DR, Schinozaki T, Beekman E, Davis J. Relationship of Arterial blood gases and pulmonary radiographs to the degree of pulmonary damage in experimental pulmonary contusion. *J Trauma* 1971;11:689–694.

53 Lynch AM, O'Toole TE, Respess M. Transfusion practices for treatment of dogs hospitalized following trauma: 125 cases (2008–2013). *J Am Vet Med Assoc* 2015;247:643–649.

54 Stillion JR, Fletcher DJ. Admission base excess as a predictor of transfusion requirement and mortality in dogs with blunt trauma: 52 cases (2007–2009). *J Vet Emerg Crit Care* 2012;22(5):588–594.

55 Lisciandro G, Lagutchik MS, Mann KA, et al. Evaluation of an abdominal fluid scoring system determined using abdominal focused assessment with sonography for trauma in 101 dogs with motor vehicle trauma. *J Vet Emerg Crit Care* 2009;19(5):426–437.

56 Schmiedt C, Tobia KM, Otto CM. Evaluation of abdominal fluid:peripheral blood creatinine and potassium ratios for diagnosis of uroperitoneum in dogs. *J Vet Emerg Crit Care* 2001;11:275–280.

57 Aumann M, Worth LT, Drobatz KJ. Uroperitoneum in cats: 26 cases (1986–1995). *J Am Anim Hosp Assoc* 1998;34:315–324.

58 Boysen SR, Rozanski EA, Tidwell AS. Evaluation of a focused assessement with sonography for trauma protocol to detect free abdominal fluid in dogs involved in motor vehicle accidents. *J Am Vet Med Assoc* 2004;225(8):1198–1204.

59 Hoffberg JE, Koenigshof AM, Guiot LP. Retrospective evaluation of concurrent intra–abdominal injuries in dogs with traumatic pelvic fractures: 83 cases (2008–2013). *J Vet Emerg Crit Care* 2016;26(2):288–294.

60 Ludwig LL, McLoughlin MA, Graves TK, Crisp MS. Surgical treatment of bile peritonitis in 24 dogs and 2 cats: a retrospective study (1987–1994). *Vet Surg* 1997;26(2):90–98.

61 Dennler R, Grundmann S. Traumatic rupture of the common bile duct in a dog. *Schweiz Arch Tierheikd* 2003;145(4):181–187.

62 Peddle GD, Carberry CA, Goggin JM. Hemorrhagic bile pleuritic and peritonitis secondary to traumatic common bile duct rupture, diaphragmatic tear, and rupture of the spleen in a dog. *J Vet Emerg Crit Care* 2008;18(6):631–638.

63 Barnhardt MD, Rasmussen LM. Pleural effusion as a complication of extrahepatic biliary tract rupture in the dog. *J Am Anim Hosp Assoc* 1996;32(5):409–412.

64 Perel P, Roberts I, Ker K. Colloids versus crystalloids for fluid resuscitation in critically ill patients. *Cochrane Database Syst Rev* 2013;2:CD000567.

65 Finfer S, Bellomo R, Boyce N, et al. A comparison of albumin and saline for fluid resuscitation in the intensive care unit. *N Engl J Med* 2004;350:2247–2256.

66 Annane D, Siami S, Jaber S, et al. Effects of fluid resuscitation with colloids versus crystalloids on mortality in criticall ill patients presenting with hypovolemic shock the CRISTAL randomized trial. *J Am Vet Med Assoc* 2013;310(17):1809–1817.

67 Silverstein DS, Aldrich J, Haskins SC, Drobatz KJ, Cowgill LD. Assessment of changes in blood volume in response to resuscitative fluid administration in dogs. *J Vet Emerg Crit Care* 2005;15(3):185–192.

68 Bauer M, Kortgen A, Hartog C, et al. Isotonic and hypertonic crystalloid solutions in the critically ill. *Best Pract Res Clin Anaesthesiol* 2009;23:173–181.

69 James MF, Michell WL, Joubert IA. Resuscitation with hydroxyethyl starch improves renal function and lactate clearance in penetrating trauma in a randomized controlled study: the FIRST trial (fluids in resuscitation of severe trauma). *Br J Anaesth* 2011;107(5):693–702.

70 Treib J, Hass A, Pindur G. Coagulation disorders caused by hydroxyethyl starch. *Thromb Haemost* 1997;78:974–983.

71 Petroianu GA, Liu J, Malek WH, Mattinger C, Bergler WF. The effect of in vitro hemodiluation with gelatin, dextran, hydroxyethyl starch, or Ringer's solution on the thromboelastograph. *Anesth Analg* 2000;90:795–800.

72 Yozova ID, Howard J, Adamik KN. Retrospective evaluation of the effects of administration of tetrastarch (hydoxyethyl starch 130/0.4) on plasma creatinine concentration in dogs (2010–2013): 201 dogs. *J Vet Emerg Crit Care* 2016;26(4):568–577.

73 Kramer GC, Elgjo GI, Poli de Figueiredo LF, Wade CE. Hyperosmotic-hyperoncotic solutions. *Baillière's Clin Anesthesiol* 1997;11:143–60.

74 Rocha E, Silva M. Hypertonic saline resuscitation: a new concept. *Baillière's Cin Anaesthesiol* 1997;11:127–142.

75 Rizoli SB, Rhind SG, Shek PN, et al. The immunomodulatory effects of hypertonic saline resuscitation in patients sustaining traumatic hemorrhagic shock: a randomized, controlled, double blinded trial. *Ann Surg* 2006;243:47–57.

76 Luostarinen T, Niija T, Schramko A, Rosenberg R, Niem T. Comparison of hypertonic saline and mannitol on whole blood coagulation in vitro assessed by thromboelastometry. *Neurocrit Care* 2011;14(2):238–243.

77 Tan TS, Tan KH, Ng HP, Loh MW. The effects of hypertonic saline solution (7.5%) on coagulation and fibrinolysis: an in vitro assessment using thromboelastography. *Anaesthesia* 2002;57(7):644–648.

78 Wilder DM, Reid TJ, Bakaltcheva IB. Hypertonic saline resuscitation and blood coagulation: in vitro comparison of several hypertonic solutions for their action on platelets and plasma coagulation. *Thromb Res* 2002;107(5):255–261.

79 Hanke AA, Maschler S, Schochl H, et al. In vitro impairment of whole blood coagulation and platelet function by hypertonic saline hydroxyethyl starch. *Scand J Trauma Resus Emerg Med* 2011;19:12.

80 Adamik KN, Butty E, Howard J. In vitro effects of 3% hypertonic saline and 20% mannitol on canine whole blood coagulation and platelet function. *BMC Vet Res* 2015;11:242.

81 Bickell WH, Bruttig SP, Millnamow GA, et al. Use of hypertonic saline/dextran versus lactated Ringer's solution as a resuscitation fluid after uncontrolled hemorrhage in anesthetized swine. *Ann Emerg Med* 1992;21:1077–1085.

82 Shaftan GW, Chiu CJ, Dennis C, Harris B. Fundamentals of physiologic control of arterial hemorrhage. *Surgery* 1965;58:851–856.

83 Bickell WH, Bruttig SP, Millnamow GA, et al. The detrimental effects of intravenous crystalloid after aortotomy in swine. *Surgery* 1991;110:529–536.

84 Bickell WH, Wall MJ, Pepe PE, et al. Immediate versus delayed fluid resuscitation for hypotensive patients with penetrating torso injuries. *N Engl J Med* 1994;331:1105–1109.

85 Dutton RP, Mackenzie CF, Scalea TM. Hypotensive resuscitation during active hemorrhage: impact on in-hospital mortality. *J Trauma* 2002;52:1141–1146.

86 Hammond TN, Holm JL, Sharp CR. A pilot comparison of limited versus large volume fluid resuscitation in canine spontaneous hemoperitoneum. *J Am Anim Hosp Assoc* 2014;50(3):1–8.

87 Stanworth SJ, Davenport R, Curry N, et al. Mortality from trauma hemorrhage and opportunities for improvement in transfusion practice. *Br J Surg* 2016;103(4):357–65.

88 Frith D, Brohi K. The pathophysiology of trauma-induced coagulopathy. *Curr Opin Crit Care* 2012;18(6):631–636.

89 Frith D, Davenport R, Brohi K. Acute traumatic coagulopathy. *Curr Opin Anaesthesiol* 2012;25(2):229–234.

90 CRASH-2 Trial Collaborators, Shakur H, Roberts I, et al. Effects of tranexamic acid on death, vascular occlusive events, and blood transfusion in trauma patients with significant hemorrhage (CRASH-2): a randomized, placebo-controlled trial. *Lancet* 2010;376(9734):23–32.

91 Marin LM, Iazbik MC, Zaldivar-Lopez S, et al. Epsilon aminocaproic acid for the prevention of delayed postoperative bleeding in retired racing greyhounds undergoing gonadectomy. *Vet Surg* 2012;41(5):594–603.

92 Marin LM, Iazbik MC, Zaldivar-Lopez S, et al. Retrospective evaluation of the effectiveness of epsilon aminocaproic acid for the prevention of postamputation bleeding in retired racing Greyhounds with appendicular bone tumors:46 cases (2003–2008). *J Vet Emerg Crit Care* 2012;22(3):332–340.

93 Davis M, Bracker K. Retrospective study of 122 dogs that were treated with the antifibrinolytic drug aminocaprioic acid: 2010–2012. *J Am Anim Hosp* 2016;52:144–148.

94 Kelmer E, Marer K, Bruchim Y, et al. Retrospective evaluation of the safety and efficacy of tranexamic acid (Hexakapron®) for the treatment of bleeding disorders in dogs. *Isr J Vet Med* 2013;68(2):94–100.

161

Trauma Center Registry

Kelly Hall, DVM, MS, DACVECC

ACVECC-Veterinary Committee on Trauma, Stillwater, MN, USA

Veterinary Trauma Initiative

Cats and dogs sustaining traumatic injury present frequently to hospitals, and have an overall very high survival rate [1–4]. Despite a high frequency of positive outcomes, trauma is the second leading cause of death in dogs and there remains an acute drop-off in survivability for more severely injured animals [4–6]. Data support a significant drop-off in survivability of dogs with an Animal Trauma and Triage (ATT) score greater than 5 [4,5,7]. There is enormous opportunity to improve outcome and reduce co-morbidities in the veterinary trauma population.

Established in 2010, and subsequently recognized as an *ad hoc* committee by the American College of Veterinary Emergency and Critical Care (ACVECC), the Veterinary Committee on Trauma (VetCOT) has a vision to create a network of lead hospitals that seed development of trauma systems. These hospitals work collaboratively to define high standards of care and disseminate information that improves trauma patient management efficiency and outcome. In order to achieve this vision, veterinary trauma centers (VTCs) contribute to a trauma registry that allows for continued advancement of trauma patient care.

The four aims of the trauma initiative are:

- enhancement of trauma patient care
- enhancement and promotion of research collaborations
- expansion and formalization of education on veterinary trauma
- enhancement of the visibility of veterinary specialty colleges.

Trauma Registries: History and Purpose

In the United States, formation of trauma centers and systems for human trauma patient care was initiated in the 1970s through the American College of Surgeons Committee on Trauma (ACS-COT). Trauma registries began development at the same time. In its first large-scale study (Major Trauma Outcome Study), 139 North American hospitals submitted data on >80 000 cases over a 5-year period (1982–1987). This study became the springboard for further development of trauma registries, and established the importance of utilizing trauma registries for individual hospital and trauma system quality assurance as well as informing performance improvement programs [8]. Today, the National Trauma Data Bank (NTDB) houses the largest aggregation of trauma registry data ever assembled and is utilized by hospitals and researchers alike to improve trauma patient care [9].

The objectives of trauma registries are to [10]:

- assess and improve patient care
- identify opportunities for injury prevention initiatives
- document the medical, economical, and social effects of trauma
- develop and test research hypotheses.

In 2013, the VetCOT-Registry Subcommittee (VetCOT-RS) recommended the use of REDCap [11] to house the first ever multicenter veterinary trauma registry. In September of that year, nine VTCs started entering prospectively obtained data on trauma cases presenting to their hospital. In the first year, data from >3000 trauma cases were entered into the database. With 13 additional VTCs entering their trauma cases beginning January 2015, and five additional centers in August 2015, the veterinary trauma registry grew to >10 000 cases by October 2015. This makes the VetCOT-housed trauma registry the largest trauma-specific medical database in veterinary medicine.

Trauma Registry: The Future

In January 2015, the VetCOT Registry subcommittee, in collaboration with the full VetCOT and VTC leads, finalized the "Registry Guidelines for Data Use and Authorship," outlining the mechanisms for accessing and evaluating data from the veterinary trauma database [12]. As of this writing, the first two projects that were approved are in process, and a further calls for applicants are expected. It is anticipated that the results of these, and future studies, will be presented at the annual Veterinary Trauma and Critical Care Conference and published in peer-reviewed journals. Studies of this magnitude are rare in veterinary medicine, and the ability to apply findings to improve current patient care and inform development of future clinical research is enhanced by the statistical power possible with large, multicenter study cohorts.

The VetCOT-RS anticipates publishing an open-access annual summary of the epidemiological data in the veterinary trauma registry modeled after the NTDB annual report [9]. It is hoped that this information will inform development of interventional clinical research, which is particularly sparse in veterinary trauma literature. Volume resuscitation of the severely hemorrhaging patient, damage control surgery, management of traumatic brain and spinal injury, maximizing triage tool application, improving survival for the most severely injured patients and cost-effective care for all patients are just a few of the areas where opportunity exists in improving veterinary trauma patient care. Additionally, given the similarities between human and canine trauma, opportunity exists to utilize naturally occurring trauma in dogs as a pre-phase I and pre-phase II model for interventions being evaluated for human trauma patient care [13]. This advantage, supported by registry data, can potentially help researchers obtain funding for clinical trials and research that would ultimately benefit both veterinary and human trauma patients.

Acknowledgments

Significant admiration, gratitude, and appreciation to the VetCOT members and particularly the Registry Subcommittee (Manuel Boller, Soren Boysen, Jamie Hoffberg, Marie Holowaychuk, Maureen McMichael, Marc Raffe, Lauren Sullivan) as well as the VTC leads and teams, ACVECC Regents, and collaborating allied specialty groups.

Excerpts of this chapter were paraphrased from similar resources generated by the author (Hall) and collaborators:

- Hall K, de Laforcade A. Veterinary trauma centers. J Vet Emerg Crit Care 2013;23(4):373–375.
- Hall K, Sharp C. The veterinary trauma initiative: why bother? J Vet Emerg Crit Care 2014;24(6):639–641.

References

1 Hayes G, Mathews K, Doig G, et al. The acute patient physiologic and laboratory evaluation (APPLE) score: a severity of illness stratification system for hospitalized dogs. *J Vet Intern Med* 2010;24(5):1034–1047.

2 Hayes G, Mathews K, Doig G, et al. The feline acute patient physiologic and laboratory evaluation (Feline APPLE) score: a severity of illness stratification system for hospitalized cats. *J Vet Intern Med* 2011;25(1): 26–38.

3 Hall KE, Sharp, CR, Reineke E, Cooper E, Koenigshof A, Drobatz K. A multi-center prospective cohort study of feline patients sustaining trauma: interim analysis. *J Vet Emerg Crit Care* 2013;23(S1):S7.

4 Hall KE, Holowaychuk MK, Sharp CR, Reineke E. Multicenter prospective evaluation of dogs with trauma. *J Am Vet Med Assoc* 2014;244(3):300–308.

5 Rockar RA, Drobatz KS, Shofer FS. Development of a scoring system for the veterinary trauma patient. *J Vet Emerg Crit Care* 1994;4(2):77–83.

6 Fleming JM, Creevy KE, Promislow DE. Mortality in North American Dogs from 1984 to 2004: an investigation into age-, size-, and breed-related causes of death. *J Vet Intern Med* 2011;25(2):187–198.

7 Abelson AL, O'Toole TE, Johnston A, Respess M, de Laforcade AM. Hypoperfusion and acute traumatic coagulopathy in severely traumatized canine patients. *J Vet Emerg Crit Care* 2013;23(4):395–401.

8 Champion HR, Copes WS, Sacco WJ, Lawnick MM, Keast SL, Frey CF. The Major Trauma Outcome Study: establishing national norms for trauma care. *J Trauma Acute Care Surg* 1990;30(11):1356–1365.

9 American College of Surgeons, Committee on Trauma. National Trauma Data Bank (NTDB). Available at: www.facs.org/quality-programs/trauma/ntdb/docpub (accessed 13 February 2018).

10 Zehtabchi S, Nishijima DK, McKay MP, Clay Mann N. Trauma registries: history, logistics, limitations, and contributions to emergency medicine research. *Acad Emerg Med* 2011;18(6):637–643.

11 Harris PA, Taylor R, Thielke R, Payne J, Gonzalez N, Conde JG. Research electronic data capture (REDCap) – a metadata-driven methodology and workflow process for providing translational research informatics support. *J Biomed Informat* 2009;42(2):377–381.

12 Veterinary Committee on Trauma. Registry. Available at: https://sites.google.com/a/umn.edu/vetcot/registry (accessed 13 February 2018).

13 Hall KE, Sharp CR, Adams CR, Beilman G. A novel trauma model: naturally occurring canine trauma. *Shock* 2014;41(1):25–32.

162

High-Rise Syndrome

Yekaterina Buriko, DVM, DACVECC

Matthew J. Ryan Veterinary Hospital, University of Pennsylvania, Philadelphia, PA, USA

Definition and Pathophysiology

High-rise syndrome (HRS) refers to the constellation of injuries sustained after falling from a certain height. By convention, in veterinary medicine a high-rise injury is defined as vertical fall from two stories or higher, which is a distance of about 24 feet. Animals that reside in urban areas are particularly predisposed to this condition. It appears to be a disease of young animals, likely due to the fact that they are more curious and more likely to explore, but all ages have been represented [1,2]. Sexually intact animals may be more likely to suffer from HRS, potentially due to increased propensity for roaming [1,2]. HRS has been reported to occur in warmer months, as it is likely the time when most people open windows, providing the animals with access to the outdoors [1,2].

During a fall from a height in atmospheric environment, the velocity of the fall is dependent on the distance fallen, as well as body mass and shape due to air resistance. These are likely the major determinants of injury severity. Distance fallen is a major predictor of injury severity and mortality in people [3], with head and chest injuries being significantly associated with mortality. Other factors that may play a role are objects encountered during the fall, the surface type encountered upon impact, as well as the body parts that hit the surface first [1,2,4].

It appears that dogs and cats behave differently when falling from a height. Dogs behave more like humans in that injury severity and life-threatening injuries were directly proportional to the height of the fall [2]. Conflicting evidence exists in cats. Some studies report that survival is negatively associated with the height of the fall [5], and injury scores increase in animals that have fallen over seven stories [6]. Others conclude that the injury rates ceased to increase and fracture numbers decreased in cats that fell from a height of over seven stories [1]. It is

speculated that during the fall, due to air resistance, their small size, natural dexterity and ability to stretch their body to increase the surface area, thus enhancing drag, cats achieve a terminal velocity of 100 kilometers per hour after a fall of about five stories, after which acceleration ceases and they continue falling at a constant speed [1]. Prior to reaching terminal velocity, it is postulated that cats reflexively extend their limbs, and if the fall is under five stories, the limbs absorb the impact of the fall. After the terminal velocity is reached, the cat assumes a more horizontal position, flexes its limbs, and if contact happens at any point during that time, the impact of the deceleration is more evenly distributed, potentially leading to more truncal injuries [1,5]. This is corroborated by the study by Vnuk, in which the percentage of fractures decreased and the percentage of thoracic injuries went up in falls higher than seven stories [6]. Other studies do not report any particular pattern, but uncover a complex relationship between the number of floors fallen and the types and extent of injuries sustained by cats [5]. This is likely due to the multifactorial nature of the cause of damage to the body in HRS.

The landing surface may play a significant role in the morbidity of cases of high-rise injury. In addition, objects encountered during the fall may enhance or mitigate sustained trauma. One study evaluated injury association with the landing surface and did not detect a difference in the severity of injury for cats [1]. However, landing onto spiked metal railings resulted in severe life-threatening penetrating injuries to three cats in one case series [4]. Gordon et al. reported that dogs landing on hard surfaces suffered more total injuries [2].

Clinical Signs

The first priority upon triage and initial assessment of the patient that has experienced HRS is establishing

Textbook of Small Animal Emergency Medicine, First Edition. Edited by Kenneth J. Drobatz, Kate Hopper, Elizabeth Rozanski and Deborah C. Silverstein.
© 2019 John Wiley & Sons, Inc. Published 2019 by John Wiley & Sons, Inc.
Companion Website: www.wiley.com/go/drobatz/textbook

whether any life-threatening injuries have occurred (see Chapter 2). The stabilization effort should be directed to rapidly identifying and addressing these. A complete physical examination is imperative; previous reports of HRS identified that head, thoracic, and extremity injuries have been reported most commonly [1,2,6], and an effort should be made to thoroughly inspect those areas.

A substantial number of animals present in shock, which could be due to hemorrhage, distributive shock secondary to massive tissue damage, or hypoxia [1,5,6] (see Chapters 152, 153, and 155). Signs of shock may include dull mentation, poor pulse quality, and pale mucous membranes. Hypothermia may be associated with poor perfusion and has been documented in cats with shock in one study [5]. It is of the utmost importance that animals in shock are identified as such, so immediate resuscitation can be initiated.

Acute traumatic coagulopathy (ATC) is a condition described in both severely injured human and veterinary patients and is characterized by impairment of hemostasis that can ensue independent of exogenous factors, such as fluid resuscitation, acidemia, and hypothermia [7–10] (see Chapters 70 and 163). The exact etiology is not well described, but is likely in part due to endogenous hyperfibrinolysis and elevated levels of protein C [7,9]. It is probable that acute traumatic coagulopathy exists in the subset of more severely injured high-rise cases, particularly those with massive tissue damage and shock on presentation [7]. These animals are possibly more likely to experience ongoing hemorrhage. Therefore, it is prudent to identify the patients most at risk for ATC, so that careful monitoring and re-evaluation may be implemented.

Thoracic trauma is an essential component of the HRS in dogs and cats [1,2,5,6] (see Chapters 48 and 49). Respiratory signs range from normal exam and auscultation to severe dyspnea. Pneumothorax and pulmonary contusions are very frequent findings in both dogs and cats and may be present in cats that are eupneic on physical examination [1] (see Chapter 44). Diaphragmatic hernia is an infrequent but significant sequela of HRS, and has been documented in about 2% of feline cases in several case series [1,6] (see Chapter 47). Thoracic auscultation may reveal increased lung sounds or crackles in the event of pulmonary contusions or decreased lung sounds in the event of pneumothorax, hemothorax or diaphragmatic hernia. Palpation of the chest may reveal pain or crepitus, if rib fractures are present.

Injuries to the head and face are a significant cause of morbidity in dogs and cats affected by HRS, and up to 67% patients may have these injuries [1,2,5,6] (see Chapter 19). Common signs include facial swelling, abrasions and wounds, epistaxis, pain upon manipulation of the jaw and possible bony instability if the fractures have

occurred. A complete evaluation of the facial area, palpation for fractures and thorough evaluation of the oral cavity for wounds, fractured or displaced teeth and fractures, including the hard palate for fractures and soft palate for tears, is paramount (Figure 162.1). Ophthalmological examination is important to rule out ocular injury, specifically intraocular hemorrhage, which may result in loss of sight (see Chapter 12).

Even though facial injuries are common in animal HRS, the incidence of significant traumatic brain injury is significantly smaller than that in people, with reported numbers of 7% in cats and 5% in dogs [2,5]. However, a detailed neurological examination should be undertaken as the patient's condition permits, and the animal should be frequently reassessed after stabilization to gain a more complete clinical picture and detect any changes.

Abdominal injuries are not as common as thoracic injuries in HRS but represent a significant threat to life and may require extensive care. Physical examination may reveal body wall defects, if a traumatic body wall hernia occurred. Pain upon palpation of the abdomen may be present with abdominal injury and should prompt a closer investigation of the abdominal cavity [5]. Hematuria may be present as well [1,2]. Studies that evaluated abdominal injuries found that 15% of dogs and 1–17% of cats had significant abdominal injuries, including hemoperitoneum secondary to splenic rupture (see Chapter 84), uroperitoneum secondary to rupture of the urinary bladder or other conduits (see Chapter 103), and diaphragmatic hernia [1,2,5,6]. Moreover, pancreatic rupture and traumatic pancreatitis are rare complications of HRS that have been documented in cats and may result in severe systemic inflammation, multiorgan failure and death [8,9] (see Chapter 86). Clinical signs of pancreatic rupture may not be evident immediately upon evaluation and may take several days after initial injury to fully manifest [11,12].

Skeletal injuries are a major component of HRS in both dogs and cats, with up to 50% of animals sustaining at least one fracture or ligamentous injury [1,2,5,6]. Reported distributions of injuries vary slightly, but generally are similar in frequency between forelimbs and hindlimbs. Animals with skeletal injuries may present with a range of symptoms ranging from lameness to non-ambulation with elicited pain upon manipulation of the affected site. Some injuries may be readily apparent, while others may require a thorough examination to pinpoint. In addition, cardiovascular and respiratory instability may delay diagnosis of the skeletal injury, and a thorough physical exam should be undertaken after the patient is stable.

Spinal cord and canal injuries are reported in 2–13% of cats suffering from HRS and up to 15% of dogs [1,2,5] (see Chapter 24). Signs may be similar to animals with other skeletal injuries and include difficulty ambulating

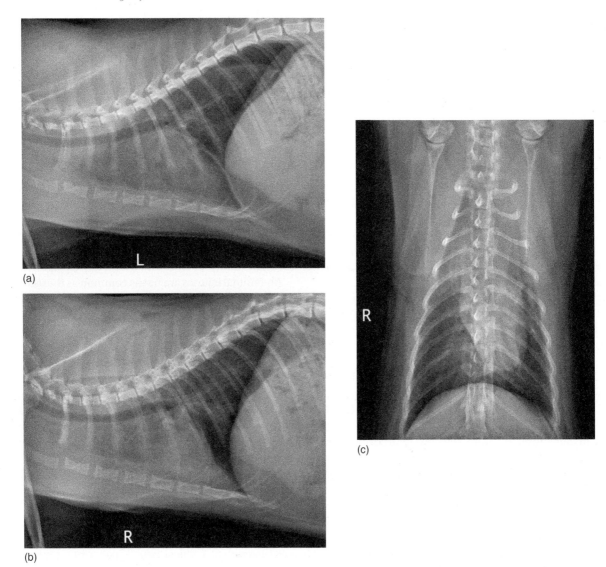

(a)

(b)

(c)

Figure 162.1 (a–c) Pulmonary contusions and a mild pneumothorax in a cat who suffered from HRS but appeared eupneic on presentation to the hospital.

or inability to ambulate, ataxia and neurological deficits, dependent on the anatomical location of the injury. As the focus tends to be on the more obvious abnormalities and fractures of the extremities, spinal injuries may be easily missed, but can change the prognosis and alter the course of treatment, if significant. Similarly to evaluation of skeletal injuries, a full neurological examination should be undertaken once the patient is stable.

Diagnostics

In addition to a thorough physical examination, the initial diagnostic database should be tailored to the needs of the individual animal and the severity of injuries sustained.

Most commonly, values collected upon triage should include a rectal temperature, a blood pressure measurement, pulse oximetry, electrocardiogram and point-of-care bloodwork, which includes a packed red blood cell volume (PCV), blood glucose and ideally a venous blood gas with a lactate (see Chapter 2). Serial evaluations of physical exam parameters, PCV, and lactate measurements will be useful in guiding resuscitation.

Due to the high incidence of thoracic injuries, imaging of the chest cavity (see Chapter 182) should be undertaken in all animals exhibiting signs of respiratory tract dysfunction. Animal stability should never be compromised to obtain imaging; if severe dyspnea is present, stabilization measures should be undertaken first, including oxygen supplementation, minimizing stress, adequate pain control and possibly diagnostic thoracentesis, in case clinically significant pleural space disease is present (see Chapters 181, 183 and 193). Variable incidence of thoracic trauma has been documented, and the need for thoracic radiographs in animals without obvious abnormalities referable to the respiratory tract is questioned. Some animals, notably cats, have been documented to be eupneic while thoracic injuries were present [1] (see Figure 162.1). Many of these animals will be sedated or anesthetized for additional procedures and surgeries, and therefore routine imaging of the thorax may be advisable.

Veterinary abdominal and thoracic focused assessment with sonography for trauma (FAST) has been increasingly utilized and can be an invaluable bedside tool in evaluation of high-rise patients, especially those that are too unstable to be moved for radiographs [14] (see Chapter 182). aFAST is a rapid non-invasive way of evaluating for abdominal effusion, and tFAST may be used for evaluation of pleural effusion, as well as for pneumothorax, although the learning curve for recognition of pneumothorax is higher than for fluid recognition. Ultrasound may aid in timely diagnosis of hemorrhage and rupture of the urinary or gastrointestinal tracts, and could be instrumental in better stabilization and treatment of high-rise patients.

Blood analysis should be considered in high-rise patients, especially if they are scheduled to undergo general anesthesia for repair of any of the sustained injuries. Complete blood cell count may reveal an elevated neutrophil count and possibly anemia, if significant hemorrhage has taken place. Serum chemistry may reveal a number of abnormalities, including elevated liver enzymes, azotemia, and altered protein levels in the event of significant shock, hypoxemia, and hemorrhage. Azotemia may also be present if rupture of the urinary tract has occurred. In cats, species-specific pancreatic lipase monitoring may be advisable, especially in animals with evidence of significant abdominal injuries [11,12] (see Chapter 86). Coagulation testing, including thromboelastography, should be considered in severely traumatized animals with or without clinically apparent hemorrhage to rule out hemostatic disturbances, including coagulopathy of trauma.

After initial stabilization and treatment, evaluation of the facial and orthopedic injuries should be undertaken, if the patient's condition dictates. Orthopedic radiographs may be able to be performed with good pain management and possibly light sedation; however, for full evaluation of the facial and dental injuries, dental radiographs may be necessary, which typically require general anesthesia. Such procedures should be delayed as long as necessary for stabilization of the cardiovascular, respiratory and nervous systems, which may take up to several days of hospitalization.

Treatment

Treatment of animals with HRS should firstly focus on achieving acceptable ventilation, oxygenation, and cardiovascular stability. This is referred to as the primary survey and initial resuscitation (see Chapter 2). Airway patency should be evaluated and established immediately upon presentation, with intubation if necessary. Breathing and circulation should be evaluated and addressed next. Oxygen supplementation should be provided, and immediate thoracocentesis should be performed as a diagnostic and therapeutic step in severely dyspneic patients.

Cardiovascular stabilization is achieved via intravenous catheterization and administration of intravenous fluids, which may include isotonic crystalloids, colloids and a combination of blood products for hemorrhagic shock (see Chapters 167–169, and 176). Judicious but not restrictive fluids should be used in patients with pulmonary contusions to limit fluid extravasation and worsening hypoxemia [15]. Higher ratios of plasma to red blood cells are recommended in human medicine and should be considered; however, this is controversial [16]. Antifibrinolytic medications may be considered in animals with suspect acute traumatic coagulopathy [7] (see Chapter 163).

Pain management is imperative in animals with significant injuries, and may include systemic and local analgesia, as well as a multimodal approach using different types of analgesics, such as a combination of opioids and non-steroidal anti-inflammatory drugs when appropriate and safe (see Chapter 193).

If traumatic brain injury is suspected, hyperosmolar solutions should be used to improve cerebral blood flow (see Chapter 19). Hypertonic saline may also be used as small-volume resuscitation in polytrauma patients to improve perfusion.

After initial stabilization, a full physical examination and definitive repair should be pursued, if indicated. This is called the secondary survey. Any imaging or full bloodwork is performed at this juncture. Depending on the type of injury requiring repair, definitive fixation could be delayed up to several days after the initial insult to allow for organs like the brain and pulmonary parenchyma to return to normal or near-normal function. This may not be possible if surgical intervention is necessary for intractable hemorrhage or severe thoracic or abdominal wounds that require urgent exploration. Rupture of the urinary conduit can be managed with an abdominal drain prior to pursuing surgery for definitive repair (see Chapter 103).

When anesthesia is deemed to be safe, repair of the orthopedic and facial injuries should be pursued. Vertebral and appendicular skeleton fractures

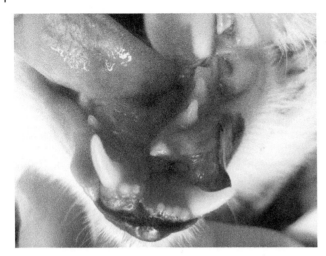

Figure 162.2 Mandibular symphyseal and left body fracture in a cat.

can be managed conservatively or surgically, according to imaging, clinician discretion, and individual animal characteristics, such as age, disposition and co-morbidities, as well as owner compliance and finances. Facial soft tissue injuries and fractures may be treated conservatively or surgically, depending on clinician preference and the nature of the injury (Figure 162.2). Hard palate fractures are a hallmark of HRS in cats, and significant controversy exists over whether

they should be managed medically or if surgical repair should be pursued (Figure 162.3). Oronasal fistula is a complication of untreated and medically managed hard palate fractures and may be a challenge to address once it develops. Therefore, some authors recommend surgical closure of the initial defect [17] (Figure 162.4).

Prognosis

Overall prognosis for animals with HRS is good, with mortality ranging from 6% to 17%, including both euthanized cases and those that died [1,2,5,6]. Two studies in cats reported 100% survival in animals surviving the first 36 hours of hospitalization [1,6]. Animals that require surgery predictably have longer duration of hospitalization (median 2.7 days without surgery, 5 days with surgery in one study in dogs) [2]. Severity of injuries is directly proportional to the number of floors in most studies [2,5,6]. In many studies of feline HRS, mortality was associated with thoracic injuries and shock [5]. One study found that hypothermia at presentation was positively associated with death, and likely with shock [5]. In addition, this study found that mortality of cats with abdominal injuries was 2.5 times higher compared to the other cats with HRS. The authors concluded that presence of abdominal trauma signifies more severe injury and should be regarded as a negative prognostic indicator in feline HRS.

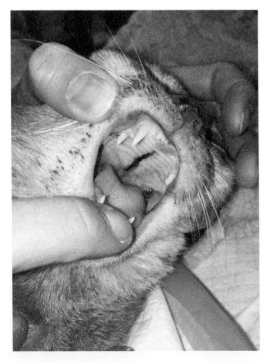

Figure 162.3 Hard palate fracture in a cat due to HRS.

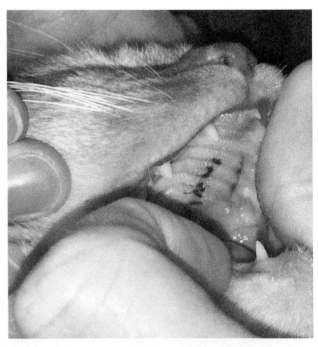

Figure 162.4 Surgical fixation of a hard palate fracture in a cat.

References

1 Whitney W, Mehlhaff C. High-rise syndrome in cats. *J Am Vet Med Assoc* 1987;191(11):1399–1403.

2 Gordon L, Thacher C, Kapatkin A. High-rise syndrome in dogs: 81 cases (1985–1991). *J Am Vet Med Assoc* 1993;202(1):118–122.

3 Lapostolle F, Gere C, Borron S, et al. Prognostic factors in victims of falls from height. *Crit Care Med* 2005;33(6):1239–1242.

4 Pratschke K, Kirby B. High rise syndrome with impalement in three cats. *J Small Anim Pract* 2002;43(6):261–264.

5 Merbl Y, Milgram J, Bibring U, Perry D, Arch I. Epidemiological, clinical and hematological findings in feline high rise syndrome in Israel: a retrospective case-controlled study of 107 cats. *Isr J Vet Med* 2013;68(1):28–37.

6 Vnuk D. Feline high-rise syndrome: 119 cases (1998–2001). *J Feline Med Surg* 2004;6(5):305–312.

7 Davenport R, Brohi K. Cause of trauma-induced coagulopathy. *Curr Opin Anaesthesiol* 2016;29: 212–219.

8 Theusinger O, Madjdpour C, Spahn D. Resuscitation and transfusion management in trauma patients. *Curr Opin Crit Care* 2012;18(6):661–670.

9 Holowaychuk M, Hanel R, Darren Wood R, Rogers L, O'Keefe K, Monteith G. Prospective multicenter evaluation of coagulation abnormalities in dogs following severe acute trauma. *J Vet Emerg Crit Care* 2014;24(1):93–104.

10 Abelson A, O'Toole T, Johnston A, Respess M, de Laforcade A. Hypoperfusion and acute traumatic coagulopathy in severely traumatized canine patients. *J Vet Emerg Crit Care* 2013;23(4):395–401.

11 Liehmann L, Dorner J, Hittmair K, Schwendenwein I, Reifinger M, Dupre G. Pancreatic rupture in four cats with high-rise syndrome. *J Feline Med Surg* 2012;14(2):131–137.

12 Zimmermann E, Hittmair K, Suchodolski J, Steiner J, Tichy A, Dupré G. Serum feline-specific pancreatic lipase immunoreactivity concentrations and abdominal ultrasonographic findings in cats with trauma resulting from high-rise syndrome. *J Am Vet Med Assoc* 2013;242(9):1238–1243.

13 Duhautois B, Pucheu B, Juillet C. High-rise syndrome ou syndrome du chat parachutiste: études rétrospectives et comparatives de 204 cas. *Bul de l'Ac Vét France* 2010;1:167.

14 Lisciandro G. Abdominal and thoracic focused assessment with sonography for trauma, triage, and monitoring in small animals. *J Vet Emerg Crit Care* 2011;21(2):104–122.

15 Cohn S, DuBose J. Pulmonary contusion: an update on recent advances in clinical management. *World J Surg* 2010;34(8):1959–1970.

16 Rajasekhar A, Gowing R, Zarychanski R, et al. Survival of trauma patients after massive red blood cell transfusion using a high or low red blood cell to plasma transfusion ratio. *Crit Care Med* 2011;39(6):1507–1513.

17 Bonner SE, Reiter AM, Lewis JR. Orofacial manifestations of high-rise syndrome in cats: a retrospective study of 84 cases. *J Vet Dent* 2012;29(1):10–18.

163

Trauma-Associated Coagulopathy

Alex Lynch, BVSc (Hons), DACVECC, MRCVS[1] and Robert Goggs, BVSc, DACVECC, DECVECC, PhD, MRCVS[2]

[1] *North Carolina State University, Raleigh, NC, USA*
[2] *College of Veterinary Medicine, Cornell University, Ithaca, NY, USA*

Introduction

Acute hemorrhage is the most important reversible cause of death in people following trauma [1–3]. The consequences of acute hemorrhage, including cardiovascular collapse, compromised tissue oxygen delivery, impaired organ function, and secondary sepsis, are widely recognized [4]. Until recently, therapeutic strategies for patients with acute traumatic hemorrhage involved restoration of intravascular volume with crystalloid and colloid fluids and augmentation of oxygen-carrying capacity via red blood cell transfusion [5,6] efforts have been made to optimize resuscitative and operative strategies for the management of traumatic hemorrhage [7,8]. Our understanding of the role hemostatic dysfunction plays in exacerbating traumatic injury has grown significantly over the last 15 years, such that two major contributors to traumatic hemorrhage are now recognized in people – the trauma and resultant shock itself and our resuscitation efforts [9,10]. There has been a consequent paradigm shift in the way human trauma patients are resuscitated in the prehospital setting, in the emergency department, and in operating rooms [11–13]. A corresponding evolution of understanding and management is also in veterinary trauma.

Pathogenesis

Trauma-associated coagulopathy (TAC) is the preferred term for any coagulopathy identified in traumatized patients. TAC encompasses both the endogenous coagulopathy that develops early in severely traumatized individuals with concurrent tissue hypoperfusion – acute coagulopathy of trauma-shock (ACOTS) – and the syndrome that occurs later and is exacerbated by resuscitation practices – resuscitation-associated coagulopathy (RAC).

Resuscitation-Associated Coagulopathy

Until recently, coagulopathy in trauma patients was considered to result from the "bloody vicious cycle" of dilution, acidosis, and hypothermia secondary to the effects of tissue damage, hemorrhage, hypoperfusion, and crystalloid resuscitation [14–16]. In the clinical setting, the additive effects of dilution, acidosis, hypothermia, and hypocalcemia on coagulation status are likely more important than any individual component alone. Indeed, using thromboelastography, it has been shown that acidosis in isolation has minimal impact on coagulation, while more profound hypocoagulability ensues with combined acidosis and hypothermia [17].

The administration of crystalloid fluids contributes to TAC via clotting factor dilution and induction of hypofibrinogenemia [18,19], thereby directly impeding clot formation and lowering resultant clot strength. The degree of coagulopathy may be dose dependent, but large-volume resuscitation has not consistently resulted in coagulopathy development in people [20,21]. The choice of resuscitation fluid undoubtedly has significant consequences for trauma patients [22]. In particular, the inhibitory effects of hydroxyethyl starch solutions on coagulation factor activity, platelet function, and hemostasis have been extensively documented in humans and small animals, raising important questions about their use in fluid resuscitation [23] (see Chapter 168) Although the impact on canine trauma patients is unknown, dilution does occur in traumatized dogs following resuscitation. In one study, volume resuscitation resulted in a 10% reduction in packed cell volume (PCV) and a 1.0 g/dL fall in serum protein concentration [24].

The development of acidosis in traumatized patients is multifactorial. Hyperlactatemia associated with high concentrations of circulating catecholamines and impaired tissue oxygenation, the administration of chloride-rich fluids, and accumulation of citrate from blood products could act individually or in combination to induce metabolic acidosis [16]. The presence of hypoalbuminemia following hemorrhage and fluid resuscitation may also hinder traditional interpretation of acid–base status, increasing the likelihood that the presence and potential impact of acidemia on coagulation will be overlooked [25]. Simplistically, the coagulation cascade involves sequential activation of enzymes leading to the generation of thrombin. Enzymes function optimally within a narrow range of environmental conditions (e.g. pH and temperature), and any deviations from normality adversely affect enzyme function. In the context of hemostasis, this could lead to impaired thrombin generation and a hypocoagulable phenotype. A reduction in pH from 7.4 to 7.0 reduces the activity of factor VIIa by more than 90%, and the FXa/FVa complex by 70%, and hence impairs thrombin generation [26].

Acidosis has also been associated with enhancing fibrinogen breakdown and impairing the interaction between coagulation factors and the surface of activated platelets [27]. Although severe acidemia was uncommon in one canine trauma retrospective [24], two studies have documented that metabolic acidosis and hyperlactatemia are associated with outcome in traumatized dogs [28,29]. While causation cannot currently be confirmed, there is an association between hemorrhage and acidosis in traumatized dogs, since those dogs requiring a packed red cell transfusion have significantly larger base deficits [29].

Hypothermia can occur in people after trauma due to environmental exposure, large-volume resuscitation with room temperature fluids, soft tissue exposure during surgery, and administration of vasodilating anesthetic agents that impair thermoregulation. Hypothermia may negatively affect hemostasis by inducing platelet dysfunction [30], reducing coagulation factor activity [31], slowing clot formation [32], and limiting thrombin generation [33]. Fibrinolytic activity appears to be minimally affected by hypothermia, however, which may contribute to development of a fibrinolytic phenotype [34]. Hypothermia appears to be an uncommon finding in dogs with trauma [24,35] but may occur in more severely injured dogs and those requiring massive transfusion [36–38]. This mirrors the human situation, where the degree of heat loss varies with injury severity and patient age [39,40].

The downstream effects of unintentional hypothermia should always be considered in any traumatized patient requiring urgent anesthesia and surgery [41]. Given the potential impact of hypothermia on hemostasis, some advocate performing hemostatic assays at a temperature equivalent to the patient's core body temperature, in addition to the conventional 37 °C, in an attempt to uncover the true *in vivo* hemostatic potential [42].

Calcium is an important co-factor for hemostasis *in vivo*, so ionized hypocalcemia could induce hemostatic dysfunction [43]. Hypocalcemia is commonly identified in dogs receiving massive transfusion, likely associated with excessive administration of citrate in blood products [38]. The level at which hypocalcemia interferes with coagulation is unclear, however, with one human study suggesting hemostatic function is preserved with ionized calcium concentrations as low as 0.56 mmol/L [44].

Acute Coagulopathy of Trauma-Shock

Although the iatrogenic effects of trauma resuscitation undoubtedly contribute to TAC, it is now clear that people suffer a separate and early coagulopathy characterized by hypocoagulability with hyperfibrinolysis that occurs independent of and prior to resuscitation [9,10]. Patients that develop ACOTS have higher transfusion requirements, spend longer in the hospital, develop multiple organ dysfunction more frequently, and are four times more likely to die [9,10]. The exact mechanism underlying the development of ACOTS is debated, but its development requires both the presence of severe tissue injury and hemorrhagic shock [45,46].

Central to the current hypothesis of ACOTS development is increased generation of anticoagulant activated protein C by high concentrations of the thrombin-thrombomodulin complex (Figure 163.1). The activation of the protein C pathway requires the combination of severe injury, tissue hypoperfusion, and sympathoadrenal activation, hence the term ACOTS [47,48]. In patients with mild-to-moderate trauma where increases in catecholamines are minimal, increased systemic thrombin generation and blood hypercoagulability are balanced by catecholamine-induced release of tissue-type plasminogen activator (tPA) and activation of the protein C (PC) pathway, such that ACOTS does not result [49,50].

Following severe trauma, widespread tissue injury and excessive plasma catecholamines cause generalized endothelial activation (Figure 163.2). Consequently, there is expression and release of thrombomodulin [45], systemic coagulation activation, and consumption of clotting factors and platelets [51]. Procoagulant thrombin, once bound to thrombomodulin, activates protein C

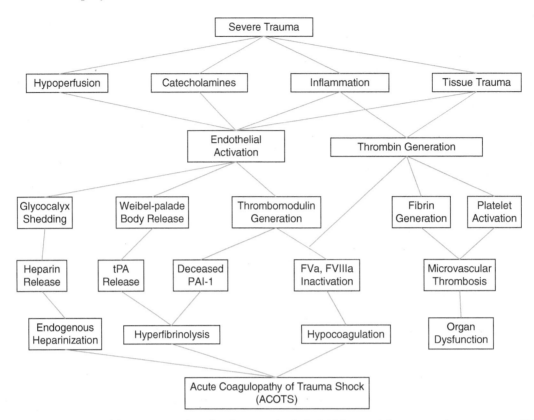

Figure 163.1 The pathogenesis of the acute coagulopathy of trauma-shock. An initial severe injury causes tissue trauma and blood loss that result in hypoperfusion, inflammation, and a sympathoadrenal response. In turn, these generate thrombin to aid hemostasis and activate the endothelium. If the injury and the body's responses are sufficiently profound then the high concentrations of thrombin-thrombomodulin mediate the inhibition of FVa and FVIIIa and the inhibition of PAI-1. This results in hypocoagulation and potentiates fibrinolysis, while endothelial activation and damage releases endogenous heparin-like compounds. The result of these three processes is the acute coagulopathy of trauma-shock.

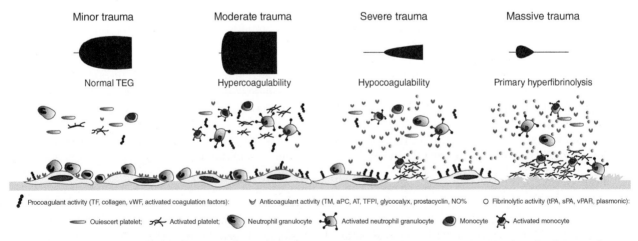

Figure 163.2 A schematic illustration of the hemostatic response to increasing trauma severity as assessed by thromboelastography (TEG). The variable hemostatic responses occurring in the bloodstream and endothelium with increasing trauma severity are depicted. The hypothesized pathogenesis is that the combined effects of tissue injury, associated shock, and the catecholamine responses promote a switch from hypercoagulability to hypocoagulability and hyperfibrinolysis, generating the acute coagulopathy of trauma-shock (ACOTS). *Source:* Adapted with permission from Johansson PI, Ostrowski SR. Medical Hypotheses 2010;75:564–567.

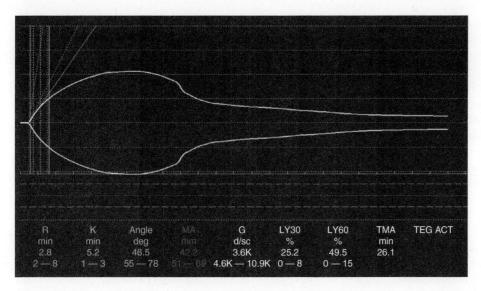

R min	K min	Angle deg	MA mm	G d/sc	LY30 %	LY60 %	TMA min	TEG ACT
2.8	5.2	46.5	42.2	3.6K	25.2	49.5	26.1	
2 — 8	1 — 3	55 — 78	51 — 69	4.6K — 10.9K	0 — 8	0 — 15		

Figure 163.3 Kaolin-activated thromboelastography (TEG) tracing from a 20 kg 3-year-old CM pit bull mix dog hit by a car 60 minutes before; the dog had received 500 mL of lactated Ringer's solution prior to obtaining blood for this assay. The TEG tracing demonstrates a hyperfibrinolytic profile, suggesting that this dog has suffered significant injury.

[50,52], a potent endogenous anticoagulant that inhibits factors Va and VIIIa. Activated protein C also inhibits plasminogen activator inhibitor 1 (PAI-1) and thrombin activatable fibrinolytic inhibitor concurrently, inducing hyperfibrinolysis [53–55]. Soluble thrombomodulin inhibits further thrombin generation [56], tipping the scales further in favor of hypocoagulability. The sympathoadrenal response following trauma is also integral to ACOTS development. Severe trauma can induce a catecholamine surge that can damage the endothelial glycocalyx [57]. This glycocalyx damage results in a shift towards a local procoagulant effect, with shedding and release of endogenous anticoagulants (e.g. heparan sulfate) and profibrinolytic agents (e.g. tPA) into the systemic circulation. This results in systemic anticoagulation and hyperfibrinolysis.

There is equipoise regarding the differentiation of ACOTS from disseminated intravascular coagulation (DIC) characterized by a fibrinolytic phenotype [58]. The Educational Initiative on Critical Care Bleeding in Trauma (EICBT) concluded that ACOTS is distinct from DIC [59] while the Scientific and Standardization Committee on DIC of the International Society on Thrombosis and Haemostasis (ISTH) suggests that ACOTS represents a variation of DIC [60]. Traditionally, early DIC has been considered a hypercoagulable condition with *de novo* tissue factor expression favoring thrombin generation and PAI-1-mediated inhibition of fibrinolysis. Over time, this early prothrombotic and antifibrinolytic tendency wanes and progresses to a consumptive hypocoagulable and fibrinolytic state characterized by clinically relevant bleeding. In simpler terminology, the early stages of DIC can be considered non-overt/thrombotic/antifibrinolytic and the latter stages are overt/hemorrhagic/fibrinolytic. In contrast, ACOTS

may be considered as a process that limits thrombin generation early on in its course via the action of thrombombodulin/activated protein C pathway. Some human trauma victims exhibit hypercoagulability identified using thromboelastography prior to resuscitation (Figure 163.3), a finding that complicates our mechanistic understanding of ACOTS and suggests that further work is required to clarify the similarities and difference between DIC and ACOTS [61].

Platelet dysfunction occurs in some people shortly after trauma and may also contribute to ACOTS [62–64]. The origin of platelet dysfunction in naturally occurring trauma is also multifactorial. In people following trauma, retention of hypofunctional platelets may occur, contributing to hemostatic dysfunction [65]. Widespread release of ADP following tissue trauma in patients with shock may prematurely activate platelets, leading to their exhaustion and then retention in the circulation [66]. This phenomenon may also occur in dogs. In a canine hemorrhage model, where dogs were bled to 80% and 60% of their blood volumes, a progressive but mild hypocoagulability identified using traditional and viscoelastic coagulation tests. Platelet dysfunction can also be identified in this model using impedance aggregometry despite largely unchanged platelet counts [67]. Further work focused on the incidence and impact of platelet dysfunction in naturally occurring canine trauma is warranted, since this may offer a therapeutic solution in some situations (e.g. platelet-containing transfusions).

Trauma-Associated Coagulopathy in Dogs

To date, there are only a handful of publications in the veterinary literature focused on the coagulation defects in dogs following trauma [24,35,36,68,69]. Prior to evaluating the evidence provided by these studies, the potential impact of analysis timing in relation to resuscitation should be considered. Hemostatic defects identified before fluid administration may more closely resemble the ACOTS phenomenon described in people, while in comparison, coagulopathy identified in dogs after treatment may more accurately reflect RAC or a combined phenomenon.

Several publications have specifically evaluated coagulation status in traumatized dogs prior to fluid administration. One study aimed to evaluate severely injured dogs by utilizing an Animal Trauma Triage (ATT) score ≥5 to stratify patients [36]. In this study, 33% of dogs were considered hypercoagulable based on the thromboelastography-derived G value; no hypocoagulable or hyperfibrinolytic tracings were obtained. The finding of hypercoagulability in these dogs echoes some studies in people [70–72] but the lack of convincing evidence for hypocoagulability and hence ACOTS begs the question about the true injury severity of these dogs. Since most dogs in the study had ATT < 10, the inclusion criteria may have been too liberal to identify ACOTS in dogs. Further work on severely injured dogs with evidence of shock prior to fluid administration will be necessary to characterize TAC in dogs and to determine if ACOTS does indeed occur in our patients. In this regard, we must recognize that the most severely injured dogs may be euthanized or die naturally before an opportunity arises to analyze their coagulation status, which may hinder our progress in identifying ACOTS in this species.

Two studies report comprehensive coagulation analyses of 30 dogs that sustained trauma prior to treatment [68,69]. The analyses performed included platelet enumeration and measurement of prothrombin time (PT), activated partial thromboplastin time (aPTT), fibrinogen, FDP concentrations, and activities of coagulation factors, protein C, antithrombin, plasminogen and alpha-2 plasmin inhibitor. Thrombocytopenia and factor deficiencies were commonly identified, as were increased soluble fibrin concentrations, reflecting intravascular thrombin generation. Resonance thrombography, a viscoelastic method of coagulation assessment, was also performed. The resonance thrombography results were suggestive of delayed fibrin formation, but there was overlap with controls sufficient to make it insensitive compared to conventional tests.

Two further studies reported data from traumatized dogs that received treatment prior to blood collection for coagulation testing. A large retrospective study of blunt trauma reported coagulation tests performed commonly in emergency practice [24]. Mild-to-moderate prolongations of PT and aPTT were identified in 20.8% and 47.2% of dogs tested, respectively.

Coagulation parameters were not significantly different in dogs that survived to discharge compared to non-survivors. Disseminated intravascular coagulation was only recognized in 2% of the dogs in this study. In a second study involving 40 dogs treated at two institutions, 70% of dogs received crystalloids before blood sampling, making an iatrogenic influence on hemostasis likely. Mild-to-moderate coagulation abnormalities were recognized commonly in these dogs, with hemostatic abnormalities impacting the likelihood of survival, presence of body cavity hemorrhage, and outcome [35]. In this study, coagulation deficits also correlated with indicators of tissue hypoperfusion (i.e. lactate and blood pressure) [35].

Hemostatic Testing for Trauma

The availability of hemostatic assays in emergency practice is hospital dependent. Based on review of the veterinary literature, there is useful information to be gleaned from traditional coagulation tests, including platelet count, PT, and aPTT, when evaluating dogs that have sustained trauma. In human medicine, there are compelling data to suggest a clinical utility for viscoelastic monitoring in the assessment of trauma victims and, in particular, in the prediction of transfusion requirements [73,74]. In veterinary medicine, an additional potential advantage of viscoelastic monitoring is the ability to recognize hyperfibrinolysis, since this offers a potential therapeutic intervention (antifibrinolytics) [75], but more work is required in veterinary patients to establish whether antifibrinolytic drug administration to trauma patients will impart the survival advantage identified in people [76].

Conclusion

Trauma-associated coagulopathy has been described in dogs, but the mechanisms of the observed phenomena are less certain. Currently, there is little evidence to suggest that ACOTS occurs in dogs presenting to emergency rooms following trauma but more work is required to characterize the coagulopathy present in severely injured dogs prior to treatment. The emergency clinician should be cognizant of complicating iatrogenic factors, including dilution, acidosis, and hypothermia, that may worsen pre-existing coagulopathy and negatively affect outcome. Resuscitation strategies for veterinary patients should be based on available data from dogs and until further evidence is available, we can rationally incorporate the early hemostatic transfusion principles developed for people.

References

1 Cothren CC, Moore EE, Hedegaard HB, Meng K. Epidemiology of urban trauma deaths: a comprehensive reassessment 10 years later. *World J Surg* 2007;31(7):1507–1511.

2 Riskin DJ, Tsai TC, Riskin L, et al. Massive transfusion protocols: the role of aggressive resuscitation versus product ratio in mortality reduction. *J Am Coll Surg* 2009;209(2):198–205.

3 Evans JA, van Wessem KJ, McDougall D, et al. Epidemiology of traumatic deaths: comprehensive population-based assessment. *World J Surg* 2010;34(1):158–163.

4 Muir W. Trauma: physiology, pathophysiology, and clinical implications. *J Vet Emerg Crit Care* 2006;16(4):253–263.

5 Driessen B, Brainard B. Fluid therapy for the traumatized patient. *J Vet Emerg Crit Care* 2006;16(4):276–299.

6 Cohen MJ. Towards hemostatic resuscitation: the changing understanding of acute traumatic biology, massive bleeding, and damage-control resuscitation. *Surg Clin North Am* 2012;92(4):877–891, viii.

7 Holcomb JB, Jenkins D, Rhee P, et al. Damage control resuscitation: directly addressing the early coagulopathy of trauma. *J Trauma* 2007;62(2):307–310.

8 Cotton BA, Gunter OL, Isbell J, et al. Damage control hematology: the impact of a trauma exsanguination protocol on survival and blood product utilization. *J Trauma* 2008;64(5):1177–1182; discussion 82–83.

9 Brohi K, Singh J, Heron M, Coats T. Acute traumatic coagulopathy. *J Trauma* 2003;54(6):1127–1130.

10 MacLeod JB, Lynn M, McKenney MG, Cohn SM, Murtha M. Early coagulopathy predicts mortality in trauma. *J Trauma* 2003;55(1):39–44.

11 Holcomb JB, del Junco DJ, Fox EE, et al. The prospective, observational, multicenter, major trauma transfusion (PROMMTT) study: comparative effectiveness of a time-varying treatment with competing risks. *JAMA Surg* 2013;148(2):127–136.

12 Holcomb JB, Pati S. Optimal trauma resuscitation with plasma as the primary resuscitative fluid: the surgeon's perspective. *Hematology Am Soc Hematol Educ Program* 2013;2013:656–659.

13 Holcomb JB, Tilley BC, Baraniuk S, et al. Transfusion of plasma, platelets, and red blood cells in a 1:1:1 vs a 1:1:2 ratio and mortality in patients with severe trauma: the PROPPR randomized clinical trial. *JAMA* 2015;313(5):471–482.

14 Kashuk JL, Moore EE, Millikan JS, Moore JB. Major abdominal vascular trauma – a unified approach. *J Trauma* 1982;22(8):672–679.

15 Schreiber MA. Damage control surgery. *Crit Care Clin* 2004;20(1):101–118.

16 Thorsen K, Ringdal KG, Strand K, et al. Clinical and cellular effects of hypothermia, acidosis and coagulopathy in major injury. *Br J Surg* 2011;98(7):894–907.

17 Dirkmann D, Hanke AA, Gorlinger K, Peters J. Hypothermia and acidosis synergistically impair coagulation in human whole blood. *Anesth Analg* 2008;106(6):1627–1632.

18 Fries D, Martini WZ. Role of fibrinogen in trauma-induced coagulopathy. *Br J Anaesth* 2010;105(2):116–121.

19 Howard BM, Daley AT, Cohen MJ. Prohemostatic interventions in trauma: resuscitation-associated coagulopathy, acute traumatic coagulopathy, hemostatic resuscitation, and other hemostatic interventions. *Semin Thromb Hemost* 2012;38(3):250–258.

20 Maegele M, Lefering R, Yucel N, et al. Early coagulopathy in multiple injury: an analysis from the German Trauma Registry on 8724 patients. *Injury* 2007;38(3):298–304.

21 Frith D, Brohi K. The pathophysiology of trauma-induced coagulopathy. *Curr Opin Crit Care* 2012;18(6):631–636.

22 Brummel-Ziedins K, Whelihan MF, Ziedins EG, Mann KG. The resuscitative fluid you choose may potentiate bleeding. *J Trauma* 2006;61(6):1350–1358.

23 Adamik KN, Yozova ID, Regenscheit N. Controversies in the use of hydroxyethyl starch solutions in small animal emergency and critical care. *J Vet Emerg Crit Care* 2015;25(1):20–47.

24 Simpson SA, Syring R, Otto CM. Severe blunt trauma in dogs: 235 cases (1997–2003). *J Vet Emerg Crit Care* 2009;19(6):588–602.

25 Hopper K, Epstein SE, Kass PH, Mellema MS. Evaluation of acid-base disorders in dogs and cats presenting to an emergency room. Part 1: comparison of three methods of acid–base analysis. *J Vet Emerg Crit Care* 2014;24(5):493–501.

26 Meng ZH, Wolberg AS, Monroe DM 3rd, Hoffman M. The effect of temperature and pH on the activity of factor VIIa: implications for the efficacy of high-dose factor VIIa in hypothermic and acidotic patients. *J Trauma* 2003;55(5):886–891.

27 Martini WZ, Holcomb JB. Acidosis and coagulopathy: the differential effects on fibrinogen synthesis and breakdown in pigs. *Ann Surg* 2007;246(5):831–835.

28 Hall KE, Holowaychuk MK, Sharp CR, Reineke E. Multicenter prospective evaluation of dogs with trauma. *J Am Vet Med Assoc* 2014;244(3):300–308.

29 Stillion JR, Fletcher DJ. Admission base excess as a predictor of transfusion requirement and mortality in dogs with blunt trauma: 52 cases (2007–2009). *J Vet Emerg Crit Care* 2012;22(5):588–594.

30 Watts DD, Trask A, Soeken K, et al. Hypothermic coagulopathy in trauma: effect of varying levels of hypothermia on enzyme speed, platelet function, and fibrinolytic activity. *J Trauma* 1998;44(5):846–854.

31 Wolberg AS, Meng ZH, Monroe DM 3rd, Hoffman M. A systematic evaluation of the effect of temperature

on coagulation enzyme activity and platelet function. *J Trauma* 2004;56(6):1221–1228.

32 Taggart R, Austin B, Hans E, Hogan D. In vitro evaluation of the effect of hypothermia on coagulation in dogs via thromboelastography. *J Vet Emerg Crit Care* 2012;22(2):219–224.

33 Waibel BH, Schlitzkus LL, Newell MA, et al. Impact of hypothermia (below 36 degrees C) in the rural trauma patient. *J Am Coll Surg* 2009;209(5):580–588.

34 Martini WZ, Cortez DS, Dubick MA, Blackbourne LH. Different recovery profiles of coagulation factors, thrombin generation, and coagulation function after hemorrhagic shock in pigs. *J Trauma Acute Care Surg* 2012;73(3):640–647.

35 Holowaychuk MK, Hanel RM, Darren Wood R, et al. Prospective multicenter evaluation of coagulation abnormalities in dogs following severe acute trauma. *J Vet Emerg Crit Care* 2014;24(1):93–104.

36 Abelson AL, O'Toole TE, Johnston A, Respess M, de Laforcade AM. Hypoperfusion and acute traumatic coagulopathy in severely traumatized canine patients. *J Vet Emerg Crit Care* 2013;23(4):395–401.

37 Ateca LB, Drobatz KJ, King LG. Organ dysfunction and mortality risk factors in severe canine bite wound trauma. *J Vet Emerg Crit Care* 2014;24(6):705–714.

38 Jutkowitz LA, Rozanski EA, Moreau JA, Rush JE. Massive transfusion in dogs: 15 cases (1997–2001). *J Am Vet Med Assoc* 2002;220(11):1664–1669.

39 Gregory JS, Flancbaum L, Townsend MC, Cloutier CT, Jonasson O. Incidence and timing of hypothermia in trauma patients undergoing operations. *J Trauma* 1991;31(6):795–798; discussion 798–800.

40 Bernabei AF, Levison MA, Bender JS. The effects of hypothermia and injury severity on blood loss during trauma laparotomy. *J Trauma* 1992;33(6):835–839.

41 Peterson NW, Buote NJ, Barr JW. The impact of surgical timing and intervention on outcome in traumatized dogs and cats. *J Vet Emerg Crit Care* 2015;25(1):63–75.

42 Goggs R, Brainard B, de Laforcade AM, et al. Partnership on Rotational ViscoElastic Test Standardization (PROVETS): evidence-based guidelines on rotational viscoelastic assays in veterinary medicine. *J Vet Emerg Crit Care* 2014;24(1):1–22.

43 Ho AM, Karmakar MK, Dion PW. Are we giving enough coagulation factors during major trauma resuscitation? *Am J Surg* 2005;190(3):479–484.

44 Ho KM, Leonard AD. Concentration-dependent effect of hypocalcaemia on mortality of patients with critical bleeding requiring massive transfusion: a cohort study. *Anaesth Intensive Care* 2011;39(1):46–54.

45 Brohi K, Cohen MJ, Ganter MT, et al. Acute coagulopathy of trauma: hypoperfusion induces systemic anticoagulation and hyperfibrinolysis. *J Trauma* 2008;64(5):1211–1217; discussion 1217.

46 Chesebro BB, Rahn P, Carles M, et al. Increase in activated protein C mediates acute traumatic coagulopathy in mice. *Shock* 2009;32(6):659–665.

47 Cohen MJ, Call M, Nelson M, et al. Critical role of activated protein C in early coagulopathy and later organ failure, infection and death in trauma patients. *Ann Surg* 2012;255(2):379–385.

48 Johansson PI, Ostrowski SR. Acute coagulopathy of trauma: balancing progressive catecholamine induced endothelial activation and damage by fluid phase anticoagulation. *Med Hypotheses* 2010;75(6):564–567.

49 von Kanel R, Dimsdale JE. Effects of sympathetic activation by adrenergic infusions on hemostasis in vivo. *Eur J Haematol* 2000;65(6):357–369.

50 Esmon CT. The protein C pathway. *Chest* 2003;124(3 Suppl):26S–32S.

51 Hess JR, Brohi K, Dutton RP, et al. The coagulopathy of trauma: a review of mechanisms. *J Trauma* 2008;65(4):748–754.

52 Brohi K, Cohen MJ, Ganter MT, et al. Acute traumatic coagulopathy: initiated by hypoperfusion: modulated through the protein C pathway? *Ann Surg* 2007;245(5):812–818.

53 Palmer L, Martin L. Traumatic coagulopathy – part 1: pathophysiology and diagnosis. *J Vet Emerg Crit Care* 2014;24(1):63–74.

54 Brohi K, Cohen MJ, Davenport RA. Acute coagulopathy of trauma: mechanism, identification and effect. *Curr Opin Crit Care* 2007;13(6):680–685.

55 Davenport R. Pathogenesis of acute traumatic coagulopathy. *Transfusion* 2013;53(Suppl 1):23S–27S.

56 Takahashi Y, Hosaka Y, Imada K, et al. Species specificity of the anticoagulant activity of human urinary soluble thrombomodulin. *Thromb Res* 1998;89(4):187–197.

57 Ostrowski SR, Johansson PI. Endothelial glycocalyx degradation induces endogenous heparinization in patients with severe injury and early traumatic coagulopathy. *J Trauma Acute Care Surg* 2012;73(1):60–66.

58 Davenport R, Manson J, De'Ath H, et al. Functional definition and characterization of acute traumatic coagulopathy. *Crit Care Med* 2011;39(12):2652–2658.

59 Bouillon B, Brohi K, Hess JR, et al. Educational initiative on critical bleeding in trauma: Chicago, July 11–13, 2008. *J Trauma* 2010;68(1):225–230.

60 Gando S, Wada H, Thachil J, Scientific and Standardization Committee on DICotISoT and Haemostasis. Differentiating disseminated intravascular coagulation (DIC) with the fibrinolytic phenotype from coagulopathy of trauma and acute coagulopathy of trauma-shock (COT/ACOTS). *J Thromb Haemost* 2013;11(5):826–835.

61 Schreiber MA. Coagulopathy in the trauma patient. *Curr Opin Crit Care* 2005;11(6):590–597.

62 Wohlauer MV, Moore EE, Thomas S, et al. Early platelet dysfunction: an unrecognized role in the acute coagulopathy of trauma. *J Am Coll Surg* 2012;214(5):739–746.

63 Solomon C, Traintinger S, Ziegler B, et al. Platelet function following trauma. A multiple

electrode aggregometry study. *J Thromb Haemost* 2011;106(2):322–330.

64 Jacoby RC, Owings JT, Holmes J, et al. Platelet activation and function after trauma. *J Trauma* 2001;51(4):639–647.

65 Kutcher ME, Redick BJ, McCreery RC, et al. Characterization of platelet dysfunction after trauma. *J Trauma Acute Care Surg* 2012;73(1):13–19.

66 Pareti FI, Capitanio A, Mannucci L, Ponticelli C, Mannucci PM. Acquired dysfunction due to the circulation of "exhausted" platelets. *Am J Med* 1980;69(2):235–240.

67 Lynch AM, de Laforcade AM, Meola D, et al. Assessment of hemostatic changes in a model of acute hemorrhage in dogs. *J Vet Emerg Crit Care* 2016;26(3):333–343.

68 Mischke R. Alterations of the global haemostatic function test 'resonance thrombography' in spontaneously traumatised dogs. *Pathophysiol Haemost Thromb* 2003-2004;33(4):214–220.

69 Mischke R. Acute haemostatic changes in accidentally traumatised dogs. *Vet J* 2005;169(1):60–64.

70 Kaufmann CR, Dwyer KM, Crews JD, Dols SJ, Trask AL. Usefulness of thrombelastography in assessment of trauma patient coagulation. *J Trauma* 1997;42(4):716–720; discussion 720–722.

71 Schreiber MA, Differding J, Thorborg P, Mayberry JC, Mullins RJ. Hypercoagulability is most prevalent early after injury and in female patients. *J Trauma* 2005;58(3):475–480; discussion 80–81.

72 Ostrowski SR, Sorensen AM, Larsen CF, Johansson PI. Thrombelastography and biomarker profiles in acute coagulopathy of trauma: a prospective study. *Scand J Trauma Resusc Emerg Med* 2011;19:64.

73 de Jager P, Burgerhof JG, van Heerde M, et al. Tidal volume and mortality in mechanically ventilated children: a systematic review and meta-analysis of observational studies. *Crit Care Med* 2014;42(12):2461–2472.

74 Vogel AM, Radwan ZA, Cox CS Jr, Cotton BA. Admission rapid thrombelastography delivers real-time "actionable" data in pediatric trauma. *J Pediatr Surg* 2013;48(6):1371–1376.

75 Fletcher DJ, Blackstock KJ, Epstein K, Brainard BM. Evaluation of tranexamic acid and epsilon-aminocaproic acid concentrations required to inhibit fibrinolysis in plasma of dogs and humans. *Am J Vet Res* 2014;75(8):731–738.

76 Shakur H, Roberts I, Bautista R, et al. Effects of tranexamic acid on death, vascular occlusive events, and blood transfusion in trauma patients with significant haemorrhage (CRASH-2): a randomised, placebo-controlled trial. *Lancet* 2010;376(9734):23–32.

164

Metabolic Consequences of Trauma

Leo Roa, DVM and Elizabeth M. Streeter, DVM, DACVECC

Iowa Veterinary Referral Center, Des Moines, IA, USA

Introduction

Trauma is defined as tissue injury caused by violence or accident that occurs suddenly and includes physical damage to the body [1]. Traumatic injury is a common occurrence in veterinary medicine. Kolata et al. reported that the incidence of patients seen for trauma at an urban veterinary teaching hospital was approximately 11–13% [2]. Trauma may result from penetrating wounds or blunt forces.

The metabolic consequences of trauma have been well documented in human medicine but less so in veterinary medicine. Several have described the "ebb and flow" phenomenon following trauma [3]. After the traumatic insult occurs, there is initially a decrease in metabolism secondary to a hypovolemia and hypoperfusion. This results in activation of several compensatory physiological mechanisms which attempt to restore hemodynamic stability. As treatment ensues and restoration of volume status takes place, the "flow" state occurs and hypermetabolism and inflammatory changes are seen. These metabolic changes occur via multiple mechanisms which are discussed in more detail below.

Sympathoadrenal Activation

Catecholamine activation after traumatic injury can occur via different mechanisms. One mechanism occurs via loss of blood or fluids leading to hypovolemia. This decrease in blood volume is sensed via baroreceptors located in the carotid bodies and aortic arch. Also, pain can cause catecholamine activation by stimulation of the hypothalamus. Once sympathetic nervous system activation occurs, the adrenal medulla is stimulated and epinephrine and norepinephrine are released. These catecholamines mediate several functions including increasing heart rate, increases in cardiac contractility,

and peripheral vasoconstriction. These effects result in increased cardiac output and help to restore blood pressure.

Neuroendocrine Activation

After the initial sympathetic activation occurs, an additional hormonal response is seen. This response is more long standing and slower in activation but strives for the same goals as the sympathetic response with increased hemodynamic parameters. This response is mediated via release of adrenocorticotropic hormone (ACTH) and growth hormone. Antidiuretic hormone (ADH) is also released in times of hypovolemia. These hormones result in antidiuresis and help to restore vascular volume. In addition, decreased cardiac output detected by baroreceptors and/or increased sodium levels sensed by chemoreceptors result in activation of the renin-angiotension-aldosterone system. Renin is transformed to angiotensin in the liver and causes vasoconstriction of the peripheral vasculature, shunting blood centrally to more vital organs. Angiotensin activation also stimulates the release of aldosterone, as does sodium concentration and ACTH levels. Aldosterone acts to retain sodium and minimize water loss with additional antidiuretic effects.

Hyperglycemia

Glucose is the main nutrient source for the neurons and red blood cells and results from carbohydrate breakdown [4]. Circulating glucose levels are normally balanced via the interaction of insulin and glucagon. Any excess in carbohydrates is converted to glycogen and stored within the liver. When the level of carbohydrates decreases below normal, moderate quantities of glucose can be formed from amino acids, the glycerol portion of

Textbook of Small Animal Emergency Medicine, First Edition. Edited by Kenneth J. Drobatz, Kate Hopper, Elizabeth Rozanski and Deborah C. Silverstein.
© 2019 John Wiley & Sons, Inc. Published 2019 by John Wiley & Sons, Inc.
Companion Website: www.wiley.com/go/drobatz/textbook

fat, and lactate; this process is called gluconeogenesis [4]. Glycogen breakdown also helps maintain normal levels of glucose. This process is known as glycogenolysis [4].

After trauma, patients will have elevation in blood glucose secondary to the release of counterregulatory hormones, such as glucagon, cortisol, growth hormone, and catecholamines. Epinephrine leads to proteolysis, glycogenolysis, and inhibition of insulin-mediated glucose uptake by the muscle [5], whereas cortisol release promotes gluconeogenesis, inhibits insulin activity, and exacerbates the effects of glucagon and epinephrine [4,5].

Hyperglycemia has been associated with outcome in human patients. In veterinary medicine, elevated blood glucose has not been associated with outcome, but dogs and cats with hyperglycemia after head trauma did have more significant injury [6]. In these patients, elevated blood glucose levels can increase free radical production and excitatory amino acid release and worsen cerebral edema and acidosis.

Hyperlactatemia

Hyperlactatemia is described as an increase in plasma lactate. Post trauma, lactate levels become elevated as a result of poor tissue perfusion and anaerobic metabolism secondary to hypovolemia and fluid losses. In normal aerobic conditions, pyruvate is converted into ATP via the tricarboxylic acid cycle (TCA), resulting in 36 moles of ATP. During anaerobic metabolism, pyruvic acid is converted into lactic acid; during this process 2 moles of ATP are formed. Even though this seems like a small amount of ATP, glycolysis is fast enough that this may satisfy tissue demands temporarily. The production of $NADH^+$ and lactate promotes metabolic acidosis and subsequent vasodilation. This alternative energy pathway is essential for preserving cellular function during times of shock and hypoxia. As the shock state resolves and aerobic metabolism returns, lactate is recycled into the TCA cycle and the hyperlactatemia resolves.

Acid–Base Disorders

The most common acid–base disorder seen in trauma patients is metabolic acidosis [7]. Metabolic acidosis is identified in a venous blood gas sample via the presence of low bicarbonate, low CO_2 and blood pH less than 7.35. Metabolic acidosis occurs secondary to the presence of hydrogen ions, lactate, uremic acid, ketoacids, phosphates, and other unmeasured anions. Acidosis is one component of the "triad of death" seen in trauma patients; the other components are hypothermia and coagulation disturbances. Metabolic acidosis can

contribute to coagulopathy and cellular and enzymatic disruptions (see Chapter 163). The degree of acidosis has been shown to be prognostic in some human patients.

The ideal crystalloid for correction of metabolic acidosis is a balanced electrolyte solution (see Chapter 167). Drobatz and Cole revealed a faster correction of acid–base in severely acidotic cats with urethral obstruction when a balanced electrolyte solution was implemented [8]. Sodium chloride has an acidifying effect and it is not recommended in cases with severe metabolic acidosis. Also, fluids with high chloride volume may worsen metabolic acidosis via the Stewart method, resulting in a hyperchloridemic metabolic acidosis. Rarely, bicarbonate is necessary to correct the metabolic acidosis (see Chapter 174). The bicarbonate provided will be converted to CO_2 which later needs to be exhaled. If the patient has concurrent respiratory disease then CO_2 will build up, which may result in worsening hypercapnia and acidosis. Fluid therapy to address underlying hypovolemia is usually sufficient to correct acidosis.

Body Temperature

Decreases in body temperature are commonly seen after traumatic injury. The cause of this decrease may be the traumatic injury and exposure or it may occur during initial resuscitation. The hypothermia may be the result of loss of vasomotor tone and subsequent vasodilation. Also, traumatic injury may alter central thermoregulation and affect the body's ability to respond to decreased temperatures. The shivering response often does not take place in states of hypotension and has been shown to occur at lowered temperatures in injured animals [9].

As hypothermia persists, the renal system becomes affected (see Chapter 148). The primary effects are known as cold diuresis, which is triggered by the sense of increased blood volume induced by peripheral vasoconstriction [10,11]. Also, there is a decrease in response to antidiuretic hormone, which results in poor water reabsorption. The water loss contributes to further hypovolemia, which further reduces cardiac output and renal perfusion, leading to azotemia and renal dysfunction. The decreased renal perfusion results in accumulation of hydrogen ions and metabolic acidosis.

The decreases in temperature can affect coagulation systems and can also contribute to traumatic coagulopathy (see Chapter 163). Decreases in body temperature affect platelet function by decreasing production of thromboxane B_2 and platelet adhesion molecules. Also, lowered temperature can affect coagulation enzymatic activity and fibrinolysis.

Hypothermia, despite its many potential adverse reactions, has also been shown to improve outcome in certain populations. Hypothermia has been advocated in patients with traumatic brain injury due to decreases in metabolic rate, thereby decreasing oxygen consumption and improving ischemic injury to the brain (see Chapter 19). Also, patients undergoing cardiac and transplant surgery have had similar potential improved outcomes with hypothermia. Despite these reports, evidence remains conflicted and due to the potential detrimental consequences, further research is needed to confirm any beneficial effects of hypothermia in trauma.

Gastrointestinal Injury

Secondary to the shock state, hypoperfusion of splanchnic tissues occurs due to shunting of blood in order to preserve perfusion to more vital structures such as the heart, brain, and lungs. This decrease in blood supply leads to cell injury and death and increased gastrointestinal permeability is seen. This increase in intestinal permeability may result in bacteria translocation, leading to exacerbation of inflammation, and possibly predispose to multiple organ failure and death.

Studies have been performed in both people and dogs showing increases in intestinal permeability up to 48 hours after trauma that improve as recovery from the insult occurs [12,13]. While this change has been documented, not all patients with increases in intestinal permeability go on to develop sepsis or systemic inflammation (see Chapter 159). These discrepancies in pathological changes and clinical effects likely represent differences in immune system ability to clear offending organisms.

Gastrointestinal injury manifests as vomiting, diarrhea, ileus, gastrointestinal ulceration, and bleeding. Prevention is aimed at improvement in shock states. Early enteral nutrition has also been shown to improve GI tract viability and health [14–16]. Enteral feeding should be instituted in trauma patients as soon as possible. Prophylactic antibiotics are controversial and should be used only in cases of confirmed sepsis (see Chapter 200). Use of other medications, such as H_2 blockers, proton pump inhibitors, etc., is also controversial. While these may improve intestinal health, prevent stress ulcers, and decrease incidence of bacterial translocation, altered intestinal flora may also occur and predispose to resistant infection if bacterial translocation takes place. Evidence regarding many of these therapies is conflicting.

Systemic Inflammation

In most traumatic injuries, tissue disruption occurs. This cellular injury, in addition to ischemia and vascular disruption, can lead to an inflammatory response. The activation of cytokines and release of inflammatory mediators such as interleukin (IL)-6, TNF alpha, and IL-1B occur following the tissue injury. Once released into the bloodstream, these mediators can cause widespread inflammation and possible organ failure. Vascular activation can also occur, leading to coagulation abnormalities as well.

In many patients, this inflammatory response may be mild and self-limiting with appropriate support of vascular and respiratory systems. In other patients, it may be more severe and lead to more widespread complications. One possible contributor to the disparity in degrees of inflammation may be the "two hit" theory. In this explanation, the initial inflammatory response seen after trauma predisposes to a severe inflammatory response. In patients with a second inflammatory trigger, such as surgical repair of the original injury, systemic inflammatory response syndrome (SIRS) and possible multiple organ failure can result (see Chapter 159). In a recent publication reviewing organ dysfunction and mortality in dogs with bite wounds, patients with prolonged anesthesia were more likely to develop multiorgan dysfunction syndrome (MODS) and disseminated intravascular coagulation (DIC), and had a higher mortality rate [17]. Also patients with extensive wounds have a significant risk of developing SIRS.

Treatment or prevention of systemic inflammatory activation is aimed at support of cardiovascular and respiratory systems with appropriate intravenous fluid resuscitation, oxygen therapy, and other vascular support if needed.

Activation of the Coagulation Cascade

Trauma patients commonly have alteration of normal coagulation pathways (see Chapter 163). This change is multifactorial and occurs via several mechanisms. The inflammatory response, as discussed above, can lead to activation of the clotting cascade and initially a hypercoagulable state. As coagulation factors and platelets are consumed, a hypocoagulatory state can then follow. This syndrome (disseminated intravascular coagulation or DIC) has been associated with significant increases in morbidity and mortality in both human and veterinary populations [17–19].

Traumatic injury can result not only in DIC and resultant coagulopathy but coagulopathy via other mechanisms. In trauma patients, acute traumatic coagulopathy (ATC) has been seen (see Chapter 163). Acute traumatic coagulopathy can develop within 30 minutes post trauma and may be seen even before fluid therapy is initiated. In the past, hemodilution was suspected to be an important factor in development of this condition but over the last 10 years it has been demonstrated that ATC is independent of dilution or consumption of coagulation factors and thrombocytopenia [20,21]. Tissue injury and hypoperfusion appear to be the two main initiators of ATC, which can worsen patient outcomes and impair response to treatment. Early identification and correction of coagulopathy, acidosis, hypothermia, and hypovolemia are essential for successful treatment of ATC.

Conclusion

Trauma is a common occurrence in veterinary medicine and these injuries can trigger widespread metabolic changes. Understanding the pathophysiology behind these changes is essential in determining the appropriate therapies used for successful patient outcomes. Also, knowledge of these metabolic changes helps to guide the clinician in selecting appropriate monitoring and treatment goals for patients with traumatic injuries.

References

1 Muir W. Trauma: physiology, pathophysiology and clinical implications. *J Vet Emerg Crit Care* 2006;16:253–263.

2 Kolata RJ, Kraut NH, Johnston DE. Patterns of trauma in urban dogs and cats: a study of 1,000 cases. *J Am Vet Med Assoc* 1974;164:499–502.

3 Desborough JP. The stress response to trauma and surgery. *Br J Anaesth* 2000;85:109–117.

4 Guyton AC, Hall JE. Lipid metabolism. In: *Textbook of Medical Physiology*, 11th edn (eds Guyton AC, Hall JE). Elsevier Saunders, Philadelphia, 2006, pp. 840–851.

5 Koenig A. Hypoglycemia. In: *Small Animal Critical Care Medicine*, 2nd edn (eds Silverstein DC, Hopper K). Elsevier Saunders, St Louis, 2015, pp. 352–356.

6 Syring RS, Otto CM, Drobatz KH. Hyperglycemia in dogs and cats with head trauma:122 cases (1997–1999). *J Am Vet Med Assoc* 2001;7:1124–1129.

7 Kaplan LJ, Frangos S. Clinical review: acid base abnormalities in the intensive care unit Part II. *Crit Care* 2005;9(2):198–203.

8 Drobatz KJ Cole SG. The influence of crystalloid type on acid–base and electrolyte status of cats with urethral obstruction. *J Vet Emerg Crit Care* 2008;184:355–361.

9 Tsuei BJ, Kearney PA. Hypothermia in the trauma patient. *Injury* 2004;35:7–15.

10 Armstrong SR. Perioperative hypothermia. *J Vet Emerg Crit Care* 2005;15:32.

11 Mallet ML. Pathophysiology of accidental hypothermia. *QJM* 2002;95:775.

12 Langkamp-Henken B, Donovan TB, Pate L, et al. Increased intestinal permeability following blunt and penetrating trauma. *Crit Care Med* 1995;23:660–664.

13 Streeter EM, Zsombor-Murray E, Moore K, et al. Intestinal permeability and absorption in dogs with traumatic injury. *J Vet Intern Med* 2002;16:669–673.

14 Chen Z, Wang S, Yu B, Li A. A comparison study between early enteral nutrition and parenteral nutrition in severe burn patients. *Burns* 2007;33(6):708–712.

15 Jiang XH, Li N, Li JS. Intestinal permeability in patients after surgical trauma and effect of enteral nutrition versus parenteral nutrition. *World J Gastroenterol* 2003;9(8):1878–1880.

16 Mohr AJ, Leisewitz AL, Jacobson L, et al. Effect of early enteral nutrition on intestinal permeability, intestinal protein loss, and outcome in dogs with severe parvoviral enteritis. *J Vet Intern Med* 2003;17:791–798.

17 Ateca LB, Drobatz KJ, King LG. Organ dysfunction and mortality risk factors in severe canine bite wound trauma. *J Vet Emerg Crit Care* 2014;24(6):705–714.

18 Gando S, Otomo Y. Local hemostasis, immunothrombosis and systemic disseminated intravascular coagulation in trauma and shock. *Crit Care* 2015;19(1):72.

19 Beck JJ, Staatz AJ, Pelsue D, et al. Risk factors associated with short-term outcome and development of perioperative complications in dogs undergoing surgery because of gastric dilatation-volvulus: 166 cases (1992–2003). *J Am Vet Med Assoc* 2002;229(12):1934–1939.

20 Estrin MA, Wehausen CE, Jessen C, Lee J. Disseminated intravascular coagulation in cats. *J Vet Intern Med* 2006;20:1334–1339.

21 Palmer L, Martin L. Traumatic coagulopathy part 1: pathophysiology and diagnosis. *J Vet Emerg Crit Care* 2014;24(1):63–74.

165

Traumatic Orthopedic Emergencies

Marian E. Benitez, DVM, MS, DACVS-SA[1] and Spencer A. Johnston, VMD, DACVS[2]

[1] *Virginia-Maryland College of Veterinary Medicine, Blacksburg, VA, USA*
[2] *College of Veterinary Medicine, University of Georgia, Athens, GA, USA*

General Considerations for the Trauma Patient

Orthopedic emergencies include a small group of traumatic injuries and joint infections. Most orthopedic injuries are not an immediate threat to life, the exceptions being skull and vertebral trauma.

While addressing immediate life-threatening concerns based on initial triage (see Chapter 2), a covering and/or immobilizing bandage can be applied to the affected limb(s). After the patient is hemodynamically stable, the animal should be helped to a standing position. If possible, the patient is walked and general proprioception assessed, followed by a complete orthopedic examination. Gentle palpation of the limbs, along with assessment of range of motion and stability of the joints, should allow localization of fractures or luxations. A digital rectal examination is done to assess pelvic integrity. A complete neurological examination should be performed to assess for concomitant neural injury, which may help dictate prognosis for repair. Radiographs of bones should be delayed until the animal is stable.

Analgesics should be administered but the potential adverse effects of analgesics should be considered in light of the patient's overall condition (see Chapter 190).

Fractures

Under normal circumstances, bones are subjected to multiple forces during daily use. When forces applied to a bone exceed its physiological capacity, traumatic orthopedic injury results, often in the form of a fracture.

Different types of forces or loads applied to bones can result in differences in fracture configuration and energy release. When loaded in compression, bone fails along the lines of the highest shear stress. This leads to an oblique fracture of a long bone. Tensile forces tend to result in simple transverse fractures perpendicular to the load applied. Bending forces combine both compressive and tensile forces. When a bending force is applied, the convex side of the bone is under tension and the concave side is under compression. Because bone is weaker in tension, the bone fractures perpendicular to its long axis and the fracture propagates towards the compressive side of the bone. Torsional forces generally result in spiral fractures. When multiple forces are applied concurrently, combinations of fracture configurations occur.

Due to the viscoelastic properties of bone, the rate at which a load is applied influences the fracture configuration. Rapid loading results in high-energy storage and much greater damage to the bone in the form of comminution. Whether a fracture is closed or open is determined by the energy released and the amount of soft tissue surrounding the bone. High-energy fractures in the proximal region of the limb, where soft tissues are more plentiful, tend to be closed, while a similar injury toward the distal part of the limb, where soft tissues are less robust, may result in an open fracture. Both regions, however, may sustain substantial soft tissue trauma associated with the fracture.

Closed Fractures

Closed fractures are not addressed initially and repair should be delayed until the patient is stable for general anesthesia. Fractures of the distal extremities may be temporarily splinted. This allows for fracture immobilization, prevents further swelling, keeps a closed fracture from becoming an open fracture, and helps prevent additional soft tissue trauma. Fracture immobilization also increases patient comfort and facilitates movement. Immobilization is best accomplished by including the joint above and below the fracture in a splint. Effective coaptation of fractures involving bones proximal to the elbow and stifle joints is difficult and requires placement of a spica splint for immobilization of the shoulder and hip, respectively.

Open Fractures

Open fractures are typically the result of high-energy trauma. Open fractures with associated severe wounds should receive initial therapy to control blood loss and limit further contamination (see Chapter 166). Significant bleeding vessels should be isolated and ligated to stop ongoing hemorrhage. The primary goal of open fracture management is to limit acute infection and prevent osteomyelitis. Tissue should be collected or deep tissues swabbed for initial culture and sensitivity to help direct initial antimicrobial therapy. Early use of broad-spectrum antimicrobials is warranted in the treatment of open fractures [1].

Open fractures are classified into groups that describe the degree of soft tissue damage present. The most commonly used in veterinary medicine is the Gustilo–Anderson classification scheme (Table 164.1) [2,3]. Wound care with daily evaluation serves as important management of open fractures because bone healing is associated with soft tissue health and overall wound healing. Gross tissue contamination should be removed as soon as possible to avoid continued bacterial growth [4]. If the wound will be managed open, an absorbent bandage should be used. A splint can be incorporated into the bandage to limit bone movement if it can be applied without further compromise to the injured tissues; alternatively, external skeletal fixation allows wound treatment while providing bone stability. Once the debridement stage of wound healing is completed, non-adherent bandages should be placed over the wound.

Table 165.1 Gustilo–Anderson open fracture classification scheme.

Type	Classification
I	Open fracture with wound <1 cm; mild to moderate soft tissue bruising
II	Open fracture with wound >1 cm without extensive soft tissue damage
III	Open fractures with extensive soft tissue damage
IIIa	Extensive trauma with adequate tissue covering remaining, irrespective of wound size
IIIb	Extensive trauma with soft tissue loss, periosteal stripping, and bone exposure
IIIc	Extensive trauma associated with arterial blood supply injury

The decision to close a wound is dependent on a variety of factors including time from injury, wound appearance, bacterial load, and mechanism of injury (see Chapter 166). Early closure of infected tissue may worsen cellulitis, lead to systemic sepsis, and/or result in osteomyelitis. The time from initial injury to definitive surgical repair of open fractures varies; definitive fracture repair should be postponed until the patient is a good anesthetic candidate and the soft tissues are sufficiently healthy for closure, grafting, or continued open wound therapy.

Decision Making for Fracture Repair

Fracture repair is performed only after concomitant injuries are treated and the patient is considered a stable anesthetic candidate. Goals of repair include anatomical alignment, fragment apposition, fracture stabilization, prevention of infection, repair of soft tissue damage, and restoration of normal function.

Closed reduction and external coaptation of incomplete or closed simple fractures can be performed under general anesthesia. This is rarely an option for open fractures as daily wound evaluation is needed. Radiographs are necessary after coaptation to verify adequate fracture reduction.

Open reduction is the treatment of choice for most fractures. Both internal and external skeletal fixation methods have been used for the treatment of open and closed fractures in veterinary medicine [5–10]. In general, the simplest method that maximizes the stability of fracture fragments while allowing access to soft tissue injuries and minimizing disruption to the soft tissues and blood supply should be chosen. The surgical approach for open reduction of open fractures should be selected in an area away from the initial wound if possible.

Internal fixation with bone plates, pins, cerclage wires, and interlocking nails has been used successfully in the treatment of closed and type I open fractures. Type II open fractures, when managed appropriately, can also be treated with a variety of internal fixation methods. The use of internal fixation is questioned, however, in areas of contamination or infection, particularly with type III open fractures. Articular fractures usually require internal fixation to achieve anatomical alignment, fragment apposition, and fragment stabilization. If damage is too severe to allow reconstruction and stabilization, salvage procedures (joint replacement or arthrodesis) or amputation may be preferred treatment options.

Fractures involving the growth plate of young dogs should be evaluated immediately. If possible, such fractures should be repaired within 3 days of the injury [11]. Although not evident at the time of injury, owners should be made aware that disturbance in growth of long bones can lead to future angular limb deformities and joint incongruity.

Advancements of internal fixation include minimally invasive techniques that incorporate the theory of biological osteosynthesis. This theory places less emphasis on mechanical factors and greater emphasis on preservation of blood supply and tissue biology during fracture repair. Employing this theory, there is little disruption at the fracture site in efforts to promote rapid secondary bone healing. Both biological osteosynthesis and traditional methods of open reduction and internal fixation have been used in the management of open and closed fractures in veterinary medicine [5–16].

External skeletal fixation is an option to avoid implants adjacent to potentially contaminated or infected areas. External skeletal fixation can be performed with minimal disruption of the surrounding soft tissues and can be removed once fracture stability is achieved. This helps avoid long-term implant-associated complications. Placement of an external skeletal fixator allows easy access for open wound management, which is particularly useful when treating an open fracture [17]. Complications of this technique include pin loosening, drainage from the area around transfixation pins, pin tract infection, implant failure, delays in fracture healing, and non-union.

After repair, patients should be strictly prohibited from strenuous activity for 6–8 weeks. Additional radiographs are recommended at 4–8-week intervals to assess fracture healing. Patients with open wounds should be assessed regularly until wound closure is complete. Alternatively, skin reconstruction techniques can be used to facilitate wound healing (see Chapter 166).

Traumatic Joint Injuries

Penetrating Injuries

Injury involving entry into the joint space should be treated promptly in a manner similar to treatment of open wounds involving bone. Delay of treatment can lead to deep infection and septic arthritis. Although cases of infective arthritis may occur from penetrating traumatic injuries, infective arthritis can also develop from hematogenous spread, or local spread from adjacent tissues, especially after a previous surgery. Arthrotomy or arthroscopy is indicated for complete joint exploration, removal of foreign debris or devitalized bone or cartilage, and lavage. The integrity of intra- and extra-articular structures should be assessed. Tissue samples should be obtained and submitted for bacterial culture and susceptibility testing. Severe injuries should remain open, packed with sterile gauze, and immobilized for daily

wound care and coaptation prior to closure. Very mild penetrating joint injuries with minimal soft tissue damage warrant joint exploration with irrigation and may be closed primarily. Patients should be placed on empiric antimicrobial therapy until targeted antimicrobial selection can occur based on culture and susceptibility testing results (see Chapter 200).

Traumatic Joint Luxation

Joint luxation occurs as a result of damage to the supporting ligaments, tendons, joint capsule, and other soft tissue structures surrounding the joint. Reduction of a joint luxation should occur as soon as possible after the patient is adequately stabilized from the initial trauma. Orthogonal radiographic views are required to determine the degree of injury as well as the direction of luxation and to allow visualization of concurrent fractures. When chosen as the treatment method, closed reduction should be performed under general anesthesia for patient comfort and to allow adequate muscle relaxation; however, occasionally heavy sedation is adequate. Indications for open reduction are listed in Box 165.1.

After reduction, immobilization or support of the joint to limit weight-bearing forces is generally indicated for several weeks until the support structures surrounding the joint are healed or until periarticular fibrosis develops.

Hip Luxation

The hip joint is the joint most commonly luxated in small animals, with the femoral head luxated in the craniodorsal direction. When craniodorsal luxation occurs, the affected limb may appear shortened, adducted, and externally rotated. Radiographs should confirm the presence and direction of luxation and identify concurrent acetabular fractures, slipped capital epiphysis, femoral head and neck fractures, and the presence of hip dysplasia. The presence of hip dysplasia precludes success with most closed and open reduction techniques. In those circumstances, a salvage procedure (e.g. total hip

---

Box 165.1 Indications for open reduction after traumatic joint luxation.

Unsuccessful attempts at closed reduction
Joint reluxation
Chronic luxation
Concurrent intra-articular fractures
Internal stabilization is necessary for adjacent long bone fractures
Neurological injury suspected and exploration warranted

replacement or femoral head and neck ostectomy) is recommended.

Closed reduction is ideally performed within 12–48 hours of injury, prior to muscle contraction and further cartilage damage. Once reduced, the joint should be manipulated through a full range of motion to displace blood clots and other soft tissues from the joint space. Joint stability is assessed during manipulation. An Ehmer sling should be applied for 1–2 weeks for craniodorsal luxations to limit movement and prevent reluxation (Figure 165.1). Reduction should be documented radiographically with orthogonal views before and after sling placement. Reported failure rates following closed reduction may be as high as 50% [18–20]. Failures should be treated with open reduction techniques or salvage joint procedures.

Elbow Luxation

Luxation of the elbow joint occurs most frequently with the olecranon displaced in the lateral direction due to the size and shape of the humeral condyle. Patients are generally non-weight bearing with the elbow joint held slightly flexed with the antebrachium abducted and externally rotated. Orthogonal radiographic views are needed to confirm the diagnosis and rule out additional fractures involving the humerus, radius, or ulna.

Closed reduction is generally successful when performed soon after injury. After reduction, the joint should be tested for collateral ligament stability. External coaptation (e.g. spica splint; Figure 165.2) with the elbow joint in 140° of extension can be maintained for 7–10 days depending on the severity of the injury. Orthogonal radiographic views are obtained to document reduction. If ligament integrity is questionable and instability persists, internal fixation is recommended.

Miscellaneous Joint Injury

Shear injuries to the carpus, tarsus, and digits are common and often treated with open wound therapy with or without the need for internal fixation, arthrodesis, digit amputation, and/or skin reconstructive techniques.

Traumatic stifle derangements and luxations have been reported [21,22]. Salvage procedures or ligament reconstruction techniques can be performed. Temporary stabilization and referral to an orthopedic specialist are recommended.

Skull and Maxillofacial Trauma

Most skull, maxillofacial, and mandible fractures are a result of traumatic injury such as blunt trauma from a vehicular accident, high-impact forces or kicks, or falling from high elevations [23]. These injuries require prompt diagnosis and treatment due to concurrent life-threatening injury to the central nervous system and the reader is referred to Chapter 19 for additional

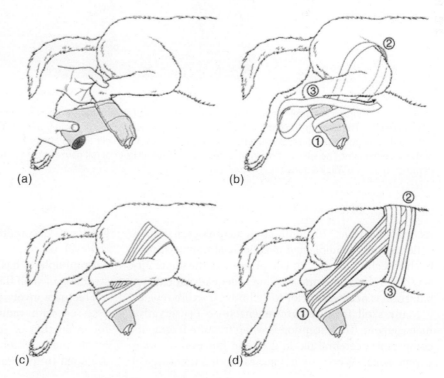

Figure 165.1 Ehmer sling application. (a) Begin with application of cotton padding on the plantar metatarsal surface of the foot. (b) Use roll gauze or adhesive tape wrapped from medial to lateral around the metatarsus to cover the soft cotton padding. Next, bring the bandage material from the lateral aspect of the metatarsus to the medial aspect of the flexed stifle (1) and bring the bandage over the cranial aspect of the thigh (2). In a figure-of-8 pattern, continue the bandage towards the medial aspect of the distal tibia and around the plantar aspect of the paw (3). The hock and stifle joints should be flexed with the limb internally rotated at the level of the hip joint. (c) This process is repeated with additional layers of adhesive tape onto the skin or hair. (d) Modification of this bandage includes incorporation of the bandage with adhesive tape around the caudal abdomen. Avoid the preputial sheath in male dogs and shave the hair if necessary to keep bandage from slipping. Reproduced with permission of Elsevier.

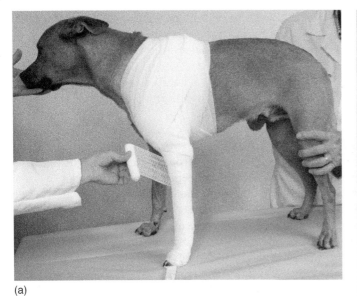
(a)

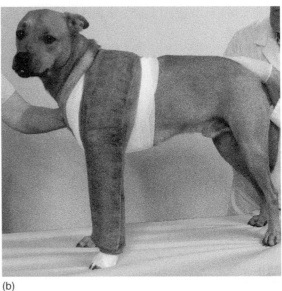
(b)

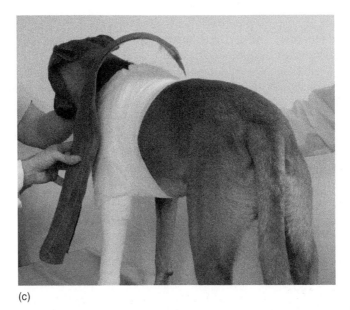
(c)

Figure 165.2 Thoracic spica splint application. (a) Several layers of cast padding with a layer of roll gauze are placed to incorporate the distal extremity. The bandage is continued over the dorsum to include the thorax in front of and behind the limb. (b) A fiberglass splint is made that begins at the digits and extends over the dorsum. (c) The splint should be broad enough to cover the craniolateral aspect of the shoulder joint. The splint is held in place with an additional layer of roll gauze and an outer protecting layer. Reproduced with permission of John Wiley & Sons.

recommendations. In addition to neurological injury, patients with mandible and maxillofacial trauma should be thoroughly assessed for compromise of the upper airway due to facial and oral swelling. Adequate patient stabilization is necessary prior to definitive fracture repair.

Many skull fractures are amenable to conservative management. The exception is when fracture fragments compromise cerebral blood flow and function or brain parenchyma. When such injuries occur, the surgical goal is to decompress the surrounding tissue through removal of comminuted fragments. Internal fixation with miniplates has been reported for advanced reconstruction of skull fractures [24].

Fractures involving the mandible and maxilla can be assessed with radiographs or computed tomography for evaluation of fracture configuration, location, and involvement of tooth roots. Most mandible fractures are open to the oral cavity and the discontinuity in the gingiva or bone is easily palpated or visible on physical examination.

Proper dental occlusion is the goal of fracture stabilization. Removal of teeth is not advised unless involved teeth are fractured, loose, or cannot be stabilized [25]. Removal of teeth may disrupt the blood supply, cause damage to adjacent tissues, further displace fracture fragments, eliminate occlusal landmarks, and/or eliminate available structures for fixation. If the viability of the tooth is uncertain, continue with fracture repair and have the tooth re-evaluated during and after fracture healing.

Fixation techniques include intraosseous and interdental wiring, plates, and external skeletal fixation [26,27]. Interdental wiring and intraoral splinting with acrylic or other composite material is a useful non-invasive technique for alignment of relatively stable fractures rostral to the first molar. Maxillomandibular fixation (bonding the maxilla to the mandible) can be applied to the teeth to maintain alignment and occlusion of minimally displaced fractures of the mandible caudal to the canine teeth.

Symphyseal separation or fracture of the mandible is commonly seen in cats and can be repaired with circumferential wiring using orthopedic wire (Figure 165.3). The wire is generally re-evaluated and removed in 4–6 weeks.

Incomplete fractures or minimally displaced fractures with little effect on occlusion can be managed with support using a muzzle. The muzzle is applied tight enough to maintain occlusion and dental interlock, but loose enough to permit tongue movement for prehension of gruel or liquid food and water. If concurrent injuries will delay definitive treatment of unstable fractures, nutritional support should be provided via an esophagostomy or gastrostomy tube.

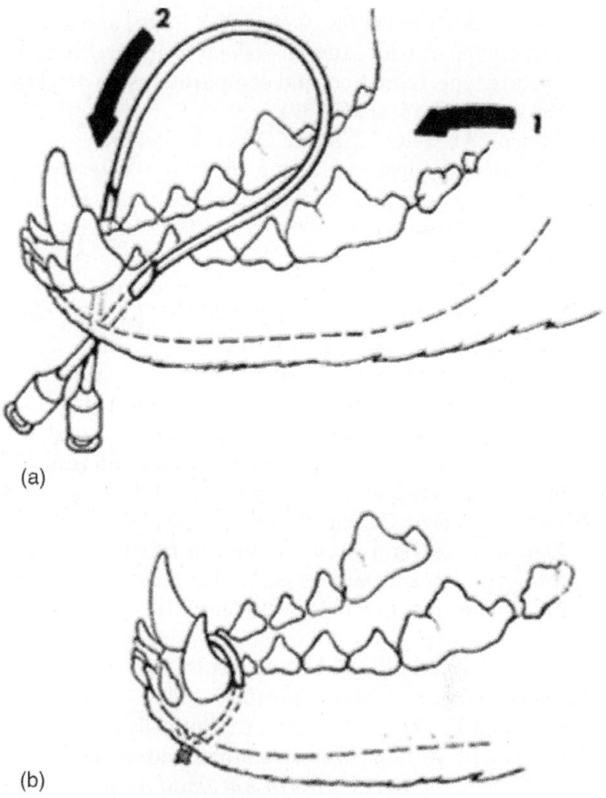

(a)

(b)

Figure 165.3 Circumferential symphyseal wiring. (a) Direct two 16 gauge hypodermic needles from the ventral midline through the gingival soft tissues to exit lateral to the right and left mandibular bodies. Stay against bone to avoid incorporation of excess tissue. Direct 20 gauge cerclage wire through one needle (1) and redirect the wire to exit the needle on the opposite site (2). (b) Both needles are removed and with the wire seated behind the canine teeth, it is tightened ventrally until no vertical shearing motion can be produced. Close the mouth to ensure adequate dental occlusion prior to final tightening. Reproduced with permission of Elsevier.

References

1 Patzakis MJ, Wilkins J. Factors influencing infection rate in open fracture wounds. *Clin Orthop Relat Res* 1989;243:36–40.

2 Gustilo RB, Anderson JT. Prevention of infection in the treatment of one thousand and twenty-five open fractures of long bones: retrospective and prospective analyses. *J Bone Joint Surg Am* 1976;58:453–458.

3 Gustilo RB, Mendoza RM, Williams DN. Problems in the management of type III (severe) open fractures: a new classification of type III open fractures. *J Trauma* 1984;24:742–746.

4 Tripuraneni K, Ganga S, Quinn R, Gehlert R. The effect of time delay to surgical debridement of open tibia shaft fractures on infection rate. *Orthopedics* 2008;31(12):1–5.

5 Dudley M, Johnson AL, Olmstead M, Smith CW, Schaeffer DJ, Abbuehl U. Open reduction and bone plate stabilization, compared with closed reduction and external fixation, for treatment of comminuted tibial fractures: 47 cases (1980–1995) in dogs. *J Am Vet Med Assoc* 1997;211(8):1008–1012.

6 Boone EG, Johnson AL, Montavon P, Hohn RB. Fractures of the tibial diaphysis in dogs and cats. *J Am Vet Med Assoc* 1986;188(1):41–45.

7 Walter MC, Lenehan TM, Smith GK, Matthiesen DT, Newton CD. Treatment of severely comminuted diaphyseal fractures in the dog, using standard bone plates and autogenous cancellous bone graft to span fracture gaps: 11 cases (1979–1983). *J Am Vet Med Assoc* 1986;189:457–462.

8 Johnson AL, Kneller SK, Weigel RM. Radial and tibial fracture repair with external skeletal fixation: effects of fracture type, reduction, and complications on healing. *Vet Surg* 1989;18(5):367–372.

9 Johnson AL, Seitz SE, Smith CW, Johnson JM, Schaeffer DJ. Closed reduction and type-II external fixation of comminuted fractures of the radius and tibia in dogs: 23 cases (1990–1994). *J Am Vet Med Assoc* 1996;209(8):1445–1448.

10 Lincoln JD. Treatment of open, delayed union, and nonunion fractures with external skeletal fixation. *Vet Clin North Am Small Anim Pract* 1992;22(1):195–207.

11 Cook JL, Tomlinson JL, Reed AL. Fluoroscopically guided closed reduction and internal fixation of fractures of the lateral portion of the humeral condyle: prospective clinical study of the technique and results in ten dogs. *Vet Surg* 1999;28(5):315–321.

12 Pozzi A, Hudson CC, Gauthier CM, Lewis DD. Retrospective comparison of minimally invasive plate osteosynthesis and open reduction and internal fixation of radius-ulna fractures in dogs. *Vet Surg* 2013;42(1):19–27.

13 Beale MS, McCally R. Minimally invasive plate osteosynthesis: tibia and fibula. *Vet Clin North Am Small Anim Pract* 2012;42(5):1023–1044.

14 Hudson CC, Lewis DD, Pozzi A. Minimally invasive plate osteosynthesis in small animals: radius and ulna fractures. *Vet Clin North Am Small Anim Pract* 2012;42(5):983–996.

15 Pozzi A, Risselada M, Winter MD. Assessment of fracture healing after minimally invasive plate osteosynthesis or open reduction and internal fixation of coexisting radius and ulna fractures in dogs via ultrasonography and radiography. *J Am Vet Med Assoc* 2012;241(6):744–753.

16 Boero Baroncelli A, Peirone B, Winter MD, Reese DJ, Pozzi A. Retrospective comparison between minimally invasive plate osteosynthesis and open plating for tibial fractures in dogs. *Vet Comp Orthop Traumatol* 2012;25(5):410–417.

17 Ness MG. Treatment of inherently unstable open or infected fractures by open wound management and external skeletal fixation. *J Small Anim Pract* 2006;47(2):83–88.

18 Duff SRI, Bennet D. Hip luxation in small animals: an evaluation of some methods of treatment. *Vet Rec* 1982;111(7):140–143.

19 McLaughlin RM. Traumatic joint luxations in small animals. *Vet Clin North Am Small Anim Pract* 1995;25(5):1175–1196.

20 Evers P, Johnston GR, Wallace LJ, Lipowitz AH, King VL. Long term results of treatment of traumatic coxofemoral joint dislocation in dogs: 64 cases (1973–1992). *J Am Vet Med Assoc* 1997;210:59–64.

21 Keeley B, Glyde M, Guerin S, Doyle R. Stifle joint luxation in the dog and cat: the use of temporary intraoperative transarticular pinning to facilitate joint reconstruction. *Vet Comp Orthop Traumatol* 2007;20(3):198–203.

22 Bruce WJ. Stifle joint luxation in the cat: treatment using transarticular external skeletal fixation. *J Small Anim Pract* 1999;40(10):482–488.

23 Mulherin BL, Snyder CJ, Soukup JW, Hetzel S. Retrospective evaluation of canine and feline maxillomandibular trauma cases. A comparison of signalment with non-maxillomandibular traumatic injuries (2003–2012). *Vet Comp Orthop Traumatol* 2014;27(3):192–197.

24 Arzi B, Verstraete FJ. Internal fixation of severe maxillofacial fractures in dogs. *Vet Surg* 2015;44(4):437–442.

25 Gerbino G, Tarello F, Fasolis M, de Gioanni PP. Rigid fixation with teeth in the line of mandibular fractures. *Int J Oral Maxillofac Surg* 1997;26(3):182–186.

26 Kitshoff AM, Rooster H, Ferreira SM, Steenkamp G. A retrospective study of 109 dogs with mandibular fractures. *Vet Comp Orthop Traumatol* 2013;26:1–5.

27 Kitshoff AM, Rooster H, Ferreira SM, Steenkamp G. The comparative biomechanics of the reinforced interdental crossover and the Stout loop composite splints for mandibular fracture repair in dogs. *Vet Comp Orthop Traumatol* 2013;26:461–468.

166

Wound Management Principles

F.A. (Tony) Mann, DVM, MS, DACVS, DACVECC

Veterinary Health Center, University of Missouri, Columbia, MO, USA

Introduction

Trauma patients frequently have external wounds of varying degrees of complexity. Oftentimes, these wounds must be addressed after more life-threatening injuries are managed to (see Chapter 2). However, prompt attention to wounds and early appropriate wound management can make the difference between uncomplicated healing and a protracted course of wound complications. What the emergency doctor does to treat an acutely acquired traumatic wound can make a huge difference in the course of wound healing. A comprehensive review of wound management is beyond the scope of this chapter, and can be found in standard surgical textbooks [1–3]. The purpose of this chapter is to guide the emergency clinician in wound management decisions that will optimize healing and minimize patient morbidity. To that end, a basic understanding of wound healing is reviewed as a basis for making treatment decisions. Then, a stepwise organized approach to early wound management is described, incorporating probing questions to stimulate a problem-solving effort in wound management.

Phases of Wound Healing

Wound healing is the process by which tissue continuity is re-established, and this process occurs through co-ordinated cellular and biochemical events. These events can be explained in phases where activation of different cellular elements and specific signaling molecules takes place. The reader is referred to surgical texts [1–3] for detailed information of the cellular and biochemical processes of wound healing, but a basic understanding of wound healing phases, as follows, is important for decision making in wound management.

Wound healing processes are interwoven and a distinct point of transition from one phase to another is not identifiable but, for discussion purposes, the three broad phases of wound healing are: (1) inflammation and debridement, (2) repair (also called proliferation), and (3) maturation.

Inflammation and Debridement Phase

Immediately after injury, the wound fills with blood and the clot becomes the first barrier to the outside environment. Transient (5–10 min) local vasoconstriction occurs in response to catecholamines and mast cell products (serotonin and bradykinin) to temporarily decrease blood loss. Then, local vasodilation occurs in response to histamine and interleukin-8 (IL-8), allowing plasma and intravascular cellular components to reach the extravascular space. Platelets and clotting factors gain access to the wound via the damaged blood vessels and are activated to generate fibrin, forming a blood clot. The extracellular matrix created by fibrin in association with fibronectin and activated factor XIII provides a scaffold for cell migration and early collagen deposition in the next phase of wound healing.

Inflammation ensues via migration of leukocytes from the intravascular space into the wound bed. Initially, neutrophils populate the wound, but their numbers are soon exceeded by macrophages. Tissue macrophages and mast cells activated at the time of injury promote the release of prostaglandins and leukotrienes, which attract neutrophils to the wound. Macrophages also produce IL-1, which stimulates endothelial cells to produce IL-8, another chemoattractant for neutrophils. The neutrophils and macrophages gain access to the injured tissue by margination, attachment, and diapedesis. At the wound site, neutrophils release superoxide radicals that kill bacteria and proteinases that help degrade necrotic tissue. Although these actions are important, neutrophils are not essential for wound healing. The neutrophils degenerate and die very soon and, mixed with degraded tissue and wound fluid, form the wound exudate known as pus.

Textbook of Small Animal Emergency Medicine, First Edition. Edited by Kenneth J. Drobatz, Kate Hopper, Elizabeth Rozanski and Deborah C. Silverstein.
© 2019 John Wiley & Sons, Inc. Published 2019 by John Wiley & Sons, Inc.
Companion Website: www.wiley.com/go/drobatz/textbook

Monocytes from the blood differentiate into macrophages in the wound, and it is the macrophage that is the essential inflammatory cell for wound healing. Macrophages produce cytokines that enhance the immune response. They also produce fibronectin and growth factors that stimulate mitosis and are essential for cell proliferation. Growth factors and cytokines produced by macrophages stimulate fibroblasts to produce and eventually modify the provisional matrix which becomes granulation tissue in the next phase of wound healing. Because macrophages are capable of phagocytosis of large particles, they are also vital to the debridement process.

As the wound becomes free of bacteria and necrotic tissue, the number of macrophages decreases. Fewer macrophages result in lower production of prostaglandins, leukotrienes, and cytokines and, therefore, fewer cells are attracted to the wound bed. However, macrophages will persist in chronic wounds, especially those containing foreign material. These macrophages can coalesce and become very large and multinucleated (referred to as epithelioid macrophages).

The duration of the inflammatory phase of wound healing is generally considered to be 48–72 hours, but the amount of injured tissue and bacterial load can influence the need for neutrophils and macrophages. Greater injury and higher bacterial contamination can prolong this phase, delay the next phase, or result in greater overlap of the phases. Some areas of the wound might have prolonged inflammation while other areas progress to the repair phase.

Repair (Proliferative) Phase

The four prominent processes in the repair phase of wound healing are angiogenesis, fibroplasia, wound contraction, and epithelialization. The end of the inflammatory phase and beginning of the repair phase are marked by the appearance of increased numbers of fibroblasts. One of the hallmarks of the repair phase of open wound healing is the presence of granulation tissue, which is typically evident by 3–5 days after initial wounding. The large numbers of fibroblasts combined with the formation of new capillaries give the granulation tissue its red fleshy and granular appearance. Granulation tissue markedly increases the wound's resistance to infection, serves as a surface for epithelial cell movement, and provides myofibroblasts for wound contraction.

Angiogenesis, the formation of new capillaries from vessels present at the limits of the wound, results from the migration and proliferation of endothelial cells in response to cytokines and growth factors produced by macrophages. This is regulated by the extracellular matrix. Proteins present in the extracellular matrix are responsible for apoptosis of endothelial cells and the decrease in the number of capillaries as wound healing progresses. As capillaries die, the wound takes on a pale appearance characteristic of old granulation tissue.

Fibroplasia is the proliferation of wound fibroblasts and the resultant production of collagen. Fibroblasts are attracted to the wound by growth factors, and fibroblast migration is influenced by proteins (integrin receptors) in the extracellular matrix. Integrin receptors expressed on the cell's surface guide the movement of both fibroblasts and epithelial cells to cover the wound. Fibroblasts produce collagen and change the predominant type of collagen in the wound. Initially, collagen type III predominates, but collagen type I takes over as the most common type of collagen when the new fibroblasts fill the wound. The height of collagen deposition occurs between 7 and 14 days after wounding. Then, as the numbers of fibroblasts and new capillaries decrease, the collagen content stabilizes and the granulation tissue becomes a relatively acellular scar. The wound continues to gain tensile strength over time as collagen fibers align according to the tension of applied forces during the next phase of wound healing, although the scar tissue never achieves the strength of the original unwounded tissues.

Wound contraction, the process primarily responsible for decreasing the size of a wound, is achieved by the migration of myofibroblasts towards the center of the wound. As the wound contracts, the surrounding skin stretches and the wound changes configuration, often taking on a stellate appearance. Contraction of the wound ceases when the tension on the surrounding skin equals the contracting forces or when epithelialization is complete. The end result of contraction is usually beneficial by decreasing the diameter of the wound and making closure less reliant upon epithelialization. If the opposing forces limit the amount of wound contraction, incomplete closure or an extremely thin layer of epithelium may result. When excessive contraction occurs around tubular structures and joints, strictures and gait abnormalities, respectively, may result. The result of excess wound contraction is termed contracture. Early closure of wounds around tubular structures and joints is desired to avoid contracture and its consequences.

Epithelialization, the covering of the wound with new epithelial cells, begins with mobilization and migration of epithelial cells from the wound edges. Epithelialization begins almost immediately in partial-thickness skin wounds with mobilization of epithelial cells from the wound edges and skin appendages. In full-thickness skin wounds, granulation tissue is necessary for epithelialization to take place. Epithelial cells at the wound edges change their phenotype and disconnect from neighboring cells to migrate across the wound surface. When migrating cells come in contact with each other, movement ceases (contact inhibition), the phenotypic changes reverse, and a new basement membrane is formed. Concurrent wound contraction minimizes the amount of epithelial migration needed to close the wound, but in large open wounds, where complete contraction does not occur, epithelialization continues. In such cases, a thin layer of epithelial cells covers the wound. This thin layer of epithelium is easily traumatized, and repetitive trauma may prevent epithelialization from being complete.

The duration of the repair phase of wound healing varies because of variable depths and dimensions of wounds, but one might expect this phase to last 1–3 weeks in most cases. Overlap of phases may occur at this juncture, just as there is overlap between inflammatory and repair phases. Some portions of the wound may begin to mature before all repair is complete.

Maturation Phase

Maturation, the phase of wound healing characterized by progressive gain of tissue strength, revolves around collagen deposition. Collagen deposition and gain in tissue strength are marked in the first 7–14 days after wounding, and then the rates of deposition and strength gain decrease. Despite the initial rapid gain in strength, most wounded tissues achieve only 20% of their final strength in the first 3 weeks after wounding. Tissue strength improves by rearrangement and increased cross-linkage of collagen fibers. Maturation may take months or years, but still, the final tensile strength of the scar is only 70–80% of normal tissue. In fact, the process of wound maturation continues for the life of the animal, with only two tissues (urinary bladder and bone) capable of returning to 100% of the tissue's unwounded strength.

Wound Closure

Local wound factors, concurrent injuries, co-morbidities, and time elapsed since the creation of the wound must be considered prior to wound closure in order to increase the chances of uncomplicated healing. Knowledge of how the wound was induced (incision by a sharp blade, gunshot, car accident, etc.) is of the utmost importance in determining the expected amount of tissue trauma and degree of wound contamination and necrosis.

Wounds can be managed by primary closure, delayed primary closure, secondary closure, and second intention healing. First intention healing refers to surgical closure of a wound with the intent of having the apposed wound edges heal to each other without the need for epithelium to migrate across a granulation bed. All three of the above-mentioned closures are performed to achieve first intention healing, whereas second intention healing does not involve surgical apposition of wound edges.

Primary closure is closure of a wound soon after it is created. A planned surgical incision is the most obvious example of a wound suitable for primary closure. Clean wounds can be managed by wound cleaning and primary closure if within a few (preferably 6) hours of wound creation. In such wounds, there should be minimal, if any, need for debridement. At wound evaluation, the veterinarian must decide that the chances of additional loss of tissue viability and infection will be minimal after closure. In addition, primary closure should result in minimal tension on wound edges in order to minimize the chances for dehiscence.

Delayed primary closure is closure of a wound after a delay to determine wound viability but before the onset of granulation tissue. Delayed primary closure is employed when there is minimal to moderate tissue damage, but the chances of contamination progressing to infection are significant. Cleaning, debridement, and bandaging are performed until the wound is suitable for closure. Delayed primary closure is performed within 3 days after wound creation, prior to the presence of granulation tissue. Local or distant tissue (tissue flaps) may be required for wound closure.

Secondary closure is wound closure after the onset of granulation tissue. Wounds with extensive tissue loss or necrosis, severe contamination, or marked presence of debris are good candidates for secondary closure. In such wounds, extensive cleaning is usually necessary due to the presence of large amounts of foreign material (dirt, asphalt, feces, etc.). Debridement of necrotic tissue should be performed daily until additional necrosis is not detected and a healthy bed of granulation tissue covers the wound (usually at least 5 days after wounding). Advancement of local skin with walking sutures, skin flaps, or skin grafts may be required for closure.

Second intention healing is non-closure of a wound. Closure is achieved naturally as previously described. Second intention healing is dependent on wound contraction and epithelialization. Small uncomplicated wounds or wounds where local or distant tissues are not available for closure may be suitable for second intention healing. Second intention healing should be avoided in wounds adjacent to tubular structures (perianal wounds) and in periarticular wounds, due to the risk of stricture and decrease in range of motion, respectively.

Management of Acute Traumatic Wounds and Deciding When and How to Close Them

Emergency practitioners are often presented with wounds that have just occurred, and what veterinarians do to initially manage these wounds may dictate the ultimate outcome of the definitive treatment. The remainder of this chapter is written to stimulate the reader to think about the decisions involved in acute wound management and accompanying antibiotic therapy that may (or may not) be indicated. Answers to the questions posed below are somewhat incomplete in order to promote an active thought process when managing any particular wound.

Initial Wound Care

Early management of acutely inflicted wounds greatly influences healing and ultimate outcome. When shock or other injuries take priority over wound management, an attempt should be made to quickly cover wounds with clean (preferably sterile) material to provide a barrier to the environment until the wounds can be addressed. As soon as patient conditions permit, the following procedures should be carried out in order, to promote optimal results: prompt and efficient wound inspection, lavage, appropriate debridement, and aseptic bandaging. It is debatable whether topical medications are indicated and, if so, what topical medications should be used. Generally speaking, topical medications, other than lavage solutions, are rarely needed in acute wound management. A "cookbook" approach to the steps in wound management discussed below will inevitably result in an undesirable outcome at an unexpected time. Therefore, thoughtful consideration of the questions below should be part of the wound management process each time a veterinarian is presented with an acute wound to manage.

Wound Inspection

A thorough examination of the wound is essential for determining the immediate course of action, the possibilities for closure, and initial prognosis for success of treatment. Consider the necessity of the various components of wound inspection. Why is adequate clipping of hair around the wound important? How does one protect the wound from clipped hair during the process of clipping, and why is it important to provide this protection? Why are sterile gloves and sterile instruments used to inspect acute traumatic wounds? Is it really necessary that the gloves and instruments are sterile given that these wounds are already contaminated?

Here are some answers: Generous hair removal is important for adequate visualization, optimal decontamination, and general hygiene. Protection of the wound from clipped hair is accomplished by packing the wound with sterile gauze and/or sterile jelly. This protection is necessary to avoid foreign body (hair) contamination of the wound. Sterile gloves and instruments are used to avoid iatrogenic contamination. The wound needs to be protected from contamination by micro-organisms

in the hospital environment that could lead to serious nosocomial infection by resistant bacteria.

Lavage

It is generally accepted that wounds should be irrigated (lavaged) during inspection and treatment, but why should this happen? And what solutions are appropriate for wound lavage? List one advantage and one disadvantage of pressurizing the lavage. What is the optimal lavage pressure and how can this pressure be achieved? Should puncture wounds be lavaged? Why or why not?

Here are some answers: Wounds are lavaged to hydrate them. Remember the old adage that "moist tissues are happy tissues." Also, another old adage states that "dilution is the solution to pollution." As such, lavage is performed to remove small debris and to "dilute" the bacteria that are likely present. Removal of all foreign matter, even the particulate variety, will make the wound environment less conducive to bacterial growth, and copious lavage will help "wash away" bacteria as well. Depending on the solution used for lavage, some bacteria may even be killed.

A number of solutions have been used to lavage acute traumatic wounds. A balanced electrolyte solution with a physiologically acceptable pH (such as lactated Ringer's solution) is ideal. Other solutions that have been successfully used for wound lavage include normal saline, 0.05% chlorhexidine, 0.1% povidone-iodine, and tap water, the latter typically reserved for wounds that are excessively covered with environmental dirt and grime. When antiseptics are used, solutions should be used; scrubs (detergents) should not be applied to wounds.

Some prefer to pressurize the lavage to facilitate removal of foreign matter in the wound. A disadvantage of pressurized lavage is the potential to drive bacteria into the tissues rather than washing them away. The optimal lavage pressure has been taught to be 7–8 psi achieved using an 18 or 19 gauge hypodermic needle attached to a 35 mL syringe. However, in one study a 35 mL syringe and 16 gauge hypodermic needle produced approximately double that amount of pressure [4]. Lavage of puncture wounds can be detrimental. Doing so could introduce fluid into the subcutaneous tissues, and it is likely that all of the introduced fluid will not be retrieved, ultimately resulting in "iatrogenic" edema. Therefore, it is recommended to not lavage puncture wounds, but rather to surface cleanse them.

Surgical Debridement

Debridement is the "removal of debris," the removal of dead tissue and foreign material. The proper English pronunciation (dǐ-brēd'mǝnt) is recommended to emphasize that debris, not living tissue, is being removed. How does debridement differ from "freshening wound edges"? Why would "freshening edges" ever be indicated?

Describe appropriate anesthesia/restraint for surgical debridement. Why are sterile drapes, instruments, and gloves important for debridement?

Here are some answers: The technique of freshening wound edges involves incision until bleeding is witnessed; therefore, freshening removes viable tissue. Debridement does not remove viable tissue. Freshening edges has no role in surgical debridement of wounds. Freshening is occasionally done during wound closure (see "Freshening Wound Edges" below), but only when necessary for cosmesis or to avoid burying epithelium. The most appropriate restraint for surgical debridement is general anesthesia (see Chapter 190). The actual protocol should be tailored to the individual patient but in most cases, thorough debridement is best done with an intubated patient and inhalant anesthesia. Sterile drapes, instruments, and gloves are important for surgical debridement to avoid iatrogenic contamination.

Aseptic Bandaging

Bandaging a wound after surgical debridement can be beneficial, if appropriately applied, or detrimental, if errantly applied. What wounds require bandaging? What wounds require splinted bandaging? What wounds do not require bandaging? Why is it important for the contact layer of the bandage to be sterile? What is the purpose of a wet-to-dry dressing? When is a dry-to-dry dressing used? When is it appropriate to switch from an adherent to a non-adherent dressing?

Here are some answers: Ideally, all wounds should be bandaged after surgical debridement. Unfortunately, bandaging is not always practical. Essentially, all wounds in hospitalized patients should be bandaged if at all possible in order to minimize the chance of nosocomial wound infection. Splinted bandages are required for wounds around joints or wounds that are otherwise subjected to excessive movement. Wounds that can be safely left unbandaged are those that are covered by healthy granulation tissue and are going to be managed at home and not in the hospital environment. The contact layer of bandages is sterile in order to protect against iatrogenic contamination. Wet-to-dry dressings are used when continued debridement is required. A dry-to-dry dressing is used when the wound is already wet due to exudation, and, like the wet-to-dry dressing, the dry-to-dry dressing is used for debridement. Wet-to-dry and dry-to-dry dressings are adherent to the wound. A switch from adherent to non-adherent dressing is done once there is a granulation bed to protect the granulation tissue from being disrupted during bandage changes.

Negative pressure wound therapy (also called vacuum-assisted wound closure) [5,6] is a nice option for open wound management in preparation for secondary wound closure. However, this option is frequently delayed 12–24 hours after acute wounds have been managed as described above. This delay is to ensure that no additional surgical debridement is necessary.

Topical Medications/Ointments

There seems to be an innate tendency for veterinarians to apply medications to wounds, and wound care products seem to be widely available. What ointments are appropriate for application to wounds? What ointments may delay wound healing? What ointments may enhance wound healing? List the reason(s) for using any justifiable ointment (is the ointment used for antimicrobial effect, enzymatic debridement, and/or direct enhancement of healing?).

Here are some answers: Any of a number of available topical wound medications may be deemed appropriate. Some for which the author has found appropriate use include triple antibiotic ointment, gentamicin ointment, silver sulfadiazine cream, sugar, and unpasteurized honey. However, the author typically avoids topical wound treatments unless a specified purpose is desired and likely to be achieved with the ointment. Further, one must consider potential detrimental effects of ointments. For example, some ointments will trap exudates in the wound, thereby contributing to bacterial growth rather than combating it. And many ointments will have some negative effect on wound healing. Petrolatum, a base found in some ointments, delays the epithelial stage of wound healing. On the other hand, some topical wound medications enhance wound healing. Notable examples of products that optimize wound healing are sugar and unpasteurized honey. Whenever a topical agent is applied to a wound, a justifiable reason (antimicrobial effect, enzymatic debridement, and/or direct enhancement of healing) should be evident.

Deciding on Wound Closure

Options for wound closure (as detailed above) are primary closure, delayed primary closure, secondary wound closure, and second intention healing. Primary wound closure is closure performed immediately after wounding (within the first few hours). Delayed primary closure is closure of the wound after allowing enough time to ascertain vascular compromise (usually 18–24 hours, but definitely before the onset of granulation tissue). Secondary wound closure is closure after the appearance of granulation tissue within the wound. The presence of granulation tissue signals that the wound is reasonably resistant to infection and therefore safe to close. Second intention healing is non-closure where, instead of closing the wound, the processes of contraction and epithelialization are allowed to progress naturally to afford eventual closure.

Deciding which method of closure is best for any individual patient requires analysis of multiple factors, such as wound classification, timing of the injury, cause of the injury, and the owner's financial limitations. Relying only on any one of these four factors for determining the method of wound closure is flirting with failure. Box 166.1 gives an outline of the four factors used to determine the most appropriate type of wound closure and discussion of each factor.

Wound Classification

Clean wounds are rare with acute injury. The best example of a clean wound is a surgical incision in aseptically prepared skin that does not penetrate a contaminated lumen such as the alimentary or respiratory tract. Clean-contaminated wounds are wounds with minimal contamination. The best example of a clean-contaminated wound is a surgical incision in an aseptically prepared patient in which the alimentary or respiratory tract is entered. Acute traumatic wounds with minimal environmental debris and absence of necrotic tissue may also be considered to be clean-contaminated wounds. Primary wound closure can be performed with minimal risk of ensuing infection in clean and clean-contaminated wounds (after appropriate wound inspection and lavage). Contaminated wounds are non-surgical wounds (or surgical wounds with major breaks in aseptic technique) where large bacterial load is likely, but there are no gross signs of infection. Contaminated wounds can be closed by primary or delayed primary wound closure if they are converted to clean-contaminated wounds through the processes of lavage and debridement (Figure 166.1).

Dirty/infected wounds are wounds with foreign debris and/or gross evidence of infection (such as purulent exudate). These wounds might also contain necrotic tissue. For a wound to be infected, enough time must have passed to allow proliferation of bacteria to the concentration of 10^5 bacteria per gram of tissue (or per mL of tissue fluid). Primary wound closure is rarely performed for dirty/infected wounds, but theoretically could be done if the wound can be converted to a clean-contaminated state through the processes of lavage and debridement.

Timing of Injury

Assuming all other factors support primary wound closure, such closure is safer if performed within 6 hours of the injury, because by 6 hours bacteria have had enough time to multiply to numbers capable of causing infection (10^5 bacterial organisms per gram of tissue or per mL of tissue fluid for most bacteria). Wounds older than 6 hours would ideally be managed as open wounds and have delayed primary or secondary wound closure once it is certain that infection is not developing or after an infection that develops is eliminated.

Cause of Injury

Puncture wounds are not typically closed because the amount of subcutaneous trauma is difficult to determine, and the punctures allow for drainage. In general,

---

Box 166.1 Four factors used to determine appropriate type of wound closure.

Wound classification
1. Clean
2. Clean-contaminated
3. Contaminated
4. Dirty/infected

Timing of injury
1. Within 6 hours of injury
2. Beyond 6 hours of injury

Cause of injury
1. Puncture wound
2. Sharp laceration
3. Sharp laceration with tissue loss (anatomical degloving)
4. Blunt injury (physiological degloving)

Owner's financial limitations
1. Is second intention closure really more economical than surgical closure?
2. Is primary closure ever warranted if dehiscence is likely?

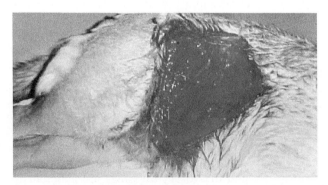

Figure 166.1 Acutely acquired wound on the right flank of 4-year-old female mixed breed dog. The wound was presumably sustained by running into a fence in the owner's back yard a few hours prior to presentation. Because of the unwitnessed and therefore unknown exact nature of the injury, delayed primary closure was performed approximately 8 hours after presentation to the emergency service to allow time to assess tissue viability.

puncture wounds are not surgically explored unless there is a known foreign object that must be retrieved. Probing of puncture wounds is warranted during the inspection stage of wound management in order to determine if the wound should be extended or modified in some way to facilitate drainage.

Sharp lacerations offer the best opportunity for primary wound closure (see Figure 166.1), whereas sharp laceration with tissue loss (anatomical degloving) and open wounds due to blunt injury (physiological degloving) require some time to determine the health of the tissue. Delayed primary closure is more appropriate than primary closure for anatomical and physiological degloving wounds. In some cases, secondary wound closure is best for degloving wounds. If there is any doubt about the degree of tissue injury or bacterial load, waiting for the onset of granulation tissue before closure (i.e. secondary wound closure) is wise (Figure 166.2).

Owner's Financial Limitations

The owner's desire for a fiscally conservative approach may make second intention healing or primary wound closure more appealing than delayed primary or secondary wound closure. However, the wrong closure choice could result in more financial burden than if the wound was managed most appropriately in the first place. Second intention healing may necessitate wound management and bandaging for a protracted period of time, resulting in accumulation of more financial investment than if surgical closure (at the appropriate time) was performed. Likewise, closing a wound before it is ready could result in infection and/or dehiscence and the added costs of dealing with those complications.

"Freshening Wound Edges"

During wound closure, one is often tempted to "freshen the wound edges." This is contraindicated because it offsets the advantage of the secondary wound phenomenon (i.e. accelerated healing due to already present and active fibroblasts). When might one justify "freshening the edges" of a wound? Perhaps edges should be trimmed if an exquisite cosmetic effect is desired (and in the best interests of the patient). During secondary wound closure, epithelium that has begun migration over the granulation bed may require excision to prevent its burial under the surgically advanced skin edges. One might consider excision of this advancing epithelium to be "freshening of the wound edge." Freshening is not indicated in acute wound management because discarding viable tissue may complicate ultimate wound closure by removing skin that would have been useful to achieve a tension-free closure. Of course, selective trimming of wound edges might facilitate some closures when the shape of the wound is inopportune.

Managing Wound Drainage

Wound drainage can be expected in most traumatic wounds. How is wound drainage managed in open

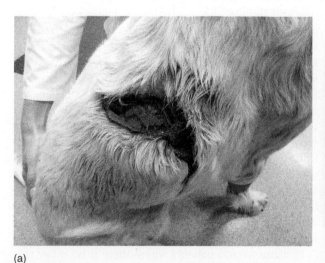
(a)

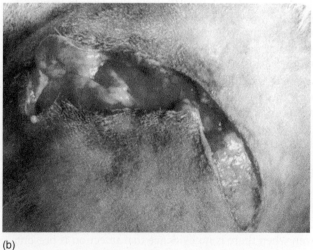
(b)

Figure 166.2 Acutely acquired wound (a) prior to and (b) after wound inspection and lavage on the upper right flank of a 6-year-old female Llewellin setter. The wound was sustained as the dog was running under a trailer less than 6 hours prior to presentation to the emergency service. Despite the ability to quickly address this wound, secondary wound closure was chosen because of the depth of the wound and suspected physiological degloving associated with the blunt trauma. (Caudal is to the lower left and cranial is to the upper right in both images.)

wounds? Drainage must be controlled in wounds that are surgically closed. Methods for drainage control include obliteration of dead space and incorporation of a passive or active wound drain. Describe a wound in which no surgical drain is necessary. Describe the proper method of dead space obliteration. When would a passive or active wound drain be indicated? Identify some particular types of passive drains. Identify some particular types of active drains. What are the advantages and disadvantages of a passive wound drain? What are the advantages and disadvantages of an active wound drain?

Here are some answers: Drainage in open wounds is achieved through the wounds themselves. Ideally, open wounds are bandaged so that wound fluids are absorbed into the bandage material and removed during bandage changes. With negative pressure wound therapy, wound fluid is drawn through the wound contact material (gauze or open cell polyurethane ether foam) and collected in a canister. Drains can be omitted in surgically closed wounds if dead space is obliterated. Dead space is obliterated with careful placement of sutures similar to walking sutures. It can also be obliterated with bandaging, but bandage obliteration of dead space is more readily achieved on limbs than on other areas of the body.

When it is not possible to effectively obliterate dead space with suture or bandage, a passive or active wound drain is recommended. A commonly used passive drain is the Penrose drain. A commonly used active drain is the Jackson–Pratt drain. Passive drains are economical and easily placed, but ideally should be bandaged to collect drainage and protect from ascending infection. Also, passive drains must be maintained for 5 days before removal to ensure that the tissues have sealed to obliterate dead space. A passive drain that can be removed prior to 5 days is probably unnecessary. Active drains pull tissues together, causing early obliteration of dead space and permitting early drain removal (typically 2–3 days after surgery). Further, active suction and the closed nature of the drain help protect against ascending infection. The major disadvantage of active drains is that they are more expensive than passive drains; however, their effectiveness may offset the expense.

Antibiotic Therapy in Wound Management

There is a tendency to prescribe antibiotic therapy for animals with wounds to provide a "cover" for infection, even when there is no evidence that infection is present or likely (see Chapter 200). However, indiscriminate use of antibiotics is potentially harmful. And, as a profession, if we do not curtail inappropriate use of antibiotics, governmental restrictions could limit, or prevent altogether, access to certain antimicrobial drugs for veterinary use.

When managing a wound, certain questions should come to mind regarding antibiotic therapy. Answering these questions is much preferred to the simpler "knee jerk" response of prescribing an antibiotic or applying an antimicrobial ointment. The reader is encouraged to carefully consider the following questions before prescribing systemic or topical antibiotics in the treatment of wounds.

Acute Wounds

The mere presence of a laceration is not an indication for emergency administration of antibiotic therapy. However, the acutely traumatized patient may require antibiotic therapy for other reasons. List some potential indications for antibiotic therapy in acutely traumatized patients. How might antibiotic administration affect the wound?

Infected Wounds

Most clinicians feel that antibiotic therapy is indicated for infected wounds. If that is the case, what antibiotic should be used? By what route should the antibiotic be given? How long should the duration of antibiotic therapy be? What factors guide the choice of antibiotic? Should antibiotic therapy be guided by culture and susceptibility? If so, when and how should the bacteriology sample be obtained? What would be some disadvantages of antibiotic administration in the management of open wounds?

Here are some answers: Patients with traumatic wounds often have concurrent injuries or co-morbidities, and some of the co-existing problems may warrant antibiotic therapy. If the patient is at risk for sepsis, systemic antibiotic therapy is unquestionably warranted. In most cases, such therapy will not adversely affect the wound; however, one must consider that wound infections have been shown to be more common in wounds of patients treated inappropriately with antibiotics than when no antibiotics were used at all [7], and the wrong choice for the wound could exacerbate a resistant infection. In human beings, antibiotic therapy for non-bite wounds treated in the emergency room has been shown to offer no protection against development of wound infection [8]. Furthermore, a lack of advantage has been demonstrated with antibiotic usage in human beings with gunshot wounds [9–12].

In acute wound patients where there is no other reason for antibiotic therapy, a rational approach would be to not use antibiotic therapy unless signs of infection ensue, or to employ perioperative intravenous antibiotics if primary or delayed primary closure is employed, similar to what is done with planned surgical procedures that warrant antibiotic prophylaxis. If the urge to administer antibiotics as part of wound management is strong, then secondary wound closure would be more appropriate than primary closure.

Choice of empirical antibiotic for the wound itself should be based on the most likely contaminant given the situation. Culture and susceptibility is the ideal method for antibiotic choice; however, the bacteria in the wound at the time of wounding are not always the bacteria responsible for the ultimate infection [13,14], and not all culture-positive wounds result in clinical infection [15]. Therefore, it is most prudent to wait for gross evidence of infection before performing culture and

susceptibility. To optimize accuracy of the culture, tissue from the wound should be obtained rather than merely swabbing the wound. The wrong antibiotic choice can lead to a wound with a resistant infection that is difficult to treat; therefore, wise empirical choices and choices based on appropriately timed cultures of wound tissue are important for optimal results. Intravenous antibiotics are recommended when initiating antibiotic therapy, but a switch to oral medications can often be done to finish a proper course of antibiotics (5–7 days after the last gross evidence of infection). In wounds with established infection, reculturing before secondary wound closure is often warranted.

References

1 Tobias KM, Johnson SA. *Veterinary Surgery: Small Animal.* Elsevier Saunders, St Louis, 2012.
2 Fossum TW. *Small Animal Surgery*, 4th edn. Elsevier Mosby, St Louis, 2013.
3 Mann FA, Constantinescu GM, Yoon H. *Fundamentals of Small Animal Surgery.* Wiley-Blackwell, Ames, 2011.
4 Gall TT, Monnet E. Evaluation of fluid pressures of common wound-flushing techniques. *Am J Vet Res* 2010;71:1384–1386.
5 Demaria M, Stanley BJ, Hauptman JG, et al. Effects of negative pressure wound therapy on healing of open wounds in dogs. *Vet Surg* 2011;40:658–669.
6 Ben-Amotz R, Lanz OI, Miller JM, et al. The use of vacuum-assisted closure therapy for the treatment of distal extremity wounds in 15 dogs. *Vet Surg* 2007;36:684–690.
7 Brown DC, Conzemius MG, Shofer F, Swann H. Epidemiologic evaluation of postoperative wound infections in dogs and cats. *J Am Vet Med Assoc* 1997;210:1302–1306.
8 Cummings P, del Beccaro MA. Antibiotics to prevent infection of simple wounds: a meta-analysis of randomized studies. *Am J Emerg Med* 1995;13:396–400.
9 Dickey RL, Barnes BC, Kearns RJ, Tullos HS. Efficacy of antibiotics in low-velocity gunshot fractures. *J Orthop Trauma* 1989;3:6–10.
10 Howland WS, Ritchey SJ. Gunshot fractures in civilian practice. *J Bone Joint Surg* 1971;53-A:47–55.
11 Patzakis MJ, Harvey JP, Ivler D. The role of antibiotics in the management of open fractures. *J Bone Joint Surg* 1974;56-A:532–541.
12 Knapp TP, Patzakis MJ, Lee J, et al. Comparison of intravenous and oral antibiotic therapy in the treatment of fractures caused by low-velocity gunshots. A prospective, randomized study of infection rates. *J Bone Joint Surg* 1996;78-A:1167–1171.
13 Valenziano CP, Chattar-Cora D, O'Neill A, et al. Efficacy of primary wound cultures in long bone open extremity fractures: are they of any value? *Arch Orthop Trauma Surg* 2002;122:259–261.
14 Lee J. Efficacy of cultures in the management of open fractures. *Clin Orthop Rel Res* 1997;339:71–75.
15 Ireifej S, Marino DJ, Loughin CA, et al. Risk factors and clinical relevance of positive intraoperative bacterial cultures in dogs with total hip replacement. *Vet Surg* 2012;41:63–68.

168

Colloid Fluid Therapy

Marie K. Holowaychuk, DVM, DACVECC

Critical Care Vet Consulting, Calgary, AB, Canada

Introduction

Colloids are large molecular weight (MW) p[ ]
remain dispersed in liquid due to their size a[ ]
charge. Colloids are too big to pass through [ ]
lar endothelial membrane and exert an oncot[ ]
that pulls additional fluid into the vascular [ ]
the interstitial fluid compartment [1]. These [ ]
make colloid solutions desirable during fluid [ ]
tion because of their rapid and efficient int[ ]
volume expansion and relatively long-lastii[ ]
However, colloid solutions are not without si[ ]
which tend to occur in a dose-dependent man[ ]

Colloid Osmotic Pressure

Colloid osmotic pressure (COP) is the oncoti[ ]
exerted by proteins or protein-like substanc[ ]
context of the intravascular compartment, pla[ ]
tends to pull fluid into the vasculature in opp[ ]
hydrostatic pressure, thus limiting extravasatic[ ]
into the interstitium [2].

Starling's equation has been used to desc[ ]
movement across the vascular wall:

$$J_v = K[(P_c - P_i) - \sigma(\pi_c - \pi_i)]$$

where J_v is the difference between hydrostatic (P_c[ ]
oncotic ($\pi_c - \pi_i$) gradients, P_c is the intravascul[ ]
lary) hydrostatic pressure, P_i is the interstitial hy[ ]
pressure, π_c is the intravascular oncotic pressur[ ]
is the interstitial oncotic pressure. K is the filtrat[ ]
ficient that represents the ease with which flui[ ]
across the membrane, whereas σ is the reflectic[ ]
cient that represents the pore size or permeabili[ ]
membrane [2].

In healthy animals, albumin accounts for 80% o[ ]
COP, while other proteins such as immunoglobu[ ]

shown to result in the development of fluid overload in up to 67% of patients at 24 hours [21]. Fluid overload and a positive fluid balance following the initial resuscitation period have been shown to result in significantly increased mortality in sick dogs [22]. Positive fluid balance can result in impaired microcirculation and organ dysfunction (of primary concern in critically ill small animal patients are kidney, lung, and GI dysfunction).

Consideration should be given to resuscitating patients according to an individualized physiology-based approach. A conservative fluid therapy approach, aiming to achieve negative fluid balance or at least avoid a positive fluid balance, may be warranted. Additionally, based on recent evidence showing that earlier use of norepinephrine is associated with improved outcome and lower cumulative fluid balance in critically ill people, small animals may benefit from earlier vasopressor support rather than continued fluid boluses to patients that are not responding [23].

Crystalloid Fluids for Rehydration and Maintenance

Following treatment of hypovolemia, continued crystalloid fluid therapy may be indicated to address dehydration and any ongoing losses or maintenance requirements.

To determine the volume of fluid required for rehydration, the typical formula used is body weight (kg) × % dehydration × 1000 (see Table 167.2). For example, if a 20 kg dog is assessed as 10% dehydrated, the overall fluid requirement to rehydrate that patient would be 2 liters of fluid.

Maintenance fluid requirements vary according to the age, size, and body condition of a given animal, but estimates of 2–4 mL/kg/h are commonly used initially. Very

small (<2 kg) or giant breeds (>50 kg) may benefit from a body surface area calculation of daily fluid requirements using: body weight $(kg)^{0.75} \times 70$. Any calculated fluid deficit is typically added to maintenance fluid requirements and corrected over 6–24 hours in stable patients. Ongoing losses may be quantified (for example, weighing vomitus or diarrhea), but this is a rough calculation. As such, ongoing losses are often estimated at 2–4 mL/kg per episode of vomiting or diarrhea. Any estimate of ongoing losses is added to the calculated deficit and maintenance fluid requirements.

Continued monitoring and reassessment of a patient is of the utmost important during the replacement phase of fluid therapy. Monitoring of physical examination parameters, clinical pathology, and body weight should be performed frequently in all patients receiving intravenous fluid therapy. Body weight monitoring can be particularly useful, as any rapid change in body weight is likely to reflect changes in water weight in the patient. Other physical examination variables and clinical pathology parameters that should be serially monitored are presented in Table 167.1.

Complications of Crystalloid Fluid Therapy

While fluid therapy is often considered relatively benign, it is not without risk. The benefits versus risks associated with the use of crystalloid fluids should always be considered, as with use of any other drug administered to a patient. Complications that can develop associated with the use of crystalloids include volume overload and associated complications; heart failure; development of pulmonary edema; rapid changes in serum sodium concentrations which may result in immediate or delayed neurological signs; and/or development of other electrolyte or acid–base derangements.

References

1 Awad S, Allison SP, Lobo DN. The history of 0.9% saline. *Clin Nutr* 2008;27(2):179–188.
2 DiBartola SP (ed.). *Fluid, Electrolyte, and Acid–Base Disorders in Small Animal Practice*. Elsevier Saunders, St Louis, 2012.
3 Silverstein DC, Hopper K (eds). *Small Animal Critical Care Medicine*, 2nd edn. Elsevier Saunders, St Louis, 2015.
4 Davis H, Jensen T, Johnson A, et al. 2013 AAHA/AAFP Fluid Therapy Guidelines for Dogs and Cats. *J Am Anim Hosp Assoc* 2013;49(1):149–159.
5 Rudloff E, Kirby R. Fluid therapy: crystalloids and colloids. *Vet Clin North Am Small Anim Pract* 1998;28(2):297–328.
6 Kien ND, Kramer GC, White DA. Acute hypotension caused by rapid hypertonic saline infusion in anesthetized dogs. *Anesth Analg* 73(5):597–602.
7 Silverstein DC, Aldrich J, Haskins SC, et al. Assessment of changes in blood volume in response to resuscitative fluid administration in dogs. *J Vet Emerg Crit Care* 2005;15(3):185–192.
8 Chappell D, Jacob M, Hofmann-Kiefer K, et al. A rational approach to perioperative fluid management. *Anesthesiology* 2008;109:723–740.
9 Cazzolli D, Prittie J. The crystalloid-colloid debate: consequences of resuscitation fluid selection in veterinary critical care. *J Vet Emerg Crit Care* 2015;25(1):6–19.

10 Silverstein DC, Kleiner J, Drobatz KJ. Effec intravenous fluid resuscitation in the emer for treatment of hypotension in dogs: 35 ca 2010). *J Vet Emerg Crit Care* 2012;22(6):66

11 Yozova ID, Howard J, Adamik KN. Effects maize-derived 6% tetrastarch (hydroxyethy 130/0.4) on plasma creatinine levels in dog retrospective analysis (2010–2013). *J Vet E Care* 2014;24:S31.

12 Gauthier V, Holowaychuk MK, Kerr CL, et of synthetic colloid administration on hemo and laboratory variables in healthy dogs an with systemic inflammation. *J Vet Emerg C* 2014;24(2):251–258.

13 Dellinger RP, Levy MM, Rhodes A, et al. Su Sepsis Campaign: International Guidelines Management of Severe Sepsis and Septic Sl *Intens Care Med* 2013;39(1):165–228.

14 Morgan TJ. The ideal crystalloid – what is 'l *Curr Opin Crit Care* 2013;19(4):299–307.

15 Chowdhury AH, Cox EF, Francis ST, et al. A randomized, controlled, double-blind cross on the effects of 2-L infusions of 0.9% saline Plasma-Lyte® 148 on renal blood flow veloci cortical tissue perfusion in healthy voluntee *Surg* 2012;256(1):18–24.

16 Raghunathan K, Shaw A, Nathanson B, et al Association between the choice of IV crysta in-hospital mortality among critically ill adu sepsis. *Crit Care Med* 2014;42(7):1585–1591

Types of Colloid Solutions

Colloid solutions can be classified as natural or synthetic. Natural colloids are blood products that contain albumin, which is largely responsible for COP. Examples include whole blood, plasma components, or concentrated albumin. Synthetic colloids contain high MW particles manufactured from other substances that are suspended in crystalloid solutions. Examples include dextrans, gelatin, and hydroxyethyl starch (HES) solutions. Use of natural versus synthetic colloids, as well as the type of synthetic colloid solution, varies geographically based on what is available or approved by the country's drug administration program [7].

Natural Colloids

The characteristics of commonly administered natural colloids are summarized in Table 168.1. Because natural colloids are blood products, they often have the inconvenience of a shorter shelf-life, need for specialized storage equipment (e.g. temperature-controlled refrigerator) and administration sets (e.g. filters), as well as requirements for pretransfusion recipient screening (e.g. blood typing and/or cross-matching) [8]. Likewise, blood products are sometimes in short supply or unavailable at the time of need. More information regarding the administration of blood products can be found in Chapter 176.

Whole Blood

Whole blood contains all components of circulating blood, including red and white blood cells, platelets, clotting factors, globulins, and albumin, which exerts the majority of COP. Whole blood is considered *fresh* if stored briefly (<8 h) at room temperature prior to transfusion, whereas *stored* whole blood can be refrigerated for up to 30 days depending on the anticoagulant preservative solution used [8]. Whole blood is typically used as a colloid in patients experiencing life-threatening hemorrhage.

Plasma

Plasma components are prepared from whole blood by centrifugation and are available from most commercial blood banks or in-hospital blood donor programs. Plasma is available as fresh frozen plasma (stored in a -18 °C freezer within 6–8 hours of collection), frozen plasma (fresh frozen plasma stored for longer than 1 year or plasma frozen more than 24 hours after collection), or liquid plasma (never frozen and refrigerated for up to 5 days) [9]. While these components vary in terms of their clotting factor activity, they all contain equal amounts of albumin and thus have a similar ability to increase COP and be used as a colloid. However, this is not generally an efficient use of blood products since a large volume of plasma is necessary to increase the albumin by a significant amount.

Plasma components are typically used to correct clotting factor deficiencies in patients with congenital or acquired bleeding disorders, as well as for support of hemostasis in patients with severe hemorrhagic shock and/or undergoing massive transfusion [10]. Plasma can be administered as a colloid in hypoproteinemic patients, but large volumes (20–25 mL/kg) are required to raise the albumin by 0.5 g/dL, assuming no major ongoing losses [8].

Albumin

Concentrated albumin solutions are of a uniform molecular size according to the species of origin and are

Table 168.1 Composition, colloid osmotic pressure, and storage recommendations for natural colloids (blood products) used in veterinary patients [8,34].

Blood product	Composition	COP (mmHg)	Storage
Whole blood	RBCs, WBCs, platelets, albumin, globulin, all clotting factors	21–25	Refrigerated for <30 days
Fresh frozen plasma	Albumin, globulin, all clotting factors	17	< –18 °C for 1 year
Frozen plasma	Albumin, globulin, clotting factors II, VII, IX, X, XI, XII	17	< –18 °C for 5 years
Cryopoor plasma	Albumin, globulin, clotting factors II, VII, IX, X, XI, XII	17	< –18 °C for 5 years
Liquid plasma (<5 days old)	Albumin, globulin, all clotting factors	17	Refrigerated for <5 days
Human serum albumin	Albumin	>200 (25%) 23 (5%)	Room temperature
Canine-specific albumin	Albumin	Unpublished	Room temperature or refrigeration

COP, colloid osmotic pressure; RBC, red blood cell; WBC, white blood cell.

therefore monodisperse colloid solutions. Colloid support in the form of concentrated albumin solutions can be considered for critically ill, hypoalbuminemic patients (i.e. serum albumin < 1.5–2.0 g/dL). Examples include patients with vasculitis, systemic inflammatory response syndrome (SIRS), or sepsis [11]. Unfortunately, patients with ongoing or refractory protein loss (e.g. protein-losing enteropathy or nephropathy) are ultimately going to lose any albumin that is administered and are less likely to benefit.

Human Serum Albumin

Human serum albumin (HSA) is available as 5% or 25% solutions. Dosing regimens are extrapolated from human studies and generally recommended as 2 mL/kg over 2 hours, followed by 0.1–0.3 mL/kg/h. A total daily dose of 2 g/kg should not be exceeded (typically 2.5–5 mL/kg of the 25% HSA solution) [12–14]. Alternatively, some advocate the use of 5% HSA given to dogs at a rate of 2 mL/kg/h over 10 hours, repeated daily as needed to maintain serum albumin concentrations [15].

The possibility of severe and potentially fatal type III hypersensitivity reactions after initial or repeated exposure to HSA has been reported [16–18] even though many hospitalized patients have been given HSA without significant adverse effects. Delayed hypersensitivity reactions have also been reported so repeated administration after 48–72 hours is not recommended.

Canine-Specific Albumin

Canine-specific albumin (CSA) is a lyophilized product that is available in a 5 g vial that can be reconstituted with 0.9% NaCl or 5% dextrose in water (D5W) to a 5% (considered iso-oncotic), 10%, or 16% concentration. A dose of 450 mg/kg is expected to raise the serum albumin concentration by 0.5 g/dL but a maximum daily dosage has not been determined [19]. CSA administration has been reported in hospitalized dogs recovering from septic peritonitis with minimal adverse effects [20]. Theoretically, CSA is non-antigenic in dogs, so repeat transfusions should not elicit reactions.

Synthetic Colloids

The characteristics of commonly administered synthetic colloids are summarized in Table 168.2. Synthetic colloids are readily available fluid solutions that can be stored at room temperature for extended periods of time. They do not require specialized equipment for administration, nor do they require any form of recipient screening. They are simply administered as an IV fluid, with adjustments in dosing compared with crystalloid solutions, in order to ameliorate the side-effects.

Dextrans

Dextrans are composed of glucose polymers suspended in D5W or 0.9% NaCl. They are polydisperse colloid solutions, meaning they have a broad range of molecules with different MWs, for example, dextran-40 (average MW 40 kDa) and dextran-70 (average MW 70 kDa) [2]. Because a large percentage of the molecules are below the renal threshold for clearance, these colloid solutions have a short half-life and have been associated with acute kidney injury (AKI). They also impair platelet adhesion and factor VIII/von Willebrand factor complex formation [2]. As such, their use and availability have markedly decreased.

Gelatins

Gelatins are colloid solutions derived from bovine gelatin, a derivative of collagen. The forms most commonly used include urea-linked gelatins (polygeline) or succinylated gelatin (modified fluid gelatin). Gelatins are polydisperse colloid solutions and more than 75% of the

Table 168.2 Properties and maximum recommended daily dose of synthetic colloid solutions [24,33,34].

Product	Conc.	Carrier fluid	MW (kDa)	Molar substitution	C2:C6 ratio	COP (mmHg)	Maximum daily dose (mL/kg/day)
Dextran-70	6%	0.9% NaCl	70	NA	NA	62	20
Succinylated fluid gelatin	4%	0.9% NaCl	30	NA	NA	34	Unspecified
Urea cross-linked gelatin	3.5%	0.9% NaCl	35	NA	NA	15	Unspecified
Hespan	6%	0.9% NaCl	600	0.75	4-5:1	26	20
Hextend	6%	LRS	670	0.75	4:1	31	20
Pentaspan	10%	0.9% NaCl	200	0.4–0.5	4-5:1	66	30
Voluven	10%	0.9% NaCl	130	0.38–0.45	9:1	70–80	50
Voluven/ VetStarch	6%	0.9% NaCl	130	0.38–0.45	9:1	36	50

Conc., concentration; COP, colloid osmotic pressure; LRS, lactated Ringer's solution; MW, weight-average molecular weight; NA, not applicable.

molecules are < 30 kDa [2]. Therefore, while the small molecules exert a powerful initial COP, the effect is relatively short-lived as the molecules are rapidly cleared. Anaphylactoid reactions have been reported following administration of gelatins. They are manufactured and used mostly in Europe.

Hydroxyethyl Starch Solutions

Hydroxyethyl starch solutions are the most commonly used synthetic colloid in veterinary practice and are the focus of this chapter. First-generation HES solutions were introduced to the United States market in the 1970s. Concerns regarding AKI, hemostatic impairment, tissue deposition, and persistent pruritus in people led to the development of newer generation HES solutions that were initially considered safer. However, these products, which are simply modifications of former HES solutions, have the same side-effects as the older HES solutions [21].

Physiology and Classification

Hydroxyethyl starch solutions contain a polymer of glucose units derived from amylopectin and modified by substituting hydroxyethyl for hydroxyl groups at C2, C3, and C6 positions on the glucose units [22]. HES solutions are polydisperse and classified according to the concentration, MW, molar substitution, carrier fluid, and type of starch molecule. The concentration (e.g. 6% HES) refers to the concentration of HES in solution (i.e. 6 g HES/100 mL).

Hydroxyethyl starch solutions are categorized as first-, second-, or third-generation products relative to their average MW [1]. First-generation HES solutions include high MW products (HES 450/0.7, HES 550/0.7, and HES 670/0.75), second-generation HES solutions include medium MW products (HES 200/0.5), and third-generation HES solutions include low MW products (HES 130/0.4 and HES 130/0.42).

Hydroxyethyl starch solutions are also classified according to their molar substitution or the average number of hydroxyethyl residues per glucose unit, from which the terminology of hetastarch (0.7), hexastarch (0.6), pentastarch (0.5), and tetrastarch (0.4) is derived [22]. HES solutions exist in a variety of carrier solutions, including 0.9% NaCl and balanced/buffered crystalloids (e.g. lactated Ringer's solution).

The starch molecule is either waxy maize (e.g. 6% HES 130/0.4) or potato (e.g. 6% HES 130/0.42), which have small differences in the molar substitution. Potato starch HES solutions have a slightly larger negative charge, which is theorized to contribute to the formation of complexes between HES molecules and endogenous lipid molecules, but with unclear clinical effects [23].

Metabolism and Excretion

Most HES molecules are metabolized by alpha-amylase in the plasma and then cleared by renal excretion or tissue uptake. Small HES (<45–60 kDa) are not metabolized, but simply filtered by the glomerulus and excreted [22]. The rate of metabolism by alpha-amylase is slower with high MW and high molar substitution HES molecules. Likewise, HES molecules with a higher ratio of constituent glucose units hydroxylated at C2 to C6 (i.e. larger C2:C6 ratio) also have a slower rate of metabolic breakdown in the plasma [22].

If not metabolized or excreted, HES molecules are recognized by the reticuloendothelial system as foreign and taken up by monocytes, macrophages, endothelial cells, proximal tubule (renal epithelial) cells, liver parenchymal cells, Schwann cells, and keratinocytes and incorporated into lysosomes where they are resistant to degradation [22]. Smaller HES molecules are hypothesized to be more likely to undergo pinocytosis into cells leading to tissue accumulation, which might explain why recent clinical trials have failed to demonstrate a safety benefit of the low MW and lower molar substitution HES solutions. HES molecules have been detected in the skin, muscle, intestines, and kidneys more than 12–50 months after intravenous infusion in people [22].

Side-Effects

Large randomized controlled trials in the human medical field demonstrate safety concerns with all generations of HES solutions, namely an increased risk of AKI requiring dialysis, coagulopathies, volume overload, and allergic reactions [24]. However, serious adverse effects are largely unreported in small animals.

Suggested mechanisms causing AKI include osmotic nephrosis (i.e. proximal renal tubular vacuolization and swelling), tubular plugging due to hyperviscous urine, attenuation or cessation of glomerular filtration rate, and inflammation of the kidney interstitium [1,24]. A retrospective cohort study investigated the association between HES 250/0.5 administration and AKI or mortality in dogs admitted to a tertiary referral hospital intensive care unit. AKI was defined as a ≥ 2-fold increase in baseline creatinine or new onset of oliguria or anuria lasting ≥ 12 hours. After adjusting for illness severity, admission type, and concurrent administration of blood products, HES administration was found to be an independent risk factor for AKI and in-hospital mortality, with a number needed to harm of 6 [25]. A prospective investigation of HES administration in canine patients is warranted to confirm these findings.

Coagulopathies are thought to occur secondary to a dilutional coagulopathy, platelet dysfunction, and increased fibrinolysis, as well as decreased concentrations of von Willebrand factor (vWF) and factor VIII

(FVIII) [23]. Veterinary studies investigating the *in vitro* effect of HES solutions on coagulation in canine blood suggest that HES solutions decrease platelet function and fibrinogen in a dose-dependent manner, but there is controversy as to whether these findings are clinically relevant [26–29]. *In vivo* canine studies also demonstrate alterations in coagulation after HES boluses (10–40 mL/kg) and constant-rate infusions (1–2 mL/kg/h), but with no documentation of clinical bleeding [30–32].

Indications

Hydroxyethyl starch solutions can be administered to patients requiring volume resuscitation (i.e. hypovolemic shock) or colloid support, especially those with concurrent hypoproteinemia or hypoalbuminemia (e.g. SIRS or sepsis) that are unresponsive to conventional fluid resuscitation with crystalloids [11,24,33]. HES solutions have also been advocated for hypercoagulable human patients at risk of venous thrombosis [24].

Dose Recommendations

Hydroxyethyl starch solutions should be given in combination with isotonic balanced/buffered crystalloids

and dosed to effect based on goal-directed cardiovascular parameters. Typical IV bolus doses are 5–20 mL/kg (dogs) or 2–10 mL/kg (cats), administered over 15–20 minutes. Alternatively, HES solution administration has been used for COP support at a constant-rate infusion of 20–30 mL/kg/day [24].

Contraindications – Human Medicine

In 2013, marketing authorizations for HES solutions were suspended in Europe. Since then, the United States Food and Drug Administration has stated that HES solutions are contraindicated in critically ill patients, patients with sepsis, severe liver disease, AKI or kidney dysfunction, as well as oliguria or anuria not related to hypovolemia [24].

Conclusion

Hydroxyethyl starch solutions are relatively widely used colloids in veterinary practice with possible side-effects in canine patients that are similar to those in humans. As such, caution should be exercised when using HES solutions in veterinary patients until further prospective studies can be performed.

References

1 Argalious M. Colloid update. *Curr Pharm Des* 2012;18:6291–6297.
2 Vercueil A, Grocott MP, Mythen MG. Physiology, pharmacology, and rationale for colloid administration for the maintenance of effective hemodynamic stability in critically ill patients. *Transfus Med Rev* 2005;19:93–109.
3 Chan DL, Rozanski EA, Freeman LM, Rush JE. Colloid osmotic pressure in health and disease. *Compendium Contin Educ Vet* 2001;23:896–904.
4 Woodcock TE, Woodcock TM. Revised Starling equation and glycocalyx model of transvascular fluid exchange: an improved paradigm for prescribing intravenous fluid therapy. *Br J Anaesth* 2012;108:384–394.
5 Odunayo A, Kerl ME. Comparison of whole blood and plasma colloid osmotic pressure in healthy dogs. *J Vet Emerg Crit Care* 2011;21:236–241.
6 Jackson ML, Kerl ME, Tynan B, Mann FA. Comparison of whole blood and plasma colloid osmotic pressure in healthy cats. *J Vet Emerg Crit Care* 2014;24:408–413.
7 Finfer S, Lui B, Taylor C, et al. Resuscitation fluid use in critically ill adults: an international cross-sectional study in 391 intensive care units. *Crit Care* 2010;14:R185.
8 Davidow B. Transfusion medicine in small animals. *Vet Clin North Am Small Anim Pract* 2013;43:735–756.
9 Kakaiya R, Aronson CA, Julleis J. Whole blood processing and component processing at blood

collection centers. In: *Technical Manual and Standards for Blood Banks and Transfusion Services*, 17th edn (eds Roback JD, Grossman BJ, Harris T, et al). AABB, Bethesda, 2011, pp. 187–226.
10 Roback JD, Caldwell S, Carson J, et al. Evidence-based practice guidelines for plasma transfusion. *Transfusion* 2011;50:1227–1239.
11 Mazzaferro E, Powell LL. Fluid therapy for the emergent small animal patient: crystalloids, colloids, and albumin products. *Vet Clin North Am Small Anim Pract* 2013;43:721–734.
12 Mathews K, Barry M. The use of 25% human serum albumin: outcome and efficacy in raising serum albumin and systemic blood pressure in critically ill dogs and cats. *J Vet Emerg Crit Care* 2005;15:110–118.
13 Trow A, Rozanski E, de Laforcade A, et al. Evaluation of the use of human albumin in critically ill dogs: 73 cases (2003–2006). *J Vet Intern Med* 2008;233:607–612.
14 Horowitz FB, Read RL, Powell LL. A retrospective analysis of 25% human serum albumin supplementation in hypoalbuminemic dogs with septic peritonitis. *Can Vet J* 2015;56:591–597.
15 Vigano F, Perissinotto L, Bosco V. Administration of 5% human serum albumin in critically ill small animal patients with hypoalbuminemia: 418 dogs and 170 cats (1994–2008). *J Vet Emerg Crit Care* 2010;20:237–243.

Table 169.2 Nomenclature and classification of various available hydroxyethyl starch solutions.

Generation	MW/MS	Concentration	Classification	C2/C6 ratio	Carrier solution	Trade name
First	670/0.75	6%	Hetastarch	4.5:1	Balanced	Hextend®
	600/.07	6%	Hetastarch	5:1	Saline	Hespan®
	480/0.7	6%	Hetastarch	5:1	Saline	Plasmasteril®
Second	200/0.62	6%	Hexastarch	9:1	Saline	Elohes®
	200/0.5	6% or 10%	Pentastarch	5:1	Saline	Pentaspan®
	70/0.5	6%	Pentastarch	3:1	Balanced	Hemohes®
Third	130/0.42	6% or 10%	Tetrastarch	9:1	Saline	Tetraspan®
						Vetstarch®
						Voluven®
	130/0.42	6% or 10%	Tetrastarch	9:1	Balanced	Volulyte®

MS, molar substitution; MW, molecular weight.

The integrity of the ESL is thought to play a critical role in the fluid flux between the IVS and the interstitium. In healthy euvolemic patients with an intact ESL, colloids are retained in the IVS and maintain intravascular volume better than crystalloids [1]. A veterinary study evaluated blood volume (BV) expansion by different solution infusions in healthy dogs, and synthetic colloidal solutions (Dextran-70 and 6% HES) generated the largest cumulative effects, with BVs that continued to increase beyond the administration interval [21]. However, damage to the ESL is common in critical illness and can occur secondary to systemic inflammation, FO and hypoalbuminemia itself [32]. When the EG becomes degraded and capillary hydrostatic pressures are low, increased vascular permeability and capillary leak ensue and allow for extravasation of both proteins and synthetic colloids [1]. Under these conditions, crystalloids may be as effective as colloids in volume-expanding capacity. A comparative veterinary research study evaluated the effect of tetrastarch administration on hemodynamic and laboratory variables in healthy dogs and dogs with lipopolysaccharide (LPS)-induced systemic inflammation, compared with an equal volume of saline. Despite the provision of oncotic support, no significant beneficial effect on hemodynamic stabilization (HDS) in the LPS-treated dogs was demonstrated with tetrastarch over normal saline [58].

Under ongoing debate is the utility of colloids for the treatment of hypovolemia and anesthetic-induced hypotension. Clinical data have supported a hemodynamic advantage of colloid administration over crystalloids in the acute phase of hypovolemic resuscitation. Data from large RCTs in human intensive care have shown that resuscitation with HES solutions, compared to crystalloids alone, provided more rapid HDS, reduced vasopressor doses, and significantly higher central venous pressures [40,41,59,60]. There are smaller human trials which have favored the use of colloids over crystalloids in the treatment of trauma and hypovolemic shock [60,61]. These studies have shown trends towards improved outcome, with insufficient study populations to demonstrate an outcome advantage. Similar to other larger clinical trials, although time to HDS was expedited and initially more efficient with the use of HES, a sustainable volume-sparing effect was not documented. Meta-analyses have failed to show an outcome advantage with the use of HES in any patient cohort [42,43].

Experimental veterinary trials have shown an advantage with HES resuscitation over crystalloids for anesthetic-induced hypotension. In one of these trials, hypovolemia was induced via blood draw in isoflurane-anesthetized dogs, and resuscitation with HES was more effective than LRS at achieving HDS [62]. A second trial evaluating isoflurane-induced hypotension in normovolemic dogs also found HES to be superior to LRS at restoration of HDS. These authors recommended colloid administration in lieu of crystalloid for anesthetic hypotension, particularly in the face of ongoing surgical blood loss [63]. Given the short duration and low volume of HES administered in the perioperative setting, it is possible that some of the described adverse effects of HES use may be avoided in this patient population. However, robust safety data in veterinary patients are lacking, and vigilance is warranted.

Adverse Effects of HES

Safety concerns with HES products have made their continued use controversial. The most significant adverse effects are coagulopathies, AKI, tissue accumulation, and trends towards increased mortality [1]. Increased postoperative bleeding tendencies and transfusion requirements have been documented in people treated with HES.

The etiology of HES-associated coagulopathy is multi-factorial. Administration of HES leads to platelet dysfunction, reduced von Willebrand factor (vWF) and factor VIII (fVIII) activity, and an acquired fibrinogen deficiency or dysfunction in both animals and people [64]. Hypotheses that more modern HES solutions (tetrastarches) would be devoid of hemostatic impairment remain unsubstantiated. Recent data evaluating these solutions in both people and animals have shown reduced, but not absent, HES-associated coagulation abnormalities and clinical bleeding tendencies. The hemostatic effects and clinical bleeding associated with 6% HES (600/.75), compared with LRS, in healthy dogs anesthetized for orthopedic surgery were evaluated. Although there was a significant prolongation of prothrombin time and buccal mucosal bleeding time at 1 hour post infusion in both groups, there was no significant difference between groups in vWF antigen concentration, fVIII activity, platelet aggregation or clinical bleeding [65]. Numerous other experimental and *in vitro* veterinary studies have confirmed the coagulopathic effects of HES, with hypocoagulable changes demonstrated via platelet function tests and thromboelastographic analyses [66–70]. It has yet to be determined whether these hemostatic changes translate into an increased risk of clinical bleeding in veterinary patients.

Several RCTs in critically ill human patients have demonstrated an association between HES administration and AKI and increased need for RRT. Proposed pathophysiologies are hyperviscosity-mediated ischemic injury, HES uptake by the renal interstitial reticuloendothelial system (a property unique to HES over other synthetic colloids), and osmotic nephrosis [71–74]. The CHEST and S6 trials were two highly influential RCTs that showed an increased incidence of AKI and need for RRT in patients randomized to receive HES solutions [40,41]. Similarly, a recent Cochrane review specifically evaluated the effect of HES on kidney function, compared with any other fluid therapy. This meta-analysis concluded that all HES products increase the risk of AKI and RRT across patient populations and that a safe volume of any HES solution has yet to be determined [43]. The use of HES solutions is currently banned in Europe and Surviving Sepsis Campaign guidelines recommend against the use of HES for fluid resuscitation of patients with severe sepsis and septic shock (grade 1B) [75].

The incidence or risk of HES-induced AKI in the veterinary population has been less well investigated. A recent retrospective study evaluated the incidence of AKI in dogs treated with 10% HES 250/0.5 and found that dogs treated with this HES solution had an overall increased risk of in-hospital death and AKI [76]. This risk persisted after adjustment for confounding variables, and appeared to be dose dependent. A small prospective study investigated the presence of neutrophil gelatinase-associated

lipocalin (NGAL), an early biomarker of AKI, in 15 dogs with sepsis requiring laparotomy. Dogs that were treated with HES had significantly higher NGAL levels than dogs that did not receive HES across all time points in the study, suggesting a contribution to kidney injury [77]. Conversely, a second retrospective study evaluated creatinine levels in dogs admitted to a university ICU and found no increase in creatinine in dogs treated with HES compared with those treated with crystalloids alone [78]. Large RCTs are needed to better assess the risk of these products in veterinary patients.

Summary

The only clearly defined role for (natural) colloids in ECC patients is for treatment of coagulopathy. Preferential selection of colloids for treatment of shock and/or maintenance of plasma COP in sick animals cannot be recommended based on current literature. The incorporation of artificial colloids into LFVR strategies for short-duration use in low doses (e.g. for traumatic shock- or anesthesia-associated hypotension) may prove to be safe and of therapeutic value. However, at this time their role remains unclearly defined.

Fluids: Strategies, Dosages, and Endpoints

Undeniably, fluids play a fundamental role in shock reversal. However, overzealous or indiscriminate fluid administration can result in patient harm. When designing a fluid strategy individualized for a sick patient, consideration must be given to injury type, severity, and stage.

For shock patients, fluid resuscitation can be divided into four stages: Rescue (or salvage); Optimization; Stabilization; and De-escalation (ROS-D) [79,80]. During the Rescue stage, patients typically require aggressive early IV fluid therapy to restore effective circulating volume and prevent multiple organ failure (the ebb phase of shock) [80]. In both human and veterinary patients, early goal-directed therapy (EGDT) has been shown to improve patient outcomes [81,82]. Fluid accumulation and a positive fluid balance may be anticipated and are accepted during this early resuscitative stage.

Fluid resuscitation from shock can be accomplished utilizing isotonic and/or hypertonic crystalloids, with consideration being given to incorporation of non-protein colloids to achieve prolonged expansion of the intravascular space with less total volume infused (as part of LFVR). Fluids are administered as boluses (typically one-fourth of the total shock volume, or 1 blood volume), and these are repeated as needed to meet desired endpoints (Table 169.3). Asanguinous fluids are not substitutes for blood products, which may be incorporated into a patient's resuscitation protocol for treatment of anemia, coagulopathy or massive blood loss. Vasopressor therapy is indicated in shock patients that fail to respond to fluid challenges and demonstrate clinical and laboratory parameters consistent with ongoing tissue hypoperfusion.

Implementation of EGDT may not be suitable for all shock patients, however. Aggressive fluid therapy may exacerbate bleeding in trauma patients with uncontrolled hemorrhage, and fluid restriction in the forms of delayed and hypotensive resuscitation strategies has been investigated in both experimental animal and human trials evaluating this patient subset (exclusive of TBI patients) [18,24,83–86]. The former strategy was found to be beneficial in selected human patients, but these positive effects do not appear generalizable across human patient cohorts or to clinical veterinary

Table 169.3 Initial fluid strategy for shock resuscitation: choices and dosages.

	Dosages
Isotonic crystalloid (lactated Ringer's, Plasma-Lyte)	**10–20 mL/kg over 10–15 min**

- Assess for clinical response; repeat boluses with same fluid type as needed to achieve desired endpoints.
- Shock dose (avoid fluid overload by titrating as above): 90 mL/kg (dog); 50–60 mL/kg (cat).
- Consider the addition of synthetic colloids and/or hypertonic crystalloids in selected cases as part of limited fluid volume resuscitation (e.g. large-breed dog; traumatic brain injury; severe burn injury).

Hydroxyethyl starch solutions (HES)	**5–10 mL/kg over 15–30 min: maximum daily dose, 20–50 mL/kg**
7–7.5% Hypertonic saline (HTS)	**4–6 mL/kg over ~ 15 min**
HTS + synthetic colloid (HES) (Turbostarch)	**4 mL/kg IV over 4–5 min**

Turbostarch "cheat sheet":

Weight in kg (lb)	23.4% HT (mL)	6% HES (mL)
1 (2)	1.3	2.7
2 (5)	2.6	5.5
4.5 (10)	6	12
7 (15)	9	18
9 (20)	12	24
11 (25)	15	30
14 (30)	19	38
16 (35)	21	42
18 (40)	24	48
20.5 (45)	27	54
23 (50)	31	62
25 (55)	33	66
27 (60)	36	72
29.5 (65)	39	78
32 (70)	43	86
34 (75)	45	90
36 (80)	48	96
38.5(85)	51	102
41 (90)	55	110
43 (95)	57	114
45.5 (100)	61	122

Blood component therapy as indicated:	15 mL/kg will increase packed cell volume (PCV) by 10%; over 4–6h
Packed red blood cells	20–30 mL/kg will increase PCV by 10%; <6h
Fresh whole blood	10–20 mL/kg over 4–6h for clinically significant coagulopathy
Fresh frozen plasma	

patients [24,83]. Hypotensive resuscitation involves targeting lower than normal BP (mean arterial BP and systolic BP of 50–60 mmHg and 80–90 mmHg, respectively) that support vital organ perfusion but are less likely to exacerbate bleeding from dilution or clot dislodgement. While sustained hypotension (>120 min) can increase tissue hypoxia and organ damage, experimental animal models have found that shorter periods of permissive hypotension result in improved patient survival [84,85].

The effect of fluids on patient outcome may be influenced by hemorrhage severity [85]. In animal trials, fluid resuscitation following severe hemorrhage reduced risk of death. Alternatively, withholding resuscitation fluids from patients with less severe hemorrhage conferred a survival advantage, possibly by prevention of hemodilution and blood clot disruption [85]. While there are several RCTs and observational studies which have shown that permissive hypotension reduces morbidity and mortality in bleeding human trauma patients, other investigators and meta-analyses have failed to replicate this findings. Larger prospective RCTs are necessary [86–89].

During the Optimization stage of resuscitation, the patient is in compensated shock, and responses to fluid challenges are assessed to guide continued fluid resuscitation and avoid excessive fluid accumulation. Patients are categorized as "responders" or "non-responders" based on increased (10–15%) or unchanged stroke volume following fluid infusion, respectively. Giving fluids to non-responders (reportedly > 50% hemodynamically unstable patients) will not improve perfusion but only exacerbate tissue edema [90,91].

Patients overcoming severe injury will experience restoration of homeostatic mechanisms and hemodynamic stability, and re-establishment of adequate tissue perfusion (the flow phase of shock). These patients are in the Stabilization stage, and require fluid only for ongoing fluid losses and maintenance of hydration.

In severely ill human patients hospitalized for several days, conservative late fluid management (CLFM) and fluid De-escalation (de-resuscitation) have been shown to confer a survival advantage [90,92–94]. Conservative late fluid management is defined as achievement of an even-to-negative fluid balance at least two consecutive ICU days during the first week in the hospital (accomplished via fluid restriction, diuretic administration, and/or hemodialysis) [90]. Achievement of CLFM has been shown to be an independent predictor of survival in patients with septic shock and in critically ill, mechanically ventilated patients. Patients with global increased permeability syndrome (GIPS) demonstrate continued positive fluid balance, progressive capillary leak and organ dysfunction, and increased mortality [90,92].

The concept of "the best fluid may be the one that has not been given to the patient" was most dramatically demonstrated in the FEAST trial, which found that boluses of either albumin or saline (versus no bolus) to severely ill and hypotensive African children increased 48-hour mortality [95]. The investigators postulated that reversal of blood shunting to vital organs and/or reperfusion injury could, in part, explain these findings in this very specific patient population. These results, while absolutely not generalizable to other ECC patient cohorts, do demonstrate that fluid plans should be patient and disease specific. Optimal individualized fluid plans target replenishment of body fluid compartments while minimizing unnecessary fluid loading. For shock patients, early goal-directed fluid therapy endpoints include normalization of perfusion parameters, blood lactate, base excess, central venous oxygenation saturation, and/or shock index (heart rate/BP), among other parameters [96–100]. For patients with interstitial and/or intravascular dehydration, fluids are discontinued when hydration is restored and ongoing losses have ceased. A single ideal fluid likely does not exist. Judicious and attentive use of any selected fluid is advocated with incorporation of CLFM to mitigate detrimental effects. Due to the concerns for toxicity associated with HES solutions and isotonic saline, their role in critically ill human and veterinary patients requires further investigation and definition [101,102].

References

1 Raghunathan K, Shaw AD, Bagshaw SM. Fluids are drugs: type, dose and toxicity. *Curr Opin Crit Care* 2013;19(4):290–298.

2 Kortbeek JB, Al Turki SA, Ali J, et al. Advanced Trauma Life Support, 8th edition, the evidence for change. *J Trauma* 2008;64(6):1638–1650.

3 Stewart PA. Modern quantitative acid-base chemistry. *Can J Physiol Pharmacol* 1983;61(12):1444–1461.

4 Chowdbury AH, Cox EF, Francis ST, et al. A randomized, controlled double-blind crossover study on the effects of 2-L infusions of 0.9% saline and Plasma-Lyte 148 on renal blood flow velocity and renal cortical tissue perfusion in healthy volunteers. *Ann Surg* 2012;256(1):18–24.

5 Yunos NM, Bellomo R, Hegarty C, et al. Association between a chloride-liberal vs chloride-restictive intravenous fluid administration strategy and kidney injury in critically ill adults. *JAMA* 2012;308(15):1566–1572.

6 Shaw AD, Bagshaw SM, Goldstein SL, et al. Major complications, mortality, and resource utilization after

open abdominal surgery: 0.9% saline compared to Plasma-lyte. *Ann Surg* 2012;255(5):821–829.

7 Raghunathan K, Shaw A, Nathanson B, et al. Association between choice of IV crystalloid and in-hospital mortality among critically ill adults with sepsis. *Crit Care Med* 2014;42:1585–1591.

8 Wilcox CS. Regulation of renal blood flow by plasma chloride. *J Clin Invest* 1983;7(3):726–735.

9 Powell-Tuck J, Gosling P, Lobo DN, et al. *British Consensus Guidelines on Intravenous Fluid Therapy for Adult Surgical Patients (GIFTASUP)*. NHS National Library of Health, London, 2011.

10 Lira A, Pinsky MR. Choices in fluid type and volume during resuscitation: impact on patient outcomes. *Ann Intensive Care* 2014;4:38.

11 Rose RJ. Some physiological and biochemical effects of the intravenous administration of five different electrolyte solutions in the dog. *J Vet Pharm Ther* 1979;2(4):279–289.

12 Drobatz K, Cole S. The influence of crystalloid type on acid-base and electrolyte status in cats with urethral obstruction. *J Vet Emerg Crit Care* 2008;18(4):355–361.

13 Cunha MGMC, Freitas GC, Carregaro AB, et al. Renal and cardiovascular effects of treatment with lactated Ringer's solution or physiologic saline (0.9% NaCl) solution in cats with experimentally induced urethral obstruction. *Am J Vet Res* 2010;71:840–846.

14 Ince C, Groeneveld J. The case for 0.9% NaCl: is the undefendable, defensible? *Kidney Int* 2014;86(6): 1087–1095.

15 Guidet B, Soni N, Della Rocca G, et al. A balanced view of balanced solutions. *Crit Care* 2010;14:325–336.

16 Mazzaferro E, Powell LL. Fluid therapy for the emergent small animal patient: crystalloids, colloids and albumin products. *Vet Clin Small Anim Pract* 2013;43:721–734.

17 DiBartola SP, Bateman S. Introduction to fluid therapy. In: *Fluid, Electrolyte, and Acid–Base Disorders in Small Animal Practice*, 3rd edn (ed. DiBartola SP). Elsevier Saunders, St Louis, 2006, pp. 325–344.

18 Driessen B, Brainard B. Fluid therapy for the traumatized patient. *J Vet Emerg Crit Care* 2006;16(4):276.

19 Hammond TN, Holm JL. Limited fluid volume resuscitation. *Compendium* 2009;31(7):309–321.

20 Schertel ER, Allen DA, Muir WW, et al. Evaluation of a hypertonic saline-dextran solution for treatment of dogs with shock induced by gastric dilatation-volvulus. *J Am Vet Med Assoc* 1997;210:226–230.

21 Silverstein DC, Aldrich J, Haskins SC, et al. Assessment of changes in blood volume in response to resuscitative fluid administration in dogs. *J Vet Emerg Crit Care* 2005;15(3):185–192.

22 Strandvik GF. Hypertonic saline in critical care: a review of the literature and guidelines for use in hypotensive states and raised intracranial pressure. *Anaesthesia* 2009;64:990–1003.

23 Kyes J, Johnson JA. Hypertonic saline solutions in shock resuscitation. *Compend Contin Educ Vet* 2011;33(3):E1–E8, quiz E9.

24 Santry HP, Alam HB. Fluid resuscitation: past, present, and the future. *Shock* 2010;33(3):229–241.

25 Bunn F, Roberts I, Tasker R, et al. Hypertonic versus near isotonic crystalloid for fluid resuscitation in critically ill patients. *Cochrane Database Syst Rev* 2007;3:CD002045.

26 Perel P, Roberts I. Colloids versus crystalloids for fluid resuscitation in critically ill patients. *Cochrane Database Syst Rev* 2013;2:CD000567.

27 Van Den Berghe G, Wouters R, Weekers F, et al. Intensive insulin therapy in critically ill patients. *N Engl J Med* 2001;345(19):1359–1367.

28 *Committee on Trauma. Advanced Trauma Life Support Manual*. American College of Surgeons, Chicago, 1997, pp. 103–112.

29 Lowell JA, Schifferdecker C, Discoll D, et al. Postoperative fluid overload: not a benign problem. *Crit Care Med* 1990;18(7):728–733.

30 Chappel D, Jacob M, Hofmann-Kieffer K et al. A rational approach to perioperative fluid management. *Anesthesiology* 2008;109:723–740.

31 Alphonsus CS, Rodseth RN. The endothelial glycocalyx: a review of the vascular barrier. *Anaesthesia* 2014;69(7):777–784.

32 Cotton BA, Guy JS, Morris JA, et al. The cellular, metabolic, and systemic consequences of aggressive fluid resuscitation strategies. *Shock* 2006;26(2):115–121.

33 Holte K, Sharrock NE, Kehlet H. Pathophysiology and clinical implications of perioperative fluid excess. *Br J Anaesth* 2002;89(4):622–632.

34 Muir WW. Rethinking your approach to perioperative fluid therapy. Available at: http://veterinarymedicine. dvm360.com/rethinking-your-approach-perioperative-fluid-therapy (accessed 19 February 2018).

35 National Heart, Lung, and Blood Institute Acute Respiratory Distress Syndrome (ARDS) Clinical Trials Network. Comparison of two fluid management strategies in acute lung injury. *N Engl J Med* 2006;354(24):2564–2575.

36 Godin M, Bouchard J, Mehta RL. Fluid balance in patients with acute kidney injury: emerging concepts. *Nephron Clin Pract* 2013;123:238–245.

37 Bouchard J, Soroko SB, Chertow GM, et al. Fluid accumulation, survival and recovery of kidney function in critically patients with acute kidney injury. *Kidney Int* 2009;76:422–427.

38 Grams ME, Estrall MM, Coresh J, et al. Fluid balance, diuretic use, and mortality in acute kidney injury. *Clin J Am Soc Nephrol* 2011;6:966–973.

39 Bellomo R, Cass A, Cole L, et al. An observational study fluid balance and patient outcomes in the randomized evaluation of normal vs. *augmented level of replacement therapy trial. Crit Care Med* 2012;40:1753–1760.

40 Perner A, Haase N, Guttormsen AB, et al. Hydroxyethyl starch 130/0.42 verses Ringer's acetate in severe sepsis. *N Engl J Med* 2012;367(2):124–134.

41 Myburgh JA, Finfer S, Bellomo R, et al. Hydroxyethyl starch or saline for fluid resuscitation in intensive care. *N Engl J Med* 2012;367(20):1901–1911.

42 Zarychanski R, Abou-Setta AM, Turgeon AF, et al. Association of hydroxyethyl starch administration with mortality and acute kidney injury in critically ill patients requiring volume resuscitation: a systematic review and meta-analysis. *JAMA* 2013;309(7):678–688.

43 Mutter TC, Ruth CA, Dart AB. Hydroxyethyl starch (HES) verses other fluid therapies: effects on kidney function. *Cochrane Database Syst Rev* 2013;7:CD007594.

44 Mazzaferro EM, Rudloff E, Kirby R. The role of albumin replacement in the critically ill veterinary patient. *J Vet Emerg Crit Care* 2002;12(2):113–124.

45 Tocci LJ. Transfusion medicine in small animal practice. *Vet Clin North Am Small Anim Pract* 2010;40(3):485–494.

46 SAFE Study Investigators. A comparison of albumin and saline for fluid resuscitation in the intensive care unit. *N Engl J Med* 2004;350(22):2247–2256.

47 Caironi P, Tognoni G, Masson S, et al. Albumin replacement in patients with severe sepsis or septic shock. *N Engl J Med* 2014;370(15):1412–1421.

48 Mathews KA, Barry M. The use of 25% human serum albumin: outcome and efficacy in raising serum albumin and systemic blood pressure in critically ill dogs and cats. *J Vet Emerg Crit Care* 2005;15(2):110–118.

49 Trow AV, Rozanski EA, de Laforcade AM, et al. Evaluation of the use of human albumin in critically ill dogs: 73 cases (2003–2006). *J Am Vet Med Assoc* 2008;223(4):607–612.

50 Vigano F, Perissinotto L, Bosco VR. Administration of 5% human serum albumin in critically ill small animal patients with hypoalbuminemia: 418 dogs and 170 cats (1994–2008). *J Vet Emerg Crit Care* 2010;20(2):237–243.

51 Francis AH, Martin LG, Haldorson GJ, et al. Advrese reactions suggestive of type III hypersensitivity in six healthy dogs given human albumin. *J Am Vet Med Assoc* 2007;230(6):873–879.

52 Cohn LA, Kerl ME, Lenox CE, et al. Response of healthy dogs to infusions of human serum albumin. *Am J Vet Res* 2007;38(6):657–663.

53 Powell C, Thompson L, Murtaugh RJ. Type III hypersensitivity reaction with immune complex deposition in 2 critically ill dogs administered human serum albumin. *J Vet Emerg Crit Care* 2013;23(6): 598–604.

54 Martin LG, Luther TY, Alperin DC, et al. Serum antibodies against human albumin in critically ill and healthy dogs. *J Am Vet Med Assoc* 2008;232(7):1004–1009.

55 Craft EM, Powell LL. The use of canine-specific albumin in dogs with septic peritonitis. *J Vet Emerg Crit Care* 2012;22(6):631–639.

56 Westphal M, James MF, Kozek-Langenecker S, et al. Hydroxyethyl starches: different products – different effects. *Anesthesiology* 2009;111(1):187–202.

57 Zhi-Yong P, Kellum JA. Perioperative fluids: a clear road ahead. *Curr Opin Crit Care* 2013;19:353–358.

58 Gauthier V, Holowaychuk MK, Kerr CL, et al. Effect of sythetic colloid administration on hemodynamic and laboratory variables in healthy dogs and dogs

with systemic inflammation. *J Vet Emerg Crit Care* 2014;24(3):251–258.

59 Guidet B, Martinet O, Boulain T, et al. Assessment of hemodynamic efficacy and safety of 6% hydroxyethyl starch 130/0.4 vs 0.9% NaCl fluid replacement in patients with severe sepsis: the CRYSTMAS study. *Crit Care* 2012;16(3):R94.

60 Annane D, Siami S, Jaber S, et al. Effects of fluid resuscitation with colloids vs crystalloids on mortality in critically ill patients presenting with hypovolemic shock. *JAMA* 2013;310(17):1809–1817.

61 James MF, Michell WL, Joubert IA, et al. Resuscitation with hydroxyethyl starch improves renal function and lactate clearance in penetrating trauma in a randomized controlled study: the FIRST trial (Fluids in Resuscitation of Severe Trauma). *Br J Anaesth* 2011;107(5):693–702.

62 Muir WW, Wiese AJ. Comparison of lactated Ringer's solution and a physiologically balanced 6% hetastarch plasma expander for the treatment of hypotension induced via blood withdrawal in isoflurane-anesthetized dogs. *Am J Vet Res* 2004;65(9):1189–1194.

63 Aarnes TK, Bednarski RM, Lerche P, et al. Effect of intravenous administration of lactated Ringer's solution or hetastarch for the treatment of isoflurane-induced hypotension in dogs. *Am J Vet Res* 2009;70(11): 1345–1353.

64 Kozek-Langenecker SA. Effects of hydoxyethyl starch solutions on hemostasis. *Anesthesiology* 2005;103(3):654–660.

65 Chohan AS, Greene SA, Grubb TL, et al. Effects of 6% hetastarch (600/0.75) or lactated Ringer's solution on hemostatic variables and clinical bleeding in healthy dogs anesthetized for orthopedic surgery. *Vet Anaesth Anal* 2011;38(2):94–102.

66 Smart L, Kass PH, Wierenga JR, et al. The effect of Hetastarch (670/0.75) in vivo on platelet closure time in the dog. *J Vet Emerg Crit Care* 2009;19(5):444–449.

67 Blong AE, Epstein KL, Brainard BM. In vitro effects of three formulations of hydroxyethyl starch solutions on coagulation and platelet function in horses. *Am J Vet Res* 2013;74(5):712–720.

68 Classen J, Adamik KN, Weber K, et al. In vitro effect of hydroxyethyl starch 130/0.42 on canine platelet function. *Am J Vet Res* 2012;73(12):1908–1912.

69 Wierenga JR, Jandrey KE, Haskins SC, Tablin F. In vitro comparison of the effects of two forms of hydroxyethyl starch solutions on platelet function in dogs. *Am J Vet Res* 2007;68(6):605–609.

70 Epstein KL, Bergren A, Giguère S, Brainard BM. Cardiovascular, colloid osmotic pressure, and hemostatic effects of 2 formulations of hydroxyethyl starch in healthy horses. *J Vet Intern Med* 2014;28(1):223–233.

71 Schortgen F, Brochard L. Colloid-induced kidney injury: experimental evidence may help to understand mechanisms. *Crit Care* 2009;13(2):130.

72 Siegemund M. 10% Hydroxyethylstarch impairs renal function and induces interstitial proliferation,

macrophage infiltration and tubular damage. *Crit Care* 2009;13(4):413.

73 Huter L, Simon TP, Weinman L, et al. Hydroxyethylstarch impairs renal function and induces interstitial proliferation, macrophage infiltration, and tubular damage in an isolated renal perfusion model. *Crit Care* 2009;13(1):R23.

74 Simon TP, Schuerholz T, Huter L, et al. Impairment of renal function using hyperoncotic colloids in a two hit model of shock: a prospective randomized study. *Crit Care* 2012;16(1):R16.

75 Dellinger RP, Levy MM, Rhodes A, et al. Surviving Sepsis Campaign: international guidelines for management of severe sepsis and septic shock. *Crit Care Med* 2013;41(2):580–637.

76 Hayes G, Benedicenti L, Mathews K. Retrospective cohort study on the incidence of acute kidney injury and death following hydroxyethyl starch (HES 10% 250/0.5/5:1) administration in dogs (2007–2010). *J Vet Emerg Crit Care* 2016;26(1):35–40.

77 Cortellini S, Pelligand L, Syme H, et al. Neutrophil gelatinase-associated lipocalin in dogs with sepsis undergoing emergency laparotomy: a prospective case-control study. *J Vet Intern Med* 2015;29:1595–1602.

78 Yozova ID, Howard J, Adamik KN. Retrospective evaluation of the effects of administration of tetrastarch (hydroxyethyl starch 130/0.4) on plasma creatinine concentration in dogs (2010–2013): 201 dogs. *J Vet Emerg Crit Care* 2016;26(4):568–577.

79 Vincent JL, de Backer D. Circulatory shock. *N Engl J Med* 2013;369:1726–1734.

80 Hoste EA, Maitland K, Burdney CS, et al. Four phases of intravenous fluid therapy: a conceptual model. *Br J Anaesth* 2014;113(5):740–747.

81 Rivers E, Nguyen B, Havstad S, et al. Early goal-directed therapy in the treatment of severe sepsis and septic shock. *N Engl J Med* 2001;345(19):1368–1377.

82 Silverstein DC, Kleiner J, Drobatz KJ. Effectiveness of intravenous fluid resuscitation in the emergency room for treatment of hypotension in dogs: 35 cases (2000–2010). *J Vet Emerg Crit Care* 2012;22(6):666–673.

83 Bickell WH, Wall MJ, Pepe PE, et al. Immediate versus delayed fluid resuscitation for hypotensive patients with penetrating torso injuries. *N Engl J Med* 1994;331:1105–1109.

84 Li T, Zhu Y, Hu Y, et al. Ideal permissive hypotension to resuscitate uncontrolled hemorrhagic shock and the tolerance time in rats. *Anesthesiology* 2011;114(1):111–119.

85 Mapstone J, Roberts I, Evans P. Fluid resuscitation strategies: a systematic review of animal trials. *J Trauma* 2003;55:571–589.

86 Morrison CA, Carrick MM, Norman MA, et al. Hypotensive resuscitation strategy reduces transfusion requirements and severe postoperative coagulopathy in trauma patients with hemorrhagic shock: preliminary results of a randomized controlled trial. *J Trauma* 2011;70(3):652–663.

87 Dutton RP, MacKenzie CF, Scalea TM. Hypotensive resuscitation during active haemorrhage: impact on in-hospital mortality. *J Trauma* 2002;52:1141–1146.

88 Kwan I, Bunn F, Roberts I. Timing and volume of fluid administration for patients with bleeding. *Cochrane Database Syst Rev* 2003;3:CD002245.

89 Wang CH, Hesih WH, Chou HC, et al. Liberal versus restricted fluid resuscitation strategies in trauma patients: a systematic review and meta-analysis of randomized controlled trials and observational studies. *Crit Care Med* 2014;42:954–961.

90 Malbrain M, Marik PE, Witters I, et al. Fluid overload, de-resuscitation, and outcomes in critically ill or injured patients: a systematic review with suggestions for clinical practice. *Anaesthesiol Intensive Ther* 2014;46(5):361–380.

91 Marik PE, Monnet X, Teboul JL. Haemodynamic parameters to guide fluid therapy. *Ann Intensive Care* 2011;1(1):1.

92 Cordemans C, de Laet I, Regenmortel NV, et al. Fluid management in critically ill patients: the role of extravascular lung water, abdominal hypertension, capillary leak, and fluid balance. *Ann Intensive Care* 2012;2(Suppl 1):S1.

93 Murphy CV, Schramm GE, Doherty JA, et al. The importance of fluid management in acute lung injury secondary to septic shock. *Chest* 2009;136:102–109.

94 Alsous F, Khamiees M, DeGirolamo A, et al. Negative fluid balance predicts survival in patients with septic shock: a retrospective pilot study. *Chest* 2000;117:1749–1754.

95 Maitland K, Kiguli S, Opoka RO, et al. Mortality after fluid bolus in African children with severe infection. *N Engl J Med* 2011;364(26):2483–2495.

96 Prittie J. Optimal endpoints of resuscitation and early goal-directed therapy. *J Vet Emerg Crit Care* 2006;16(4):329–339.

97 Stevenson CK, Kidney BA, Duke T, et al. Serial blood lactate concentrations in systemically ill dogs. *Vet Clin Pathol* 2007;36(3):234–239.

98 Stillion JR, Fletcher DJ. Admission base excess as a predictor of transfusion requirement and mortality in dogs with blunt trauma: 52 cases (2007–2009). *J Vet Emerg Crit Care* 2012;22(5):588–594.

99 Young BC, Prittie JE, Fox P, et al. Decreased central venous oxygen saturation despite normalization of heart rate and blood pressure post shock resuscitation in dogs. *J Vet Emerg Crit Care* 2014;24(2):154–161.

100 Porter AE, Rozanski EA, Sharp CR, et al. Evaluation of the shock index in dogs presenting as emergencies. *J Vet Emerg Crit Care* 2013;23(5):538–544.

101 McDermid RC, Raghunathan K, Romanovsky A, et al. Controversies in fluid therapy: type, dose, and toxicity. *World J Crit Care Med* 2014;3(1):24–33.

102 Severs D, Hoorn EJ, Rookmaaker MB. A critical appraisal of intravenous fluids: from the physiologic basis to clinical evidence. *Nephrol Dial Transplant* 2015;30:178–187.

170

Management of Hemorrhagic Shock

Andrew Linklater, DVM, DACVECC

Lakeshore Veterinary Specialists, Glendale, WI, USA

Signalment/History

The signalment and history may present information regarding the etiology of hemorrhage to help direct immediate care and obtain a definitive diagnosis. Young patients are at risk for trauma, congenital coagulopathies, infectious disease, and toxin ingestion (anticoagulant rodenticides), while older patients are at risk for spontaneous hemorrhage associated with neoplasia. Any age patient undergoing emergency or elective surgery or invasive procedures is at risk for significant hemorrhage and critically ill patients are at risk for development of secondary coagulopathies (e.g. DIC). Collection of a complete history may have to be delayed while urgent care is initiated; an attempt may be made to quantify external blood loss if evident. Dogs are far more frequently affected by hemorrhagic shock than cats.

Physical Examination

The physical examination of a patient with hemorrhage varies substantially depending upon the location and severity of blood loss. External hemorrhage is immediately apparent, but internal hemorrhage may not be as obvious.

Patients will demonstrate signs of shock when as little as 15–20% of their blood volume is lost [1]: approximately 15–20 mL/kg in the dog or 10–15 mL/kg in the cat. Quantifying blood loss is challenging unless a patient has a bandage that can be weighed, a drain tube in place, or is in surgery with available suction; a 4×4 inch gauze can hold approximately 10 mL of blood when fully saturated [2,3].

Hemorrhage leads to decreased cardiac output, intravascular volume and blood hemoglobin concentration, resulting in decreased delivery of oxygen (DO_2). With a significant enough decrease, the DO_2 is unable to meet the body's oxygen consumption demands (VO_2), resulting in signs of cardiovascular shock. Patients that present with signs of poor perfusion (shock) warrant immediate resuscitation (see Chapter 152). Physical signs of shock can be rapidly assessed and include alterations of heart rate, blood pressure, mucous membrane color, capillary refill time, respiratory rate, pulse quality, and level of consciousness. Patients under general anesthesia may not have the same physiological compensatory mechanisms due to cardiovascular effects of anesthetic drugs; these patients should be monitored closely with ECG, blood pressure, pulse oximetry, end-tidal CO_2, and an experienced veterinary technician (e.g. VTS-anesthesia) or ideally an anesthesiologist. Temperature assessment is important as both severe hyper- and hypothermia can affect normal coagulation.

Abnormal heart sounds may indicate anemia, arrhythmias or location-specific hemorrhage. Increased respiratory rate, effort or altered breathing pattern along with abnormal lung sounds may indicate pulmonary or pleural hemorrhage. Patients with abdominal hemorrhage may have a fluid wave or positive ballotment, but this may not be apparent until hemorrhage is significant (40 mL/kg) [4].

Soft tissue swelling or bruising may be present with soft tissue bleeding. Measuring a swollen area with a tape measure may help monitor progression. The mucous membranes, skin, retina, and rectum should be closely examined for evidence of petechia, ecchymoses or frank blood. Hemorrhage into specific locations, such as the retroperitoneal space, pharyngeal area or airways, or around neurological tissues has specific localizing signs and presents additional therapeutic and diagnostic challenges. Evidence of hemorrhage at more than one location without a history of trauma is supportive of coagulopathy [5] (see Chapters 69 and 70).

Textbook of Small Animal Emergency Medicine, First Edition. Edited by Kenneth J. Drobatz, Kate Hopper, Elizabeth Rozanski and Deborah C. Silverstein.
© 2019 John Wiley & Sons, Inc. Published 2019 by John Wiley & Sons, Inc.
Companion Website: www.wiley.com/go/drobatz/textbook

Point-of-Care Diagnostics

Point of care (POC) diagnostics support evidence of hemorrhage and poor perfusion, identify coagulopathy, and help identify hemorrhage location(s).

Laboratory Testing

Consideration should be given to the location, method, and frequency of blood collection. Patients with a potential coagulopathy should have blood collected from peripheral sites where hemorrhage can be controlled with a bandage; frequency of blood collection should be minimized to avoid repeated phlebotomy; and only the smallest sample necessary should be collected to minimize iatrogenic blood loss. Resuscitation should begin before results are obtained.

Emergency Database

An emergency database, including PCV/TS, electrolytes, glucose, blood gases, lactate, and BUN, is important for immediate diagnostics. A normal or even elevated PCV with a disproportionate decrease in total solids may reflect acute hemorrhage in the dog, as the PCV is preserved through sympathoadrenal splenic contraction [6,7]. The PCV and TS will both decrease with ongoing fluid resuscitation and continued blood loss.

Any bloody fluid collected from a cavity should also have a PCV/TS performed. Active hemorrhage is supported by PCV from cavitary fluid within 5% of peripheral blood. In more long-standing hemorrhage, the PCV of the fluid may be higher than the periphery (see Chapter 84).

Gastrointestinal tract hemorrhage (see Chapter 77), poor renal perfusion, renal failure or urinary obstruction can elevate the BUN; a low BUN suggests hepatic dysfunction, prior PU/PD or IV fluid therapy.

Lactate provides a monitor of restoration of DO_2 (see Chapter 156). Canine studies of hemorrhagic shock and critically ill and injured dogs have demonstrated that an increase in lactate is correlated with a worse prognosis after blood loss and a lack of lactate normalization is associated with an increase in morbidity and mortality. Normalization of lactate is an indicator of adequate resuscitative efforts [8–14] (see Chapter 156).

Blood gas data and central venous oxygenation ($ScvO_2$) may help identify metabolic acidosis from hypoperfusion and oxygen extraction status. Acidemia can have detrimental effects on coagulation; if pH is < 7.200, bicarbonate therapy should be considered (see Chapter 174). A study of dogs suffering blunt force trauma found that an admission base excess cut-off of −6.6 was 88% sensitive and 73% specific for later transfusion requirement and

a cut-off of −7.3 was 81% sensitive and 80% specific for survival with no difference in admission PCV between survivors and non-survivors [15].

Coagulation Assessment (see Chapters 69 and 70)

Assessment of coagulation should occur in patients with concern for coagulopathy or prior to invasive procedures. The results of coagulation testing should always be interpreted with the clinical picture of the patient (signs of blood loss, PCV/TS, etc.). If an intervention is deemed necessary (transfusions, etc.), it is appropriate to recheck these values to ensure the therapeutic benefit has been achieved.

The prothrombin time (PT) reflects both the function and quantity of the coagulation factors in the extrinsic (factor VII, tissue factor) and common (factors I, II, V, and X) coagulation pathways. The activated partial thromboplastin time (aPTT) reflects the function and quantity of coagulation factors in the intrinsic (factors VIII, IX, XI, XII) and common pathways. A decrease of > 70% of one or more of these clotting factors is necessary for the PT or aPTT to be prolonged. Prolonged aPTT in dogs that have sustained trauma has been correlated with non-survival [16]. PT and aPTT testing does require specific equipment that is widely available and affordable [17].

A machine count and manual platelet estimate should be performed in patients with signs of thrombocytopenia. The feathered edge of the blood smear is examined for platelet clumping and morphology [18]. Patients are typically at risk for spontaneous hemorrhage when platelet counts are less than 30 000–50 000/uL. Buccal mucosal bleeding time is an uncommon method of evaluating *in vivo* platelet function. It may be run in patients with concern for a primary platelet disorder and normal platelet numbers, such as Dobermans with unknown vWF status.

Other coagulation testing may include thromboelastography (TEG) or thromboelastometry (also called rotational thromboelastography, ROTEM); these viscoelastic methods assess many aspects of coagulation.

Radiography and Ultrasound

Radiographs and ultrasound are both useful to identify free fluid, hemorrhage into tissues or other disease processes. Although radiographs are less sensitive for detection of free fluid in the abdomen, they are useful for assessment of pulmonary patterns, mineralized tissues, and free air. Animals can be quickly evaluated for abdominal, thoracic (or pulmonary), and pericardial fluid with the focused assessment with sonography technique (FAST) (see Chapter 182) [19]. The abdominal and thoracic FAST (aFAST and tFAST) are simple, inexpensive POC diagnostic tests which most emergency clinicians can perform and are recommended as an assessment and monitoring tool [20]. The presence of free fluid warrants centesis as a diagnostic measure (PCV/TS, etc.), and potentially a therapeutic measure, reliving respiratory distress and collecting fluid for potential autologous blood transfusion (ABT) (see Chapters 183 and 186).

Ultrasound can also be used to evaluate ventricular chamber and vessel size to assess intravesicular volume. An experience operator can detect changes in volume status and contractility [21–23]. Small inferior vena cava diameter during inspiration (<2 cm) has been shown to be an indicator of poor prognosis in human trauma patients and acute surgical patients [24]. A collapse index has also been investigated and is associated with shock and increased CO when fluids are administered, but this has yet to be investigated in veterinary patients [25].

Other diagnostics such as CBC, blood smear evaluation, serum biochemistry, and urinalysis are simple, widely available tests that may give insight into underlying disease processes. Other tests such as platelet assays, antithrombin levels, D-dimers, activated protein C, toxin quantification, individual clotting factors tests, and others may be important for definitive diagnosis and long-term therapy but are not often immediately available.

Treatment

Rapid identification and correction of hemorrhage are critical to prevent systemic consequences and death. Initial stabilization requires rapid, appropriate, and potentially aggressive intervention. Therapy may need to be initiated prior to collection and interpretation of any diagnostics due to the life-threatening nature of hemorrhage.

Providing supplemental oxygen during resuscitation can increase oxygen transport by ensuring that the blood hemoglobin is fully saturated and by raising the quantity of oxygen carried in solution in the plasma [26] (see Chapter 181). Most patients will require rapid placement of an IV or IO catheter for administration of fluids, blood products, and medications or to facilitate sedation or anesthesia.

Patients with location-specific hemorrhage (such as airway or pharynx) may require rapid-sequence induction of anesthesia with intubation or tracheostomy (see Chapter 191). If hemorrhage into the pleural or pericardial space is identified, a therapeutic centesis may be required (see Chapter 183). Blood collected from a patient via centesis should be collected in a sterile fashion and preserved for analysis (PCV/TS, lactate, glucose, cytology if indicated) and for potential ABT [27,28].

Patients with signs of hypoperfusion require fluid resuscitation and internal hemorrhage often requires more invasive diagnostics and therapeutics as outlined below (see Chapter 153).

Limiting External Blood Loss

External sources of hemorrhage should immediately have a compression bandage or digital pressure applied with a gloved hand to limit further blood loss while the patient is prepared for definitive care.

External coaptation with pressure can be placed easily on some body parts to minimize blood loss temporarily. Tourniquets are generally not recommended as they limit blood flow, which may delay healing and can exacerbate blood loss from the venous system; tourniquets should be removed within 10 minutes.

Many external sources of hemorrhage (such as arterial bleeding, or bleeding from the tongue or nasal cavity) may not be amenable to direct compression, in which case, the patient will require rapid-sequence induction of anesthesia with an injectable agent, and maintenance of anesthesia as deemed appropriate to allow hemostasis; this may include application of hemostatic agents, surgical correction (tissue or vessel ligation), local packing or local or distant source control (arterial ligation).

There are a variety of external and internal hemostatic agents available to assist in arresting hemorrhage (Table 170.1); these work through obstructing blood flow, providing a framework for clotting, absorbing water to increase effectiveness of natural clotting, or stimulating the coagulation cascade. Many are absorbable and do not need to be removed, but should be used with care in surgical wounds as they may inhibit healing [29]. These are commonly used in surgery in conjunction with thermal coagulation units. Administration of epinephrine into a nasal cavity is often ineffective as it is rapidly diluted by ongoing hemorrhage.

Fluid Resuscitation

The concept of damage control resuscitation (DCR) involves a combination of techniques to minimize derangements that commonly occur in the actively hemorrhaging patient (acidosis, coagulopathy, and hypothermia). DCR involves a combination of permissive hypotension, early use of blood products, limitation of crystalloid therapy, and minimizing surgical time to avoid these systemic complications and this has led to improved mortality [32–35].

Permissive hypotension uses small-volume fluid infusion techniques (discussed below) with low-normal resuscitation endpoints; this avoids potentially dislodging a fragile clot, hypothermia and dilution of

Table 170.1 Examples of hemostatic agents by category [30,31]. Reproduced with permission of John Wiley & Sons.

Category/ mechanism	Examples	Manufacturer	Notes
Caustic agents: coagulate proteins, tissue necrosis, eschar formation			
	Aluminum Cl, ferric sulfate, silver nitrate, Zn Cl	Many manufacturers including Vet One (GF Health Products, Atlanta, GA), Kwik-Stop (ARC Laboratories, Atlanta, GA)	Silver nitrate will cause pigmentation, Zn Cl is uncommonly used; often applied with an applicator stick or powder; external use only
Non-caustic agents: primarily create a physical mesh facilitating platelet aggregation and amplification and propogation of coagulation			
	Gelatins; provide a matrix for clot formation, activated thrombin	Gelfoam (Pfizer, Memphis, TN) Vetspon (Ethicon, Somerville, NJ)	Requires blood in field, not a sealing agent
	Microporous polysaccharide hemospheres (MPH) from potato starch; hydrophilic and concentrate blood	Hemablock (Abbott, Abbott Park, IL)	Increase in volume of the spheres
	Oxidized regenerated (methyl) cellulose (plant cellulose) – physical barrier for clotting, provides a matrix for clotting	Surgicell (Ethicon, Somerville, NJ)	Acidic and therefore bacteriocidal
	Microfiber collagen (bovine collagen) – aggregation and degranulation of platelets	Instat (Ethicon, Somerville, NJ), Helistate (Integra, Plainsboro, NJ)	Wound should be dried and product applied with pressure using gauze
	Physiological hemostatics (fibrin, thrombin, platelet gels, antifibrinolytics)	Aminocaproic acid (Hospira, Lake Forest, IL), others	Topical use may not be effective; few reported data
	Fibrin glue – activates conversion of fibrinogen to fibrin	Tisseel/Tissucol (Baxter),Hemaseel (Haemacure), Evisel (Ethicon)	Dry field preferred, spray delivery
	Glutaraldehyde adhesives – cross-linking cell to cell proteins	Bioglue (Cryolite)	Dry field preferred
	Waxes; malleable and form physical block as well as clotting surface	Bone wax (Aesculap, Center Valley, PA)	Difficult to apply to flat surface, may delay healing
Hemostatic dressings: used as wound dressings to prevent bleeding			
	Alginate dressing – seaweed protein, absorbs fluids through ion exchange reaction, releases calcium	Sorbosan (UDL Laboratories, Rockford, IL)	Not effective in high-pressure bleeding nor for intracavitary use
	Mineral zeolite – kaolin impregnanted polyester gauze, kaolin immediately activates XII, XI; absorbs water	Quickclot (Z-Medica, Wallingford, CT)	Foreign body reaction; early products were exothermic
	Chitin (chitosan) dressing, from crab exoskeletons, adheres to and seals wounds	Celox gauze and powder (Medtrade, Crewe, UK)	May also be antimicrobial

clotting factors [32]. Low normal endpoints of resuscitation include a patient with normal physical perfusion parameters (BAR, HR 80–140 bpm dog and >160 bpm cat, pale or pale pink mucous membrane color, with a capillary refill time <2 sec, strong synchronous pulses, a normal body temperature, and an adequate, but conservative blood pressure (systolic >90 mmHg and mean 60–80 mmHg)) [33]. Other parameters include normalization of $ScvO_2$ and lactate (see Chapter 153).

Fluid resuscitation is most often initiated with a combination of crystalloids and colloids, while the need for blood products is assessed (see Chapters 167–169).

Balanced isotonic crystalloids such as Plasma-Lyte-A, Normosol-R or lactated Ringer's are the most common initial choice. Small-volume resuscitation utilizes 10–20 mL/kg of a crystalloid with or without 2–5 mL/kg of a colloid, administered over 10–15 minutes, at which point the patient is reassessed (see Chapter 167).

Colloids (see Chapter 168) such as hydroxyethyl starch solutions have been known to exacerbate coagulopathies through dilution of coagulation proteins, coating platelets and interference with normal clotting factor activity [36]; some solutions have been associated with acute kidney injury and increased mortality, although further research is indicated [37]. Hypertonic solutions may be considered in patients that are not dehydrated; benefits of decreased neutrophil function, increased inotropy, and other effects have been reported [38–43], but these solutions may also worsen normal coagulation [44].

Transfusion of Blood Products

Patients experiencing a significant amount of hemorrhage will require blood products; early administration in clinical and hemorrhagic models has demonstrated improved outcome in some studies [32–35]. The type of blood product required depends on the underlying disease process and availability of blood products. A guide

for selection of products along with dose is provided in Table 170.2 and in Chapter 176.

Massive transfusion (see Chapters 177 and 190) predisposes patients to electrolyte (K, Ca, Mg) abnormalities, coagulopathies, thrombocytopenia, hypothermia, metabolic acidosis, delayed wound healing, and increased infection rates [45–52].

Alternatives to Blood Products

If species-specific stored or fresh blood is not available, alternatives may be considered and include autologous blood and xenotransfusions. Hemoglobin-based oxygen-carrying solutions (HBOCs) are not currently available, but may be useful in the future (see Table 170.2).

Autologous Blood Transfusion (ABT)
Patients with surgical or cavitary losses of blood that can be collected in a sterile fashion can be given ABTs. Advantages of ABT include immediate availability and

Table 170.2 Choice of product, indications, and dose for small animal transfusions [4]. Reproduced with permission of John Wiley & Sons.

Product	Indication	Suggested dose
Fresh whole blood (FWB)	Acute hemorrhage, anemia with hypoproteinemia, coagulopathy	2 mL/kg to raise PCV 1% (often 10–20 mL/kg) titrated to effect until stable
Stored whole blood	Same as FWB; NOT factor V or VIII deficiency	Same as FWB
Autologous blood	Volume resuscitation or RBC administration	Entire salvaged volume can be infused, avoid volume overload if given with concurrent additional blood products
Frozen plasma	Hypoproteinemia, coagulation factor deficiency (NOT V, VIII), augment COP	Coagulopathy: 6–20 mL/kg PRN to stop hemorrhage
		Hypoalbuminemia: 45 mL/kg to raise albumin 1 g/dL
Fresh frozen plasma	Coagulopathy of many etiologies without anemia, augment COP	Same as frozen plasma
Packed red blood cells	Anemia, without coagulopathy	1 mL/kg to raise PCV 1% or until PCV supports sufficient DO_2
Platelet concentrate	Thrombocytopenia with life-threatening hemorrhage	1 unit/10 kg PRN to arrest bleeding or until platelet count ≥ 30–50 000 platelets/mL
Platelet-rich plasma	Thrombocytopenia with life-threatening hemorrhage	1 unit/3 kg
Cryopreserved or lyphophilized platelets	Thrombocytopenia	Limited data; estimated that 2–3 times as many units needed as platelet-rich plasma to achieve same effect
Cryoprecipitate	Von Willebrand's disease, hemophilia A, hypofibrinogen	1 unit/10 kg
Hemoglobin-based oxygen carriers	Anemia when allogenic blood is not available, may help with concurrent hypotension	Dog 1–5 mL/kg, titrated to effect
		Cat 0.5–1 mL/kg, titrated to effect
		Constant-rate infusion 0.8 mL/kg/h

COP, colloid oncotic pressure; PCV, packed cell volume; PRN, as needed (*pro re nata*); RBC, red blood cell.

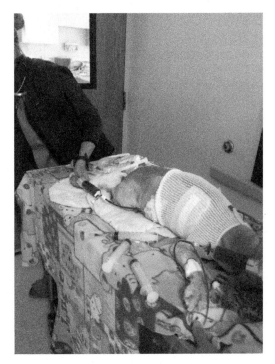

Figure 170.1 A patient that developed life-threatening pleural hemorrhage after lung lobectomy. This patient is being given an autologous blood transfusion (ABT) while being transferred back to the surgical suite. Note the syringe on the left removing blood from the thoracostomy tube and the syringe on the right administering the same blood IV through a filter. Reproduced with permission of John Wiley & Sons.

compatibility, normothermic blood products, lack of infectious agents, higher levels of RBC 2,3-DPG than stored blood and decreased overall cost [53]. Studies in humans undergoing oncological surgery have demonstrated no worse outcome in patients with ABT compared to banked blood [54,55]. If the ABT has GI contamination, culture, susceptibility, and antibiotic therapy are warranted. Blood that has been in a peritoneal cavity for prolonged periods may contain inflammatory mediators that could contribute to systemic inflammation, warranting careful monitoring for SIRS. ABT has been reported in veterinary patients with vascular injury (from trauma and GDV and after ovariohysterectomy), neoplasia, and anticoagulant rodenticide intoxication [28] (Figure 170.1).

Xenotransfusion

A xenotransfusion is the transfusion of blood from one species to another. In veterinary medicine, this specifically refers to canine blood administered to a cat. There is some evidence to support the use of xenotransfusion and it may be considered as a one-time option if type-specific (allogenic or autologous) feline blood is not available and the cat is suffering life-threatening anemia or hemorrhage [56].

Limiting Internal Hemorrhage

Internal hemorrhage may be severe enough that additional measures may be necessary prior to and during definitive (surgical) intervention.

External abdominal counterpressure may be used to help increase abdominal pressure and minimize blood loss from organs in trauma patients or patients with normal coagulation for which surgery is not an option. It is described in Box 170.1 and pictured in Figure 170.2 [4].

Many cases of internal abdominal (and occasionally thoracic) hemorrhage require surgical intervention; most commonly this occurs from blunt or penetrating trauma, bleeding tumor, organ torsions or recent surgical cases with uncontrolled hemorrhage (such as recent gonadectomy or other surgery; see Figure 170.1). In these cases, it is best to try to stabilize the animal as discussed above

---

Box 170.1 Application of external abdominal and hindlimb counterpressure* [4]. Reproduced with permission of John Wiley & Sons.

1. Provide sedation and analgesia.
2. Place urinary catheter if time allows.
3. Place patient in lateral recumbency.
4. Place rolled towel between the hindlegs for padding.
5. Place a rolled towel along ventral midline from xiphoid to pubis.
6. Wrap towels, cotton roll or disposable pads tightly around the circumference of the feet in a spiral pattern, ascending the limbs, over the pelvis and around the abdomen to the xiphoid.
7. Assess degree of tamponade – should be snug but allow a hand to slide between abdomen and bandage. Adequate ventilation should be allowed.
8. Place duct tape or stretch bandage in a spiral pattern from toes to xiphoid to secure position of bandage.
9. Monitor physical perfusion parameters, ventilation efforts, urine output, blood pressure, PCV and TS for evidence of ongoing hemorrhage.
10. Allow bandage to remain in place until patient has stabilized for >4 hours or until aseptic preparation needed for surgical intervention begins.
11. Release the tape first, section by section, in the direction from xiphoid to toes and monitor for decompensation for at least 5 minutes per section. This may be performed more rapidly if the patient is going to surgery.
12. Loosen and remove the towels or cotton slowly in the direction of xiphoid to toes, but leave in place in case counterpressure needs to be reapplied. Monitor for decompensation.

*Patients with hindlimb or pelvic fractures may not be able to tolerate this procedure without general anesthesia or epidural analgesia.

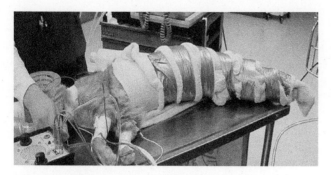

Figure 170.2 Abdominal and hindlimb counterpressure in a patient with a traumatic hemoabdomen. Reproduced with permission of John Wiley & Sons.

prior to anesthesia and surgical intervention (this may not be possible in all patients). For patients that require surgery, it is important to be as prepared as possible prior to anesthetic induction (Table 170.3) (see Chapter 191). Penetrating foreign objects should not be removed until the patient is stable enough to receive definitive surgical care. An experienced surgeon with rapid technique is essential; multiple challenging procedures may be necessary to control hemorrhage. Steps for emergency surgery are discussed in Box 170.2.

Internal Abdominal Pressure and Damage Control

With blunt force trauma, it may not be possible to arrest or remove all the sources of hemorrhage (such as diffuse crush injury to the liver). Damage control techniques (see Chapter 189) are necessary: blood may be collected for ABT, then further hemorrhage is limited by internally packing the abdomen with sterile towels or laparotomy sponges in a brief surgical procedure [4], with definitive surgical care delayed until the patient can tolerate prolonged anesthesia.

Additional Therapy for Specific Conditions

Patients with liver failure (see Chapter 90), DIC, acute traumatic coagulopathy (see Chapter 163), anticoagulant rodenticide intoxication (see Chapter 130), and other disease may also benefit from additional medical therapy (Table 170.4). The liver is responsible for making factors I, II, V, VII, IX, X, and XI. Vitamin K1 is an important co-factor for the carboxylation of factors II, VII, IX, and X, making administration of plasma products and vitamin K1 necessary for patients suffering from hemorrhage from these conditions.

Table 170.3 Preparation checklist for patients with significant hemorrhage which require surgical hemostasis.

To be set up prior to emergency surgery	Notes
Anesthesia machine	Ensure tubes connected, oxygen connected, appropriate size reservoir bag, sufficient volatile agent, leak test, appropriate ventilator settings
Anesthesia	Preoxygenate patient if time allows. Premedications calculated and administered; balanced/multimodal anesthesia/analgesia used; induction agents should allow rapid-sequence induction and intubation
Monitors to set up	Ensure adequate monitors in area and ready to go: CVT, ECG, ETCO$_2$, blood pressure, SpO$_2$, etc.
Monitoring patient	Prepared anesthetic monitor record is printed, with anesthetic and emergency drugs precalculated based on patient weight. Drugs drawn up and/or nearby
Surgical preparation area	Monitors and anesthetic machine as above, endotracheal tube size, check cuffs for leaks, laryngoscope, ET tubes, cuff syringe, pressure monitor and tie-in, eye lube, warming units, clippers, vacuum, scrub
Surgical area	Monitors and anesthetic machine as above, warming unit, ventilator, second scrub ready, suction unit, thermal or cautery units ready
Surgical equipment ready	Gloves, gowns, caps, masks, instruments, suture, lavage, blades, cautery, retractors, sterile suction, laparotomy pads, light handles, warmed lavage fluids, etc.
Patient preparation	IV catheter(s), analgesia, presurgical bloodwork, shave prior to induction (may need to shave both abdominal and thoracic cavity)
Blood administration	Type and cross-match if possible, allogenic blood or materials for ABT, blood filters, correction of coagulopathy (see below)
Additional staff	To assist with anesthetic or surgical challenges
Coagulation status	Check coagulation parameters if indicated and time allows. Administer blood products or medications to treat coagulopathy if present

ABT, autologous blood transfusion; CVT, certified veterinary technician; ECG, electrocardiogram; ET, endotracheal; ETCO$_2$, end-tidal carbon dioxide; IV, intravenous; SpO$_2$, peripheral capillary oxygen saturation.

Box 170.2 Steps for emergency surgery for abdominal hemorrhage. Reproduced with permission of John Wiley & Sons.

1. Have personnel, equipment, and medications (doses calculated) ready at time of induction (see also Table 170.3).
2. Clip and aseptically prepare patient prior to anesthetic induction.
3. Use multimodal analgesia and anesthesia that supports blood pressure.
4. Make 10-15 cm incision on midline below xiphoid to allow digital compression of anterior aspect of aorta for immediate hemostasis (compression for 10 minutes maximum).
5. Collect free peritoneal blood aspectically in sterile suction container for ABT if necessary.
6. Extend midline incision caudally to pubis.
7. Pack abdomen with sterile laparotomy pads to provide hemostasis by tamponade.
8. Explore each quadrant and control hemorrhage as indicated using local or source vessel compression or ligation, use of surgical instruments, organ removal or other hemostatic equipment, supplies or techniques.
9. Control bleeding from massive crush injuries by placing large surgical towels or laparotomy pads to pack off organs, limit hemorrhage and contamination and apply internal abdominal pressure (called damage control technique).
10. Close the abdomen with towels or pads in place, applying internal tamponade to oozing organs.
11. Re-explore in 12-36 hours for definitive therapy.

Acute traumatic coagulopathy (ATC) (also called trauma-induced coagulopathy and acute coagulopathy of trauma shock) is a severe coagulopathy described in human and veterinary trauma patients (see Chapter 163). A combination of key factors is the driving force in the initiation and propagation of ATC: tissue damage, inflammation, hypoperfusion, hemodilution, hypothermia, and acidosis [57,58]. Animals experiencing ATC may benefit from antifibrinolytic therapy (tranexamic acid or epsilon-aminocaproic acid), but further investigation is warranted (see Chapter 68) [57,58]. The use of tranexamic acid has been investigated in human medicine and has demonstrated positive effects in human patients [59]. One study evaluated 68 dogs with bleeding disorders treated with blood products and tranexamic acid (Hexakapron; mean dosage of 8.6 ± 2.2 mg/kg q6–8h) [60]. The dogs given tranexamic acid received fewer blood transfusions and a lower blood component dose with minimal adverse effects. Patients with acidosis or hypothermia should have those abnormalities corrected.

Patients predisposed to specific coagulopathies may benefit from administration of additional drugs (see Table 170.4). Greyhounds may suffer from hyperfibrinolysis and benefit from administration of aminocaproic acid in the perioperative period [61]. Patients with von Willebrand's or hemophilia will benefit from the administration of plasma products (see Table 170.1) and/or desmopressin. Desmopression may also alleviate clinical sings of bleeding secondary to aspirin administration [62] (i.e. prior to emergency therapy).

Table 170.4 Medications that may be administered for patients with hemorrhage. Reproduced with permission of John Wiley & Sons.

Medication	Indication	Dose
Vincristine	Thrombocytopenia	0.5 mg/m^2 IV through new IV catheter as delivery outside the vein causes tissue sloughing
Antivenom/antivenin	Snake bites	1–10 vials as directed and indicated based on coagulopathy, pain and clinical judgment
DDAVP (desmopressin)	Von Willebrand's disease, platelet inhibitory drugs, FVIII deficiency	Intranasal product 1–4 mg/kg SC to control bleeding or preoperatively; parenteral product should be given slowly and at lower doses, 0.3–1 mg/kg SC or IV
hrVIIa	Bleeding from coagulopathies, sepsis, DIC	90 ug/kg bolus q2h until hemostasis; little information to support use
Epsilon-aminocaproic acid	Hyperfibrinolysis, greyhounds	50–100 mg/kg IV loading then 15 mg/kg/h CRI q8h or 15–40 mg/kg IV followed by 500–1000 mg PO q8h
Ca-gluconate	Hypocalcemia (may be secondary to multiple or massive transfusion)	50–150 mg/kg (0.5–1.5 mL/kg of 10% solution) slow IV, monitor ECG, stop infusion with bradyarrhythmia
Vitamin K1	Liver disease, anticoagulant drugs or toxicity	2.5–5 mg/kg SC or PO q12–24h
Protamine sulfate	Heparin toxicity	1 mg for every 100 U heparin slow IV
Tranexamic acid	Hyperfibrinolysis	10–15 mg/kg SC IM, slow IV q6–8h
Human IV immunoglobilulin	Immune thrombocytopenia	0.5–1 g/kg IV over 6–12h once
Yunnan Baiyao	Neutraceutical but may be helpful with prolonged bleeding	Dog: <15 kg, 1 capsule PO q12h; 15–30 kg, 2 capsules PO q12h; >30 kg, 2 capsules PO q8h
		Cats: ½ capsule PO q12h

Anecdotal reports support the use of Yunnan Baiyao for veterinary bleeding disorders; some reports support topical and oral use in humans [63,64]. Other products such as recombinant human (or canine) factor VII (hrFVII) and activated protein C have yet to demonstrate substantial benefit; cost and availability and immune reactions will likely limit the role of these medications as well.

Investigation and treatment of the concurrent injuries and/or underlying disease leading to patient hemorrhage is essential, but beyond the scope of this chapter. The author recommends that any critically ill patient should have the Patient's Rule of 20 assessed twice daily (see Supplemental Reading).

References

1 Ferreira RR, Gopegui RR, De Matos AJ. Volume-dependant hemodynamic effects of blood collection in canine donors – evelution of 13% and 15% of total blood volume depletion. *An Acad Bras Cienc* 2015;87(1):381–388.

2 Kolb KS, Day T, McCall WG. Accuracy of blood loss termination by health care professionals. *Clin Forum Nurse Anaesth* 1999;10:170–173.

3 Larsson C, Saltvedt S, Wiklund I, Pahlen S, Andolf E. Estimation of blood loss after cesarean section and vaginal delivery has low validity with a tendency to exaggeration. *Acta Obstet Gynaecol Scand* 2006;85:1448–1452.

4 Herold L, Devey J, Kirby R, Rudloff E. Clinical evaluation and management of hemoperitoneum in dogs. *J Vet Emerg Crit Care* 2008;18(1):40–53.

5 Hackner SG. Bleeding disorders. In: *Small Animal Critical Care Medicine* (eds Silverstein DC, Hopper K). Elsevier Saunders, Philadelphia, 2014, pp. 507–514.

6 Greenway CV, Stark RD. Vascular response of the spleen to rapid haemorrhage in the anaesthetized cat. *J Physiol* 1969;204(1):169–179.

7 Ramlo JH, Brown JR. Mechanism of splenic contraction produced by severe hypercapnia. *Am J Physiol* 1959;197:1079–1082.

8 Jacobson S, Lobetti RG. Glucose, lactate, and pyruvate concentrations in dogs with babesiosis. *Am J Vet Res* 2005;66(2):244–250.

9 Nel M, Lobetti RG, Keller N, Thompson PN. Prognostic value of blood lactate, blood glucose, and hematocrit in canine babesiosis. *J Vet Intern Med* 2004;18(4):471–476.

10 Green T, Tonozzi C, Kirby R, Rudloff E. Evaluation of initial plasma lactate as a predictor of gastric necrosis and initial and subsequent plasma lactate values as a predictor of survival in dogs with gastric dilatation-volvulus: 84 dogs (2003–2007). *J Vet Emerg Crit Care* 2011;21(1):36–44.

11 Zacher LA, Berg J, Shaw AP, et al. Association between outcome and changes in plasma lactate concentration during presurgical treatment in dogs with gastric dilation-volvulus: 64 cases (2002–2008). *J Am Vet Med Assoc* 2010;236(8):892–897.

12 Mooney E, Raw C, Hughes D. Plasma lactate concentration as a prognostic biomarker in dogs with gastric dilatation and volvulus. *Top Compan Anim Med.* 2014;29(3):71–76.

13 Holahan ML, Brown AJ, Drobatz KJ. The association of blood lactate concentration without come in dogs with idiopathic immune-mediated hemolytic anemia: 173 cases (2003–2006). *J Vet Emerg Crit Care* 2010;20(4):413–420.

14 Stevenson CK, Kidney BA, Duke T, et al. Serial blood lactate concentrations in systemically ill dogs. *Vet Clin Pathol* 2007;36(3):234–239.

15 Stillion JR, Fletcher DJ. Admission base excess as a predictor of transfusion requirement and mortality in dogs with blunt trauma: 52 cases (2007–2009). *J Vet Emerg Crit Care* 2012;22(5):588–594.

16 Holowaychuk MK, Hanel RM, Darren Wood R, et al. Prospective multicenter evaluation of coagulation abnormalities in dog following severe acute trauma. *J Vet Emerg Crit Care* 2014;24(1):93–104.

17 Harrell K. Activated clotting time. In: *Blackwell's Five-Minute Veterinary Consult: Laboratory Tests and Diagnostic Procedures, Canine and Feline* (eds Vaden SL, Knoll JS, Franks WK, Tilley LP). Wiley-Blackwell, Ames, 2009, pp. 24–25.

18 Taki K, Takamura M, Sotani H, Wakusawa R. Management of the acid–base balance by the red blood cell carbonic anhydrase (RCA). *I. Correlation of the RCA activity and acid-base balance in the in vitro and in vivo experiments. Tohoku J Exp Med* 1983;139(4):339–348.

19 Boysen SR, Lisciandro GR. The use of ultrasound for dogs and cats in the emergency room: AFAST and TFAST. *Vet Clin North Am Small Anim Pract* 2015;43(4):773–797.

20 Lisciandro GR. The abdominal FAST3 (AFAST3) exam. In: *Focused Ultrasound Techniques for the Small Animal Practitioner* (ed. Lisciandro GR). Wiley-Blackwell, Ames, 2014, pp. 14–17.

21 Roscoe A, Strang T. Echocardiography in intensive care. *Cont Educ Anaesth Crit Care Pain* 2008;8(2):46–49.

22 Durkan SD, Rush JE, Rozanski EA, et al. Echocardiographic findings in dogs with hypovolemia. Proceedings of the International Veterinary Emergency and Critical Care Congress Atlanta, Georgia, 2005. *J Vet Emerg Crit Care* 2005;15:S4.

23 DeFrancesco T. Focused or coast³ – echo (heart). In: *Focused Ultrasound Techniques for the Small Animal Practitioner* (ed. Lisciandro GR). Wiley-Blackwell, Ames, 2014, pp.189–205.

24 Ferrada P, Vanguri P, Anand RJ, et al. Flat inferior vena cava: indicator of poor prognosis in trauma and acute care surgery patients. *Am Surg* 2012;78(12):1396–1398.

25 Airapetian N, Maizel J, Alyamani O, et al. Does inferior vena cava respiratory variability predict fluid responsiveness in spontaneously breathing patients? *Crit Care* 2015;19(1):400–408.

26 Batement NT, Leach RM. Acute oxygen therapy. *Br Med J* 1998;317(7161):798–801.

27 Higgs V, Rudloff E, Kirby R, Linklater A. Autologous blood transfusion in 24 dogs with thoracic and/or abdominal hemorrhage. *J Vet Emerg Crit Care* 2015;25(6):731–738.

28 Linklater A, Higgs V. Treatment of acute hemoabdomen in a dog. *Clin Brief* 2013;11(1):13–15.

29 Anderson DM. Surgical hemostasis. In: *Veterinary Surgery: Small Animal*, vol. 1 (eds Tobais KM, Johnston SP). Elsevier Saunders, St Louis, 2012, pp. 214–220.

30 Glick JB, Kaur RR, Siegel D. Achieving hemostasis in dermatology – Part II: Topical hemostatic agents. *Indian Dermatol Online J* 2013;4(3):172–176.

31 Galanakis I, Vasdev N, Soomro N. A review of current hemostatic agents and tissue sealants used in laparoscopic partial nephrectomy. *Rev Urol* 2011;13(3):131–138.

32 Chatrath V, Kheterpal R, Ahuja J. Fluid management in patients with trauma: restrictive versus liberal approach. *J Anaesthesiol Clin Pharmacol* 2015;31(3):308–316.

33 Hammond TN, Holm JL, Sharp CR. A pilot comparison of limited versus large fluid volume resusciation in canine spontaneous hemoperitoneum. *J Am Anim Hosp Assoc* 2014;50(3):159–166.

34 Bogert JN, Harvin J, Cotton BA. Damage control resuscitation. *J Intensive Care Med* 2016;31(3):177–186.

35 Hughes NT, Burd RS, Teach SJ. Damage control resuscitation: permissive hypotension and massive transfusion protocols. *Pediatr Emerg Care* 2014;30(9):651–656.

36 Glover PA, Rudloff E, Kirby R. Hydroxyethylstarch: a review of pharmacokinetics, pharmacodynamics, current products, and potential clinical risks, benefits and use. *J Vet Emerg Crit Care* 2014;24(6):642–661.

37 Hayes G, Benedicenti L, Mathews K. Retrospective cohort study on the incidence of acute kidney injury and death following hydroxyethyl starch (HES 10% 250/0.5/5:1) administration in dogs (2007–2010). 2016;26(1):35–40.

38 Wildenthal K, Mierzwiak DS, Mitchell JH. Acute effects of increased serum osmolality on left ventricular performance. *Am J Physiol* 1969;216:898–904.

39 Kien ND, Kramer GC. Cardiac performance following hypertonic saline. *Braz J Med Biol Res* 1989;22:245–248.

40 Rosengren S, Henson PM, Worthen GS. Migration-associated volume changes in neutrophils facilitate the migratory process in vitro. *Am J Physiol* 1994;267(6 Pt 1):C1623–1632.

41 Coimbra R, Junger WG, Liu FC, Loomis WH, Hoyt DB. Hypertonic/hyperoncotic fluids reverse prostaglandin E2 (PGE2)- induced T-cell suppression. *Shock* 1995;4(1):45–49.

42 Wolf MB. Plasma volume dynamics after hypertonic fluid infusing in nephrectomized dog. *Am J Physiol* 1971;221:1392–1395.

43 Li M, Chen T, Chen SD, Cai J, Hu YH. Comparison of equimolar doses of mannitol and hypertonic saline for the treatment of elevated intracranial pressure after traumatic brain injury. *Medicine* 2015;94(17):e736.

44 Wurlod VA, Howard J, Francey T, et al. Comparison of the in vitro effect of saline, hypertonic hydroxyethyl starch. *J Vet Emerg Crit Care* 2015;25(4):474–487.

45 Jutkowitz LA, Rozanski EA, Moreau J, et al. Massive transfusion in dogs: 15 cases (1997–2002). *J Am Vet Med Assoc* 2002;220(11):1664–1669.

46 Meikle A, Milne B. Management of prolonged QT interval during a massive transfusion: calcium, magnesium, or both? *Can J Anaesth* 2000;47(8):792–795.

47 Ho KM, Leonard A. Risk factors and outcomes associated with hypomagnesemia in massive transfusion. *Transfusion* 2011;51(2):270–276.

48 Wilson RF, Mammen E, Walt AJ. Eight years of experience with massive transfusion. *J Trauma* 1971;11(4):275–285.

49 Reiss RF. Hemostatic defects in massive transfusion: rapid diagnosis and management. *Am J Crit Care* 2000;9(3):158–165.

50 Cosgriff N, Moore EE, Sauaia A, et al. Predicting life–threatening coagulopathy in the massively transfused trauma patient: hypothermia and acidosis revisited. *J Trauma* 1997;42(5):857–861.

51 Argarwal N, Murphy JG, Cayten CG, et al. Blood transfusion increases the risk of infection after trauma. *Arch Surg* 1993;128(2):171–176.

52 Ford CD, van Moorleghem G, Menlove RF. Blood transfusion and postoperative wound infections. *Surgery* 1993;113(6):603–607.

53 Purvis D. Autotransfusion in the emergency patient. *Trans Med* 1995;25(6):1291–1304.

54 Ubee S, Kumar M, Athmanathan N, et al. Intraoperative red blood cell salvage and autologous transfusion during open radical retropubic prostatectomy: a cost-benefit analysis. *Ann R Coll Surg Engl* 2011;93(2):157–161.

55 Brewster DC, Ambrosino JJ, Darling R, et al. Intraoperative autotransfusion in major vascular surgery. *Am J Surg* 1979;137(4):507–513.

56 Bovens C, Gruffydd-Jones T. Xenotransfusion with canine blood in the feline species: review of the literature. *J Feline Med Surg* 2103;15(2):62–67.

57 Palmer L, Martin L. Traumatic coagulopathy – Part 1: Pathophysiology and diagnosis. *J Vet Emerg Crit Care* 2014;24(1):63–74.

58 Palmer L, Martin L. Traumatic coagulopathy – Part 2: Resuscitative strategies. *J Vet Emerg Crit Care* 2014;24(1):75–92.

59 Ausset S, Glassberg E, Nadler R, et al. Tranexamic acid as part of remote damage-control resuscitation in the prehospital setting: a critical appraisal of the medical

literature and available alternatives. *J Trauma Acute Care Surg* 2015;78(6 Suppl 1):S70–S75.

60 Kelmer E, Marer K, Bruchim Y, et al. Retrospective evaluation of the safety and efficacy of tranexamic acid (Hexakapron) for the treatment of bleeding disorders in dogs. *Israel J Vet Med* 2013;68(2):94–100.

61 Marin LM, Iazbik MC, Zaldivar-Lopez S, et al. Epsilon aminocarpoic acid for the prevention of delayed postoperative bleeding in retired racing Greyhounds undergoing gonadectomy. *Vet Surg* 2012;41(5):594–603.

62 Di Mauro FM, Holowaychuk MK. Intravenous administration of desmopressin acetate to reverse acetylsalicylic acid-induced coagulopathy in three dogs. *J Vet Emerg Crit Care* 2013;23(4):455–458.

63 Tang ZL, Wang X, Yi B, et al. Effects of the preoperative administration of Yunnan Baiyao capsules on intraoperative blood loss in bimaxillary orthognathic surgery: a prospective, randomized, double-blind, placebo-controlled study. *Int J Oral Maxillofac Surg* 2009;38(3):261–266.

64 Ladas EJ, Karlik JB, Rooney D, et al. Topical Yunnan Baiyao administration as an adjunctive therapy for bleeding complications in adolescents with advanced cancer. *Support Care Cancer* 2012;20(12):3379–3383.

Supplemental Reading

Herold L, Devey J, Kirby R, Rudloff E. Clinical evaluation and management of hemoperitoneum in dogs. *J Vet Emerg Crit Care* 2008;18(1):40–53.

Linklater AK, Kirby R. *Monitoring and Intervention for the Critically Ill Patient: Kirby's Rule of 20*. Wiley-Blackwell, St Louis, 2016.

Palmer L, Martin L. Traumatic coagulopathy – Part 1: Pathophysiology and diagnosis. *J Vet Emerg Crit Care* 2014;24(1):63–74.

Palmer L, Martin L. Traumatic coagulopathy – Part 2: Resuscitative strategies. *J Vet Emerg Crit Care* 2014;24(1):75–92.

171

Management of Dehydration

Ashley E. Allen-Durrance, DVM, DACVECC and Samantha Campos, VMD

College of Veterinary Medicine, University of Florida, Gainesville, FL, USA

Introduction

Water is vital to homeostasis in the body. It forms the body's blood supply, carries substrates across cellular membranes, evaporates to assist with thermoregulation, and functions as the universal solvent of the body. The healthy animal maintains an essential balance between fluid loss into the gastrointestinal tract, urine, and insensible losses and fluid gain through oral hydration [1].

Changes in the volume and distribution of water in the body can affect patient outcome. Significant water loss can lead to life-threatening alterations of blood pressure, temperature regulation, neurological function, and electrolyte abnormalities. However, excess body water can also cause fluid accumulation inside organs and body cavities, leading to impaired organ function and potentially fatal complications [2,3].

Definition of Dehydration

Dehydration is a state of reduced body water content resulting from either decreased intake or increased loss. Bodily fluid losses can occur through the gastrointestinal tract, urinary system, respiratory system, wounds, sweat, or a combination thereof, resulting in dehydration. Clinically, dehydration is specific to the interstitial and intracellular compartments, but if severe enough can affect the intravascular compartment [4].

The type of fluid lost from the body and the tonicity or effective osmolality of the remaining body fluid can further classify dehydration as hypertonic dehydration, isotonic dehydration, or hypotonic dehydration. Tonicity or effective osmolality can be estimated by the following formula: $2(Na)+glucose/18$ [5]. Note that effective osmolality is simply the calculated plasma osmolality $[2(Na)+BUN/2.8+glucose/18]$ minus the effect of blood urea nitrogen (BUN) because BUN freely distributes in total body water, whereas sodium and glucose are impermeant solutes and do not readily distribute across cell membranes. Pure water loss and hypotonic fluid loss (e.g. uncontrolled diabetes insipidus, fever, small intestinal obstruction, etc.) cause hypertonic dehydration. Isotonic fluid loss (e.g. some types of diarrhea, vomiting, hemorrhage) results in isotonic dehydration because sodium and water are lost in equivalent ratios from the body. Hypertonic fluid loss or isotonic fluid loss with free water replacement (e.g. water deprivation, iatrogenic) results in hypotonic dehydration [5].

Estimating Dehydration

On physical examination, the minimal degree of dehydration detectable is 5% of body weight; see Table 171.1 for more details [5,6]. At approximately 5–6% dehydrated, a very subtle loss of skin elasticity is detected. After 6–8% dehydration, a prolonged capillary refill

Table 171.1 Physical examination and approximate percent interstitial dehydration [4].

Approximate percent dehydration	Physical exam findings
<5	Undetectable, history of fluid loss
5–6	Tacky mucous membranes
6–8	Decreased skin turgor
	Dry mucous membranes
8–10	Retracted globes within orbits
10–12	Persistent loss of skin tent
	Evidence of hypovolemia
>12	Hypovolemic shock
	Death

Textbook of Small Animal Emergency Medicine, First Edition. Edited by Kenneth J. Drobatz, Kate Hopper, Elizabeth Rozanski and Deborah C. Silverstein.
© 2019 John Wiley & Sons, Inc. Published 2019 by John Wiley & Sons, Inc.
Companion Website: www.wiley.com/go/drobatz/textbook

time, sunken eyes, dry mucous membranes, and tented skin become apartment. At approximately 10–12% dehydrated, the intravascular compartment is affected and the above clinical signs are present with the addition of signs associated with hypovolemic shock such as tachycardia, weak pulses, tachypnea, and dull mentation. A poor prognosis is associated with greater than 12% dehydration [5,6].

A decrease in body weight may be the most practical and even most accurate method to determine loss of total body water over a short period of time. Discrepancies in variable scales, patient positioning, and accuracy of scales may limit the ability to use weights reliably when patients present to the emergency room. In order to use weights appropriately, the scale should be calibrated and zeroed prior to placing the patient on the scale. If done properly, weights over the duration of hospitalization can be used as an indication of fluid loss or gain, which can then be converted to an estimation of dehydration because 1 kg is equivalent to 1 L of fluid.

Unfortunately, often we do not have the known prior accurate weights of dogs and cats presenting for emergency treatment unless medical records are presented with the owner and the scale discrepancies are minimal. In addition, one must consider a change in weight with the disease process of the patient. For example, weight gain in a postoperative septic abdomen patient could be due to interstitial, intracellular, or intravascular volume changes or third-spacing of fluid into the abdominal compartment (see Chapter 159). Often, on initial assessment, we rely on physical examination findings and clinicopathological values [6]. Clinicopathological parameters such as packed cell volume (PCV), total solids (TS), and urine specific gravity (USG) may help to clarify hydration status. The PCV and TS increase with all fluid losses excluding situations when splenic contraction occurs (e.g. acute hemorrhage, acute stress). The USG should be high in a dehydrated animal with normal renal function. Other diseases that also alter the USG and make its use

as a measure of hydration status inappropriate include liver disease, pyelonephritis, diabetes mellitus, pyometra, central or peripheral diabetes insipidus, hyper- or hypoadrenocorticism, and hypercalcemia [7].

Additionally, it is important to note that serum sodium concentration may or may not be helpful in evaluating dehydrated patients. Hypernatremia develops with excess sodium intake, retention, or administration (such as through salt poisoning, hyperaldosteronism, hyperadrenocorticism, or hypertonic saline therapy), inadequate water intake, and hypotonic fluid loss such as gastrointestinal losses (vomiting, diarrhea), third space losses (peritonitis, pancreatitis), and cutaneous losses (burns) [5].

Total Body Water

The total body water in the intracellular and extracellular compartments is 0.6 L/kg or 60% of body mass in adult animals. In neonatal or pediatric patients, total body water is increased at 80% of body weight [8,9]. Total body water has been estimated as approximately 534–660 mL/kg in healthy adult dogs and cats [10]. In addition, total body water is typically decreased in perioperative patients and those with systemic inflammatory conditions (i.e. sepsis, major trauma, burns) due to changes in vascular permeability [11,12] (see Chapter 159).

The intracellular compartment is approximately 0.4 L/kg or 66% of total body water and represents the largest water compartment [8]. The extracellular component is 0.2 L/kg or 33% of the total body water. The extracellular compartment is further broken down into interstitial (75% of the extracellular fluid) and intravascular (25% of the extracellular fluid) [11] (Figure 171.1). The majority of the intravascular volume is plasma which is about 42–58 mL/kg in adult dogs and 37–49 mL/kg in adult cats [8]. Dehydration is typically referred to as a loss of fluid in the extracellular fluid compartment and, more specifically, in the interstitial space [4,5,12].

Figure 171.1 Division of total body water.

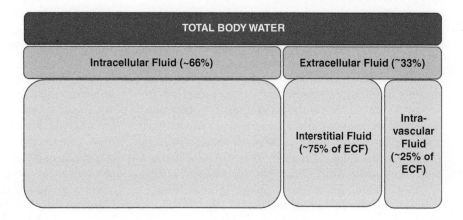

Body water is distributed across two compartmentalizing membranes: endothelium (intravascular from interstitial space) and the cell membranes separating the intracellular from extracellular space. Osmosis regulates the movement of water in the direction of higher solute concentration as shown in Starling's law [13]. A modified Starling's equation takes into account the role of the endothelial glycocalyx in the control of transvascular fluid movement [14].

Fluctuations in total body water vary depending on hormonal mechanisms to control water and sodium balance through the renin-angiotensin-aldosterone system, thirst mechanisms, and ADH hormone secretion from the pituitary [8].

Interstitial changes can be evaluated by monitoring the moistness of mucous membranes, skin tent response, eye position, and corneal position. All of these changes equilibrate within the intravascular space such that dogs and cats with evidence of interstitial dehydration will also have some degree of hypovolemia. Interstitial overrhydration leads to increased turgor of the skin and tissue, gelatinous appearance, peripheral or ventral pitting edema, chemosis, and/or clear nasal discharge. Frequent monitoring of a patient's respiratory status is important as tachypnea and cough often occur before clinical signs of chemosis and nasal discharge [13]. With severe fluid overload, organ edema can occur and impair oxygenation of the tissues [13].

Intravascular changes are assessed by perfusion parameters such as mucous membrane color, capillary refill time, heart rate, pulse quality, temperature, and mentation. Rapid intravascular losses, such as occur with acute hemorrhage, result in hypovolemia without causing clinical changes in interstitial dehydration. Acute, severe intravascular fluid loss will progress to hypovolemic shock [12]. In contrast, hypervolemia leads to jugular venous distension, increased central venous pressure, and eventually the most obvious clinical sequelae of tachypnea or cough due to pulmonary edema. This is particularly true in the lungs when pulmonary capillary pressures exceed 25 mmHg [13].

Intracellular changes cannot be readily identified on physical exam. However, the clinician must rely on changes in effective osmolality [2(Na)+glucose/18] of the extracellular fluid to determine changes in cell volume [4,5]. With decreases in effective blood osmolality, movement of water into the intracellular compartment increases the volume in the cell. This is evident in cases of hyponatremia in which overzealous correction of the hyponatremia results in central pontine myelinolysis characterized by progressive neurological abnormalities [15]. Alternatively, with increases in extracellular effective osmolality, there will be decreased intracellular volume. This can result in tissue shrinkage and vascular trauma [15,16].

Mechanism of Thirst

Thirst is regulated by an area in the anterior wall in the third ventricle of the hypothalamus, known as the thirst center [17,18]. Fluctuation in osmolality is sensed by osmoreceptors in the circumventricular organs, which lack the blood–brain barrier and can therefore rapidly respond to minute, acute changes in osmolality [18]. This area of the hypothalamus (also known as the Verney receptor) provides the drive for water intake by the dog or cat and also controls excretion of water into the urine [17,19].

Plasma osmolality (primarily sodium concentration) is the most potent driving force for thirst. When plasma osmolality increases around the osmoreceptors, animals will seek out water to return plasma osmolality to normal [17]. In addition, vasopressin (also known as antidiuretic hormone, ADH) is released from the supraoptic nuclei which stimulates reabsorption of water in the renal collecting duct by binding to V2 receptors, ultimately triggering insertion of aquaporin-2 channels in the apical membrane to rapidly increase renal water reabsorption [18,19]. Dogs and cats with an ineffective thirst mechanism or unavailable supply of water are at risk for severe dehydration.

Rehydration

Correction of dehydration involves pre-emptively planning the route of administration and type of fluid to administer, calculating the estimated fluid deficit, determining the time interval to correct the fluid deficit, incorporating maintenance fluid requirements, estimating ongoing losses, and monitoring for progression or resolution of dehydration (Table 171.2) [20,21]. In addition to the initial fluid therapy plan, one must also preconceive how the patient will be monitored for resolution of dehydration, ongoing dehydration, or overhydration. Each clinical situation will vary in the appropriate fluid therapy plan, and ultimately many different plans may be efficacious for each patient.

Fluid can be administered via the following routes of administration: oral, subcutaneous, intravenous, intraosseous, intraperitoneal, or rectal. In the emergency room setting, any route can be appropriate, depending on the clinical scenario. Oral administration of fluid should not be used if the patient is regurgitating, vomiting, or cannot physically drink enough water to account for ongoing losses. Most commonly, the intravenous route is preferred in critically ill patients. Fluid with an osmolality of 600 mOsm/L or less can be safely administered through a peripheral intravenous catheter, whereas a central venous catheter should be used if the osmolality is greater than 600 mOsm/L [21].

Table 171.2 Rehydration fluid therapy plan.

Routes of administration	Intravenous (most common)
	Oral
	Subcutaneous
	Intraosseous
	Intraperitoneal
	Rectal
Type of fluid to administer	Isotonic crystalloids (most common)
	Lactated Ringer's solution (273 mOsm/L)
	Plasma-Lyte 148 (295 mOsm/L)
	Normosol-R (295 mOsm/L)
	0.9% sodium chloride (308 mOsm/L)
Estimated fluid deficit	Weight (kg) × percent dehydration = L fluid to replace
Length of time to replace deficit	Typically 6–24 hours
Maintenance fluid requirements	Dog/cat: [70 × (body weight$_{kg}$)$^{0.75}$]/24h [21]
	[30 × body weight$_{kg}$ + 70]/24h [21]
	(40–60 mL/kg)/24h [21]
	Dogs: [132 × (body weight$_{kg}$)$^{0.75}$]/24h [14,20]
	2–6 mL/kg/h [14]
	Cats: [80 × (body weight$_{kg}$)$^{0.75}$]/24h [14,20]
	2–3 mL/kg/h [14]
	Neonate/pediatric: 80–120 mL/kg/day [23]
Estimated ongoing losses	Estimate or measure (preferred) vomit, regurgitation, diarrhea, urine, fluid from wounds, fluid from any indwelling tubes
Monitoring plan	Body weight, physical examination, urine output, packed cell volume, total solids, blood urea nitrogen, urine specific gravity, and osmolality

Isotonic crystalloids, also known as replacement fluids, are the most commonly used type of fluids to rehydrate a dog or cat. Clinically, most cases of dehydration are due to isotonic fluid loss resulting in interstitial dehydration [4]. Therefore, isotonic crystalloids such as lactated Ringer's solution, Plasma-Lyte 148, Normosol-R, or isotonic saline are the most commonly used fluids (see Chapter 167). Normal osmolality in the dog is 290–310 mOsm/L and in the cat is 311–322 mOsm/L, whereas the commonly used isotonic crystalloids have an osmolality of 270–310 mOsm/L [5,22]. Clinical situations in which dehydration is treated with hypotonic or hypertonic fluids, with or without addition of isotonic fluids, typically involve those with chronic sodium disorders in which plasma osmolality needs to be slowly adjusted to minimize central nervous system consequences (cerebral edema or central pontine myelinolysis). A thorough

discussion of the treatment of sodium disorders is beyond the scope of this chapter, but further details can be found in Chapter 108.

Approach to the fluid plan for rehydration is, at best, an estimation of the animal's fluid deficit and maintenance fluid requirements. Clinical signs of dehydration, discussed above, are subjective evaluations. In general, the fluid deficit is calculated by multiplying the estimated percent dehydration by the animal's body weight in kilograms which will yield a number in kilograms. One kilogram of water is equivalent to 1 L of water so the number obtained is converted to liters and multiplied by 1000 to obtain milliliters [9,20]. For example, if a 20 kg dog is estimated to be 7% dehydrated, then the deficit will be 1.4 L or 1400 mL. After calculating the fluid deficit, one must then decide how fast to replace the deficit. Many advocate replacing the deficit over 6–24 hours in cardiovascularly stable patients, depending on how quickly dehydration developed [9].

In any fluid plan, beyond simply replacing a deficit, provision of maintenance fluid requirements is needed. Insensible (fecal, cutaneous, respiratory; 13–20 mL/kg/day) and sensible (urine output; 27–40 mL/kg/day) losses are incorporated into the maintenance fluid requirements and do not need to be calculated separately [20]. Daily fluid requirements parallel daily resting caloric requirements so calculation of an animal's resting energy requirement (RER) will provide an estimate of daily fluid requirements because 1 kcal of energy is equivalent to 1 mL water [29,21]. Neonatal (0–21 days) and pediatric (<6 months) patients have higher maintenance fluid requirements (80–120 mL/kg/day) and are highly susceptible to dehydration [23].

Many different formulae exist for calculating daily maintenance fluid requirements (see Table 171.2). One must keep in mind that the formulae for maintenance fluid requirements pertain to healthy animals with normal renal function. If the animal is polyuric and/or polydipsic (e.g. uncontrolled diabetes, hyperadrenocorticism, chronic kidney disease), then the formulae are inherently inaccurate and so clinical judgment and history must be used when creating a fluid plan.

Replacement isotonic crystalloids have little or no added potassium, so maintenance potassium supplementation should be incorporated into the overall fluid plan and the animal's measured serum potassium will guide supplementation (see Chapter 173). It is important to remember that when adding potassium to any fluid, the bag should be thoroughly agitated to prevent iatrogenic hyperkalemia and the total rate of potassium administration should not exceed 0.5 mEq/kg/h without ECG monitoring [24]. Some advocate administering two types of fluids, an isotonic replacement fluid and a maintenance fluid, simultaneously, with a goal of replacing the dehydration deficit with an isotonic crys-talloid while providing a lower sodium, higher potassium maintenance fluid to prevent excessive sodium admin-istration. More commonly, many replace the deficit and provide maintenance with an isotonic replacement solu-tion appropriately supplemented with potassium.

Ongoing losses (also known as contemporary losses) can be estimated subjectively or objectively [20]. When the rehydration plan is initiated, ongoing losses are always a subjective estimate based on the animal's history. With inpatient monitoring, more objective estimates of ongoing losses can be obtained. Fluid losses which can be measured include vomitus, diarrhea, urine output, wound drainage, fluid collected from indwelling drains, and blood loss [9]. Many hospitals use diaper pads to absorb fluid in kennels; thus, weighing the pad after a patient has vomited, regur-gitated, or had diarrhea can enable conversion to a quanti-tative fluid amount (diaper pad with bodily fluids – diaper pad dry weight = kg × 1000 = mL contemporary loss). Alter-natively, if an indwelling tube (urinary catheter, nasogastric tube, chest tube, abdominal drain, wound drain, etc.) is in place, the fluid collected is easily measured in milliliters and can be added to the ongoing losses estimate. Ongoing losses are likely to change during the course of hospitalization and the daily fluid plan should account for these changes.

Complications of rehydrating an animal can be asso-ciated with the route of administration, iatrogenic fluid overload, persistent dehydration, and acid–base or electrolyte abnormalities. Most commonly, emergency patients are rehydrated with intravascular fluids, so phlebitis, hemorrhage, thrombosis, catheter embolism, or infection (catheter-related bloodstream infection, endocarditis) are possible [13,20]. Intravenous cathe-ters should be placed aseptically and maintained prop-erly. Patients should be evaluated several times per day for fever, new-onset cardiac murmurs, or swelling, heat, or pain around the catheter. If the aforementioned signs occur, the catheter should be promptly removed with subsequent cultures taken from the tip of the catheter or serial blood cultures from the patient [20].

Animals should be monitored daily for signs of fluid overload or persistent dehydration. Weighing the animal can be quite helpful, keeping in mind the considerations discussed above. Iatrogenic fluid overload manifests clinically as tachypnea, cough, pulmonary crackles, clear nasal discharge, serous nasal discharge, chemosis, edema (especially around the hock), diarrhea, gelatinous subcu-taneous tissues, and shivering [13,20]. Decrease in PCV, TS, BUN, urine osmolality, and urine specific gravity can also be associated with fluid overload; however, this must be evaluated in context with the animal's condition and concurrent diseases [4].

Fluid overload has been associated with increased morbidity and mortality in humans and clinically asso-ciated with impaired cognition, impaired pulmonary gas exchange, decreased lung compliance, increased work of breathing, ileus, gastrointestinal bacterial translocation, malabsorption, impaired cardiac contractility, cardiac conduction abnormalities, poor wound healing, wound infection, acute kidney injury, salt and water retention, cholestasis, and impaired hepatic synthetic function [25].

Frequent, diligent daily monitoring of the animal is essential and once dehydration is corrected, fluid should be adjusted or discontinued, accordingly. If fluid over-load occurs, exogenous fluid administration should be discontinued and diuretics considered [25].

Conclusion

Management of dehydration in the emergency room setting starts with the history of the patient and assess-ment of the clinical level of dehydration. Once these fac-tors are known, a fluid plan can be designed to replace the fluid deficit while supplying maintenance fluids and correcting ongoing losses. Isotonic replacement fluids are the most commonly used fluid type to correct inter-stitial dehydration. As with any therapeutic interven-tion, complications must be considered and monitored for regularly. In veterinary medicine, frequent physical examinations, assessment of urine output, trends in clin-icopathological variables, trends in patient weight, and evaluation of ongoing losses are recommended to moni-tor the rehydration plan. Iatrogenic fluid overload is not without potentially serious clinical consequences and rehydration must be monitored vigilantly.

References

1 Reineke E, Walton K, Otto C. Evaluation of an oral electrolyte solution for treatment of mild to moderate dehydration in dogs with hemorrhagic diarrhea. *J Am Vet Med Assoc* 2013;243(6):851–857.
2 Rudloff E, Kirby R. Colloid and crystalloid resuscitation. *Vet Clin North Am Small Anim Pract* 2001;31(6):1207–1229.
3 Lee J, Rozanski E, Anastasio M, et al. Water intoxication in two cats. *J Vet Emerg Crit Care* 2013;23(1):53–57.
4 Rudloff E. Assessment of hydration. In: *Small Animal Critical Care Medicine*, 2nd edn (eds Silverstein DC, Hopper K). Elsevier Saunders, St Louis, 2015, pp. 307–311.

5 DiBartola SP. Disorders of sodium and water: hypernatremia and hyponatremia. In: *Fluid, Electrolyte and Acid–Base Disorders in Small Animal Practice*, 4th edn (ed. DiBartola SP). Elsevier Saunders, St Louis, 2012, pp. 57–75.

6 Hensen B, DeFrancesco T. Relationship between hydration estimate and body weight change after fluid therapy in critically ill dogs and cats. *J Vet Emerg Crit Care* 2002;12(4):235–243.

7 Waldrop JE. Urinary electrolytes, solutes, and osmolality. *Vet Clin North Am Small Anim Pract* 2008;38:503–512.

8 Wellman ML, DiBartola SP, John CW. Applied physiology of both fluids in dogs and cats. In: *Fluid, Electrolyte and Acid–Base Disorders in Small Animal Practice*, 4th edn (ed. DiBartola SP). Elsevier Saunders, St Louis, 2012, pp. 2–12.

9 Mazzaferro E, Powell L. Fluid therapy for the emergency small animal patient. *Vet Clin North Am Small Anim Pract* 2013;43:721–734.

10 Edelman IS, Leibman J, O'Meara MP, et al. Interrelations between serum sodium concentration, serum osmolarity and total exchangeable sodium, total exchangeable potassium and total body water. *J Clin Invest* 1958;37(9): 1236–1256.

11 Maxwell MH, Kleeman CR, Narins RG. *Clinical Disorders of Fluid and Electrolyte Metabolism*. McGraw-Hill, New York, 1987.

12 Boller E, Boller M. Assessment of fluid balance and the approach to fluid therapy in the perioperative patient. *Vet Clin North Am Small Anim Pract* 2015;45: 895–915.

13 Mazzaferro E. Complications of fluid therapy. *Vet Clin North Am Small Anim Pract* 2008;38:607–619.

14 Chohan AS, Davidow EB. Clinical pharmacology and administration of fluid, electrolyte, and solutions. In: *Veterinary Anesthesia and Analgesia*, 5th edn

(eds Grimm K, Lamont AA, Tranquili WJ, et al.). John Wiley & Sons, Ames, 2015, pp. 386–407.

15 Sterns RH. Disorders of plasma sodium – causes, consequences, and correction. *N Engl J Med* 2015;372:55–65.

16 Marks S, Taboada J. Hypernatremia and hypertonic syndromes. *Vet Clin North Am Small Anim Pract* 1998;28(3):533–543.

17 Hall JE. Cerebral cortex, intellectual functions of the brain, learning, and memory. In: *Guyton and Hall Textbook of Medical Physiology*, 12th edn (ed. Hall JE). Saunders Elsevier, Philadelphia, 2011, p. 716.

18 Arai S, Stotts N, Puntillo K. Thirst in critically ill patients: from physiology to sensation. *Am J Crit Care* 2013;22(4):328–335.

19 Park EJ, Kwon TH. A minireview on vasopressin-regulated aquaporin-2 in kidney collecting duct cells. *Electrolyte Blood Press* 2015;13(1):1–6.

20 DiBartola SP, Bateman S. Introduction to fluid therapy. In: *Fluid, Electrolyte and Acid–Base Disorders in Small Animal Practice*, 4th edn (ed. DiBartola SP). Elsevier Saunders, St Louis, 2012, pp. 331–350.

21 Silverstein DC, Santoro-Beer K. Daily intravenous fluid therapy. In: *Small Animal Critical Care Medicine*, 2nd edn (eds Silverstein DC, Hopper K). Elsevier Saunders, St Louis, 2015, pp. 316–321.

22 Dugger DT, Mellema MS, Hopper K, et al. Comparative accuracy of several published formulae for the estimation of serum osmolality in cats. *J Small Anim Pract* 2013;54(4):184–189.

23 Macintire DK. Pediatric fluid therapy. *Vet Clin North Am Small Anim Pract* 2008;38:621–627.

24 Hoehne SN, Hopper K, Epstein SE. Accuracy of potassium supplementation of fluids administered intravenously. *J Vet Intern Med* 2015;29(3):834–839.

25 Ogbu OC, Murphy DJ, Martin GS. How to avoid fluid overload. *Curr Opin Crit Care* 2015;21(4):315–321.

172

Maintenance Fluid Therapy

Travis Lanaux, DVM, DACVECC

College of Veterinary Medicine, University of Florida, Gainesville, FL, USA

Introduction

In veterinary medicine, the term *maintenance fluid(s)* has several different meanings. Maintenance fluid(s) may refer to the daily fluid requirement of a patient to maintain normal physiological processes or a type of fluid resembling the usual fluid and electrolyte losses of a given patient throughout the day [1]. It is important to distinguish between calculation of a patient's "maintenance" fluid requirements versus using a crystalloid with a composition classified as a maintenance fluid (or both). These concepts will be explained in more detail throughout this chapter.

Estimation of a Patient's "Maintenance" Fluid Requirement

Fluid requirements in health and disease may vary substantially between patients and may even have significant variability in the same patient over a period of time. There are several methods of estimating the patient's daily maintenance fluid requirements. Regardless of the method chosen, the most important part of any fluid plan is frequent reassessment of the patient's fluid balance.

Disease states such as kidney disease/injury, diabetes insipidus, diabetes mellitus, hyperadrenocorticism, endotoxemia, trauma, and many others may greatly increase the daily fluid requirement of a patient. Within these disease states, common etiologies of increased fluid loss include hemorrhage, panting, inability to concentrate urine, exudative wounds or burns, and increased fecal fluid excretion (e.g. diarrhea). Adding another level of complexity is the composition of the fluid that is being lost. For example, panting and certain causes of polyuria may lead to excessive water loss without a significant loss of electrolytes such as sodium, whereas other disease processes, such as wounds and diarrhea, may cause fluid losses with a composition closer to that of normal serum or plasma.

Calculating the estimated daily fluid requirement of a patient will help the clinician determine the starting rate of fluids for a given patient, but often requires alterations during treatment based on serial evaluations of the patient.

The following are common methodologies employed to estimate daily fluid requirements in dogs and cats.

- Use of a resting energy requirement calculation and substituting milliliters of water per day for calculated kilocalories per day [2–4].
- Cats: $80 \times$ body weight $(kg)^{0.75}$ [5].
- Dogs: $132 \times$ body weight $(kg)^{0.75}$ [5].
- General estimates based on species and size of the patient.

Adult cats generally have lower fluid requirements than dogs due to their lower blood volume, slower metabolic rate, and greater ability to concentrate urine and conserve water. As a generalization, young animals or dogs with a larger surface area to body weight ratio, as well as smaller or lean animals, will tend to require greater fluid supplementation to maintain adequate hydration states than obese or large animals with decreased surface area to body weight ratios [2–4].

Commonly suggested estimations include the following.

- Cats: 40–50 mL/kg/day
- Giant-breed dogs: 30–40 mL/kg/day
- Large-breed dogs: 50 mL/kg/day
- Medium/small-breed dogs: 60 mL/kg/day
- Puppies and kittens: 80–90 mL/kg/day
- Neonates: 100–140 mL/kg/day

Estimation of maintenance fluid requirements does not take into account the hydration status of the patient or potential additional ongoing losses such as vomiting and diarrhea. It is important to develop a more

Textbook of Small Animal Emergency Medicine, First Edition. Edited by Kenneth J. Drobatz, Kate Hopper, Elizabeth Rozanski and Deborah C. Silverstein.
© 2019 John Wiley & Sons, Inc. Published 2019 by John Wiley & Sons, Inc.
Companion Website: www.wiley.com/go/drobatz/textbook

comprehensive fluid plan for patients with pre-existing or ongoing losses.

Having decided upon an estimation and initiated maintenance fluid therapy, reassessment of the patient is critical. Serial physical examinations may be used to assess hydration status. In addition, once hydration is deemed corrected, monitoring the patient's body weight is another simple method of assessing fluid loss or gain. A patient should be weighed every 4–6 hours to monitor for weight gain or weight loss. For example, if the patient loses 0.2 kg over a 4-hour period, remembering that 1 kilogram is equal to 1000 mL of fluid, then the patient has lost a total of 200 mL of fluid or an average of 50 mL of fluid per hour. When using this method, it is important to use the same scale and methodology such as taking measurement of weight after a short walk to allow the animal to urinate and defecate.

Composition of a Maintenance Fluid

Crystalloids are often classified as maintenance or replacement fluids based on their sodium and potassium content. Maintenance fluids are indicated in patients that are not eating or drinking, but also do not suffer from hypovolemia, hypotension or excessive ongoing fluid losses. Maintenance fluids typically resemble fluid loss during normal processes such as sweating, panting, normal urination, and defecation. Often, these fluid losses are lower in sodium (hypotonic) and higher in potassium relative to patient serum composition. Most maintenance fluids will have a sodium content in the 50–70 mEq/L range and a potassium content in the 10–20 mEq/L range [6].

Many maintenance fluids also contain dextrose in order to supplement basal energy requirements and increase the osmolality of the fluid. When administered at conservative rates, the amount of dextrose added to common commercial fluid preparations supplies only a small percentage of the daily caloric requirements and is of little clinical utility in maintaining a patient's daily energy requirements [6]. However, if dextrose was not added to maintenance fluids, most of the preparations would have a dangerously low tonicity and osmolality compared with plasma. It is important to note that water distributes freely across all body compartments and dextrose is metabolized to water and carbon dioxide. Therefore, the dextrose in maintenance fluids does not affect the patient's plasma osmolality unless the patient becomes hyperglycemic.

The major differences between the various maintenance fluids available are addition of other electrolytes (such as calcium and magnesium) and type of buffer contained within the fluid (see Table 172.1).

The major buffers encountered in commercially prepared fluids include lactate, gluconate, and acetate. These commonly used buffers form salts of a weak acid when combined with sodium ions found in fluid preparations. The pKa of many of these buffers is near the pH of the patient and when administered intravenously, the salt will disassociate, resulting in a sodium ion and an acid anion (lactate, acetate, gluconate). The resulting acid anion will act as a weak base by binding hydrogen ions, producing bicarbonate during metabolism. Buffers help to offset the acidifying effect of sodium chloride-containing fluids. Generally, patients will not develop a significant metabolic alkalosis as excess bicarbonate is excreted by the kidneys [6].

Use of Maintenance Fluids

Maintenance fluids are primarily intended for use at conservative fluid rates and not for bolus therapy or aggressive fluid resuscitation in patients with a normal sodium concentration. Major electrolyte imbalances such as hyponatremia and hyperkalemia may occur with rapid or chronic administration due to the lower sodium content and higher potassium content of maintenance fluids. In addition, red blood cell lysis may occur with rapid intravenous administration of a hypotonic fluid as water moves into the red blood cells according to the sodium gradient.

Table 172.1 Composition of maintenance fluids.

Fluid	Na⁺ (mEq/L)	K⁺ (mEq/L)	Glucose (g/L)	Cl⁻ (mEq/L)	Ca²⁺ (mEq/L)	Mg²⁺ (mEq/L)	Buffer	Osmolarity (mOsmol/L)
0.45% NaCl	77	0	0	77	0	0	0	154
2.5% dextrose in 0.45% NaCl	77	0	25	77	0	0	0	280
Normosol-M in 5% dextrose*	40	13	50	40	0	3	Acetate 16 mEq/L	363
Plasma-Lyte 56 in 5% dextrose†	40	13	50	40	0	3	Acetate 16 mEq/L	363

*Hospira, Inc., Lake Forest, IL.
†Baxter Healthcare Pty Ltd., Toongabbie, NSW.

The major advantage of using a maintenance fluid to supplement daily fluid requirement is that the composition is closer to the actual typical daily fluid losses of patients. Use of replacement fluids, which are higher in sodium, may lead to natriuresis or sodium overload in some animals. Sodium is a major determinant of water balance within the body and excess body sodium may lead to hypervolemic states. Other potential uses of maintenance fluids include correction of electrolyte disturbances and rehydration or maintenance of hydration in patients with disease processes that predispose them to sodium overload (e.g. congestive heart failure, liver cirrhosis, and nephrotic syndrome). For example, management of a dehydrated patient with a history of significant heart disease and congestive heart failure can be challenging. Patients with congestive heart failure retain sodium due to decreased cardiac output, arterial underfilling, and poor renal perfusion leading to excessive activation of the renin-angiotensin-aldosterone system [7–9]. Hypovolemia and increased angiotensin II levels result in vasopressin release from the pituitary gland which leads to water retention via aquaporin-2 channels in the kidney [10–15]. Due to excess water retention, in addition to sodium retention, the patient plasma sodium level is often low due to a dilutional effect; however, there is still a total body excess of sodium.

While fluids are not typically administered to patients with congestive heart failure, occasionally, a patient with significant heart disease may become dehydrated and require fluid therapy. A maintenance fluid with lower sodium content is often the preferred fluid choice for use in these patients, although alternative fluid plans such as lower rates of isotonic crystalloids and free access to water may be more logical in hypovolemic or dehydrated patients. Typically, the patient is administered a conservative rate of maintenance fluids, the hydration status is frequently reassessed, and the fluids discontinued when the patient is rehydrated. During fluid administration, the patient must be closely monitored for signs of congestive heart failure such as an increased respiratory rate or effort, coughing, crackles on lung auscultation, or development of a gallop rhythm (predominantly in cats).

Lower sodium fluids are also indicated for resuscitation of patients suffering from chronic hyponatremia (>48h) in order to prevent a rapid increase in the sodium concentration (see Chapter 108). Rapid correction of a chronic hyponatremia may lead to permanent paralysis or death due to osmotic demyelination or central pontine myelinolysis [16–19]. Often, the duration of hyponatremia is difficult to ascertain and a reasonable precaution would be to manage all patients with an unknown duration of hyponatremia as if they were chronically affected. It is important to realize that even with a fluid containing a lower or similar sodium concentration to that of a patient's serum, the patient's sodium concentration may rise rapidly and frequent monitoring is necessary. If the patient's sodium concentration rises too quickly, it is recommended that the sodium rapidly be lowered down to a safer range using 5% dextrose in water solution.

Management of hypernatremia will also often require the use of lower sodium-containing fluids. Animals with mild elevations in sodium may benefit from treatment with hypotonic maintenance fluids rather than isotonic replacement fluids, but high fluid rates may lead to a rapid decline in blood sodium concentrations. During states of hypernatremia, the brain will form idiogenic osmoles to maintain normal cellular volume and prevent cell shrinkage and dehydration (see Chapter 108). If hypernatremia is corrected too quickly, the low serum sodium concentration will lead to a net movement of water into the cells of the brain, causing cerebral edema and potentially brain herniation. It is recommended to not exceed a change in the patient's serum sodium of greater than 0.5 mEq/L/h or 12 mEq/L in 24 hours [20,21].

Conclusion

In conclusion, it is important to develop a fluid plan that is tailored to the individual patient based on hydration, electrolyte status, and concurrent disease processes. The developed plan should be reassessed on a regular and consistent basis to ensure that hydration is maintained and that no acute dramatic shifts in fluid and electrolyte concentrations are experienced.

References

1 Wellman ML, DiBartola SP, Kohn CW. Applied physiology of body fluids in dogs and cats. In: *Fluid, Electrolyte, and Acid–Base Disorders in Small Animal Practice*, 3rd edn (ed. DiBartola SP). Elsevier, St Louis, 2006, pp. 3–26.
2 Harrison JB, Sussman HH, Pickering DE. Fluid and electrolyte therapy in small animals. *J Am Vet Med Assoc* 1960;137:637–645.
3 Haskins SC. Fluid and electrolyte therapy. *Compend Contin Educ Pract Vet* 1984;6:244–260.
4 Haskins SC. A simple fluid therapy planning guide. *Semin Vet Med Surg* 1988;3:227–236.
5 Davis H, Jensen T, Johnson A, et al. 2013 AAHA/AAFP fluid therapy guidelines for dogs and cats. *J Am Anim Hosp Assoc* 2013;49:149–159.

6 DiBartola SP, Bateman S. Introduction to fluid therapy. In: *Fluid, Electrolyte, and Acid–Base Disorders in Small Animal Practice*, 3rd edn (ed. DiBartola SP). Elsevier, St Louis, 2006, pp. 325–344.

7 Farmakis D, Filippatos G, Parissis J, Kremastinos DT, Gheorghiade M. Hyponatremia in heart failure. *Heart Fail Rev* 2009;14:59–63.

8 Sica DA. Hyponatremia and heart failure – pathophysiology and implications. *Congest Heart Fail* 2005;11:274–277.

9 Schrier RW. Water and sodium retention in edematous disorders: role of vasopressin and aldosterone. *Am J Med* 2006;119:S47–S53.

10 Brooks VL, Keil LC, Reid IA. Role of the renin-angiotensin system in the control of vasopressin secretion in conscious dogs. *Circ Res* 1986;58:829–838.

11 Schrier RW, Berl T, Anderson RJ. Osmotic and nonosmotic control of vasopressin release. *Am J Physiol* 1979;236:F321–F332.

12 Funayama H, Nakamura T, Saito T, et al. Urinary excretion of aquaporin-2 water channel exaggerated dependent upon vasopressin in congestive heart failure. *Kidney Int* 2004;66:1387–1392.

13 Kumar S, Rubin S, Mather PJ, Whellan DJ. Hyponatremia and vasopressin antagonism in congestive heart failure. *Clin Cardiol* 2007;30:546–551.

14 Nielsen S, Kwon TH, Christensen BM, Promeneur D, Frøkiaer J, Marples D. Physiology and pathophysiology of renal aquaporins. *J Am Soc Nephrol* 1999;10:647–663.

15 Radin JM, Yu M, Stoedkilde L, et al. Aquaporin-2 regulation in health and disease. *Vet Clin Pathol* 2012;41:455–470.

16 Sterns RH. Severe symptomatic hyponatremia: treatment and outcome. A study of 64 cases. *Ann Intern Med* 1987;107:656–664.

17 Sterns RH, Cappuccio JD, Silver SM, Cohen EP. Neurologic sequelae after treatment of severe hyponatremia: a multicenter perspective. *J Am Soc Nephrol* 1994;4:1522–1530.

18 Karp BI, Laureno R. Pontine and extrapontine myelinolysis: a neurologic disorder following rapid correction of hyponatremia. *Medicine* 1993;72:359–373.

19 Sterns RH, Riggs JE, Schochet SS Jr. Osmotic demyelination syndrome following correction of hyponatremia. *N Engl J Med* 1986;314:1535–1542.

20 DiBartola SP. Disorders of sodium and water: hypernatremia and hyponatremia. In: *Fluid, Electrolyte, and Acid–Base Disorders in Small Animal Practice*, 3rd edn (ed. DiBartola SP). Elsevier, St Louis, 2006, pp. 47–79.

21 Sterns RH, Spital A, Clark EC. Disorders of water balance. In: *Fluids and Electrolytes* (eds Kokko JP, Tannen RL). WB Saunders, Philadelphia, 1996, p. 63.

173

Potassium Supplementation
Jillian DiFazio, DVM, DACVECC

Veterinary Emergency and Referral Group, Brooklyn, NY, USA

Introduction

Hypokalemia is a common electrolyte disorder. Extrapolation from the human literature would support a relatively high incidence, with 20% of hospitalized patients affected by this derangement [1]. As the major intracellular cation, potassium is essential for the maintenance of a normal resting cell membrane potential. Hypokalemia results in a more negative resting membrane potential, thereby hyperpolarizing the cell, and contributes to muscle weakness, electrocardiographic changes, and arrhythmias [2]. Therefore, potassium supplementation is a crucial aspect of fluid therapy for the hospitalized, and particularly critically ill, patient.

Potassium Physiology

Knowledge of the role of potassium in generating the resting membrane potential is essential in understanding the importance of supplementation in hypokalemic states. The majority of body potassium (roughly 98%) is located intracellularly with concentrations of approximately 140 mEq/L intracellularly and 4 mEq/L extracellularly. This normal relationship is maintained by cellular membrane Na/K-ATPase that pumps sodium ions out of and potassium ions into a cell in a 3:2 ratio. This results in a concentration gradient for potassium to flow extracellularly.

Because the cell membrane is impermeable to most intracellular anions, a net electrical difference is generated across the cell membrane with potassium outward flow. This electrical difference or resting cell membrane potential is crucial in the generation of action potentials in excitable tissues (i.e. cardiac muscle, skeletal muscle, nerves). Hypokalemia, by increasing the concentration difference across the cell membrane, results in a more negative resting membrane potential and hyperpolarization

of the cell. It is therefore readily apparent that while the absolute amount of potassium is important, the ratio of the potassium concentration intracellularly relative to the concentration extracellularly is perhaps more important when considering the clinical implications of hypokalemia. Generally, extracellular (and therefore plasma) concentrations of potassium are reflective of total body potassium stores. In certain conditions, as will be discussed below, this is not always the case [2,3].

Normal potassium levels are maintained by intake (namely the diet) and output (approximately 90–95% via the kidneys, the remainder via the gastrointestinal tract). An additional aspect of potassium balance is the normal distribution of potassium between the cells and the extracellular fluid. At the cellular level, potassium balance is mainly affected by the upregulation of Na/K-ATPase by insulin and beta-2 adrenergic stimulation. Additionally, acid–base status has an impact on potassium distribution with acidosis, typically resulting in the movement of potassium extracellularly and alkalosis leading to intracellular movement [2,3].

Causes of Hypokalemia

When considering causes of hypokalemia, it is important to distinguish total body potassium depletion and extracellular (or plasma) measured hypokalemia. Total body potassium depletion is typically a consequence of excessive loss from the kidneys and gastrointestinal tract. Excessive renal loss occurs with chronic kidney disease, postobstructive diureses, dialysis, mineralocorticoid excess, and treatment with drugs (namely loop diuretics). Other processes that result in a primary or secondary polyuria also can result in hypokalemia, due to increased tubular flow and decreased renal reabsorption. Excessive gastrointestinal loss occurs primarily as a consequence of vomiting [2].

Textbook of Small Animal Emergency Medicine, First Edition. Edited by Kenneth J. Drobatz, Kate Hopper, Elizabeth Rozanski and Deborah C. Silverstein.
© 2019 John Wiley & Sons, Inc. Published 2019 by John Wiley & Sons, Inc.
Companion Website: www.wiley.com/go/drobatz/textbook

Anorexic patients that are not experiencing excessive gastrointestinal or renal loss of potassium are usually normokalemic. However, when treated with intravenous fluid therapy not containing potassium supplementation, these patients can frequently develop an iatrogenic dilutional hypokalemia [2].

A measured plasma hypokalemia in spite of normal total body potassium levels occurs in conditions that cause increased translocation of potassium from extracellular to intracellular fluid. Conditions include alkalemia, administration of insulin, glucose-containing fluids or other insulin-inducing products, medications or states (i.e. xylitol, oral hypoglycemic medications, refeeding syndrome), catecholamines (as a result of beta-2 agonist stimulation), hypothermia, albuterol overdose, thyrotoxicosis, barium toxicosis, and hypokalemic periodic paralysis of Burmese cats [4–7].

Potassium supplementation is an important consideration in all patients, but in patients with excessive loss or those with conditions predisposing to increased intracellular translocation of potassium, supplementation becomes critical.

Clinical Signs of Hypokalemia

Many patients with hypokalemia do not have any clinical signs. Muscle weakness, polyuria, and polydipsia are the most common clinical signs reported. It is important to remember that there is individual variation in the potassium level at which clinical signs of hypokalemia develop. This occurs for two primary reasons. As discussed previously, the effect of hypokalemia is dependent predominantly upon the degree to which there is a similar change in intracellular potassium concentration. The measured plasma potassium is not always an accurate reflection of alterations in the intracellular:extracellular potassium ratio. Additionally, membrane excitability is determined by factors other than potassium, including calcium concentration and blood pH, that may result in clinical signs independent of potassium derangements [3].

Muscle weakness typically develops when serum potassium is less than 3 mEq/L, increases in creatine kinase occur when potassium decreases to less than 2.5 mEq/L, and rhabdomyolysis may occur when potassium decreases to less than 2 mEq/L. Hindend weakness and plantigrade stance may be seen in dogs and cats with hypokalemia. Cervical ventroflexion is commonly observed in hypokalemic cats. Hypokalemia also can result in respiratory muscle weakness, potentially necessitating ventilatory support [2].

Hypokalemia also can result in cardiac arrhythmias (see Chapter 53), by delaying ventricular repolarization and increasing the duration of the action potential and automaticity. Generally, this does not occur until potassium levels are less than or equal to 2.5 mmol/L [1]. ECG changes are inconsistently seen in veterinary patients, but can occur. Supraventricular and ventricular arrhythmias occur more frequently than ECG changes. ECG alterations associated with hypokalemia include blunted T-waves, ST segment depression, and U-waves. Additionally, hypokalemia can decrease the clinical response to class I antiarrhythmic medications [2].

Hypokalemia also can result in hypokalemic nephropathy, characterized by renal vasoconstriction leading to a decrease in renal blood flow and glomerular filtration rate. Polyuria and polydipsia occur because of impaired responsiveness to antidiuretic hormone [2].

Potassium Supplementation

It is important to remember that the clinical guidelines for potassium supplementation are merely guidelines. Due to the inconsistent relationship of measured plasma potassium levels with total body potassium levels and intracellular:extracellular ratio and independent factors that impact translocation, serial monitoring is imperative. This monitoring is particularly important in patients with severe hypokalemia, those that are demonstrating clinical signs of hypokalemia and those that have factors affecting translocation (i.e. treatment with insulin, significant acid–base derangements, treatment with beta-blockers or beta-agonist toxicity). Please see Table 173.1 for commonly used guidelines for potassium supplementation.

Maintenance potassium supplementation to account for dilutional effects of intravenous fluid therapy (particularly in the anorexic animal) is roughly 0.05 mEq/kg/h. Frequently, it is recommended to limit potassium supplementation to <0.5 mEq/kg/h. However, there are also reports of supplementation with 0.5–0.9 mEq/kg/h in cases of life-threatening hypokalemia [8,9]. Due to concerns for life-threatening complications that can occur with supplementation greater than 0.5 mEq/kg/h,

Table 173.1 Guidelines for intravenous potassium supplementation in dogs and cats [2].

Serum potassium concentration (mEq/L)	mEq KCl to add to 1 L	Maximal fluid infusion rate* (mL/kg/h)
<2.0	80	6
2.1–2.5	60	8
2.6–3.0	40	12
3.1–3.5	28	18
3.6–5	20	25

*So as to not exceed 0.5 mEq/kg/h.

continuous electrocardiographic assessment should be performed to ensure that these do not occur. ECG changes that may be seen with too rapid infusion of potassium include tented T-waves, shortening of the QT interval, prolongation of the PR interval, widening of the QRS complex, shortening or absence of P-waves, development of pronounced bradycardia with sinoventricular rhythm, merging of the QRS complex with the T-wave creating a sine wave appearance, ventricular fibrillation, and finally ventricular asystole [10]. It is also important to remember that higher concentrations of potassium supplementation (i.e. greater than 60 mEq/L) should be infused via a central line due to higher concentrations potentially resulting in phlebitis when administered peripherally [3].

For patients that remain refractory hypokalemic despite high-level supplementation, it is important to consider supplementation of magnesium. Hypomagnesemia can result in secondary potassium depletion. This occurs because potassium secretion from the cells of the thick ascending limb of the loop of Henle and the cortical collecting tubule is mediated by ATP-inhibitable luminal potassium channels. Hypomagnesemia leads to a decrease in intracellular magnesium which can result in decreased ATP levels. Decreased ATP causes loss of inhibition of potassium secretion. Supplementation of magnesium in these cases in necessary to correct hypokalemia. Magnesium can be supplemented as magnesium sulfate in D5W, administered at 0.75–1 mEq/kg/day as a CRI with gradual taper as dictated by serial measurements [11].

Supplementation of potassium intravenously typically involves the use of KCl (2 mEq K/mL) and potassium phosphate (4.4 mEq K/mL). Potassium chloride is typically used in patients who do not have concurrent hypophosphatemia. Potassium chloride is generally recommended over potassium phosphate because chloride supplementation is also useful in managing the metabolic alkalosis that many patients concurrently demonstrate. Chloride depletion can exacerbate potassium depletion by enhancing urinary loss of potassium [2]. If both potassium chloride and potassium phosphate are being administered to a patient, potassium supplementation rates of both preparations should be calculated to ensure appropriate rates of administration.

Even with supplementation, it is not uncommon to see a decrease prior to increase in serum potassium concentrations as a result of dilution and increased tubular flow rates and/or increased cellular uptake if dextrose or insulin is being administered [12]. This should be kept in mind when considering supplementation rates.

It is also possible to enterally supplement potassium and there have been many recent studies in human medicine comparing parenteral versus enteral supplementation with some evidence to support that enteral supplementation or a combination of the two

may in some cases be preferable [13–15]. Potassium gluconate (Tumil-K) or potassium citrate (not potassium chloride or potassium bicarbonate) is recommended for oral supplementation. Doses for oral potassium supplementation are extremely variable and serial monitoring is recommended to achieve an optimal oral dose [2].

Support for enteral supplementation of potassium is relevant in patients that continue to have clinically relevant electrolyte derangements in spite of improvement/resolution in the underlying disease process, are off intravenous fluid therapy and are otherwise able to be discharged from the hospital successfully. Additionally, there is some risk in potassium supplementation, particularly when considering the inconsistencies of supplementation and the effect inadequate mixing can have on delivered rates of potassium supplementation. A recent study evaluated potassium supplementation in bags of fluids delivered to hospitalized patients (intended versus measured) and the effects of adequate/inadequate mixing on rates of supplementation. The disparities were profound, with measured potassium in hospitalized patients being significantly higher than intended potassium concentrations (mean difference was 9.0 mmol/L with a range of 6.5 to >280 mmol/L, P < 0.0001). In 28% of samples the potassium difference between actual measured and intended concentrations was ≥5 mmol/L [16].

There is additional evidence to support oral supplementation in patients with hypokalemia secondary to diuretic therapy. A recent study in human medicine evaluated survival benefit in patients empirically supplemented with potassium at the initiation of loop diuretic therapy. This was found to be associated with improved survival, with greater benefit seen with patients supplemented with higher diuretic dosages [17].

Diabetic Ketoacidosis (see Chapter 113)

Diabetic ketoacidosis (DKA) is likely the condition most commonly associated with clinically significant hypokalemia in veterinary medicine. While historically a prevalent issue in human medicine, a recent study documented that hypokalemia was less common than previously reported [18].

Hypokalemia occurs as a result of both the underlying condition (with total body potassium depletion occurring) as a result of osmotic diuresis due to glucosuria and ketonuria, lack of insulin (required for normal reabsorption of potassium at the renal tubules) and gastrointestinal losses), fluid therapy (dilution effect) and the need for insulin supplementation. It is also important to remember that frequently plasma concentrations of potassium are generally increased in the diabetic ketotic/ketoacidotic patient relative to total body concentrations and that with initiation of treatment, plasma concentrations largely decrease. Extracellular or plasma concentrations are increased as a result of the volume expansion effects of hyperglycemia with associated tendency for potassium shifts from the intracellular to extracellular compartment. Decreased glomerular filtration rates with volume depletion that occurs as a result of osmotic diuresis can result in eventual renal losses. With initiation of fluid therapy and associated volume expansion and insulin supplementation, true total body potassium deficits become reflected in plasma concentrations [11].

The largest study examining clinical findings in canine patients with DKA revealed that intake hypokalemia was documented in 45% of patients and 84% of patients developed a hypokalemia with treatment, resulting in an overall incidence of 92% of cases [19]. Hypokalemia was

also documented to be a common electrolyte derangement in cats with DKA [20]. As a consequence of this, it is generally recommended to delay insulin administration until volume expansion and adequacy of potassium concentrations are achieved. In human medicine, this is considered to be ≥3.3 mmol/L [21].

There is some evidence advocating earlier initiation of insulin therapy in veterinary patients [22]. Therefore, higher supplementation rates than standard would be administered for rapidity of correction. With higher rates of supplementation, more frequent serial evaluations should be performed. After starting fluid or insulin therapy, serum electrolyte concentrations ideally should be re-evaluated 1–2 hours later and then every 4–6 hours until normal hydration and adequate glycemic control are achieved [11].

References

1 Weir MR, Espaillat R. Clinical perspectives on the rationale for potassium supplementation. *Postgrad Med* 2015;127(5):539–548.
2 DiBartola SP, de Morais HA. Disorders of potassium: hypokalemia and hyperkalemia. In: *Fluid, Electrolyte and Acid–Base Disorders*, 4th edn (ed. DiBartola SP). Elsevier Saunders, St Louis, 2012, pp. 92–119.
3 Rose BD. Hypokalemia. In: *Clinical Physiology of Acid–Base and Electrolyte Disorders*, 5th edn (ed. Rose BD). McGraw-Hill, New York, 2001, pp. 836–887.
4 Fryers A, Elwood C. Hypokalemia in a hyperthyroid domestic shorthair cat with adrenal hyperplasia. *J Feline Med Surg* 2014;16(10):853–857.
5 Mackenzie SD, Blois S, Hayes G, et al. Oral thermal injury associated with puncture of a salbutamol metered-dose inhaler in a dog. *J Vet Emerg Crit Care* 2012;22(4):494–497.
6 McCown J, Lechner E, Cooke K. Suspected albuterol toxicosis in a dog. *J Am Vet Med Assoc* 2008;8:1168–1171.
7 Adam FH, Noble PJ, Swift ST, et al. Barium toxicosis in a dog. *J Am Vet Med Assoc* 2010;237(5):547–550.
8 Hamill RJ, Robinson LM, Wexler HR, et al. Efficacy and safety of potassium infusion therapy in hypokalemic critically ill patients. *Crit Care Med* 1991;19(5):694–699.
9 O'Brien MA. Diabetic emergencies in small animals. *Vet Clin North Am Small Anim Pract* 2010;40(2):317–333.
10 Tag TL, Day TK. Electrocardiographic assessment of hyperkalemia in dogs and cats. *J Vet Emerg Crit Care* 2008;18(1):61–67.
11 Boysen SR. Fluid and electrolyte therapy in endocrine disorders: diabetes mellitus and hypoadrenocorticism. *Vet Clin North Am Small Anim Pract* 2008;38(3):699–717.
12 Dow SW, LeCouteur RA, Fettman MJ, et al. Hypokalemia in cats: 186 cases (1984–1987). *J Am Vet Med Assoc* 1989;194:1604.
13 Merchant Q, Rehman Siddiqui NU, Rehmat A, et al. Comparison of enteral versus intravenous potassium supplementation in postcardiac surgery paediatric cardiac intensive care patients: prospective open label randomized control trial (EIPS). *BMJ Open* 2014;4(9):1–22.
14 Moffett BS, McDade E, Rossano JW, et al. Enteral potassium supplementation in pediatric cardiac intensive care unit: evaluation of practice change. *Pediatr Crit Care Med* 2011;12(5):552–554.
15 Hainsworth AJ, Gatenby PA. Oral potassium supplementation in surgical patients. *Int J Surg* 2008;6(4):287–288.
16 Hoehne SN, Hopper K, Epstein SE. Accuracy of potassium supplementation of fluids administered intravenously. *J Vet Intern Med* 2015;29(3):834–839.
17 Leonard CE, Razzaghi H, Freeman CP, et al. Empiric potassium supplementation and increased survival in users of loop diuretics. *Publ Libr Sci One* 2014;9(7):1–22.
18 Jang TB, Chauhan V, Morchi R, et al. Hypokalemia in diabetic ketoacidosis is less common than previously reported. *Intern Emerg Med* 2015;10(2):177–180.
19 Hume DZ, Drobatz KJ, Hess RS. Outcome of dogs with diabetic ketoacidosis: 127 dogs (1993–2003). *J Vet Intern Med* 2006;20(3):547–555.
20 Bruskiewicz KA, Nelson RW, Feldman EC, et al. Diabetic ketosis and ketoacidosis in cats: 42 cases (1980–1995). *J Am Vet Med Assoc* 1997;211(2):188–192.
21 Kitabchi A, Umpierrez G, Murphy M, et al. Hyperglycemic crises in diabetes. *Diabetes Care* 2004;27(1):S94–102.
22 DiFazio J, Fletcher DJ. Retrospective comparison of early- versus late- insulin therapy regarding effect on time to resolution of diabetic ketosis and ketoacidosis in dogs and cats: 60 cases (2003-2013). *J Vet Emerg Crit Care* 2016;26(1):108–115.

174

Administration of Sodium Bicarbonate
Jennifer E. Waldrop, DVM, DACVECC

BluePearl Veterinary Specialty and Emergency Pet Hospital, Seattle, WA, USA

Introduction

Sodium bicarbonate (SB) has been studied extensively in multiple disease states including cardiopulmonary resuscitation, renal disease, intoxications, and acidosis. Despite a large body of research, the therapeutic role of SB and its efficacy are still in doubt [1–6]. Still, some evidence for SB use persists and will be discussed here. Other injectable buffers do exist, including carbicarb (not commercially available at this time) and THAM (significant concern for side-effects) [7,8]. SB is considered CO_2 generating, whereas these other buffers are considered CO_2 consuming and may have some advantages that have not been clearly validated [9]. This chapter will focus only on IV SB; oral SB therapy and SB use in dialysis will not be covered.

Bicarbonate is an important buffer in the body, combining with protons to form CO_2 and water via carbonic anhydrase in two steps. Ventilation and renal compensation then waste excess acid. The role of the lungs and kidneys in acid–base homeostasis cannot be overemphasized since the pK for the bicarbonate buffering system is well below normal pH of the extracellular fluid (pH 5.1–7.1) although the pH in cells is usually lower than serum (7.1–7.3). Bicarbonate is also an important blood transport molecule for CO_2 as it returns from cells [10]. The complexity of the physiological role of bicarbonate and CO_2 likely explains the variable experimental results seen so often.

Sodium bicarbonate is a convenient buffer as it has no requirement for metabolism to alkalinize. Therefore, unlike buffers such as lactate and acetate used in balanced electrolyte solutions, SB is able to have immediate effect. For example, in normal, non-acidotic dogs, infusion of 6.6 mEq/kg SB over 30 minutes produced transient alkalemia, hypercapnia, and reduction in H+ ions as predicted. These changes were sustained for greater than 180 minutes after starting the infusion [11]. Cats

administered variable doses (0.5–4 mEq/kg) over 1 minute had dose- and time-dependent increases in pH, PCO_2, and HCO_3 but to a smaller magnitude than dogs [12]. The ability of SB to raise the pH of the intracellular fluid (pHi) has been harder to consistently document. This may be due to separate compartments with differing permeabilities throughout the body and the fact that bicarbonate is "not an independent determinant of blood pH" [9]. SB has varying effects on pHi of the myocardium, CSF, liver, and skeletal muscle from study to study but the majority of studies document no change or a fall in pHi [9].

Sodium bicarbonate is a hypertonic solution with a sodium concentration similar to common hypertonic saline solutions (Table 174.1). SB also contains dissolved CO_2 and may have a PCO_2 as high as 200 mmHg [5]. After IV administration of SB, 10–15% is immediately metabolized to CO_2; therefore, hypoventilation and an impaired ability to change ventilation (e.g. sedation or obtundation) are both contraindications for SB use [13]. Hypernatremia, hypokalemia, and hypocalcemia (ionized and total) may also result from bolus injections but not always in a clinically significant amount [14,15]. Other possible but variably evident complications of SB include impairment of tissue oxygenation, diffusion of PCO_2 across cell membranes more quickly than the charged HCO_3^- ion, causing intracellular acidosis, paradoxical cerebrospinal fluid acidosis, and lowering of blood pressure, presumably from the vasoactive properties of a hypertonic solution [13,16]. Excessive use

Table 174.1 Comparison of hypertonic saline (HS) and sodium bicarbonate (SB).

	7.2% HS [69,70]	SB 8.4% [13,17]
[Na] meQ/L	1232	1000
Osmolarity mOsm/L	2464	2000
Dose (bolus)	4 mL/kg over 2–10 min	1–4 mL/kg over 5–10 min

Textbook of Small Animal Emergency Medicine, First Edition. Edited by Kenneth J. Drobatz, Kate Hopper, Elizabeth Rozanski and Deborah C. Silverstein.
© 2019 John Wiley & Sons, Inc. Published 2019 by John Wiley & Sons, Inc.
Companion Website: www.wiley.com/go/drobatz/textbook

of SB, as with other hypertonic solutions, can cause a hyperosmolar state and possible fluid overload so SB is contraindicated with hypernatremia and heart failure [17,18].

Major uses of SB in clinical medicine are to buffer acidic blood, treat significant bicarbonate-rich fluid loss, elevate urinary pH to increase solubility of certain weak acids and toxins and possibly in hyperkalemic conditions (see Chapter 109).

Metabolic Acidosis (see Chapter 107)

It is generally agreed that SB is indicated in the treatment of metabolic acidosis from bicarbonate loss, including severe diarrhea or renal tubular acidosis [8,13,16] (see Chapter 107 for an extensive discussion of acid–base disorders). Common clinical disorders causing acidosis in small animal practice include lactic, uremic, and diabetic ketoacidosis.

Is Acidosis Harmful?

Both beneficial and harmful side-effects of acidosis have been found in clinical and experimental models. Severe acidemia (pH <7.20) may decrease CO, MAP, myocardial contractility, and hepatic and renal blood flow. Acidemia may shift potassium out of cells in exchange for protons but this effect is variable and mild hyperkalemia could occur [13]. Metabolic effects include a decreased response to catecholamines, insulin resistance, and reduced lactate clearance by the liver [8]. Acidemia causes arterial vasodilation, venoconstriction and shifts the oxyhemoglobin curve to the right, increasing tissue off-loading of oxygen (Bohr effect) [19]. Initially, the right shift can be of benefit, offloading more oxygen to the tissues, but over 6–8 hours the body normalizes with a decrease in 2,3-DPG to shift the oxyhemoglobin curve back to the left. There is some evidence that an increase in ionized calcium occurs due to a shift of albumin, calcium's carrier in blood; this effect may increase myocardial contractility, countering the direct effects of acidosis to a degree [19]. While in some studies, acidosis had other protective effects including delayed apoptosis and limiting myocardial infarct size, other studies noted increased apoptosis [9,19].

Part of the problem in assessing the detrimental effects of low arterial pH (pHa) is a lack of correlation with the pH of the venous or pulmonary circulation, especially in low- or no-flow states [20]. This discrepancy extends to pHi in which both the mitochondrial and cytoplasmic pH may differ and vary in resulting pathology [9,19]. For many patients, it is difficult to isolate the effect of acidemia from the detrimental effect of their underlying disease (e.g. sepsis, renal failure). Severe acidemia is generally well tolerated in mechanically ventilated patients with permissive hypercapnia [9]. Persistent hyperlactatemia is a known risk for mortality independent of pH.

Uremic Acidosis

Acute or acute-on-chronic renal failure presents commonly in the ER and is usually accompanied by a moderate-to-severe acidosis. Treatment with buffered IV fluids (lactated Ringer's, Normosol) is generally sufficient to steadily correct uremic metabolic acidosis. No veterinary studies have been performed on the use of SB in uremic patients, to the author's knowledge. Contraindications to SB treatment found in uremic patients could include hypernatremia, dehydration, decreased mentation and poor renal excretion of excess alkali. Therapy with dialysis is indicated in humans with continued acidosis in renal failure.

Diabetic Ketoacidosis (see Chapter 113)

The acidosis of DKA may be solely due to ketoacids, beta-hydroxybutyrate, and acetoacetate, which deplete bicarbonate [21]. Commonly, it is a mixed disorder due to volume depletion and impaired tissue perfusion with lactate production and acute kidney injury, combined with the effects of any concurrent disorders (e.g. infection, pancreatitis) [22,23].

According to the medical literature, treatment of DKA with SB has not been successful and has been associated with hypokalemia, intracellular acidosis, and worsened tissue hypoxia. Two studies reported a paradoxical worsening of ketonemia, while others reported no improvement in insulin requirement or resolution of ketosis [22]. Treatments with standard therapy (IV fluids, insulin, electrolytes) will convert ketoacids to bicarbonate without the need for SB. Some clinicians still treat the subset of humans with a pH of <6.9 with SB until pH is greater than 6.9, but it is not clear that SB is useful even in the most severely acidotic patients [21].

In a retrospective study of 127 DKA dogs, Hume et al. noted the use of SB in 34%. Dogs treated with bicarbonate had lower pH and longer hospitalization and were less likely to be discharged. Treatment with SB likely reflected a higher severity of illness [23]. Oster et al. induced ketoacidosis in dogs with injections of beta-hydroxybutyrate. Treatment with SB improved pH and decreased potassium to a small degree [24]. Bureau et al. induced ketosis in diabetic dogs and found that SB worsened CSF PO_2 and pH. Dogs treated with SB progressively deteriorated after the study and demonstrated worsening mentation and vomiting. The authors compared this decline to cerebral edema in DKA humans observed 4–16 hours after starting treatment [25]. Interestingly, in a study of DKA rats, SB treatment improved arterial pH and pHi of myocardial cells but increased lactate and beta-hydroxybutyrate and worsened blood pressure [26]. Clinical prospective studies are lacking, but the general recommendation for SB in DKA animals is to limit use to patients with pHa < 7.0 or 7.1 despite IV fluids and insulin [13,27,28].

Lactic Acidosis (see Chapter 156)

There are no clinical studies in small animals regarding naturally occurring lactic acidosis (LA) and treatment with SB. Experimental studies have been performed in dogs by injecting compounds to increase lactate without tissue hypoxia (type B) or by reducing inspired oxygen concentration or blood volume to induce hypoxic LA (type A). In two studies of type B LA, SB was ineffective in changing pHa [29] or actually decreased pHa [30], increased arterial lactate, and decreased pHi in liver and RBCs [29]. In other animal models of type B LA, researchers have found similar results and increases in mortality with SB [31].

Hypoxic LA was investigated in four canine models all of which documented an increase in arterial lactate after SB treatment [31–34]. No study documented an improvement in pHa (two unchanged [32,33], two lower [31,34]), cardiovascular parameters, or pHi of liver or myocardial cells. All four studies lacked resuscitation efforts and were performed entirely under hypoxic conditions and therefore are difficult to compare to normal clinical situations. Without oxygen and adequate ventilation, anaerobic metabolism dominates and SB treatment may shunt pyruvate to more lactate by disinhibition of PFK. Intracellular acidosis inhibits PFK to limit production of pyruvate and, in energy-depleted cells, pyruvate shunting to lactate [31,35].

Iberti et al. studied a canine hemorrhagic shock model comparing saline and SB without resuscitation. They observed no change in pHa or HCO_3 but lactate did increase [36]. Benjamin et al. resuscitated dogs with induced hemorrhagic shock for 30 minutes after treatment with SB or hypertonic saline and found that SB did increase pHa and bicarbonate, but severely elevated PCO_2 and increased lactate. Improvements in MAP and cardiac output seen with SB were similar to hypertonic saline controls [37].

The medical literature echoes the findings in animal studies. One study of severely ill and lactic acidotic humans found that SB use was an independent risk factor for mortality [38]. Currently, SB is not recommended for LA regardless of pHa. Treatment of LA should focus on treatment of the underlying disease [8]. Dialysis may be the next treatment option for LA when standard treatments are not successful.

Cardiopulmonary Cerebral Resuscitation
(see Chapter 150)

Quality cardiopulmonary cerebral resuscitation (CPCR) with ventilation with oxygen, support of tissue perfusion and high-quality chest compressions to restore some cardiac output, and rapid return of spontaneous circulation (ROSC) are the mainstays of restoring acid–base balance during cardiac arrest [2]. The current American Heart Association (AHA) guidelines do not recommend SB in CPCR except under special circumstances, including cocaine and antiarrhythmic (Ia and Ic) overdose and hyperkalemia [1,2]. The RECOVER guidelines echo that sentiment; SB is not recommended routinely but can be considered in prolonged CPCR >10–15 minutes without ROSC [39,40].

There is no doubt that cardiopulmonary arrest causes significant mixed acidosis (hypoxic, lactic, hypercapnic) by itself and some patients may have a pre-existing acidosis. In a recent review of acid–base and electrolyte abnormalities in CPCR in dogs and cats, 88% were acidemic (median pH 6.79), hypercapnic (median PCO_2 64 mmHg), and hyperlactatemic (median 16 mmol/L) [41]. Despite documented acidosis in arrest, when CPCR treatment modalities were compared for impact on ROSC in a large university study of CPCR, SB administration was not significant [42].

The debate over SB in CPCR is understandable when you consider the puzzling results found in similarly devised studies. There are many canine studies examining SB and its impact on ROSC, fibrillation threshold, pHi, mortality, and neurological outcome. Most of these studies are in models of induced ventricular fibrillation (VFIB). In our limited CPCR literature, VFIB is the documented arrest rhythm in 7–20% [42–44].

The appropriate treatment for VFIB is timely defibrillation [2,39]. AHA guidelines recommend vasopressors only after multiple unsuccessful defibrillation attempts. With >4 minutes of arrest, a brief period of CPCR prior to defibrillation is suggested but the benefit of more prolonged CPCR is unclear [2]. After excluding one study that preloaded SB prior to prolonged arrest [45], there are four survival studies with improved outcomes using bolus SB [46–49]. Significant improvements in ROSC (77–90% of dogs) and survival (66–73%) were seen after 10–15 minutes of VFIB arrest. Two studies noted good neurological outcomes in survivors [46,48], one did not comment [47], and one reported poor outcomes for all dogs [49]. All studies employed some CPCR per AHA guidelines, including epinephrine in four studies, atropine in two, and ventilation to maintain normocapnia in all four.

The importance of efficient CPCR is highlighted in a short arrest study by Minuck and Sharma in which both

SB and control animals were defibrillated and resuscitated quickly with open chest CPCR and ventilation. Of note, in that study no adverse effects of SB treatment were reported (alkalemia or hypercapnia) [50]. Two studies in canine VFIB arrest could not identify SB-induced paradoxical CSF acidosis [51,52] and in one of those, SB maintained pHi brain over control [51].

Many of the canine VFIB and SB studies cited as "associated with worse outcome" [39] in CPCR have designs that hamper the drawing of clear conclusions. For example, three studies by Bleske et al. in short arrest (<5 min) used variable timing of SB and varied protocols (SB bolus versus CRI, ±epinephrine), treated mildly acidotic and non-acidotic dogs with SB (pH >7.32 in all studies), and the experiments induced arrest serially in the same dogs for multiple studies [53–55]. Study design complicated interpretation of results in additional VFIB canine research by using arrest dogs multiple times as their own controls [56], treating only moderate acidemia (pHa >7.2) [15,57,58], short arrest (≤4 min) [15,57,58], and late defibrillation (>18 min post arrest) [59]. One study documenting paradoxical CSF acidosis in short-arrest, non-defibrillated dogs administered SB when they were not acidotic (pHa mean 7.4) and used large, repeated doses of SB, a protocol chosen by the authors because it "frequently culminate[s] in metabolic alkalosis" [58].

There is evidence in the medical literature that SB should be reconsidered in specific arrest conditions: prolonged good CPCR without ROSC (>10–15 min), documented acidemia, and out-of-hospital arrests [60–62]. Empirical use of SB is not advocated for witnessed arrest or short arrests as overshoot alkalemia may occur [63].

Hyperkalemia (see Chapter 109)

Recommendations for treatment of life-threatening hyperkalemia have generally included SB administration [1,13,27,64,65]. Calcium is administered first to immediately stabilize the myocardial cell membrane, then insulin/glucose to increase an influx of K (in exchange for Na) into cells. The effect of insulin/glucose occurs within 10–20 minutes, lasts 4–6 hours and can be expected to decrease K 0.6–1.0 mEq/L [66]. SB has been thought to act similarly until recently. New evidence in dialysis patients calls into question the ability of SB to cause intracellular influx of K. In multiple studies, SB administration alone has not effectively lowered potassium in dialysis patients [8,66–68]. It is theorized that the modest potassium-lowering effect of SB is instead due to enhanced renal excretion of potassium and is dependent on intact renal function [66]. The current medical recommendation is to avoid SB use for treatment of hyperkalemia unless the patient is also severely acidotic [8,66–68].

In small animal medicine, common causes of hyperkalemia include urinary tract obstruction or rupture, hypoadrenocorticism, and acute kidney injury (AKI). Most will respond to IV fluid therapy and restoration of renal perfusion, treatment of the underlying disorder (e.g. "unblocking," DOCP), and use of calcium or insulin/glucose as necessary. The hyperkalemia of AKI may necessitate dialysis treatment.

Dosage and Administration

As discussed above, it is difficult to make specific recommendations for SB given the lack of clear efficacy and clinical indications. Clinicians have many choices among recommendations for dose and administration timing as there is no clear consensus in the medical or veterinary literature, other than "not too fast and not too much" (Table 174.2). Many sources recommend dosing based on bicarbonate deficit and titrating to an acceptable pH but this can be difficult given that the

Table 174.2 Administration strategies for intravenous sodium bicarbonate [13,40,53,65].

Disease state	Clinical caveats	Dosage	Time of administration
CPCR	Prolonged CPCR without ROSC (>10–15 min)	1 mEq/kg	5–10 min or
	Documented metabolic acidosis		0.1 mEq/kg/min
Hyperkalemia	After calcium and insulin/glucose	1–2 mEq/kg	Variable, 10–15 min
	Ensure adequate urine output		
	Documented metabolic acidosis		
Metabolic acidosis	First address underlying disease	Calculate desired [HCO_3]	Variable, 1–24 h, recheck bloodwork prior to readministration
	Contraindicated in LA	Titrate	
		Increase pH only to 7.1 or 7.2	

CPCR, cardiopulmonary cerebral resuscitation; LA, lactic acidosis; ROSC, return of spontaneous circulation.

volume of distribution (Vd) of SB is highly variable (0.2–0.5×body weight) and treating to "normal" can lead to alkalemia [27,65]. Another strategy is to calculate to an "acceptable" $[HCO_3]$ of 10 or 12 mEq/L as follows: body weight (kg)×(Vd)×(desired $[HCO_3]$ – current $[HCO_3]$) [13,19]. For example, a 10 kg dog with a current $[HCO_3]$ of 6 mEq/L could be given 15–30 mEq of SB (10×(0.25–0.5)×(12–6)).

References

1 Vanden Hoek TL, Morrison LJ, Shuster M, et al. Part 12: Cardiac arrest in special circumstances: 2010 American Heart Association guidelines for cardiopulmonary resuscitation and emergency cardiovascular care. *Circulation* 2010;122(Suppl 3):S829–S861.

2 Neumar RW, Otto CW, Link MS, et al. Part 8: Adult advanced cardiovascular life support: 2010 American Heart Association guidelines for cardiopulmonary resuscitation and emergency cardiovascular care. *Circulation* 2010;122(Suppl 3):S729–S767.

3 Zaritsky A. Bicarbonate in cardiac arrest: the good, the bad, and the puzzling. *Crit Care Med* 1995;23:429–431.

4 Arieff AI. Efficacy of buffers in the management of cardiac arrest. *Crit Care Med* 1998;26:1311–1313.

5 Marion PL, Sutin KM. Organic acidosis. In: *The ICU Book*, 3rd edn. Lippincott Williams and Wilkins, Philadelphia, 2007, pp. 551–552.

6 Graf H, Arieff AI. The use of sodium bicarbonate in the therapy of organic acidosis. *Intensive Care Med* 1986;12:285–288.

7 Boothe DM. *Small Animal Clinical Pharmacology and Therapeutics*, 2nd edn. Elsevier Saunders, St Louis, 2012.

8 Kline JA, Weisber LS. Acid–base, electrolyte, and metabolic abnormalities. In: *Critical Care Medicine: Principles of Diagnosis and Management in the Adult* (eds Parillo JE, Dellinger RP). Elsevier, Philadelphia, 2014, pp. 993–1028.

9 Forsythe SM, Schmidt GA. Sodium bicarbonate for the treatment of lactic acidosis. *Chest* 2000;117:260–267.

10 Guyton AC, Hall JE. *Textbook of Medical Physiology*, 9th edn. WB Saunders, Philadelphia, 1996.

11 Hartsfield SM, Thurmon JC, Corbin JE, Bensone GJ, Aiken T. Effect of sodium acetate, bicarbonate and lactate on acid-base status in anaesthetized dogs. *J Vet Pharmacol Ther* 1981;4:51–61.

12 Chew DJ, Leonard M, Muir WW 3rd. Effect of sodium bicarbonate infusion on serum osmolality, electrolyte concentrations, and blood gas tensions in cats. *Am J Vet Res* 1991;52:12–17.

13 DiBartola SP. Metabolic acid–base disorders. In: *Fluid, Electrolyte and Acid–Base Disorders in Small Animal Practice*, 4th edn (ed. DiBartola SP). Elsevier, St Louis, 2012, pp. 253–286.

14 Chew DJ, Leonard M, Muir WW 3rd. Effect of sodium bicarbonate infusions on ionized calcium and total calcium concentrations in serum of clinically normal cats. *Am J Vet Res* 1989;50:145–150.

15 Salerno DM, Elsperger KJ, Helseth P, Murakami M, Chepuri V. Serum potassium, calcium and magnesium after resuscitation from ventricular fibrillation: a canine study. *J Am Coll Cardiol* 1987;10:178–185.

16 Adeva-Andany MM, Fernandez-Fernandez C, Mourino-Bayolo D, Castro-Quintela E, Dominguez-Montero A. Sodium bicarbonate therapy in patients with metabolic acidosis. *Sci World J* 2014;2014: 627–673.

17 Sodium Bicarbonate 8.4%. Drug monograph. Hospira Inc, Lake Forest, 2005.

18 Sodium Bicarbonate 8.4%. Drug monograph. AFT Pharmaceuticals Ltd Auckland, 2013.

19 Kraut JA, Madias NE. Treatment of acute metabolic acidosis: a pathophysiologic approach. *Nat Rev Nephrol* 2012;8:589–601.

20 Rose BD, Post TW. *Clinical Physiology of Acid–Base and Electrolyte Disorders*, 5th edn. McGraw-Hill, New York, 2001.

21 Laufgraben M, Kaufman ST. Acute diabetic emergencies, glycemic control and hypoglycemia. In: *Critical Care Medicine: Principles of Diagnosis and Management in the Adult* (eds Parillo JE, Dellinger RP). Elsevier, Philadelphia, 2014, pp. 1029–1046.

22 Chua HR, Schneider A, Bellomo R. Bicarbonate in diabetic ketoacidosis – a systematic review. *Ann Intensive Care* 2011;1:23.

23 Hume DZ, Drobatz KJ, Hess RS. Outcome of dogs with diabetic ketoacidosis: 127 dogs (1993–2003). *J Vet Intern Med* 2006;20:547–555.

24 Oster JR, Alpert HC, Rodriguez GR, Vaamonde CA. Effect of acute reversal of experimentally-induced ketoacidosis with sodium bicarbonate on the plasma concentrations of phosphorous and potassium. *Life Sci* 1988;42:811–819.

25 Bureau MA, Begin R, Berthiaume Y, et al. Cerebral hypoxia from bicarbonate infusion in diabetic acidosis. *J Pediatr* 1980;96:968–973.

26 Beech JS, Williams SC, Iles RA, et al. Haemodynamic and metabolic effects in diabetic ketoacidosis in rats of treatment with sodium bicarbonate or a mixture of sodium bicarbonate and sodium carbonate. *Diabetalogia* 1995;38:889–898.

27 Schaer M. Feline Metabolic Emergencies. VIN Internal Medicine Lecture Notes. April 2003

28 Boysen SR. Fluid and electrolyte therapy in endocrine disorders: diabetes mellitus and hypoadrenocorticism. *Vet Clin North Am Small Anim Pract* 2008;38:699–717.

29 Arieff AI, Leach W, Park R, Lazarowitz VC. Systemic effects of NaHCO3 in experimental lactic acidosis in dogs. *Am J Physiol* 1982;242:F586–F591.

30 Minot AS, Dodd K, Saunders JM. The acidosis of guanidine intoxication. *J Clin Invest* 1934;13:917–932.

31 Graf H, Leach W, Arieff AI. Evidence for a detrimental effect of bicarbonate therapy in hypoxic lactic acidosis. *Science* 1985;27:754–756.

32 Graf H, Leach W, Arieff AI. Metabolic effects of sodium bicarbonate in hypoxic lactic acidosis in dogs. *Am J Physiol* 1985;249:F630–F635.

33 Rhee KH, Toro LO, McDonald GG, Nunnally RL, Levin DL. Carbicarb, sodium bicarbonate, and sodium chloride in hypoxic lactic acidosis. *Chest* 1993;104:913–918.

34 Bersin RM, Arieff AI. Improved hemodynamic function during hypoxia with Carbicarb, a new agent for the management of acidosis. *Circulation* 1988;77:227–233.

35 Brandis K. 8.7 Use of bicarbonate in metabolic acidosis. Acid–Base Physiology. Available at: www.anaesthesiamcq.com/AcidBaseBook/ab8_7.php (accessed 19 February 2018).

36 Iberti TJ, Kelly KM, Gentill DR, et al. Effects of sodium bicarbonate in canine hemorrhagic shock. *Crit Care Med* 1988;16:779.

37 Benjamin E, Oropello JM, Abalos AM, et al. Effects of acid–base correction on hemodynamics, oxygen dynamics, and resuscitability in severe canine hemorrhagic shock. *Crit Care Med* 1994;22:1616–1623.

38 Kim HJ, Son YK, An WS. Effect of sodium bicarbonate administration on mortality in patients with lactic acidosis: a retrospective analysis. *PLoS One* 2013;8:e65283.

39 Rozanski EA, Rush JE, Buckley GJ, Fletcher DJ, Boller M. RECOVER evidence and knowledge gap analysis on veterinary CPR. Part 4: Advanced life support. *J Vet Emerg Crit Care* 2012;22(S1):44–64.

40 Fletcher DJ, Boller M, Brainard BM, et al. RECOVER evidence and knowledge gap analysis on veterinary CPR. Part 7: Clinical guidelines. *J Vet Emerg Crit Care* 2012;22(S1):102–131.

41 Hopper K, Borchers A, Epstein SE. Acid base, electrolyte, glucose, and lactate values during cardiopulmonary resuscitation in dogs and cats. *J Vet Emerg Crit Care* 2014;24:208–214.

42 Hofmeister EH, Brainard BM, Egger CM, Kang S. Prognostic indicators for dogs and cats with cardiopulmonary arrest treated by cardiopulmonary cerebral resuscitation at a university teaching hospital. *J Am Vet Med Assoc* 2009;235:50–57.

43 Rush JE, Wingfield WE. Recognition and frequency of dysrhythmias during cardiopulmonary arrest. *J Am Vet Med Assoc* 1992;200:1932–1937.

44 McIntyre RL, Hopper K, Epstein SE. Assessment of cardiopulmonary resuscitation in 121 dogs and 30 cats at a university teaching hospital (2009–2012). *J Vet Emerg Crit Care* 2014;24:694–704.

45 Sanders A, Kern KB, Fonken S, Otto CW, Ewy GA. The role of bicarbonate and fluid loading in improving resuscitation from prolonged cardiac arrest with rapid manual chest compression CPR. *Ann Emerg Med* 1990;19:1–7.

46 Vukmir RB, Bircher NG, Radovsky A, Safar P. Sodium bicarbonate may improve outcome in dogs with brief or prolonged cardiac arrest. *Crit Care Med* 1995;23:515–532.

47 Leong EJC, Bendall JC, Boyd AC, Einstein R. Sodium bicarbonate improves the chance of resuscitation after 10 minutes of cardiac arrest in dogs. *Resuscitation* 2001;51:309–315.

48 Redding JS, Pearson JW. Resuscitation from ventricular fibrillation. *Drug therapy. J Am Med Assoc* 1968;203:255–260.

49 Bar-Joseph G, Weinberger T, Castel T, et al. Comparison of sodium bicarbonate, Carbicarb and THAM during cardiopulmonary resuscitation in dogs. *Crit Care Med* 1998;26:1397–1408.

50 Minuck M, Sharma GP. Comparison of THAM and sodium bicarbonate in resuscitation of the heart after ventricular fibrillation in dogs. *Anaesth Analg* 1977;56:38–45.

51 Eleff SM, Sugimoto H, Shaffner H, Traystman RJ, Koehler RC. Acidemia and brain pH during prolonged cardiopulmonary resuscitation in dogs. *Stroke* 1995;26:1028–1034.

52 Rosenberg JM, Martin GB, Paradis NA, et al. The effect of CO2 and non-CO2-generating buffers on cerebral acidosis after cardiac arrest: a ^{31}P NMR study. *Ann Emerg Med* 1989;18:341–347.

53 Bleske BE, Chow MSS, Zhao H, Kluger J, Fieldman A. Effects of different dosages and modes of sodium bicarbonate administration during cardiopulmonary resuscitation. *Ann J Emerg Med* 1992;10:525–532.

54 Bleske BE, Rice TL, Warren EW. An alternative sodium bicarbonate regimen during cardiac arrest and cardiopulmonary resuscitation in a canine model. *Pharmacotherapy* 1994;14:95–99.

55 Bleske BE, Warren EW, Rice TL, Gilligan LJ, Tait AR. Effect of high-dose sodium bicarbonate on the vasopressor effects of epinephrine during cardiopulmonary resuscitation. *Pharmacotherapy* 1995;15:660–664.

56 Blecic S, DeBacker D, Deleuze M, Vachiery JL, Vincent JL. Correction of metabolic acidosis in experimental CPR: a comparative study of sodium bicarbonate, Carbicarb, and dextrose. *Ann Emerg Med* 1991;20:235–238.

57 Bishop RL, Weisfeldt ML. Sodium bicarbonate administration during cardiac arrest. *J Am Med Assoc* 1976;235:506–509.

58 Berenyi KJ, Wolk M, Killip T. Cerebrospinal fluid acidosis complicating therapy of experimental cardiopulmonary arrest. *Circulation* 1975;52:319–324.

59 Guerci AD, Chandra N, Johnson E, et al. Failure of sodium bicarbonate to improve resuscitation from ventricular fibrillation in dogs. *Circulation* 1986;74(6 Pt 2):IV 75–79.

60 Bar-Joseph G, Abramson NS, Kelse SF, et al. Improved resuscitation outcome in emergency medical systems

with increased usage of sodium bicarbonate during cardiopulmonary resuscitation. *Acta Anaesthesiol Scand* 2005;49:6–15.

61 Vukmir RB, Katz L. Sodium bicarbonate improves outcome in prolonged prehospital cardiac arrest. *Am J Emerg Med* 2006;24:156–161.

62 Davis J. Balanced equations: sodium bicarbonate as treatment for cardiac arrest. *J Emerg Med Servs* 2010;35:48–52.

63 Geraci MJ, Klipa D, Heckman MG, Persoff J. Prevalence of sodium bicarbonate-induced alkalemia in cardiopulmonary arrest patients. *Ann Pharmacother* 2009;42:1245–1250.

64 DiBartola SP, de Morais HA. Disorders of potassium: hypokalemia and hyperkalemia. In: *Fluid, Electrolyte and Acid–Base Disorders in Small Animal Practice*, 4th edn (ed. DiBartola SP). Elsevier, St Louis, 2012, pp. 92–119.

65 Langston C. Managing fluid and electrolyte disorders in renal failure. In: *Fluid, Electrolyte and Acid–Base Disorders in Small Animal Practice*, 4th edn (ed. DiBartola SP). Elsevier, St Louis, 2012, pp. 554–556.

66 Parham WA, Mehdirad AA, Biermann KM, Fredman CS. Hyperkalemia revisited. *Tex Heart Inst J* 2006;3: 40–47.

67 Shingarev R, Allon M. A physiologic-based approach to the treatment of acute hyperkalemia. *Am J Kidney Dis* 2010;56:578–584.

68 Allon M, Shanklin N. Effect of bicarbonate administration on plasma potassium in dialysis patients: interactions with insulin and albuterol. *Am J Kid Dis* 1996;28:508–514.

69 Hypertonic Saline 7.2%. Drug monograph. Aspen Veterinary Resources. Available at: aspenveterinaryresources.com (accessed 19 February 2018).

70 Kyes J, Johnson JA. Hypertonic saline solutions in shock resuscitation. *Compend Contin Educ Vet* 2011;33(3):E1–E8, quiz E9.

175

Continuous-Rate Infusion

Andrea M. Steele, MSc, RVT, VTS(ECC)

Ontario Veterinary College, Health Sciences Centre, University of Guelph, Guelph, ON, Canada

Preparing Drug Solutions for Infusions

There is considerable room for error when making admixtures, and it is vitally important to ensure proper technique is used. Use the following tips to reduce errors.

- Use the closest syringe size for the volume of initial drug concentration (whether full strength or previously diluted) you need for the admixture.
- Choose a compatible carrier fluid; use the product monograph or a drug compatibility chart.
- Instill only the volume measured in the syringe, not the remaining volume in the syringe hub and needle. "Flushing" the hub and needle can lead to considerable error in dosing.
- Ensure adequate mixing of the bag, syringe or buretrol after addition of each drug. Currently, four inversions are recommended for complete mixing of bags or syringes. In burettes, inversion is not recommended, as fluid delivery can be affected if the filter at the top gets wet. Swirl the contents to mix.

Fluid Bag Delivery

Delivery of one or more medications in the fluid bag with maintenance fluids is a very simple method of delivering a CRI. There are some drawbacks that should be mentioned, however.

- *Less flexibility in dosing*: If the CRI is running with the maintenance fluids, there is less flexibility in dosing without changing the amount of fluids the patient is receiving. This method is ideal for CRIs that maintain a standard dose over a long period, for example metoclopramide.
- *More wastage*: The bag method is best for patients that will use the entire bag in a 24-hour period, such as large dogs or patients with higher fluid rates. Using

smaller fluid bags such as 100, 250, or 500 mL may help alleviate wastage, but these bags are typically more expensive/mL than their 1 L counterparts. Light sensitivity and long-term compatibility with the carrier fluid must be investigated.

- *Overfilling of fluid bags leads to inaccuracies*: Fluid bags are overfilled ~10% by the manufacturer. When stored for long periods, bags lose volume due to evaporative losses and may contain less than stated on the label. This will cause the concentration of the bag to be different from that expected. Likely, this will not cause concern but it is important to be aware of this source of error. Because of overfill and evaporative losses, human compounding pharmacies will not provide CRI medication in an IV bag, as the concentration cannot be guaranteed (the exception being if the drug and the fluid in measured quantities are added to an empty, sterile bag). Prefilled IV bags are only used for drug admixtures when they are providing a set number of milligrams, by using the entire contents of the bag in a short period of time (for example, diluting 500 mg of ampicillin in 50 mL of saline and giving over 30 min), where the final concentration is not as important as knowing the number of milligrams being administered. For this reason alone, CRI delivery in a fluid bag should be considered the least desirable method of administering analgesic drugs.
- *The 10% Rule*: This is a rule that hospital pharmacies use to ensure consistency in the final admixture product. If the medication to be added to the bag is 10% or more of the volume in the bag, then the same volume should be removed from the bag prior to addition of the medication. For example, to make a 5% dextrose solution using 50% dextrose, in a 1 L bag of fluid, 100 mL of dextrose must be added to the container. In this case, 100 mL of fluid should be removed from the bag before the addition. In the case of 2.5% dextrose solution, 50 mL must be added to 1 L. As this

Textbook of Small Animal Emergency Medicine, First Edition. Edited by Kenneth J. Drobatz, Kate Hopper, Elizabeth Rozanski and Deborah C. Silverstein.
© 2019 John Wiley & Sons, Inc. Published 2019 by John Wiley & Sons, Inc.
Companion Website: www.wiley.com/go/drobatz/textbook

is < 10% of the volume in the fluid bag, there is no need to remove 50 mL prior to addition. By ensuring that all parties are following the 10% Rule in your practice, you can be assured that if the solution is made up correctly, the final concentration should be similar from person to person.

- *Mixing*: After addition of an admixture drug, it is important to invert the bag at least four times to ensure adequate mixing.
- *Adjust based on patient response*: Knowing that the final concentration of a drug in a fluid bag can never be guaranteed due to the overfill of the bag, it is important that the veterinarian and veterinary technicians understand that the dose delivered per hour may not be exactly what is expected. This highlights the importance of assessing the patient for response to therapy and adjusting the dosing accordingly.

Drug Infusions Using a Burette

A burette is an inexpensive tool for IV fluid therapy and is an inline, graduated volume cylinder that allows for accurate portioning of IV fluids into a smaller volume. Adjustments to drug dose rate are easily made by adding more fluid (decrease concentration) or more drug (increase concentration), or simply emptying the burette and adding fresh solution. Typically, burettes hold 150 mL and have an IV spike at the top that is attached to the IV fluid bag. A roller clamp allows for fluid entry into the burette, and a standard solution set is either permanently attached or spiked into the bottom of the burette to attach to the patient. Drug infusions in a burette should always be administered using an IV fluid pump for accuracy.

There is an injection port at the top of the burette for medication additions. It is important to note that on some models (usually needleless port types), there is a large amount of deadspace within the injection port. Following addition of small volumes of medication, it is advisable to instill ~1 mL of a sterile fluid (NaCl or fluid drawn aseptically from the fluid bag into a syringe) to flush out the port and ensure that the entire dose has been instilled in the burette. Ensure the mixture is adequately mixed by swirling.

Preparation of Drug Infusions for Bag/Burette

To prepare medications for infusion in a fluid bag or burette, there are several key pieces of information required.

- The dose to be provided per hour
- The initial concentration of the drug
- The weight of the patient
- The volume of the fluid bag OR the actual or desired volume of the buretrol
- The fluid rate/h at which to deliver

Using the provided dose, calculate the number of mL/h of drug that is required.

Example 1: Dexmedetomidine CRI, at 0.5 μg/kg/h for a 20 kg dog, delivered by burette.

$$0.5 \, \mu g/kg/h \times 20 \, kg = 10 \, \mu g/h$$

Dexmedetomidine is 500 μg/mL (0.5 mg/mL) concentration:

$$10 \, \mu g/h / 500 \, \mu g/mL = 0.02 \, mL/h$$

Next, determine how many hours of fluid will fit in the burette, if the hourly rate is 30 mL/h and the burette holds 150 mL.

$$150 \, mL / 30 \, ml/h = 5h$$

Finally, how many mL of dexmedetomidine are needed for 5 hours?

$$5h \times 0.02 \, mL/h = 0.1 \, mL \text{ of dexmedetomidine is needed}$$

Example 2: The exact same calculation is performed for delivery in a fluid bag.

Using a 500 mL 0.9% NaCl bag, calculate how much metoclopramide should be added to deliver 2 mg/kg/day to a 30 kg dog receiving 75 mL/h. Calculate the number of mL/h of metoclopramide required.

$$2 \, mg/kg/day \times 30 \, kg = 60 \, mg/day/24h = 2.5 \, mg/h$$

Metoclopramide is 5 mg/mL, so:

$$2.5 \, mg/h / 5 \, mg/mL = 0.5 \, mL/h$$

Next, calculate the number of hours, assuming an actual volume of 500 mL.

$$500 \, mL / 75 \, mL/h = 6.7h$$

Finally, how much metoclopramide do we need?

$$6.7h \times 0.5 \, mL/h = 3.3 \, mL$$

Since 3.3 mL is < 10% of the volume of the bag, we simply add it to the bag, and invert to mix.

Labeling the Drug Infusion

It is very important to appropriately label the drug infusion, not only to accurately identify the contents but to

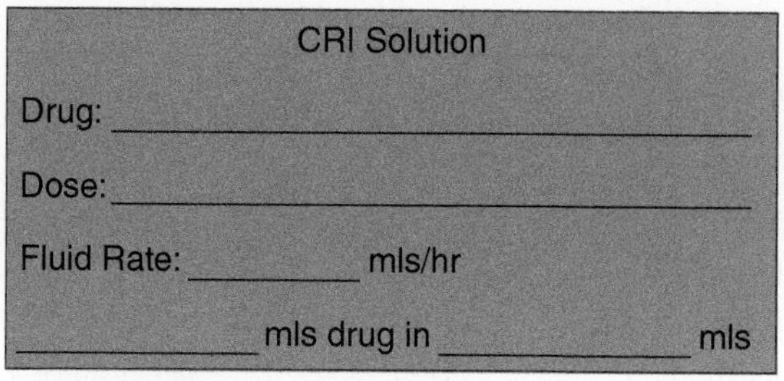

```
┌─────────────────────────────────────────┐
│               CRI Solution               │
│                                           │
│   Drug: _____  │
│                                           │
│   Dose: _____  │
│                                           │
│   Fluid Rate: _____ mls/hr           │
│                                           │
│   _____ mls drug in _____ mls   │
└─────────────────────────────────────────┘
```

Figure 175.1 Label for drug infusion.

ensure consistency or in some cases, an error in the previous drug calculation may be identified. The admixture should be recalculated as a verification each time a new solution is made.

A simple label can be made for you at the local print shop (Figure 175.1).

Standardized Concentration Infusions

As mentioned above, some veterinarians prefer to use standardized concentrations of analgesics, delivered on a sliding scale based on patient weight. These infusions do have some benefits.

- *Less likely to have calculation errors*: The same amount of drug is added to the same size bag each time it is made up, reducing the chance of an error due to calculations.
- *Less likely to have administration errors*: Likewise, there is less chance of an administration error when the dose is standardized. If prescribed at 1 mL/kg/h, this is simply the body weight of the patient entered into the pump.
- *Recipes can be used to make multidrug bags*: Fairly advanced CRIs can be created using a standard recipe. This delivers each drug at a set rate. Commonly, morphine-lidocaine-ketamine infusions are prepared in this manner.
- *Flexibility in dosing*: While the standard recipe may be delivered at 1 mL/kg/h, increasing or decreasing the hourly rate will allow titration. For multidrug bags, the infusion of each medication is increased or decreased.

Just as there are some benefits, and ease of use for the veterinary staff, there are some drawbacks.

- *Additional fluid line and pump required*: Often the mL/h supplied with the standardized concentration method is not sufficient to meet the individual patient's hourly requirements. Therefore, an additional line and bag with maintenance crystalloid may be required.
- *Wastage*: Wastage can be significant with this method, as the patient may not use the entire bag of medication. Consider recipes for 100/250/500/1000 mL bags to adjust for patient size.

- *Lack of individualization:* Especially with multidrug bags, this method allows increasing or decreasing the dosage of all drugs, but not each drug individually. Often, finding the right level of each drug for the patient is a challenge, and this type of system makes it a little more difficult.

All things considered, the standardized infusion bag is an acceptable method of providing a CRI, and may be preferable in veterinary clinics with a limited number of fluid pumps available.

Preparing a standardized infusion bag is as simple as following a recipe. Several organizations offer recipes and CRI calculators online, which make set-up extremely easy. To produce your own customized recipe, the following information is needed.

- Volume of fluid bag
- Concentration of each drug
- Desired dose for each drug

For example, ketamine has a typical dose range as a CRI of 0.1–1.0 mg/kg/h. Ideally, starting at the middle of the dose for the standardized bag to deliver at 1 mL/kg/h of fluid will allow for some flexibility. The dose can be decreased or increased by changing the fluid rate, so that 0.5 mL/kg/h will reduce the dose to 0.25 mg/kg/h. Doubling the fluid rate to 2 mL/kg/h will deliver ketamine at 1 mg/kg/h. Therefore, calculate based on 0.5 mg/kg/h.

Initial concentration of ketamine is 100 mg/mL. Desired dose of 0.5 mg/kg/h in 1 mL/kg/h of final concentration. Therefore, we want 0.5 mg in every mL of fluid. For a 1 litre bag of fluid:

0.5 mg/mL × 1000 mL = 500 mg of ketamine or 5 mL to add to the bag

For alternate bag sizes: 0.5 mL/100 mL, 1.25 mL/250 mL, 2.5 mL/500 mL.

To add fentanyl at 3 μg/kg/h to the same bag at the same 1 mL/kg/h rate:

3 μg delivered in 1 mL/h of fluids = 3 μg / mL of final solution

For 1000 mL bag, need 3000 μg. Fentanyl is 50 μg/mL, therefore:

3000 μg / 50 μg / mL = 60 mL of fentanyl to a 1000 mL bag

For alternate bag sizes: 6.0 ml/100 ml, 15 ml/250 ml, 30 ml/500 ml. Keep in mind that due to overfill/evaporative losses, the actual concentration may vary by ± 10%.

Drug Infusions Using a Syringe Pump

Syringe pumps are becoming much more widely available, and are ideal to administer CRIs. One distinct advantage is the ability to adjust drug dose rate with just a few simple clicks. The drug can be prepared full strength but if very small hourly volumes are required, some syringe pumps may struggle with accuracy, making dilution of the drug a necessity. Many syringe pumps offer onboard programs that allow the manager to create drug libraries and set the concentration, dose range, dosing limits for the drug (min/max), and program boluses. Some basic syringe pumps will be programmed simply with mL/h, and in some cases, pumps are programmed using a chart that converts mL/h for each possible syringe size and manufacturer to mm/h. These latter pumps are very inexpensive but care must be taken to ensure training is sufficient to avoid errors.

An example of a drug that may be administered via syringe pump is midazolam. Midazolam may also be administered via the other methods described above.

Midazolam has a dose rate of 0.25–1 mg/kg/h. To calculate this for a syringe pump, the following information is needed.

- Patient weight
- Desired dose
- Concentration

For a 34 kg dog, to receive 0.5 mg/kg/h of midazolam, the following calculation is used:

$$\text{Patient weight (kg)} \times \text{dose} = 34 \text{ kg} \times 0.5 \text{ mg/kg/h}$$
$$= 17 \text{ mg/h}$$

To calculate mL/h:

$$17 \text{ mg/h} / 5 \text{ mg/mL} = 3.4 \text{ mL/h}$$

The syringe pump will be set to deliver 3.4 mL/h.

Table 175.1 Common continuous-rate infusion (CRI) dosages.

Drug (CRI)	Dose	Units
Butorphanol	0.1–0.4	mg/kg/h
Dexmedetomidine	0.25–1.0	µg/kg/h
Diazepam	0.5–1.0	mg/kg/h
Diltiazem	1–5	µg/kg/min
Dobutamine	5–20	µg/kg/min
Dopamine	5–20	µg/kg/min
Epinephrine	0.025–0.3	µg/kg/min
Fentanyl	2–5	µg/kg/h
Furosemide	0.1–1.0	mg/kg/h
Hydromorphone	0.01–0.03	mg/kg/h
Ketamine	0.1–1.0	mg/kg/h
Lidocaine	25–75	µg/kg/min
Metoclopramide	1–2	mg/kg/day
Midazolam	0.25–1	mg/kg/h
Morphine	0.1–0.5	mg/kg/h
Nitroprusside	1–10	µg/kg/min
Norepinephrine	0.1–1.0	µg/kg/min
Procainamide	25–50	µg/kg/min
Propofol	25–300	µg/kg/min
Vasopressin	1–5	mU/kg/min

Table 175.1 provides CRI doses for commonly used drugs.

Acknowledgment

Some of this work concurrently appears in Analgesia and Anesthesia for the Critically Ill or Injured Dog and Cat by Matthews, Sinclair, Steel, and Grub, published by Wiley.

176

Transfusion of Red Blood Cells and Plasma

Raegan J. Wells, DVM, MS, DACVECC[1] and Brandi L. Mattison, DVM, DACVECC[2]

[1]Phoenix Veterinary Emergency and Referral, Emergency Animal Clinic, Phoenix, AZ, USA
[2]Arizona Veterinary Emergency and Critical Care Center, Gilbert, AZ, USA

Transfusion Therapy

Transfusion therapy has been a life-saving intervention for many years, with a dog-to-dog blood transfusion being the first known documented transfusion event in medical history [1]. Many advances have been made since the incorporation of small animal transfusion medicine into veterinary practice in the 1950s. Navigating the complex landscape of blood component therapy, pretransfusion screening, and potential complications can become an overwhelming task for the busy emergency room clinician. This chapter summarizes key points in canine and feline transfusion medicine, using an evidence-based yet practical approach when available. Red blood cell and plasma transfusion will be discussed. Expanded component therapy is beyond the scope of this chapter.

Donor and Recipient Screening

Blood products are obtained from donor animals and thus are a limited resource in hospital settings. For the busy emergency practice, it is recommended that commonly used blood component therapy products be stocked. For the canine patient, the most common and practical components include fresh frozen plasma and packed red blood cells. Dependent upon caseload and patient acuity, feline blood products may not be a practical inventory investment. In a very busy setting, it is prudent to keep feline packed red blood cells and fresh frozen plasma available. Many hospitals still manage a feline blood donor program, with the intent of using fresh whole blood on an as-needed basis.

Each hospital must evaluate its practice needs in order to direct which, if any, blood products will be stocked on site.

Blood type of donors and recipients is relevant to unit selection and prevention of hemolytic blood transfusion reactions. Hemolytic transfusion reactions occur when the recipient has existing antibodies that are specific for antigens on the donor erythrocytes. The dog erythrocyte antigen (DEA) system is applied to canine blood types. The canine blood type of most clinical importance is the DEA 1 system (DEA 1.1, DEA 1.2, DEA 1.3), as DEA 1 is highly antigenic. A DEA 1-negative dog that receives a DEA 1-positive transfusion is likely to mount a strong alloantibody response, resulting in sensitization, so that a future DEA 1-positive transfusion may cause a catastrophic hemolytic transfusion reaction. Dogs do not have pre-existing alloantibodies to the DEA 1 system. Although natural antibodies have been demonstrated in some dogs for DEA 3, DEA 5, and DEA 7, these are considered "weak antibodies" and not capable of causing a hemolytic transfusion reaction [2]. The Dal red blood cell antigen is present in most dogs, but lacking in some Dalmatians. As such, a canine patient without the Dal antigen may become sensitized and experience a hemolytic crisis upon future transfusion of Dal-positive red blood cells [3]. The current universal canine blood donor phenotype is DEA 1.1, 1.2, 3, 5, and 7 negative but positive for DEA 4.

A practical approach to stored blood products for most emergency hospitals is to inventory primarily universal donor blood (DEA 1.1 negative). If both DEA 1.1 positive and negative blood is stocked, canine typing systems designed for in-house use are available to screen for DEA 1, for pretransfusion recipient screening. The two most common in-house testing systems available utilize monoclonal anti-DEA 1.1 antibodies. These are the DMS card test (CARD, DMS Laboratories, NJ) and the Quick-test DEA 1.1 (CHROM, Alvedia, France). Autoagglutination will not interfere with the ability to read results with the Alvedia test. Donor screening should be sent to a reference laboratory for gold standard methodology and if comprehensive typing beyond the DEA 1 system is desired.

The system applied to cats is the AB blood group. Cats are type A, type B or, rarely, type AB. Feline type A is dominant over type B. As such, cats with the type A phenotype are genetically a/a or a/b. In order to demonstrate the type B phenotype, cats must be genetically b/b. The rare cat with type AB phenotype has a genotype with a third allele allowing expression of both A and B substances on the surface of their red blood cells [4]. The geographic distribution of these blood types varies, but the highest reported incidence of type B has been in Australia at 36% [5]. In the north-east region of the United States, the percentage of type B cats has been reported to be between 0.3% and 8% [6]. The United Kingdom reports that 68% of non-pedigree cats are type A, 30% type B, and 2% type AB [7]. All Siamese cats are type A, while type A and B blood has been reported in other exotic cat breeds such as the Devon rex, British short-hair, Cornish rex, exotic short-hair, and Scottish fold. Domestic short-hair cats are also known to have type B blood [8]. The *Mik* red blood cell antigen has been identified in some domestic short-hair cats. Cats that lack the *Mik* antigen may have preformed alloantibodies that can result in transfusion reactions [9].

All donors and recipients should be blood typed. Xenotransfusion of cats with canine blood has been reported, but is not recommended due to a high rate of reaction and the advances made in feline blood transfusion medicine [10]. However, in certain critical circumstances, if feline blood is not available canine blood may be considered [11].

All type A and B cats have preformed natural alloantibodies, and are at risk of hemolytic transfusion reactions if given an incompatible transfusion. Type B cats have strong anti-A antibodies and may experience a fatal transfusion reaction if given as little as 1 mL of type A blood [12]. Type B blood administered to a type A cat is unlikely to cause a fatal reaction, but will result in shortened lifespan of the transfused cells. Type AB cats do not have alloantibodies to either A or B antigens, and should receive either type AB or type A blood if transfusion is needed. The two most common in-house feline blood typing systems available are the CARD Rapid®-VetH Feline (DMS Laboratories, Flemington, NJ) and the Quick-test A+B (Alvedia, France). Type B and AB cats should be confirmed by sending to an outside laboratory [13]. Cats should always receive type-specific plasma.

Cross-Matching

Ideally, all patients should have a cross-match performed prior to transfusion of red blood cells. A major cross-match tests the recipient's serum for alloantibodies against donor blood cells. The minor cross-match tests the donor's serum for alloantibodies against recipient blood cells. It is reasonable to skip a cross-match in a dog receiving its first blood transfusion, as they do not have pre-existing alloantibodies. Some clinicians recommend that dogs with immune-mediated hemolytic anemia ideally be cross-matched prior to all transfusions. The authors recommend a cross-match in all feline transfusion events, as this is the most reliable bedside method to assess for inaccurate blood typing, incompatibilities due to *Mik* cell antigens, or possibly other unrecognized antigens. A cross-match should also be performed in all patients that have received a blood transfusion greater than 5–7 days prior to the planned transfusion, or have experienced hemolysis with prior transfusion.

Commercial kits are available for in-house cross-matching. In the event that an emergency transfusion is needed prior to the completion of a cross-match, a crude, rapid bedside method for testing AB compatibility in cats is to mix a single drop of donor and recipient blood, then evaluate for agglutination.

Blood Product Administration

Transfusion administration technique will impact recipient safety, efficacy, and efficient use of hospital resources. Red blood cells do not need to be warmed prior to administration but this may be considered when the recipient is a very small patient. Frozen plasma products should be placed in a sealed plastic bag, then warmed in a water bath until thawed. A microwave should not be used to thaw frozen blood products. Use of peristaltic pumps to deliver red blood cell transfusions has been shown to cause damage and decrease survival of transfused red blood cells [14,15]. As such, the authors recommend gravity flow and standard blood filter set (170–260 micron) for canine blood product transfusions. Unfortunately, the priming volume of these sets is too large for cats and small dogs. A human neonatal syringe filter set with a 150 micron filter or a syringe pump with Hemo-Nate (18 micron) filter can be used for these patients. Plasma transfusions should also be administered via a standard blood filter set.

The blood product volume to be transfused is best guided by goal-directed therapy. The most straightforward formula used to calculate volume of pRBCs to transfuse is [16]:

$$\text{pRBC volume to transfuse} = \text{desired \% PCV increase} \times 1.5 \times \text{kg body weight}$$

See Table 176.1 for commonly used doses for blood products.

Table 176.1 Commonly used doses of blood products available at most ER practices. Note that many more blood products and components are available that are beyond the scope of this chapter.

Blood product	Contents	Indications	Common dose (mL/kg)
Packed red blood cells (pRBC)	Red blood cells +/− white blood cells Anticoagulant (CPDA) +/− preservative (Optisol, Nutricel)	Anemia with clinical signs of decreased oxygen delivery (DO_2) despite optimization of preload and contractility	10–15 mL/kg
Fresh whole blood	Red blood cells White blood cells Plasma (coag. factors) Platelets Anticoagulant (CPDA)	Anemia with clinical signs of decreased DO_2 despite optimization of preload and contractility if pRBCs not available Need for multiple components – severe hemorrhage	20–22 mL/kg
Stored whole blood	Red blood cells White blood cells Plasma (coag. factors) Anticoagulant (CPDA)	Anemia with clinical signs of decreased DO_2 despite optimization of preload and contractility if pRBCs not available Need for multiple components (red cells and stable coagulation factors)	20–22 mL/kg
Fresh frozen plasma	Coagulation factors Antithrombin Albumin Globulins	Hypocoagulability with hemorrhage due to coagulation factor deficiency	10–20 mL/kg

The administration rate of the blood product is dependent upon the status of the patient. In patients with acute severe hemorrhage, blood components may need to be administered as quickly as possible. Patients at risk for fluid overload, such as those with congestive heart failure, may need transfusions administered at a conservative rate. For the typically anemic but relatively stable patient, a common method of product transfusion is to begin the transfusion at 0.25 mL/kg/h for 5 minutes and observe for evidence of a transfusion reaction. If no reaction is appreciated based on patient observation and comparing vital signs to baseline vitals, the rate is increased for the transfusion to be delivered over the time desired.

It is generally recommended that blood products are not left at room temperature for more than 4–6 hours to prevent bacterial growth, although one study found no bacterial growth in canine stored whole blood after 24 hours room temperature [17,18]. If fresh frozen plasma is thawed but not used, refreezing within 1 hour is acceptable and does not appear to have deleterious effects on hemostatic protein activity [19]. Additional freeze-thaw cycling has not been evaluated and should be avoided.

Transfusion Reactions

Multiple types of transfusion reactions can occur from administering blood products as component therapy or whole blood. Overall, the transfusion reaction rate is low, reportedly 3.3–15% of recipients [20–23]. Using compatible blood products from screened donors, replacing only the necessary component(s), careful consideration of the necessity of the transfusion, and appropriate administration are the most effective means of limiting the frequency of transfusion reactions.

Monitoring for transfusion reactions is accomplished by close observation of the patient during and after the transfusion. Multiple transfusion administration patient monitoring protocols exist with the common goal of prompt recognition of a reaction. A common method of transfusion monitoring is to obtain baseline vital signs of temperature, pulse, respiration, and capillary refill time prior to administration. Five minutes following administration of the blood product, the baseline vital signs are re-evaluated. If no reaction has occurred, evaluation of vital signs is performed at 15 minutes, 30 minutes, and then every 60 minutes throughout the transfusion. In addition to these parameters, the patient should be

Table 176.2 Common transfusion reactions, symptoms, and suggested actions.

Product	Clinical signs	Response
Acute immunological reactions		
Red blood cells	Febrile non-hemolytic reactions. Other signs may include tachycardia, tachypnea, vomiting and/or diarrhea	Stop or slow transfusion rate
	Hemolytic reactions – signs may include fever, tachycardia, tachypnea, vomiting and/or diarrhea, cardiovascular collapse, pigmenturia	Discontinue transfusion
Plasma	Pruritus, urticaria, facial edema	Diphenhydramine, stop transfusion, may resume transfusion slowly
	Transfusion-related acute lung injury – most commonly reported after plasma transfusions in people	Usually develops 6–24h following transfusion
Acute non-immunological reactions		
All products	Transfusion-associated circulatory overload	Furosemide trial
	Citrate toxicity	Calcium gluconate or calcium chloride
Delayed immunological reactions		
Red blood cells (RBC)	Shortened RBC lifespan, hemolysis	Type and cross-match all future transfusions
All products	Transfusion-related immunomodulation	None
Delayed non-immunological reactions		
All products	Infectious disease transmission	Use screened donors
		Treat underlying disease

observed for vomiting, restlessness, increased respiratory effort, and/or pigmenturia (Table 176.2). In cases of life-threatening hemorrhage, rapid administration of blood products is necessary and transfusion protocols are not utilized. Chapters 170 and 177 discuss rapid administration of blood products in more detail.

Transfusion reactions can be divided into two broad categories: immunological and non-immunological. These categories can be further divided into acute (up to 48h) and delayed reactions (beyond 48h) [23,24]. Acute immunological transfusion reactions include hemolysis, fever, and urticaria. Examples of acute non-immunological reactions include transfusion-associated circulatory overload (TACO), vomiting, acute respiratory distress, and infectious disease transmission or citrate toxicity.

Red blood cell transfusion can cause two main acute immunological reactions: febrile non-hemolytic reactions and hemolytic reactions. Hemolytic reactions are the most severe transfusion reactions and can be fatal. If a reaction is suspected in patients receiving red blood cells, the transfusion should be stopped and the patient assessed for hemolysis. If hemolysis is evident, the transfusion should be discontinued immediately and the patient monitored and supported closely. Using blood from a compatible cross-match should prevent hemolytic transfusion reactions. Febrile non-hemolytic reactions are much more common. They are the result of cytokines and white blood cells in the donor unit.

The transfusion can usually be completed in the face of a febrile non-hemolytic reaction although the administration rate may need to be slowed. Premedication with glucocorticoids or antihistamine drugs will not prevent either of these transfusion reactions and is not recommended [25].

Plasma transfusion (either as component therapy or as part of whole blood) can cause acute hypersensitivity reactions manifested by urticaria and pruritus. Antihistamine administration may be of benefit for these patients. Citrate toxicity may occur with transfusion of anticoagulated blood products. Citrate chelates ionized calcium, resulting in ionized hypocalcemia. This can cause tremors, facial pruritus, hypotension, arrhythmias or any combination thereof. Citrate toxicity is treated with administration of IV calcium, in a separate line from the blood product.

The clinician must carefully evaluate the risk:benefit relationship in any potential transfusion recipient. Transfusion of red blood cells has been associated with activation of the immune system and secondary transfusion-related immunomodulation (TRIM), TACO, and transfusion-related acute lung injury (TRALI). Each of these poses serious potential risks and must be carefully considered prior to transfusion of any blood products. Use of clinical endpoints of resuscitation, such as heart rate, blood pressure, mentation, and lactate, should be emphasized over solely evaluating the HCT, PCV, or hemoglobin.

References

1 Lower R. The success of the experiment of transfusing the blood of one animal into another. *Philos Trans R Soc Lond B Biol Sci* 1665;1:352.

2 Kessler RJ, Reese J, Chang D, et al. Dog erythrocyte antigens 1.1, 1.2, 3, 4, 7 and Dal blood typing and cross-matching by gel column technique. *Vet Clin Pathol* 2010;39(3):306–316.

3 Blais MC, Berman L, Oakley DA, et al. Canine Dal blood type: a red cell antigen lacking in some Dalmatians. *J Vet Intern Med* 2007;21(2):281–286.

4 Griot-Wenk ME, Giger U. Feline transfusion medicine: feline blood types and their clinical importance. *Vet Clin North Am Small Anim Pract* 1995;25:1305.

5 Malik R, Griffin DL, White JD, et al. The prevalence of feline A/B blood typs in the Sydney region. *Aust Vet J* 2005;83(1–2):38–44.

6 Giger U, Kilrain CG, Filippich LJ, et al. Frequencies of feline blood groups in the United States. *J Am Vet Med Assoc* 1989;195(9):1230–1232.

7 Forcada Y, Guitian J, Gibson G. Frequencies of feline blood types at a referral hospital in the south east of England. *J Small Anim Pract* 2007;48:570–573.

8 Giger U, Bucheler J, Patterson DF. Frequency and inheritance of A and B blood types in feline breeds of the United States. *J Hered* 1991;82(1):15–20.

9 Weinstein NM, Blais MC, Harris K, et al. A newly recognized blood group in domestic shorthair cats: the Mik red cell antigen. *J Vet Intern Med* 2007;21(2):287–292.

10 Bovens C, Gruffydd-Jones T. Xenotransfusion with canine blood in the feline species: review of the literature. *J Feline Med Surg* 2012;15(2):62–67.

11 Klainbart S, Oron L, Lenchner I, et al. Canine-to-feline xenotransfusions: a case series of 9 clinical cases. *J Vet Emerg Crit Care* 2015;25(S1):S6.

12 Giger U, Bucheler J. Transfusion of type-A and type-B blood to cats. *J Am Vet Med Assoc* 1991;198(3):411–418.

13 Vap LM. An update on blood typing, crossmatching, and doing no harm in transfusing dogs and cats. *Vet Med* 2010:447–458.

14 McDevitt RI, Ruaux CG, Baltzer WI. Influence of transfusion technique on survival of autologous red blood cells in the dog. *J Vet Emerg Crit Care* 2011;21(3):209–211.

15 Heikes B, Ruaux C. Syringe and aggregate filter administration does not affect survival of transfused autologous feline red blood cells. *J Vet Emerg Crit Care* 2014;24(2):162–167.

16 Short JL, Diehl S, Seshadri R, et al. Accuracy of formulas used to predict post-transfusion packed cell volume rise in anemic dogs. *J Vet Emerg Crit Care* 2012;22:428–434.

17 Day MJ, Barbara K (eds). *BSAVA Manual of Canine and Feline Haematology and Transfusion Medicine*, 2nd edn. British Small Animal Veterinary Association, Gloucester, 2012.

18 Beymer JS, Rudloff E, Kirby R, et al. Serial blood cultures from canine stored whole blood held at room temperature for 24 h. *Comp Clin Pathol* 2009;18(3):279–281.

19 Yaxley P, Beal MW, Jutkowitz L. Comparative stability of canine and feline hemostatic proteins in freeze-thaw-cycled fresh frozen plasma. *J Vet Emerg Crit Care* 2010;20(5):472–478.

20 Callan MB, Oakley DA, Shofer FS, et al. Canine red blood cell transfusion practice. *J Am Anim Hosp Assoc* 1996;32:303–311.

21 Assarasakorn S, Niwetpathomwat A. A retrospective study of blood transfusion in dogs from a veterinary hospital in Bangkok, Thailand. *Comp Clin Pathol* 2006;15:191–194.

22 Kerl ME, Hohenhaus AE. Packed red blood cell transfusions in dogs: 131 cases (1989). *J Am Vet Med Assoc* 1993;202(9):1495–1499.

23 Bruce JA, Kriese-Anderson L, Bruce AM, et al. Effect of premedication and other factors on the occurrence of acute transfusion reactions in dogs. *J Vet Emerg Crit Care* 2015;25(5):620–630.

24 Prittie JE. Triggers for use, optimal dosing, and problems associated with red cell transfusions. *Vet Clin North Am Small Anim Pract* 2003;33(6):1261–1275.

25 Marti-Carvajal AJ, Sola I, Gonzalez LE, et al. Pharmacological interventions for the prevention of allergic and febrile non-hemolytic transfusion reactions. *Cochrane Database Syst Rev* 2010;6:CD007539.

177

Massive Transfusion

Kari Santoro Beer, DVM, DACVECC¹ and Amanda Thomer, VMD, DACVECC²

¹*Oakland Veterinary Referral Services, Bloomfield Hills, MI, USA*
²*ACCESS Specialty Animal Hospitals, Culver City, CA, USA*

Introduction

In cases of severe hemorrhage, patients may require large volumes or rapid infusions of blood products to achieve hemodynamic stabilization. This resuscitation strategy is termed *massive transfusion*, and is most commonly defined as receiving one blood volume or more of blood products within 24 hours. Receiving 50% of one blood volume within 3 hours, 150% of one blood volume regardless of time, or 1.5 mL/kg/min of blood products for 20 minutes have also been considered massive transfusion. In veterinary patients, blood volumes are approximately 80–90 mL/kg in canines and 40–60 mL/kg in felines [1].

In human and veterinary medicine, classic resuscitation strategies for patients with severe hemorrhage include crystalloid fluids followed by red blood cell transfusion, and plasma products if hypocoagulability is documented. More recently, in human medicine, review articles suggest a change in this approach, with the focus redirected at rapid surgical correction of bleeding, prevention and treatment of acidosis and hypothermia, transfusion of plasma, platelets and red blood cells in a 1:1:1 ratio, early use of fibrinogen, potential use of recombinant activated factor VII (rFVIIa), and decreased emphasis on excessive crystalloid and RBC use [2]. Some of these strategies have been incorporated into veterinary medicine in recent years, and the evidence for their use will be discussed.

Patients requiring massive transfusion are often severely affected or critically ill, and survival rates in human medicine (25–84%) and veterinary medicine (4/15 dogs in one study, 27%) reflect this [1]. Given the cost and resources associated with massive transfusion strategies, it is important to be aware of treatment recommendations and possible complications of massive transfusion to ensure the best possible outcomes.

Common Conditions Requiring Massive Transfusion

In human patients, massive transfusion is rare and is most commonly employed following hemorrhage from trauma in cases of combat. Other less common conditions requiring massive transfusion include aortic aneurysm, liver transplant, and obstetric catastrophes. In veterinary patients, data are limited and based primarily on a single retrospective study of 15 dogs [3]. In this small population, underlying causes of hemorrhage included abdominal neoplasia with resultant hemoabdomen (n=6), traumatic hemoabdomen (3), gastrointestinal hemorrhage (3), gastric dilation-volvulus (2), and septic peritonitis with severe intra-abdominal hemorrhage (1).

Diagnosis/Prediction

Patients presenting with a requirement for massive transfusion will likely demonstrate signs of severe hypovolemic shock secondary to decreased tissue perfusion and cellular hypoxia (see Chapter 153). Left untreated, hemodynamic instability will lead to organ damage and death [4]. Pale mucous membranes, prolonged capillary refill time, tachycardia (or bradycardia in cats), poor peripheral pulses, tachypnea, weakness, and mental obtundation are the classic signs of hypovolemia, but not all patients with tissue hypoperfusion as the result of massive hemorrhage present with obvious signs of shock.

Signs of blood loss may be external or may be detected via initial assessment with ultrasound (FAST scan; see Chapter 182) or rectal examination in the case of gastrointestinal hemorrhage [5]. Initial blood database should consist of packed cell volume (PCV) and total solids (TS), with a venous blood gas if possible. While low PCV and TS are supportive of hemorrhage due to loss of both red blood cells and protein from the intravascular space, splenic contraction can lead to an increase in PCV and discordant PCV/TS (normal PCV/low TS) early on following blood loss, especially in dogs. Venous blood gas results will often be suggestive of a lactic acidosis due to tissue hypoperfusion, although other changes are possible depending on the patient's clinical signs (see Chapter 156). If hemorrhage is suspected based on history, physical exam or laboratory findings, the lack of a specific diagnosis in terms of source of bleeding should not delay resuscitation.

While hypotension (historically defined as a systolic blood pressure ≤90 mmHg) has classically been considered an indicator of shock, early compensation by the cardiovascular system may allow patients to maintain a relatively normal blood pressure despite significant blood loss. As such, the shock index (SI), defined as the ratio of heart rate (HR) to systolic blood pressure (SBP), has been developed in people to attempt to recognize shock earlier, during this compensatory phase. In healthy adults, normal SI ranges from 0.5 to 0.7, and human studies have identified a prehospital SI > 0.9 as a risk factor for massive transfusion [6]. Shock index has recently been evaluated in a small retrospective study of canine patients with blunt trauma requiring transfusion [7]. In that study, a SI > 1.43 was 71% accurate for predicting the need for transfusion, and the authors concluded that SI may have some utility in predicting transfusion needs following blunt trauma in dogs, although further studies are warranted (see Chapter 152).

In addition to the SI, a scoring system exists in human medicine to attempt to predict the need for massive transfusion. The Trauma-Associated Severe Hemorrhage (TASH) score takes into account a number of variables including hemoglobin concentration, base excess, systolic blood pressure, heart rate, the presence of free abdominal fluid, the presence of clinically unstable pelvic fractures or open/dislocated femur fractures, as well as gender, and calculates a score to determine the probability of massive transfusion [8]. Higher scores increase the probability of massive transfusion. No such scores have been developed for veterinary patients.

Pre-Resuscitation Complications/Acute Traumatic Coagulopathy

Even before resuscitation with fluids and blood products, patients with severe hemorrhage and shock necessitating massive transfusion are prone to coagulation abnormalities that may predispose them to further bleeding. While it was initially hypothesized that this coagulopathy was due to blood loss, hemostatic dysfunction and/or

hemodilution of coagulation factors and platelets, more recent evidence has shown that this acute traumatic coagulopathy (ATC) can occur as quickly as within 30 minutes post trauma, and is characterized by anticoagulation and hyperfibrinolysis (see Chapter 163) [9–11]. This coagulopathy occurs before resuscitation is instituted, and in human patients, its severity appears to be positively correlated with the severity of injury and degree of shock. In human trauma patients, the presence of ATC is an independent risk factor for death, and is associated with a four-fold higher risk of multiple organ dysfunction syndrome (MODS) and death [9,12].

While the exact mechanisms of ATC are not fully understood, current hypotheses include a disseminated intravascular coagulation (DIC) process with hyperfibrinolysis, an enhanced thrombomodulin-thrombin-protein C pathway, and catecholamine-induced endothelial damage from exuberant sympathoadrenal stimulation [9,11]. Hypothermia, acidosis, hemodilution, and systemic inflammation may further contribute to what has been termed a "bloody vicious cycle," in which "bleeding leads to resuscitation, resuscitation leads to dilution and hypothermia, dilution and hypothermia lead to coagulopathy, and coagulopathy leads to bleeding" [13]. Hypothermia may worsen coagulation by inhibiting platelet function, reducing synthesis, inhibiting function of coagulation factors, and increasing fibrinolysis. In addition, acidosis impairs coagulation factor function [1,14].

In human patients with trauma, the incidence of ATC is 10–30% [15]. The incidence in veterinary medicine remains unknown, but several studies have documented the occurrence of a hypocoagulable state in canine patients with trauma. In one prospective study, spontaneously traumatized dogs had a significant reduction in all measured hemostatic factors and significant prolongations of aPTT and PT compared to a healthy control group [16]. In another study of dogs with trauma, ATC was identified in 15% of patients, and there was a correlation between prolonged aPTT times and non-survival [14].

Treatment

In human medicine, the standard treatment approach to hemorrhagic shock and those patients requiring massive transfusion historically included administration of liberal amounts of crystalloids and pRBCs followed by the administration of plasma and platelets based on coagulation testing [17,18]. Damage control resuscitation is now recommended, the purpose of which is to try to stop the "vicious bloody cycle" in which the triad of hypothermia, acidosis, and coagulopathy leads to continued hemorrhage [11,13,19,20].

Damage control resuscitation includes hypotensive resuscitation, decreased use of crystalloids, administration of fresh frozen plasma, platelets and packed red blood cells (FFP:plt:pRBC) in a 1:1:1 ratio, use of other hemostatic agents as needed, heat support, and early surgical intervention [21–23]. Based on a recent prospective observational study, the PROMMTT trial, and a prospective randomized controlled clinical trial, the PROPPR trial, it is now recommended that blood products, FFP:plt:pRBC, be administered early on in resuscitation and in a 1:1:1 ratio in human medicine to improve survival and decrease transfusion requirements [21,22]. In veterinary medicine, no studies currently exist examining blood product component therapy and transfusion ratios. However, based on the human evidence, it may be advisable to consider plasma and platelet transfusions early on in patients requiring massive transfusion, or administering whole blood when available [11,12,15,19,24].

Other blood products utilized in human medicine for massive transfusion resuscitation include cryoprecipitate, fibrinogen concentrate, rFVIIa, prothrombin complex, and antifibrinolytics [10,17,20,25–27]. Cryoprecipitate or fibrinogen concentrate is indicated when fibrinogen levels are below 100 mg/dL [17,25,27]. The fibrinogen goal is 150–200 mg/dL with the ideal range being >200 mg/dL [27]. Tranexamic acid, an antifibrinolytic, has been shown to decrease mortality in human trauma patients when used within the first 3 hours; no evidence currently exists to support the use of antifibrinolytics in veterinary patients requiring massive transfusion (see Chapter 68) [10].

Damage control resuscitation should be implemented in veterinary patients receiving or expected to receive a massive transfusion. It is recommended to optimize the use of blood products and administer them sooner to decrease the dilutional effect of large amounts of crystalloids. Transfusions should be given as needed and it is recommended that for each pRBC transfusion that is administered, a FFP transfusion be given as well. The recommended dose for FFP is 10–20 mL/kg and the dose for pRBC is 15 mL/kg to raise the PCV by 10% [28,29]. If whole blood is available, the recommended starting dose is 20–30 mL/kg. If fibrinogen is able to be measured and is low, then cryoprecipitate can be given. Tranexamic acid or aminocaproic acid can also be considered. If possible, synthetic colloids should be avoided given their reduction in fVIII and vWf activity (see Chapter 168).

Usually, it is recommended to administer a blood product transfusion slowly within a 4-hour period [30]. In stable, resuscitated patients that are meeting the criteria of massive transfusion, this recommendation should be followed (see Chapter 176). However, in unstable patients requiring massive transfusion due to hemorrhagic shock, it is the authors' recommendation to administer blood products as fast as necessary in order to stabilize the patient as the benefit of preventing death outweighs the risk of a transfusion reaction. In the authors' experience, patients in hemorrhagic shock can be bolused pRBC transfusions within minutes without experiencing significant transfusion reactions. Hypotensive resuscitation should be implemented with a systolic blood pressure target of 90 mmHg during the early resuscitation period until hemostasis can be achieved. Additional treatments should include heat support and early surgical intervention.

Complications

Electrolyte Abnormalities

Possible electrolyte abnormalities secondary to massive transfusion include hypocalcemia, hypomagnesemia, and hyperkalemia (see Chapters 109 and 110). Citrate from pRBC units can bind to ionized calcium, causing hypocalcemia [11,13,20]. Common signs of hypocalcemia include muscle tremors, excitation, disorientation, hypersensitivity to stimuli, and facial rubbing [31]. Echocardiographic and ECG abnormalities may include evidence of decreased cardiac output, decreased contractility, arrhythmias, and a prolonged QT interval [31]. Patients with hypocalcemia showing clinical signs should be treated with calcium gluconate at a dose of 0.5–1.5 mL/kg IV administered slowly and to effect. Hypomagnesemia can also occur secondary to citrate binding [11]. Common signs are muscle fasciculations, muscle weakness, and seizures. ECG findings include arrhythmias and a prolonged QT interval [32]. Magnesium sulfate should be administered if clinical signs are present. The recommended magnesium dose for life-threatening arrhythmias is 0.15–0.3 mEq/kg diluted in 5% dextrose or normal saline and administered intravenously over 5–60 minutes [33].

Hyperkalemia can occur secondary to increased potassium levels in the pRBC supernatant [11,13]. Potassium levels increase with each day of pRBC storage and by 42 days of storage, there can be a significant amount of potassium in a unit, with studies citing 45–77 mEq/L [11,13,34]. Hyperkalemia from pRBC transfusion is thought to be less of a problem in veterinary medicine as dogs have less potassium in their red blood cells compared to humans; however, in cases of massive transfusion, potassium levels should be monitored closely [1]. If hyperkalemia occurs, it is usually transient, and resolves as potassium is redistributed in the body [34].

However, there is evidence in human medicine that cardiac arrest can occur from hyperkalemia during a pRBC transfusion [11,34]. In addition to measuring potassium levels periodically, ECG monitoring should occur continuously in patients requiring massive transfusion. Signs of hyperkalemia on an ECG in veterinary medicine include peaked T-waves, widened QRS, atrial standstill, sinoventricular rhythm, and ventricular fibrillation [35].

Methods used to prevent hyperkalemia in human patients requiring massive transfusion include administering fresher blood, washing pRBCs to remove extracellular potassium, using in-line potassium filters, and administering insulin [13,34].

Hypothermia (see Chapter 148)

Patients in hypovolemic shock and requiring massive transfusion are likely to be hypothermic on presentation secondary to impaired tissue perfusion, and this hypothermia can be exacerbated by administering cold blood products. Complications of hypothermia include decreases in hepatic metabolism, citrate metabolism, acute-phase protein production, clotting factor production, and drug clearance [11]. Therefore, it is important to aggressively warm patients. Hypothermia should be treated with heat support, increasing the ambient room temperature, using commercial blood and fluid warmers, and humidifying air in intubated patients. Body temperature should be monitored carefully in patients with hypothermia so as not to overshoot during the rewarming process.

Acid–Base Disorders (see Chapter 107)

Both metabolic alkalosis and metabolic acidosis can develop from pRBC transfusion. A metabolic alkalosis can occur when the citrate from the pRBC unit is metabolized to bicarbonate [11,13]. Alternatively, metabolic acidosis can occur when transfusing units that are low in pH or when transfusing patients with liver dysfunction [11]. The pH of stored pRBC units can reach 6.4–6.6 due to increasing lactate and pyruvate concentrations from glucose metabolism [13]. Liver dysfunction can contribute to acidosis due to decreased ability to metabolize citrate to bicarbonate and decreased ability to metabolize

lactate [11]. Patients requiring massive transfusion should have venous or arterial blood gas values monitored regularly.

Transfusion Reactions (see Chapter 176)

Transfusion reactions, such as multiple organ failure (MOF), transfusion-related acute lung injury (TRALI), acute respiratory distress syndrome (ARDS), and transfusion-associated cardiac overload (TACO), can occur from blood product administration, and adverse events may be increased in patients requiring massive transfusion due to the increased amount of blood products administered. In human medicine, blood transfusion is an independent risk factor for MOF, and massive transfusion is independently associated with death [2]. Blood transfusion and increased total blood volume infused in human trauma patients are associated with increased incidence of SIRS and mortality [11].

In the single veterinary study on massive transfusion, the complications found among the population included hypocalcemia (10/10 dogs), hypomagnesemia (9/9), hyperkalemia (2/10), metabolic acidosis, thrombocytopenia (5/5), prolonged PT/aPTT (7/10), and transfusion reactions. The transfusion reactions were fever (3), delayed hemolysis (3), vomiting (1), and facial swelling (1) [3].

Prognosis

The prognosis for veterinary patients receiving massive transfusion is guarded and depends on the underlying cause. In the authors' opinion, prognosis is guarded to poor if hemorrhage is secondary to underlying disease, whereas patients requiring massive transfusion secondary to trauma may have a guarded to fair prognosis. In the veterinary study mentioned above, the mortality rate was 73% and no dog with a PT/PTT>150% prolonged survived [3]. However, these results should be interpreted with caution as more recent advances in recognition of the need for transfusion and treatments may help to improve outcomes.

References

1 Jutkowitz LA. Massive transfusion. In: *Small Animal Critical Care Medicine*, 2nd edn (eds Hopper KA, Silverstein DC). Saunders Elsevier, St Louis, 2015, pp. 337–342.
2 Spinella PC, Perkins JG, Grathwohl KW, et al. Effect of plasma and red blood cell transfusions on survival in patients with combat related traumatic injuries. *J Trauma* 2008;64:S69–S78.
3 Jutkowitz LA, Rozanski EA, Moreau JA, et al. Massive transfusion in dogs:15 cases (1997–2001). *J Am Vet Med Assoc* 2002;220:1664–1669.
4 Gutierrez G, Reines HD, Wulf-Gutierrez ME. Clinical review: hemorrhagic shock. *Crit Care* 2004;8:373–381.
5 Lisciandro GR. Abdominal and thoracic focused assessment with sonography for trauma, triage, and

monitoring in small animals. *J Vet Emerg Crit Care* 2011;21(2):104–122.

6 Vandromme MJ, Griffin RL, Kerby JD, et al. Identifying risk for massive transfusion in the relatively normotensive patient: utility of the prehospital shock index. *J Trauma* 2011;70:384–390.

7 Gonzalez A, Thawley V, Drobatz K. Evaluation of shock index as a predictor of transfusion requirement in dogs with blunt trauma. *J Vet Emerg Crit Care* 2015;25:S5.

8 Maegele M, Lefering R, Wafaisade W, et al. Revalidation and update of the TASH Score: a scoring system to predict the probability for massive transfusion as a surrogate for life-threatening haemorrhage after severe injury. *Vox Sang* 2011;100:231–238.

9 Palmer L, Martin L. Traumatic coagulopathy Part 1: Pathophysiology and diagnosis. *J Vet Emerg Crit Care* 2014;24(1):63–74.

10 Shakur H, Roberts I, Bautista R, et al. Effects of tranexamic acid on death, vascular occlusive events, and blood transfusion in trauma patients with significant haemorrhage (CRASH-2): a randomised, placebo-controlled trial. *Lancet* 2010;376:23–32.

11 Sihler KC, Napolitano LM. Complications of massive transfusion. *Chest* 2010;137(1):209–220.

12 Sperry JL, Ochoa JB, Gunn Sr, et al. An FFP:PRBC transfusion ratio ≥1:1.5 is associated with a lower risk of mortality after massive transfusion. *J Trauma* 2008;65:986–993.

13 Hess JR, Zimrin AB. Massive blood transfusion for trauma. *Curr Opin Hematol* 2005;12:488–492.

14 Holowaychuk M, Hanel R, O'Keefe K, et al. Prognostic value of coagulation parameters in dogs following trauma (abstract). *J Vet Emerg Crit Care* 2011;21:S6.

15 Zink KA, Sambasivan CN, Holcomb JB, et al. A high ratio of plasma and platelets to packed red blood cells in the first 6 hours of massive transfusion improves outcomes in a large multicenter study. *Am J Surg* 2009;197(5):565–570.

16 Mischke R. Acute hemostatic changes in accidentally traumatized dogs. *Vet J* 2005;169:60–64.

17 Hardy J, de Moerloose P, Samama C, et al. Massive transfusion and coagulopathy: pathophysiology and implications for clinical management. *Can J Anaesth* 2006;53:S40–S58

18 Pham HP, Shaz BH. Update on massive transfusion. *Br J Anaesth* 2013;111 (S1):i71–i82.

19 Gonzalez E, Moore F, Holcomb J, et al. Fresh frozen plasma should be given earlier to patients requiring massive transfusion. *J Trauma* 2007;62:112–119.

20 Elmer J, Wilcox S, Raja A. Massive transfusion in traumatic shock. *J Emerg Med* 2013;44:829–838.

21 Holcomb J, del Junco D, Fox E, et al. The prospective, observational, multicenter, major trauma transfusion (PROMMTT) study: comparative effectiveness of a time-varying treatment with competing risks. *JAMA Surg* 2013;148:127–136.

22 Holcomb J, Tilley B, Baraniuk S, et al. Transfusion of plasma, platelets, and red blood cells in a 1:1:1 vs a 1:1:2 ratio and mortality in patients with severe trauma: the PROPPR Randomized Clinical Trial. *JAMA* 2015;313:471–482.

23 Holcomb J, Jenkins D, Rhee P, et al. Damage control resuscitation: directly addressing the early coagulopathy of trauma. *J Trauma* 2007;62:307–310.

24 Holcomb J, Zarzabal L, Michalek J, et al. Increased platelet:RBC ratios are associated with improved survival after massive transfusion. *J Trauma* 2011;71:S318–S328.

25 Levy JH. Massive transfusion coagulopathy. *Semin Hematol* 2006;43:S59–S63.

26 Spinella P, Perkins J, McLaughlin D, et al. The effect of recombinant activated factor VII on mortality in combat-related casualties with severe trauma and massive transfusion. *J Trauma* 2008;64:286–294.

27 Nienaber U, Innerhofer P, Westermann I, et al. The impact of fresh frozen plasma vs coagulation factor concentrates on morbidity and mortality in trauma-associated haemorrhage and massive transfusion. *Injury* 2011;42:697–701.

28 Short L, Diehl S, Seshadri R, Serrano S. Accuracy of formulas used to predict post–transfusion packed cell volume rise in anemic dogs. *J Vet Emerg Crit Care* 2012;22:428–434.

29 Balakrishnan A, Silverstein DC. Shock fluids and fluid challenge. In: *Small Animal Critical Care Medicine*, 2nd edn (eds Hopper KA, Silverstein DC). Saunders Elsevier, St Louis, 2015, pp. 321–327.

30 Sullivan L, Hackett TB. Transfusion medicine: best practices. In: *Small Animal Critical Care Medicine*, 2nd edn (eds Hopper KA, Silverstein DC). Saunders Elsevier, St Louis, 2015, pp. 309–313.

31 Green TA, Chew DJ. Calcium disorders. In: *Small Animal Critical Care Medicine*, 2nd edn (eds Hopper KA, Silverstein DC). Saunders Elsevier, St Louis, 2015, pp. 274–280.

32 Martin LG, Allen-Durrance AE. Magnesium and phosphate disorders. In: *Small Animal Critical Care Medicine*, 2nd edn (eds Hopper KA, Silverstein DC). Saunders Elsevier, St Louis, 2015, pp. 281–288.

33 Palme LE, Martin LG. Approach to hypomagnesemia and hypokalemia. In: *Small Animal Critical Care Medicine*, 2nd edn (eds Hopper KA, Silverstein DC). Saunders Elsevier, St Louis, 2015, pp. 248–253.

34 Vraets A, Lin Y, Callum JL. Transfusion-associated hyperkalemia. *Transfus Med Rev* 2011;184–196.

35 Riordan LL, Schaer M. Potassium disorders. In: *Small Animal Critical Care Medicine*, 2nd edn (eds Hopper KA, Silverstein DC). Saunders Elsevier, St Louis, 2015, pp. 269–273.

Section 6

Emergency Room Procedures

178

Vascular Access

Matthew W. Beal, DVM, DACVECC

College of Veterinary Medicine, Michigan State University, East Lansing, MI, USA

Introduction

Patients presented to veterinarians on an emergency basis often have severe physiological derangements necessitating rapid access to vascular structures in order to deliver fluids, blood products, and potentially life-saving medications. Vascular access devices can also provide valuable monitoring information about intravascular pressures on both the venous and arterial sides of the circulation. Gaining efficient vascular access using appropriate devices facilitates the rapid delivery of care and thus contributes to positive outcomes in this often unstable patient population. The following pages will describe various methods and devices for venous and arterial access that may be utilized on an emergency basis.

Venous Access

Considerations for Venous Access

Patients presenting on an emergency basis are often under extreme stress due to their underlying condition(s), pain, transportation, and the emergency room environment. In this patient population, venous access must be performed efficiently while causing as little discomfort and stress to the patient as possible. Despite the availability of devices that are placed using creative techniques and advanced technology, "keeping it simple" is a guiding principle when dealing with this patient population. Placing short, over-the-needle IV catheters in easily accessed (cephalic, saphenous) veins meets these requirements. Concurrent administration of oxygen (see Chapter 181) in patients with cardiorespiratory compromise and the judicious use of analgesics and sedatives will also help minimize stress (see Chapter 193).

Vascular access sites are a potential source of hospital-acquired infection in veterinary patients [1].

While rapid acquisition of vascular access is important in the patient population that presents on an emergency basis, adherence to strict asepsis may help minimize the chance of catheter-related complications in the days following admission. The proposed vascular access site should be clipped very widely, allowing for a large sterile area within which to work. Full surgical preparation in accordance with institutional guidelines is indicated. Use of sterile gloves and a sterile drape during placement of routine peripheral venous access devices is indicated. However, at minimum, examination gloves should be utilized. All measures of sterile technique (sterile surgical gowns, caps, masks, sterile gloves, and wide draping) further minimize the chance of contamination and should be used in more complex access procedures (central venous access, dialysis access).

The access site should be evaluated critically at least once daily and the vein proximal to the site should be evaluated multiple times daily for evidence of thrombophlebitis (redness, pain, swelling, thrombosis).

Choice of vascular access site and device type placed on an emergency basis is determined by numerous factors including, but not limited to, the pathophysiology of major problems (need for rapid infusion, presence of hemostatic abnormalities, etc.), ease of device placement, need for ability to monitor central venous pressures, need for ability to reliably sample, and patient stability.

Hypovolemia is one of the most common cardiovascular derangements encountered on an emergency basis (see Chapter 153). The ability to rapidly infuse large volumes of crystalloid fluids or blood products is often needed for the management of this condition.

The vascular access device and placement location can have significant influence on the maximum rate of fluid administration. Flow of fluid through rigid tubes is governed by the Hagan–Poiseuille equation [2]. Although the IV infusion system, IV catheter, and vasculature

Textbook of Small Animal Emergency Medicine, First Edition. Edited by Kenneth J. Drobatz, Kate Hopper, Elizabeth Rozanski and Deborah C. Silverstein.
© 2019 John Wiley & Sons, Inc. Published 2019 by John Wiley & Sons, Inc.
Companion Website: www.wiley.com/go/drobatz/textbook

are not rigid tubes, the equation still provides valuable insights into the physics of flow. Flow (Q) is determined by the pressure differential across the tube ($P_{in} - P_{out}$), the radius of the tube (raised to the fourth power, r^4), the length of the tube (L), and viscosity of the fluid flowing through the tube (μ) according to the equation below

$$\text{Flow rate}(Q) = \frac{(P_{in} - P_{out})\Pi r^4}{8\mu L}$$

Simply stated, this equation indicates that increasing pressure at the inlet of a tube (squeezing or elevating an IV fluid bag), increasing the radius of the "tube" (larger bore IV placed in large vessels), infusing fluids with low viscosity (for example, diluting with saline and warming packed red blood cells), and minimizing length of the system (not choosing long central venous catheters when rapid infusion is needed) will facilitate rapid infusion of IV fluids and blood products. Of note, the radius of the "tube" has greatest influence on flow as it is raised to the fourth power. Simply doubling radius results in a 16-fold increase in flow rate.

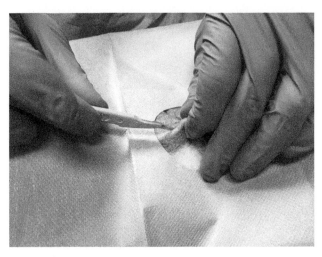

Figure 178.1 Percutaneous facilitative approach to the jugular vein in a dog. A small skin defect is created using a sharp instrument such as a #11 scalpel blade through which the IV catheter is placed. When performing the percutaneous facilitative technique, the skin should be tented over the vessel prior to incision to minimize the chance of underlying vascular injury.

Approaches and Techniques for Venous Access

Venous catheters may be placed via three major approaches.

The percutaneous approach is most commonly utilized. In this technique, the IV catheter is placed directly through the skin into the venous structure.

The percutaneous facilitative technique involves creation of a small skin defect of similar diameter to the IV catheter using a sharp instrument such as a #11 scalpel blade through which the IV catheter is placed. When performing the percutaneous facilitative technique, the skin should be tented over the vessel prior to incision to minimize the chance of underlying vascular injury (Figure 178.1). The percutaneous facilitative technique decreases resistance caused by the skin during attempts to penetrate it and advance a catheter through it while also decreasing the chance of trauma to the catheter itself while penetrating the skin. The facilitative technique is very useful in thick-skinned patients and in areas of the body with thicker skin, including the cervical region. The technique should always be used when placing larger diameter access devices.

The third approach is a surgical cut-down. Cut-down may need to be performed on an emergency basis when no other access device can be placed and immediate patient stability hinges on gaining vascular access. The emergency cut-down procedure involves creation of a generous incision slightly lateral or medial to the anatomical location of the preferred vein. In peripheral sites (cephalic or saphenous vein), after incision, the skin may

be rolled slightly to facilitate visualization of the vein (Figure 178.2a). The IV catheter is then placed (preferably) through the skin distal to the cut-down site, into the site, and then into the vein (Figure 178.2b). This allows the cut-down site to be closed without the IV catheter penetrating through the incision.

The author finds that in the most urgent situations when an emergency cut-down is needed, the jugular vein provides a very reliable access site that allows for the placement of a large-bore venous access device. The anatomical location of the jugular vein is easily determined by identifying the angle of the mandible and drawing a line between it and the thoracic inlet (Figure 178.3a). Cut-down over the jugular vein is performed as described above for a peripheral vein, but some blunt dissection will be necessary to strip away subcutaneous fat and adventitial tissue from the vessel itself to optimally visualize the vessel (Figure 178.3b). Dissection around the vessel allows for placement of a monofilament suture or silicone vessel loop for facilitating control of the vessel prior to catheter placement (Figure 178.3c).

The emergency cut-down procedure should be performed with adherence to strict asepsis. However, on an emergency basis, if the situation precludes adherence to strict asepsis, then after resuscitation, alternative sterile access should be attained and the catheter placed via emergency cut-down should be removed.

The aforementioned approaches may be utilized for the placement of a variety of types of catheters using a

Figure 178.2 (a) Cut-down just
medial to the cephalic vein. After
incision, the skin is rolled slightly
to facilitate visualization of the
vein. (b) The IV catheter is placed
through the skin distal to the
cut-down site, into the site, and
then into the vein. This allows the
cut-down site to be closed without
the IV catheter penetrating through
the incision.

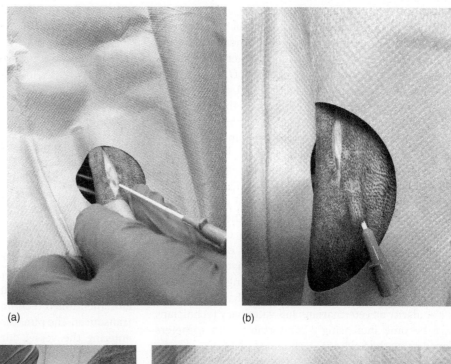

(a) (b)

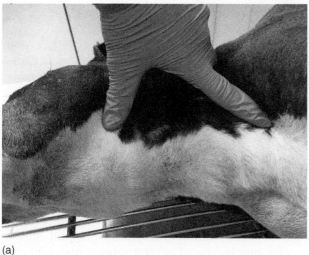

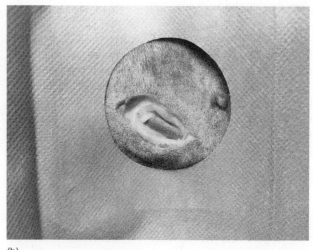

(a) (b)

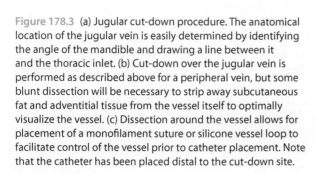

(a)

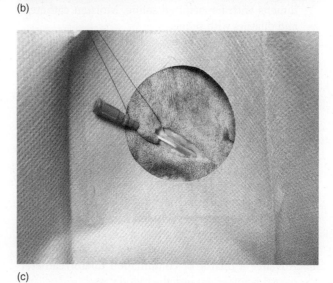

Figure 178.3 (a) Jugular cut-down procedure. The anatomical
location of the jugular vein is easily determined by identifying
the angle of the mandible and drawing a line between it
and the thoracic inlet. (b) Cut-down over the jugular vein is
performed as described above for a peripheral vein, but some
blunt dissection will be necessary to strip away subcutaneous
fat and adventitial tissue from the vessel itself to optimally
visualize the vessel. (c) Dissection around the vessel allows for
placement of a monofilament suture or silicone vessel loop to
facilitate control of the vessel prior to catheter placement. Note
that the catheter has been placed distal to the cut-down site.

(c)

variety of techniques. As previously mentioned, the most commonly utilized catheters in the small animal emergency room are over-the-needle IV catheters placed in peripheral vessels. These catheters are generally placed using direct visualization and palpation of the target vessel. The over-the-needle catheter is directed into the target vessel at approximately a 20° angle to the skin. When a flash of blood is visualized in the chamber of the needle, the entire system is advanced 1–3 mm and then the catheter is fed over the needle into the vessel and secured and dressed using standard techniques.

Through-the-needle catheters were once used for the placement of a variety of types of central venous catheters and peripherally inserted central catheters (PICCs). These catheters are economical but they create a larger defect in the vessel than the catheter occupies after placement and, as a result, may be associated with more hemorrhage than catheters placed using other techniques. Through-the-needle catheters have decreased in popularity as veterinarians and veterinary technicians have become increasingly comfortable with catheters placed using the Seldinger technique.

The Seldinger or modified Seldinger techniques are also called "over-the-wire" techniques. They are utilized for the placement of a variety of types of catheters but most commonly, central venous catheters and PICCs use this technique [3]. The author uses this technique for the placement of large catheter introducers (also called sheath introducers) in the jugular vein of patients with severe hypovolemia, allowing for extremely rapid volume expansion.

The following are the major steps in the Seldinger technique.

1. Surgical preparation.
2. +/− Local anesthetic infiltration.
3. Prepare the IV catheter for insertion. Flush all lumens with heparinized saline. Moisten catheters and dilators with saline.
4. Make a small 2–4 mm incision with a #11 blade over the vessel (percutaneous facilitative approach). Note that this step may be performed or the incision may be expanded after step 6.
5. Insert the needle or catheter into the blood vessel. Blood should flow freely from the needle/catheter.
6. Feed a flexible "J-tip" guidewire or other soft tip guidewire through the needle into the blood vessel. For all future steps, the guidewire should be held by the operator to eliminate the chance of dislodgment or inadvertent loss in the patient.
7. Withdraw the needle/catheter over the guidewire. Mild hemorrhage may be noted. Direct pressure can be applied after needle/catheter withdrawal.
8. Advance a dilator or combination dilator/catheter over the guidewire into the blood vessel.
9. Remove the dilator over the guidewire and advance a prepared catheter (step 3) over the wire into the vessel.
10. Remove the guidewire.
11. All ports should then be flushed with saline or heparinized saline.
12. Suture the catheter in place and apply a sterile dressing.

Advanced imaging techniques may be useful for gaining vascular access. Ultrasound-guided vascular access is especially useful in patients in which the vessel to be punctured cannot be visualized or palpated [4]. The author uses this technique most often to access the jugular, maxillary, or femoral veins in patients with deep vessels, obesity, or edema. Briefly, a high-frequency, linear array transducer with a sterile cover is used to identify the target vessel and is placed over it and in a longitudinal plane. Vessel puncture is performed using one of the aforementioned techniques behind (upstream from) the transducer. The puncture needle or catheter is visualized entering the vessel during placement. The ultrasound transducer is then removed and catheter placement proceeds according to manufacturer instructions.

Fluoroscopy-assisted vascular access in the emergency room is most often utilized during placement of dialysis catheters for intermittent hemodialysis or continuous renal replacement therapy (CRRT) in patients with acute renal injury. Fluoroscopy allows for optimal positioning of the catheter tip during placement.

Locations for Venous Access

As previously stated, venous access locations should be chosen to minimize stress to the patient while meeting the given goal of the access device (administration of medications only versus rapid fluid infusion, versus monitoring of central venous pressure, etc.). Peripheral veins are the most common sites for venous access, with the cephalic vein, accessory cephalic vein, and saphenous vein most often utilized. Using these sites allows the patient to remain sternal which is often helpful when there is respiratory compromise. Box 178.1 indicates peripheral venous access sites that may be considered.

The use of highly mobile sites such as the auricular vein or common digital veins will require the utilization of a splint. Securing the IV catheter to the pinna with rolled gauze placed beneath it is helpful for auricular venous access. A simple spoon splint will help immobilize the carpus when utilizing the common digital veins.

Central venous access is not often utilized in the initial minutes after a patient presents on an emergency basis. However, central venous access is often performed soon thereafter in patients in which central venous pressure

Cephalic vein
Accessory cephalic vein
Medial saphenous vein
Lateral saphenous vein
Dorsal common digital vein
Auricular vein
Jugular vein

monitoring is indicated and in those which require a highly reliable catheter for repeated blood sampling. Some central venous catheters allow for the monitoring of central venous oxygen saturation which has potential as a monitoring tool in the emergency room and intensive care unit.

The jugular vein is the most commonly utilized site for central venous access, but a catheter placed in the saphenous vein (or rarely cephalic) can be advanced into the central circulation (PICC). The author also utilizes the maxillary vein in dogs that have a temporary tracheostomy and require central venous access. In these patients, the jugular vein is in close proximity to the temporary tracheostomy site and thus puts a catheter placed in this location at significant risk for contamination.

When considering utilizing the jugular or maxillary veins for central venous access, hemostasis should be assessed (platelet count and coagulation through assessment of ACT or PT/aPTT). Significant hemostatic abnormalities are a contraindication to jugular, maxillary, and femoral vein access.

Intraosseous Access

Considerations for Intraosseous Access

Intraosseous access to the rich sinusoidal network of the marrow cavity allows for the delivery of fluids, blood products, and medications in patients in which venous access is not possible or is technically challenging. This may include patients that are extremely small (neonates) and those with severe chronic vascular injury or severe hypovolemia where venous access is challenging. Intraosseous access can often be achieved very rapidly. Most often, intraosseous access is used until traditional venous access can be acquired. Contraindications to placement of IO devices include fracture of the proposed insertion bone, injury or disease at the proposed insertion site, and sepsis. This being said, access is needed and IO catheters may be placed despite the possibility of sepsis, especially in neonatal patients.

Approaches and Techniques for Intraosseous Access

Spinal needles or standard hypodermic needles (20–22 G) in neonates and Jamshedi bone biopsy/bone marrow aspiration needles in larger patients are commonly utilized for IO access. The stylet in these devices (except hypodermic needles) prevents bone spicules from clogging the needle itself.

Briefly, the proposed insertion site is aseptically prepared and aseptic technique is practiced. Most patients requiring IO access are moribund and local anesthesia is not utilized. However, in the more alert patient, local infusion of 1 mg/kg lidocaine in the skin and down to the periosteum is indicated if time permits. If using the intertrochanteric fossa of the femur, the greater trochanter is palpated and the needle is directed through the skin and onto the greater trochanter. Then, the needle is simply "walked" medially until it falls into the fossa (Figure 178.4). This technique may help avoid injury to the sciatic nerve. Short 90° oscillations of the needle are applied while gentle pressure is directed down the axis of the femur. Palpation of the medial aspect of the femur helps identify unintended penetration of the medial cortex. The stylet is removed and the catheter is gently flushed to ensure patency. If not patent, rotate the catheter 90° to ensure that the bevel is not closely apposed

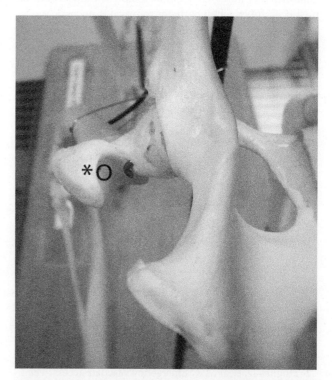

Figure 178.4 Intraosseous landmarks for IO catheter insertion at the intertrochanteric fossa of the femur. The greater trochanter is palpated and the needle is directed through the skin and onto the greater trochanter (*). Then, the needle is simply "walked" medially until it falls into the fossa (O).

to the inner cortex. If fluid accumulates subcutaneously at the insertion site, an alternative site should be considered. Once in place, a sterile dressing should be applied. The author secures these catheters in place using a tape butterfly and sutures.

Alternative devices, including spring-loaded impact penetration devices and powered drivers, are commercially available for very rapid placement of IO catheters (Veterinary BIG, WaisMed Ltd, Rosh Ha'Ayin, Israel; EZ-IO by Vidacare, Mila International, Erlanger, KY, USA). These devices most often utilize the flat, proximal aspect of the tibia or the proximal humerus at the level of the greater tubercle. Collectively, they allow for very rapid, successful placement of IO catheters in non-neonatal dogs and cats [5].

Arterial Access

Arterial access is acquired in the emergency room for monitoring of direct arterial blood pressure and for sampling for analysis of arterial blood gases. The dorsal pedal artery is most commonly utilized in veterinary patients for arterial access because it is superficial and peripheral. The puncture site is usually just distal to where the artery dives between metatarsals II and III (Figure 178.5). The anatomy facilitates easy compression should access be unsuccessful or when catheter removal is necessary.

Alternative peripheral sites for arterial puncture include the radial artery and auricular artery. More proximal sites for arterial access include the femoral artery and brachial artery. These sites, especially the femoral artery, are easily accessed, but high motion makes catheter dislodgment a problem in mobile patients. The author only uses proximal arterial sites for access in patients that are moribund or immobilized (ventilator-dependent patients, CRRT patients) and only longer catheters should be utilized to minimize the chance of dislodgment with motion. Proximal arterial access sites are difficult to compress should placement be unsuccessful or when catheter removal is necessary, making bleeding a significant risk of placement.

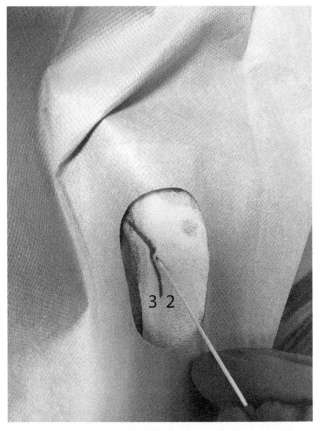

Figure 178.5 Path of the dorsal pedal (metatarsal) artery of the right pelvic limb. The catheter indicates the direction of puncture. Numbers 2 and 3 indicate the location of the proximal aspect of the second and third metatarsals.

Hemostasis should be completely assessed if proximal arterial access sites are chosen.

Over-the-needle catheters are most often placed for arterial access. However, kits that utilize the Seldinger technique are also available. Aseptic technique should be adhered to during placement and similar monitoring should proceed as described above for venous access. Arterial catheters are optimally connected to a continuous blood pressure monitoring system which provides a continuous low-volume heparinized saline flush to the system.

References

1 Sequela J, Pages JP. Bacterial and fungal colonization of peripheral intravenous catheters in dogs and cats. *J Small Anim Pract* 2011;52:531–535.

2 Hughes D, Beal MW. Emergency vascular access. *Vet Clin North Am Small Anim Pract* 2000;30:491–507.

3 Beal MW, Hughes D. Vascular access: theory and techniques in the small animal emergency patient. *Clin Tech Small Anim Pract* 2000;15:101–109.

4 Chamberlin SC, Sullivan LA, Morley PS, et al. Evaluation of ultrasound-guided vascular access in dogs. *J Vet Emerg Crit Care* 2013;23:498–503.

5 Olsen D, Packer BE, Perrett J, et al. Evaluation of the bone injection gun as a method for intraosseous cannula placement for fluid therapy in adult dogs. *Vet Surg* 2002;31:533–540.

179

Intraosseous Catheters

Alison Allukian, DVM[1] and Amanda Abelson, DVM, DACVAA, DACVECC[2]

[1]*Angell Animal Medical Center, Jamaica Plain, MA, USA*
[2]*Cummings School of Veterinary Medicine, North Grafton, MA, USA*

Introduction

The ability to obtain rapid vascular access in an emergency setting is of paramount importance to allow for the administration of resuscitative drugs and fluids. Obtaining prompt intravenous access can be difficult, especially in patients that present with cardiovascular collapse. Other challenges such as small patient size, trauma to commonly used vascular sites, obesity, or peripheral edema can also hinder gaining rapid intravenous access. Multiple attempts at gaining intravenous access lead to delays in treatment, and can increase morbidity and mortality.

There are several ways to gain vascular access percutaneously, ultrasound guided, or surgically (see Chapter 178). When intravenous access is not possible, intraosseous (IO) catheterization is a viable alternative to obtain vascular access [1–11]. In fact, due to IV access limitations in small patients, the IO catheter in avian, exotic mammals, and some reptile patients is well utilized [12].

Human medicine now widely accepts IO catheterization when IV access is not obtainable and several IO insertion devices (automated bone injection guns) have been developed to allow for rapid IO catherization [2,4,5,7,8]. It has been demonstrated that when using an automated bone injection gun in pediatric patients, it takes between 10 seconds to 1 minute to place an IO catheter with 70–80% success rate [6]. In adults requiring resuscitation from trauma, one study showed that the IO catheterization success rate was 85% on first attempt with a mean of 2.0 minutes, compared to 60% success rate and a mean of 8.0 minutes for central line placement [7]. Due to the speed with which an IO catheter can be placed, the American Heart Association finds the use of an IO catheter a reasonable alternative if venous access cannot be obtained peripherally [4,5].

At the time of writing, there is limited information on the use of IO catheters in veterinary patients. Olsen et al. demonstrated that the placement of an IO catheter in dogs using an automated bone injection gun provided reliable vascular access [13], and another study using feline cadavers identified that the use of a bone injection gun to facilitate IO catheter placement allowed for rapid placement [14]. Both studies suggest that the use of an IO catheter in animals suffering from cardiac arrest may be a viable alternative to an IV catheter.

Physiology

The rationale that IO catheterization provides rapid accessible vascular access is due to the rigid nature of bone which prevents bone marrow vessels from collapsing [1,2,15]. Administration of drugs and fluids into bone marrow is effective because bone marrow has a well-defined venous system that empties quickly into the systemic circulation [3]. Intraosseous infusions achieve similar onset of action time to peripherally or centrally administered fluids or drugs [15].

Blood analysis can also be performed from the bone marrow aspirate and studies have shown that in comparison to peripheral blood analysis (electrolytes, blood gas, blood typing), the values are similar, especially if drawn at time of insertion; however, blood gas and electrolyte levels may not be accurate if the sample has been collected after the administration of fluids or drugs.

Indications

The indications for IO catheterization have been extrapolated from human medicine as there are no veterinary studies documenting the impact of IO placement. The American Heart Association recommends a central line during resuscitation because it allows for higher peak drug concentrations and shorter circulation times. However, due to its time-consuming nature, peripheral access is recommended. Often, peripheral access is not obtainable, so an IO catheter is a reasonable alternative in these settings.

An IO catheter is indicated when a critically ill patient of any age requires intravascular access that cannot be secured in a timely fashion. Common conditions where an IO catheter might be warranted include life-threatening cardiovascular collapse (cardiopulmonary arrest, shock, sepsis), unique patient conformation (edematous or obese states or small/neonate patients), and thrombosis, trauma or severe burns or skin disease at conditional catheter sites.

Contraindications

There are few contraindications to intraosseous catheterization. The primary one is if the IO site has a fractured bone or one suspected to be fractured because infused medication or fluids may not make it to the systemic circulation and it may also lead to compartment syndrome or extravasation.

Medications

Most drugs that can be administrated intravenously can also be safely administered intraosseously (Table 179.1), although certain drugs, mostly limited to hyperosmolar drugs, can cause tissue necrosis if extravasation occurs [16].

Methods

Intraosseous catheter sites that are easily accessible in dogs and cats include the humeral head, the flat medial surface of the proximal tibia, and the trochanteric fossa of the femur. The skin is clipped and aseptically prepared as it would be for placement of an intravenous catheter. The bone is palpated for a flat spot and the limb is supported so that it will not move under pressure. The needle is then drilled into the bone either manually or through the use of an insertion device. In the avian species, care must be taken to avoid insertion of an IO into pneumatic bones.

Devices for IO placement range from the traditional manually placed hypodermic needle to battery-operated automatic drills. A variety of needles can be utilized for IO catheterization including butterfly, spinal, standard, and bone marrow needles. Additionally, there are commercially available IO needles that come with a stylet to avoid occlusion of the catheter with bone material in

Table 179.1 Medications that can be given via the intraosseous route.

Therapy	Limitations
Medication	
Adenosine	
Amiodarone	
Atropine	
Bretylium	
Calcium chloride	
Cisatracurium	
Dextrose	Reported tissue necrosis with extravasation
Dobutamine	
Dopamine	
Epinephrine	
Etomidate	
Fentanyl	
Heparin	
Insulin	
Lidocaine	
Naloxone	
Norepinephrine	
Phenytoin	
Propofol	
Rocuronium	
Sodium bicarbonate	Reported tissue necrosis with extravasation
Succinycholine	
Tenecteplase	
Vasopressin	
Vecuronium	
Fluid therapy	
Albumin	
Fresh frozen plasma	
Hypertonic saline	Reported tissue necrosis
Lactated Ringer's solution	
Normal saline	
Packed erythrocytes	

adults; however, regular hypodermic needles (18–20 G) will suffice for the soft bony cortex of neonates or small dogs or cats. Needles of smaller size often bend under the strain of insertion and can become occluded during placement.

In addition to standard needles and commercially available needles, other devices have been manufactured that improve ease and shorten access times, such as the bone injection gun (BIG, WaisMEd, Houston, TX), drill (EZ-IO, Vidacare, San Antonio, TX), and sternal IO device (FAST1, Pyng Medical, Richmond, Canada). The BIG is a spring-loaded needle with a pre-fixed depth that is propelled at high speed into the bone marrow. It was found to be significantly faster at gaining IO access than a Jamshidi bone marrow needle in a dog tibia [13].

The EZ-IO is a small, battery-powered drill that has needles of varying length. The needle hub is secured on the drill and penetrates through the cortex into the bone marrow. The stylet is then removed. A study using feline cadavers identified that the use of a EZ-IO gun to facilitate IO catheter placement allowed for rapid placement compared to the BIG and manual IO needle placement, while a dog cadaver study found that the EZ-IO gun facilitated faster IO catheter placement compared to a jugular venous cut-down technique regardless of experience level of the operative [12,17].

There are a variety of ways to ensure proper placement of an IO catheter. The needle should be well implanted so that it moves in the same motion if the limb is moved forward and backward. It should also stand on its own because when properly seated in the medulla, it is laterally supported by the rigid cortex. Along with this maneuver, correct placement can be verified by infusion of fluid and monitoring for extravasation.

Possible Complications

Complications after proper IO catheterization are rare, with a low overall incidence of <1% [18]. They include:

- extravasation
- fracture
- osteomyelitis
- skin abscess
- cellulitis
- fat embolism.

The primary complication of intraosseous catheters is extravasation of infusions (drugs, fluids, blood, etc.) into the soft tissue which infrequently leads to compartment syndrome [19]. Osteomyelitis reports are rare (incidence of 0.6%) and it most likely occurs subsequent to leaving an IO catheter in for greater than 24 hours, poor aseptic technique or multiple IO attempts at the same location [2,18]. Other complications include cellulitis and skin abscesses [20]. The longer an IO catheter is left in place, the higher the chance of adverse events. For this reason, it is recommended to replace the IO catheter with a peripheral or central catheter as soon as possible, but as standard within 24 hours. There have been no ill effects for bone deformity/growth arrest secondary to intraosseous placement in patients as evidenced by long-term follow-up [21].

Intraosseous Catheter Care

Alternative IV access should be sought as soon as feasible. While in place, the site should be kept clean and standard hand hygiene for handling the catheter should be employed. Flushing of the catheter should be performed as with an IV catheter with either heparinized or saline solutions. Securement or wrapping of the IO may or may not be feasible, depending on the IO site and the patient's size or critical state.

References

1 Otto CM, Kaufman GM, Crowe DT. Intraosseous infusion of fluids and therapeutics. *Compend Cont Educ Pract Vet* 1989;11:421–430.

2 Day MW. Intraosseous devices for intravascular access in adult trauma patients. *Crit Care Nurse* 2011;31(2):76–89.

3 Voigt J, Waltzman M, Lottenberg L. Intraosseous vascular access for in-hospital emergency use. A systemic clinical review of the literature and analysis. *Pediatr Emerg Care* 2012;28(2):185–199.

4 American Heart Association. Guidelines for Cardiopulmonary Resuscitation and Emergency Cardiovascular Care. *Circulation* 2010;122:S729–S767.

5 American Heart Association. Guidelines for Cardiopulmonary Resuscitation and Emergency Cardiovascular Care. *Circulation* 2005;112(Suppl 1):58–66.

6 Horton MA, Beamer C. Powered intraosseous insertion provides safe and effective vascular access for pediatric emergency patients. *Pediatr Emerg Care* 2008;24:347–350.

7 Leidel BA, Kirchoff C, Bogner V, et al. Comparison of intraosseous versus central venous vascular access in adults under resuscitation in the emergency department with inaccessible peripheral veins. *Resuscitation* 2011;83:40–45.

8 Leidel BA, Kirchoff C, Bogner V, et al. Is the intraosseous access route fast and efficacious compared to conventional central venous catheterization in adult patients under resuscitation in the emergency department? A prospective observational pilot study. *Patient Safety Surg* 2009;3:24.

9 Hamed RK, Hartmans S, Gausche-Hill M.. Anesthesia through an intraosseous line using an 18-gauge intravenous needle for emergency pediatric surgery. *J Clin Anesth* 2013;25(6):447–451.

10 Smith R, Davis N, Bouamra O, Lecky F. The utilisation of intraosseous infusion in the resuscitation

of paediatric major trauma patients. *Injury* 2005;36(9):1034–1038; discussion 1039.

11 Abe KK, Blum GT, Yamamoto LG. Intraosseous is faster and easier than umbilical venous catheterization in newborn emergency vascular access models. *Am J Emerg Med* 2000;18(2):126–9.

12 Allukian AR, Abelson A, Babyak J, Rozanski E. Comparison of time to obtain intra-osseous versus jugular venous catheterization in dog cadavers. *J Vet Emerg Crit Care* 2017;27:506–511.

13 Olsen D, Packer BE, Perrett J, et al. Evaluation of the bone injection gun as a method for intraosseous cannula placement for fluid therapy in adult dogs. *Vet Surg* 2002;31:533–540.

14 Bukoski A, Winter M, Bandt C, et al. Comparison of three intraosseous access techniques in cats. *J Vet Emerg Crit Care* 2010;20(4):393–397.

15 Orlowski JP, Porembka DT, Gallagher JM, Lockrem JD, van Lente F. Comparison study of intraosseous, central intravenous, and peripheral intravenous infusions of emergency drugs. *Am J Dis Child* 1990;144:112–117.

16 Anson JA. Vascular access in resuscitation: is there a role for the intraosseous route? *Anesthesiology* 2014;120:1015–1031.

17 Bukoski A, Winter M, Bandt C, et al. Comparison of three intraosseous techniques in cats. *J Vet Emerg Crit Care* 2010;20(4):393–397.

18 Rosetti VA, Thompson BM, Miller J, Mateer JR, Aprhamian C. Introsseous infusion: an alternative route of pediatric intravascular access. *Ann Emerg Med* 1985;14;885–888.

19 Simmons CM, Johnson NE, Perkin RM, van Stralen D. Introsseous extravasation complication rates. *Ann Emerg Med* 1994;23:363–366.

20 Fiser DH. Intraosseous infusion. *N Engl J Med* 1990;322:1579–1581.

21 Iserson KV. Intraosseous infusions in adults. *J Emerg Med* 1989;7:587–591.

180

Airway Management

Elizabeth Rozanski, DVM, DACVIM (SAIM), DACVECC

Cummings School of Veterinary Medicine, Tufts University, North Grafton, MA, USA

Introduction

Airway management may be broadly defined as ensuring that the patient has a patent airway from nose to alveoli; methods of oxygen supplementation are discussed in Chapter 181. Oxygen therapy is theoretically not required with airway obstruction, but may decrease the work of breathing and limit upper airway swelling associated with increased inspiratory efforts. The emergency specialist should be familiar with indications and techniques to identify and maintain the airway.

The airways may be divided into the upper and lower airway, with the thoracic inlet being the dividing point. Upper airway obstruction causes difficulty on inspiration due to collapse associated with negative inspiratory pressure, while lower airway obstruction causes obstruction on expiration (see Chapters 28 and 30–32). Normal expiration is passive but with obstruction, there may be active expiratory "push." Most of airway management involves treatment of upper airway obstruction and/or maintenance of a tracheostomy tube. Animals with airway obstruction have increased inspiratory effort and typically loud breathing. Hyperthermia may develop due to increased respiratory efforts and the inability to effectively cool, but it is possible that aspiration pneumonia may have developed as well. The possibility of pneumonia should be considered if temperature fails to normalize after respiratory efforts improve, or as a possible cause of exacerbation of stable upper airway disease.

The decision to manage the airway should be made early; often the recommendation is that if you consider intubation, you should do it! In general, outside routine general anesthesia for diagnostics or therapy, intubation is performed for dynamic upper airway obstruction or to provide for positive pressure ventilation (PPV) for either respiratory or ventilatory failure. A tracheostomy may be required to bypass a fixed upper airway obstruction or in a patient with dynamic collapse such as severe laryngeal collapse or cervical tracheal collapse (see Chapters 30 and 32).

Healthy Dog or Cat

Normal dogs and cats may require airway management if they are sedated or anesthetized for diagnostics or treatment. Clients often perceive sedation to be "safer" than general anesthesia; this is not always true. While light sedation may be inadequate to permit orotracheal intubation, it is still essential to carefully monitor heavily sedated patients until they are able to adequately maintain sternal recumbency. Airway occlusion/obstruction is considered to be a principal cause of unexpected death during the perianesthesia period. Brachycephalic dogs should always be intubated and monitored closely until recovery; they often tolerate endotracheal tubes even after they are able to sit sternal and occasionally even walk around (see Chapter 28). Oxygen helmets, high-flow oxygen or heliox may facilitate anesthetic recovery when available (see Chapter 181) [1–3].

Upper Airway Obstruction (see Chapters 28 and 30–32)

Upper airway obstructions (UAOs) are more frequently dynamic in dogs and fixed in cats. Common UAOs in dogs include brachycephalic syndrome, tracheal collapse, and laryngeal paralysis. In cats, UAO is

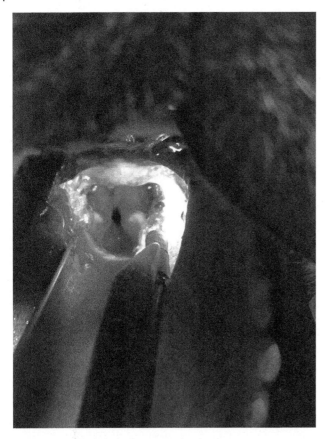

Figure 180.1 Oral view of a nasotracheal catheter.

often harder to appreciate initially due to lower inspiratory flow rates and subsequently less upper airway noise. Cats may have a wheeze associated with a fixed UAO which is commonly mistaken for bronchoconstriction associated with asthma. Emergency clinicians should recall that feline asthma rarely develops late in life in cats.

The decision to intubate a patient with UAO should be made confidently, but ideally with a plan in mind for follow-up for patient care. Follow-up will depend on what is identified at the point of oral examination but may include surgical palliation, biopsy, temporary tracheostomy or other supportive care. In particular, in cats with suspected laryngeal masses, the need for a temporary tracheostomy is very common, and should be discussed with the family *before* undertaking an oral examination under heavy sedation.

Nasal oxygen alone is rarely helpful in the treatment of airway obstruction as the obstruction is not bypassed. Nasotracheal intubation is commonly performed in people and in larger animals such as horses,

but it is difficult to place a tube to provide an adequate airway via the nasal route in small animals. However, nasotracheal tubes may be placed for provision of supplemental oxygen, which may prevent the need for intubation or help a patient with a compromised airway recover from surgery [4]. Nasotracheal tubes require anesthesia and direct visualization of the glottis for placement. From an emergency room perspective, nasotracheal oxygen may prevent the need for intubation or a temporary tracheostomy in animals with upper airway obstruction although intubation may be practically easier!

In order to place the nasotracheal tube, the patient needs to be under anesthesia or otherwise obtunded enough to permit oropharyngeal manipulation. The nasotracheal tube is placed by passing a red rubber catheter through the nasal cavity and then retrieving it with hemostats and then directing it down the trachea, approximately to the level of the carina (Figure 180.1). Successful placement can be verified by direct visualization and by confirmation of the presence of end-tidal CO_2.

Difficult Intubation

If adequate oxygenation and ventilation cannot be achieved with sedation/anxiolysis and supplemental oxygen, intubation and/or tracheostomy may be considered. However, if respiratory arrest is imminent, then intubation should be urgently attempted. However, if time permits, collection of supplies before efforts are made is useful for cases of suspected difficult intubation. Dogs with laryngeal masses or severe brachycephalic syndrome are most commonly associated with intubation difficulty, so the clinician should be prepared to "capture the airway" by a variety of methods as the clinical course dictates.

Prior to efforts to intubate, it is prudent to have a variety of supplies available including a number of tube sizes, as well as a guidewire (or long polypropylene catheter for a guidewire exchange-based intubation), and surgical instruments and supplies in case tracheostomy becomes necessary. If direct visualization of the laryngeal lumen is not possible, it may be possible to digitally palpate and introduce an endotracheal tube in larger dogs. Endoscopic assistance may also be used, although this technique is best accomplished after some prior practice. Finally, before a tracheostomy is performed, if preferred, retrograde tracheal intubation may be performed by placing a needle into the trachea and then directing a guidewire orally to permit placement of an endotracheal tube over the guidewire or alternatively, supplemental oxygen may be provided via a long catheter directed towards the carina.

Laryngeal mask airways (LMAs) are used occasionally in small animals and may be a useful tool to provide ventilation [5,6]. LMAs are composed of a standard tube with an inflatable "mask" which is designed to preferentially cover the larynx in order to provide oxygen and inhalational anesthetic agents. LMAs are also useful for intubation of smaller species such as rabbits, or in cases where it is difficult to open the mouth adequately to directly visual the larynx. In the emergency setting, LMAs are useful to have in stock, particularly in practice settings with fewer personnel or less comfort with surgical airways. As with any airway, ensuring adequate oxygenation and ventilation is important.

Following successful intubation in a patient with a difficult airway, it is essential to determine what the next steps in patient care should include. It may be that successful extubation is possible if a foreign object is removed or that surgical intervention is required to facilitate restoration of an airway lumen. Pharyngeal abscesses are common in dogs, particularly in stick chewers, and these may result in airway impingement and require temporary tracheostomies until resolution of the swelling. Percutaneous drainage may result in immediate improvement.

Tracheostomy

Temporary tracheostomy is commonly performed in the emergency room, and while a discussion of the specific procedure is beyond the scope of this chapter, it is essential that an ER clinician understands how to perform the procedure urgently and does not need to review the procedure in the event of an airway occlusion. Key tips include staying on midline, making a long incision, and placing labeled stay sutures to permit easy replacement of the tube if it is dislodged.

Permanent tracheostomy is rarely performed in the emergency room, but it may be wise for the ER clinician to discuss permanent tracheostomies as a possible endpoint for therapy in order to have owners consider the implications and commitment required.

Management of the Tracheostomy Tube

Patients that have a tracheostomy tube in place should be closely observed as occlusion or dislodgment can prove fatal. Unless the patient is undergoing mechanical ventilation or lacks a gag reflex, the cuff should not be inflated in case the lumen of the tube becomes occluded with secretions. All personnel working in an ER should be trained in managing or replacing a tracheostomy tube. Supplies for replacement of the tube, suction, cotton swabs, and propofol should be kept close to the cage or run.

The lumen of the tube may be easily occluded by mucus or blood/blood clots. As the role of the upper airway includes humidification of inspired air, tracheal tubes are prone to becoming obstructed. Obstruction may build up slowly and then result in apparent acute blockage. Tracheostomy tubes should be suctioned and/or changed as needed. Routine suctioning is not required.

When the airway obstruction has resolved, the tracheostomy tube may be removed and the site allowed to heal by second intention. It is important not to close the skin, as until the tracheal incision heals, closing the skin will permit the development of subcutaneous emphysema. It is uncommon in the emergency room to both place and remove the tracheostomy tube unless it was urgently placed to remove a foreign body.

Pharmacological Therapy

No medical therapy exists to directly help dilate the upper airway. Theophylline and albuterol/terbutaline have no direct benefit for any upper airway obstruction. Dogs are not thought to develop naturally occurring bronchoconstriction, so bronchodilators are usually of no benefit, although additional effects (mucus clearance, diaphragmatic strength) may be helpful in some dogs with generalized lower airway disease, although not tracheal collapse. Cats do suffer from bronchoconstriction so in cats with true asthma, bronchodilators are useful.

Anxiolytics may be helpful to decrease the anxiety associated with respiratory distress. Acepromazine is widely used in the emergency setting, and butorphanol may also have some benefit from this perspective. Trazadone has been gaining popularity as a mild sedative/anxiolytic and may help some dogs with more minor airway obstruction. Doxepin has been proposed as an adjuvant therapy for dogs with laryngeal paralysis. At the time of this writing (June 2016), there is an ACVIM Foundation/Zoetis-funded grant by Rishniw evaluating the efficacy of this therapy in a randomized clinical trial.

Glucocorticoids are the mainstay therapy for lower airway obstruction and may help with upper airway obstruction associated with swelling, such as with brachycephalic airway obstruction or tracheal collapse. Laryngeal paralysis does not benefit from glucocorticoids unless severe swelling is observed.

References

1 Byers CG, Romeo K, Johnson AS, et al. Helium-oxygen gas-carrier mixture (heliox): a review of physics and potential applications in veterinary medicine. *J Vet Emerg Crit Care* 2008;18:586–593.

2 Keir I, Daly J, Haggerty J, et al Retrospective evaluation of the effect of high flow oxygen therapy delivered by nasal cannula on PaO2 in dogs with moderate-to-severe hypoxemia. *J Vet Emerg Crit Care* 2016;26(4):598–602.

3 Staffieri F, Crovace A, de Monte V, et al. Noninvasive continuous positive airway pressure delivered using a pediatric helmet in dogs recovering from general anesthesia. *J Vet Emerg Crit Care* 2014;24(5):578–585.

4 Senn D, Sigrist N, Forterre F, et al. Retrospective evaluation of postoperative nasotracheal tubes for oxygen supplementation in dogs following surgery for brachycephalic syndrome: 36 cases (2003–2007). *J Vet Emerg Crit Care* 2011;21(3):261–267.

5 Kazakos GM, Anagnostou T, Savvas I, et al. Use of the laryngeal mask airway in rabbits: placement and efficacy. *Lab Anim* 2007;36:29–34.

6 Braz JR, Martins RH, Mori AR, Luna SP. Investigation into the use of the laryngeal mask airway in pentobarbital anesthetized dogs. *Vet Surg* 1999;28:502–505.

181

Oxygen Therapy

Christine L. Guenther, DVM, DACVECC

Pittsburgh Veterinary Specialty and Emergency Center, Pittsburgh, PA, USA

Introduction

Oxygen supplementation is widely used in veterinary medicine to relieve hypoxia and increase oxygen delivery to the tissues. For patients presenting to the emergency room who are triaged with signs of respiratory distress, oxygen administration during the assessment process can be beneficial and even life saving to the patient. As there are few contraindications to short-term oxygen administration, oxygen supplementation should be initiated in patients presenting with signs of respiratory distress until the status of the patient's respiratory system can be determined.

Oxygen therapy increases the fraction of inspired oxygen (FiO_2) delivered to the alveoli. Causes of respiratory distress and decreased delivery of oxygen to the tissues are often multifactorial in the patient presenting to the emergency room (see Chapter 4). Whatever the cause of respiratory distress, an increase in FiO_2 to the patient can be beneficial. The oxygen content in arterial blood (CaO_2) along with cardiac output (CO) is a major determinant of oxygen delivery (DO_2) to the tissues. CaO_2 is defined as $(Hb \times 1.34 \times SaO_2) + (PaO_2 \times 0.003)$ which factors in the amount of hemoglobin (Hb), the arterial oxygen saturation of hemoglobin (SaO_2), and the amount of oxygen dissolved in plasma. An increase in FiO_2 will lead to an increase in SaO_2 in most situations. With supplemental oxygen, there is an increase in the partial pressure of arterial oxygen (PaO_2) and a subsequent shift of the oxyhemoglobin dissociation curve to the left, facilitating the binding of oxygen to hemoglobin and leading to a subsequent increase in SaO_2 [1]. The increase in SaO_2 is more profound with primary pulmonary disease or injury causing a defect in gas exchange versus disease or injury causing anemia or a decrease in binding of oxygen to hemoglobin such as carbon monoxide poisoning (see Chapter 139). In the emergency setting, whether the effect of oxygen therapy is large or small, oxygen administration is an important part of stabilization in patients presenting with signs of respiratory distress.

Non-Invasive Oxygen Therapy

Non-invasive oxygen delivery methods are readily available in most emergency clinics. These methods vary in the ease of oxygen administration to the patient and patient tolerance. They also vary greatly with regard to the FiO_2 delivered to the patient. Most of these oxygen delivery methods are inexpensive and are easy to set up and use. Prior to the initiation of non-invasive oxygen therapy, the patency of the upper airway must be assessed. If a partial or complete upper airway obstruction is present, a patent airway must be quickly established with intubation or, if unable to intubate, emergent tracheostomy (see Chapter 180). The patient's ability to ventilate also needs to be quickly established. The non-breathing or hypoventilating patient should be immediately intubated and resuscitation methods started.

Flow-By Oxygen

Flow-by oxygen is delivered via a tube placed in the vicinity of the patient's nose or mouth. The tube is connected to an oxygen source such as oxygen tank, wall-mounted oxygen or an anesthesia machine. A humidifier can be placed in circuit to provide humidified air. Oxygen flow rates are set by the clinician and can deliver an FiO_2 of 25–40% [2]. Benefits of flow-by oxygen are ease of use and quick implementation. Disadvantages include variable FiO_2, oxygen waste, and patient tolerance. Providing flow-by oxygen can be labor intensive in that an assistant is required to remain by the patient's side at all times holding the tube to the patient's face for oxygen administration. Because of the ease and speed with which flow-by oxygen can be administered, it is a reasonable

Textbook of Small Animal Emergency Medicine, First Edition. Edited by Kenneth J. Drobatz, Kate Hopper, Elizabeth Rozanski and Deborah C. Silverstein.
© 2019 John Wiley & Sons, Inc. Published 2019 by John Wiley & Sons, Inc.
Companion Website: www.wiley.com/go/drobatz/textbook

first line of oxygen therapy for the emergency patient presenting with signs of respiratory distress, allowing for an immediate increase in FiO_2 during assessment, stabilization, and placement of IV catheter. Flow-by oxygen therapy is a temporary delivery method that can be utilized until a method of long-term oxygen therapy can be implemented.

Face Mask

A face mask can be attached to an oxygen source for delivery of higher FiO_2 compared to flow-by oxygen. Oxygen delivery with face mask provides for a variable FiO_2 of 35–60%, depending on how tight fitting the mask is around the face [2]. With a face mask, oxygen administration flow rates are typically set at 200 mL/kg/min but can be set higher. Oxygen delivery with a face mask is easy to use and quick to set up, providing an immediate increase in FiO_2 to the emergency patient presenting in respiratory distress (Figure 181.1). Patient tolerance of the face mask, especially a tight-fitting mask, can be a limiting factor with this oxygen delivery method. Care should be taken when using a face mask on patients presenting with facial trauma. With a tight-fitting face mask there is a risk of rebreathing of CO_2 and hyperthermia. Use of a non-rebreathing circuit with a face mask can prevent rebreathing of CO_2 and limit hyperthermia.

Due to its quick implementation and ease of use, oxygen delivery by face mask is a good first-line method of oxygen therapy in the emergency setting. Like flow-by oxygen, face mask oxygen delivery requires the constant presence of an assistant for administration in the awake and alert patient. For long-term oxygen delivery, face mask administration is usually only tolerated in the obtunded patient. Face mask oxygen delivery is

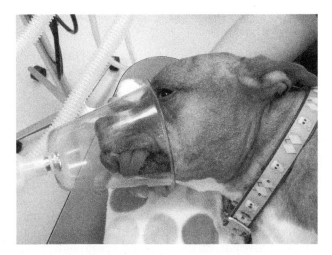

Figure 181.1 Canine patient receiving oxygen via a loose-fitting face mask.

a reasonable first line oxygen delivery method in the patient presenting to the emergency room with signs of respiratory distress but most patients will require other delivery methods if long-term oxygen support is needed.

Oxygen Hood

An oxygen hood can be constructed using an Elizabethan collar and covering the opening 75–90% with clear plastic wrap. An oxygen source is placed within the collar and secured to the patient. Use of an oxygen hood can deliver an FiO_2 of 30–40% with flow rates of 1–2 L/min once the hood has been flooded with oxygen [3]. With an oxygen hood, there must be a sufficient opening to allow for escape of CO_2 and heat. This method of oxygen delivery is well tolerated by most patients, can be used for long-term oxygen therapy, and does not require specialized equipment.

Nasal Oxygen

Delivery of oxygen through a nasal cannula is a common supplementation method in veterinary patients. This method of oxygen delivery is well tolerated and can be used for long-term administration. Oxygen delivery through a nasal cannula is technically easy, inexpensive, limits oxygen waste, is well tolerated and can provide a FiO_2 of up to 70% [4–6]. However, the FiO_2 delivered to the patient can be variable and is influenced by flow rates, panting, and respiratory rate [6,7]. Patients receiving nasal oxygen are readily accessible to the clinician for assessment and diagnostics without disruption of oxygen therapy.

Nasal cannula placement can be unilateral or bilateral. Nasal cannulae are usually placed up to the level of the medial canthus of the eye although they can be placed into the pharyngeal region at the level of the ramus of the mandible. Nasal prongs are also available for oxygen administration and do not require advancement into the nasal cavity. Prongs most likely delivery a comparable FiO_2 to nasal cannula oxygen but no studies have evaluated their use in oxygen delivery. The nasal cannula or nasal prong size should be no more than half the diameter of the nares. A humidification source such as a bubbler humidifier is recommended to prevent drying of the nasal mucosa.

Contraindications for nasal oxygen include facial trauma or other nasal obstruction precluding placement of nasal cannula or prongs. Recommended flow rate through each nasal cannula is 100 mL/kg/min. At higher oxygen flow rates the nasal mucosa are unable to adequately heat and humidify the incoming air. This can lead to patient discomfort, drying of the nasal mucosa and a decrease in pulmonary compliance and conductance [6].

Oxygen Cage

Oxygen cages are a stress-free method of oxygen supplementation. Emergency patients presenting in respiratory distress can be quickly triaged and placed in an oxygen cage, allowing for immediate delivery of a FiO_2 up to 60% [5,7]. Oxygen cages can range from expensive commercial cages that control FiO_2, CO_2, heat, and humidity to a simple plastic-wrapped cage door, pet carrier or incubator with an external oxygen source. When using an oxygen cage that does not control heat and CO_2, care must be taken to prevent hyperthermia and rebreathing of CO_2. A commercial CO_2 monitor and thermometer can be placed in the oxygen cage with the patient to monitor temperature and carbon dioxide levels.

The ease and stress-free nature of oxygen administration using an oxygen cage is appealing and often necessary in the patient presenting in respiratory distress. However, the clinician should be cautioned that cage oxygen administration severely limits hands-on access to the patient. Opening of an oxygen cage causes a precipitous drop in FiO_2 that can be detrimental to the patient. Emergency patients present with varying degrees of pulmonary injury and disease and can quickly decompensate with a sudden drop in oxygen levels. The clinician must weigh the benefits of oxygen cage use against the inability to interact with the patient and provide basic stabilization. In the emergency patient requiring immediate cage oxygen support, careful visual monitoring of the patient is necessary to monitor for signs of decompensation. The use of continuous electrocardiogram, pulse oximetry, and blood pressure connected to a monitoring device may aid the clinician with monitoring of patient status and response to therapy. A step-wise plan for the stabilization and assessment of these patients should be organized and implemented as soon as possible.

Advanced Oxygen Delivery Methods

When conventional oxygen delivery methods are not adequate for relief of hypoxia or if the patient has facial injury or deformities precluding conventional therapies, advanced non-invasive oxygen delivery methods should be considered. Advanced non-invasive oxygen delivery methods are popular in people failing conventional oxygen therapies as these methods can avoid intubation which comes with increased risk for morbidity and mortality [8,9]. Advanced oxygen delivery methods such as transtracheal oxygen and high-flow nasal cannula have been used with success in veterinary patients failing conventional therapies and may be useful when escalation of oxygen therapy in patients presenting to the emergency room in respiratory distress is required.

Transtracheal Oxygen Administration

Oxygen administration through a transtracheal catheter (TTC) can be considered in patients requiring oxygen support where a nasal cannula cannot be placed or for those patients failing conventional oxygen therapies. The main benefit of transtracheal oxygen delivery over conventional therapies is that the placement of the TTC into the lower airways bypasses a significant portion of the upper airway. This limits the mixing of oxygen with deadspace and delivers an increased FiO_2 of up to 80% compared to nasal oxygen at similar flow rates [10]. TTCs are reported to be well tolerated by both dogs and cats and allow for easy clinician access to the patient [10]. They require expertise to be placed and injury to the trachea and surrounding tissues has been reported [7].

Oxygen flow rates using TTCs have been reported to be lower than with nasal cannulae. The recommended starting oxygen flow rate for a TTC is 50 mL/kg/min which is comparable to an oxygen flow rate of 100 mL/kg/min through a nasal cannula [10]. The use of TTCs completely bypasses the upper airway, allowing for delivery of cold, dry air directly to the lungs, so proper humidification of oxygen is recommended. Reported complications with use of a TTC include kinking of the catheter, tracheitis, subcutaneous emphysema, catheter dislodgment, and obstruction of catheter with secretions [7,10]. Because a TTC can deliver a FiO_2 of greater than 60%, oxygen toxicity is a concern.

High-Flow Nasal Cannula

High-flow nasal cannula (HFNC) has been used in people since the early 2000s as an advanced oxygen delivery method to avoid intubation. More recently, HFNC has found utility in the human emergency setting when convention oxygen therapies fail and escalation of oxygen therapy is needed [11,12]. High-flow nasal cannula accurately delivers humidified and heated oxygen via nasal prongs to the patient, allowing for safe delivery of higher oxygen flow rates. The delivery system humidifies the air to 99% relative humidity, allows for adjustment of the gas temperature and for adjustment of FiO_2 from 21% to 100%. Oxygen flow rates vary with the system used and the size of the nasal prongs, ranging from 1 to 60 L/min.

The proposed mechanism for the improvement in oxygenation and ventilation parameters seen with HFNC is based on the higher flow rates achieving deadspace wash-out [13]. With complete deadspace wash-out, the desired FiO_2 is delivered to the lungs without any mixing of end-expiratory gas. Studies in people have also shown a potential pressure benefit with HFNC which can vary with flow rate and open or closed mouth [14].

There are limited studies in veterinary medicine looking at the use of HFNC and none specifically looking at the use of high-flow oxygen therapy in veterinary patients presenting to the emergency room for respiratory distress [15,16]. One study reported the use of HFNC in a dog presenting to the emergency room with polytrauma including pneumothorax, severe pulmonary contusions, and pelvic fractures after a motor vehicle accident. The pneumothorax was continuous, necessitating chest tube placement prior to initiation of HFNC but remained continuous for several days until oxygen flow rates were less than 10 L/min [16]. The use of HFNC therapy in patients with existing pneumothorax should be undertaken with caution.

Advantages to the use of HFNC in the emergency patient include possible avoidance of intubation in those failing conventional oxygen therapies, patient comfort with higher oxygen flow rates, ease of use comparable to conventional nasal oxygen administration and delivery of higher and accurate FiO_2. Disadvantages includes expense of equipment, risk of oxygen toxicity with $FiO_2 > 60\%$, and risk of exacerbation of pneumothorax.

Invasive Oxygen Delivery Methods

Patients presenting with severe work of breathing, hypoxemia ($PaO_2 < 60$ mmHg or $SpO_2 < 90\%$) or hypercapnia ($PaCO_2 > 60$ mmHg) unresponsive to non-invasive oxygen support may require intubation and positive pressure ventilation (PPV) (see Chapter 188). In addition, previously stable patients presenting to the ER may decompensate and require invasive oxygen support. Invasive oxygen administration involves intubation of the patient. Intubation has been associated with an increase in morbidity and mortality due to loss of normal airway defense mechanisms, risk of pneumonia and prolonged immobility secondary to heavy sedation required for intubation [1,17]. Despite these risks, in the severely unstable patient, intubation and PPV can be life saving until the patient can be stabilized.

Positive Pressure Ventilation

Positive pressure ventilation can help improve hypoxemia in dogs and cats with severe hypoxemia unresponsive to conventional oxygen support (see Chapter 188). Overall, in dogs and cats undergoing mechanical ventilation for pulmonary pathology, regardless of the cause, reported survival rates are 20–30% [18,19]. Caution should be exercised when using PPV in veterinary trauma patients with existing pneumothorax or who are at risk for pneumothorax. PPV can worsen an existing pneumothorax or cause a pneumothorax requiring continuous suction while the patient is being ventilated (see Chapter 44). Constant attention to patient pulmonary function is of the utmost importance

and pneumothorax should be highly considered in any patient receiving PPV that undergoes acute desaturation.

The use of PPV requires a level of expertise to operate, expensive equipment, and intensive patient care and monitoring. Complications associated with PPV include ventilator-acquired pneumonia, pneumothorax, and effects of prolonged sedation and immobility.

Hyperbaric Oxygen

With the increasing availability of portable hyperbaric oxygen chambers specifically engineered for veterinary patients, hyperbaric oxygen (HBO) is finding utility in veterinary medicine. The utility of HBO in improving oxygen delivery is based on the effect of pressure on the various gas laws (Fick, Henry, Boyle) [20,21]. Hyperbaric oxygen leads to changes in oxygen solubility and pressure. By increasing atmospheric pressure beyond 1 atmosphere (1 atm), more oxygen can be dissolved in and transported by plasma. In addition, the increased amount of oxygen dissolved in blood will increase the partial pressure of oxygen as measured by PaO_2. This allows for improved diffusion of oxygen into the tissues compared to oxygen being transported by hemoglobin. And indeed, it has been proposed that at 2.5 × atmospheric pressure (2.5 atm) with an FiO_2 of 100%, the amount of dissolved oxygen in plasma is adequate to meet the resting requirement of the tissues without the need for hemoglobin [20,21]. In people, hyperbaric oxygen is used in the treatment of carbon monoxide poisoning, wound healing, gas bubble reduction, enhancement of antimicrobial function, modulation of inflammation, and angiogenesis. Veterinary publications on the use of hyperbaric oxygen therapy in small animals are mostly limited to case reports and to date no controlled studies have been published.

Complications with HBO include oxygen toxicity, barotrauma, decompression sickness, and oxygen-induced seizures [20,21]. While patients are undergoing HBO therapy, the clinician does not have hands-on access and in an emergency it can take several minutes to decompress the chamber. Monitoring equipment is generally not available in veterinary HBO chambers. In the veterinary emergency setting, HBO may have a utility in smoke inhalation, post cardiopulmonary arrest, envenomations, and sepsis [22,23].

Monitoring Response to Oxygen Therapy

When starting supplemental oxygen therapy, regardless of the cause, the patient must be carefully and continuously monitored for response to therapy. Lack of patient response to therapy must be quickly recognized and requires an escalation to more advanced or invasive methods of oxygen administration.

Response to oxygen therapy can be monitored using several methods. The easiest and less stressful method is continuous visual monitoring of the patient. This is particularly important for the patient in an oxygen cage or in severe distress. For a patient in an oxygen cage, any intervention that requires opening of the cage door can lead to a detrimental decrease in FiO_2. For this reason, observation of response to therapy is key for these patients. In addition, patients in severe respiratory distress may not tolerate blood draws for arterial blood gas or application of a pulse oximetry probe.

In the author's opinion, visual inspection of the patient is one of the most useful and non-stressful tools for evaluation of response to oxygen therapy. Attention should be paid to the patient's respiratory rate and effort and color of the gums or tongue. Patients which are showing a positive response to oxygen therapy should have a decrease in their respiratory rate and improvement in their respiratory effort. Patients with cyanosis responding to oxygen therapy should have improvement in the color of their gums or tongue. Patients responding to oxygen therapy should be willing to lie down and sleep as well as eat and drink. Other vital parameters such as heart rate and blood pressure should normalize with response to oxygen therapy. Persistent signs of respiratory distress warrant escalation of oxygen therapy.

Pulse oximetry is a non-invasive monitoring method which, using spectrophotometry, detects the saturation of hemoglobin with oxygen (SpO_2). SpO_2 readings of less than 92% with continued signs of respiratory distress indicate the need for escalation of oxygen therapy. Inaccuracies associated with pulse oximetry can be seen with patient motion, pigmented skin, hypothermia, vasoconstriction, bright lights, and poor cardiac output (Editors' note: Carbon monoxide toxicity can result in inaccurate pulse oximetry readings). The probe is typically placed on the tongue or gums but can also be placed on the pinna, webbing of the toes, prepuce or vulva. SpO_2 readings are a useful tool for monitoring response to oxygen therapy but do not give information regarding the efficiency of gas exchange or ventilation [24].

Arterial blood gas monitoring is the gold standard for determining oxygenation and ventilation parameters. This requires blood sampling from an arterial vessel. The dorsal pedal artery in the hind foot is typically used for arterial blood sampling but arterial blood can also be sampled from the femoral, auricular, lingual and digital arteries of the front foot (see Chapter 178).

For patients receiving oxygen therapy, a PaO_2 of less than 70 mmHg with continued signs of respiratory distress requires escalation of oxygen therapy. A $PaCO_2$ of greater than 50 mmHg indicates hypoventilation and mechanical ventilation should be considered for these patients.

Oxygen Toxicity

Oxygen is directly toxic to the pulmonary epithelium secondary to the formation of free oxygen radicals. The degree of damage to the lungs is related to both the duration of oxygen therapy and the FiO_2. In animals receiving 100% oxygen for 4 days almost total destruction of type I epithelial cells was seen. In contrast, exposure of animals to 60% oxygen for 7 days produced few morphological changes to the lungs [25]. Sensitivity to oxygen toxicity varies between species and between neonates and adults. Neonates seem more resistant to oxygen toxicity compared to adults of the same species [26].

To avoid oxygen toxicity, FiO_2 should be kept below 50% whenever possible. The majority of the oxygen delivery methods available in veterinary medicine are not able to consistently delivery a FiO_2 of more than 60% to the patient. However, transtracheal oxygen, high-flow nasal cannula and intubation with or without positive pressure ventilation have the capacity to consistently deliver an FiO_2 of greater than 60% and consideration must be given to the development of oxygen toxicity.

Conclusion

Oxygen supplementation should be administered to all tachypneic patients presenting to the emergency room. For initial triage and stabilization, flow-by and face mask oxygen can be rapidly instituted to provide an increase in FiO_2 to the patient. An oxygen cage can be used as a fast and stress-free method of oxygen delivery in the patient presenting in respiratory distress but lack of hands-on access needs to be weighed against the ease of use. Hood oxygen and nasal oxygen are reasonable long-term oxygen delivery methods in patients requiring ongoing oxygen support.

In patients failing these conventional oxygen delivery methods, oxygen supplementation via transtracheal catheter can be considered. High-flow nasal cannula is a novel oxygen delivery method in veterinary medicine and may be useful for providing oxygen support to emergency patients failing conventional therapies. With severe respiratory distress not responsive to other methods of oxygen supplementation or with hypoventilation, intubation and positive pressure ventilation should be considered.

The emergency clinician must carefully monitor patient response to oxygen therapy and be prepared for escalation of oxygen therapy if improvement is not seen.

References

1 West JB. *Respiratory Physiology: The Essentials*, 8th edn. Lippincott Williams and Wilkins, Baltimore, 2008.

2 Loukopoulos PRW. Comparative evaluation of oxygen therapy techniquues in anaesthetized dogs:face mask and flow-by techniques. *Aust Vet Pract* 1997;27(1): 34–39.

3 Loukopoulos PRW. Comparative evaluation of oxygen therapy techniques in dogs: intranasal catheter and Elizabethan collar canopy. *Aust Vet Pract* 1996;26(4):199–205.

4 Marks SL. Nasal oxygen insufflation. *J Am Anim Hosp Assoc* 1999;35(5):366–367.

5 Camps-Palau MA, Marks SL, Cornick JL. Small animal oxygen therapy. *Comp Contin Educ Pract Vet* 2000;21(7):587–598.

6 Dunphy ED, Mann FA, Dodam JR, et al. Comparison of unilateral versus bilateral catheters for oxygen administration in dogs. *J Vet Emerg Crit Care* 2002;12(4):245–251.

7 Drobatz KJ, Powell S. Oxygen supplementation. In: *Current Veterinary Therapy XII: Small Animal Practice* (ed. Bonagura JD). WB Saunders, Philadelphia, 1995.

8 Klompas M, Kleinman K, Murphy MV. Descriptive epidemiology and attributable morbidity of ventilator-associated events. *Infect Control Hosp Epidemiol* 2014;35(5):502–510.

9 Levine SA, Niederman MS. The impact of tracheal intubation on host defenses and risks for nosocomial pneumonia. *Clin Chest Med* 1991;12(3):523–543.

10 Mann FA, Wagner-Mann C, Allert JA, Smith J. Comparison of intranasal and intratracheal oxygen administration in healthy awake dogs. *Am J Vet Res* 1992;53(5):856–860.

11 Lenglet H, Sztrymf B Leroy C, et al. Humidified high flow nasal oxygen during respiraotry failure in the emergency department: feasibility and efficacy. *Respir Care* 2012;57(11):1873–1878.

12 Rittayamai N, Tscheikuna J, Praphruetkit N, Kijpinyochai S. Use of high-flow nasal cannula for acute dyspnea and hypoxemia in the emergency department. *Respir Care* 2015;60:1377–1382.

13 Dysart K, Miller T, Wolfson MR, Shaffer TH. Research in high flow therapy: mechanisms of action. *Respir Med* 2009;103(10):1400–1405.

14 Frizzola M, Miller T, Rodriguez ME, et al. High-flow nasal cannula:impact on oxygenation and ventilation in an acute lung injury model. *Pediatr Pulmonol* 2011;46(1):67–74.

15 Daly JL, Keir I, Guenther CL. Evaluation of high flow oxygen therapy in normal dogs: a pilot study. *J Vet Emerg Crit Care* 2014;24(S1):S5.

16 Keir I, Daly J, Haggerty J, Guenther CL. High flow oxygen therapy delivery by nasal cannula improves paO2 in dogs with severe hypoxemia. *J Vet Emerg Crit Care* 2016;26:598–602.

17 Haskins SC. *Positive Pressure Ventilation*. Saunders, St Louis, 2004.

18 Hopper K, Haskins S, Kass PH, Rezende M, Aldrich J. Indications, management and outcome of long-term positive pressure ventilation in dogs and cats:148 cases (1990–2001). *J Am Vet Med Assoc* 2007;230(1):64–75.

19 Bruchim Y, Aroch I, Sissi A, et al. A retrospective study of positive pressure ventilation in 58 dogs: indications, prognostic factors and outcome. *J Small Anim Pract* 2014;55:314–319.

20 Edwards ML. Hyperbaric oxygen therapy. Part 1: history and principles. *J Vet Emerg Crit Care* 2010;20(3):284–288.

21 Edwards ML. Hyperbaric oxygen therapy. Part 2: application in disease. *J Vet Emerg Crit Care* 2010;20(3):289–297.

22 Elkins A. Hyperbaric oxygen therapy: potential veterinary applications. *Comp Contin Educ Pract Vet* 1997;19(5):607–612.

23 Crowe D. Hyperbaric oxygen therapy in veterinary medicine: a case series at Carson–Tahoe veterinary hospital. *Hyperbaric Med Today* 2000;1(3):13–15.

24 Hackett T. Pulse oximetry and end tidal carbon dioxide monitoring. *Vet Clin North Am Small Anim Pract* 2002;32(5):1021–1029.

25 Crapo JD. Morphologic changes in pulmonary oxygen toxicity. *Annu Rev Physiol* 1986;48:721–731.

26 Frank L, Bucher J, Roberts R. Oxygen toxicity in neonatal and adult animals of various species. *J Appl Physiol Respir Environ Exerc Physiol* 1978;45(5): 699–704.

182

Sonography in the Emergency Room
Gregory R. Lisciandro, DVM, DABVP, DACVECC

Hill Country Veterinary Specialists and FASTVet.com, Spicewood, TX, USA

Terminology

The terminology for standardized focused and complete veterinary ultrasound examinations and ultrasound signs and terms used during global FAST is shown in Table 182.1.

Abdominal Focused Assessment of Sonography for Trauma (FAST)

Target-Organ Approach

The use of the target-organ approach (naming abdominal FAST (aFAST) views by internal anatomy rather than external sites) maximizes the amount of clinical information gained during aFAST far beyond a simplistic approach of fluid positive or fluid negative (Figure 182.1) [1–6]. The author's recommended way to perform each aFAST view, their respective strengths, weaknesses, pearls, and pitfalls have been described [3,4]. Each aFAST view should be imaged in a standardized manner with dogs and cats placed in lateral recumbency (right generally preferred) [1–6] by fanning away and toward the table top in longitudinal orientation (same as sagittal) followed by rocking the probe cranially at each respective view [3,4]. The use of transverse orientation is likely unnecessary based on the landmark publication by Boysen et al. in which 397/400 views matched comparing longitudinal to transverse orientation when fluid was detected [7]. Lastly, pleural and pericardial effusion may be detected via the FAST diaphragmatico-hepatic (DH) view and all sonographers performing aFAST should make it habitual to look beyond the diaphragm into the thorax [3,4,6–9]. Goal-directed templates for recording aFAST findings keep veterinarians on task, give clinical value to initial and serial examinations, and provide a means for ultrasound program surveillance (detecting strengths and weaknesses in training) [2–4,6,8–10].

Abdominal Fluid Scoring System

The abdominal fluid scoring (AFS) system was developed to better characterize bleeding dogs because of the higher rate of hemoabdomen than previously reported pre-FAST (pre-FAST ~20% compared to a FAST rate of 45%) [1]. The scoring system is simple (0–4 scale) for dogs and cats placed in either lateral recumbency (see Figure 182.1) and includes positive intra-abdominal fluid (retroperitoneal fluid is not scored) [1]. Importantly, low-scoring dogs and cats (abdominal fluid score of 1,2) will *not* become anemic from their intra-abdominal bleed as long their AFS *remains* 1,2 on serial exams [1–3,11]. Therefore, if an AFS 1,2 dog or cat is anemic or becomes anemic, then pre-existing anemia was present or bleeding is occurring at another site (another space or cavity, gastrointestinal tract, reproductive tract, fracture site(s), or externally), respectively (or there is hemodilution due to large volumes of intravenous fluids) [1–3,11].

Conversely, higher-scoring dogs with AFS 3,4 will predictably become anemic and ~20–25% of bluntly traumatized dogs with AFS 3,4 will become anemic enough to require blood transfusion(s) [1–3] and, uncommonly, surgical exploratory surgery [1–3,6,7]. In contrast, higher scoring AFS 3,4 dogs bleeding postinterventionally or from penetrating trauma or ruptured tumors generally require resuscitation and exploratory surgery to stop the bleeding [3]. Exceptions would include coagulopathic dogs, including those with anaphylaxis [3,12]. These same principles likely hold true for cats, but felines are less likely to survive acute large-volume blunt trauma-induced bleeds (hemoabdomen FAST rate of 14% compared to dogs FAST rate of 27–45%) [5,11]. A similar human scoring system also aids in decision making (blood transfusion, exploratory surgery) [13] and any positive AFS should always be considered as major intra-abdominal injury until proven otherwise.

Textbook of Small Animal Emergency Medicine, First Edition. Edited by Kenneth J. Drobatz, Kate Hopper, Elizabeth Rozanski and Deborah C. Silverstein.
© 2019 John Wiley & Sons, Inc. Published 2019 by John Wiley & Sons, Inc.
Companion Website: www.wiley.com/go/drobatz/textbook

Table 182.1 Terminology for standardized focused and complete veterinary ultrasound examinations and ultrasound signs and terms used during global FAST.

Terminology for standardized ultrasound exams

Abdominal FAST	aFAST
Thoracic FAST	tFAST
Veterinary bedside lung ultrasound exam	Vet BLUE
Global FAST	aFAST, tFAST and Vet BLUE combined
Complete abdominal ultrasound	
Complete echocardiography	

Ultrasound signs and characterizations used during global FAST

A-lines	Hyperechoic horizontal equidistant lines extending from the pulmonary-pleural line representing a strong air interface
Caudal vena cava (CVC) characterization	Bounce: expected ~35–50% dynamic changes in CVC diameter during inspiration and expiration
	Flat: lacks dynamic change in CVC diameter (<10%) during inspiration and expiration having an abnormally small diameter
	FAT: lacks dynamic change in CVC diameter (<10%) during inspiration and expiration having an abnormally large diameter
B-lines (also called ultrasound lung rockets)	Hyperechoic vertical lines originating from the pulmonary surface that extend through the far field and swing in synchronization with inspiration and expiration, obliterating A-lines representing strong acoustic impedance between air and fluid at the lung surface
Bull's eye sign	Sign indicative of pericardial effusion at the right tFAST PCS view (directing the probe toward the sternum) through the observation of the heart's apex rounded by free fluid contained within the pericardial sac
Cardiac bump	Observation at the FAST DH view in which the muscular apex of the heart beating and indenting along the diaphragm is observed; helps rule in or out pericardial effusion
Gall bladder halo sign	Occurs with the presence of gall bladder wall edema and supports the diagnosis of anaphylaxis (flat CVC) vs right-sided heart failure/generalized systolic dysfunction, pericardial effusion (FAT CVC) vs right-sided volume overload (FAT CVC) in collapsed, weak, hypotensive dogs
	Note: There are other causes for gallbladder wall edema
Glide sign	Observation of the to-and-fro motion of the lung sliding along the thoracic wall at the pulmonary-pleural interface in concert with inspiration and expiration; also called lung sliding
Lung point	Transition point where lung recontacts the thoracic wall evidenced most commonly by the observation of either the glide sign or B-lines (ultrasound lung rockets) ventrally (or toward the sternum) and lack of both dorsally (or toward the spine); the lung point increases the sensitivity for the diagnosis of pneumothorax and semi-quantitates/allows tracking of the degree of pneumothorax by its distance from the chest tube site
Nodule sign	Observation of a round anechoic structure off the pulmonary surface that has a hyperechoic far border often with air reverberation artifact appearing as a B-line (ULR) through the far field; most commonly represents neoplastic abscess and granulomatous conditions
Racetrack sign	Sign indicative of pericardial effusion at the FAST DH view through the observation of the heart's apex rounded by free fluid contained within the pericardial sac
Shred sign	Observation of irregularities along the normal expected linear continuity of the pulmonary surface with variable degrees of echogenicity and hyperechoic foci contained within, representing lung consolidation with air bronchograms
Tissue sign	Observation of irregularities along the normal expected linear continuity of the pulmonary surface with variable degrees of echogenicity often appearing like soft tissue (liver-like) without hyperechoic foci, representing severe lung consolidation without an air bronchogram
Tree trunk sign	Observation of distended hepatic veins as they drain into a distended (FAT) caudal vena cava (abnormal finding); represents conditions impeding blood flow from the liver to the right heart (most commonly right-sided failure, pericardial effusion)
Ultrasound lung rockets (ULRs) (also called B-lines)	Hyperechoic vertical lines originating from the pulmonary surface that extend through the far field and swing in synchronization with inspiration and expiration, obliterating A-lines representing strong acoustic impedance between air and fluid at the lung surface
Urinary bladder volume estimation formula (mL)	$Length (cm) \times Width (cm) \times Height (cm) \times 0.2 \times Pi (0.625)$

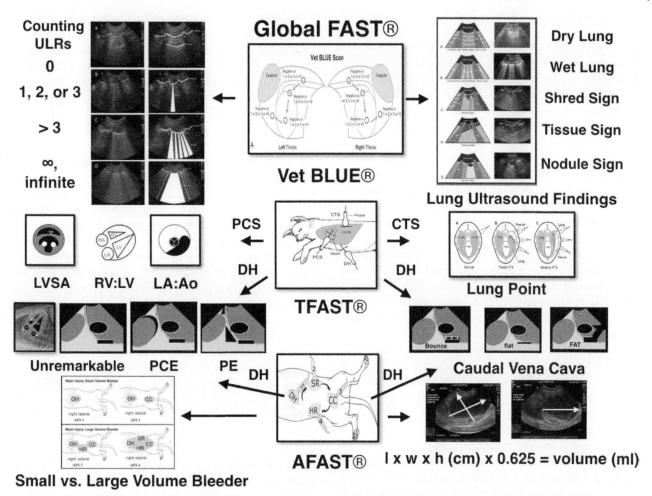

Figure 182.1 Clinical information acquired through Global FAST. (a) Vet BLUE protocol showing four acoustic windows (eight total views) on both hemithoraces. (b) How ultrasound lung rockets (ULRs, also called B-lines) are counted (0, 1, 2, 3, > 3 and infinity (∞)) .The scoring from lowest to highest is shown from the top to the bottom. (c) Five basic lung ultrasound signs from top to bottom: dry lung (A-lines with a glide sign); wet lung (ULRs); shred sign (air bronchogram); tissue sign; and nodule sign. (d) tFAST is now a five-point (view) exam with bilateral chest tube sites, bilateral pericardial sites, and a single diaphragmatico-hepatic (DH) view. (e) The three tFAST echo views to be mastered which include the left ventricular short-axis so-called "mushroom" view for volume and contractility; the long-axis four-chamber view for the right ventricular to left ventricular ratio (RV:LV) to screen for right-sided heart problems; and the left atrial to aortic (LA:Ao) to screen for left-sided heart problems. (f) How to characterize the degree of pneumothorax by looking for the lung point as a partial pneumothorax versus a massive pneumothorax. The distance of the lung point from the chest tube site with dogs and cats in sternal or standing position allows tracking of the worsening and resolution of pneumothorax. (g) How imaging through the DH view into the thorax images the heart and screens for pericardial and pleural effusion. (h) How the DH view may be used to assess the caudal vena cava as normal (bounce), flat (hypovolemia [low CVP]) and FAT (hypervolemia [high CVP]). (i) aFAST consists of four basic views which include the diaphragmatico-hepatic (DH), spleno-renal (SR), cysto-colic (CC), and hepato-renal (HR) view. aFAST is shown in right lateral recumbency but may be performed in left lateral recumbency or modified sternal recumbency. Dorsal recumbency should not be used as it is dangerous for hemodynamically fragile dogs and cats. (j) Showing the abdominal fluid scoring system and abdominal fluid scores (AFS) of 1, 2, 3, and 4. AFS of 1, 2 will not become anemic from intra-abdominal bleeds if they remain an AFS 1, 2 on serial exams (so if an AFS 1, 2 is anemic, it was pre-existing or bleeding is occurring at another site); and AFS 3, 4 will become anemic with 20–25% becoming transfusion candidates or needing exploratory laparotomy to stop the bleeding or both, depending on the patient subset. (k) Measurements taken during aFAST at the CC view to estimate urinary bladder volume (L×W×H×0.2×Pi) [0.625]. Images for TFAST, the Lung Point, AFAST and the Abdominal Fluid Scoring System. Reproduced with permission of John Wiley & Sons Ltd.

Lastly, the AFS system is invaluable as a monitoring tool (serial exams) for any bleeding patient or any dog or cat with other abdominal effusions for determining whether the condition is worsening (increasing AFS) or improving (decreasing AFS) [2,3,6]. Once bleeding stops in dogs (unknown in cats but likely the same), blood is rapidly absorbed from the abdominal cavity in < 48 hours [2,3,6]. If free fluid is safely accessible, abdominocentesis and fluid analysis should be performed in order to accurately characterize the effusion (ultrasound cannot reliably characterize free fluid) [2,3,5,6].

Blunt Versus Penetrating Trauma

There are gross differences in the coagulation cascade that occur between blunt trauma, in which blood is rapidly defibrinated by the mesothelial cells (and thus seen during aFAST as black anechoic triangulations), versus penetrating trauma, in which the crushing, tearing or shearing of tissue result in clotted blood (and thus is often missed during aFAST since clotted blood appears like adjacent soft tissue) [3,6,14]. In time, however, clotted blood will defibrinate and thus be apparent as free fluid and detected during serial aFAST [3,6,14]. Likewise, ruptured abdominal viscera will in time leak their contents and be detectable during serial aFAST (septic, exudative effusions) [15] and vascular injuries may in time, with cicatrization, lead to portal and hepatic hypertension (transudate/modified transudate) [16–19]. In other words, serial aFAST allows for the detection of a wide range of intra-abdominal injury when free fluid is not initially present, and detected free fluid may be characterized for a diagnosis and decision making regarding medical versus surgical conditions [2]. For these reasons, the liberal use of serial exams and serial aFAST for up to 24–48 hours is imperative for all at-risk dogs and cats [2,3,6,14,15,20,21], and 4-hour postadmission FAST exams have been standard of care since 2001 in human medicine [22] and are recommended for dogs and cats [2,3,6,11].

In summary, the recommended approach is to rehydrate, resuscitate, and re-evaluate with serial aFAST exams [2,3,6]. It is important to record the AFS in a systematic method because dogs and cats with small-volume bleeding or suspect for ruptured abdominal viscous (acute abdomen), especially when dehydrated, often develop marked effusions over the next 2–6 hours when placed on even modest intravenous fluid rates [2,3,6]. If free fluid becomes safely accessible, then abdominocentesis and fluid analysis are recommended in order to accurately characterize the effusion (ultrasound cannot reliably characterize free fluid) [2,3,5,6].

Triage or Non-Trauma Subsets: Collapsed, Weak, Hypotensive

The use of FAST formats for triage (non-trauma) subsets of dogs and cats as a first-line screening test has been advocated for several years [2,3,6]. In a recent clinical study, it was found that 75% of unstable and 9% of stable dogs and cats undergoing the combination of aFAST and tFAST had clinically relevant findings that helped direct care and diagnostics [5]. In another non-trauma study, pericardial effusion was detected in dogs at a much higher frequency when aFAST and tFAST were applied at triage than prior to using FAST (28 cases in 2011 versus three cases in 2005) [9].

In addition to detecting free fluid in the peritoneal cavity and retroperitoneal space, and in the pleural cavity and pericardial sac, the observation of gallbladder wall edema (so-called gallbladder halo sign) alerts the sonographer to the possibilities for anaphylaxis [23] in dogs, and right-sided heart conditions (dysfunction, failure/volume overload, pericardial effusion) in dogs [3,24] and, although rare, cats [24]. Importantly, anaphylactic dogs not uncommonly develop hemoabdomen that range from low-scoring AFS 1,2 to high-scoring AFS 3,4 with variable findings on traditional coagulation times (PT, aPTT) [3,12]. The pathogenesis has not been sorted out but is likely a combination of severe hepatic venous congestion from massive histamine release, coupled with heparinization from mast cells and the subsequent effects of tryptae and bradykinin resulting in diapedesis of blood into the peritoneal cavity. Mistaking an anaphylactic hemoabdomen for a surgical case will likely lead to a fatal patient outcome [12].

Moreover, the target-organ approach lends itself to detecting incidental and unexpected findings triggering continued imaging and diagnostics for many conditions, including as examples: DH view – liver (masses, cysts), gallbladder (choleliths, sludge, mucoceles); SR view – spleen (masses), left kidney (cortical cysts, pyelectasis/hydronephrosis, nephroliths); CC view – urinary bladder (thrombus, intraluminal debris, wall abnormalities); HR view – splenic masses, midabdominal masses, pyometra, right kidney (same as left kidney). In a human FAST study, ~8% of patients undergoing FAST had clinically relevant incidental findings detected [25]. Published aFAST goal-directed templates have a "comments section" to record suspect incidental findings [2–4,6,10].

Thoracic FAST

Thoracic FAST is a five-point exam that includes bilaterally applied chest tube sites (CTS) for rapid detection of pneumothorax (PTX) (highest point to which air would rise) and pulmonary contusions; bilaterally applied pericardial sites (PCS) for echocardiographic views of the left and right heart, pleural effusion (PE), and pericardial effusion (PCE); and singly applied diaphragmatico-hepatic (DH) view for PE and PCE, volume status (caudal vena cava and hepatic veins), and a deep window into the lung (see Figure 182.1) [2,6,8,26]. tFAST views, their strengths, and the clinical information garnered from them are listed in Table 182.2.

Thoracic FAST PCS and DH Views

Pericardial Effusion
The gold standard for the diagnosis of PCE is ultrasound [9]. For non-radiologist and non-cardiologist

Table 182.2 Thoracic FAST: how to perform, strengths, pearls, and pitfalls.

tFAST views	How to perform	Strengths	Pearls	Pitfalls
Left and right chest tube site (CTS) *Air rises	1. Place probe directly above xiphoid in upper 1/3 of the thorax either in lateral or standing or sternal recumbency where the cap of air would rise if PTX was present 2. With the probe perpendicular to the long axis of the ribs, establish the gator sign orientation to identify the lung line (pulmonary-pleural interface) 3. The glide sign is best observed by scattering the echoes by placing the rib head in the middle of the field (one-eyed gator) or oblique the echoes by fanning the probe to make the lung line less bright white and more gray	Diagnosis of PTX by A-lines without a glide sign	1. A-lines with a glide sign rule out PTX 2. ULRs (also called B-lines) rapidly rule out PTX 3. ULRs support the present of pulmonary contusions 4. If suspected PTX then search for the lung point generally evidenced by the resumption of the glide sign, ULRs, but also any lung signs including shred and tissue	1. Imaging too far caudally over the abdomen 2. Imaging too far dorsally over the hypaxial muscles 3. Rapid shallow breathing makes it difficult to see the glide sign 4. Safe sedation such as butorphanol slows the breathing to better search for the glide sign
Left pericardial site (PCS) *Fluid falls to the most gravity-dependent sites	1. Left PCS in right lateral recumbency – palpate for the apical beat with your left hand with your fingers on the right thoracic wall and your thumb on the left thoracic wall 2. Your thumb on the left thoracic wall will guide you on where to place the probe 3. Image the heart with the marker toward the elbow 4. Increase depth to be able to see the bright pericardium in the far field so the heart is clearly seen in its entirety	Diagnosis of pleural effusion *Diagnosis of PCE better via the right PCS riew and the DH View	1. Moving the probe closer to the sternum and directing toward the heart helps avoid air interference from lung 2. One view is no view – use multiple views to diagnose PE and PCE	1. Mistaking the major fluid-filled structure in the thorax, the heart, for free fluid, leading to the most catastrophic of mistakes – performing centesis on a heart chamber
Right pericardial site (PCS) *Fluid falls to the most gravity-dependent sites	1. Right PCS in right lateral recumbency – palpate for the apical beat with your left hand with your fingers on the right thoracic wall 2. Where your middle 2 fingers palpate the apical beat guides you on right thoracic wall to where to place the probe 3. Increase depth to be able to see the bright pericardium in the far field so the heart is clearly seen in its entirety 4. Image the heart with the marker toward the elbow for the short-axis view 5. Image the heart with the marker toward the spine for the long-axis view	1. Diagnosis of PE and PCE 2. Volume and contractility via the left ventricular short-axis mushroom view 3. Left-sided hypertension (LA:Ao ratio) 4. Right-sided hypertension (RV:LV ratio)	1. Only diagnose PCE if (a) imaging toward the muscular apex of the heart (bull's eye sign) or (b) imaging the long-axis 4-chamber view if all 4 chambers are clearly identified or (c) using the DH view (racetrack sign) *The pericardium attaches at one atrium and then rounds the apex of the heart to attach at the other atrium	1. Mistaking the major fluid-filled structure in the thorax, the heart, for free fluid, leading to the most catastrophic of mistakes – performing centesis on a heart chamber

(Continued)

Table 182.2 (*Continued*)

tFAST views	How to perform	Strengths	Pearls	Pitfalls
Diaphragmatico-hepatic (DH) view	1. Place the probe immediately caudal to the xiphoid and direct the probe toward the head of the patient 2. The curvilinear white line indicating the diaphragmatic–air-filled lung interface should be observed 3. Increase depth to be able to see into the thorax (25–33% of the far field) for PE 4. Rock the probe toward the sternum (parallel to it) to observe the "cardiac bump" (the muscular apex of the heart indenting into the diaphragm) to be able to interrogate for PCE 5. Fan through the gall bladder in both directions to observe for free intra-abdominal fluid 6. Look for the CVC for volume status as a bright white equals sign (=) made by the near and far CVC walls as the CVC traverses the diaphragm	1. Diagnose PE and PCE 2. Diagnose free intra-abdominal fluid 3. Volume status via the CVC 4. Gall bladder edema (halo sign) for anaphylaxis or right-sided heart conditions 5. DH view has less air interference than PCS views 6. The DH view performed similarly in sternal or standing as in lateral recumbency with imaging of the gall bladder, cardiac bump, and CVC	1. May be used as a single diagnostic view for PCE because the view interrogates the muscular apex of the heart making it much less likely to mistake a heart chamber for PCE 2. Mirror image artifact along the diaphragm immediately rules out PE	1. Mirror image artifact (created by the strong air–soft tissue interface of air-filled lung and diaphragm) can be a major confounder especially when free intra-abdominal fluid, the gall bladder, and the hepatic venous system are reflected into the thorax 2. Gall bladder wall edema (halo sign) is *not* pathognomonic for anaphylaxis

Ao, aorta; CVC, caudal vena cava; LA, left atrium; LV, left ventricle; PCE, pericardial effusion; PE, pleural effusion; PTX, pneumothorax; RV, right ventricle; ULR, ultrasound lung rocket.

sonographers, it is imperative to know how to properly diagnose PCE without mistaking the heart, the major fluid-filled structure in the thorax, for free fluid (Table 182.3) [6,8,9,27]. Such a misdiagnosis of a heart chamber for PCE (or PE) potentially leads to the most catastrophic of mistakes – performing centesis on the heart [6,8,9].

To maximize a correct diagnosis of PCE, the sonographer should adhere to the following tenets:

- image the heart at the right PCS view in its entirety with adequate depth to visualize the bright (hyperechoic [white]) pericardium in the far field [6,8,9,27]
- image toward the muscular apex of the heart where no fluid-filled heart chambers are likely to be mistaken for free fluid (bull's eye sign at the right PCS view, race-track sign at the DH view) [8,9]
- use the long-axis four-chamber view only if all four heart chambers are clearly identified [9,27,28].

The sonographer should know that the pericardium is attached at one atrium and then courses toward and

around the muscular apex of the heart to attach to the other atrium [8,9,27,28]. Adhering to the sage axiom that "one view is no view," using combinations of the aforementioned strategies also prevents mistakes.

Finally, the diagnosis of PCE should never be made solely on short-axis views other than by imaging toward the muscular apex of the heart because it is easy to mistake the right ventricle (or other heart chambers/structures) for free fluid [8,9].

If a diagnosis cannot be made, then a cardiologist or radiologist should be consulted.

Pleural Effusion

The gold standard for the diagnosis of PE is debatable and suggestions have included thoracoscopy, ultrasound, and computed tomography (CT) [29]. The diagnosis of PE follows the tenets for diagnosing PCE (see Table 182.3) [6,8,27]. However, in contrast to PCE in which the free fluid is contained within the pericardial sac, PE is uncontained and unrestrained unless compartmentalization is

Table 182.3 Diagnosis of pericardial and pleural effusion.

Diagnosis of pericardial effusion

The gold standard for the diagnosis of pericardial effusion is ultrasound

Radiography is poor

Pericardial effusion is contained in the pericardial sac that attaches at one atrium and rounds the apex of the heart to attach to the other atrium

Imaging strategy	FAST DH view	tFAST PCS view
Image toward the muscular apex of the heart where no heart chambers can be mistaken for free fluid	FAST DH view – racetrack sign	tFAST right PCS view – bull's eye sign
Long-axis 4-chamber view where all 4 chambers are identified		tFAST right PCS view
Increase depth to view the heart in its entirety using the bright white (hyperechoic) pericardium in the far field as a landmark		

Diagnosis of pleural effusion

The gold standard for the diagnosis of pleural effusion is computed tomography

Radiography is generally good

Pleural effusion is uncontained and unrestrained unless compartmentalized

Imaging strategy	FAST DH view	tFAST PCS view
Increase depth to image the heart in its entirety using the bright white pericardium in the far field as a landmark		tFAST right and left PCS – anechoic (black) triangulations
Image toward the muscular apex of the heart where no heart chambers can be mistaken for free fluid	FAST DH view – anechoic (black) triangulations	

DH, diaphragmatico-hepatic; PCS, pericardial site; tFAST, thoracic FAST.

present [6,8,27]. At the left and right PCS views, depth should be increased so the heart is clearly imaged in its entirety by observing the bright (hyperechoic [white]) pericardium in the far field [6,8,27]. The diagnosis of PE on PCS views is made by observing free fluid outside the heart and its pericardium.

The DH view is advantageous because it is much more difficult to mistake the heart for free fluid when compared to the transthoracic PCS views [8,9]. At the DH view, PE is observed as anechoic triangulations (in contrast to the rounding of PCE and its racetrack sign) [6,8,9]. Pitfalls of the DH view include mistaking the caudal vena cava for PE as it traverses the diaphragm [4]. However, by fanning through the diaphragm with a more liberal use of the DH view, the diagnosis of PE may be more confidently made, and the savvy sonographer knows that a mirror image artifact at the DH view immediately rules out PE along that plane.

Finally, PE on ultrasound may look like a large-volume effusion when in fact the effusion is minimal (and sonographers should be familiar with the centimeter scale on their machine). In questionable cases, thoracic radiography, although less sensitive, is a readily available modality to perform on stable patients [30].

If a diagnosis still cannot be made, then a cardiologist or radiologist should be consulted.

FAST DH View and CVC for Estimating Volume Status

The DH view is part of both tFAST and aFAST and eyeball characterization estimates central venous pressure (CVP) at the point where the caudal vena cava (CVC) traverses the diaphragm (see Figure 182.1) [2,3,26,27,31]. The CVC is characterized as having a normal bounce (~50% variation in diameter with phases of respiration), being flat with <10% change and small sized (volume depleted (low CVP)), or being FAT with <10% change and enlarged (volume overloaded (high CVP)) [27,31–34]. The hepatic veins should likewise be characterized as unremarkable (typically only evident in patients with high CVP) or distended (tree trunk sign) [3,6,8,31,33,34]. Distension of hepatic veins should concurrently have a FAT CVC [3,8,27,31,34]. Whenever a FAT CVC and hepatic venous distension are observed on admission prior to volume resuscitation, right-sided heart problems, PCE, or vascular obstruction between the diaphragm and the pulmonary outflow track should be suspected [3,6,8,26,27,31,33,34]. When a FAT CVC and hepatic venous distension occur following fluid resuscitation or while dogs and cats are receiving intravenous fluid therapy during hospitalized care, right heart volume overload is present until proven otherwise [26,27,31,33–35].

tFAST Basic Echo Views

Three views at the right PCS view are taught: the short-axis left ventricular view (so-called mushroom view), the short-axis quick-peek LA:Ao view, and the long-axis four-chamber view (RV:LV) (see Figure 182.1) [6,26,27,35]. These views provide information regarding volume and contractility, and left-sided and right-sided hypertension, respectively [26,27,34–36]. The eyeball approach generally gives ample information during patient resuscitation and monitoring when complete echocardiography is not readily available or is too risky for an unstable patient [6,8,26,27,33–37]. The eyeball approach (subjective assessment) has been shown to reliably give similar information as obtained by more technically challenging measurements using M-mode and color flow Doppler [37]. If concern regarding cardiac function and volume overload persists, then complete echocardiography should be performed by a sonographer with advanced training (cardiologist or radiologist). When echocardiography views are too risky or indeterminate, then the fallback strategy of using Vet BLUE for left-sided failure/overload and the caudal vena cava and hepatic venous congestion for right-sided failure/overload should be used (see Figure 182.1).

tFAST CTS Views

Pneumothorax and Lung Point

The CTS is designated as the highest point on the thorax to which the cap of air would rise when free air (pneumothorax (PTX)) is present within the pleural space (see Figure 182.1) [2,8,27,38]. The observation of either the glide sign or ultrasound lung rockets (ULRs), also called B-lines, rules out PTX at that specific point along the thoracic wall [2,8,38].Thus, if the glide sign or ULRs are observed at the highest point to which air would rise in that positioning, then PTX is ruled out [2,8,38]. If A-lines without a glide sign are observed, then PTX is likely and with the patient in sternal or standing position, the sonographer should search for the lung point [2,8,26,39].

The lung point is the location where lung recontacts the thoracic wall and is most often evidenced through either observation of the glide sign or presence of ULRs (see Figure 182.1) [2,8,26,39]. The lung point increases the sensitivity for the diagnosis of PTX, semi-quantitates its degree (partial versus massive), and serially allows for tracking worsening or resolving PTX [39]. When the lung point is in the middle one-third or midthorax from the CTS to the sternum or further ventrally, thoracocentesis generally should be performed.

Pulmonary Contusions

The presence of ULRs rapidly rules out PTX at the CTS view but the presence of ULRs supports the diagnosis of pulmonary contusions (PCs) [2,8,40,41]. Numbers of ULRs likely correlate with severity of PCs and through the use of Vet BLUE, the total number of ULRs is used to assign the patient a "pulmonary contusion score" [2,8,40]. Serial exams allow for tracking PCs as worsening (increasing ULRs) or resolving (decreasing ULRs). In severe PCs, additional lung ultrasound signs of consolidation, referred to as the shred sign and the tissue sign, are observed (see Figure 182.1) [8,40,42,43].

Vet BLUE

Vet BLUE (bedside lung ultrasound exam) should be considered as an extension from the CTS to better characterize patient respiratory status (see Figure 182.1) [6,40,42,44–46]. Using lung ultrasound (LUS) and the Vet BLUE pattern-based approach screens for respiratory conditions and developing complications during hospitalized care [26,44–48]. Dogs and cats should have dry LUS profiles (infrequent to no ULRs) during Vet BLUE [44,45]. LUS findings may include the following: dry lung (A-lines with a glide sign; normal patients), wet lung (ULRs, also called B-lines; patients with interstitial lung fluid), shred sign (analogous to air bronchograms), tissue sign (consolidation with no aeration, referred to as hepatization [30]), and nodule sign (nodular infiltration) (see Figure 182.1) [2,40,43,49,50]. The wedge sign is a subset of the shred sign and strongly suggests the presence of pulmonary thromboembolism (vascular infarction) [42].

Assumptions, Strengths, and Weaknesses of Lung Ultrasound

Lung ultrasound has been shown to be diagnostically more sensitive than both lung auscultation and chest radiography for common respiratory conditions in human patients [49,51]. The LUS assumption is that acute pathology makes it peripherally to the outer 1–3 mm of lung, and thus may be detected by LUS [40,43–47,49,51,52]. Conversely, if the pathology does not make it to peripheral lung then abnormalities will be missed [49,51,52]. However, most acute respiratory conditions in people, and apparently with dogs and cats, extend to peripheral lung and may be detected using LUS [44–47,49,51]. Serial Vet BLUE exams should be used in suspect cases [26,35,40].

Importantly, ULRs are non-specific LUS findings and generally represent a fluid–air interface at the lung periphery [2,40,43–47,49,51]. Conditions associated with the presence of ULRs include cardiogenic and non-cardiogenic pulmonary edema, hemorrhage, pneumonia, and inflammation [2,8,40,41,44–47,49,51]. Thus, a Vet BLUE pattern-based approach best characterizes the likely diagnosis, for example cardiogenic edema is more dorsal or generalized with bacterial bronchopneumonia being more ventral [30,42,44–46]. ULRs are counted $(1, 2, 3, > 3, \text{infinity } (\infty))$ over a representative single intercostal space during Vet BLUE (see Figure 182.1) [40,44–46,48]. ULRs are counted because their numbers correlate with the degree of alveolar-interstitial edema on CT [53]. Recently, a simplistic strong positive approach of having two or more positive sites (positive being > 3 or infinity ULRs) on both hemithoraces was shown to have comparable sensitivity and specificity to thoracic radiography for the diagnosis of left-sided congestive heart failure in cats [46].

Vet BLUE is advantageous over radiography because it is point of care, requires minimal to no restraint, and is rapid (<60–90 sec) [40,44–46]. Through use of the Vet BLUE pattern-based approach and proper LUS training for learning additional LUS signs (shred sign, wedge sign, tissue sign, and nodule sign), a more accurate LUS conclusion may be drawn [40,42,43,49,50,54].

Finally, atelectic lung may result in ULRs, shred sign or tissue sign [30,48,55,56] but in most instances, these LUS findings resolve within 2 hours post-sedation anesthesia [56].

Global FAST

Global FAST for Patient Monitoring

Through the use of aFAST, its fluid scoring system, and the cystocolic view urinary bladder volume estimation formula [57,58], tFAST and Vet BLUE patient surveillance for developing complications and volume status may be better ascertained and should be included in daily rounds following physical examination (see Figure 182.1) (Table 182.4) [6,26,27,54–56,59,60]. Global FAST evaluates volume status and cardiac contractility, left-sided heart status (Vet BLUE (ULRs) and LA:Ao), right-sided heart status (CVC and hepatic veins), the possibility of

Table 182.4 Use of global FAST for rapid assessment and monitoring of the critical dog and cat modified from the RUSH exam [33].

Global FAST evaluation	Hypovolemic shock	Cardiogenic shock	Obstructive shock	Distributive shock
Pump – how contracting? **Inotropy**	**Works** Hypercontractile heart Small chamber size Dry lung	**Deficient** Hypocontractile heart Dilated heart Wet lung	**Works –Overloaded** Hypercontractile heart PCE/tamponade RV strain (increased RV:LV) when PTE, cardiac thrombus Dry >> wet lung	**Works – Deficient** Hypercontractile heart (early sepsis) Hypocontractile heart (late sepsis) Dry > wet lung
Tank – how full? **Volume**	**Empty** Flat CVC Flat jugular veins Dry lung	**Overfilled** Distended CVC Distended jugular vein ULRs (lung edema) Wet lung	**Overfilled** Distended CVC Distended jugular PTX (A-lines and no glide sign) Dry or wet lung	**Empty or Overfilled** Normal or small CVC (early sepsis) Peritoneal fluid (exudate/ sepsis source) PE (exudate/ sepsis source) Dry or wet lung
Pipes – leaky?	**Leaky** Peritoneal fluid (loss) PE (loss) Splenic or other intra-abdominal bleeding tumor	**Normal** Peritoneal fluid (ascites) PE	**Obstructed** Thromboembolism	**Leaky or Distended** ARDS Third spacing
Comments	Use Vet BLUE and AFS	Use Vet BLUE and AFS	Vet BLUE can detect PTE	Vet BLUE and tFAST can detect non-cardiogenic edema

AFS, abdominal fluid scoring; ARDS, acute respiratory distress syndrome; BLUE, bedside lung ultrasound exam; CVC, caudal vena cava; LV, left ventricle; PCE, pericardial effusion; PE, pleural effusion; PTE, pulmonary thromboembolism; PTX, pneumothorax; RV, right ventricle; ULR, ultrasound lung rocket.

drug reactions (dogs and the gallbladder halo sign), and assessment for effusions in four spaces (abdominal, retroperitoneal, pleural, and pericardial) plus lung edema [7,26,27,35,56,59,60]. The abdominal fluid scoring system allows for predicting the need for blood transfusion by differentiating small-volume bleeders (AFS 1,2) from large-volume bleeders (AFS 3,4) [2,3,6]. The cystocolic view urinary bladder volume estimation formula allows for estimating urine output when measurements are performed over time (see Figure 182.1)[57,58].

Lastly, global FAST may be performed with the abdominal preset and a single microconvex probe in < 5–7 minutes by properly trained veterinarians [2,6,26,59,60] and global FAST accomplishes many of the same objectives as the combined use of FAST and the RUSH exam used by physicians (see Table 182.4) [26,33,59,60].

Global FAST for CPR and Advanced Life Support

When dogs and cats have unexplained hypotension, appear close to cardiopulmonary arrest (CPA) or have experienced CPA, minutes count and global FAST rapidly screens for potentially treatable conditions,

Table 182.5 Use of global FAST for rapidly ruling out your Hs and Ts in patients nearing cardiopulmonary arrest and during cardiopulmonary resuscitation. Source: Modified from AHA CPR guidelines.

The Hs	The Ts
Evaluated for using venous blood gas, physical exam, vital signs	Evaluated for using global FAST
Hypothermia	Tension pneumothorax
Hypotension	Trauma, hemorrhage
Hyperkalemia, hypokalemia	Thromboembolism
Hypoglycemia	Tamponade, pericardial effusion
Hydrogen ion (acidosis)	Toxin, anaphylaxis

including tension PTX, pulmonary thromboembolism, internal hemorrhage, pericardial effusion/tamponade, and anaphylaxis (Table 182.5) [6,26,54,59,60]. Moreover, global FAST serves as a monitoring tool directing fluid resuscitation and inotropic and vasopressor therapy through principles previously discussed and as shown in people (see Figure 182.1) [26,33,59–62].

References

1 Lisciandro GR, Lagutchik MS, Mann KA, et al. Evaluation of an abdominal fluid scoring system determined using abdominal focused assessment with sonography for trauma in 101 dogs with motor vehicle trauma. *J Vet Emerg Crit Care* 2009;19(5):426–37.
2 Lisciandro GR. Abdominal and thoracic focused assessment with sonography for trauma, triage, and monitoring in small animals. *J Vet Emerg Crit Care* 2011;21(2):104–122.
3 Lisciandro GR. The abdominal FAST[3] (AFAST[3]) exam. In: *Focused Ultrasound for the Small Animal Practitioner* (ed. Lisciandro GR). Wiley-Blackwell, Ames, 2014, pp. 17–43.
4 Lisciandro GR. Abdominal (AFAST[3]) Scan and Thoracic (TFAST[3]) and Vet BLUE Scan Techniques for Trauma, Triage and Tracking (Monitoring) Lab Manual. Hill Country Veterinary Specialists, Spicewood, Texas.
5 McMurray J, Boysen S, Chalhoub S. Focused assessment with sonography in nontraumatized dogs and cats in the emergency and critical care setting. *J Vet Emerg Crit Care* 2016;26(1):64–73.
6 Boysen SR, Lisciandro GR. The use of ultrasound in the emergency room (AFAST and TFAST). *Vet Clin North Am Small Anim Pract* 2013;43(4):773–797.
7 Boysen SR, Rozanski EA, Tidwell AS, et al. Evaluation of focused assessment with sonography for trauma protocol to detect abdominal fluid in dogs involved in motor vehicle accidents. *J Am Vet Med Assoc* 2004;225(8):1198–1204.
8 Lisciandro GR. The thoracic FAST[3] (TFAST[3]) exam. In: *Focused Ultrasound for the Small Animal Practitioner* (ed. Lisciandro GR). Wiley-Blackwell, Ames, 2014, pp. 140–165.
9 Lisciandro GR. The use of the diaphragmatico-hepatic (DH) views of the abdominal and thoracic focused assessment with sonography for triage (AFAST/TFAST) examinations for the detection of pericardial effusion in 24 dogs (2011–2012). *J Vet Emerg Crit Care* 2016;26(1):125–1231.
10 Available free of charge at www.facebook.com/fastvet or FASTVet.com.
11 Lisciandro GR. Evaluation of initial and serial combination focused assessment with sonography for trauma (CFAST) examination of the thorax (TFAST) and abdomen (AFAST) with the application of an abdominal fluid scoring system in 49 traumatized cats. *J Vet Emerg Crit Care* 2012;22(2):S11.
12 Lisciandro GR. Abdominal FAST (AFAST)-detected hemorrhagic abdominal effusion in 11 dogs with acute collapse and gallbladder wall edema (Halo Sign) with presumed anaphylaxis. *J Vet Emerg Crit Care* 2016;26(S1):S8–9.
13 Sirlin CB, Casola G, Brown MA, et al. Quantification of fluid on screening ultrasonography for blunt abdominal

trauma: a simple scoring system to predict severity of injury. *J Ultrasound Med* 2001;20(4):359–364.

14 Udobi KF, Rodriguez A, Chiu WC, et al. Role of ultrasonography in penetrating abdominal trauma: a prospective clinical study. *J Trauma* 2001;50: 475–479.

15 Mohammadi A, Ghasemi-Rad M. Evaluation of gastrointestinal injury in blunt abdominal trauma "FAST is not reliable": the role of repeated ultrasonography. *World J Emerg Surg* 2012;7(1):2.

16 Cornelius L, Mahaffey M. Kinking of the intrathoracic caudal vena cava in five dogs. *J Small Anim Pract* 1985;26:67–80.

17 Crowe DT, Lorenz MD, Hardie EM, et al. Chronic peritoneal effusion due to partial caudal vena caval obstruction following blunt abdominal trauma: diagnosis and successful surgical management. *J Am Anim Hosp Assoc* 1984;20:231–238.

18 Lisciandro GL, Harvey HJ, Beck KA. Automobile-induced obstruction of the caudal vena cava in a dog. *J Small Anim Pract* 1995;36(8):368–372.

19 Fine DM, Olivier NB, Walshaw R, et al. Surgical correction of late onset Budd–Chiari-like syndrome in a dog. *J Am Vet Med Assoc* 1998;212(6):835–837.

20 Bilello JF, Davis JW, Lemaster D, et al. Prehospital hypotension in blunt trauma identifying the "crump factor." *J Trauma* 2011;70(5):1038–1042.

21 Blackbourne LH, Soffer D, McKenney M, et al. Secondary ultrasound examination increases the sensitivity of the FAST exam in blunt trauma. *J Trauma* 2004;57(5):934–938.

22 American College of Emergency Physicians. ACEP emergency ultrasound guidelines 2001. *Ann Emerg Med* 2001;38:470–481.

23 Quantz JE, Miles MS, Reed AL, et al. Elevation of alanine transaminase and gallbladder wall abnormalities as biomarkers of anaphylaxis in canine hypersensitivity patients. *J Vet Emerg Crit Care* 2009;19(6):536–544.

24 Lisciandro GR. Case series: gallbladder wall edema (halo sign) as a marker for right-sided heart failure and pericardial effusion. Unpublished data, 2016.

25 Sgourakis G, Lanitis S, Korontzi M, et al. Incidental findings in focused assessment with sonography for trauma in hemodynamically stable blunt trauma patients: speaking about cost to benefit. *J Trauma* 2011;71(6):123–127.

26 Lisciandro GR, Armenise A. Focused or COAST[3] – cardiopulmonary resuscitation (CPR), global FAST (GFAST[3]) and the FAST-ABCDE exam. In: *Focused Ultrasound for the Small Animal Practitioner* (ed. Lisciandro GR). Wiley-Blackwell, Ames, 2014, pp. 269–285.

27 DeFrancesco TC. Focused or COAST[3] – echo (heart). In: *Focused Ultrasound for the Small Animal Practitioner* (ed. Lisciandro GR). Wiley-Blackwell, Ames, 2014, pp. 189–205.

28 de Madron E. Pericardial diseases. In: *Clinical Echocardiography of the Dog and Cat* (eds Chetboul V, Bussadori C, de Madron E). Elsevier, St Louis, 2012, p. 261.

29 Sikora K, Perera P, Mailhot T, et al. Ultrasound for the detection of pleural effusions and guidance for the thoracocentesis procedure. *ISRN Emerg Med* 2012; article ID 676524.

30 Hecht S. Thorax. In: *Atlas of Small Animal Ultrasonography* (eds Penninck D, d'Anjou MA). Wiley-Blackwell, Ames, 2008, p. 141.

31 Nelson NC, Drost WT, Lerche P, et al. Noninvasive estimation of central venous pressure in anesthetized dogs by measurement of hepatic venous blood flow velocity and abdominal venous diameter. *Vet Radiol Ultrasound* 2010;51(3):313–323.

32 Ferrada P, Vanguri P, Anand RJ, et al. Flat inferior vena cava: indicator of poor prognosis in trauma and acute care surgery patients. *Am Surg* 2012;78(12):1396–1398.

33 Perera P, Mailhot T, Riley D, Mandavia D. The RUSH exam: Rapid Ultrasound in SHock in the evaluation of the critically ill. *Emerg Med Clin North Am* 2010;28(1):29–56.

34 Tchernodrinski S, Arntfield R. Inferior vena cava. In: *Point of Care Ultrasound* (eds Soni N, Arntfield R, Kory P). Elsevier, Philadelphia, 2015, pp. 135–141.

35 Acquah S, Arntfield R. Right ventricular function. In: *Point of Care Ultrasound* (eds Soni N, Arntfield R, Kory P). Elsevier, Philadelphia, 2015, pp. 110–118.

36 Arntfield R, Soni N, Kory P. Left ventricular function. In: *Point of Care Ultrasound* (eds Soni N, Arntfield R, Kory P). Elsevier, Philadelphia, 2015, pp. 103–109.

37 Ferrada P, Evans D, Wolfe L, et al. Findings of a randomized controlled trial using limited transthoracic echocardiogram (LTTE) as a hemodynamic monitoring tool in the trauma bay. *J Trauma Acute Care Surg* 2014;76(1):31–37.

38 Lisciandro GR, Lagutchik MS, Mann KA, et al. Accuracy of Focused Assessment with Sonography for Trauma (FAST) to detect pneumothorax in 145 dogs with blunt and penetrating trauma. *J Vet Emerg Crit Care* 2008;18(3):258–269.

39 Lichtenstein D, Meziere G, Biderman P, Gepner A. The "lung point": an ultrasound point specific to pneumothorax. *Intensive Care Med* 2000;26(10): 1434–1440.

40 Lisciandro GR. The Vet BLUE lung scan. In: *Focused Ultrasound for the Small Animal Practitioner* (ed. Lisciandro GR). Wiley-Blackwell, Ames, 2014, pp. 166–188.

41 Soldati G, Testa A, Silva FR, et al. Chest ultrasonography in lung contusion. *Chest* 2006;130(2):533–538.

42 Lisciandro GR. Establishing Vet BLUE profiles for common respiratory conditions of dogs and cats (400 cases). Unpublished data, 2016.

43 Lee P, Tofts R, Kory P. Lung Ultrasound Interpretation. In: *Point of Care Ultrasound* (eds Soni N, Arntfield R, Kory P). Elsevier, Philadelphia, 2015, pp. 59–69.

44 Lisciandro GR, Fosgate GT, Fulton RM. Frequency and number of ultrasound lung rockets (B-lines) using a

regionally based lung ultrasound examination named vet BLUE (veterinary bedside lung ultrasound exam) in dogs with radiographically normal lung findings. *Vet Radiol Ultrasound* 2014;55(3):315–322.

45 Lisciandro GR, Fulton RM, Fosgate GT, Mann KA. Frequency of B-lines using a regionally-based lung ultrasound examination (the Vet BLUE protocol) in 49 cats with normal thoracic radiographical lung findings. *J Vet Emerg Crit Care* 2017;27(3):267–277.

46 Ward JL, Lisciandro GR, Tou SP, Keene BW, DeFrancesco TC. Accuracy of point-of-care lung ultrasound (Vet BLUE protocol) for the diagnosis of cardiogenic pulmonary edema in dogs and cats with acute dyspnea. *J Am Vet Med Assoc* 2017;250(6):666–675.

47 Rademacher N, Pariaut R, Pate J, et al. Transthoracic lung ultrasound in normal dogs and dogs with cardiogenic pulmonary edema: a pilot study. *Vet Radiol Ultrasound* 2014;55:447–452.

48 Lisciandro GR, Romero LA, Bridgeman CH. Pilot Study: Vet BLUE profiles pre- and post-anesthesia in 31 dogs undergoing surgical sterilization. *J Vet Emerg Crit Care* 2015;25(S1):S7–8.

49 Lichtestein DA, Meziere GA. Relevance of lung ultrasound in the diagnosis of acute respiratory failure: the BLUE protocol. *Chest* 2008;134(1):117–125.

50 Kulhavy DA, Lisciandro GR. Use of a lung ultrasound examination called Vet BLUE to screen for metastatic lung nodules in the emergency room. *J Vet Emerg Crit Care* 2015;25(S1):S14.

51 Volpicelli G, Elbarbary M, Blaivas M, et al. International evidence-based recommendations for point-of-care lung ultrasound. *Intensive Care Med* 2012;38:577–591.

52 Soldati G, Sher S, Testa A. Lung and ultrasound: time to "reflect." *Eur Rev Med Pharmacol Sci* 2011;15(2):223–227.

53 Jambrik Z, Monti S, Coppola V, et al. Usefulness of ultrasound lung comets as a nonradiologic sign of extravascular lung water. *Am J Cardiol* 2004;93: 1265–1270.

54 Squizzato A, Galli L, Gerdes VE. Point-of-care ultrasound in the diagnosis of pulmonary embolism. *Crit Ultrasound J* 2015;27:7.

55 Acosta CM, Maidana GA, Jacovitti D, et al. Accuracy of transthoracic ultrasound for diagnosing anesthesia-induced atelectasis in children. *Anesthesiology* 2014;120(6):1370–1379.

56 Lisciandro GR. Use of Vet BLUE protocol for the detection of lung atelectasis and sonographic gallbladder wall evaluation for anaphylaxis and volume overload in 63 dogs undergoing general anesthesia. *In review*, 2017.

57 Lisciandro GR, Fosgate GT. AFAST cysto-colic view urinary bladder measurements to estimate urinary bladder volume in dogs and cats. *J Vet Emerg Crit Care* 2015;25(1):S8.

58 Lisciandro GR, Fosgate GT. Use of AFAST cysto-colic view urinary bladder measurements to estimate urinary bladder volume in dogs and cats. *J Vet Emerg Crit Care* 2017;27(6):713–717.

59 Lisciandro GR. The Global FAST (GFAST) triad for patient monitoring and CPR. Proceedings of the American College of Veterinary Internal Medicine Symposium, Indianapolis, IN, 2015.

60 Lisciandro GR. Ultrasound in animals. In: *Critical Care Ultrasound* (eds Lumb P, Karakitsos D). Elsevier, St Louis, 2014, pp. 290–293.

61 Breitkreutz R, Price S, Steiger HV, et al. Focused echocardiographic evaluation in life support and peri-resuscitation of emergency patients: a prospective trial. *Resuscitation* 2010;81(11):1527–1533.

62 Breitkreutz R, Walcher F, Seeger FH, et al. Focused echocardiographic evaluation in resuscitation management (FEER): concept of an advanced life support-conformed algorithm. *Crit Care Med* 2007;35(S5):S150–161.

183

Thoracocentesis

Melissa Bucknoff, DVM, DACVECC[1] and Meghan Respess, DVM, DACVECC[2]

[1] *School of Veterinary Medicine, Ross University, Bassetterre, St Kitts, West Indies*
[2] *BluePearl Veterinary Partners, Brooklyn, NY, USA*

Introduction

Thoracocentesis is a straightforward procedure that is widely performed in veterinary practice, particularly in the emergency setting. Indications include the alleviation of respiratory distress due to pleural space disease, as well as to aid diagnosis. The procedure is rapid, relatively technically simple, and usually associated with minimal complication. Thoracocentesis does not require highly specialized equipment. It can be performed with or without ultrasound guidance and under light sedation and/or local anesthesia.

Recently, a veterinary thoracocentesis simulator model was validated for training purposes as part of an entry-level clinical skill set checklist [1]. Such simulator-based training has been demonstrated to significantly improve an individual's performance and level of comfort with the procedure [2]. However, most clinicians will learn to perform thoracocentesis on patients, either during veterinary school or in the early days of practice.

Indications

The goals of thoracocentesis may be therapeutic, diagnostic, or both. Animals with signs of respiratory difficulty due to pleural space disease are candidates for therapeutic thoracocentesis and animals with an unclear diagnosis and pleural effusion may have a thoracocentesis performed for diagnostic purposes, specifically to look for infection or neoplasia. Pleural space disease is typically suspected on physical examination and confirmed by point-of-care ultrasound or radiography (see Chapter 182). Dogs and cats being supported by positive pressure mechanical ventilation are also at increased risk of barotrauma, which may result in pneumothorax; this is more commonly a concern in longer duration ventilation (see Chapter 188).

Diagnostic thoracocentesis can be performed in patients with pleural space disease in the absence of significant respiratory signs. These patients usually have smaller volume effusions and do not require a therapeutic procedure. However, in any patient which undergoes thoracocentesis, it is important that samples are collected for fluid analysis (to include cell and protein counts), cytology, and bacterial culture and susceptibility if indicated. Brief in-house cytology is useful and can, for instance, aid in making the presumptive diagnosis of pyothorax if intracellular bacteria are present in the sample or neoplasia, such as lymphoma, in a cat with a mediastinal mass. If chylothorax is suspected, triglyceride and cholesterol concentrations should be submitted on both the fluid and serum for definitive diagnosis.

Contraindications

Thoracocentesis can exacerbate clinical bleeding in cases of coagulopathy, severe thrombocytopenia, or thrombocytopathia. In young dogs with pleural effusion, the clinician should be sure to rule out anticoagulant rodenticide toxicity prior to thoracocentesis as pleural hemorrhage is a common site for bleeding in such cases (see Chapter 130). Additionally, fractious or anxious patients must be adequately sedated and safely restrained to minimize risks of procedure (see Chapter 192).

Preparation and Considerations

Preparedness is strongly advocated in all aspects of clinical medicine, and may be life-saving in the event of fulminant pleural space disease, particularly if a tension pneumothorax is present (see Chapter 44, Pneumothorax). Emergency thoracocentesis set-ups, or "chest-tap kits" (Figure 183.1),

Textbook of Small Animal Emergency Medicine, First Edition. Edited by Kenneth J. Drobatz, Kate Hopper, Elizabeth Rozanski and Deborah C. Silverstein.
© 2019 John Wiley & Sons, Inc. Published 2019 by John Wiley & Sons, Inc.
Companion Website: www.wiley.com/go/drobatz/textbook

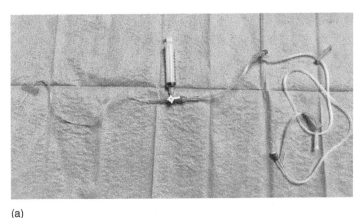
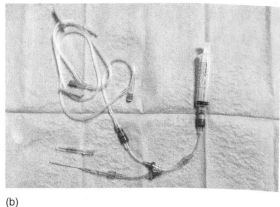

(a)   (b)

Figure 183.1 (a,b) Example of an emergency chest tap set-up which can be stored on a crash cart where it can be easily accessed, accompanied by butterfly catheter set-up.

should be assembled and stocked in easily accessible locations, such as within a crash cart or in a drawer next to the main triage area, as well as in the intensive care units. Sedation and analgesics may be indicated to reduce anxiety, treat pain, and minimize movement during the procedure (see Chapter 193). Local anesthesia may also be used.

Procedure

Gather supplies and prepare the patient (see Table 183.1 and Box 183.1 for a thoracocentesis procedure checklist and equipment options). Ensure anyone assisting with the procedure is comfortable with patient restraint, monitoring, and basic equipment handling (e.g. aspirating syringe, managing three-way stopcock). An area over

the appropriate rib spaces is clipped, typically between the seventh and ninth intercostal spaces, and aseptically prepped. This location over the thorax is chosen in order to avoid the heart and to avoid inadvertent sampling of the abdominal cavity. Ideal positioning will be somewhat

Table 183.1 Thoracocentesis procedure equipment options.

	Pros	Cons
Needle with extension tubing	Allows rapid penetration of check wall without tissue drag, does not kink	Risks laceration of lung or blood vessels
Butterfly catheter	Ideal for small patients	May not be long enough for use in larger patients, risks laceration of lung or blood vessels
Over-the-needle catheter	Removal of stylet reduces risk of intrathoracic laceration, attachment of active suction for drainage of large-volume or chronic effusions	Often kinks once stylet removed, risks tissue drag through skin with wider bore catheters (≥16 G)

Box 183.1 Thoracocentesis equipment checklist.

Clippers

Aseptic scrub for prepping thorax

Sterile gloves

#11 scalpel blade (optional); only if large-gauge catheter use planned

Syringes (10–60 mL; may depend on size of animal and volume of effusion)

Three-way stopcock or smart "Y" bi-clave adapter

Sterile needle, over-the-needle IV catheter or butterfly catheter

Sterile extension tubing

Collection bowl for fluid

Supplies for fluid sample submission:
    Red- and lavender-top tubes for fluid sample submission
    Culturettes (aerobic and anaerobic)
    Glass slides for cytology

Oxygen (flow-by mask and/or cage for recovery)

Assistant(s):
    Help with restraint
    Administer sedation as needed
    Operate syringe and three-way stopcock

Ultrasound machine (optional)

Sedation or local anesthesia if desired

dictated by what is most comfortable for the patient. If a pneumothorax is present, air will rise to the top of the chest, making sternal or lateral recumbency acceptable. Conversely, effusion is gravity dependent and accumulates ventrally, making sternal recumbency better; dogs may stand if preferred. However, as the mediastinum is not complete in dogs and cats, fluid and air may usually be aspirated successfully from any location. Inadvertent abdominocentesis is more common if there is a large amount of ascites which results in the forward displacement of the diaphragm. Care must be taken to prevent undue stress caused by restraining a patient in lateral recumbency that is having difficulty breathing.

Identify Anatomical Landmarks

The point of entry for draining pleural effusion is just above the costochondral junction at approximately the seventh or eighth intercostal space. A more dorsal approach may be needed if treating pneumothorax, about halfway between the spine and the costochondral junction between the eighth and ninth intercostal space (Figure 183.2). The intercostal blood vessels run along the caudal border of the ribs and should be avoided.

Once the point of entry is identified, a local anesthetic block can be administered if desired and applied to the depth of the pleura. In unstable patients with the need to evacuate the chest urgently, this step should be skipped. Local anesthetics do cause a sting at the site of administration, and this additional stress may be counterproductive to the procedure. One part sodium bicarbonate may be mixed with nine parts lidocaine to reduce injection discomfort when used to block the intended thoracocentesis site.

Sterile gloves are often used for the procedure to permit palpation of the thoracic wall prior to thoracocentesis. The

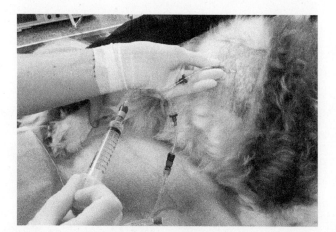

Figure 183.2 Thoracocentesis procedure performed with polypropylene over-the-needle catheter and a smart "Y" adapter instead of a three-way stopcock.

point of entry site is palpated and the needle is advanced through the skin cranial to the adjacent rib to avoid lacerating intercostal vessels running caudally. For thoracocentesis, a 20 or 22 gauge needle with an attached extension set, a butterfly catheter or over-the-needle IV catheter may be used based upon clinician preference (see Figure 183.1). In cats, a butterfly catheter (21 gauge) is most commonly used, with the exception of large cats, where a 1.5" needle may be required to gain access to the pleural space.

For cases with large-volume effusions, the extension tubing may be attached directly to an active suction unit to expedite drainage. Since negative pressure will not be detected with this method, the collection canister is monitored and once fluid production ceases, the suction unit is switched off and a final attempt at hand aspiration is made. If pleural evacuation endpoints are unattainable in the presence of a large-volume pneumothorax, or if repeated thoracocentesis is required within a short period of time, thoracostomy tube placement and continuous suction are likely indicated.

Complications

In general, thoracocentesis is a low-risk procedure, but complications can occur. The most common acute complication is iatrogenic pneumothorax due to laceration of the pulmonary parenchyma or excessive generation of negative intrathoracic pressure and subsequent ripping of unexpandable lung [3]. While iatrogenic laceration is easy to understand, the concept of unexpandable lung is perhaps less so. In this scenario, long-standing effusion results in small restricted lungs, covered with fibrotic pleura. In people, unexpandable lung is further divided into trapped lung and entrapped lung. Entrapped lung occurs during active pleural disease, and trapped lung develops following recovery from prior pleural space disease. Increasing pleural effusion results in a positive intrathoracic pressure. As this fluid is drained, the pressure in the chest becomes increasingly more negative, and this will result in the formation of pleural–pneumo fistulae that permit air leakage. Iatrogenic hemorrhage from laceration of intrathoracic blood vessels can occur, but is usually mild and self-limiting. Occasionally, stress caused by restraint may lead to rapid decompensation and even death from respiratory arrest in unstable patients. It is important to note that *more* complications are associated with not performing thoracocentesis and permitting persistent respiratory distress.

Postprocedure Monitoring

Patients should be monitored closely following thoracocentesis for signs of new or progressive respiratory distress. Such signs may represent an iatrogenic complication, such as pneumothorax or hemothorax, or re-expansion pulmonary edema (less common). Postprocedure thoracic FAST can be used to reassess the residual volume of effusion, aid in detection of pneumothorax, and help guide the deci-sion on whether or not to re-tap (see Chapter 182). Additionally, postprocedure radiographs may be obtained and compared with baseline images to opti-mize detection of soft tissue mass lesions that may have been obscured by the presence of effusion prior to thoracocentesis.

References

1 Williamson JA. Construct validation of a small-animal thoracocentesis simulator. *J Vet Med Educ* 2015;42(5):384–389.

2 Jiang G, Chen H, Wang S, et al. Learning curves and long-term outcome of simulation-based thoracentesis training for medical students. *BMC Med Educ* 2011;22:11–39.

3 Doelken P. Clinical implications of unexpandable lung due to pleural disease. *Am J Med Sci* 2008;335(1): 21–25.

184

Thoracostomy Tube Placement

Alex Lynch, BVSc (Hons), DACVECC, MRCVS[1] and Samantha Campos, VMD[2]

[1] North Carolina State University, Raleigh, NC, USA
[2] College of Veterinary Medicine, University of Florida, Gainesville, FL, USA

Indications for Thoracostomy Tubes

Thoracostomy tubes, also referred to as chest tubes or thoracic drains, are used to remove air and/or fluid from the pleural space [1]. The evacuation of the pleural space may be a life-saving intervention, specifically when the continuous presence of air or effusion cannot be managed by intermittent thoracocentesis alone. In practice, this may include cases in which frequent intermittent thoracocentesis is necessary (e.g. > 3 thoracocentesis procedures performed in 12–24h). In these cases, the presence of an indwelling thoracostomy tube may be associated with improved patient comfort and welfare compared to performing repeated thoracocentesis procedures. Thoracostomy tubes may also be utilized therapeutically for locoregional analgesia and pleurodesis. Pleurodesis involves the delivery of a substance (e.g. whole blood, chemotherapy) via a thoracostomy tube into the pleural space with the intention of artificially obliterating the space by promoting adhesion of the pleural membranes.

Pneumothorax

Pneumothorax may be considered spontaneous [2–5], traumatic [6] or iatrogenic [7] (e.g. during mechanical ventilation or following thoracocentesis) (see Chapter 44). Intermittent thoracocentesis may be sufficient for the management of non-recurrent and low-volume pneumothorax in animals. Thoracostomy tubes are indicated when there is large-volume and/or rapid accumulation of air in the pleural space causing respiratory embarrassment. This typically occurs in animals with spontaneous pneumothorax (e.g. secondary to ruptured pulmonary bullae) and in patients recovering from thor-

acotomies rather than in cases of traumatic pneumothorax [8]. Local analgesia can also be provided safely via thoracostomy tubes (i.e. interpleural block) in patients recovering from lateral thoracotomies and following trauma [9]. Alternative approaches to analgesia in these patients, including subcutaneous wound soaker catheters, intercostal analgesia, and systemic analgesia, may also be reasonable depending on specific patient considerations and clinician preference (see Section 7).

Thoracostomy tubes can be used for autologous blood patch in cases of recurrent spontaneous pneumothorax or persistent pneumothorax in the patient recovering from pneumectomy [10]. This technique has been described in dogs with persistent pneumothorax with a reported good success [10], although it is likely inferior to definitive surgical treatment of spontaneous pneumothorax in most cases.

Pleural Effusion (see Chapter 45)

Pleural effusion, irrespective of the etiology, may benefit from thoracostomy tube placement if the effusion is persistent, rapidly accumulating or necessitating frequent thoracocentesis procedures. Continued drainage is additionally beneficial in some specific situations such as pyothorax [11], where drainage of infected material helps with source control. The presence of the thoracostomy tube in specific patients following surgery may also be advantageous. For instance, a thoracostomy tube in a dog recovering from an esophagotomy enables the clinician to monitor the characteristics of any pleural effusion (e.g. cellularity, presence of bacteria) in a minimally invasive way. In this example, the thoracostomy tube may enable the clinician to identify dehiscence of the surgical site definitively if new septic suppurative effusion develops.

Textbook of Small Animal Emergency Medicine, First Edition. Edited by Kenneth J. Drobatz, Kate Hopper, Elizabeth Rozanski and Deborah C. Silverstein.
© 2019 John Wiley & Sons, Inc. Published 2019 by John Wiley & Sons, Inc.
Companion Website: www.wiley.com/go/drobatz/textbook

Thoracostomy tubes can also be used for the delivery of chemotherapy drugs (e.g. cisplatin, carboplatin) into the pleural space in cases of chronic, recurrent malignant pleural effusions [12,13].

Preparation for Placement

Thoracostomy tubes are usually placed under sedation or general anesthesia [8] (see Chapters 190–193). It is advisable to have the patient intubated when using large-bore trocar type tubes to allow temporary intermittent positive pressure ventilation and brief apnea. The patient should not receive any assisted breaths during the insertion and advancement of the thoracostomy tube. The lateral aspect of the thorax should be clipped between the sixth and 10th intercostal spaces and aseptically prepared. Systemic opioids and locoregional analgesia (e.g. intercostal block) can be considered prior to placement of the tube. Preoxygenation is advisable prior to induction of anesthesia.

Tube Types

Several tubes can be considered for use in small animals: trocar type, small-bore wire-guided tubes placed using the Seldinger technique [14], and red rubber catheter tubes. Thoracostomy trocar tubes are stiffer than the wire-guided and red rubber catheters, so are less prone to kinking. Stiffer tubes are associated with increased discomfort and do require general anesthesia for placement.

Tube size will depend on patient size and is roughly comparable to the diameter of the mainstem bronchi [8]. A 14–16 French tube is suitable for cats and small dogs, while large dogs can take a 24–26 French tube. Other items required include Christmas tree connectors, tubing with a Luer-Lok, a non-collapsing extension set, and a three-way stopcock [11]. A pack with the aforementioned materials, blades (both number 10 and 15), sterile thoracostomy tubes, sterile gauze, instrument set consistent with a hemostat, needle holder, scalpel holder, suture scissors, and tube clamp should all be readily available for use [11].

Tube Placement Techniques

Trocar Tubes

Trocar tubes should be placed under general anesthesia (see Chapter 191). The patient is placed in lateral recumbency and an assistant pulls the skin cranially. A midthoracic area should be clipped and aseptically prepared.

Different techniques can be used for the placement of these tubes. One technique involves making a full-thickness incision at approximately the 10th to 11th intercostal space. The trocar tube is advanced through the skin incision and then advanced to the level of the seventh or eighth intercostal space.

An alternative technique involves the use of a Kelly hemostat to bluntly dissect through a partial-thickness intercostal space incision. The tube should be gripped with the non-dominant hand close to the distal end of the tube to prevent accidental overadvancement into the thoracic cavity.

Once the thoracostomy tube is in place, it can then be reorientated so it may be advanced off in a cranioventral direction. Once in place, the assistant can stop pulling the skin forward, enabling the skin to retract back and thus creating a tunnel for the tube. A connector with three-way stop cock and syringe can be attached to ensure air and/or fluid is collected, depending on the underlying disease. Postprocedural thoracic radiographs are recommended to verify tube position. The tube can be secured with a purse-string suture around its base and then further secured with a finger trap pattern [11].

Wire-Guided Tube

These tubes are becoming increasing popular in small animal emergency practice given the technical ease with which they can be placed compared to trocar style tubes. These smaller bore tubes also appear to be less painful compared to the larger bore tubes.

A small incision can be made in the skin using a #11 blade in the skin overlying the intended intercostal space (e.g. seventh to ninth). A standard over-the-needle style catheter is inserted through this incision into the pleural space. The stylet is removed from the catheter, enabling passage of a guidewire into the pleural space. The catheter is then removed over this guidewire, allowing for the insertion of a pliable thoracostomy tube over the guidewire. Once the tube is in the pleural space, the guidewire can be removed, a closed valve attachment is applied to the end of the tube, and the tube is secured to the external chest wall. A specific plastic butterfly attachment included in the thoracostomy tube kit is usually secured to the tube itself. This enables the placement of nylon skin sutures through the attachment securing the tube to the skin.

Red Rubber Catheter

A simple sterile red rubber catheter may also be used as a chest tube if no other options are available. To make it more functional as a chest tube, additional fenestrations can be added to the end of the catheter. The tube can be placed in a similar fashion to the trocar tube by making a skin incision over the appropriate intercostal space. A tunnel can be created with blunt dissection using a Carmalt or Kelly forceps, allowing passage of the catheter to about the level of the seventh intercostal space.

Thoracostomy Tube Maintenance and Care

Strict aseptic care of the thoracostomy tube is required after placement, although prophylactic antibiotics are uncommonly recommended. A barrier over the tube itself (e.g. body stocking, self-adhesive bandage) can be considered and changed daily if used. A tubing clamp is usually recommended in addition to the three-way stopcock. An e-collar should be used to prevent patient interference. Analgesia is essential for these patients as well as close monitoring of respiratory rate and effort (see

Chapter 193). Chest tubes should be removed as soon as they are no longer needed [1]. For cases of pneumothorax, usually no or very mild air production is necessary before a tube is removed. In cases of pleural effusion, it should be remembered that the presence of the tube itself will be associated with some mild effusion. In these instances, a low volume of effusion that is not causing respiratory distress is usually acceptable.

Complications

Thoracostomy tubes are usually well tolerated but potential complications include infection, hemorrhage, visceral injury during placement, and re-expansion pulmonary edema [1]. Additionally, the clinician should recall that the presence of a thoracostomy tube does not exclude clinically significant pleural space disease, as a tube may kink or become occluded.

References

1 Sigrist NE. Thoracostomy tube placement and drainage. In: *Small Animal Critical Care Medicine*, 2nd edn (eds Silverstein DC, Hopper K). Elsevier, St Louis, 2014.

2 Puerto DA, Brockman DJ, Lindquist C, et al. Surgical and nonsurgical management of and selected risk factors for spontaneous pneumothorax in dogs: 64 cases (1986–1999). *J Am Vet Med Assoc* 2002;220:1670–1674.

3 Lipscomb VJ, Hardie RJ, Dubielzig RR. Spontaneous pneumothorax caused by pulmonary blebs and bullae in 12 dogs. *J Am Anim Hosp Assoc* 2003;39:435–445.

4 Mooney ET, Rozanski EA, King RG, et al. Spontaneous pneumothorax in 35 cats. *J Feline Med Surg* 2012;14(6):384–391.

5 Liu DT, Silverstein DC. Feline secondary spontaneous pneumothorax: a retrospective study of 16 cases (2000–2012). *J Vet Emerg Crit Care* 2014;24(3):316–325.

6 Shaw SP. Thoracic trauma. In: *Kirk's Current Veterinary Therapy XIV*, 14th edn (eds Bonagura JD, Twedt DC). Saunders/Elsevier, St Louis, 2009, pp. 272–277.

7 Hopper K, Powell LL. Basics of mechanical ventilation for dogs and cats. *Vet Clin North Am Small Anim Pract* 2013;43(4):955–969.

8 Tobias KM. Thoracostomy tube placement. In: *Manual of Small Animal Soft Tissue Surgery*. Wiley-Blackwell, Ames, 2010, pp. 461–471.

9 Thompson SE, Johnson JM. Analgesia in dogs after intercostal thoracotomy. A comparison of morphine, selective intercostal nerve block, and interpleural regional analgesia with bupivacaine. *Vet Surg* 1991;20:73–77.

10 Oppenheimer N, Klainbart S, Merbl Y, et al. Retrospective evaluation of the use of autologous blood-patch treatment for persistent pneumothorax in 8 dogs (2009–2012). *J Vet Emerg Crit Care* 2014;24(2):215–220.

11 Kirsch TD, Mulligan P. Tube thoracostomy. In: *Clinical Procedures in Emergency Medicine* (eds Roberts JR, Hedges JR). Saunders, Philadelphia, 2004.

12 Moore AS, Kirk C, Cardona A. Intracavitary cisplatin chemotherapy experience with six dogs. *J Vet Intern Med* 1991;5(4):227–231.

13 Charney SC, Bergman PJ, McKnight JA, et al. Evaluation of intracavitary mitoxantrone and carboplatin for treatment of carcinomatosis, sarcomatosis and mesothelioma, with or without malignant effusions: a retrospective analysis of 12 cases (1997–2002). *Vet Comp Oncol* 2005;3(4):171–181.

14 Valtolina C, Adamantos S. Evaluation of small-bore wire-guided chest drains for management of pleural space disease. *J Small Anim Pract* 2009;50(6): 290–297.

185

Pericardiocentesis

Kursten V. Pierce, DVM, DACVIM and John E. Rush, DVM, MS, DACVIM, DACVECC

Cummings School of Veterinary Medicine, Tufts University, North Grafton, MA, USA

Etiology and Indications for Pericardiocentesis

Pericardial effusion can be caused by cardiac neoplasia such as hemangiosarcoma, chemodectoma, lymphoma, ectopic thyroid carcinoma, mesothelioma, and several non-neoplastic disorders such as idiopathic pericarditis, constrictive pericardial disease, congestive heart failure, left atrial tear, hypoproteinemia, and infection [1–3]. Causes of pericardial effusion are described in greater detail in Chapter 54.

Pericardiocentesis is warranted when pericardial effusion is causing cardiac tamponade (Figure 185.1). The European Society of Cardiology (ESC) has established guidelines for management of pericardial diseases in people as well as indications for pericardiocentesis; cardiac tamponade is considered a class I indication (i.e. very strong recommendation) [4,5]. Cardiac tamponade occurs when intrapericardial pressure exceeds the

pressure within the right atrium and/or right ventricle during diastole, leading to reduced right heart filling and a resultant decrease in cardiac output. Cardiac tamponade can occur with either a large or small volume of pericardial effusion, so the volume of effusion should not be the main trigger for pericardiocentesis. Cardiac tamponade is present when hemodynamic compromise is evident; clinical signs consistent with tamponade include hypotension, jugular venous distension, tachycardia, tachypnea, and cardiogenic shock [6–8]. Signs of right-sided congestive heart failure such as ascites may be identified and may indicate chronic cardiac tamponade. The degree of hemodynamic compromise depends upon both the volume of effusion and the rate of fluid accumulation, with acutely developing effusions causing tamponade with relatively small volumes of effusion.

Cardiac tamponade can be suspected based on clinical examination findings such as pulsus paradoxus, tachycardia, muffled heart sounds, jugular venous distension, or mucous membrane pallor [7,8]. Electrocardiographic signs that may be observed include sinus tachycardia, low-voltage QRS complexes, electrical alternans, or ST segment changes, and radiographic findings can include cardiomegaly with globoid cardiac silhouette or a distended caudal vena cava [7,8]. Confirmation of cardiac tamponade is usually made by assessment with echocardiography with classic findings of an anechoic or hypoechoic space between the pericardium and epicardium and collapse of the right atrial and/or right ventricular wall (Video Clip 185.1). A complete echocardiogram is ideally performed prior to pericardiocentesis as cardiac masses are easier to visualize with the pericardial effusion still present, but in unstable cases pericardiocentesis should be done immediately.

Pericardiocentesis may be performed to relieve tamponade or in order to obtain a diagnostic sample for fluid analysis and cytology. It is less frequently indicated in cats for tamponade, and should be performed with caution as

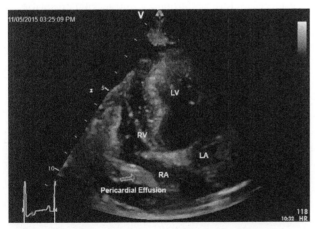

Figure 185.1 Still image of echocardiogram from the left apical view depicting presence of pericardial effusion and collapse of the right atrial wall (*arrow*) consistent with cardiac tamponade.

the space between the pericardium and the epicardium can be less than 0.5 cm, increasing the chance for cardiac trauma during pericardiocentesis.

Contraindications

Pericardiocentesis is contraindicated or relatively contraindicated in animals with active hemorrhage into the pericardial sac and those with coagulopathy. The most common situation where active bleeding might preclude pericardiocentesis is cardiac tamponade secondary to left atrial splitting/left atrial rupture (Video Clip 185.2). The typical example might be a geriatric, small-breed dog with degenerative mitral valve disease, pericardial effusion, thrombus in the pericardial space, and signs of hemodynamic compromise. If a left atrial tear is suspected then pericardiocentesis should be withheld, except in animals with cardiogenic shock at risk for cardiopulmonary arrest in which case the benefits of pericardiocentesis might outweigh the concerns of hemorrhage into the thoracic cavity after pericardiocentesis. Suspected or known coagulopathy is another relative contraindication for pericardiocentesis (e.g. vitamin K rodenticide intoxication). Finally, if pericardial effusion is secondary to congestive heart failure (CHF), then the effusion might resolve with treatment of CHF and pericardiocentesis might not be required (especially in cats).

Sedation (see Chapter 192)

Sedation may be indicated to perform pericardiocentesis and should be assessed on a case-by-case basis. Evaluation of the patient's stability, alertness, temperament, and potential for sudden movements may determine whether sedation is indicated and to what degree. In severely ill or decompensated patients, sedation is often not required. The authors prefer to use an opioid or a combination of an opioid with a benzodiazepine (e.g. butorphanol 0.2 mg/kg with midazolam 0.2 mg/kg). Drugs that might compromise hemodynamic situation such as alpha-2 agonists should be avoided.

A local anesthetic block can be performed within the intercostal space with lidocaine or bupivacaine. Sodium bicarbonate can be added to the local block to neutralize the acidic pH and reduce discomfort associated with the block (1 part sodium bicarbonate to 9 parts lidocaine).

Equipment

Supplies for pericardiocentesis can vary based on clinician preference and availability of certain equipment. In most situations, necessary supplies include clippers and antiseptic solution(s) for aseptic skin preparation, sterile gloves, #11 scalpel blade for stab skin incision, catheter with stylet for pericardiocentesis (e.g. 16 gauge × 5½ inch IV catheter with stylet, large-bore trocar catheter, or a specific centesis catheter), three-way stopcock, extension set, syringes of varying sizes to aspirate the effusion, sample collection tubes (red top tube and EDTA tube), and a container to collect fluid. The size of the syringes may be based on clinician preference, size of patient, and volume of pericardial effusion present. If indicated in a cat, pericardiocentesis is typically performed using a smaller catheter or needle (e.g. 18 or 20 gauge 1.5 inch needle or catheter).

Ideally, ultrasound imaging is available for ultrasound-guided pericardiocentesis and electrocardiographic monitoring.

Procedure

Ideally, pericardiocentesis would be performed in a quiet setting or environment to avoid sudden movement secondary to loud stimuli. The patient should be sedated if indicated, local anesthetic block drawn up, electrocardiographic (ECG) monitoring hooked up to observe for cardiac arrhythmias, the patient properly positioned, and all supplies gathered and readily accessible. The patient should have a peripheral intravenous catheter already in place to allow for administration of sedation and venous access in case emergency antiarrhythmic or resuscitation drugs are indicated. A defibrillator should be readily accessible if possible.

Positioning

The patient can be positioned in sternal or lateral recumbency as determined by clinician preference. A right-sided approach is preferred, between the third and fifth intercostal spaces, typically at the left fifth intercostal space. Patients with dyspnea may prefer to be positioned in sternal recumbency. A right-sided approach is preferred based on anatomy as the cardiac window (cardiac notch) is larger on the right hemithorax [8,9]. Approach via the left hemithorax is less desirable due to the anatomical location of the coronary arteries and risk of vascular damage with the catheter or needle.

Procedural Monitoring

Prior to performing the pericardiocentesis, ECG monitoring should be established to identify baseline arrhythmias and observe for ventricular arrhythmias during the procedure. A 2 mg/kg dose of lidocaine should be drawn up and on hand in case it is required during the procedure. Arrhythmias may indicate that the catheter tip is in contact with the myocardium and when noted they should trigger a relocation of the catheter or a temporary termination of aspiration on the syringe. Typically, patients with cardiac tamponade are tachycardic and as the tamponade is relieved, the heart rate should decrease and return to normal. ECG monitoring should be continued in the postprocedural period as arrhythmias may develop post pericardiocentesis.

Technique

The right hemithorax is shaved and a location for the pericardiocentesis is chosen between the third and fifth intercostal spaces, ideally based on ultrasonic guidance (Figure 185.2). A mental note of this location can be made or it can be demarcated with a permanent marker. A local anesthetic block can be administered, and the chest should be prepped in an aseptic fashion.

Sterile gloves should be worn and the syringe can be attached to the extension tubing and three-way stopcock.

At the desired site for centesis, a #11 blade is used to make a hole in the skin large enough to accept the stylet and catheter, such that the catheter is not burred as it advances through the skin. With the stylet advanced all the way into the catheter, the catheter and stylet are advanced through the skin and subcutaneous tissues, through the intercostal space and into the pleural space. Occasionally, a "pop" is felt as the catheter enters the

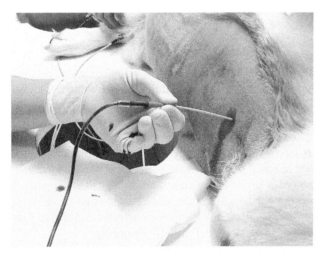

Figure 185.2 Image depicts a pericardiocentesis being performed at the level of the fifth intercostal space. Patient is positioned in left lateral recumbency with the right hemithorax clipped and aseptically prepared. ECG leads are attached to the patient. The clinician is wearing sterile gloves to hold the catheter in place. A hemorrhagic effusion is being aspirated and visualized within the extension tubing.

thoracic cavity and/or the pericardial space. This deliberate puncture should be slow but continuous as the catheter is inserted ~2.5–5 cm into the thoracic cavity. As the catheter is being inserted and enters the pericardial space, the stylet should be removed from within the catheter. After puncture and flashback, the position of the needle can be confirmed via agitated saline under echocardiographic guidance [6]. A modified transudate of pleural effusion may be seen before pericardial effusion is noted.

A syringe, three-way stopcock, and extension tubing are attached to the catheter and gentle negative pressure is applied to obtain samples for fluid analysis and assessment of clotting of the effusion. If ventricular arrhythmia is observed on the ECG or if it feels as though there is tissue against the catheter tip, the catheter should be slightly pulled outward.

If there is uncertainty whether the catheter is appropriately located within the pericardial space, the ultrasound probe can be placed near the catheter and a contrast echocardiogram can be performed. Ultrasonography can be used to assess if the amount of effusion is reduced and whether there is resolution of cardiac tamponade. Femoral pulses and mucous membrane color should be assessed for improvement post pericardiocentesis. Clinical improvement, ultrasonographic evidence of improvement, lack of additional fluid being obtained, or resistance at the catheter tip may all be used to determine that the catheter should be retracted from the thoracic cavity.

Samples to Obtain and Submit

At a minimum, the pericardial effusion obtained from the pericardiocentesis should be placed in an EDTA lavender top for cytology and fluid analysis and within a non-additive red top tube. The effusion placed within a non-additive tube should be assessed for the presence of clotting versus non-clotting hemorrhagic effusion during pericardiocentesis. Fluid obtained from within the pericardial sac should be non-clotting in most cases, and if the fluid does clot then this is indicative of an intracardiac puncture or active ongoing bleeding from the source (i.e. a mass). If clotting of the aspirated fluid occurs then the catheter should be immediately retracted and the animal should be re-evaluated.

Postprocedure Monitoring

Within the 12–36 hour post pericardiocentesis, continuous ECG (telemetry) monitoring is advised to evaluate for ventricular arrhythmias, which are sometimes severe enough to require treatment. The mucous membrane color and refill time, heart rate, respiratory rate, and femoral pulse quality should be monitored to assess for evidence of recurrent effusion. Serial ultrasound evaluation should be performed if recurrence is suspected or if hemodynamic instability develops. Pleural effusion may develop if ongoing bleeding from the heart leaks from the hole made in the pericardial space and into the pleural cavity. Volume support with administration of intravenous fluids may be indicated, based on clinical signs or clinician preference.

Complications

Potential complications resulting from pericardiocentesis include ventricular arrhythmias, sudden death, laceration or perforation of the myocardium or great vessels, hemorrhage into the pleural space or recurrent pericardial effusion, pneumothorax, or introduction of infection into the pericardial space.

The rate of major complications following pericardiocentesis using ultrasonic guidance in people is 1.3–1.6% compared to 20.6% rate of life-threatening complications with an unguided, blind approach [9]. For veterinary patients, ultrasound guidance, if available, is recommended in order to minimize the risk of complications and determine the best window for pericardiocentesis.

In a study by Humm et al., the incidence of adverse events was 10.7% within 1 hour of pericardiocentesis and 15.2% (17 out of 85 dogs) within 48 hours, based on retrospective evaluation of 85 dogs (112 episodes of pericardiocentesis) with varying etiologies of pericardial effusion [3]. The most commonly observed complication was arrhythmia requiring drug therapy in 11 out of the 17 patients with observed complications, followed by cardiopulmonary arrest in four patients, and continued bleeding into the pericardium which resulted in euthanasia in three out of 17 cases. There was no significant difference between frequency of pericardiocentesis and etiology of pericardial effusion in relation to the risk of adverse events in this study [3].

Pearls of Wisdom

Ultrasound-guided pericardiocentesis is preferred to determine the most appropriate window with the least chance for cardiac trauma or perforation. During pericardiocentesis, if there is concern regarding location of the needle or catheter, contrast echocardiography can help to determine whether they are within the pericardial space. Injection of a small volume of agitated saline through the catheter should result in visualization of microbubbles within the pericardial sac via ultrasonography.

References

1 Stafford Johnson M, Martin M, Binns S, et al. A retrospective study of clinical findings, treatment and outcome in 143 dogs with pericardial effusion. *J Small Anim Pract* 2004;45(11): 546–552.

2 Berg JR, Wingfield W. Pericardial effusion in the dog: a review of 42 cases. *J Am Anim Hosp Assoc* 1983;20:721–730.

3 Humm KR, Keenaghan-Clark MA, Boag AK. Adverse events associated with pericardiocentesis in dogs: 85 cases (1999–2006). *J Vet Emerg Crit Care* 2009;19(4):352–356.

4 European Society of Cardiology. Guidelines on the diagnosis and management of pericardial diseases. *Eur Heart J* 2004;25:587–610.

5 Imazio M, Adler Y, Ristić AD, et al. A new scoring system for the triage of cardiac tamponade. *Expert Rev Cardiovasc Ther* 2015;13 (3):237–238.

6 Gluer R, Murdoch D, Haggani HM, et al. Pericardiocentesis – how to do it. *Heart Lung Circ* 2015;24(6):621–625.

7 Gidlewski J, Petrie JP. Therapeutic pericardiocentesis in the dog and cat. *Clin Tech Small Anim Pract* 2005;20:151–155.

8 Cote E. Pericardiocentesis. In: *Clinical Veterinary Advisor: Dogs and Cats* (ed. Cote E). Mosby Elsevier, St Louis, 2007, pp. 1298–1299.

9 Loukas M, Walters A, Boon JM, et al. Pericardiocentesis: a clinical anatomy review. *Clin Anat* 2012;25:872–881.

186

Abdominocentesis

Karl E. Jandrey, DVM, MAS, DACVECC

School of Veterinary Medicine, University of California, Davis, CA, USA

Introduction

The decision to take a patient with abdominal disease to emergency surgery is predicated on the accuracy of the diagnosis. The challenge is to determine when surgery is indicated based on vague abdominal signs. Besides serial physical examinations for the assessment of increasing abdominal size or progressive pain, samples of peritoneal fluid obtained by abdominocentesis or diagnostic peritoneal lavage can yield the specific diagnosis of an abdominal disease process and lead to focused surgical or medical intervention.

Indications

Indications for abdominocentesis are listed in Box 186.1 [1]. In general, blind abdominocentesis is considered when free abdominal fluid is suspected or unknown abdominal disease is present. Periumbilical ecchymosis (Cullen's sign) may be associated with hemorrhage in the peritoneum or retroperitoneum and can be an indication

---

Box 186.1 Indications for abdominocentesis [1].

- Radiographic loss of serosal detail
- Free abdominal fluid detected on ultrasound
- Abdominal injury without obvious peritoneal entry wounds
- Shock, multiple injuries, or signs of abdominal injury after blunt trauma
- Head or spinal injury precluding reliable abdominal examination
- Persistent abdominal pain or fluid distension of unknown cause
- Postoperative complications possibly caused by leakage from an enterotomy or anastomotic site

---

for abdominocentesis. Relative contraindications to abdominocentesis include coagulopathy, organomegaly, and distension of abdominal viscera. Intestinal or uterine penetration is rare unless the viscus is dilated and/or adherent to the abdominal wall [2]. Ultrasound-guided abdominocentesis allows directed aspiration of abdominal free fluid. With ultrasound-guided techniques, the risk of abdominocentesis is considered far less than blind techniques. Proper technique attempts to prevent the introduction or spread of infection, laceration of an organ, or hemorrhage from a punctured vessel.

Technique

Abdominocentesis is completed using a single paracentesis (open or closed needle technique) or a four-quadrant approach. Ultrasound guidance can highlight a smaller accumulation of fluid and allow for a more directed approach. The site for blind single paracentesis lies caudal to the umbilicus to avoid the falciform fat. Four-quadrant abdominocentesis encircles the umbilicus. Use of ultrasound may more directly guide the best location based on the size and accessibility of the fluid pocket within the peritoneum.

Focused Assessment with Sonography for Trauma (see Chapter 182)

The focused assessment with sonography for trauma (FAST) protocol was studied in dogs to prove that it is a rapid and simple technique to allow veterinary clinicians with minimal previous ultrasound experience to detect free abdominal fluid in the emergency room [3]. This technique scans four regions (caudal to the xyphoid process, midline over the urinary bladder, and each flank) in longitudinal and transverse planes of the abdomen with

---

Textbook of Small Animal Emergency Medicine, First Edition. Edited by Kenneth J. Drobatz, Kate Hopper, Elizabeth Rozanski and Deborah C. Silverstein.
© 2019 John Wiley & Sons, Inc. Published 2019 by John Wiley & Sons, Inc.
Companion Website: www.wiley.com/go/drobatz/textbook

patients in lateral recumbency. If free abdominal fluid is detected, ultrasound-guided abdominocentesis may be indicated.

Preparation of the Patient

Patient positioning in left lateral recumbency may be most effective to avoid puncture of the spleen. This is particularly relevant to blind abdominocentesis. Restraint may be completed manually or with the use of sedatives and analgesics (see Chapters 192 and 193). Prior to penetration of the abdomen, a wide surgical clip and preparation of the site using aseptic technique must be completed in the region identified for paracentesis. If using a blind technique, this will be along the ventral midline centered at the umbilicus. Alternatively, if an abdominal ultrasound has identified a focal pocket of fluid, a standard aseptic clip and preparation at that location is prudent.

Closed-Needle Abdominocentesis

A closed-needle diagnostic abdominocentesis can be completed using a 22 or 24 gauge needle attached directly to a 3, 6 or 12 ml syringe, or attached to a syringe via an extension set. Local anesthetic infusion of 2% lidocaine may be used at the abdominocentesis site. With a blind approach, penetration of the abdominal cavity can be completed on the midline, caudal to the umbilicus. The location of abdominocentesis is ideally determined by ultrasound guidance.

The needle is gently inserted completely at this site and further movement of the needle tip is avoided to prevent laceration of internal structures. The syringe is aspirated to remove peritoneal fluid. If the fluid is hemorrhagic it should be observed for the formation of clots. Ideally, the hemorrhagic fluid should be placed in a glass container such as a plain blood tube to evaluate for clot formation. Free fluid within the abdominal cavity should not clot while hemorrhagic fluid obtained from puncture of the spleen, liver or any vessel will readily clot. If clotting of the abdominal fluid is observed, the needle should be removed and abdominocentesis attempted in another location. Cytological, biochemical analysis and culture of the abdominal fluid should be performed, as indicated, on the collected fluid.

The advantages of the closed needle technique include greater ability to avoid contamination of the fluid sample or abdominal cavity. It may also require less manipulation of the needle while it is in the abdomen so it may be less likely to be traumatic. Free gas should not be evident on radiographs after a closed-needle abdominocentesis.

A closed-needle abdominocentesis can also be used for therapeutic removal of peritoneal fluid. Therapeutic removal of large volumes of fluid may be indicated if the abdominal distention impairs diaphragmatic motion, increases intra-abdominal pressure impeding blood flow to the visceral organs, or is painful for the patient. To maintain a closed system, a three-way stopcock can be placed between the syringe and extension set. Another extension set placed on the stopcock can be directed into a bowl or graduated cylinder. A large over-the-needle catheter may be preferable to the use of a hypodermic needle as it may reduce the risk of internal organ injury.

Open-Needle Abdominocentesis

An open-needle abdominocentesis is an alternative method for blind abdominocentesis. It is completed in a similar fashion to that described for a closed-needle technique, except the needle alone is inserted into the peritoneal cavity. Fluid from the peritoneum is allowed to flow freely through the needle into a container or sample submission tube. Rotation of the needle hub may facilitate flow. This technique may help prevent occlusion with or aspiration of omentum or intestinal viscera. It may be a more successful technique as false-negative results are more likely to occur if suction is applied during paracentesis [4]. Free abdominal gas on radiographs is possible after this procedure.

Four-Quadrant Abdominocentesis

A modification of the open-needle technique is the four-quadrant abdominocentesis. Instead of one open needle, four open needles are placed simultaneously in each quadrant surrounding the umbilicus. Gravity dependency or changes in transabdominal pressure between the needles may increase the likelihood of obtaining fluid. One study using a four-quadrant technique in dogs showed that fluid was obtained in 78 of 100 needle paracenteses when 5.2–6.6 mL of abdominal fluid/kg body weight was present [5].

Alternative Techniques for Abdominocentesis

The use of a peritoneal dialysis catheter for abdominocentesis has been shown to detect 1.0–4.4 mL of abdominal fluid/kg body weight, so it may increase the sensitivity of a blind technique [6]. A larger diameter and multiple fenestrations make this apparatus more reliable for detecting smaller volumes of peritoneal fluid compared to a standard needle or catheter. Commercial peritoneal dialysis catheters work well, but over-the-needle catheters can be carefully fenestrated and used with good results. The use of a 14 or 16 gauge, over-the-needle catheter with multiple, small fenestrations placed manually using a #10 scalpel blade can increase the surface area for drainage. There are also commercially available, fenestrated paracentesis catheters available for this purpose. The use of a fenestrated catheter increases the likelihood of fluid collection compared to needle abdominocentesis alone [7]. A fenestrated catheter can also be a useful technique for therapeutic abdominal fluid removal.

Diagnostic Peritoneal Lavage

Diagnostic peritoneal lavage (DPL) is performed when alternative diagnostic methods such as sonography are unavailable, or when the patient's condition does not allow other diagnostics or imaging to be performed. Patient positioning, use of sedatives, and preparation of the site are similar to abdominocentesis. Local anesthetic infusion of 2% lidocaine should be placed at the puncture site either at the umbilicus or 2–3 cm lateral to it to avoid the falciform fat.

A small stab incision is made in the skin with the #11 scalpel blade at the site of local anesthetic infusion. The fenestrated catheter, such as a commercially available peritoneal dialysis catheter, is introduced through the incision completely into the abdomen. Slow gentle rotation of the closed-end, dialysis catheter is needed to overcome considerable resistance from fascial planes and the linea alba. If a fenestrated over-the-needle catheter is used, the catheter is advanced completely off the stylet once the tip of the catheter has penetrated the peritoneal cavity. A syringe may be attached to the catheter at this point. If no peritoneal fluid is obtained, saline is infused into the abdomen through the catheter. A volume of 22 mL/kg of warm, sterile 0.9% sodium chloride is infused by gravity through a drip set attached to the catheter. The abdomen is gently massaged or the patient is rolled without dislodging the catheter to distribute the saline throughout the abdomen. A syringe is attached and gently aspirated or fluid is allowed to flow by gravity into a collection container or back into the drip set and fluid bag.

Large volumes of fluid are generally not obtained due to the wide dispersion throughout the abdomen. Any amount retrieved should be submitted for biochemical and cytological evaluation including culture and sensitivity testing. Fluid samples from a DPL must be interpreted in light of the dilution effect of this collection method.

Abdominal Fluid Analysis

Paracentesis Sample

Packed cell volume (PCV), total protein (TP), creatinine, glucose concentration, and blood urea nitrogen (BUN) should be measured from the peritoneal fluid sample. Potassium and lactate are other biochemical markers that can be tested to add diagnostic value to the fluid sample. If the PCV of the peritoneal fluid exceeds the peripheral PCV, it is suggestive of parenchymal organ laceration or large vascular disruption. Hemodilution with urine may cause a decreased PCV of abdominal fluid in patients with both abdominal hemorrhage and urological injury. Uroabdomen can be diagnosed from simultaneous measurement of creatinine and potassium in both the abdominal fluid and peripheral blood. Because of its high molecular weight, a creatinine concentration in the abdominal fluid higher than twice that of peripheral blood is highly suggestive of free urine in the abdominal cavity [8]. An increased ratio of potassium in the abdominal fluid compared to peripheral blood (greater than 1.4:1) also suggests urological injury [8]. Rapid assessment and comparison of the BUN in abdominal fluid and peripheral blood can be completed using reagent strip technology. However, BUN can readily equilibrate across the peritoneal lining and is less reliable for the diagnosis of uroabdomen.

Cytological Analysis

Cytological analysis of cellular effusions is always recommended and culture of abdominal fluid with susceptibility testing should be submitted if sepsis is possible. Emergency cytological analysis often assists the clinician in initiating appropriate therapy. In many cases, the decision for medical versus surgical therapy can be readily apparent before official clinical pathological analysis.

The gross appearance of the fluid should be examined. An abdominal fluid sample that is completely clear and colorless makes the diagnosis of peritonitis, severe intra-abdominal injury or perforation, and leakage from the gastrointestinal tract less likely [4]. Fluid that appears opaque, cloudy, or flocculent should be examined immediately. Since accurate hemocytometer analyses are less commonly completed in practice, the cell concentration must be estimated. The higher the cellularity (>10 000/μL) and protein concentration (>3.5 g/dL), the more likely the fluid is an exudate; surgical therapy may be indicated, especially if the microscopic analysis shows intracellular bacteria. The lowest cell (<2500/μL) and protein concentrations (<2 g/dL) may be transudates; therefore, continued therapy is more likely to be medical. Modified transudates may have more cells and a lower protein concentration (or fewer cells and a higher protein). Other clinical data may be needed in these cases to more clearly direct the next therapeutic step

A direct smear that has been dried and stained appropriately can be examined at low power for large particulate material such as plant material or crystals. High-power magnification is used to identify bacteria, fungi, and blood cells. Intracellular bacteria (with or without extracellular bacteria) and degenerate neutrophils characterize a septic effusion. Surgical intervention should be considered and undertaken immediately if this is found, often prior to confirmation by a reference laboratory. Surgery is not necessarily indicated when only extracellular bacteria are found in the fluid sample.

Glucose and lactate measurements on peritoneal fluid can also aid in the diagnosis of septic peritonitis. In one prospective analysis of 18 dogs with septic effusion, peritoneal fluid glucose concentration was always lower than the blood glucose concentration [9]. A blood-to-peritoneal fluid glucose difference >20 mg/dL was 100% sensitive and 100% specific for the diagnosis of septic peritoneal effusion in dogs.

With gall bladder or common bile duct injury, the clinical signs of icterus may be delayed. A dark green to black or dark amber color of peritoneal fluid suggests the presence of bile pigments. Peritoneal fluid can be analyzed for total bilirubin. If the abdominal fluid bilirubin is significantly greater than peripheral bilirubin, then bile peritonitis is present.

Diagnostic Peritoneal Lavage Samples

Cytological characteristics of the white cells are more meaningful than absolute cell counts due to dilutional consequences of a DPL [2,10]. In a study comparing pre- and postoperative DPL samples, recent surgery increased the white blood cell count from normal (1000 cells/mm^3) to usually less than 10 000 cells/mm^3 [11]. Elevations in the peritoneal white blood cell count in response to sepsis occur over variable time periods [5] that overlap these normal ranges. Due to dilution, the PCV of the DPL fluid cannot be directly compared with the peripheral blood PCV. It has been reported that a PCV of the DPL fluid of greater than 5% is indicative of significant hemorrhage [10]. Serial assessments of the abdominal fluid with increasing PCVs may more clearly define continuing hemorrhage.

Creatinine and potassium elevations in the lavage fluid are more difficult to interpret due to dilutional effects of the 0.9% NaCl. Excretory urography, retrograde contrast cystourethrography or surgical intervention may be indicated.

Conclusion

Serial physical examinations and diagnostic studies are required to decide when acute abdominal disease should be surgically explored versus treated medically. Blunt abdominal trauma cases are challenging diagnostic problems because the clinical manifestations may be delayed for hours or days. Abdominocentesis is a valuable tool to obtain a sample for laboratory and cytological analysis in the emergency room or intensive care unit. A diagnostic peritoneal lavage may be indicated in a patient where significant abdominal injury has occurred but no diagnostic sample was identified by FAST or obtainable via abdominocentesis.

References

1 Saxon WD. The acute abdomen. *Vet Clin North Am Small Anim Pract* 1994;24(6):1207–1224.
2 Swann H, Hughes D. Diagnosis and management of peritonitis. *Vet Clin North Am Small Anim Pract* 2000;30(3):603–615.
3 Boysen SR, Rozanski EA, Tidwell AS, et al. Evaluation of a focused assessment with sonography for trauma protocol to detect free abdominal fluid in dogs involved in motor vehicle accidents. *J Am Vet Med Assoc* 2004;225(8):1198–1204.
4 Crowe DT, Crane SW. Diagnostic abdominal paracentesis and lavage in the evaluation of abdominal injuries in dogs and cats: clinical and experimental investigations. *J Am Vet Med Assoc* 1976;168(8):700–705.
5 Giacobine J, Siler VE. Evaluation of diagnostic abdominal paracentesis with experimental and clinical studies. *Surg Gynecol Obstet* 1960;110:676–686.
6 Kolata RJ. Diagnostic abdominal paracentesis and lavage: experimental and clinical evaluations in the dog. *J Am Vet Med Assoc* 1976;168(8):697–699.

7 Glickman LT, Glickman NW, Perez CM, et al. Analysis of risk factors for gastric dilatation and dilatation-volvulus in dogs. *J Am Vet Med Assoc* 1994;204(9):1465–1471.
8 Schmiedt C, Tobias KM, Otto CM. Evaluation of abdominal fluid:peripheral blood creatinine and potassium ratios for diagnosis of uroperitoneum in dogs. *J Vet Emerg Crit Care* 2001;11:275–280.
9 Bonczynski JJ, Ludwig LL, Barton LJ, et al. Comparison of peritoneal fluid and peripheral blood pH, bicarbonate, glucose, and lactate concentration as a diagnostic tool for septic peritonitis in dogs and cats. *Vet Surg* 2003;32(2):161–166.
10 Mann F. Acute abdomen: evaluation and emergency treatment. In: *Current Veterinary Therapy XIII* (ed. Bonagura JD). WB Saunders, Philadelphia, 2000, pp. 160–164.
11 Bjorling DE, Latimer KS, Rawlings CA, et al. Diagnostic peritoneal lavage before and after abdominal surgery in dogs. *Am J Vet Res* 1983;44(5):816–820.

187

Urethral Catheterization (Including Urohydropulsion)

Sean Smarick, VMD, DACVECC

Avets, Monroeville, PA, USA

Introduction

Placing a catheter into the urethra via the urethral opening is indicated in a number of emergent conditions (Box 187.1). The condition will often dictate if single, intermittent, or indwelling urethral catheterization is required and therefore determine the type of catheter used. Species and sex differences play a role in catheter selection and placement technique. Catheter selection and placement technique also can limit complications such as lower urinary tract trauma and catheter-associated urinary tract infections.

Indications for Urethral Catheterization

Urinary retention is a common emergent presentation and can be caused by anatomical pathologies, such as physical obstructions to include urolithiasis, neoplasia, inflammation, and trauma, or functional pathologies,

---

Box 187.1 Indications for urethral catheterization.

Relief of urinary retention
    Anatomical
    Functional
Contrast imaging study of the lower urinary tract
Monitoring of critically ill patients
    Urine output
    Intra-abdominal pressure
Keep urinary bladder decompressed or empty
    Perioperative
        Urogenital surgery
        Prolonged surgery or possible large intraoperative
            urinary output
    Intoxications
    Selected patients that are immobilized

---

such as myogenic neurological or dyssynergic pathologies. One-time, intermittent or indwelling catheterization may be needed to relieve the urinary retention, but care must be taken to prevent trauma to lower urinary structures [1–3]. A catheter should not be used directly to dislodge calculi; instead, use retrograde urohydropropulsion, which uses water pressure via the catheter to dilate the urethra and move the obstruction into the bladder [4].

Contrast diagnostic imaging may be useful in assessing urinary retention or trauma to the lower urinary tract. This may be a one-time catheterization and the catheter is fed just into the urethra for a urethrocystogram or advanced into the bladder for a cystogram [5].

Indwelling catheterization may be warranted in critically ill patients to monitor urine output, determine fractional excretions (e.g. of free water), or measure intra-abdominal pressure [6,7].

Bladder decompression and maintenance of urine output may be considered in a number of conditions. In surgeries of the urinary tract or associated structures, prolonged procedures or in anesthetized patients with increased urine output, an indwelling catheter may be warranted [1,2]. Additionally, keeping the bladder empty via an indwelling urinary catheter will hasten elimination of toxins (e.g. methylxanthines) that are reabsorbed from the bladder [8]. While urethral catheterization should not be a substitute for nursing care, it is reasonable to utilize one intermittently or long term in cases where the benefits in patients who are immobilized or who have wounds that would be compromised with normal urination outweigh the risks [1,2,9,10].

Although urine samples may be obtained from an indwelling urethral catheter, urethral catheterization should not be performed for the sole purpose of routine urine sampling as cystocentesis yields a superior sample and free-catch sampling avoids the risks of catheterization [11].

Risks of Urethral Catheterization

Urethral catheterization carries the risk of trauma to the lower urinary tract or catheter-associated urinary tract infection (CAUTI).

Stylets, stiff catheters (e.g. polypropylene), excessive force, lack of lubrication, and diseased tissue can lead to urethral or bladder trauma (see Chapter 100). Stylets should be designed for urethral catheter use and not extend outside the catheter. Excessive force should also be avoided if an anatomical obstruction is encountered, but even with appropriate placement technique and when indicated to obtain cytological samples, diseased tissue may be more friable [3,4,12]. In one retrospective study, the most common cause of urethral tears in cats was secondary to catheterization in patients with urethral obstruction [13]. Lower urinary tract tears should be recognized as a potential complication of urethral catheterization, especially when localized pathology is suspected.

The length of catheter to be inserted into the urethra should be premeasured prior to placement to limit trauma to the bladder. Additionally, this step can prevent overinsertion resulting in the catheter kinking, knotting or folding back onto itself and traveling antegrade down the urethra. If the catheter has folded onto itself, advancing another catheter alongside the original and applying gentle traction under anesthesia may successfully remove the catheter in these instances; otherwise, surgery is indicated [12].

Microorganisms may be introduced into the urinary tract during catheter placement and one study reported a 20% incidence of a UTI in a one-time catheterization of female dogs [14] (see Chapter 96) Subsequently, microorganisms may migrate along the external or internal surface of the catheter with biofilm, thus offering resistance to the host defenses. Veterinary studies have reported the incidence of CAUTIs to be up to 55% with indwelling urinary catheters. As with any intervention, the risks must be weighed against the benefits. Placing a catheter only when it is indicated, using it for only as long as necessary and following aseptic placement and maintenance protocols will limit complications. Studies utilizing this approach have reported the incidence of CAUTI in veterinary intensive care units in patients with an indwelling urethral catheter >24 hours to be as low as 10% [9,10,15–22].

Catheter Considerations

Urethral catheters are made from various materials and available in different diameters and lengths, and with balloon tips.

Size

Urinary catheters diameters are expressed in French (Fr) scale. The French scale value divided by 3 is the outside diameter of the catheter in millimeters; so, a 6 Fr catheter would have an outside diameter of 2 mm. Cats generally need a 3.5–5 Fr, female dogs a 3.5–14 Fr, and male dogs a 3.5–10 Fr. Especially in dogs, males require a longer catheter than females. Some catheters may be too short to reach the bladder in large male dogs and therefore premeasurement to the center of the bladder or desired location in the urethra should be made to ensure the catheter on hand is of adequate length.

Materials

Urinary catheters are made from a variety of materials that affect stiffness, urethral reactivity, and resistance to bacterial swarming and biofilm formation. While commonly available urethral catheters can be used for a single (in and out) catheterization, indwelling catheters are ideally soft for patient comfort and to decrease the potential for urethral trauma, biologically inert to limit urethral inflammation, and resistant to biofilm and bacterial adherence to reduce CAUTIs. Silicone and polyurethane catheters are therefore preferred for long-term indwelling catheters. Other commonly used materials include hydrogel, siliconized and Teflon-coated latex, latex, red rubber, and plastic/polypropylene. Antimicrobial and antiseptic-coated urethral catheters are available to reduce CAUTIs but they are reserved as a supplemental intervention in long-term catheterizations due to their increased cost, potential to induce reactions and effectiveness of primary interventions such as hand washing and placement and maintenance protocols [1,2,23,24].

Foley Catheters

In 1934, Dr Frederic Foley developed a balloon-tipped catheter with a distal port. Modern veterinary versions include smaller diameters and longer lengths to address anatomical differences from humans. They offer the advantage of anchoring the catheter within the bladder with the balloon inflated near the distal end. This eliminates the need to secure the catheter at the vulva or prepuce. They are ideal when an indwelling catheter is needed but the balloon offers the potential for some unique considerations. The balloon should ideally be filled with a sterile solution (versus air or tap water) as it is non-compressible and stays in the balloon longer compared to air and prevents contamination in case of balloon leakage or rupture. There is some debate between sterile water and saline as the ideal filling solution; sterile water has been proposed to be the preferred solution as it maintains balloon inflation longer and avoids the potential of balloon valve or lumen occlusion due to salt crystals. Proper inflation volumes indicated on the catheter should be observed. Overfilling the balloon can lead to occlusion of the catheter lumen from the balloon itself or contact with the bladder wall or even balloon rupture. Underfilling the balloon can lead to displacement from the bladder [24,25].

Placement Technique

Universal

While there are technical differences in the placement of urethral catheters, a universal protocol emphasizing asepsis is the foundation to limit complications, namely CAUTIs (Box 187.2) [18,20]. Considerations for technique are also based on patient signalment and cardiopulmonary stability.

Male Dogs

Male dogs tend to tolerate catheterization with simple restraint and comforting: sedation may not be necessary. The urethral opening in a male is at the distal penis and is easily accessed by extruding the penis from the prepuce. After clipping and scrubbing the distal prepuce and surrounding area, the penis is extruded, wiped of gross contamination and the internal prepuce is flushed with a 0.05% chlorhexidine solution. With the penis still extended (and barrier drapes in place), the catheter is guided into the urethral opening and advanced to the desired location.

Female Dogs

Female dogs present an anatomical challenge of identifying the urethral papilla which is usually on the ventral floor at the junction of the vaginal vestibule and vault. The author prefers to perform urethral catheterization in lateral recumbency with the pelvic limbs in a neutral position using a digital technique. It requires no

---

Box 187.2 Universal protocol for urethral catheterization.

1. Premeasure length of catheter needed by estimating the length from the urethral opening to the bladder or intended distal tip, following the path of the urethra.
2. Assemble needed supplies (+/− sedatives PRN).
   a. Sterile drapes/barrier for work area and patient
   b. Sterile urinary catheter
      – If Foley catheter, syringe and sterile water for balloon, test balloon
   c. Clippers
   d. Gauze sponges
   e. Chlorhexidine surgical scrub and water rinse
   f. Lidocaine or water-based lubricant (single use)
   g. Sterile gloves
   h. Solution of 6.25 mL of 2% chlorhexidine in 250 mL sterile water (0.05% solution)
   i. Syringe for flushing prepuce
   j. If performing urohydropropulsion:
      Sterile lubricant mixed with sterile saline 1:1 in a syringe
      Exam/sterile gloves for transrectal/vaginal urethral palpation
      Syringes (depending on signalment, 1–60 cc)
      Flush solution (saline for irrigation, isotonic IV solutions)
      Assistant(s) as this is a team effort
      Additional urinary catheters for urohydropropulsion or indwelling
   k. If indwelling, closed collection system
      Collection bag (appropriate size for animal)

   If bag does not have tubing, aspiration port or male adapter for catheter:
      Male (referring to adapter) connector for urinary catheter
      Extension tubing (1 or 2)
      Three-way Luer-Lok stopcock
      Infusion plug
   Cable tie(s) and application gun
   l. If non-Foley indwelling catheter
      Skin forceps
      Needle drivers/hypodermic needle
      Scissors
      Suture, e.g. 3-0 nylon
      Commercial "butterfly" adapter or tape
3. Wash hands (before and after procedure).
4. Clip a 3–5 cm border of hair from the catheter insertion site, i.e. the preputial or vulvar area.
5. Utilize a chlorhexidine scrub and tap water solution to prepare the area with three washes and subsequent rinses.
6. Flush the area of the urethral opening (vaginal vestibule or prepuce) with a 0.05% chlorhexidine solution five times.
7. Use a sterile barrier drape, gloves, and single-use water-based lubricating jelly to aseptically place urethral catheter.
8. Once the catheter is successfully in the urethral opening, it is advanced until the premeasured length or resistance is encountered.
9. Secure the catheter if indwelling.

specialized equipment and is an easy technical skill to learn. Keeping the digit, hand, and forearm in line and along with the catheter parallel to the work surface, the initial approach is at an angle to access the vaginal vestibule then straighten to approach the urethral papilla. Others prefer visualization of the urethral papilla with the patient in dorsal recumbency with the caudal extremities elevated cranially or in ventral recumbency with the caudal extremities hanging off the work surface.

The external genital area is clipped and scrubbed (gently) and the vestibule is flushed with 0.05% chlorhexidine solution. The urethral papilla may be palpated digitally or directly visualized with a light source and vaginal speculum or a sterilized otoscope. Once the papilla is identified, the catheter is advanced into the urethral opening. Successful placement is confirmed by following the catheter from the vulva and hitting a rim of tissue. Sedation is often warranted for female patients; flushing the area of the urethral papilla with lidocaine (injectable) solution or jelly (not to exceed 4 mg/kg) with a lubricated syringe (without a needle) has anecdotally been suggested for patient comfort. When a patient is too small to accommodate a digit or equipment as above, a blind technique where the catheter is advanced along the ventral midline of the vaginal vestibule is utilized.

Male Cats (see Chapter 98)

Male cats are rarely amenable to urethral catheterization without sedation unless the cat is obtunded. Placement in male cats is like that of dogs, keeping in mind that the penis in cats has a more caudal angle than dogs and extrusion should follow suit, that is the prepuce is retracted craniodorsally. Gentle caudoventral traction of the penis may further facilitate catheterization.

Female Cats

Female cats are also rarely amenable to urethral catheterization and sedation is warranted unless the cat is obtunded. Unless the cat can accommodate a digit or viewing device, the blind technique is utilized as described above.

In all cases, if the catheter is advanced into the bladder, urine should flow; alternatively, flushing sterile saline and subsequent aspiration, radiography (with or without contrast), and ultrasound can be used to assess catheter placement. Once the catheter is in place, it should be connected to a closed collection system and secured.

Retrograde Urohydropropulsion

If the catheter is being placed to relieve an anatomical obstruction due to a urethral plug or calculus, it is advanced to the area of obstruction under general anesthesia or heavy sedation (see Chapter 191). Injecting a sterile physiological solution through the catheter to dilate the urethra and move the obstruction towards the bladder is referred to as retrograde urohydropropulsion. It is preferred to using the catheter to physically move or bypass the obstruction to minimize the risk of urethral trauma, including tearing or subsequent stricture formation. If urohydropropulsion is unsuccessful, using the catheter to manipulate or bypass the obstruction should be weighed carefully against repeated decompressive cystocentesis or a tube cystotomy until definitive surgery can be performed (see Chapter 106).

Decompressive cystocentesis to a modest residual volume is recommended in cases of bladder overdistension prior to retrograde urohydropropulsion as it decreases the pressure against the obstruction, accommodates the volume of flushing solution, provides for a pure urine sample, and relieves the pathologies associated with an overdistended bladder and obstructive uropathy.

Once the catheter tip is just distal (with respect to the urethra) to the area of the obstruction, a sterile 1:1 solution of isotonic saline (or other physiological solution) and water-based lubricant is injected. Palpation and retrograde manipulation of the stone can be attempted via the rectum, vagina or transabdominal palpation while this lubricating solution is being injected. In anticipation of flushing the catheter with physiological solution, an assistant applies digital pressure in appropriate sized patients via the rectum or vagina to the urethra, either distal to the obstruction (with respect to the urethra) to prevent backflow and promote urethral dilation or proximal to the obstruction to dilate the segment of the urethra with the obstruction and when pressure is released abruptly, carry the stone or plug to the bladder. The urethral opening at the penis may be occluded around the catheter in males. A Foley catheter with the balloon inflated may substitute for or complement digital occlusion [4]. The author has found that 1 cc syringes generate the pressure needed to relieve obstructions due to plugs in male cats when larger syringes have failed. Once the obstruction is relieved, a new indwelling catheter may be considered if urethral catheterization is warranted.

Indwelling Catheter Care

If a catheter is to be left in place, a closed collection system is utilized. Closed collection systems are commercially available and contain a sampling port and distal emptying spigot or one can be constructed from a collection bag, tubing, three-way stopcock, injection caps and adapters, all ideally sterile. Cable ties and the associated "gun" are available at home improvement stores to secure connections in either case.

It has been suggested that a used IV catheter bag that contained dextrose-free solutions can be used as the collection bag if it is capped with a sterile plug and stored for <7 days in a cabinet. However, this requires that the closed collections system be "broken" for emptying of the bag. This "open" system had a slightly higher incidence of CAUTI compared with a closed collection system in one study, but the difference was not significant. Limitations included an average catheterization time of 2 days, none longer than 7 days, and a relatively small sample size [20]. Regardless of the system used, contamination of any spigot or connection should be prevented; this means keeping the bag off the floor (e.g. laying it in a clean plastic container), but always lower than the patient to prevent retrograde flow [1,2].

If a Foley catheter is placed, the catheter is advanced to insure the balloon is in the bladder, then the balloon is inflated with sterile water using the volume indicated on the balloon port of the catheter. Gentle caudal traction is applied until resistance is met, insuring the catheter is seated appropriately. Non-Foley catheters are secured using two skin sutures placed into the vulva or prepuce apposed 180° utilizing a commercially available or tape-made "butterfly" encompassing the catheter. Care should be taken to ensure that the collection system is not placing tension on the urethral catheter by bandaging the collection tubing to a leg or tail. If the tail is used, distal anchoring is recommended to minimize fecal contamination.

Emergent patients with indwelling urethral catheters should undergo regular catheter care every 8 hours or when gross contamination occurs, consisting of hand washing, examination glove usage, cleaning the catheter and area with chlorhexidine scrub (and rinse) and gentle chlorhexidine flushing similar to preplacement. Once an indwelling catheter is no longer needed, it should be removed [18]. Case transfer from emergency care should include information on the indication for the catheter, catheter type, placement and care, and removal contingencies to avoid excessive time of catheterization.

References

1 Gould C V, Umscheid CA, Agarwal RK, Kuntz G, Pegues DA. Guideline for prevention of catheter-associated urinary tract infections 2009. *Infect Control Hosp Epidemiol* 2010;31(4):319–326.
2 Hooton TM, Bradley SF, Cardenas DD, et al. Diagnosis, prevention, and treatment of catheter-associated urinary tract infection in adults: 2009 International Clinical Practice Guidelines from the Infectious Diseases Society of America. *Clin Infect Dis* 2010;50(5):625–663.
3 Knapp DW. *Withrow and MacEwen's Small Animal Clinical Oncology*. Elsevier, New York, 2007, pp. 649–658.
4 Osborne CA, Lulich JP, Polzin DJ. Canine retrograde urohydropropulsion. Lessons from 25 years of experience. *Vet Clin North Am Small Anim Pract* 1999;29(1):267–281, xiv.
5 Kealy JK, McAllister H, Graham J. *Diagnostic Radiology and Ultrasonography of the Dog and Cat*. Elsevier, New York, 2005, pp. 21–171.
6 Smarick S, Hallowell TC. *Small Animal Critical Care Medicine*. Elsevier, St Louis, 2015, pp. 1001–1004.
7 Smith SE, Sande AA. Measurement of intra-abdominal pressure in dogs and cats. *J Vet Emerg Crit Care* 2012;22(5):530–544.
8 Dolder LK. *Small Animal Toxicology*. Elsevier, St Louis, 2013, pp. 647–652.
9 Bubenik L, Hosgood G. Urinary tract infection in dogs with thoracolumbar intervertebral disc herniation and urinary bladder dysfunction managed by manual expression, indwelling catheterization or intermittent catheterization. *Vet Surg* 2008;37(8):791–800.
10 Bubenik LJ, Hosgood GL, Waldron DR, Snow LA. Frequency of urinary tract infection in catheterized dogs and comparison of bacterial culture and susceptibility testing results for catheterized and noncatheterized dogs with urinary tract infections. *J Am Vet Med Assoc* 2007;231(6):893–899.
11 Comer KM, Ling GV. Results of urinalysis and bacterial culture of canine urine obtained by antepubic cystocentesis, catheterization, and the midstream voided methods. *J Am Vet Med Assoc* 1981;179(9):891–895.
12 Basdani E, Papazoglou LG, Kazakos GM, Bright RM. Spontaneous urethral catheter kinking or knotting in male dogs: four cases. *J Am Anim Hosp Assoc* 2011;47(5):351–355.
13 Anderson RB, Aronson LR, Drobatz KJ, Atilla A. Prognostic factors for successful outcome following urethral rupture in dogs and cats. *J Am Anim Hosp Assoc* 2006;42(2):136–146.
14 Biertuempfel PH, Ling GV, Ling GA. Urinary tract infection resulting from catheterization in healthy adult dogs. *J Am Vet Med Assoc* 1981;178(9):989–991.
15 Barsanti JA, Blue J, Edmunds J. Urinary tract infection due to indwelling bladder catheters in dogs and cats. *J Am Vet Med Assoc* 1985;187(4):384–388.
16 Glickman LT. Veterinary nosocomial (hospital-acquired) Klebsiella infections. *J Am Vet Med Assoc* 1981;179(12):1389–1392.
17 Ogeer-Gyles J, Mathews K, Weese JS, Prescott JF, Boerlin P. Evaluation of catheter-associated urinary tract infections and multi-drug-resistant Escherichia coli isolates from the urine of dogs with

indwelling urinary catheters. *J Am Vet Med Assoc* 2006;229(10):1584–1590.

18 Smarick SD, Haskins SC, Aldrich J, et al. Incidence of catheter-associated urinary tract infection among dogs in a small animal intensive care unit. *J Am Vet Med Assoc* 2004;224(12):1936–1940.

19 Stiffler KS, Stevenson MAM, Sanchez S, Barsanti JA, Hofmeister E, Budsberg SC. Prevalence and characterization of urinary tract infections in dogs with surgically treated type 1 thoracolumbar intervertebral disc extrusion. *Vet Surg* 2006;35(4):330–336.

20 Sullivan LA, Campbell VL, Onuma SC. Evaluation of open versus closed urine collection systems and development of nosocomial bacteriuria in dogs. *J Am Vet Med Assoc* 2010;237(2):187–190.

21 Wise LA, Jones RL. Nosocomial canine urinary tract infections in a veterinary teaching hospital. *J Am Anim Hosp Assoc* 1990;24:627.

22 Francey T, Gaschen F, Nicolet J, Burnens AP. The role of Acinetobacter baumannii as a nosocomial pathogen for dogs and cats in an intensive care unit. *J Vet Intern Med* 14(2):177–183.

23 Segev G, Bankirer T, Steinberg D, et al. Evaluation of urinary catheters coated with sustained-release varnish of chlorhexidine in mitigating biofilm formation on urinary catheters in dogs. *J Vet Intern Med* 2013;27(1):39–46.

24 Stewart E. Urinary catheters: selection, maintenance and nursing care. *Br J Nurs* 7(19):1152–1154, 1156, 1158–11561.

25 Sharpe SJ, Mann FA, Wiedmeyer CE, Wagner-Mann C, Thomovsky EJ. Optimal filling solution for silicone Foley catheter balloons. *Can Vet J* 2011;52(10): 1111–1114.

188

Mechanical Ventilation in the Emergency Room

Lisa L. Powell, DVM, DACVECC

BluePearl Veterinary Partners, Eden Prairie, MN, USA

Introduction

Intermittent positive pressure ventilation (IPPV) may be considered in dogs and cats that present to the emergency room in respiratory distress/failure or rapidly developing failure (Box 188.1). Additionally, IPPV may be considered in dogs and cats with toxicity (e.g. baclofen or ivermectin in dogs), with severe hypoventilation or for support following successful CPR. The ER efforts are unique in providing ventilation for these patients, as early initiation of ventilation (prior to CPR) may be associated with a better outcome.

Supplies Required

Ventilation may be simply provided with an Ambu bag or anesthesia machine; in fact, this is almost certainly the first line of therapy in most pets ventilated in the ER. Non-invasive ventilation, which is more commonly used in people, is poorly tolerated in conscious dogs and cats. Hi-flow oxygen therapy (see Chapter 181) may represent an additional approach to treating hypoxemia that is refractory to conventional therapy. Anesthesia ventilators are able to provide more short-term support to ventilated cases, although most frequently these are only able to provide 100% oxygen support. More long-term ventilation may be accomplished with dedicated critical care ventilators. Many ERs are associated with 24-hour ICU services as well, and in some cases it may be prudent to move a patient to the ICU before initiating long-term ventilation. In emergency hospitals not associated with 24-hour hospitals, efforts to stabilize the patient in the ER before transport to a 24-hour hospital are advised if possible.

Personnel

Most ventilated patients need at least one person dedicated to them full time, although some toxicities/hypoventilating cases are more tolerant of less intensive monitoring. Adequate staff should be available if ventilation is offered for more than a short time.

Transport

If 24-hour ventilatory support is not available and it seems likely that the patient may require more support, it may be necessary to transport the patient to a critical care hospital (Figure 188.1). This may be accomplished in a few urban areas with "animal ambulances" but in general, this is challenging unless the transport distance is short. Animals with hypoventilation may be more easily moved while being ventilated than those dogs or cats with severe hypoxemia. Small oxygen tanks may be used for transport, and in some cases, a veterinarian or veterinary technician may accompany the patient and will provide assisted ventilation during transport. The feasibility of transport should be carefully considered prior to moving a patient, and every effort should be made to avoid transport if possible. However, if the patient is declining or there is no option for ongoing support, transport should be pursued.

Box 188.1 Goals of ventilation in the ER.
• Decrease or eliminate hypoxemia and/or hypercarbia
• Reduce fear and anxiety
• Permit diagnostic tests to evaluate the underlying cause of the respiratory distress, if needed
• Initiate therapy specific for the patient's condition

Textbook of Small Animal Emergency Medicine, First Edition. Edited by Kenneth J. Drobatz, Kate Hopper, Elizabeth Rozanski and Deborah C. Silverstein.
© 2019 John Wiley & Sons, Inc. Published 2019 by John Wiley & Sons, Inc.
Companion Website: www.wiley.com/go/drobatz/textbook

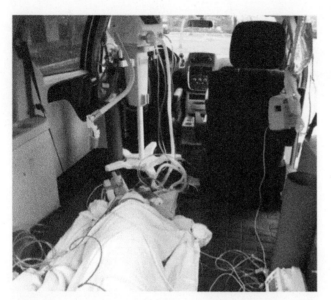

Figure 188.1 A dog being transported from an emergency hospital to a 24-hour hospital for ventilation following a coral snake attack. Source: Photo courtesy of Alex Lynch BVSc (Hons), DACVECC, University of Florida.

Owner Communication

The decision to provide a pet with IPPV is an important one; it should be based upon a strong assessment of the potential benefits and risks to that patient, as well as a discussion of the emotional and financial implications of IPPV. In some cases, ventilation will clearly be short term (e.g. some toxicities) and in other cases, the outcome will be clear quite quickly so 12–24 hours of support may be warranted and more easily undertaken. In other cases, the decision to pursue IPPV will accompany a significant medical or surgical undertaking (e.g. MRI and ventral slot) and the owner should be advised that ventilation is only a small part of the treatment and hopeful recovery of the patient.

Respiratory Distress (Hypoxemia)

Respiratory distress is common in ER patients; most animals will respond to efforts to stabilize them with oxygen, thoracocentesis, and/or medications. However, in some cases progressive respiratory failure appears imminent and in those cases, consideration should be given to providing IPPV. After a patient is anesthetized and intubated for support, additional diagnostic testing, such as diagnostic imaging or sample collection, may be more safely accomplished. Ventilation is additionally a humane option as it removes anxiety and fear associated with hypoxemia.

Recently, a small study by Edwards et al. evaluated the outcome surrounding ventilation associated with congestive heart failure (CHF) and identified 10 dogs and six cats that were supported with IPPV [1]. Overall survival to discharge was 62.5%, with a mean onset to ventilation from admission of 5.9+/−6.4 hours, suggesting that IPPV may have a role in the emergency stabilization of animals with CHF.

In dogs with pulmonary contusions (see Chapter 49), in 2000 Campbell and King evaluated 10 dogs that were supported with IPPV and found that 30% of dogs survived [2]. Interestingly, due to the changing approach to fluid therapy, with the pendulum shifting to more conservative fluids in the last 15 years, it may be that IPPV would more successful in dogs and cats treated today following initial resuscitation.

Intoxications/Envenomation

In some parts of the world (e.g. Australia), ventilation for exposure to ticks and snakes results in frequent need for short-term ventilatory support, with a good outcome [3]. Ingestion of sedative drugs, avermectins or tremorgenic toxins may result in the development of respiratory depression or decreased respirations may accompany the anesthetic agents required to control excessive muscle activity or tremors. In these cases, IPPV is very useful to support the patient as the intoxication is directly treated or is metabolized. Some intoxicants (e.g. baclofen) are amenable to hemodialysis and lipid therapy may also be used to shorten the duration of some toxicities (see Chapter 129) [4].

Post Cardiopulmonary Resuscitation

Following successful return of spontaneous circulation (ROSC), IPPV may be pursued to better support the patient during recovery from the arrest. Recurrent CPA is common in survivors of CPR (see Chapter 150), and hypopnea or apnea can be avoided with support. IPPV may negatively impact cardiac output, so close attention should be paid to monitoring cardiac function and urine output.

Tetraparesis

Tetraparesis may result from a compressive cervical lesion; while normally cervical intervertebral disk disease (IVDD) does not result in hypoventilation, in severe cases it may do so. Dogs that are ventilated for IVDD have a fair to good prognosis with surgery [5]. In the emergency setting, dogs with tetraparesis should be evaluated for hypoventilation. Pulse oximetry values of >95% while breathing room air practically exclude hypoventilation [6] but with lower values, an arterial blood gas should be obtained. Care should be taken to not provide supplemental oxygen to a patient with hypoxemia, without excluding hypoventilation, as while the PaO_2 will improve, the $PaCO_2$ may be rapidly worsened (Table 188.1). End-tidal CO_2 analysis is not helpful when assessing hypoventilation as $ETCO_2$ may only assess expired air from the anatomical deadspace. In animals with hypoxemia/hypoventilation from lower motor neuron disease (see Chapter 27), the prognosis is much more grave [7].

Ventilation

As in all cases of IPPV, care should be taken to ensure adequate sedation/analgesia, not only for patient comfort but also to decrease work of breathing and limit patient–ventilator asynchrony (see Chapter 191). Ventilatory settings should be as conservative as possible, with efforts aimed at prevention of worsening lung injury and iatrogenic complications. Tolerance of moderate amounts of hypoxemia (e.g. SpO_2 89–90%) may limit the inspiratory pressures or volumes required, which can help avoid complications.

Conclusion

Emergent mechanical ventilation can be life-preserving, allowing for support of respiration in cases of imminent

Table 188.1 Arterial blood gases from a Doberman pinscher with tetraparesis and respiratory failure associated with wobbler's syndrome. The dog was given oxygen therapy to treat the hypoxemia, without appropriate recognition of the respiratory failure. Note the effect of supplemental oxygen on PCO_2 and pH.

	On admission	After oxygen therapy
pH	7.237	7.021
PCO_2	51.3 mmHg	91.5 mmHg
PO_2	59.7 mmHg	371.4 mmHg
HCO_3	22 mmol/L	27 mmHg
BE	–2 mEq/L	+3 mEq/L
SPO_2	89% (pulse oximeter)	100% (pulse oximeter)

BE, base excess.

respiratory failure. The ER should be fully prepared to rapidly sedate and intubate these patients and, initially, manually provide positive pressure ventilation. If prolonged assisted ventilation is required, the patient can be transferred to a critical ventilator for further support within the ER or an ICU. Rapid sedation, intubation, and assisted ventilation can allow the ER veterinarian to more fully assess the patient, and educate the owners on underlying disease and prognosis. In addition, with some diseases, positive pressure ventilation, in conjunction with therapeutic medications, will provide support while the underlying insult resolves.

References

1 Edwards TH, Coleman AE, Brainard BM, et al. Outcome of positive-pressure ventilation in dogs and cats with congestive heart failure: 16 cases (1992–2012). *J Vet Emerg Crit Care* 2014;24(5):586–593.

2 Campbell VL, King LG. Pulmonary function, ventilator management, and outcome of dogs with thoracic trauma and pulmonary contusions: 10 cases (1994–1998). *J Am Vet Med Assoc* 2000;217(10):1505–1509.

3 Trigg NL, Leister E, Whitney J, et al. Outcomes of mechanical ventilation in 302 dogs and cats in Australia (2005–2013). *Aust Vet Pract* 2014;44(4): 698–703.

4 Torre DM, Labato MA, Rossi T, et al. Treatment of a dog with severe baclofen intoxication using

hemodialysis and mechanical ventilation. *J Vet Emerg Crit Care* 2008;18(3):312–318.

5 Beal MW, Paglia DT, Griffin GM, et al. Ventilatory failure, ventilator management, and outcome in dogs with cervical spinal disorders: 14 cases (1991–1999). *J Am Vet Med Assoc* 2001;218(10):1598–1602.

6 Fu ES, Downs JB, Schweiger JW, et al. Supplemental oxygen impairs detection of hypoventilation by pulse oximetry. *Chest* 2004;126:1552–1558.

7 Rutter CR, Rozanski EA, Sharp CR, et al. Outcome and medical management in dogs with lower motor neuron disease undergoing mechanical ventilation: 14 cases (2003–2009). *J Vet Emerg Crit Care* 2001;21(5): 531–554.

189

Damage Control Surgery

Steve J. Mehler, DVM, DACVS

Hope Veterinary Specialists, Philadelphia, PA, USA

Introduction

Damage control surgery (DCS) is a set of surgical techniques and principles utilized to care for critically ill patients in the emergency room setting. There is a subset of patients, etiologies, and situations that require immediate surgical intervention without the benefit of a surgeon being present or immediately accessible. The decision to switch from definitive treatment to damage control should be made early, ideally prior to entering the operative suite, as this has been associated with improved mortality [1–4].

In humans, the leading cause of death among trauma patients remains uncontrolled hemorrhage which accounts for approximately 30–40% of trauma-related deaths [1,2].

The implementation of DCS in humans emphasizes preventing the lethal triad of metabolic acidosis, hypothermia, and coagulopathy, rather than providing definitive surgical intervention and correction of the distorted anatomy.

The life-saving methodology of DCS has resulted in a significant decrease in morbidity and mortality of critically ill patients; however, it is important to remember that complications associated with DCS being undertaken by an undertrained or unprepared team will lead to fatal consequences. In human trauma patients, the procedure is generally indicated when a severe injury occurs that induces severe hemorrhage that leads to the lethal triad as a sequela [3]. The surgical approach, performed in the emergency room, would provide a limited surgical intervention in order to control both hemorrhage and contamination. This allows for the emergency clinician to focus on reversing the physiological insult and stabilizing the patient prior to definitive surgical intervention. While the temptation to perform a definitive procedure may exist, it is avoided in this situation because of the secondary deleterious effects on patients.

In small animal trauma patients, DCS can and should be employed in similar circumstances as described in the human literature, attempting to avoid and correct persistent hypothermia, metabolic acidosis, and progressive coagulopathy.

In animals with severe, acute, abdominal trauma, DCS is divided into three stages.

1. Initial laparotomy
2. Intensive care unit or postoperative resuscitation and stabilization
3. Definitive repair

Each of these three stages has to be well timed and meet specific objectives to assure a successful outcome.

Damage Control Surgery Stage 1: Initial Laparotomy

The first goal of stage 1 is controlling hemorrhage. Current human recommendations are to keep the operative time to 90 minutes or less to avoid death [2]. Control of ongoing contamination, packing of the abdomen or compartment, and placement of a closed suction drainage device are all part of stage 1. One of the most important factors in determining the outcome of a stage 1 DCS patient is to minimize the length of time spent in this phase. The ultimate outcome associated with stage 1 DCS is directly related to the ability to mobilize appropriate personnel, equipment, and the particular resources required to treat the patient. Establishing and maintaining control over hemorrhage is the most important step in this phase. The packing off of all four abdominal quadrants with radiopaque laparotomy sponges usually will allow the clinician to establish initial hemorrhagic control. Depending on the source of hemorrhage, a number of different techniques and methods are utilized.

Textbook of Small Animal Emergency Medicine, First Edition. Edited by Kenneth J. Drobatz, Kate Hopper, Elizabeth Rozanski and Deborah C. Silverstein.
© 2019 John Wiley & Sons, Inc. Published 2019 by John Wiley & Sons, Inc.
Companion Website: www.wiley.com/go/drobatz/textbook

While the patient is being prepared for anesthesia and surgery, all potential required supplies are identified and made available to the surgical team. This would include, but is not limited to, surgical packs with a variety of instrument sizes, straight and curved hemostats, Satinsky forceps, suction devices and multiple suction canisters, cell saver device or similar supplies needed for autotransfusion, abdominal retractors, a variety of suture sizes and materials, large radiopaque laparotomy pads, and radiopaque gauze squares. Topical hemostatic agents can also be used to control hemorrhage in certain situations [5]. Fibrin and thrombin topical sprays and gels, cyanoacrylate tissue glue, topical collagen, gelatin sponges, oxidized cellulose and VETIGEL (Suneris, Brooklyn, NY), a novel, rapid-acting, plant polymer topical hemostatic agent, are currently available products.

Electrosurgery is indispensable for rapid and efficient control of hemorrhage. Both monopolar and bipolar electrosurgery are indispensible when performing DCS. Attempting to control hemorrhage at any level in any tissue without electrosurgery in an unstable and potentially hypothermic and coagulopathic patient will lead to significant prolongation of anesthesia and surgery times and ultimately to the patient's demise. Electrosurgery has to be used judiciously; indiscriminate and inappropriate use will lead to thermal damage, ischemia, and delayed healing.

It is necessary to have a good light source available and often, the lighting in an emergency room is not adequate for exploration of the abdomen. A head-mounted halogen, xenon, or LED light source is recommended.

The fur of the ventral abdomen is clipped with the animal in lateral recumbency, ideally prior to providing general anesthesia. All loose and clipped fur is removed from the patient and from the surgical table with a vacuum prior to applying the surgical scrub. Once the patient is intubated and secured in dorsal recumbency, the animal is draped and the skin incision is made from the xiphoid to the pubis. One of the most common and costly mistakes in early DCS is limited exposure of the peritoneal cavity. If the skin incision is not long enough, the linea incision will be limited and so will the ability of the surgeon to identify the source of hemorrhage and control it. The linea should be incised from the xiphoid to the level of the umbilicus.

At this point, the peritoneum is still intact and blood will not be able to rapidly leave the abdominal cavity. A Poole suction tip is used to penetrate the falciform fat and peritoneum at the most caudal extent of the linea incision. The suction tip is aimed to the right and caudal in the abdomen to avoid the spleen and omentum. This technique allows for a controlled evacuation of blood from the abdomen. The blood can be immediately processed for autotransfusion (see Chapter 176). Once most

of the blood has been removed from the abdomen, the linea incision is expanded to the level of the pubis.

The most efficient method to identify the source of the hemorrhage is to have a consistent and repeatable plan for exploration that starts with evaluation of the most common sites of hemorrhage. The most common sources of hemorrhage are the spleen, liver, and retroperitoneum. If these locations do not provide the source of hemorrhage, a routine systematic abdominal exploratory is performed. Less common sites of severe hemorrhage include mesenteric vessels, the portal vein, and direct damage to the caudal vena cava or iliac veins, or the aorta and its major branches. Temporary occlusion of the aorta, caudal vena cava, or portal vein may be required. Solid organ injury should be dealt with by complete or partial resection, if possible. The spleen is rapidly evaluated for hemorrhage. If it is the source of hemorrhage, a rapid splenectomy technique is performed or the splenic hilar vessels can be clamped with hemostats or Carmalt forceps. The liver is evaluated next and exploration of all liver lobes on all surfaces is facilitated by linea incision that is extended from the xiphoid to the pubis. The liver can be retracted caudally by placing laparotomy sponges between the diaphragm and the concave cranialmost surface of the liver. This technique may also partially tamponade the hepatic veins as they leave the liver parenchyma cranially to enter the caudal vena cava. If the liver is the source of hemorrhage, it is possible to temporarily slow or cease the flow of blood to the liver. The Pringle maneuver is performed by identifying the portal vein and the hepatic artery within the hepatoduedonal ligament [5]. The hepatoduodenal ligament is the portion of the lesser omentum that attaches the liver to the descending duodenum and forms the ventral border of the epiploic foramen.

Compressing the hepatoduodenal ligament with the portal vein and hepatic artery with a vascular clamp will cease all blood flow to the liver. This technique also inadvertently occludes the bile duct. The technique can be performed intermittently as needed to identify the source of liver hemorrhage and control it. If the portion of the bleeding liver lobe can be rapidly removed with a guillotine suture technique or surgical stapling device (thoracoabdominal stapler), this can be performed at the time of DCS. If the hemorrhage cannot be immediately stopped, an encircling loop of 2-0 to 0 PDS suture is tied and secured proximal to the site of hemorrhage. This technique is unlikely to yield a permanent solution to the hemorrhage but the compression of the liver parenchyma around the intrahepatic vessels will decrease the amount of active bleeding. Laparotomy sponges are lightly moistened and packed in the cranial abdomen to assist in the tamponade of the source of the liver hemorrhage. The sponges are retained in the cranial abdomen and the incision is closed, stabilization continues, and definitive sponge removal and surgical intervention are performed at another time in the near future.

The portal vein and hepatic artery cannot be clamped for a long period of time. The abdomen should not be closed with the hepatoduodenal ligament compressed. Intermittent use of the Pringle maneuver is well tolerated intraoperatively but prolonged compression is damaging to the intestines and pancreas and rapidly induces severe portal hypertensionso its use must be limited to the DCS event.

Common sources of severe retroperitoneal hemorrhage include the kidneys and their blood supply, the phrenicoabdominal veins, and the deep circumflex iliac arteries leaving the aorta at the level of the lumbar vertebral bodies. These vessels may need to be ligated and the patient closed prior to definitive repair being performed. In cases of severe renal trauma with significant hemorrhage, the renal artery and vein can be clamped or ligated and the kidney and ureter definitively removed once the patient is more stable. Other arteries and veins directly associated with the caudal vena cava or abdominal aorta may be able to be ligated but attempts to spare the celiac and cranial mesenteric artery must be performed.

Acute ligation of the caudal vena cava distal to the renal veins can be performed but will induce significant venous obstruction to the pelvic limbs and a decrease in cardiac preload. Ligation of the cava proximal to the renal veins will lead to renal azotemia, a massive decrease in preload, and ultimate failure of the kidneys. Temporary caudal caval occlusion can be performed during DCS to identify the source of hemorrhage and repair it. The use of a Satinsky clamp is ideal to isolate a tear in the caudal vena cava. The clamp is applied parallel to the long axis of the vessel so that the damaged region is isolated but blood can still flow through the non-clamped portion of the vessel.

If the abdominal aorta or any of its major tributaries are the source of the hemorrhage, they can be clamped during DCS stage 1 for up to 30 minutes without permanent damage to the viscera.

Once hemorrhage control is achieved, one should quickly proceed to controlling intra-abdominal contamination from hollow-viscous organs. Although it may be tempting to perform an intestinal resection and anastomosis during DCS, this should not be done. The goal of DCS is to prevent continued intra-abdominal contamination without restoring normal luminal flow of the bowel. This can be undertaken with the utilization of a TA stapler to come across the bowel, or primary suture closure. Once this is complete, the abdomen should be packed. Many of these patients become coagulopathic and can develop diffuse oozing (see Chapter 163). It is important to pack not only areas of injury but also areas of surgical dissection. There are various methods that can be utilized to pack the abdomen. Packing with radiopaque laparotomy pads allows the benefit of being able to detect them via x-ray prior to definitive closure. As a rule, definitive closure should not takeplace until there has been radiological confirmation that no retained objects are present in the abdomen.

Damage Control Surgery Stage 2: ICU Resuscitation

Upon completion of the initial phase of damage control, the key is to reverse the physiological insult that has taken place. The second stage of DCL is resuscitation focused on correction of physiological derangements, acidosis, oxygen debt, coagulopathy, and hypothermia which is covered elsewhere in this book (see Section 4).

Prophylactic antibiotics should be administered preoperatively when possible as infection rates increase if given intra- or post-operatively only, and duration should be no longer than 24 hours, unless soft tissue wounds are present or if there is concurrent trauma to the abdominal viscera with secondary spillage of gastrointestinal, biliary tract, or urogenital tract contents (see Chapter 200).

Damage Control Surgery Stage 3: Definitive Reconstruction

Definitive surgical intervention and reconstruction occurs once the patient is stable and improving. This is usually within 24–48 hours after presenting to the hospital. In veterinary medicine, DCS is often performed at the primary veterinary clinic or within the emergency department of a specialty hospital. Stage 3 of DCS in small animals often involves the transportation of the patient to a referral facility for definitive surgical intervention. The patient must be stable enough to tolerate transportation without significant decompensation, impeding stage 3 DCS. In human trauma patients, stage 3 will only occur after the resolution of acidosis, hypothermia, and coagulopathy has occurred. All tamponade materials used to pack the abdomen are gently removed. If radiopaque laparotomy pads or gauze squares were used for abdominal packing, they may induce a debridement effect when removed, causing serosal damage and hemorrhage. To prevent this and to facilitate safe removal, sterile saline is used as an abdominal lavage to loosen the adhesive interaction between the packing material and the serosal surface of the viscera prior to its removal.

Immediately after removal of the packing material, a complete and thorough abdominal exploratory is performed. The goal of the re-exploratory is to identify any injuries missed during the initial laparotomy and re-evaluate the known injuries. If hemorrhage has ceased completely, no further intervention may be necessary. Once the previous source of hemorrhage is identified, evaluated, and addressed, attention is then turned to performing the necessary bowel anastomosis or other definitive repair. In many cases, the abdomen will be lavaged with 200–600 mL/kg of warm sterile saline and a closed suction drain placed and maintained for 24–48 hours.

Although there are no data supporting the use of DCS in dogs and cats, anecdotal data do exist enabling the translation of the human literature to the practice of DCS in emergency trauma small animal patients. Utilizing the lethal triad of metabolic acidosis, hypothermia, and coagulopathy in small animal trauma patients as a justification to elect DCS is reasonable. However, other factors such as financial implications, co-morbidities, and availability of emergency doctors and support staff that are comfortable with DCS stages 1 and 2 may preclude the implementation of such interventions.

References

1 Costantini T, Coimbra R. Abdominal damage control surgery and reconstruction: World Society of Emergency Surgery position paper. *World J Emerg Surg* 2013;8(1):53.
2 Jaunoo SS, Harji DP. Damage control surgery. *Int J Surg* 2009;7(2):110–113.
3 Roberts DJ, Bobrovitz N, Zygun DA, et al. Indications for use of thoracic, abdominal, pelvic, and vascular damage control interventions in trauma patients: a content analysis and expert appropriateness rating study. *J Trauma Acute Care Surg* 2015;79(4):568–579.
4 Rotondo MF, Schwab CW, McGonigal MD, et al. "Damage control": an approach for improved survival in exsanguinating penetrating abdominal injury. *J Trauma* 1993;35(3):375–382; discussion 82–83.
5 Devey JJ. Surgical considerations in the emergent small animal patient. *Vet Clin North Am Small Anim Pract* 2013;43(4):899–914.

Section 7

Anesthesia and Analgesia for the Emergency Room Patient

190

Anesthesia and Analgesia in the Emergency Room: An Overview

Lisa J. Bazzle, DVM, DACVECC[1] and Benjamin M. Brainard, VMD, DACVAA, DACVECC[2]

[1] *Animal Medical Center, New York, NY, USA*
[2] *College of Veterinary Medicine, University of Georgia, Athens, GA, USA*

Introduction

Pain is the most common presenting complaint in human emergency departments (EDs), yet treatment is consistently delayed and underdelivered. Only 20–50% of human patients presenting to the ED with acute pain receive analgesia, and the time to delivery increases with severity of illness, age, trauma, overcrowding, triage category, time of arrival, and gender [1,2]. In an Australian survey, general surgery and trauma patients were most likely to receive delayed analgesia [3].

Veterinary ED patients also encounter "oligoanalgesia," or lack of timely and adequate analgesia, with similar contributing factors. Patient pain tolerance and clinician and nurse identification and quantification (i.e. scoring) of pain are variable. Compared to anesthesiologists, veterinary students assigned lower pain scores for painful dogs, and many (58.8%) French veterinarians indicated an inadequate ability to quantify pain [4,5].

There is also a scarcity of reliable, sensitive, species-specific pain scoring systems. Most currently used scoring systems (e.g. Visual Analogue Score, Glasgow Composite-Measure Pain Scale, Simple Descriptive Scale (SDS), University of Melbourne Pain Scale) were developed and evaluated in patients already diagnosed with pain or following surgery, using an observer's interpretation of the patient's behavior and interaction with the environment to assign a score.

Beyond published pain scales, physiological responses and pain-mediated sympathetic stimulation (e.g. tachycardia, tachypnea, hypertension) are used for diagnosis of pain, but are inconsistent and neither sensitive nor specific markers [4,6,7].

While data are limited, a study conducted in a veterinary intensive care unit (ICU) found an overall 22% prevalence of pain in hospitalized dogs. Dogs on the orthopedic or neurosurgical service were more likely to

be characterized as painful, using an SDS [8]. In one veterinary ED, the prevalence of pain was estimated to be approximately 56% [9]. Unstable and under-resuscitated patients may be more susceptible to the cardiovascular and respiratory depressant side-effects of analgesic and anesthetic drugs, and in both humans and animals, clinicians are reluctant to administer pain medications to emergency patients for this reason and for concerns of masking changes in clinical condition (i.e. progression of neurological disease) [4,9–13].

Reconciling these challenges to rapidly identify and score pain in the emergent patient will allow the astute clinician to formulate and administer safe and effective analgesic or anesthetic protocol incorporating pharmacological and non-pharmacological therapies.

Origins and Sequelae of Pain

Pain sensation arises from a series of neural and electrochemical events following noxious mechanical, thermal, or chemical stimuli. These stimuli result in a release of ions, cytokines, and other substances (e.g. PGE_2) that sensitize or directly stimulate peripheral nociceptive receptors. In the periphery, this chemical stimulus is transduced to an electrochemical event that is then transmitted to the dorsal horn of the spinal cord, where it is modulated prior to its projection along the spinothalamic tracts to the brain, where it is perceived as pain.

Pain initiates a series of neuroendocrine events leading to hypothalamic-pituitary-adrenal gland axis activation with subsequent release of proinflammatory cytokines and catecholamines, resulting in altered immune function as well as cardiorespiratory changes. Pain also decreases subcutaneous oxygen tension, and may impair wound healing [14].

If nociceptor stimulation persists unmitigated, it may lead to increased responsiveness of dorsal horn neurons and promote central sensitization ("wind-up") or hyperalgesia. This may decrease the efficacy of analgesic drugs, and require the administration of higher doses of medications that may result in more pronounced side-effects.

General Approach to the Painful Patient

Triage examination to gauge cardiorespiratory, neurological, and urological stability should be performed initially (see Chapter 2), followed by appropriate volume repletion and evaluation of acid–base status and electrolyte concentrations. This can ideally occur prior to the administration of analgesic or sedative medication, but in some animals with extreme pain, analgesia should be administered along with resuscitation. Frequent monitoring of heart rate (HR), blood pressure (BP) and pulse quality, mucous membrane color, capillary refill time, rectal and distal extremity temperature, respiratory rate (RR) and effort, and mentation should be performed both initially and following resuscitation.

When assessing pain in emergency patients, the signalment of the patient, as well as evaluation of the location and type of pain (e.g. visceral, orthopedic), should be taken into consideration. The cause, duration, and severity of the pain should also be determined. Behavioral indications of pain include vocalization or protective behaviors, especially following palpation of the affected area. Serial monitoring to evaluate trends in the physiological response to pain, which is typically characterized by increased HR, BP, and RR, may be more sensitive in assessing pain and effectiveness of analgesia than focusing on single measurements of these variables alone. However, in states of high catecholamine release, patients will display a decrease in HR variability, which further reinforces the need to consider the many factors affecting pain rather than relying on only physiological parameters [15].

In Muir's study of pain in the ED, painful dogs were significantly older and heavier, and the majority had acute pain of mild-to-moderate severity that was somatic in origin (with skin and orthopedic injuries predominant). Painful cats were also significantly older, though their pain was more chronic in duration, and was visceral in origin, with pancreatitis, colitis, or obstruction (urethral or constipation) most common [16].

The implementation of triage pain protocols in the human ED has resulted in decreases in the time to analgesia administration, and increases in the number of patients receiving analgesia [17]. The incorporation of pain scores results in more consistent and timely delivery of opioid analgesia in this population [18].

Treating the Painful Emergent Patient

For the emergent patient, limited knowledge about disease and organ function promotes the selection of analgesics that are reversible and titratable, with minimal cardiorespiratory side-effects. Adverse side-effects can also be minimized by selecting synergistic combinations of analgesics that can result in adequate analgesia using lower total doses of each drug. These combinations are encompassed within the concept of multimodal analgesia, which also incorporates the use of local or regional analgesia to further decrease systemic drug side-effects. The use of local anesthetics (e.g. lidocaine) either locally or epidurally is another example of a multimodal approach that can result in significantly lower systemic drug requirements. For example, the use of a coccygeal epidural with lidocaine may allow better relaxation for urinary catheterization in cats with urethral obstruction, and require less systemic anesthesia [19].

The pharmacokinetics and pharmacodynamics of analgesic drugs, as well as the mechanism of action and associated side-effects, require careful consideration in emergency patients. Side-effects such as myocardial depression, decreased vasomotor tone, depressed mentation, impaired ventilation and respiratory drive, and prolonged duration of action (due to slower elimination because of metabolic dysfunction or organ hypoperfusion) are all possible in the critically ill patient. In addition, highly protein-bound drugs may have altered pharmacokinetics in patients with hypoalbuminemia. Hypothermic patients are more sensitive to the sedative and respiratory depressant effects of opioids and alpha-2 agonists [20]. The drugs of choice for the critically ill patient have predictable bioavailability, are reversible and titratable, and can be administered as a constant-rate infusion (CRI).

Analgesic Agents and Tranquilizers
(Figure 190.1)

Opioids are ideal analgesics for the critically ill patient; they are potent analgesics, are reversible (with the antagonist naloxone), provide variable duration of action (depending on the specific drug), and can be delivered as a CRI, facilitating fine-tuning of the medication dosage to achieve effective, individualized pain relief. Opioids have few cardiovascular side-effects, other than a vagally mediated bradycardia, which is most pronounced with the more potent opioids (e.g. fentanyl, remifentanil). Although respiratory depression is a major side-effect in human patients, gastrointestinal ileus and dysphoria are more common in veterinary species. Meperidine and morphine are associated with histamine release, which may cause decreased vasomotor tone. Some opioids

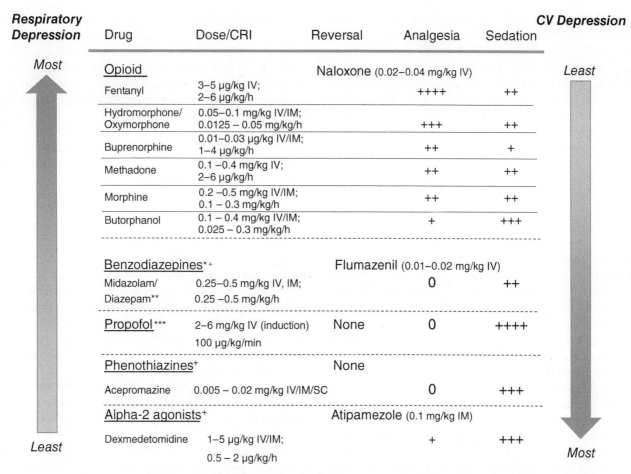

Figure 190.1 This chart demonstrates the relative sedative and analgesic qualities of various analgesic and anesthetic medications available for use in the ED. +Synergistic sedative effects when combined with an opioid. *Can cause CNS excitation if given alone. **Oral diazepam is associated with hepatic necrosis in cats, parenteral solution is hyperosmolar precluding long-term peripheral CRI infusion. ***Heinz body anemia can develop in cats after prolonged usage. CRI, constant-rate infusion; IM, intramuscular; IV, intravenous; SC, subcutaneous.

may cause emesis in dogs, and this should be taken into account in animals that present to the ED with ocular or head trauma, or with a history of vomiting. A CRI administration of fentanyl generally does not result in emesis, and is preferred in critically ill animals, as it may be easily titrated to an appropriate level of analgesia to minimize side-effects. Morphine may also be administered as a CRI. Morphine and butorphanol seem to have the most sedative effects of the opioids in dogs, and some clinicians prefer oxymorphone or methadone in cats because they may result in less excitement.

Benzodiazepines (e.g. diazepam, midazolam) are tranquilizers without analgesic properties that are used for anxiolysis and adjunctive sedation. Synergistic effects are achieved when these drugs are used in combination with opioids (neuroleptanalgesia). When given alone, these drugs can lead to unpredictable sedation or excitation. In the critical and emergent patient, benzodiazepines are

relatively safe with little cardiovascular and respiratory depression, are reversible (using flumazenil), and can be titrated and delivered as a CRI. Benzodiazepines are the drugs of choice for initial stabilization of patients with seizures (see Chapter 21 for additional information on seizure treatments).

Alpha-2 agonists (e.g. dexmedetomidine, xylazine) are tranquilizers that are generally avoided in patients with any cardiovascular instability, history of trauma, or other condition in which reduced tissue perfusion should be avoided. These drugs cause initial peripheral vasoconstriction and reflex bradycardia, which decrease cardiac output [21]. Alpha-2 agonists also increase urine output, and are relatively contraindicated in animals with urinary obstruction. These drugs do provide potent analgesia and are reversible (using atipamezole or yohimbine), but their use is restricted to cardiovascularly stable, otherwise healthy patients.

Phenothiazines (e.g. acepromazine, chlorproma-zine) should be avoided in animals with cardiovascular instability, as they are irreversible smooth muscle vasodilators (via alpha-1 antagonism) and can result in hypotension. Combined with opioids, acepromazine provides potent sedation, and this combination may be useful for sedation and anxiolysis of animals with upper airway obstruction or for sedation during short procedures.

The neuroleptic combination of an opioid and a tranquilizer is extremely important in the ED. Neuroleptanalgesia can provide sedation for brief procedures (e.g. radiography), premedication prior to anesthetic induction, and synergistic analgesia for treatment of painful conditions. The authors prefer a combination of opioid and benzodiazepine for this purpose, as they have minimal cardiorespiratory depression, and both are reversible. For more stable patients, the combination of an opioid and alpha-2 agonist provides potent sedation and analgesia that may be adequate to permit more painful procedures (e.g. splinting of fractured limbs, minor laceration repair). Hypoventilation may be more frequent using a combination of opioid and alpha-2 agonists.

Ketamine, an N-methyl-D-aspartate (NMDA) receptor antagonist, possesses moderate analgesic qualities. In addition, NMDA antagonists modulate pain at the level of the spinal cord, reducing central sensitization and wind-up. Analgesic and sedative effects are best achieved through combination with an opioid and/or benzodiazepine. Ketamine has dose-dependent sympathomimetic activity, so caution should be exercised and dose reduced in patients with cardiac disease or hypertension. Ketamine increases cerebral metabolic rate and is not recommended in patients who are or may be at risk of elevated intracranial pressure (e.g. traumatic brain injury). Ketamine causes a mild increase in intraocular pressure, which may become clinically significant in patients with ocular trauma or glaucoma [22]. Ketamine is also excreted unchanged in the urine in cats, and in situations such as a urinary blockage or urinary bladder rupture, prolonged sedation may be seen until the urine is removed from the body. The combination of low-dose ketamine in a CRI with a morphine and lidocaine has been described for both intraoperative and postoperative analgesia [23].

Non-steroidal anti-inflammatory drugs (NSAIDs) inhibit the cyclo-oxygenase enzyme, which produces prostaglandins from cell membrane arachidonic acid (AA) [24]. There are two main isoforms of cyclo-oxygenase (COX-1 and COX-2), producing prostaglandins for homeostasis (e.g. renal perfusion, mucosal blood flow; generally COX-1) and pain and inflammation (generally COX-2). NSAIDs can be non-specific or can have a more selective inhibition of the COX-2 enzyme. The COX-1 sparing NSAIDs, including carprofen, deracoxib, firocoxib, and meloxicam, inhibit some COX-1 activity, especially at high doses. NSAID side-effects can result in gastric ulceration, acute kidney injury, and platelet dysfunction. NSAIDs are contraindicated in dehydrated or hypovolemic patients, those with other organ dysfunction or co-morbidity, or those receiving other medications that can potentiate these effects (e.g. diuretics, nephrotoxic drugs, corticosteroids, other NSAIDs).

Induction Agents (see Figure 190.1)

Emergent intubation is frequently necessary in the ED. Induction drugs are generally given intravenously, resulting in rapid unconsciousness and allowing endotracheal intubation. With the exception of combinations involving ketamine or tiletamine, induction drugs are potent respiratory depressants and can result in hypotension from vasodilation. Although most induction agents provide rapid onset of anesthesia, they are not analgesic agents and should not be used as single agents for painful procedures. The combination of induction agents with neuroleptanalgesia can significantly decrease the necessary dose of induction agent for intubation, and thus decrease side-effects. This approach is recommended when intubation is necessary in unstable animals. Regardless of induction protocol, preoxygenation is recommended prior to drug administration.

Propofol is a short-acting intravenous drug that may be used for the induction and maintenance of anesthesia. In addition, it can be used as an adjunctive sedative agent in animals where a neuroleptic combination is not effective alone. Propofol administered as an IV bolus has more potent respiratory depressant and vasodilatory effects compared to its administration as a CRI. Propofol as a CRI may be used to control seizures in patients that are refractory to other therapies (see Chapter 21), and lower doses (e.g. 50–100 µg/kg/min) can be used to maintain sedation in some patients. Repeated administration of propofol can cause Heinz body anemia in cats, so prolonged usage should be avoided in this species. The benefits of anesthesia with propofol are that patients experience a rapid, smooth recovery; even those receiving long-term infusions of propofol recover relatively rapidly.

Alfaxalone is a synthetic neuroactive steroid that provides anesthesia and muscle relaxation and works in a similar matter to propofol for IV induction and maintenance of anesthesia. Alfaxalone may also be administered by an IM route. Combined with other medications, IM alfaxolone can induce anesthesia in dogs and cats [25,26].

Inhalant Anesthetics (see Figure 190.1)

In general, induction of anesthesia using inhaled agents (e.g. isoflurane, sevoflurane) is not recommended. The high doses required to induce anesthesia can result in significant hypotension and hypoventilation. In addition, the slower induction process may cause emesis during a period when the patient is unable to protect its airway, and may result in aspiration of gastrointestinal contents. In rare circumstances, very aggressive animals that must be anesthetized while breathing 100% oxygen may be induced with inhalant anesthetics. In practice, animals are placed in a plexiglass container that will allow observation during induction and into which gas and inhalant can be introduced and removed. Removal of the animal from the container will release a large amount of anesthetic into the room, and exposure of personnel should be minimized during this process. The use of a tight-fitting mask to induce anesthesia may cause stress to the animal, and carries with it the same risks of an unprotected airway, although it may be used in more tractable or sedated animals. Additional strategies for the aggressive ED patient are discussed in Chapter 199.

Conclusion

In the emergency patient, pain results from multiple pathologies, including trauma, illness, and surgery and, if left untreated, may exacerbate these same etiologies. Effective pre-emptive analgesia may mitigate central sensitization and the development of chronic pain. In humans, prompt delivery of appropriate opioid therapy to the acutely painful patient is a clinical indicator of the quality of emergency care [1,27].

Effective anesthesia and analgesia in the emergent patient relies on anticipation and prompt recognition with early and serial evaluation of pain. The use of scoring systems may make quantification of pain more practical. Analgesia should be tailored to the suspected etiology, duration, and severity of pain, taking into account the patient's overall status, history, and co-morbidities [28]. The use of neuroleptanalgesia can provide both synergistic analgesia and sedation for emergency procedures, and this and other multimodal therapeutic approaches should be employed in emergency patients.

References

1 Grant PS. Analgesia delivery in the ED. *Am J Emerg Med* 2006;24(7):806–809.

2 Stang AS, Hartling L, Fera C, Johnson D, Ali S. Quality indicators for the assessment and management of pain in the emergency department: a systematic review. *Pain Res Manag* 2014;19(6):e179–190.

3 Hansen K, Thom O, Rodda H, et al. Impact of pain location, organ system and treating speciality on timely delivery of analgesia in emergency departments. *Emerg Med Australas* 2012;24(1):64–71.

4 Hugonnard M, Leblond A, Keroack S, Cadore JL, Troncy E. Attitudes and concerns of French veterinarians towards pain and analgesia in dogs and cats. *Vet Anaesth Analg* 2004;31(3):154–163.

5 Barletta M, Young CN, Quandt JE, Hofmeister EH. Agreement between veterinary students and anesthesiologists regarding postoperative pain assessment in dogs. *Vet Anaesth Analg* 2016;43:91–98.

6 Firth AM, Haldane SL. Development of a scale to evaluate postoperative pain in dogs. *J Am Vet Med Assoc* 1999;214(5):651–659.

7 Brondani JT, Luna SP, Padovani CR. Refinement and initial validation of a multidimensional composite scale for use in assessing acute postoperative pain in cats. *Am J Vet Res* 2011;72(2):174–183.

8 Moran CE, Hofmeister EH. Prevalence of pain in a university veterinary intensive care unit. *J Vet Emerg Crit Care* 2013;23(1):29–36.

9 Wiese AJ, Muir WW 3rd, Wittum TE. Characteristics of pain and response to analgesic treatment in dogs and cats examined at a veterinary teaching hospital emergency service. *J Am Vet Med Assoc* 2005;226(12):2004–2009.

10 Dohoo SE, Dohoo IR. Factors influencing the postoperative use of analgesics in dogs and cats by Canadian veterinarians. *Can Vet J* 1996;37(9):552–556.

11 Dyson DH. Analgesia and chemical restraint for the emergent veterinary patient. *Vet Clin North Am Small Anim Pract* 2008;38(6):1329–1352, vii.

12 Manterola C, Astudillo P, Losada H, Pineda V, Sanhueza A, Vial M. Analgesia in patients with acute abdominal pain. *Cochrane Database Syst Rev* 2007;3:CD005660.

13 Brock N. Treating moderate and severe pain in small animals. *Can Vet J* 1995;36(10):658–660.

14 McGuire L, Heffner K, Glaser R, et al. Pain and wound healing in surgical patients. *Ann Behav Med* 2006;31(2):165–172.

15 Terkelsen AJ, Molgaard H, Hansen J, Andersen OK, Jensen TS. Acute pain increases HR: differential mechanisms during rest and mental stress. *Auton Neurosci* 2005;121(1–2):101–109.

16 Muir WW 3rd, Wiese AJ, Wittum TE. Prevalence and characteristics of pain in dogs and cats examined as outpatients at a veterinary teaching hospital. *J Am Vet Med Assoc* 2004;224(9):1459–1463.

17 Fosnocht DE, Swanson ER. Use of a triage pain protocol in the ED. *Am J Emerg Med* 2007;25(7):791–793.

18 Drendel AL, Brousseau DC, Gorelick MH. Pain assessment for pediatric patients in the emergency department. *Pediatrics* 2006;117(5):1511–1518.

19 O'Hearn AK, Wright BD. Coccygeal epidural with local anesthetic for catheterization and pain management in the treatment of feline urethral obstruction. *J Vet Emerg Crit Care* 2011;21(1):50–52.

20 Hansen B. Analgesia for the critically ill dog or cat: an update. *Vet Clin North Am Small Anim Pract* 2008;38(6):1353–1363, vii.

21 Kellihan HB, Stepien RL, Hassen KM, Smith LJ. Sedative and echocardiographic effects of dexmedetomidine combined with butorphanol in healthy dogs. J Vet Cardiol 2015;17(4):282–292.

22 Hofmeister EH, Mosunic CB, Torres BT, Ralph AG, Moore PA, Read MR. Effects of ketamine, diazepam, and their combination on intraocular pressures in clinically normal dogs. *Am J Vet Res* 2006;67(7):1136–1139.

23 Muir WW 3rd, Wiese AJ, March PA. Effects of morphine, lidocaine, ketamine, and morphine-lidocaine-ketamine drug combination on minimum alveolar concentration in dogs anesthetized with isoflurane. *Am J Vet Res* 2003;64(9):1155–1160.

24 Lascelles BD, McFarland JM, Swann H. Guidelines for safe and effective use of NSAIDs in dogs. *Vet Ther* 2005;6(3):237–251.

25 Rodrigo-Mocholi D, Belda E, Bosmans T, Laredo FG. Clinical efficacy and cardiorespiratory effects of intramuscular administration of alfaxalone alone or in combination with dexmedetomidine in cats. *Vet Anaesth Analg* 2016;43:291–300.

26 Tamura J, Ishizuka T, Fukui S, et al. The pharmacological effects of the anesthetic alfaxalone after intramuscular administration to dogs. *J Vet Med Sci* 2015;77(3):289–296.

27 Sokoloff C, Daoust R, Paquet J, Chauny JM. Is adequate pain relief and time to analgesia associated with emergency department length of stay? A retrospective study. *BMJ Open* 2014;4(3):e004288-2013-004288.

28 Epstein M, Rodan I, Griffenhagen G, et al. 2015 AAHA/AAFP Pain Management Guidelines for Dogs and Cats. *J Am Anim Hosp Assoc* 2015;51(2):67–84.

191

Anesthetic Concerns and Protocols for Common Conditions

Becca Reader, DVM and Amanda Abelson, DVM, DACVAA, DACVECC

Cummings School of Veterinary Medicine, Tufts University, North Grafton, MA, USA

Introduction

Prior to placing a patient under anesthesia, the clinician should obtain a minimum database that ideally consists of a packed cell volume (PCV), total protein, blood glucose, creatinine, electrolytes, lactate, and urine specific gravity. An ECG and blood pressure reading should also be obtained if indicated [1].

Before induction of anesthesia, it is highly recommended to have immediate vascular access via one or more peripheral venous catheters [1] (see Chapter 178) A laryngoscope and a range of appropriately sized endotracheal tubes should also be readily available. Many emergency patients present with a full stomach and are at risk of aspiration if they vomit or regurgitate and their airway is not adequately protected [1]. See Table 191.1 for an overview of recommendations for specific conditions.

Dystocia/Cesarean Section

(see Chapter 118)

Anesthetic protocols for cesarean section must take both the dam and neonates into consideration. Maternal lethargy and decreased neonatal vitality during the immediate postoperative period can result in decreased colostrum intake and increased neonatal mortality. Ideal protocols utilize drugs with minimal respiratory, cardiovascular, and central nervous system depression [2].

Anesthetic Concerns

Dam

- Animals that have been in active labor for a prolonged period of time may suffer from hypoglycemia and/or hypocalcemia and may require supplementation prior to anesthesia [3].

- Pregnant animals are at increased risk for regurgitation and aspiration due to a progesterone-induced decrease in lower esophageal sphincter tone and prolonged gastric emptying times [4].
- High levels of progesterone result in a 16–40% decrease in the minimum alveolar concentration (MAC) of inhalant anesthetics [3].
- The gravid uterus reduces the dam's functional residual capacity (FRC) and oxygen reserve within the lungs. This, combined with an increase in oxygen consumption associated with pregnancy, can result in hypoxemia during even short periods of apnea [3].
- Ventilation and venous return may be impeded when the dam is placed in dorsal recumbency.

Neonate
- All anesthetic drugs including inhalants cross the placental barrier, resulting in a variable amount of neonatal depression [2].
- Fetal blood flow is entirely dependent on maternal cardiac output. Anything that decreases uterine arterial flow will decrease fetal oxygen and nutrient delivery [3].
- Respiratory depression is of extreme concern in the neonate as even small changes in tidal volume and respiratory rate can result in hypoxemia [3].

Protocols

A primary goal of anesthesia for cesarean section is to minimize fetal concentrations of anesthetic drugs with respiratory, cardiovascular or central nervous system depression. Drugs that can be antagonized are ideal choices because they can be reversed in neonates after delivery [3].

Most animals undergo cesarean section without premedication, as most sedatives and tranquilizers have cardiovascular and respiratory side-effects that have been shown to increase fetal mortality. Alpha-2 agonists,

Table 191.1 Anesthetic protocols for common emergencies. Doses reflect those commonly used at Cummings School of Veterinary Medicine.

Anesthetic emergency	Premedication	Induction	Maintenance	Postoperative
Dystocia/ C-section Cat and dog	None	Propofol 6 mg/kg IV to effect Alfaxalone 1.5 mg/kg (dog), 3 mg/kg (cat) IV to effect	Isoflurane or sevoflurane Incisional block with lidocaine (1 mg/kg) and bupivacaine (1 mg/kg) Buprenorphine (0.01 mg/kg) IV after delivery	**Cat** Meloxicam 0.1 mg/kg SC once **Dog** Carprofen 2.2 mg/kg SC once Or Meloxicam 0.1 mg/kg SC once
Enucleation Cat and dog	**Opioid:** fentanyl (3–5 μg/kg), hydromorphone (0.1 mg/kg), methadone (0.3–0.5 mg), IM or IV **Phenothiazine (otherwise healthy):** acepromazine (0.01–0.05 mg/kg) IM/IV **Benzodiazepine (sick/debilitated):** midazolam (0.1–0.2 mg/kg) IV/IM, diazepam (0.1–0.2 mg/kg) IV **Anticholinergic:** atropine (0.02 mg/kg) or glycopyrrolate (0.01 mg/kg) IM/IV	Propofol 4 mg/kg IV to effect Alfaxalone 1.5 mg/kg (dog), 3 mg/kg (cat) IV to effect	Isoflurane or sevoflurane Lidocaine CRI (50 μg/kg/min, dogs only) Ketamine CRI (0.6 mg/kg/h)	**Cat** Buprenorphine (0.01 mg/kg) IV Meloxicam 0.1 mg/kg SC once **Dog** Buprenorphine (0.01 mg/kg) IV Carprofen 2.2 mg/kg SC Or Meloxicam 0.1 mg/kg SQ
Foreign body Cat and dog	**Opioid:** fentanyl (3–5 μg/kg), hydromorphone (0.1 mg/kg), methadone (0.3–0.5 mg), IM or IV **Phenothiazine (otherwise healthy):** acepromazine (0.01–0.05 mg/kg) IM/IV **Benzodiazepine (sick/debilitated):** midazolam (0.1–0.2 mg/kg) IV/IM, diazepam (0.1–0.2 mg/kg) IV	Ketamine (5.5 mg/kg) IV with diazepam or midazolam (0.28 mg/kg) IV to effect Propofol 4 mg/kg IV to effect Alfaxalone 1.5 mg/kg (dog), 3 mg/kg (cat) IV to effect	Isoflurane or sevoflurane +/– fentanyl CRI (0.1–0.5 μg/kg/min) Lidocaine CRI (50 μg/kg/min, dogs only) Ketamine CRI (0.6 mg/kg/h)	Continue pure mu-agonist opioid intermittently *or* fentanyl CRI (1–3 μg/kg/h) IV
Gastric dilation-volvulus Dog	**Opioid:** fentanyl (3–5 μg/kg), hydromorphone (0.1 mg/kg), methadone (0.3–0.5 mg), IM or IV +/–**Benzodiazepine** midazolam (0.1–0.2 mg/kg) IV/IM, diazepam (0.1–0.2 mg/kg) IV	Ketamine (5.5 mg/kg) IV with diazepam or midazolam (0.28 mg/kg) IV to effect **Recumbent/ debilitated:** Fentanyl (3 μg/kg) IV Midazolam (0.1 mg/kg) IV Ketamine (2 mg/kg) IV	Isoflurane or sevoflurane Fentanyl CRI (0.1–0.5 μg/kg/min) IV Lidocaine CRI (50 μg/kg/min, dogs only) IV Ketamine CRI (0.6 mg/kg/h) IV	Continue pure mu-agonist opioid intermittently *or* fentanyl CRI (1–3 μg/kg/h) IV

Condition	Premedication	Induction	Maintenance	Postoperative
Hemoabdomen **Dog**	**Opioid**: fentanyl (3–5 µg/kg), hydromorphone (0.1 mg/kg), methadone (0.3–0.5 mg), IM or IV +/– **Benzodiazepine** midazolam (0.1–0.2 mg/kg) IV/IM, diazepam (0.1–0.2 mg/kg) IV	Ketamine (5.5 mg/kg) IV with diazepam *or* midazolam (0.28 mg/kg) IV to effect **Recumbent/debilitated:** Fentanyl (3 µg/kg) IV Midazolam (0.1 mg/kg) IV Ketamine (2 mg/kg) IV	Isoflurane or sevoflurane Fentanyl CRI (0.1–0.5 µg/kg/min) IV Lidocaine CRI (50 µg/kg/min, dogs only) IV Ketamine CRI (0.6 mg/kg/h) IV	Continue pure mu-agonist opioid intermittently *or* fentanyl CRI (1–3 µg/kg/h) IV
Major wounds **Cat and dog**	**Opioid**: fentanyl (3–5 µg/kg), hydromorphone (0.1 mg/kg), methadone (0.3–0.5 mg), IM or IV **Otherwise healthy**: acepromazine (0.01–0.05 mg/kg) IM/IV *or* Dexmedetomidine (1–5 µg/kg) IM or IV **Sick/debilitated:** midazolam (0.1–0.2 mg/kg) IV or IM, diazepam (0.1–0.2 mg/kg) IV	Ketamine (5.5 mg/kg) IV with diazepam *or* midazolam (0.28 mg/kg) IV to effect Propofol 4 mg/kg IV to effect Alfaxalone 1.5 mg/kg (dog), 3 mg/kg (cat) IV to effect	Isoflurane or sevoflurane Lidocaine CRI (50 µg/kg/min, dogs only) IV Ketamine CRI (0.6 mg/kg/h) IV	**Cat** Continue pure mu-agonist opioid intermittently Meloxicam 0.1 mg/kg SC once *or* Robenacoxib (1 mg/kg) PO for 3 days **Dog** Continue pure mu-agonist opioid intermittently Carprofen 2.2 mg/kg SC *or* Meloxicam 0.1 mg/kg SC
Pacemaker **Dog**	**Opioid**: fentanyl (3–5 µg/kg), hydromorphone (0.1 mg/kg), methadone (0.3–0.5 mg), IM or IV +/–**Benzodiazepine** midazolam (0.1–0.2 mg/kg) IV/IM, diazepam (0.1–0.2 mg/kg) IV	**Significant heart disease/failure:** Diazepam (0.1 mg/kg) IV followed by Etomidate (1 mg/kg) IV to effect **Minimal heart disease:** Propofol 4 mg/kg IV to effect Alfaxalone 1.5 mg/kg (dog) IV to effect	Isoflurane or sevoflurane	Buprenorphine (0.01 mg/kg) IV
Urethral obstruction **Dog**	**Opioid**: fentanyl (3–5 µg/kg), hydromorphone (0.1 mg/kg), methadone (0.3–0.5 mg), IM or IV +/–**Benzodiazepine** midazolam (0.1–0.2 mg/kg) IV/IM, diazepam (0.1–0.2 mg/kg) IV	Propofol 4 mg/kg IV to effect Alfaxalone 1.5 mg/kg (dog) IV to effect	Isoflurane or sevoflurane	Buprenorphine (0.01 mg/kg) IV Carprofen 2.2 mg/kg SC *or* Meloxicam 0.1 mg/kg SC

CRI, constant-rate infusion; IM, intramuscular; IV, intravenous; PO, by mouth (*per os*); SC, subcutaneous.

particularly xylazine, should be avoided due to their association with decreased fetal survival [4]. In calm patients, intravenous catheter placement, as well as the initial clip and surgical prep, should take place prior to administration of anesthetic medications.

Due to the increased risk for regurgitation and aspiration, patients should be induced in sternal recumbency with their head elevated. Propofol and alfaxalone are ideal induction agents due to their short half-life and rapid metabolism. An incisional line block with lidocaine and bupivacaine prior to surgery can decrease response to surgical stimulation, as well as providing some intra- and postoperative analgesia [4].

It is important to avoid excessive concentrations of inhalants to minimize neonatal apnea. Inhalant anesthetics readily cross the placenta, but are rapidly cleared as long as the neonate is breathing shortly after delivery.

Buprenorphine can be administered IV or IM to the dam for pain control following delivery. Buprenorphine is selected over other opioids due to its long duration of action and minimal cardiovascular and respiratory side-effects [3]. As long as preoperative laboratory testing is normal, and mean arterial blood pressures remain greater than 60 mmHg during surgery, a single dose of carprofen or meloxicam will provide additional analgesia for the dam [4]. This opioid and postoperative NSAID combination typically provides adequate analgesia for the dam, and has minimal likelihood of interfering with her ability to care for the newborns.

Enucleation/Proptosis

Proptosis and other ocular conditions prompting emergent enucleation are typically caused by trauma. As a result, the patient should be thoroughly assessed for concurrent life-threatening injuries prior to being placed under anesthesia and an appropriate minimum database should be obtained [4].

Anesthetic Concerns

- Pressure or manipulation of the globe during surgery may elicit the oculocardiac reflex. This reflex is mediated by the trigeminal and vagus nerves, and can result in the development of dysrhythmias such as bradycardia, ventricular ectopy or asystole [3].
- Most anesthetic drugs do not affect or even decrease intraocular pressure (IOP) but common side-effects, such as vomiting, can result in a transient increase in IOP.
- Stimulation of the larynx and pharynx during intubation can transiently increase IOP [3].
- Enucleation is a painful procedure and appropriate analgesics should be administered.

Protocols

Patients with ocular trauma should be handled carefully, as even routine physical restraint or inadvertent pressure on the jugular veins can increase IOP. Intravenous catheter placement in a hindlimb may be less stressful on the patient and will also provide easier access for drug administration during the procedure.

Premedication should include an opioid in combination with a benzodiazepine or phenothiazine administered IV or IM. An anticholinergic (i.e. glycopyrrolate or atropine) can also be included in the premedication to reduce the risk of the oculocardiac reflex during surgery [4]. Induction with propofol or alfaxalone will allow for a smooth, rapid intubation. Maintenance of anesthesia can be achieved with an inhalant gas such as isoflurane or sevoflurane.

Heart rate should be monitored closely during the procedure. If there is any concern for initiation of the oculocardiac reflex, the surgeon should be asked to stop the procedure and atropine should be administered IV immediately.

Following surgery, any animal that is dysphoric can be given low-dose acepromazine or dexmedetomidine. This will provide mild sedation and help reduce the possibility of trauma to the surgical site [4]. Postoperative analgesia consists of an opioid and an NSAID to reduce swelling and pain at the surgical site [4].

Foreign Body (Esophageal, Gastric, Intestinal)

Patients with gastrointestinal foreign bodies often present with a history of vomiting, anorexia, and abdominal discomfort. These animals are typically dehydrated due to frequent vomiting and decreased fluid intake.

Preoperative laboratory testing should include a chemistry panel and complete blood count (CBC), as gastrointestinal disease often results in electrolyte and acid–base disturbances. The most common abnormalities seen include a hypochloremic metabolic alkalosis with low serum potassium values, due to loss of gastric contents secondary to vomiting (see Chapter 74). Additional laboratory testing may show evidence of dehydration, with elevated PCV, total protein, BUN, and creatinine concentrations [3].

Fluid deficits and electrolyte abnormalities should ideally be corrected with intravenous administration of balanced electrolyte solutions prior to the induction of anesthesia but with severe obstructions, chloride abnormities cannot be resolved until the obstruction is removed (see Chapter 167). Because hypokalemia can result in muscle weakness, decreased GI motility and cardiac arrhythmias, severe cases should be corrected with the intravenous administration of potassium chloride at a rate no greater than 0.5 mEq/kg/hr [3] (see Chapter 109).

Anesthetic Concerns

- Patients with gastrointestinal foreign bodies should be assumed to have a full stomach, making rapid airway capture a priority at induction in order to prevent aspiration of stomach contents.
- Body heat is rapidly lost from exposed viscera during abdominal surgery which may result in hypothermia and decreased inhalant requirements.
- For endoscopy, opioids and atropine may increase pyloric sphincter tone, making it difficult to pass the endoscope into the proximal duodenum [3].
- Overinsufflation of the stomach during endoscopy can result in decreased venous return, as well as vasovagal stimulation and bradycardia [3].

Protocols

Animals presenting for exploratory laparotomy should be premedicated with a pure mu-agonist opioid for its analgesic and MAC-sparing properties. A preanesthetic sedative may also be administered, depending on the attitude of the patient. Debilitated patients can be given a benzodiazepine and opioid combination prior to induction. More stable patients can be given low-dose acepromazine in combination with an opioid. Acepromazine is an excellent anxiolytic with central antiemetic properties, but should not be administered to dehydrated or hypovolemic patients [3].

Ketamine in combination with a benzodiazepine is an excellent induction agent for exploratory laparotomies, especially in hemodynamically compromised patients [3]. Ketamine acts as a sympathomimetic, providing cardiovascular support as well as somatic analgesia. In hemodynamically stable patients, propofol or alfaxalone are suitable alternatives, keeping in mind that neither drug provides additional analgesia.

Maintenance of anesthesia can be achieved via inhalant anesthetics such as isoflurane or sevoflurane. Nitrous oxide is contraindicated because it rapidly diffuses into gas-filled compartments, resulting in an increased volume of air trapped in the viscera [3]. For hemodynamically compromised patients, inhalant concentrations should be kept as low as possible with the use of multimodal techniques such as lidocaine, ketamine, and/or fentanyl continuous rate infusions.

Postoperative pain can be managed with intermittent dosing of a pure mu-agonist opioid or a constant-rate infusion (CRI) of an opioid. NSAIDs are contraindicated for analgesia in patients with gastrointestinal disease due to their effects on intestinal blood flow and association with gastric ulceration [3].

Gastric Dilation-Volvulus (see Chapter 82)

Gastric dilation-volvulus (GDV) is an acute, life-threatening disorder caused by distension of the stomach accompanied by a 90–360° rotation on its mesenteric axis, resulting in complete gastric outflow obstruction. Dogs with GDV often present with acute onset of abdominal distension accompanied with abdominal pain and non-productive retching. These cases can present in multiple types of shock, including obstructive, hypovolemic, and distributive [1] (see Chapter 152).

Anesthetic Concerns

- Extreme gastric distension and increased intra-abdominal pressure can compress the caudal vena cava, portal vein, and splanchnic vasculature, resulting in significant impairment of venous return to the heart [3].
- Gastric distension also prevents caudal displacement of the diaphragm, resulting in decreased pulmonary compliance and functional residual capacity [3].
- Cardiac arrhythmias are common and can include sinus tachycardia, and ventricular tachycardia [3].
- Splenomegaly can occur secondary to displacement by the rotated stomach.
- Hemoabdomen and accompanying anemia may occur as a result of tearing of the short gastric vessels [3].
- GDV is considered a painful condition and analgesics should be administered as part of the initial therapy.

Protocols

Patients with GDV require aggressive fluid resuscitation, the details of which are beyond the scope of this chapter and are discussed elsewhere (see Chapter 153) At least two large-bore catheters should be placed in both cephalic veins, or one cephalic vein and a jugular vein. Gastric decompression by trocarization or orogastric tube placement should be performed prior to induction in order to optimize cardiac output.

A pure mu-opioid, alone or in combination with a benzodiazepine, can be used as a premedication or to facilitate gastric decompression. Full mu-agonists are the drug of choice because of their MAC-sparing effects and minimal cardiovascular effects. Fentanyl, methadone, hydromorphone or oxymorphone administered IV may be less likely to cause nausea compared to other mu-agonists such as morphine [1].

Ketamine in combination with a benzodiazepine is recommended for induction in patients without significant arrhythmias or cardiovascular disease. Depressed or recumbent patients may be induced with a combination of fentanyl-midazolam-ketamine. Propofol is a less ideal induction agent in this patient population due to the potential for significant hypotension following IV administration.

Maintenance of anesthesia can be achieved via inhalant anesthetics such as isoflurane or sevoflurane. Nitrous oxide is contraindicated prior to gastric decompression because it rapidly diffuses into gas-filled compartments, resulting in organ distension and increasing intragastric volume [3]. Because inhalant anesthetics cause dose-dependent vasodilation and myocardial depression, their maintenance concentrations during surgery should be decreased as much as possible by the use of multimodal anesthetic techniques. A CRI of fentanyl or morphine may be used intraoperatively for their inhalant-sparing effects as well as additional analgesia. Lidocaine plus ketamine CRIs will provide multimodal analgesia, as well as further reducing the amount of inhalant anesthetic required. Lidocaine has the additional benefit of preventing or reducing the severity of ventricular arrhythmias [3].

An attempt should be made to place an arterial catheter in the dorsal pedal artery for invasive blood pressure monitoring, as many dogs with GDV are hypotensive (see Chapter 178). However, this attempt should not delay surgery. Fluid therapy during anesthesia should be continuously reassessed and modified on the basis of parameters such as blood pressure, PCV, total protein concentrations, heart rate, and lactate concentrations. Hypertonic saline, colloids, and blood products should be available in case hypotension refractory to isotonic crystalloid therapy occurs, or excessive bleeding and coagulopathy develop [3] (see Section 5). If necessary, inotropic drugs such as dopamine and dobutamine can be administered to maintain mean arterial pressures above 60 mmHg. In patients with hypotension refractory to fluid therapy and inotropic support, administration of vasopressor drugs such as norepinephrine, phenylephrine or vasopressin may be necessary [3].

Hemoabdomen (see Chapter 84)

Patients with a hemoabdomen often present in hypovolemic shock. Prior to undergoing anesthesia, these animals should be stabilized with administration of intravenous crystalloid solutions, hypertonic saline, and/or colloids (see Chapter 153). Resuscitation goals should include a heart rate below 150 bpm, systolic blood pressure greater than 90 mmHg, and PCV/TS of 20% and 4 g/dL, respectively, in conjunction with a decreasing lactate [4]. If blood loss exceeds 20% of the patient's estimated blood volume, or if the PCV is less than 20%, whole blood or packed RBC should be administered [4] (see Chapters 176 and 177).

Anesthetic Concerns

- The combination of pre-existing hypovolemia and administration of anesthetic agents that cause vasodilation can result in a profound hypotension.
- Cardiac arrhythmias are common and can include sinus tachycardia, and ventricular tachycardia (see Chapter 53).
- Until the source of bleeding is controlled, ongoing blood loss can occur.

Protocols

The same anesthetic protocols outlined for GDV patients apply.

Major Wounds (see Chapter 166)

Wounds that require repair under general anesthesia in the emergency room are typically the result of trauma. These patients may have severe tissue injury, inflammation, and potentially hemorrhage. Trauma patients may present in a state of shock, and stabilization prior to undergoing anesthesia is essential. Diagnostic imaging should also be performed to look for communication of wounds with the abdomen or thorax, or concurrent conditions such as pneumothorax or intracavitary effusion [3].

Anesthetic Concerns

- Pain associated with trauma is complex and can have effects on the cardiovascular and neuroendocrine systems as well as wound healing.

Protocols

Animals presenting for wound repair should be premedicated with a pure mu-agonist opioid for its analgesic and MAC-sparing properties. A preanesthetic sedative may also be administered depending on the attitude of the patient. Debilitated patients can be given a benzodiazepine and opioid combination prior to induction. More stable patients can be administered acepromazine or an alpha-2 agonist in combination with an opioid.

Ketamine in combination with a benzodiazepine is an excellent induction agent for wound repairs, as ketamine provides analgesia to the skin and muscular tissue. Propofol or alfaxalone are suitable alternatives, although neither drug provides additional analgesia to the patient.

Maintenance of anesthesia can be achieved via inhalant anesthetics such as isoflurane or sevoflurane. Whenever possible, regional anesthetic techniques with lidocaine or bupivacaine should be used to provide analgesia and reduce the amount of inhalant required [3]. Postoperative pain can be managed with the combination of an opioid and an NSAID to reduce swelling and pain at the surgical site [4].

Pacemaker

The most common reason patients present for emergency pacemaker placement is for bradyarrhythmias such as AV block (see Chapter 53). AV block is defined as the prolongation or intermittent failure of transmission of atrial depolarization through the AV node to the ventricles. First-degree AV block involves slowed conduction of depolarization through the AV node, visible as a prolongation of the P-R interval on the ECG. Second-degree AV block is characterized by intermittent failure of atrial depolarization to be conducted through the AV node, visible as one or more isolated P-waves that are not followed by a QRS complex [3].

Third-degree AV block is complete failure of AV nodal conduction and subsequent dissociation of the atria and ventricles. This is visible on an ECG as regular P-wave generation at normal sinus rate, and a ventricular escape rhythm (30–50 bpm in dogs, 60–80 bpm in cats) that has no association with the P-waves [3]. Typically, only "high-grade" second-degree and third-degree AV blocks require placement of a permanent ventricular pacemaker.

Anesthetic Concerns

- Patients with AV block already have reduced cardiac output, increasing their risk of hypotension under anesthesia.
- Introduction of the catheter and pacemaker into the heart may trigger arrhythmias.

Protocols

Animals presenting for placement of a permanent ventricular pacemaker should have temporary transthoracic pacing pads applied prior to premedication, in case drug administration results in a more severe bradycardia.

Pacemaker patients should be premedicated with a pure mu-agonist opioid for its analgesic and MAC-sparing properties. A benzodiazepine may be administered along with the opioid, depending on the temperament of the patient, and for additional MAC-sparing effects.

If there is concern for significant heart disease and/or heart failure, etomidate in combination with a benzodiazepine is the induction agent of choice. If there is no evidence of significant heart disease, propofol or alfaxalone are suitable alternatives for induction. Maintenance of anesthesia can be achieved via inhalant anesthetics such as isoflurane or sevoflurane. Arrhythmias associated with introduction of transvenous catheters or the pacemaker itself can be treated with an IV bolus of lidocaine (2 mg/kg). However, it is important that the ventricular escape beats not be confused for arrhythmias, as their suppression can result in cardiac arrest. If necessary, inotropic drugs such as dopamine or dobutamine can be administered to maintain mean arterial pressures above 60 mmHg. Postoperative pain can be managed with an opioid such as buprenorphine.

Urethral Obstruction (Canine)

Dogs presenting for urethral obstruction typically require general anesthesia for placement of a urinary catheter, since blockage usually occurs from cystic or urethral calculi. Prior to anesthesia, the patient's hydration status and electrolyte values (particularly potassium) should be assessed and abnormalities treated with IV fluids if necessary [4] (see Chapter 109).

For significant hyperkalemia (potassium > 7.5 mEq/L), calcium gluconate and dextrose (+/− regular insulin) should be administered for patient stabilization. Calcium gluconate does not directly influence serum potassium levels but stabilizes cell membranes and helps minimize cardiotoxic effects of hyperkalemia. Dextrose induces the endogenous release of insulin, which aids in the translocation of potassium out of the bloodstream and into cells. Regular insulin may also be administered in conjunction with dextrose, but requires close monitoring of the patient's blood glucose for signs of hypoglycemia [4]. Other treatment options indicated for persistent life-threatening hyperkalemia include sodium bicarbonate and beta-2 agonists.

Anesthetic Concerns

- Hyperkalemia influences the electrical excitability of the heart, and can result in bradyarrhythmias and ultimately cardiac arrest.
- Elevated serum potassium levels can be exacerbated with hypoventilation and respiratory acidosis [4].

Protocols

Dogs with urethral obstruction should be premedicated with a mu-agonist opioid for its analgesic and MAC-sparing properties. A short-acting induction agent such as propofol or alfaxalone is recommended, given that urethral catheterization should not take long once the patient is anesthetized. Maintenance of anesthesia can be achieved via inhalant anesthetics such as isoflurane or sevoflurane. Intermittent positive pressure ventilation to normocapnia ($PaCO_2$ 35–45 mmHg) should be implemented in order to prevent exacerbation of hyperkalemia by respiratory acidosis [4]. In dogs without evidence of acute or chronic kidney disease, NSAIDs can be administered postoperatively for pain management and to decrease urethral inflammation [4].

References

1 Campbell VL. Anesthetic protocols for common emergencies. *Vet Clin North Am Small Anim Pract* 2005;352005:435–453.

2 Doebeli A, Michel A, Bettschart R, et al. Apgar score after induction of anesthesia for canine caesarian section with alfaxalone versus propofol. *Theriogenology* 2013;80:850–854.

3 Snyder L, Johnson R. *Canine and Feline Anesthesia and Co-Existing Disease.* John Wiley and Sons, Chichester, 2014.

4 Cummings K, Wetmore L. Top 5 emergencies requiring anesthesia. Clinician's Brief, 2014. Available at: www.cliniciansbrief.com/article/top-5-emergencies-requiring-anesthesia (accessed 19 February 2018).

192

Sedation for the Emergency Room Patient

Stephanie R. Krein, DVM, DACVAA

Angell Animal Medical Center, Boston, MA, USA

Introduction

Emergency room clinicians commonly examine and treat animals presenting with injuries or underlying conditions requiring sedation. These animals may be painful, anxious or aggressive and may have underlying co-morbidities, making the choice of drugs used important. Unfortunately, sedation in the ER is not a one-size-fits-all scenario as one drug may be safe for one patient but may cause severe cardiovascular compromise in another. For this reason, it is important that clinicians be familiar with the pharmacology of the commonly used analgesics and sedatives and aware of the indications and contraindications for each drug.

In addition to understanding the pharmacology of the sedatives, it is important that the patient be appropriately monitored, oxygen be provided, and the patient's airway be protected when indicated. When using heavy sedation, one should always be prepared to intubate and have all necessary equipment ready, including a laryngoscope, induction agent, endotracheal tubes, and means to supply positive pressure ventilation. Monitoring during sedation procedures should include all standard monitors including end-tidal carbon dioxide (if intubated), pulse oximeter, ECG, and blood pressure. Pulse oximetry provides valuable information such as pulse rate and oxygenation, as well as an idea of whether the cardiac rhythm is normal. If at any time the oxygenation decreases or hypoventilation occurs, the patient should be intubated immediately.

Healthy Dog/Cat Emergencies

Examples of patients presenting as systemically healthy emergencies include simple laceration repairs, fractures/luxations, fractious cat examination, urinary tract issues, or patients presenting for diagnostic imaging such as radiographs or ultrasound. These patients are physiologically normal but need sedation to either diagnose or treat the presenting disease/injury.

Several different drug protocols may be chosen and used in healthy dogs and cats and should be designed based on the amount of pain expected from the procedure, the length of procedure, and the degree of sedation required. The attending clinician should evaluate the need for presedation bloodwork and treat any suspected underlying issues or electrolyte abnormalities prior to sedation.

Dog: Fast, Non-Painful Procedure (Radiographs, Blood Draws, Small Laceration Repair)

- Option 1: Butorphanol (0.2–0.4 mg/kg)+with dexmedetomidine (3–7 µg/kg)+/– midazolam (0.2–0.3 mg/kg) or ketamine (2–3 mg/kg) IM
- Option 2: Butorphanol with either acepromazine (0.02–0.05 mg/kg)+/– ketamine (3–5 mg/kg) IM
- Option 3: Butorphanol+midazolam+alfaxalone (1–2 mg/kg) IM

Cat: Fast, Non-Painful Procedure (Fractious Cat Exam, Radiographs, Blood Draws)

- Option 1: Butorphanol (0.3–0.4 mg/kg) with dexmedetomidine (5–7 µg/kg)+/– midazolam (0.3 mg/kg) or ketamine (3–5 mg/kg) IM
- Option 2: Butorphanol with either midazolam (0.2–0.3 mg/kg) or dexmedetomidine (3–5 µg/kg)+alfaxalone (1–2 mg/kg) IM

Healthy Dog: Painful Procedure (e.g. Aural Hematoma, Laceration Repair, Fracture Stabilization, Closed Hip Reduction)

- Option 1: Full mu-opioid+dexmedetomidine+/–midazolam OR ketamine IM
- Option 2: Full mu-opioid+acepromazine+/– ketamine IM

Textbook of Small Animal Emergency Medicine, First Edition. Edited by Kenneth J. Drobatz, Kate Hopper, Elizabeth Rozanski and Deborah C. Silverstein.
© 2019 John Wiley & Sons, Inc. Published 2019 by John Wiley & Sons, Inc.
Companion Website: www.wiley.com/go/drobatz/textbook

- Option 3: Full mu-opioid+midazolam+/− alfaxalone IM
- Option 4: Any of the above combinations+propofol sedation

Healthy Cat: Painful Procedure (Laceration Repair, Fracture Stabilization, Closed Hip Reduction)

- Option 1: Full mu-opioid with dexmedetomidine (5–10 µg/kg)+/− midazolam (0.3 mg/kg) or ketamine (3–5 mg/kg) IM
- Option 2: Full mu-opioid with either midazolam (0.2–0.3 mg/kg) or dexmedetomidine (3–5 µg/kg)+alfaxalone (1–2 mg/kg) IM
- Option 3: Buprenorphine (0.015–0.02 mg/kg)+dexmedetomidine (5–10 µg/kg)+/− ketamine (3–5 mg/kg) IM
- Option 4: Any of the above combinations+alfaxalone OR propofol sedation

Rapid Sedation For Upper Airway Obstruction/ Respiratory Compromise

Intubation and oxygen supplementation must be provided.

- Option 1: Butorphanol (0.2–0.3 mg/kg)+midazolam (0.2–0.3 mg/kg)+/− alfaxalone (1 mg/kg) IM
- Option 2: Butorphanol (0.1–0.2 mg/kg)+propofol (2–4 mg/kg) IV
- Option 3: Butorphanol+mixture of 2 mg/kg ketamine and 2 mg/kg propofol ("ketafol") IV

Sedation Protocols for Brachycephalic Dogs

Brachycephalics are at increased risk for upper airway obstruction, regurgitation, and aspiration pneumonia than their dolichocephalic counterparts. It is for this reason that *intubation is recommended* to provide airway protection and oxygen supplementation.

Non-Painful Procedures
Intubation highly recommended.

- Option 1: Butorphanol (0.2–0.3 mg/kg)+dexmedetomidine (3–5 µg/kg) IM OR acepromazine (0.02–0.03 mg/kg) IM+propofol (2–4 mg/kg) IV to effect
- Option 2: Substitute alfaxalone (1–2 mg/kg) for propofol in above combinations

Painful Procedures
Intubation highly recommended.

- Option 1: Methadone (0.2–0.3 mg/kg)+dexmedetomidine (3–5 µg/kg) OR acepromazine (0.02–0.03 mg/kg) IM+propofol to effect or ketafol to effect

Table 192.1 Full mu-opioid doses.

Drug	Dose range (mg/kg)
Hydromorphone	0.1 IM; 0.05 IV
Oxymorphone	0.1 IM; 0.05 IV
Methadone	0.3–0.5 IM; 0.1–0.2 IV
Morphine	0.5 IM
Fentanyl	3–5 µg/kg IV

- Option 2: Oxymorphone (0.1 mg/kg)+dexmedetomidine OR acepromazine IM+propofol OR ketafol to effect
- Option 3: Substitute alfaxalone for propofol OR ketafol in above combinations

Geriatric, Debilitated, or Hemodynamically Unstable Cat or Dog Emergencies

It is common for sick, weak, debilitated, hemodynamically unstable patients to present to the ER in need of diagnostics to aid in the proper recognition and treatment of their disease. Common presenting signs include uncontrolled hemorrhage, respiratory distress, pericardial effusion, traumatic injury, seizure activity, arrhythmias, etc. These patients need sedation protocols that will not depress their cardiac output, worsen bleeding, depress respiratory drive, or worsen seizure activity. One should always be prepared to emergently intubate these patients and reversal agents should be easily accessible.

The following protocols can be used for these patients.

- Option 1: Butorphanol (0.1–0.15 mg/kg)+midazolam (0.1–0.3 mg/kg) IV
- Option 2: Full mu-opioid (Table 192.1)+midazolam (0.1–0.3 mg/kg) IV
- Option 3: Butorphanol (0.2–0.3 mg/kg)+midazolam (0.2 mg/kg)+alfaxalone (1–2 mg/kg) IM if unable to place intravenous catheter

Sedation Agents

Opioids

Butorphanol is a mu-opioid receptor antagonist and a kappa-opioid receptor agonist used in non-painful procedures or to achieve sedation [1,2]. It is often used in animals with cardiac disease due to its lack of significant cardiovascular depression, wide therapeutic window, and short duration of action [3]. Butorphanol should not be used in painful procedures as it has been shown in several studies to be a poor analgesic drug [1,4,5].

Buprenorphine is a partial mu-opioid agonist used to provide analgesia in moderate-to-severe pain. It is commonly used in cats as it provides good analgesia with less dysphoria and hyperthermia than full mu-opioid agonists [1,6].

Full mu-opioid agonists include oxymorphone, hydromorphone, fentanyl, methadone, and morphine. These drugs are agonists at both mu-opioid and kappa-opioid receptors and exert maximal clinical response when bound to these receptors. All full mu-agonists cause centrally mediated, vagally induced bradycardia, although drugs such as methadone may do so to a greater degree than others such as morphine [7,8]. Other side-effects of full mu-agonists in dogs include panting, dysphoria, ileus, vomiting, sedation, hypothermia, miosis, respiratory depression and reduced response to carbon dioxide, and defecation [9–11]. Side-effects are similar in cats but often include central nervous system excitation instead of sedation, mydriasis, hyperthermia, and, less often defecation [9,12,13]. Hydromorphone can be used in cats but is associated with dysphoria and hyperthermia [14,15].

Methadone differs from the other full mu-opioid agonists in that it also has NMDA antagonist properties [7,16]. Owing to its unique NMDA antagonism, methadone may be useful in patients experiencing hyperalgesia or chronic pain, such as dogs presenting with cervical or thoracolumbar pain.

Full mu-opioids are useful in the ER setting because of their excellent analgesic and sedative properties.

Antagonists

Naloxone is the mu-opioid and kappa-opioid receptor antagonist and can be used to reverse all opioids [17]. Butorphanol can also be given at low doses (0.05 mg/kg IV to effect) to reverse unwanted side-effects of full mu-opioids, such as sedation, while sparing some of the analgesic effects. These agents are useful in the ER setting, as many patients need to be awake enough after procedures to be discharged quickly.

Alpha-2 Agonists

Alpha-2 agonists cause dose-dependent cardiovascular responses, including initial vasoconstriction followed by baroreceptor-mediated bradycardia and subsequent disruption of centrally mediated sympathetic outflow and an indirect reduction in cardiac output [10,18]. Alpha-2 receptors are abundant in the body and are found in the dorsal horn of the spinal cord, brain, and the periphery. They play a significant role in modulating the pain signals descending from the brain thereby reducing hyperalgesia.

Dexmedetomidine is an alpha-2 agonist commonly used in the emergency department due to its sedative and analgesic properties. Patients in which to avoid the use of dexmedetomidine include those with degenerative valvular disease or systolic dysfunction, patients with reduced cardiac output and oxygen delivery, critically ill patients, and those with bradyarrhythmias such as sick sinus syndrome or third degree AV block. The use of dexmedetomidine is controversial in cats with hypertrophic cardiomyopathy (HCM) although it has been shown to be of benefit in those with left ventricular outflow tract obstruction [19]. Adding an opioid and possibly another sedative such as midazolam or alfaxalone to the protocol will reduce the doses of dexmedetomidine needed in cats with known HCM. Patients sedated with dexmedetomidine remain noise and light sensitive and can be aroused, even under seemingly heavy sedation.

Supplemental oxygen should always be supplied to the patient to improve oxygen delivery to all tissues (see Chapter 181).

Acepromazine

Acepromazine is a phenothiazine used to provide long-lasting sedation in both cats and dogs. It must be used in conjunction with an opioid due to its lack of analgesic effects. In addition to providing sedation, acepromazine is also an antiemetic, antiarrhythmic, antihistaminic agent. Its cardiovascular side-effects include vasodilation and tachycardia. Acepromazine can be used in the ER in patients with seizures as it has not been shown to affect the seizure threshold [20,21]. It may be useful in animals in which an increase in afterload must be avoided, such as those with degenerative valvular disease or pulmonic stenosis.

Benzodiazepines

Benzodiazepines are commonly used to provide sedation and muscle relaxation and are often chosen for their lack of negative cardiorespiratory effects. The two benzodiazepines used in the ER are midazolam and diazepam, which have very similar pharmacological profiles and are often used interchangeably. Midazolam differs from diazepam in that it is water soluble and can be administered IM and has a shorter half-life, making its effects shorter lived [22]. Diazepam contains propylene glycol and should not be given IM as it will have erratic and poor absorption and can cause tissue irritation. Benzodiazepines are safe to use in patients with cardiac, respiratory, renal, or neurological disease as they cause minimal cardiorespiratory depression, maintain cardiac output and renal perfusion, and suppress seizure activity.

The use of benzodiazepines is controversial in patients with hepatic disease due to their dependence on phase I hepatic metabolism. Since the effects of benzodiazepines can be fully reversed by the antagonist flumazenil, many clinicians choose to use these drugs in animals with hepatic disease [23]. Although these drugs are often used to sedate a patient in the ER, it is not uncommon to note dysphoria and excitement in both dogs and cats [24,25].

Induction Agents Used for Sedation

Propofol

Propofol is a short-acting sedative hypnotic agent commonly used to provide procedural sedation in humans in the ER [26,27]. Propofol has a rapid onset and off-set with a smooth recovery profile. Side-effects are dose dependent and include vasodilation, respiratory depression, and reduced cardiac output [27–29]. In cats and dogs, propofol is not often used as a sedative but more commonly as an induction agent into anesthesia. If propofol is used carefully and titrated to effect, it can be given in small amounts to allow enough sedation in order to complete many procedures in a timely manner. It should always be used with adequate premedication and analgesia and not as a sole sedation agent. When using propofol as a sedative, it is imperative that supplies be in place to perform a rapid intubation if necessary. It is also mandatory that oxygen supplementation be provided and that the patient's vital signs be monitored (see Chapter 181).

Alfaxalone

Alfaxalone is a neurosteroid that enhances the actions of $GABA_A$ to produce muscle relaxation, sedation, and anesthesia. Alfaxalone comes as a clear, colorless, non-irritating, aqueous formulation and is marketed for intravenous use only, although it can be used off-label and administered IM as part of a sedation protocol. Alfaxalone has a similar pharmacodynamic profile to propofol in the dog and cat, although it may cause less vasodilation and less reduction in cardiac output [30–32]. When used as part of a sedation protocol in dogs or cats, alfaxalone can be added to an opioid and a benzodiazepine or dexmedetomidine; both combinations have been shown to provide adequate muscle relaxation and sedation to perform minor procedures [33,34]. Alfaxalone is particularly helpful in sedating aggressive animals in the ER whose underlying cardiac status is unknown [35].

Ketamine

Ketamine is a rapid-acting dissociative anesthetic used in dogs and cats to induce sedation without significant respiratory depression [36]. In addition to providing sedation, it is also used as an induction agent and as part of analgesic protocols. Ketamine is becoming more commonly used as part of procedural sedation in pediatric emergency rooms owing to its rapid effects, lack of cardiorespiratory depression, and analgesic profile [37]. Side-effects of ketamine sedation include myoclonus, dysphoria, increased intracranial pressure, and possible pain on injection. Ketamine should be avoided in patients in whom an increase in contractility and heart rate may be detrimental, such as cats with HCM or those with tachyarrhythmias and suspected or confirmed intracranial disease. Ketamine is commonly combined with an opioid and a sedative to provide sedation in the ER. Recently, ketamine and propofol have been combined (in same syringe) and used as a rapid-acting induction agent with analgesic properties.

References

1 Warne LN, Beths T, Holm M, Carter JE, Bauquier SH. Evaluation of the perioperative analgesic efficacy of buprenorphine, compared with butorphanol in cats. *J Am Vet Med Assoc* 2014;245(2):195–202.

2 Lee J, Suh S, Choi R, Hyun C. Cardiorespiratory and anesthetic effects produced by the combination of butorphanol, medetomidine, and alfaxalone administered intramuscularly in Beagle dogs. *J Vet Med Sci* 2015;77:1677–1680.

3 Ward JL, Schober KE, Fuentes VL, Bonagura JD. Effects of sedation on echocardiographic variables of left atrial and left ventricular function in healthy cats. *J Feline Med Surg* 2012;14(10):678–685.

4 Taylor PM, Kirby JJ, Robinson C, et al. A prospective multi-centre clinical trial to compare buprenorphine and butorphanol for postoperative analgesia in cats. *J Feline Med Surg* 2010;12(4):247–255.

5 Warne LN, Beths T, Holm M, Bauquier SH. Comparison of perioperative analgesic efficacy between methadone and butorphanol in cats. *J Am Vet Med Assoc* 2013;243(6):844–850.

6 Niedfeldt RL, Robertson SA. Postanesthetic hyperthermia in cats: a retrospective comparison between hydromorphone and buprenorphine. *Vet Anaesth Analg* 2006;33(6):381–389.

7 Maiante AA, Teixeira Neto FJ, Beier SL, Corrente JE, Pedroso CEBP. Comparison of the cardio-respiratory effects of methadone and morphine in conscious dogs. *J Vet Pharmacol Ther* 2009;32(4):317–328.

8 Guedes AGP, Papich MG, Rude EP, Rider MA. Pharmacokinetics and physiological effects of intravenous hydromorphone in conscious dogs. *J Vet Pharmacol Ther* 2008;31(4):334–343.

9 Mathews KA, Lamont LA. *Lumb and Jones' Veterinary Anesthesia and Analgesia*. Wiley, New York, 2010.

10 Cardoso CG, Marques DRC, da Silva THM, de Mattos-Junior E. Cardiorespiratory, sedative and antinociceptive effects of dexmedetomidine alone or in combination with methadone, morphine or tramadol in dogs. *Vet Anaesth Analg* 2014;41(6):636–643.

11 Ovbey DH, Wilson DV, Bednarski RM, et al. Prevalence and risk factors for canine post-anesthetic aspiration pneumonia (1999–2009): a multicenter study. *Vet Anaesth Analg* 2014;41(2):127–136.

12 Pypendop BH, Ilkiw JE, Shilo-Benjamini Y. Bioavailability of morphine, methadone, hydromorphone, and oxymorphone following buccal administration in cats. *J Vet Pharmacol Ther* 2014;37(3):295–300.

13 Ferreira TH, Rezende ML, Mama KR, Hudachek SF, Aguiar AJA. Plasma concentrations and behavioral, antinociceptive, and physiologic effects of methadone after intravenous and oral transmucosal administration in cats. *Am J Vet Res* 2011;72(6):764–771.

14 Posner LP, Pavuk AA, Rokshar JL, Carter JE, Levine JF. Effects of opioids and anesthetic drugs on body temperature in cats. *Vet Anaesth Analg* 2010;37(1):35–43.

15 Niedfeldt RL, Robertson SA. Postanesthetic hyperthermia in cats: a retrospective comparison between hydromorphone and buprenorphine. *Vet Anaesth Analg* 2006;33(6):381–389.

16 Ingvast-Larsson C, Holgersson A, Bondesson U, Lagerstedt AS, Olsson K. Clinical pharmacology of methadone in dogs. *Vet Anaesth Analg* 2010;37(1):48–56.

17 Freise KJ, Newbound GC, Tudan C, Clark TP. Naloxone reversal of an overdose of a novel, long-acting transdermal fentanyl solution in laboratory Beagles. *J Vet Pharmacol Ther* 2012;35 (Suppl 2):45–51.

18 Hunt JR, Grint NJ, Taylor PM, Murrell JC. Sedative and analgesic effects of buprenorphine, combined with either acepromazine or dexmedetomidine, for premedication prior to elective surgery in cats and dogs. *Vet Anaesth Analg* 2013 1;40(3):297–307.

19 Lamont LA, Bulmer BJ, Sisson DD, Grimm KA, Tranquilli WJ. Doppler echocardiographic effects of medetomidine on dynamic left ventricular outflow tract obstruction in cats. *J Am Vet Med Assoc* 2002;221:1276–1281.

20 Tobias KM, Marioni-Henry K, Wagner R. A retrospective study on the use of acepromazine maleate in dogs with seizures. *J Am Anim Hosp Assoc* 2006;42(4):283–289.

21 Drynan EA, Gray P, Raisis AL. Incidence of seizures associated with the use of acepromazine in dogs undergoing myelography. *J Vet Emerg Crit Care* 2012;22(2):262–266.

22 Schwartz M, Muñana KR, Nettifee-Osborne JA, Messenger KM, Papich MG. The pharmacokinetics of midazolam after intravenous, intramuscular, and rectal administration in healthy dogs. *J Vet Pharmacol Ther* 2013;36(5):471–477.

23 Unkel JH, Brickhouse TH, Sweatman TW, Scarbecz M, Tompkins WP, Eslinger CS. A comparison of 3 routes of flumazenil administration to reverse benzodiazepine-induced desaturation in an animal model. *Pediatr Dent* 2006;28(4):357–362.

24 Biermann K, Hungerbühler S, Mischke R, Kästner SBR. Sedative, cardiovascular, haematologic and biochemical effects of four different drug combinations administered intramuscularly in cats. *Vet Anaesth Analg* 2012;39(2):137–150.

25 Sánchez A, Belda E, Escobar M, Agut A, Soler M, Laredo FG. Effects of altering the sequence of midazolam and propofol during co-induction of anaesthesia. *Vet Anaesth Analg* 2013;40(4):359–366.

26 Sacchetti A, Senula G, Strickland J, Dubin R. Procedural sedation in the community emergency department: initial results of the ProSCED registry. *Acad Emerg Med* 2007;14(1):41–46.

27 Pershad J, Godambe SA. Propofol for procedural sedation in the pediatric emergency department. *J Emerg Med.* 2004;27(1):11–14.

28 Maney JK, Shepard MK, Braun C, Cremer J, Hofmeister EH. A comparison of cardiopulmonary and anesthetic effects of an induction dose of alfaxalone or propofol in dogs. *Vet Anaesth Analg* 2013;40(3):237–244.

29 Liehmann L, Mosing M, Auer U. A comparison of cardiorespiratory variables during isoflurane-fentanyl and propofol-fentanyl anaesthesia for surgery in injured cats. *Vet Anaesth Analg* 2006;33(3):158–168.

30 Costa D, Leiva M, Moll X, Aguilar A, Peña T, Andaluz A. Alfaxalone versus propofol in dogs: a randomised trial to assess effects on peri-induction tear production, intraocular pressure and globe position. *Vet Rec* 2015;176(3):73.

31 Psatha E, Alibhai HI, Jimenez Lozano A, Armitage Chan E, Brodbelt DC. Clinical efficacy and cardiorespiratory effects of alfaxalone, or diazepam/fentanyl for induction of anaesthesia in dogs that are a poor anaesthetic risk. *Vet Anaesth Analg* 2011;38(1):24–36.

32 Warne LN, Beths T, Whittem T, Carter JE, Bauquier SH. A review of the pharmacology and clinical application of alfaxalone in cats. *Vet J* 2015;203(2):141–148.

33 Seo JI, Han SH, Choi R, Han J, Lee L, Hyun C. Cardiopulmonary and anesthetic effects of the combination of butorphanol, midazolam and alfaxalone in Beagle dogs. *Vet Anaesth Analg* 2015;42(3):304–308.

34 Rodrigo-Mocholí D, Belda E, Bosmans T, Laredo FG. Clinical efficacy and cardiorespiratory effects of intramuscular administration of alfaxalone alone or in combination with dexmedetomidine in cats. *Vet Anaesth Analg* 2016;43:291–300.

35 Ribas T, Bublot I, Junot S, et al. Effects of intramuscular sedation with alfaxalone and butorphanol on echocardiographic measurements in healthy cats. *J Feline Med Surg* 2015;17(6):530–536.

36 Marjani M, Akbarinejad V, Bagheri M. Comparison of intranasal and intramuscular ketamine-midazolam combination in cats. *Vet Anaesth Analg* 2015;42(2):178–181.

37 Green SM, Rothrock SG, Lynch EL, et al. Intramuscular ketamine for pediatric sedation in the emergency department: safety profile in 1,022 Cases. *Ann Emerg Med* 1998;31(6):688–697.

193

Pain Management in Critical Patients

Alicia Z. Karas, MS, DVM, DACVAA

Cummings School of Veterinary Medicine, Tufts University, North Grafton, MA, USA

Pain in the Emergency Patient: Concerns and Goals

Pain has the potential to be a source of distress to the patient, the owner and caregivers, but it is also a cause of ileus and ventilatory impairment, inhibits cough and appetite, and may lead to self-injury, hypertension, and arrhythmias. Unrelieved moderate-to-severe pain is a stressor and excessive stress negatively affects health and recovery. The goal is to reduce pain to a level where the patient can cope physiologically and emotionally, not to remove all pain. Most analgesic regimens do not completely alleviate pain of tissue injury. Single-agent analgesia (e.g. fentanyl infusion) in complex pain states may not provide sufficient relief.

How Much Pain and How to Approach It

The degree and type of tissue injury, severity and extent of the inflammatory process should guide analgesia. Observation of the individual patient's response to analgesia is the only way to accurately gauge treatment success. Situational influences can greatly influence pain tolerance – fearful or anxious animals often display enhanced responses to manipulations. It can be difficult to distinguish anxiety from pain but the two have very different treatment strategies.

Pain assessment is beyond the scope of this chapter. Suffice it to say that the patient who is able to recline in a relaxed manner, is oriented and who will alert to nearby individuals, who will move with little inhibition and is easily handled is probably adequately treated for pain, and that patients who are dull, or aggressive, stiff, grimacing, and poorly able to focus on things outside their own bodies are in significant amount of distress; whether from pain or some other cause is the challenge of the veterinarian. It is more difficult to evaluate very critical patients whose behavior is inhibited by weakness, immobility or CNS depression. Continuous vocalization is, in the author's experience, less indicative of pain and more indicative of psychological abnormality; in an alert and oriented patient, it can be attributed mainly to anxiety but if there is delirium, then medication side-effects or neurological impairment are more likely to blame.

Pain can be complicated by iatrogenic damage resulting from environmental conditions, positioning, and restraint. Anesthetized or immobilized patients cannot support unstable joints or avoid positions that endanger nerves, muscle or other vulnerable structures. Thus critical patients must be handled thoughtfully and meticulously with neutral positioning. More robust patients with undertreated pain may become aggressive, struggle and resist treatment.

Drug Interactions

Adverse drug–drug interaction concerns include the following.

- *Combinations of sedative analgesics* which promote excessive central nervous system depression or inability to protect the airway.
- *Drugs which increase the risk of serotonin syndrome*: serotonin syndrome resulting from routine doses of anxiolytics and opioids is not generally thought to be a problem in veterinary medicine, but cautious prescribing is advisable.
- *Potentiation of inhalant or intravenous anesthetic action by analgesics*: when opioids, local anesthetics, ketamine, or alpha-2 agonists are used prior to or during general anesthesia, inhalant anesthetic requirements are significantly lessened. If not taken into account by minimizing anesthetic doses, extreme depression of

Textbook of Small Animal Emergency Medicine, First Edition. Edited by Kenneth J. Drobatz, Kate Hopper, Elizabeth Rozanski and Deborah C. Silverstein.
© 2019 John Wiley & Sons, Inc. Published 2019 by John Wiley & Sons, Inc.
Companion Website: www.wiley.com/go/drobatz/textbook

respiration and cardiac output and decreased elimination of drugs (e.g. intravenous lidocaine) may occur, risking morbidity or death. Decreased renal blood flow when NSAIDs are used risks nephrotoxicity.

- *Use of two drugs in succession with similar toxicities*: switching from a non-selective to COX-2-selective NSAID is thought to pose a significant GI ulceration risk.

Dose Titration, Timing, and Duration

Doses are increased when pain control requires it for opioids, alpha-2 agonists, and gabapentin. Increasing doses of NSAIDs may increase risk of organ toxicity. "Loading" doses of NSAIDs are cited for both Metacam and Deramaxx. This author recommends against use of loading doses of NSAIDs due to the potential for toxicity, accidental failure to reduce to maintenance dosing, and because the current evidence in humans is that increasing the dose of NSAID tends to increase duration rather than magnitude of effect [1].

The speed of onset of analgesia varies with the type of drug and route of administration. Approximate onset times and duration (of intermittent dosing) are listed under individual drug classes but duration generally depends on the dose. Constant-rate infusions of pure agonist opioids, alpha-2 agonists, and ketamine are preferable to intermittent injection of drug because "peaks and valleys" of effect can be avoided and the rate can be adjusted to suit the patient.

When anesthesia is planned for injured patients, ideally patients awaken from anesthesia smoothly with little discomfort; analgesia should be adequate at the time of recovery. Fear and panic, lack of orientation to surroundings, extended anesthesia time, and hypothermia lead to rough, struggling recoveries. The presence of pain potentiates fear and panic.

Pain should be expected to increase as the postinjury inflammatory response proceeds. Most humans report that pain after strenuous activity becomes evident within 12–24 hours. Thereafter, pain tends to subside over time, depending on the severity of the injury, speed of tissue repair, complicating factors, and the effectiveness of the analgesic therapy. If specific anti-inflammatory drugs (NSAIDs or corticosteroids) are contraindicated, intravenous lidocaine (dogs only) may provide anti-inflammatory effects.

Breakthrough and Unexpected Pain

Pain may episodically become more severe, especially upon or just after procedures, and is preferably pretreated with increments of additional analgesia. When pain is of greater magnitude or duration than expected despite attempts to treat it, there is reason to suspect one of several complications. These include wound infection or dehiscence, nerve impingement, fracture, ischemia, bandage or splint pain, gastric or esophageal ulceration, urinary retention, delayed gastric emptying, and pancreatitis. Trauma patients frequently suffer distressing levels of GI stasis influenced by immobility, pain, and opioid therapy. A thorough physical exam is mandatory. The author reminds practitioners that it is very difficult to bandage even your own limbs comfortably, so bandages are common significant contributions to pain.

Pharmacological Methods for Treating Acute Pain

Opioids

Advantages of opioids include safety, good evidence for dosing, rapid onset, and reversibility. While side-effects are rarely lethal, there is an increasing trend towards "opioid sparing" in medical care – using other strategies to reduce reliance on the opioid. In small animal medicine, nausea, vomiting, inappetence, ileus, and urinary retention may occur with use of opioids acting at the mu-receptor. Respiratory depression is of concern with moderate-to-severe pulmonary dysfunction, high intracranial pressure, and acidosis. Opioids are potent cough suppressants; in patients with airway compromise or vomiting/regurgitation, suppressing a cough reflex may lead to significant morbidity. Dogs receiving mu-agonist opioids have altered thermoregulatory set points, leading to what is generally a non-clinically significant hypothermia of the order of 98 °F; efforts to warm dogs who are otherwise alert and stable just risks making them feel worse. In cats, hyperthermia may occur, and hydromorphone is particularly implicated [2]. When cats appear distressed, temperature monitoring and partial reversal or a switch to buprenorphine and active cooling may be necessary.

Opioids can cause behavioral changes, including sedation, euphoria, and dysphoria. Dysphoria is a specific opioid-related syndrome (particularly with pure agonist opioids). Patients appear to be very vocal, confused and agitated, and poorly responsive to human contact; this is often mistaken for pain or anxiety [3]. The addition of tranquilizers or sedatives does not permanently resolve the condition. A dramatic response is seen following slow IV reversal of the opioid with 0.01 mg/kg naloxone or 0.1 mg/kg butorphanol. Generally within minutes, the patient becomes oriented to surroundings with more normal behavior, and does not experience more pain

[4,5]. "Weaker" opioids and adjunctive analgesics may be used to treat pain from then on.

Injectable opioids take effect within approximately 10–40 minutes (depending on the drug) when given by the intravenous or intramuscular route. Subcutaneous administration of opioids is not recommended as it produces erratic and poor analgesia [6].

Extensively studied in cats, buprenorphine is recommended to be given by the IV route when possible, and the commonly used 0.01 mg/kg dose is not thought to produce reliable analgesia as a sole analgesic. Buprenorphine has a high affinity for the mu-receptor, and is difficult to antagonize. If buprenorphine has been given prior to switching to a full mu-agonist opioid, there may be some dampening of the effect at the mu-receptor. This has led to a tendency to "withhold" morning doses of buprenorphine prior to surgery, but unfortunately this leads to a gap in analgesia coverage. As unbound mu-receptors are likely to be available, it does not represent a major limitation to continue the buprenorphine until the time that the full mu-agonist is given.

In dogs and cats, methadone does not generally cause vomiting and is also generally felt to cause less dysphoria and sedation than other common pure mu-agonists. Methadone at low doses (<0.3 mg/kg) is less suitable as an anesthetic premed as it does not spare inhalant levels as effectively as pure mu-agonists. Butorphanol is not regarded as having sufficient analgesic efficacy to treat moderate-to-severe pain.

NSAIDs

Non-steroidal anti-inflammatory drugs are extremely reliable and valuable analgesics but are insufficient as sole analgesics for moderate-to-severe pain. The impact of NSAIDs on tissue repair (COX-2 mediated) makes them unsuitable in critical situations (e.g. compromised gastric mucosal integrity), and prostaglandin inhibition is contraindicated in states of volume depletion, poor cardiac output, or with pre-existing renal compromise as the kidney relies on prostaglandins to improve renal blood flow. NSAIDs may take up to several hours for onset, regardless of route of administration. From a GI ulceration perspective, washout times of 5–7 days between administration of different NSAIDs, with the exception of aspirin (>7 days recommended), and avoiding any close overlap of corticosteroids and NSAIDs is prudent [7]. Dogs admitted to the hospital with chronic osteoarthritis or cancer pain that has been adequately treated with NSAIDs may experience disabling pain upon discontinuation; alternative methods to provide analgesia (opioids, IV lidocaine, IV microdose ketamine) must be substituted.

Local Anesthetics

Local anesthetics are very effective for acute pain control; beyond analgesia, they also have broad anti-inflammatory and antimicrobial effects [8,9]. Regional and epidural techniques require expertise to perform, and the duration of "single-shot" bupivacaine injections is limited to approximately 6–8 hours. Intravenous lidocaine (IVL) is beneficial for pain of soft tissue surgery in humans, with effects lasting beyond the duration of the infusion, leading to extrapolation of its use in veterinary patients [10]. Non-surgical pain (e.g. major trauma, burns, pancreatitis) may also benefit from IVL use. Onset of analgesia from IVL in humans with long-standing neuropathic pain began at approximately 15 minutes and was complete at 45 minutes [11]. In horses and in humans, IVL reduces the duration of post-surgical ileus [12,13]. It should be used with caution and possibly lower doses in dogs with reduced serum albumin or poor cardiac output due to increased risk of toxicity. IVL use in cats is not recommended because of poor ability to metabolize the drug [14].

Ketamine

Subanesthetic or so-called "low-dose" or "micro-dose" ketamine (0.6 mg/kg/h) is demonstrated to improve opioid sparing, prevent opioid tolerance, and reduce acute somatic and visceral pain [15–21]. Low-dose ketamine infusions are now widely used as an analgesic adjunct in dogs and cats for acute pain. Ketamine also has the potential to reduce production of proinflammatory cytokines and this may prove to be beneficial in critically ill veterinary patients, although more research is needed [22,23]. In a study of chronic (human) neuropathic pain patients, a mean 55% reduction in reported pain occurred during a 40-minute infusion, but this reduction did not persist after discontinuation of the infusion [24]. In the author's experience, when low-dose ketamine is given to anesthetized patients, the reduction in responsiveness to painful manipulation and ability to reduce the vaporizer setting occurs within 10 minutes but the onset of analgesia with administration of low-dose ketamine in dogs and cats has yet to be determined.

Dexmedetomidine

Dexmedetomidine produces sedation and, at higher doses, analgesia. As a sole agent, its analgesic effects may only occur above a dose rate of 5 μg/kg/h but when used with lidocaine and ketamine infusions, profound inhalant anesthetic-sparing effects and a level of analgesia equivalent to that of fentanyl are seen [25–27]. A major disadvantage is that it causes decreased cardiac index (CI).

At the higher doses used to facilitate minor procedures, and also at microdoses of >1 mg/kg/h, CI is reduced by 30–50%. One study suggests that at 0.5–1 µg/kg/h, CI is not appreciably depressed [28]. Above that dose range, its use is therefore recommended only in patients who would not be vulnerable to cardiovascular depression [29]. Another major advantage is that the sedative effects can be reversed, although this also reverses any analgesic effect.

Gabapentin

Gabapentin acts to reduce neuronal hyperexcitability, and has been used in humans for alleviation of neuropathic and other pain states. Recent meta-analyses have found limited support for perioperative reduction in pain or morphine requirements in humans, but there is encouraging evidence that perioperative administration of gabapentin reduces the incidence of chronic postsurgical pain [30]. Studies in dogs both support and fail to support its efficacy in reducing postoperative pain [31–33]. Several case reports supporting efficacy of gabapentin in both dogs and cats with complex chronic pain states have been published [34–36]. Gabapentin has sedative and anxiolytic properties, which the author finds useful in hospitalized patients, and may be additive with other analgesics and anesthetics. Currently, gabapentin is only available in an oral formulation.

In the dog and cat, gabapentin is relatively non-toxic even at high doses, and has been used even in critically ill or systemically impaired animals. Dose reductions in situations of hepatic or renal insufficiency should be considered. The empirically advocated doses of gabapentin in the small animal patient with acute pain are 5–20 mg/kg every 8–12 hours [37]. Gabapentin can be combined with all other analgesics and may be a useful option for sustained analgesic therapy in dogs and cats with acute pain.

Cryotherapy

Cryotherapy is typically used after recent injury or during active inflammation and is easily applicable in dogs. Cats do not tolerate cryotherapy unless they are very sedated. Cryotherapy is performed using crushed ice, frozen gel packs, or frozen alcohol/water slushes. Animals may initially find it aversive but after a few minutes the analgesic effects begin to be appreciated. Excessive cooling of skin may risk injury, and so it is to be avoided in animals with poor circulation or thin skin, and in those animals too sedates to signal severe discomfort.

References

1 McQuay HJ, Derry S, Eccleston C, et al. Evidence for analgesic effect in acute pain – 50 years on. *Pain* 2012;153:1364–1367.

2 Posner LP, Pavuk AA, Rokshar JL, et al. Effects of opioids and anesthetic drugs on body temperature in cats. *Vet Anaesth Analg* 2010;37:35–43.

3 Hofmeister EH, Herrington JL, Mazzaferro EM. Opioid dysphoria in three dogs. *J Vet Emerg Crit Care* 2006;16:44–9.

4 Maxwell LG, Kaufmann SC, Bitzer S, et al. The effects of a small-dose naloxone infusion on opioid-induced side effects and analgesia in children and adolescents treated with intravenous patient-controlled analgesia: a double-blind, prospective, randomized, controlled study. *Anesth Analg* 2005;100:953–958.

5 Gan TJ, Ginsberg B, Glass PS, et al. Opioid-sparing effects of a low-dose infusion of naloxone in patient-administered morphine sulfate. *J Am Soc Anesthesiol* 1997;87:1075–1081.

6 Steagall PV, Monteiro-Steagall BP, Taylor PM. A review of the studies using buprenorphine in cats. *J Vet Intern Med* 2014;28:762–770.

7 KuKanich B, Bidgood T, Knesl O. Clinical pharmacology of nonsteroidal anti-inflammatory drugs in dogs. *Vet Anaesth Analg* 2012;39:69–90.

8 Cassuto J, Sinclair R, Bonderovic M. Anti-inflammatory properties of local anesthetics and their present and potential clinical implications. *Acta Anaesth Scand* 2006;50:265–282.

9 Wal SE, Heuvel SA, Radema SA, et al. The in vitro mechanisms and in vivo efficacy of intravenous lidocaine on the neuroinflammatory response in acute and chronic pain. *Eur J Pain* 2016;20:655–674.

10 Barreveld A, Witte J, Chahal H, et al. Preventive analgesia by local anesthetics: the reduction of postoperative pain by peripheral nerve blocks and intravenous drugs. *Anesth Analg* 2013;116:1141.

11 Ferrante FM, Paggioli J, Cherukuri S, et al. The analgesic response to intravenous lidocaine in the treatment of neuropathic pain. *Anesth Analg* 1996;82:91–97.

12 Cook VL, Shults JJ, McDowell M, et al. Attenuation of ischaemic injury in the equine jejunum by administration of systemic lidocaine. *Equine Vet J* 2008;40:353–357.

13 McCarthy GC, Megalla SA. Impact of intravenous lidocaine infusion on postoperative analgesia and recovery from surgery. *Drugs* 2010;70:1149–1163.

14 Thomasy SM, Pypendop BH, Ilkiw JE, et al. Pharmacokinetics of lidocaine and its active metabolite,

monoethylglycinexylidide, after intravenous administration of lidocaine to awake and isoflurane-anesthetized cats. *Am J Vet Res* 2005;66:1162–1166.

15 Pypendop BH, Ilkiw JE. Assessment of the hemodynamic effects of lidocaine administered IV in isoflurane anesthetized cats. *Am J Vet Res* 2005;66: 661–668.

16 Himmelseher S, Durieux ME. Ketamine for perioperative pain management. *J Am Soc Anesthesiol* 2005;102:211–220.

17 Wagner AE, Walton JA, Hellyer PW, et al. Use of low doses of ketamine administered by constant rate infusion as an adjunct for postoperative analgesia in dogs. *J Am Vet Med Assoc* 2002;221:72–75.

18 Muir WW III, Wiese AJ, March PA. Effects of morphine, lidocaine, ketamine, and morphine-lidocaine-ketamine drug combination on minimum alveolar concentration in dogs anesthetized with isoflurane. *Am J Vet Res* 2003;64:1155–1160.

19 Galinski M, Dolveck F, Combes X, et al. Management of severe acute pain in emergency settings: ketamine reduces morphine consumption. *Am J Emerg Med* 2007;25:385–390.

20 Johansson P, Kongstad P, Johansson A. The effect of combined treatment with morphine sulphate and low-dose ketamine in a prehospital setting. *Scand J Trauma Resusc Emerg Med* 2009;17:1.

21 Jouguelet-Lacoste J, La Colla L, Schilling D, et al. The use of intravenous infusion or single dose of low-dose ketamine for postoperative analgesia: a review of the current literature. *Pain Med* 2015;16:383–403.

22 Kock M, Loix S, Lavand'homme P. Ketamine and peripheral inflammation. *CNS Neurosci Ther* 2013;19:403–410.

23 Lankveld DP, Bull S, van Dijk P, et al. Ketamine inhibits LPS-induced tumour necrosis factor-alpha and interleukin-6 in an equine macrophage cell line. *Vet Res* 2005;36:257–262.

24 Kvarnström A, Karlsten R, Quiding H, et al. The effectiveness of intravenous ketamine and lidocaine on peripheral neuropathic pain. *Acta Anaesth Scand* 2003;47:868–77.

25 Van Oostrom H, Doornenbal A, Schot A, et al. Neurophysiological assessment of the sedative and analgesic effects of a constant rate infusion of dexmedetomidine in the dog. *Vet J* 2011;190:338–344.

26 Gutierrez-Blanco E, Victoria-Mora JM, Ibancovichi-Camarillo JA, et al. Postoperative analgesic effects of either a constant rate infusion of fentanyl, lidocaine, ketamine, dexmedetomidine, or the combination lidocaine-ketamine-dexmedetomidine after ovariohysterectomy in dogs. *Vet Anaesth Analg* 2015;42:309–318.

27 Ebner LS, Lerche P, Bednarski RM, et al. Effect of dexmedetomidine, morphine-lidocaine-ketamine, and dexmedetomidine-morphine-lidocaine-ketamine constant rate infusions on the minimum alveolar concentration of isoflurane and bispectral index in dogs. *Am J Vet Res* 2013;74:963–970.

28 Pascoe PJ. The cardiopulmonary effects of dexmedetomidine infusions in dogs during isoflurane anesthesia. *Vet Anaesth Analg* 2015;42:360–368.

29 Lin GY, Robben JH, Murrell JC, et al. Dexmedetomidine constant rate infusion for 24 hours during and after propofol or isoflurane anaesthesia in dogs. *Vet Anaesth Analg* 2008;35:141–153.

30 Clarke H, Bonin RP, Orser BA, et al. The prevention of chronic postsurgical pain using gabapentin and pregabalin: a combined systematic review and meta-analysis. *Anesth Analg* 2012;115:428–442.

31 Crociolli GC, Cassu RN, Barbero RC, et al. Gabapentin as an adjuvant for postoperative pain management in dogs undergoing mastectomy. *J Vet Med Sci* 2015;77:1011.

32 Aghighi SA, Tipold A, Piechotta M, et al. Assessment of the effects of adjunctive gabapentin on postoperative pain after intervertebral disc surgery in dogs. *Vet Anaesth Analg* 2012;39:636–646.

33 Wagner AE, Mich PM, Uhrig SR, et al. Clinical evaluation of perioperative administration of gabapentin as an adjunct for postoperative analgesia in dogs undergoing amputation of a forelimb. *J Am Vet Med Assoc* 2010;236:751–756.

34 Cashmore RG, Harcourt-Brown TR, Freeman PM, et al. Clinical diagnosis and treatment of suspected neuropathic pain in three dogs. *Aust Vet J* 2009;87:45–50.

35 Vettorato E, Corletto F. Gabapentin as part of multi-modal analgesia in two cats suffering multiple injuries. *Vet Anaesth Analg* 2011;38(5):518–520.

36 Lorenz ND, Comerford EJ, Iff I. Long-term use of gabapentin for musculoskeletal disease and trauma in three cats. *J Feline Med Surg* 2013;15:507–512.

37 KuKanich B. Outpatient oral analgesics in dogs and cats beyond nonsteroidal antiinflammatory drugs: an evidence-based approach. *Vet Clin North Am Small Anim Pract* 2013;43:1109–1125.

194

Opioids

Lois A. Wetmore, DVM, ScD, DACVAA

Cummings School of Veterinary Medicine, Tufts University, North Grafton, MA, USA

Introduction

Opioids are classified based on the specific receptor(s) they bind to, their affinity for the receptor(s), and the action at the receptor(s). All opioids fall into one of the following categories.

- *Full agonist*: defined as a drug which when bound to its receptor activates the receptor to its maximal response.
- *Partial agonist*: defined as a drug which when bound to its receptor activates the receptor to a level below the maximal response. Increasing the dose of a partial agonist over the maximal therapeutic dose does not result in greater analgesia or more severe side-effects (ceiling effect).
- *Agonist/antagonist*: defined as a drug that acts simultaneously on different receptor subtypes, functioning as an agonist at one or more receptor subtypes and an antagonist at other one or more subtypes. Like partial agonists, this group of opioids also has a ceiling effect and will not induce extreme respiratory depression or bradycardia with increasing doses. Neither will they induce maximal analgesia and are not as effective at treating intense pain as are full-agonist opioids. Due to their antagonist effects, they are useful at reversing the effects of full-agonist opioids while still providing some analgesia. They are also preferred analgesics in patients where opioid side-effects can deter use.
- *Antagonist*: defined as a drug which when bound to its receptor fails to produce any stimulation of the receptor.

Opioids are also classified based in their potency and efficacy. Potency is a description of the amount of drug required to produce an effect. The potency of opioids is ranked by comparison to morphine. Morphine is given a relative potency of 1 and all other opioids are classified based on the equivalent dose required to create the same analgesia as that due to a specific dose of morphine.

Potency simply reflects a comparable mg dose and does not reflect the maximal response that an opioid can induce (efficacy). Hence, the partial agonist buprenorphine has a greater potency than morphine but is unable to effect the same maximal level of analgesia (less efficacy). As a result, it is not recommended as an effective treatment for extremely painful patients, which are best treated with a full-opioid agonist.

The efficacy of opioids is the maximal pharmacological effect that the drug can induce. It is unrelated to potency. It is determined by the intrinsic activity of a drug at its receptor. The efficacy of full agonists is greater than that due to partial agonists or agonist/antagonists. Side-effects of some full-agonist opioids, such as codeine, are severe at higher doses, thereby limiting their efficacy.

Mechanism of Action

Opioids act at specific receptors in the brain and spinal cord. In the brain, these receptors are in highest concentration in the thalamus, where they dull chronic and poorly localized pain. Opioid receptors in the limbic system, amygdala, corpus striatum, and hypothalamus, parts of the brain that modulate the emotional response to pain, are involved in euphoric responses to opioid administration. In the spinal cord, opioid receptors have been identified in the substantia gelatinosa. Here, they are found on synaptic membranes where they regulate the transmission of information from primary sensory pain afferents. Opioids also block the release of substance P, an important neurotransmitter of painful stimuli, in the dorsal horn of the spinal cord.

Based on the structure of opioid receptors and known agonists and antagonists, three different opioid receptors have been identified: kappa, mu, and delta. Kappa- (primarily located in the spinal cord and peripheral tissues), mu- (primarily located in the CNS but also present in

Textbook of Small Animal Emergency Medicine, First Edition. Edited by Kenneth J. Drobatz, Kate Hopper, Elizabeth Rozanski and Deborah C. Silverstein.
© 2019 John Wiley & Sons, Inc. Published 2019 by John Wiley & Sons, Inc.
Companion Website: www.wiley.com/go/drobatz/textbook

peripheral tissues), and delta-receptors (associated with the mu-receptor) have been shown to be associated with opioid-induced analgesia.

Opioid receptors are in the G-protein-coupled family of receptors and affect ion channels in pre- and postsynaptic nerves. Binding of an agonist to opioid receptors causes a decrease in intracellular cAMP, which results in an increase in potassium movement out of cells and a reduction in calcium movement into cells. Neurons become hyperpolarized, leading to postsynaptic neuronal inhibition and a decrease in transmission of information to the cerebral cortex. It also inhibits presynaptic neurotransmitter release. With nerve damage, opioid receptors may be lost, causing the presynaptic effect of opioids to be diminished.

Duration of Action and Administration Techniques

The duration of action of an opioid is determined by its affinity at the receptor, its rate of redistribution out of blood, its metabolic pathway (and concurrent administration of other drugs that rely on or inhibit enzymes in that pathway), and elimination from the body. Buprenorphine has a relatively high affinity for the mu-receptor and spends a greater amount of time bound to the receptor. It diffuses away from the receptor more slowly, thus prolonging its duration of action. In contrast, fentanyl is very lipophilic and has a high volume of distribution so it diffuses quickly away from receptors, thus shortening its duration of action. These drugs have similar metabolic and elimination pathways despite very different durations of action.

The route of administration may also significantly influence opioid duration of action, especially if the drug is administered in a location that delays its exposure to normal metabolic pathways. Morphine administered parenterally has a duration of action of 3–4 hours but when it is administered epidurally, even at a significantly lower dose, its duration of action is increased to 12–24 hours. This is not only due to the site of administration but to its low lipid solubility as can be demonstrated by comparison to fentanyl, an opioid as described above with high lipid solubility. Fentanyl is administered at the same dose and has the same duration of action whether given via the parenteral (IM or IV) or epidural route.

Intravenous and Epidural Administration Techniques

Intravenous (IV) administration of opioids offers the most predictable bioavailability of any possible route of administration. An opioid can be titrated to effect and then administered at regular intervals or at a constant rate of infusion (CRI) to maintain blood levels within the therapeutic range and reduce the risk of side-effects. A table listing IV and CRI doses of commonly used opioids is provided (Table 194.1).

Epidural administration can be used when the patient has pain that can be localized to the caudal half of the body. Epidural opioids do not cause motor paralysis and can be administered as a single shot or after placement of an epidural catheter. They can be administered alone or with a local anesthetic or alpha-2 agonist as part of a multimodal analgesia technique. Epidural administration of a single dose of morphine minimizes the drug's side-effects and lengthens its duration of action. Epidural administration is performed at the lumbosacral junction in the dog and cat using sterile technique and preservative-free morphine at a dose of 0.1–0.2 mg/kg (1/10th of the parenteral dose required). Other opioids such as fentanyl and oxymorphone can be administered

Table 194.1 Opioid drugs, their doses and mechanisms action.

Drug Name	Action	Opioid Receptor	IV (mg/kg) and CRI (mg/kg/hr) doses	
			Canine	Feline
Buprenorphine	Partial agonist	μ	0.005–0.02	0.01–0.02
Butorphanol	Agonist/antagonist	κ/μ	0.1–0.4	0.1–0.4
Fentanyl	Agonist	μ	0.002–0.005	0.002–0.005
			CRI: 0.001–0.006	CRI: 0.001–0.006
Hydromorphone	Agonist	μ	0.05–0.1	0.05–0.1
Methadone*	Agonist	μ	0.1–0.5	0.1–0.3
Morphine	Agonist	μ, δ	0.3–0.5	0.3–0.5
Naloxone	Antagonist	μ, κ	0.005–0.02	0.005–0.02
Oxymorphone	Agonist	μ	0.05–0.1	0.03–0.1
Remifentanil	Agonist	μ	CRI: 0.001–0.003	CRI: 0.001–0.003

* also has reported antagonist activity at the NMDA receptor and agonist activity at the Alpha 2 adrenergic receptor.

via this route but have a shorter duration of action (similar to IM administration) and require doses essentially the same as those required for parenteral administration. Epidural fentanyl is best administered as a CRI through an epidural catheter to maintain therapeutic levels for more than 1–2 hours.

Alternative Routes of Administration

Per os (PO), oral transmucosal (OTM), subcutaneous (SC), intramuscular (IM), and transdermal routes of administration are not typically used in a critical care setting. This is because this patient population often presents challenges in predicting uptake from the GI and peripheral tissues due to underlying diseases. External heating devices such as circulating water blankets and forced air warmers are often employed in these patients to maintain body temperature in the physiological range, also making uptake from transdermal patches unpredictable. However, in an emergency setting where patients may present for minor ailments, these routes of administration are advantageous, particularly when treating healthy, painful patients.

Transmucosal (oral and nasal) administration of opioids allows uptake of drug without first-pass metabolism. Drug absorption is relatively rapid (comparable to IM administration) and can be dosed similar to that administered parenterally. This route has been established as an effective and safe technique for administering buprenorphine to cats but requires the cat to have a normal (alkaline) oral pH [1]. Significant dental disease can lower the oral pH and may reduce the bioavailability of buprenorphine administered by this route. Buprenorphine is also not as bioavailable when administered transmucosally to dogs and higher doses are required to reach therapeutic levels [2].

In the US, fentanyl is the only opioid currently marketed in a transdermal formulation by veterinary distributors; however, buprenorphine patches are available in the US. Several European studies looking at the effectiveness of buprenorphine patches in cats and dogs have not shown a tremendous advantage to their use and until more favorable data are available, buprenorphine patch use in animals is not recommended. Patches must be placed in an area inaccessible to patient disruption or consumption. Hair should be clipped and the skin oil removed with minimal damage or irritation to the tissue. Fentanyl patches are dosed at 2–3 μg/kg for dogs and 12–25 μg per cat. The duration of action of these patches on dogs has been shown to be up to 72 hours whereas a fentanyl patch on a cat has been shown to maintain therapeutic drug blood levels in excess of 4 days. Owners must bring the patient to the veterinarian for patch placement.

Advantages and Side-Effects

There are many advantages to using opioids to treat pain in an intensive care setting. Opioids provide excellent analgesia with minimal cardiovascular alterations and can be antagonized in situations where they cause significant undesirable effects. The older opioids are quite reasonably priced and there are many different drugs and delivery mechanisms, allowing the veterinarian to select an analgesic that closely matches the needs of both the patient and the clinic or client. They cause sedation, which can be helpful when a patient is experiencing stress from hospitalization, can be titrated to effect and in most situations are the most innocuous and effective analgesics that can be administered, particularly when compared to non-steroidal anti-inflammatory drugs (NSAIDs) and alpha-2 agonists.

However, there are side-effects associated with their use that must be considered when making the decision to include opioids in the patient's treatment plan. Side-effects relevant to patients in a critical care setting are described below.

In most cases, reducing the dose of the opioid is an effective way to reduce the side-effects. In some situations, using an agonist/antagonist or partial agonist, which has a ceiling on the effects it causes, is an effective way to reduce side-effects but critical patients may have a profound response to these drugs and they should also be titrated to effect if used in a critical care setting. This is particularly problematic in the case of buprenorphine, which is difficult to titrate to effect due to the relatively long time (15–30 min) it takes to reach peak effect after IV administration, and its high affinity for the mu-receptor, which makes it very difficult to reverse. Because of this, the author strongly recommends buprenorphine not be used in a critical care setting until the patient has been well stabilized and is able to tolerate the effect of other opioids at standard doses.

Respiratory Effects

Opioids depress the respiratory center's responsiveness to CO_2. Patients have a dose-dependent increase in $PaCO_2$ due to a decrease in minute volume that is typically manifest as a decrease in respiratory rate although the tidal volume may also decrease. Respiratory depression is well tolerated in animals with no respiratory disease but in animals with upper airway or lung disease, the respiratory depression can cause significant hypoxemia and potentially death. Respiratory depression can also be potentially fatal in patients with pre-existing elevations in intracranial pressure (ICP) such as is associated with head trauma or brain tumors, since the rise in $PaCO_2$ will further increases ICP, potentially leading to brain herniation, coma, and death. Elevations in $PaCO_2$

will also worsen acidosis when patients have underlying metabolic disease and in patients with hyperkalemia due to renal disease, worsening acidosis further increases blood potassium levels, potentially resulting in cardiac arrhythmias and death.

In all of these groups of patients, reversible opioids can be safely administered in the presence of pre-existing pain, at low-to-moderate doses and only if proper care is taken to assure the patient is frequently assessed for complications described above. If problems are observed, opioids should be reversed with naloxone given slowly, over 2–3 minutes, IV to effect.

Administration of opioids to pregnant animals will cause both maternal and fetal respiratory depression since opioids readily cross the placenta. Although relatively well tolerated by the mother, oxygen should be concurrently supplemented to ensure that oxygen delivery to the fetus is not compromised. Neonates delivered after maternal administration of opioids should be treated with naloxone, administered either orally or IV in the umbilical vein to reverse the drug-induced respiratory depression and stimulate ventilation (see Chapter 118).

Antitussive Effects

Opioid agonists, partial agonists, and agonists/antagonists suppress the cough reflex. This effect is mediated by opioid receptors on A delta fibers that are located in or beneath the respiratory epithelium and is independent of their action on the respiratory center [3]. Opioids should be avoided in animals that are at risk for regurgitation and aspiration, particularly brachycephalic breeds with pre-existing evidence of aspiration pneumonia and/or dyspnea. Opioids should also be avoided in dogs that have undergone an arytenoidectomy or laryngeal tieback surgery because they are more likely to aspirate food or regurgitated material that enters their oral cavity.

Effects on Body Temperature

In dogs, opioids reset the thermoregulatory center in the brain, causing the patient to actively cool themselves by panting or moving away from external heat sources. Once the body temperature drops, dogs will not shiver to maintain normothermia. Hypothermic patients are more likely to be bradycardic and show signs of excessive sedation (see Chapter 148). In cats, opioid agonists, especially at higher doses, can cause elevations in body temperature. Drugs such as morphine and hydromorphone have been shown to cause hyperthermia. The SC buprenorphine formulation Simbadol, which is dosed at a higher dose than that used for IM/IV/OTM, has also been associated with hyperthermia.

All patients receiving opioids should have their body temperature regularly assessed and efforts should be made to keep their temperatures within a normal physiological range.

Opioid-Induced Hyperalgesia (OIH)

Opioids can cause hyperalgesia in patients after one or more doses due to somewhat complex cellular and molecular processes that result in the development of this condition. The most consistent finding that leads to a diagnosis of OIH is a worsening of pain in response to increasing doses of opioids. The following options have been shown to be helpful in resolving OIH: reduce the dose of opioid or rotate opioid used. Methadone is an antagonist at NMDA receptors and may be beneficial in improving analgesia due to its multimodal mechanism of action. NMDA receptor antagonists such as ketamine (0.1–0.6 mg/kg/h) or amantadine, or a low dose infusion of an alpha-2agonist (e.g. dexmedetomidine at 0.025–1 ug/kg/h) will help reduce the dose of opioid needed. A systemic infusion of lidocaine at 1–3 mg/kg/h may also reduce opioid requirements and resolve OIH.

Urine Retention

Opioids that are agonists at the mu-receptor have been reported to cause dose-related urinary retention (inability to urinate with a full bladder). Studies have demonstrated that fentanyl, buprenorphine, and, to a lesser extent, morphine alter bladder sensations and increase the residual volume in the bladder after voiding for several hours after administration. This occurs because opioids inhibit the sacral parasympathetic outflow, especially after epidural administration and after large IV doses, resulting in an increased maximal bladder capacity and detrusor muscle relaxation. Animals being treated with opioid agonists should have their urine output and bladder size assessed regularly and a urinary catheter should be placed if the bladder cannot be expressed.

Other Effects

Dysphoria
Animals may vocalize, pace, and appear anxious after opioid administration. The patient should be assessed to identify and resolve any underlying conditions such as a full bladder or a need to defecate. If none is identified, a low dose of a tranquilizer such as acepromazine or a benzodiazepine can be administered or the prescribed opioid changed to an agonist/antagonist, fentanyl or methadone, all of which are less likely to be associated with dysphoria.

Bradycardia

Central stimulation of vagal input caused by opioids may result in bradycardia. This effect is more severe in hypothermic patients.

Vomiting, Nausea, and Defecation

In opioid-naive animals, opioid administration frequently results in GI stimulation manifested as nausea, vomiting, and defecation early after the drug is administered IV, IM or SC. This usually only occurs with the first dose of an opioid. Full-agonist opioids both stimulate the chemoreceptor trigger zone (CRTZ), which causes vomiting, and depress the vomiting center which blocks input from the CRTZ. Opioids quickly reach the CRTZ but their lipid solubility determines how fast they cross the blood–brain barrier (BBB) to reach the vomiting center.

Vomiting occurs more frequently with morphine sulfate administration and less commonly with oxymorphone and fentanyl administration. This is because morphine is more water soluble than oxymorphone so crosses the BBB more slowly, allowing time for CRTZ activation to stimulate the vomiting center. Vomiting occurs rarely after administration of partial agonists and agonists/antagonists although these drugs do induce other GI effects typical of opioid administration, including delayed GI motility and increased sphincter tone.

Prior to administering opioids to any patient, it is important to ensure that the animal can open its mouth, is alert enough to position itself appropriately to avoid aspiration and is not limited by muzzles or other devices, and the oral and pharyngeal cavities are not obstructed by disease conditions (e.g. large oral foreign bodies or tumors). Avoid vomiting by administering an antiemetic such as maropitant prior to opioid dosing.

Histamine Release

Morphine and meperidine can induce histamine release when administered rapidly intravenously. To prevent or minimize this response, these two opioids should ideally not be administered intravenously. If an analgesic is immediately required, the drugs may be slowly administered intravenously (over 2–3 min) while the patient is monitored for signs of hypotension, shock or cutaneous manifestations of histamine release.

Immunosuppression

Opioids have immunomodulatory effects *in vitro* and in animal models, which are generally believed to increase the risk of infection. However, the clinical significance of opioid-induced immune suppression remains controversial, even in the critical care setting. Like other opioid-induced actions, the immune effects are reversible with administration of an opioid receptor antagonist.

Patient Management Recommendations

Opioids remain the safest and most effective analgesics for treating pain. The practitioner should follow simple guidelines to avoid using them in patients unable to tolerate the side-effects and patients receiving opioids should be monitored for significant adverse events as indicated below.

- Do not administer full agonists to any patient with an obstructed oral cavity or evidence of elevated ICP.
- Opioids may be used in patients with respiratory compromise only to facilitate correction of the problem. During this time, oxygen should be supplemented. If the problem cannot be corrected, the opioid should be reversed with naloxone, administered slowly IV, over 2–5 minutes to effect.
- Sick and debilitated patients should only receive reversible opioids.
- Monitor urine output and defecation in patients receiving opioids and take action (e.g. bladder catheterization, stool softener) if indicated.
- Giving an agonist/antagonist opioid (i.e. butorphanol) to an animal that has received a full agonist (i.e. hydromorphone, oxymorphone or fentanyl) will reverse the effects of the full agonist. This can make awake animals more painful (*bad*) or reduce side-effects in an unarousable patient showing excessive sedation after opioid administration (*good*).

References

1 Robertson SA, Taylor PM, Sear JW. Systemic uptake of buprenorphine by cats after oral transmucosal administration. *Vet Rec* 2003;152:675–678.
2 Ko JC, Freeman LJ, Barletta M, et al. Efficacy of oral transmucosal and intravenous administration of buprenorphine before surgery for postoperative analgesia in dogs undergoing ovariohysterectomy. *J Am Vet Med Assoc* 2011;238:318–328.
3 Reynolds SM, Mackenzie AJ, Spina D, Page CP. The pharmacology of cough. *Trends Pharmacol Sci* 2004;25:569–576.

195

Alpha-2 Adrenergic Agonists

Katherine A. Cummings, DVM, DACVAA

Angell Animal Medical Center, Boston, MA, USA

Introduction

The alpha-2 agonists cause dose-dependent sedation, anxiolysis, and analgesia via action at alpha-2 receptors in the CNS and peripheral tissues. Three alpha-2 receptor subtypes have been identified: alpha-2A, alpha-2B , and alpha-2C, all of which are G-protein-coupled receptors [1–3]. Important consequences of alpha-2A receptor binding include supraspinal analgesia, sympatholytic effects, and sedation with primary localization of this receptor in the CNS (cerebral cortex and locus ceruleus) [2,3]. Alpha-2B receptors are located in the spinal cord and vascular endothelium; therefore, receptor binding at this location causes the initial vasoconstriction observed with alpha-2 agonist administration, but also allows for spinal analgesia [2,3]. The alpha-2C receptor is responsible for mediating hypothermia [2].

Alpha-2 agonists used historically in small animal patients include xylazine, medetomidine, and dexmedetomidine. Medetomidine is a racemic mixture of levo- and dex-medetomidine with the L-isomer exhibiting significantly less activity than the D-isomer [1–3]. Receptor selectivity ratios (alpha-2:alpha-1) indicate that medetomidine and dexmedetomidine have higher specificity (1620:1) for the alpha-2 receptor than xylazine (160:1) [1–3].

For the purposes of this chapter, dexmedetomidine will be the drug of focus given its more widespread use in small animal patients and the limited commercial availability of medetomidine. The duration of action of dexmedetomidine in dogs and cats is approximately 1–2 hours, and the action of the drug can be effectively reversed with atipamezole.

Alpha-2 agonists should be used cautiously in emergent and critically ill patients, mainly due to their profound cardiovascular side-effects at the manufacturer's recommended dose. In patients presenting with any degree of hemodynamic instability, dexmedetomidine should be avoided, as other drug options are available with minimal to no effects on cardiovascular function.

The main physiological alterations that follow alpha-2 agonist administration include an initial increase in systemic vascular resistance and bradycardia [1–5]. The combination of these peripheral effects can reduce cardiac output up to 30–50% in dogs and cats, depending on the dosage of alpha-2 agonist administered [1–6]. A delayed central phase follows with decreased sympathetic output, causing continued bradycardia and hypotension [2,3,5]. Anticholinergics can be administered concurrently to offset dexmedetomidine-induced bradyarrhythmias; however, myocardial work and oxygen demands increase significantly so their use should be reserved for the delayed central phase only (~45-60 minutes after initial administration).

The administration of dexmedetomidine is contraindicated in patients with pre-existing heart disease, such as dilated cardiomyopathy, valvular disease, and pulmonic stenosis, as any increase in afterload and myocardial work would be detrimental [2,5] to the cardiovascular function of the patient. Similarly, patients with underlying arrhythmias should not be given alpha-2 agonists. While one study observed a positive benefit to alpha-2 agonist administration in cats with hypertrophic cardiomyopathy and left ventricular outflow tract obstruction [7], their use remains controversial; therefore, reaching for dexmedetomidine when treating the critical cat with suspected or known heart disease should be avoided [6,8,9] or the dose reduced considerably.

The presence of other underlying disease(s) also influences a patient's ability to tolerate the effects associated with alpha-2 agonist administration.

Textbook of Small Animal Emergency Medicine, First Edition. Edited by Kenneth J. Drobatz, Kate Hopper, Elizabeth Rozanski and Deborah C. Silverstein.
© 2019 John Wiley & Sons, Inc. Published 2019 by John Wiley & Sons, Inc.
Companion Website: www.wiley.com/go/drobatz/textbook

Dexmedetomidine interferes with antidiuretic hormone action at the level of the renal tubules and collecting ducts [2,3], resulting in diuresis. If administered to a patient with urinary tract obstruction, catheterization must be performed rapidly or an alternative sedative should be chosen. Furthermore, in blocked patients with pre-existing bradycardia, dehydration, and significant electrolyte abnormalities, dexmedetomidine should be avoided [10,11]. The majority of cats and some dogs will vomit following dexmedetomidine administration. Consider avoiding dexmedetomidine or administering an anti-emetic in patients with underlying ocular disease in which vomiting will result in an increase in intraocular pressure. Finally, dose-dependent and transient hypoinsulinemia and hyperglycemia can occur due to drug effect on pancreatic beta-cells.

While there are several true contraindications for alpha-2 agonist use in critically ill patients, incorporating dexmedetomidine into pain management strategies and sedation protocols in this subset of patients can be extremely beneficial. In order to optimize the positive effects and minimize the adverse effects associated with dexmedetomidine administration, a significantly *lower* dose must be administered (Table 195.1), and when possible, the drug should be administered concurrently with low doses of other sedative and analgesic drugs. Incorporating dexmedetomidine into sedation protocols in mechanically ventilated dogs and cats with adequate cardiovascular stability is prudent as administration often causes minimal to no alterations in arterial blood gas values such as pH and $PaCO_2$ [2,3]. Use of dexmedetomidine constant-rate infusion (CRI) has proven an equivalent if not superior alternative to benzodiazepines in mechanically ventilated human patients, with fewer behavioral alterations and reduced ventilator times [12].

An additional factor that can be both challenging to recognize and manage in the emergency and ICU patients is pain. Relying on multimodal pain management allows for improved patient comfort and outcome while minimizing side-effects of higher doses of single analgesic agents. This is particularly important in postoperative abdominal, thoracic, and polytrauma cases in which patient pain is multifactorial. Dexmedetomidine bolus and CRI administration has been shown to be effective in both dogs and cats given the antinociceptive properties alpha-2 agonists demonstrate at both central and peripheral levels [1–3,13–16]. Dosing strategies for dexmedetomidine will differ for dogs and cats based on the desired drug effect and route of administration (see Table 195.1).

A unique analgesic application is the use of alpha-2 agonists alongside a local anesthetic to prolong and

Table 195.1 Dexmedetomidine and atipamezole dosing strategies for critical care patients.

Indication	Dosage	Route of administration
Sedation	1–10 µg/kg (dogs)	IM*
	5–15 µg/kg (cats)	IM*
	1–3 µg/kg	IV
Pain management and postoperative sedation	1 µg/kg loading dose, then 0.25–3 µg/kg/h (dogs)	IV**
	0.5–1 µg/kg loading dose, then 0.25–2 µg/kg/h (cats)	IV**
Antisedan (drug reversal, atipamezole)	100 µg/kg	IM, IV

*The IM route of administration should be avoided in emergent and critical care patients since significant underlying disease might influence muscle perfusion and drug uptake. If combining dexmedetomidine with another sedative (e.g. opioid) for IM administration, the dose should be reduced by at least 50%.

**It is recommended to maintain constant-rate infusions in critical patients at the lowest effective dose and titrate the dose up only if needed to improve pain management and provide more adequate anxiolysis.

intensify peripheral nerve blockade [2,17,18]. While this technique requires more specialized skill and equipment (e.g. nerve stimulator, ultrasound guidance), systemic side-effects of dexmedetomidine are blunted and longer lasting analgesia is provided to the patient.

The final two positive benefits of alpha-2 agonists in the emergency room and ICU settings are immunomodulatory properties and drug reversibility. Many studies demonstrate the anti-inflammatory potential of alpha-2 agonists [19–21], which may ultimately improve patient outcome in critically ill dogs and cats.

Lastly, when any drug is administered to a critically ill patient, the ability to rapidly and completely reverse the action of that drug becomes particularly important. Once the reversal agent atipamezole has been given and taken effect, heart rate, blood pressure, and temperature will normalize [1–3,15]. The sedative and analgesic effects are also reversed by atipamezole and alternative analgesia should be provided to the patient with persisting pain. When the effects of dexmedetomidine are not life threatening, drug reversal should be carried out via the intramuscular route as rapid intravenous administration can result in hypotension. In the emergent scenario, however, intravenous administration is recommended.

References

1 Murrell JC, Hellebrekers LJ. Medetomidine and dexmedetomidine: a review of cardiovascular and antinociceptive properties in the dog. *Vet Anaesth Analg* 2005;32:117–127.

2 Tranquilli WJ, Thurmon JC, Grimm KA (eds). *Lumb and Jones' Veterinary Anesthesia and Analgesia*, 4th edn. Blackwell Publishing, Oxford, 2007, pp. 210–227.

3 Grimm KA, Tranquilli WJ, Lamont LA (eds). *Essentials of Small Animal Anesthesia and Analgesia*, 2nd edn. Wiley-Blackwell, Oxford, 2011, pp. 44–48.

4 Pascoe PJ, Raekallio M, Kuusela E, et al. Changes in the minimum alveolar concentration of isoflurane and some cardiopulmonary measurements during three continuous infusion rates of dexmedetomidine in dogs. *Vet Anaesth Analg* 2006;33:97–103.

5 Snyder LBC, Johnson RA. Canine and Feline Anesthesia and Co-existing Disease. Wiley-Blackwell, *Oxford*, 2015.

6 Robertson SA. Assessment and management of acute pain in cats. *J Vet Emerg Crit Care* 2005;15:261–272.

7 Lamont LA, Bulmer BJ, Sisson DD, et al. Doppler echocardiographic effects of medetomidine on dynamic left ventricular out-flow tract obstruction in cats. *J Am Vet Med Assoc* 2002;221:1276–1281.

8 Lamont LA, Bulmer BJ, Grimm KA, et al. Cardiopulmonary evaluation of the use of medetomidine hydrochloride in cats. *Am J Vet Res* 2001;62:1745–1749.

9 Daniel GB, Golden L, Bright JM, et al. The effects of medetomidine on cardiac function in normal cats measured by radionuclide ventriculography. *J Vet Anaesth* 1997;24(2):12–16.

10 Stafford JR, Bartges JW. A clinical review of pathophysiology, diagnosis, and treatment of uroabdomen in the dog and cat. *J Vet Emerg Crit Care* 2013;23:216–229.

11 Garcia de Carellan Mateo A, Brodbelt D, Kulendra N, et al. Retrospective study of the perioperative management and complications of ureteral obstruction in 37 cats. *Vet Anaesth Analg* 2015;42:570–579.

12 Riker RR, Shehabi Y, Bokesch PM, et al. Dexmedetomidine vs midazolam for sedation of critically ill patients: a randomized trial. *JAMA* 2009;301:489–499.

13 Valtolina C, Robben JH, Uilenreef J, et al. Clinical evaluation of the efficacy and safety of a constant rate infusion of dexmedetomidine for postoperative pain management in dogs. *Vet Anaesth Analg* 2009;36: 369–383.

14 Lervik A, Haga HA, Ranheim B, et al. The influence of a constant rate infusion of dexmedetomidine on the nociceptive withdrawal reflex and temporal summation during isoflurane anaesthesia in dogs. *Vet Anaesth Analg* 2012;39:414–425.

15 Granholm M, McKusic BC, Westerholm FC, et al. Evaluation of the clinical efficacy and safety of dexmedetomidine or medetomidine in cats and their reversal with atipamezole. *Vet Anaesth Analg* 2006;33:214–223.

16 Porters N, Bosmans T, Debille M, et al. Sedative and antinociceptive effects of dexmedetomidine and buprenorphine after oral transmucosal or intramuscular administration in cats. *Vet Anaesth Analg* 2014;41:90–96.

17 Bartel AKG, Campoy L, Martin-Flores M, et al. Comparison of bupivacaine and dexmedetomidine femoral and sciatic nerve blocks with bupivacaine and buprenorphine epidural injection for stifle arthroscopy in dogs. *Vet Anaesth Analg* 2016;43:435–443.

18 Campoy L, Read MR. *Small Animal Regional Anesthesia and Analgesia*. Wiley-Blackwell, Oxford, 2013.

19 Anderson SL, Duke-Novakovski T, Singh B. The immune response to anesthesia: Part 2 sedatives, opioids, and injectable anesthetic agents. *Vet Anaesth Analg* 2014;41:553–566.

20 Qiao H, Sanders RD, Ma D, et al. Sedation improves early outcome in severely septic Sprague Dawley rats. *Crit Care* 2009;13:R136.

21 Chen C, Zhang Z, Chen K, et al. Dexmedetomidine regulates inflammatory molecules contributing to ventilator-induced lung injury in dogs. *J Surg Res* 2014;187:211–218.

196

Non-Steroidal Anti-Inflammatory Drugs

Christopher L. Norkus, DVM, DACVAA, CVPP

Allegheny Veterinary Emergency Trauma and Speciality, Monroeville, PA, USA

Introduction

Non-steroidal anti-inflammatory drugs (NSAIDs) are the most widely used class of analgesics in veterinary medicine [1]. Additionally, they possess anti-inflammatory and antipyretic properties. Several agents are currently approved by the United States Food and Drug Administration (FDA) for use in dogs (meloxicam, carprofen, firoxocib, deracoxib, galliprant) and cats (meloxicam, robenacoxib) and are available in a wide variety of formulations including oral, injectable, and transmucosal spray. Several other NSAIDs including mavacoxib, cimicoxib, and vedaprofen are available outside the United States. Off-label usage of NSAIDs in other companion animal species such as birds, rabbits, ferrets, and pocket pets is common. While NSAIDs are the cornerstones in the treatment of osteoarthritis (OA) and other chronic painful conditions, they are generally safe and useful in many emergency room and acute pain settings as well.

Mechanisms of Action

Upon tissue injury, arachidonic acid is released from cell membrane phospholipids by the action of phospholipase A_2, resulting in a chain of events known as the arachidonic acid cascade. Two biologically and clinically important pathways are established, including 5-lipoxygenase (LOX), which metabolizes arachidonic acid into various leukotrienes, and cyclo-oxygenase (COX), which metabolizes arachidonic acid into prostaglandins, prostayclin, and thromboxanes [2]. NSAIDs exert their clinical effect predominantly by the inhibition of COX [3].

Cyclo-oxygenase is present in most tissues and two primary forms of COX have been identified: COX-1 and COX-2 [3]. Initially, COX-1 was recognized as a constitutive isoform whereas COX-2 was identified as an inducible isoform, but further studies have elucidated that both isoforms are constitutive as well as inducible [4–6]. A third isoform (COX-3), identified primarily in the canine cerebral cortex with minimal amounts found peripherally, is selectively inhibited by analgesics such as acetaminophen and metamizol (dypyrone) [7].

Cyclo-oxygenase-1 produces prostaglandin (PG) E_2 and thromboxane A_2 [3]. PGE_2 produces numerous physiological responses, including vasodilation and nociceptor sensitization, leading to both peripheral and central sensitization. PGE_2 plays a crucial role in gastrointestinal (GI) tract functioning, including generation of mucus production, increasing secretion of bicarbonate in the duodenum, decreasing gastric acid secretion, and increasing the rate of turnover of mucosal cells. The function of thromboxane A_2 results in increased platelet aggregation and vasoconstriction, leading to enhanced coagulation and blood clot formation. COX-1 is constitutively expressed in the cerebral cortex where its inhibition may contribute to the central analgesic and antipyretic effects of NSAIDs [8].

Cyclo-oxygenase-2 produces PGE_2, prostacyclin (PGI_2) and 15-epi-lipoxin A4, also known as aspirin-triggered lipoxin (ATL) [3]. PGE_2 produced by COX-2 or COX-1 results in the same physiological effects as discussed previously. PGI_2 is produced in endothelial cells and results in inhibition of platelet aggregation and vasodilation, leading to an antagonistic effect to thromboxane A_2 [3]. PGI_2 has also been identified in inflamed tissues and in the GI tract where it produces similar gastroprotective effects as PGE_2 [3].

Cyclo-oxygenase-2 is constitutively expressed in the dorsal horn of the spinal cord and contributes to the propagation of nociceptive stimuli. Inhibition of COX-2 with NSAIDs can also produce central analgesic effects [9,10]. COX-2 is increased in damaged tissue as well, producing PGE_2 and PGI_2, resulting in sensitization of peripheral nociceptors just as with COX-1 [3]. COX-2 is upregulated in endothelial cells within the hippocampus

Textbook of Small Animal Emergency Medicine, First Edition. Edited by Kenneth J. Drobatz, Kate Hopper, Elizabeth Rozanski and Deborah C. Silverstein.
© 2019 John Wiley & Sons, Inc. Published 2019 by John Wiley & Sons, Inc.
Companion Website: www.wiley.com/go/drobatz/textbook

during fever, which is a proposed mechanism of action for the antipyretic effect of some NSAIDs.

Beyond nociceptior, GI, and hemostatic functions, PGE_2 and PGI_2 alter renal physiology. They increase sodium excretion, inhibit sodium reabsorption, and alter chloride transport [3]. They also stimulate renin release and can profoundly alter total renal blood flow and regional blood flow within the kidneys of dogs [3,11].

Recently, galliprant became FDA approved for dogs as a non-COX-inhibiting NSAID. This drug uniquely targets the PGE_2 receptor EP4 with the goal of achieving anti-inflammatory and analgesic action while theoretically minimizing adverse side-effects. Clinical experience with galliprant remains in its infancy and time will tell whether or not its side-effect profile will truly differ from that of other NSAIDs.

Pharmacokinetics

Non-steroidal anti-inflammatory drugs are well absorbed after oral and injectable administration, with the exception of the licensed formulation of firocoxib which has a low oral bioavailability [12,13]. Deracoxib is best absorbed with food, but efficacy still occurs when administered to fasted dogs [14]. Most NSAIDs are highly bound to plasma proteins, but clinical implications of high protein binding are limited.

The liver is the primary organ of NSAID biotransformation, including biliary secretion, conjugation reactions, and the cytochrome P450 system [12]. Disease leading to decreased hepatic function and ability to biotransform drugs may decrease the rate of elimination and increase the terminal half-life and "area under the curve" which may lead to more total drug exposure and increase adverse effects. Some renal elimination of NSAIDs occurs and urinary alkalinization resulting in ion trapping of the weak acids may increase this elimination. A thorough review of the pharmacokinetics is available elsewhere for further reading [12].

Adverse Effects

Adverse effects of NSAIDs localize to the GI tract, kidneys, liver, and to hemostatic function.

Hemostatic Function

With the exception of aspirin, NSAIDs themselves do not appear to induce clinically significant bleeding disorders and therefore will not be a focus of this section [15–20]. The use of NSAIDs in animal patients with known bleeding disorders has not been fully investigated and

therefore they should be avoided or used with caution at this time. The effect of COX inhibition and the potential for thromboembolic occurrence have not been well studied in dogs and cats.

Gastrointestinal Effects

Gastrointestinal adverse effects are the most commonly reported adverse effect of NSAIDs [21]. Inhibition of the COX enzymes by NSAIDs leads to potential adverse effects such as delayed gastric healing, vomiting, diarrhea, lethargy, anorexia, gastroenteritis, ulceration, GI perforation, and potentially death [3,4,22–27]. NSAIDs are weak acids and can also directly irritate the GI mucosa when administered orally or following secretion in bile regardless of the route of administration [28]. GI ulcers are most commonly reported in the proximal duodenum and pylorus of dogs [27,29]. It is important to understand that when considering the most recently approved NSAIDs (carprofen, meloxicam, deracoxib, firocoxib, robenacoxib), there is no specific evidence-based literature, using controlled clinical trials, demonstrating that one drug produces a lower frequency of GI adverse effect than another.

Renal Effects

Healthy patients given approved doses of NSAIDs are at low risk for renal adverse events. However, as discussed in previous sections, PGE_2 and PGI_2 have a profound effect on the kidney. In dogs, COX-1 and COX-2 are both constitutively expressed and COX-2 is upregulated in times of renal ischemia and hypotension [30,31]. In response to volume depletion, hypotension, or hyponatremia, PGE_2 production is increased by COX-2 in dogs, resulting in alteration of renal blood flow by decreasing vascular resistance [30,32,33]. Therefore, renal injury secondary to NSAID administration may occur as a result of the inhibition of prostaglandin synthesis.

The effect of label doses of veterinary-approved NSAIDs on canine and feline renal blood flow and the distribution of blood flow within the renal cortex has not been investigated extensively. Reported cases of NSAID-induced nephropathy in dogs and cats are most commonly associated with high doses of NSAIDs or other complicating factors, including sodium depletion, dehydration, hypovolemia, poorly managed perioperative hypotension, shock, and pre-existing renal disease [32–36]. Perianesthetic hypotension should not be an unexpected risk for NSAID renal toxicity as isoflurane and sevoflurane cause a dose-dependent decrease in renal blood flow in dogs [37,38]. It should be expected that any animal undergoing anesthesia has the potential for decreased renal perfusion which may increase the risk of NSAID-induced renal toxicity. In humans, the use of NSAIDs during concurrent congestive heart failure is an additional risk factor for acute kidney injury.

The reported effect of NSAIDs on the renal function of dogs and cats with underlying chronic renal disease is unclear. It has been hypothesized that dogs with underlying renal disease have increased COX-2 expression in the renal vasculature as a compensatory mechanism and NSAID administration could lead to exacerbation of renal disease [3,39]. However, some more recent work has failed to show a detrimental effect of short- and long-term NSAIDs when given to dogs and cats in a setting of chronic kidney disease [40–43]. It is important, however, to consider that patients in these studies underwent regular monitoring and that the NSAID doses used in these studies were often lower than labeled drug doses and that some of these studies were retrospective in nature. Further research on the subject is indicated before strong conclusions can be drawn.

Hepatic Effects

Hepatic toxicity is uncommon but can occur with any pet breed or with any NSAID, and is either a dose-dependent toxicity or an idiosyncratic, dose-independent toxicity. The intrinsic, dose-dependent toxicity is typically due to massive overdosing of NSAIDs [44].

Few data describe the use of NSAIDs in animals with underlying hepatic disease and no data indicate that animals with hepatic disease are at increased risk of NSAID hepatic toxicity. However, the biotransformation and elimination of NSAIDs in these animals may be altered. It is unclear if the dose of an NSAID needs to be decreased for an animal with pre-existing hepatic disease or whether NSAIDs should be avoided all together. The precise dose adjustments in animals with hepatic disease has not been determined and, therefore, any use in animals with hepatic disease should be undertaken with caution and owner consent. Additionally, patients with liver disease may be more prone to GI ulceration and NSAID use in these cases may increase this complication [45].

Drug–Drug Interactions

Non-steroidal anti-inflammatory drugs are highly protein bound and drug displacement of other drugs from albumin can occur, although the clinical occurrence of these interactions is uncommon and low [46].

Administration of NSAIDs with corticosteroids significantly increases the risk of GI toxicity, including ulceration and perforation, and may also result in adverse effects on the kidney and with platelet function [47–50]. The concurrent administration of different NSAIDs may increase the risk for GI adverse effects [48,51]. Based on the information available, the concurrent use of two NSAIDs or an NSAID with a corticosteroid is viewed as contraindicated.

Furosemide's effect on sodium depletion may increase the risk for renal adverse effects of NSAIDs [36]. Patients receiving aminoglycosides or other potentially nephrotoxic agents may also be at higher risk for renal adverse effects. NSAIDs may affect the management of hypertension and have been shown to decrease the blood pressure-lowering effect of angiotensin converting enzyme (ACE) inhibitors and beta-blockers in humans [52,53]. Other work has suggested that the co-administration of ACE inhibitors and NSAIDs may increase the risk of renal injury in patients with impaired function [54].

Clinical Usage

Non-steroidal anti-inflammatory drugs are effective analgesic, anti-inflammatory, and antipyretic agents that are a benefit to the diverse emergency room patient population. There is little evidence to support differences in effectiveness for pain treatment when comparing all NSAIDs. NSAIDs are useful as stand-alone agents or in combination with other drugs for multimodal analgesia. When used at or below their recommended dosage, their benefits often outweigh their risks.

Prior to instituting NSAID therapy, a complete physical examination should be performed. The need for bloodwork and urinalysis should be assessed on an individual patient basis. In addition, information on recent medications, previous drug adverse reactions, and any medical conditions should be reviewed.

Non-steroidal anti-inflammatory drugs should not be administered to patients that are currently dehydrated, experiencing hypotension or systemic hypoperfusion, or have GI disease (including vomiting and diarrhea). Once these issues are resolved, an NSAID can be considered. Due to evidence in humans suggesting an increase in risk of leakage following gastrointestinal surgery, non-steroidal anti-inflammatory drugs should be avoided in dogs and cats following gastrotomy, enterotomy, or anastomosis. It is generally recommended to avoid NSAIDs in patients that are anorexic, although this practice has come into question in humans [55]. NSAIDs should be avoided or used with caution in patients with renal insufficiency, significant hyponatremeia, or hepatopathy. They are strictly contraindicated in patients that recently received or are currently on NSAIDs or corticosteroids. It is the author's opinion that NSAID administration is best withheld until the postanesthetic period to avoid concurrent administration during unexpected perianesthetic hypotension. NSAIDs are not known teratogens in people but they are typically avoided late in gestation and beyond a single dose in the nursing mother to avoid developmental changes to the fetal and newborn kidney.

Drugs such as misoprostol, famotidine, and omeprazole have been recommended for patients with increased risk of GI adverse effects or when NSAIDs are prescribed for long-term use. However, these recommendations lack comprehensive studies with strong evidence to support

their use in dogs and cats at this time. Routine hematological and biochemical analysis is recommended for patients that continue on to long-term NSAID therapy. Appropriate client education and patient selection are paramount to maximize the benefits of NSAIDs in the emergency room while reducing their risk for adverse effects.

References

1 Lascelles BDX, McFarland JM, Swann H. Guidelines for safe and effective use of NSAIDs in dogs. *Vet Ther* 2005;6:237–251.

2 Bertolini A, Ottani A, Sandrini M. Dual acting anti-inflammatory drugs: a reappraisal. *Pharmacol Res* 2001;44:437–450.

3 Simmons DL, Botting RM, Hla T. Cyclooxygenase isozymes: the biology of prostaglandin synthesis and inhibition. *Pharmacol Rev* 2004;56:387–437.

4 Wooten JG, Blikslager AT, Ryan KA, et al. Cyclooxygenase expression and prostanoid production in pyloric and duodenal mucosae in dogs after administration of nonsteroidal anti-inflammatory drugs. *Am J Vet Res* 2008;69:457–464.

5 Wooten JG, Lascelles BD, Cook VL, et al. Evaluation of the relationship between lesions in the gastroduodenal region and cyclooxygenase expression in clinically normal dogs. *Am J Vet Res* 2010;71:630–635

6 Lascelles BD, King S, Roe S, et al. Expression and activity of COX-1 and 2 and 5-LOX in joint tissues from dogs with naturally occurring coxofemoral joint osteoarthritis. *J Orthop Res* 2009;27:1204–1208.

7 Chandrasekharan NV, Dai H, Roos KL, et al. COX-3, a cyclooxygenase-1 variant inhibited by acetaminophen and other analgesic/antipyretic drugs: cloning, structure, and expression. *Proc Natl Acad Sci USA* 2002;99:13926–13931.

8 Braga PC. Ketoprofen: i.c.v. injection and electrophysiological aspects of antinociceptive effect. *Eur J Pharmacol* 1990;184:273–280.

9 Malmberg AB, Yaksh TL Antinociceptive actions of spinal nonsteroidal anti-inflammatory agents on the formalin test in the rat. *J Pharmacol Exp Ther* 1992;263:136–146.

10 Nishiyama T. Analgesic effects of intrathecally administered celecoxib, a cyclooxygenase-2 inhibitor, in the tail flick test and the formalin test in rats. *Acta Anaesthesiol Scand* 2006;50:228–233.

11 Osborn JL, Kopp UC, Thames MD, et al. Interactions among renal nerves, prostaglandins, and renal arterial pressure in the regulation of renin release. *Am J Physiol* 1984;247:F706–713.

12 Lees P. Analgesic, antiinflammatory, antipyretic drugs. In: *Veterinary Pharmacology and Therapeutics*, 9th edn (eds Riviere JE, Papich MG). Wiley-Blackwell, Ames, 2009, pp. 457–492.

13 NADA. Previcox Freedom of Information Summary. NADA, Rockville, 2007, pp. 141–230.

14 NADA. Deramax Freedom of Information Summary. NADA, Rockville, 2007, pp. 141–203.

15 Luna SPL, Basılio AC, Steagall PVM, et al. Evaluation of adverse effects of long-term oral administration of carprofen, etodolac, flunixin meglumine, ketoprofen, and meloxicam in dogs. *Am J Vet Res* 2007;68:258–264.

16 Hickford FH, Barr SC, Erb HN. Effect of carprofen on hemostatic variables in dogs. *Am J Vet Res* 2001;62:1642–1646.

17 Fresno L, Moll J, Penalba B, et al. Effects of preoperative administration of meloxicam on whole blood platelet aggregation, buccal mucosal bleeding time, and haematological indices in dogs undergoing elective ovariohysterectomy. *Vet J* 2005;170:138–140.

18 Kazakos GM, Papazoglou LG, Rallis T, et al. Effects of meloxicam on the haemostatic profile of dogs undergoing orthopaedic surgery. *Vet Rec* 2005;157: 444–446.

19 Blois SL, Allen DG, Wood RD, et al. Effects of aspirin, carprofen, deracoxib, and meloxicam on platelet function and systemic prostaglandin concentrations in healthy dogs. *Am J Vet Res* 2010;71(3):349–358.

20 Mullins KB, Thomason JM, Lunsford KV, et al. Effects of carprofen, meloxicam, and deracoxib on platlet function in dogs. *Vet Anaesth Analg* 2012;39(2):206–217.

21 Monteiro-Steagall BP, Steagall PV, Lascelles BD. Systematic review of nonsteroidal anti-inflammatory drug-induced adverse effects in dogs. *J Vet Intern Med* 2013;27(5):1011–1019.

22 Wallace JL, McKnight W, Reuter BK, et al. NSAID induced gastric damage in rats: requirement for inhibition of both cyclooxygenase 1 and 2. *Gastroenterology* 2000;119:706–714.

23 Wolfe MM, Lichtenstein DR, Singh G. Gastrointestinal toxicity of nonsteroidal antiinflammatory drugs. *N Engl J Med* 1999;340:1888–1899.

24 Whittle BJ. Mechanisms underlying intestinal injury induced by anti-inflammatory COX inhibitors. *Eur J Pharmacol* 2004;500:427–439.

25 Goodman L, Torres B, Punke J, et al. Effects of firocoxib and tepoxalin on healing in a canine gastric mucosal injury model. *J Vet Intern Med* 2009;23:56–62.

26 Fiorucci S, de Lima OM Jr, Mencarelli A, et al. Cyclooxygenase-2-derived lipoxin A4 increases gastric resistance to aspirin-induced damage. *Gastroenterology* 2002;123:1598–1606.

27 Case JB, Fick JL, Rooney MB. Proximal duodenal perforation in three dogs following deracoxib

administration. *J Am Anim Hosp Assoc* 2010;46(4): 255–258.

28 Carter GW, Young PR, Swett LR, et al. Pharmacological studies in the rat with [2-(1,3-didecanoyloxy)- propyl] 2-acetyloxybenzoate (A-45474): an aspirin pro-drug with negligible gastric irritation. *Agents Actions* 1980;10:240–245.

29 Stanton ME, Bright RM. Gastroduodenal ulceration in dogs. Retrospective study of 43 cases and literature review. *J Vet Intern Med* 1998;3:238–244.

30 Khan KN, Venturini CM, Bunch RT, et al. Interspecies differences in renal localization of cyclooxygenase isoforms: implications in nonsteroidal anti-inflammatory drug-related nephrotoxicity. *Toxicol Pathol* 1998;26:612–620.

31 Sellers RS, Senese PB, Khan KN. Interspecies differences in the nephrotoxic response to cyclooxygenase inhibition. *Drug Chem Toxicol* 2004;27:111–122.

32 Opgenorth TJ, Fiksen-Olsen MJ, Romero JC. Role of prostaglandins in the cortical distribution of renal blood flow following reductions in renal perfusion pressure. *Prostaglandins* 1987;34:591–602.

33 Rodrıguez F, Llinas MT, Gonzalez JD, et al. Renal changes induced by a cyclooxygenase-2 inhibitor during normal and low sodium intake. *Hypertension* 2000;36:276–281.

34 Data JL, Chang LC, Nies AS. Alteration of canine renal vascular response to hemorrhage by inhibitors of prostaglandin synthesis. *Am J Physiol* 1976;230:940–945.

35 Lobetti RG, Joubert KE. Effect of administration of nonsteroidal anti-inflammatory drugs before surgery on renal function in clinically normal dogs. *Am J Vet Res* 2000;61:1501–1507.

36 Surdyk K, Sloan DL, Brown AA. Evaluation of the renal effects of ibuprofen and carprofen in euvolemic and volume-depleted dogs. *Int J Appl Res Vet Med* 2001;9:129–136.

37 Hartman JC, Pagel PS, Proctor LT, et al. Influence of desflurane, isoflurane and halothane on regional tissue perfusion in dogs. *Can J Anaesth* 1992;39:877–887.

38 Takeda S, Sato N, Tomaru T. Haemodynamic and splanchnic organ blood flow responses during sevoflurane-induced hypotension in dogs. *Eur J Anaesthesiol* 2002;19:442–446.

39 Lascelles BD, McFarland JM, Swann H. Guidelines for safe and effective use of NSAIDs in dogs. *Vet Ther* 2005;6:237–251.

40 Surdyk KK, Brown CA, Brown SA. Evaluation of glomerular filtration rate in cats with reduced renal mass and administered meloxicam and acetylsalicylic acid. *Am J Vet Res* 2013;74(4):648–651.

41 Gowan RA, Lingard AE, Johnston L, et al. Retrospective case-control study of the effects of long-term dosing with meloxicam on renal function in aged cats with degenerative joint disease. *J Feline Med Surg* 2011;13(10):752–761.

42 Gowan RA, Baral RM, Lingard AE, et al. A retrospective analysis of the effects of meloxicam on the longevity of aged cats with and without overt chronic kidney disease. *J Feline Med Surg* 2012;14(12):876–881.

43 Lomas AL, Lyon SD, Sanderson MW, et al. Acute and chronic effects of tepoxalin on kidney function in dogs with chronic kidney disease and osteoarthritis. *Am J Vet Res* 2013;74(6):939–944.

44 MacPhail CM, Lappin MR, Meyer DJ, et al. Hepatocellular toxicosis associated with administration of carprofen in 21 dogs. *J Am Vet Med Assoc* 1998;212:1895–1901.

45 Stanton ME, Bright RM. Gastroduodenal ulceration in dogs. Retrospective study of 43 cases and literature review. *J Vet Intern Med* 1989;3:238–244.

46 Benet LZ, Hoener BA. Changes in plasma protein binding have little clinical relevance. *Clin Pharmacol Ther* 2002;71:115–121.

47 Dow SW, Rosychuk RA, McChesney AE, et al. Effects of flunixin and flunixin plus prednisone on the gastrointestinal tract of dogs. *Am J Vet Res* 1990;51:1131–1138.

48 Lascelles BD, Blikslager AT, Fox SM, et al. Gastrointestinal tract perforation in dogs treated with a selective cyclooxygenase-2 inhibitor: 29 cases (2002–2003). *J Am Vet Med Assoc* 2005;227:1112–1117.

49 Boston SE, Moens NM, Kruth SA, et al. Endoscopic evaluation of the gastroduodenal mucosa to determine the safety of short-term concurrent administration of meloxicam and dexamethasone in healthy dogs. *Am J Vet Res* 2003;64:1369–1375.

50 Narita T, Sato R, Motoishi K, et al. The interaction between orally administered non-steroidal anti-inflammatory drugs and prednisolone in healthy dogs. *J Vet Med Sci* 2007;69:353–363.

51 Reed S. Nonsteroidal anti-inflammatory drug induced duodenal ulceration and perforation in a mature rottweiler. *Can Vet J* 2002;43:971–972.

52 Webster J. Interactions of NSAIDs with diuretics and beta-blockers mechanisms and clinical implications. *Drugs* 1985;30:32–41.

53 Morgan T, Anderson A. The effect of nonsteroidal anti-inflammatory drugs on blood pressure in patients treated with different antihypertensive drugs. *J Clin Hypertens* 2003;5:53–57.

54 Loboz KK, Shenfield GM. Drug combinations and impaired renal function – the 'triple whammy'. *Br J Clin Pharmacol* 2005;59:239–243.

55 Rainsford, KD, Bjarnason I. NSAIDs: take with food or after fasting? *J Pharm Pharmacol* 2012;64:465–469.

197

Regional Anesthesia Techniques

Marlis L. de Rezende, DVM, PhD, DACVAA

Colorado State University, Fort Collins, CO, USA

Introduction

Regional anesthesia has been extensively used to manage intraoperative and postoperative pain. It is commonly used as part of a multimodal approach to pain management and helps reduce the use of systemic opioids and their associated side-effects. Regional anesthetic techniques provide effective and site-specific analgesia with relatively minimal adverse effects and can be a useful tool to provide analgesia and facilitate procedures in the emergency room [1–4].

Increased familiarity with the use of ultrasound as a diagnostic tool for focused assessments in human emergency rooms has facilitated the expansion of regional anesthesia in that setting, and the same is likely to happen in veterinary medicine. While regional anesthetic techniques are routinely used in veterinary anesthesia, their use in emergency medicine is still limited. Training of emergency clinicians in regional anesthesia techniques as well as clinical studies evaluating their feasibility, effectiveness, and potential benefits in the veterinary emergency room are needed to further expand the use of regional anesthesia.

Selected Regional Anesthetic Techniques

This section provides an overview of regional anesthesia techniques (Table 197.1). Selected procedures of particular interest for the emergency clinician are described in the text. For the interested reader, more specific information and excellent in-depth technique descriptions can be found in dedicated sources [5]. Please note that to perform the majority of the techniques discussed here, sedation or brief anesthesia may be required to prevent patient movement. The choice of sedation and/or anesthetic protocols should be made according to the temperament and health status of each individual patient.

Intercostal Nerve Blocks

Intercostal nerve blocks can be used to provide anesthesia and analgesia for fractured ribs, flail chest, intercostal thoracotomies, thoracocenthesis, chest tube placement or any other procedure involving the thoracic wall (see Chapters 49 and 184). This technique is easy to perform. The ribs are identified by manual palpation and ideally the block should be performed as dorsal as possible in order to maximize the desensitized area. Intercostal nerves and the associated artery and vein are located just caudal to each rib. The needle is typically directed into the lateral aspect of the rib and then walked off its caudal border and advanced slightly medial. After careful aspiration (blood or air would indicate that the needle tip was unintentionally placed in a vessel or within the pleural space), local anesthetic is injected [6].

Due to the distribution of the innervation, it is generally recommended that at least two intercostal spaces be blocked cranially and caudally to the intercostal space one wishes to desensitize. The use of electrolocation has been suggested to increase the safety of this technique in overweight patients when palpation of the ribs is difficult [5,6].

Interpleural Block

Interpleural blockade is usually used to provide analgesia for postoperative thoracotomies and other painful procedures involving the chest wall. Analgesia to the cranial abdomen (pancreas and liver) is also reported in people [7]. This technique is typically used when a chest tube is in place (a catheter could be placed in the pleural space for this purpose). It involves the blockade of intercostal nerves by the diffusion of local anesthetic administered within the interpleural space via the chest tube or catheter.

After local anesthetic injection, the animal should be placed with the side to be desensitized down (or in sternal

Table 197.1 Brief overview of selected regional anesthetic techniques, categorized by region of anatomical location.

	Desensitized area	Indications	Notes of interest	References
Head				
Maxillary block	Alveolar bone, teeth and surrounding soft tissue Hard and soft palates Upper lip Nose	Maxillary fractures Teeth extractions Upper lip lacerations Foreign body removal Rhinoscopy Biopsies	This block provides desensitization ipsilateral to the nerve blocked. A bilateral block is needed for procedures involving the entire nose, palate, and incisors. This block does not desensitize the nasal septal mucosa and additional analgesia may be required	[8,29,30]
Mandibular (inferior alveolar) block	Alveolar bone, teeth and surrounding soft tissue Lower lip/chin	Mandible fractures Teeth extractions Lower lip laceration Biopsies	This block provides desensitization ipsilateral to the nerve blocked	[8,29,30]
Auriculotemporal, great auricular, and internal auricular nerve block	Internal and external ear	Ear canal ablation Deep ear cleaning Foreign body removal Aural hematomas Laceration repair	This block has shown benefit for deep ear canal debridement but further studies are needed to verify its efficacy for other procedures of the ear	[31,32]
Thoracic limb				
Brachial plexus block	From scapula to digits (cervical paravertebral approach) From mid-humerus to digits (axillary approach)	Procedures of distal humerus, at or below the elbow, including: Fracture repair Arthroscopy Arthrodesis Wound debridement Laceration repair	The cervical paravertebral approach is difficult to perform (especially in muscular or obese dogs) and has been associated with low success rates and relatively high incidence of complications	[33–38]
Radial, ulnar, median, and musculocutaneous (RUMM) nerve block	Forelimb, distal to the elbow	Procedures distal of the elbow, including: Fracture repair Arthrodesis Wound debridement Lacerations	While the blind technique was associated with low efficacy, the use of electrolocation and ultrasound provided successful analgesia	[39,40–42]
Pelvic limb				
Combined psoas compartment block and parasacral block	The entire pelvic limb (including hemipelvis and coxofemoral joint)	Surgical procedures of the proximal pelvic limb, involving the hemipelvis and coxofemoral joint: Femur fracture repair Amputation	The techniques described to provide such proximal blocks are technically more challenging and carry a higher risk of complication. An epidural would be an alternative technique for most procedures performed under these blocks	[37,43–46]
Combined femoral and sciatic nerve blocks	From mid-femur to digits (inguinal approach for femoral and distal to the ischiatic tuberosity for sciatic nerve)	Procedures distal to mid-femur: Tibial and distal fracture repair Correction of femorotibial joint instability (TPLO, MPL, etc.)	Desensitization of the tarsal joint and distal structures can be achieved with just a sciatic nerve block (except for the first digit and the skin over the dorsomedial aspect of the tarsus, which are innervated by the femoral nerve)	[46]

MPL, medial pateller luxation; TPLO, tibial plateau leveling osteotomy.

198

Go Home Analgesics

Ashley Wiese, DVM, MS, DACVAA

MedVet Medical and Cancer Center for Pets, Cincinnati, OH, USA

Pain Assessment

Every animal presented to the emergency department should be assessed for evidence of pain using a pain scale that all staff are trained on and the pain score should be documented in the animal's medical record.

Pain assessment in animals is largely interpretation of animal behavior and understanding pain behaviors for dogs and cats [1]. Animals presenting to the emergency department are known to have a high incidence of pain, but detection of pain behaviors can be challenging in traumatized animals [2]. Generally, there is no pre-existing veterinarian–patient relationship that precludes the veterinarian from being able to develop an understanding of normal behaviors or reliable pain behaviors exhibited by this individual. Additionally, traumatized animals may not demonstrate normal pain behaviors due to the neuroendocrine response to trauma, resulting in sympathetic activation and release of endorphins and enkephalins, and endogenous opioids. Environmental factors such as traumatic events and physiological factors such as species, age, body condition, and concurrent disease may influence pain behaviors by either amplifying or tempering pain responses and should be taken into consideration when assessing animals for pain. Alternative means of assessment and an appreciation for conditions that are normally associated with pain are necessary and often an empiric approach to managing pain may be necessary in order to avoid undertreating pain in these animals [3,4].

Various pain assessment scales have been described for use in veterinary medicine, including the visual analogue scale (VAS), a simple descriptive pain scale, the numeric rating scale, and categorical pain scales [1]. Many pain scales are subjective, allow for bias, and are associated with interobserver variability. Categorical pain scales that utilize both physiological and behavior indicators of pain may be the most reliable assessment tools when acute or chronic scoring systems are used [4,5]. More

recently, owner assessment of pain in their pet through the implementation of questionnaires has been used to aid the clinical assessment of pain. Utilization of dog- and cat-specific outcome measure questionnaires introduces another level of consideration of pain assessment by questioning individuals who are most familiar with an animal's behavior [6–10].

Pathophysiology of Pain

Pain can arise from acute, high-intensity stimuli, from tissue injury or inflammation or damage of peripheral nerves. The high-intensity stimuli responsible for acute pain carry a high propensity for actual or potential tissue damage and are associated with aversive, protective behaviors (withdrawal, guarding) that are generally proportional to the intensity of the stimulus. Somatotropic localization of pain origin is usually well defined. Acute pain activates the autonomic nervous system such that these animals generate a measurable sympathetic response proportional to the stimulus intensity. In fact, autonomic responses such as heart rate variability represent a potential objective modality for acute pain assessment [11].

Pain and stress associated with tissue damage play a prominent role in the traumatized patient by triggering a neuroendocrine reaction leading to local inflammation or, if severe and progressive, systemic inflammation [12]. Tissue injury or inflammation alters the response characteristics of small afferent nerve endings that innervate inflamed tissues. Afferent nerve endings that are typically responsive only to high-intensity stimuli are now activated with lower intensity stimuli, an activation of so-called silent nociceptors. There is a disproportionate stimulus–response relationship such that there is an enhanced pain response and an increase in nerve firing given the level of stimulus applied. Characteristic of

Textbook of Small Animal Emergency Medicine, First Edition. Edited by Kenneth J. Drobatz, Kate Hopper, Elizabeth Rozanski and Deborah C. Silverstein.
© 2019 John Wiley & Sons, Inc. Published 2019 by John Wiley & Sons, Inc.
Companion Website: www.wiley.com/go/drobatz/textbook

the inflammatory pain state, there is activation of local factors and mediators that lead to the altered afferent responses described above. Release of local proinflammatory cytokines and peptides comprise this sensitizing soup [12,13]. Central spinal action of cyclo-oxygenase (COX) also plays a major role in inflammatory pain [14]. Facilitated input from afferent nerves in the setting of inflammation leads to the release of prostaglandins from the second-order neurons which bind prostanoid receptors in nerve terminals and enhance spinal excitability. Excitatory neurotransmitters, including glutamate and substance P, are released from primary afferent neurons in response to tissue injury and inflammation that cause persistent activity in small primary afferent nerves.

Damage to peripheral nerves, a condition that may or may not be associated with tissue damage, exhibits unique characteristics compared to acute or inflammatory pain. Neuropathic pain persists beyond the point at which the stimulus is removed and tissue healing occurs. Pain may be spontaneous or unprovoked and is referred to the peripheral distributions of the injured nerve. Tactile allodynia, non-painful stimuli such as light touch evoking a pain response, is a salient feature of neuropathic pain. Unlike acute pain or pain associated with tissue injury or inflammation, animals with neuropathic pain have an attenuated response to traditionally efficacious analgesics such as opioids.

Go Home Analgesics

Optimal management of pain requires a mechanistic approach to classifying pain, ultimately allowing selection of pain therapeutics targeted at specific components of the pain pathway (Table 198.1). Pain associated with trauma or emergency situations is often multimechanistic in nature, necessitating a multimodal therapeutic approach [15]. In-hospital management of pain in the emergency department is often opioid based, but transitioning to go home analgesics while accounting for all aspects of the pain syndrome often requires non-injectable formulations. Common go home analgesics are usually oral formulations although a number of non-injectable, parenteral formulations of analgesics are now available (Table 198.2).

Opioids

Opioids represent the mainstay for management of acute, physiological pain. Unfortunately, bioavailability of oral formulations is generally poor and metabolism from prodrug to active metabolites is limited in dogs and cats, leading to lack of clinical efficacy [16,17]. A study investigating codeine in dogs demonstrated

Table 198.1 Efficacy of common go home analgesics in the treatment of specific pain syndromes. Drug classes are considered effective (+), ineffective (–), or demonstrated to have questionable efficacy (+/–).

Drug class	Acute, physiological pain	Tissue injury, inflammatory pain	Nerve injury, neuropathic pain
Opioid	+	+	+/–
Non-steroidal anti-inflammatory drug	+	+	+
NMDA antagonist	–	+	+
Anticonvulsant (gabapentin)	–	+	+
Tricyclic antidepressant	–	+	+
Tramadol	+/–	+	+

NMDA, N-methyl-D-aspartate.

analgesic efficacy comparable to tramadol but rescue analgesia was required in a third of animals receiving codeine [18]. Additionally, oral opioids such as codeine, hydrocodone, morphine, oxycodone, and others may be co-formulated with acetaminophen, which poses toxicity potential and represents a significant risk for liability due to the abuse potential by owners and drug diversion.

The limited efficacy of oral opioid formulations has led to the development and utilization of parenteral formulations such as patches, transdermal creams, and injectable forms administered transmucosally. Fentanyl patches have long been utilized as a means for providing multi-day opioid therapy in the home setting despite unpredictable plasma concentrations [19–21].

Buprenorphine is available as a 0.3 mg/mL injectable formulation suitable for oral transmucosal administration in cats in the home setting and a 1.8 mg/mL solution suitable for once-daily subcutaneous administration lasting 24 hours (not to be dispensed to the owner) for the management of pain in cats [22,23].

Non-Steroidal Anti-Inflammatory Drugs

The therapeutic role NSAIDs play in treating pain associated with hypersensitivity pain states in emergency patients must be balanced with their potential adverse effects. The homeostatic functions of constitutively expressed COX isoforms are related to the adverse effects commonly encountered with this drug class. Platelet dysfunction, renal, hepatic, and gastrointestinal

Table 198.2 Common go home analgesics for dogs and cats.

Drug	Dog	Cat	Comments
Non-steroidal anti-inflammatory drugs			
Carprofen	4.4 mg/kg PO SID 2.2 mg/kg PO BID 4.4 mg/kg SC	4 mg/kg SC once	Off label in cats
Deracoxib	3–4 mg/kg PO SID (postop pain) 1–2 mg/kg PO SID (OA)		
Firocoxib	5 mg/kg PO SID	1.5 mg/kg PO once	Off label in cats
Ketoprofen	0.5–1 mg/kg PO BID	0.5–1 mg/kg PO SID 7–10 days	
Meloxicam	0.2 mg/kg PO once on day 1 then 0.1 mg/kg PO SID	0.3 mg/kg SC once	Black box warning for use in cats, lowest effective dose should be used
Robenacoxib	1 mg/kg PO SID	1–2 mg/kg PO SID up to 3 days	Do not administer with food
Tepoxalin	10–20 mg/kg PO on day 1 then 10 mg/kg SID	5–10 mg/kg	
Grapiprant	2 mg/kg PO SID (dogs)	No dose for cats	
Opioids			
Buprenorphine	–	0.01–0.03 mg/kg oral transmucosal TID	
Buprenorphine (Simbadol)	–	0.24 mg/kg SC SID	Recommend for in-hospital use prior to discharge
Fentanyl			
Transdermal patch (Duragesic)	<10 kg 25 μg/h 10–20 kg 50 μg/h 20–30 kg 75 μg/h >30 kg 100 μg/h	25 μg/h	18–24 h to peak effect in dogs 12–18 h to peak effect in cats
Analgesic adjuvants			
Amantadine	2–5 mg/kg PO SID-BID×at least 28 days	2–5 mg/kg PO SID-BID×at least 28 days	
Amitriptyline	1–2 mg/kg PO SID- BID	0.5–1 mg/kg PO SID	Not recommended to co-administer with tramadol or trazadone
Gabapentin	10–20 mg/kg PO BID-QID	10–20 mg/kg PO BID-QID	
Tramadol	2–5 mg/kg PO TID-QID	2–4 mg/kg PO BID	Unpalatable to cats

BID, twice a day (*bis in die*); OA, osteoarthritis; PO, by mouth (*per os*); QID, four times a day (*quater in die*): SC, subcutaneous; SID, once a day (*semel in die*); TID, three times a day (*ter in die*).

adverse effects constitute the primary adverse effects of NSAID therapy [24,25].

The most common side-effects of NSAIDs affect the gastrointestinal tract in dogs although more recently labeled NSAIDs, such as firocoxib, meloxicam, and carprofen, appear to have a lower incidence compared to older drugs such as aspirin, ketoprofen, etodolac, and flunixin meglumine [25–29]. It is possible that better COX-2 selectivity allowing for COX-1-mediated production of gastric prostaglandin E_2 (PGE_2) may account for the safer gastrointestinal profile in newer NSAIDs, but long-term safety studies are needed to definitively prove safety over similar but older drugs

[30]. Measures taken to minimize the risk of gastrointestinal and other side-effects of NSAIDs in dogs include ensuring they are eating and drinking normally throughout the course of therapy. Co-administration of proton pump inhibitors, H2 receptor antagonists or synthetic prostaglandin analogues such as misoprostol has limited evidence of efficacy.

The trauma patient poses the additional risk that volume depletion or hypovolemia may be present. The use of NSAIDs in volume-depleted or hypovolemic patients should be avoided until a normal circulating volume is re-established due to the risk for hypoperfusion to the gastrointestinal and renal systems [31,32].

Other animals in which NSAIDs should be avoided include pregnant or lactating animals, those with asthma or severe pulmonary disease, acute intervertebral disk herniation due to risk of worsening hemorrhage, coagulopathies, animals currently receiving NSAIDs or corticosteroids, and animals with hepatic or renal disease due to the risk for adverse effects [33].

Renal and gastrointestinal effects are the most common reported adverse effects of NSAIDs in cats. The 2010 Food and Drug Administration's addition of a Black Box Warning to the label for oral and injectable meloxicam for cats, brought about by the increased incidence of renal failure and death associated with this drug, prompted the re-evaluation of the off-label use of NSAIDs in cats. Inhibition of vasodilatory PGE_2 and PGI_2 production leading to vasoconstriction-mediated renal perfusion impairment, renal tubulointerstitial nephritis, and papillary necrosis resulting in renal failure are the primary mechanisms for renal toxicity [34]. Robenacoxib, a newer NSAID labeled for cats, appears to have a better safety and efficacy profile than meloxicam or ketoprofen [35–37]. Long-term studies evaluating safety are limited but do not suggest safety concerns for 9–30 day dosing [37–39].

Grapiprant

The priprant class of drugs act as antagonists at the target receptors for prostglandins: prostanoid (EP) receptors [40]. The E type prostaglandins, particularly PGE2, is one of the most widely produced PGs and is responsible for a variety of physiological functions, namely inflammation and pain. The target receptors whereby PGE2 exerts its effects are the EP1, EP2, EP3 and EP4 receptors [41,42]. Sensory neuron sensitization and pain are primarily mediated through activation of the EP4 receptor.

Grapiprant (Galliprant®), a selective EP4 receptor antagonist, is labeled for use in the United States to treat pain and inflammation associated with osteoarthritis in dogs. Grapiprant has been demonstrated to be effective in reducing owner and veterinarian-assessed pain in dogs with naturally occurring osteoarthritis administered 2 mg/kg orally for 28 days [43]. Most common side-effects, vomiting or diarrhea, are mild, with relatively low incidence rate – 17% and 12% respectively [43]. While not yet labeled for use in cats, early pharmacokinetic data appears similar to dogs [40].

Adjunctive or Alternative Analgesics

Tramadol

Tramadol is not a traditional opioid but has mu-opioid receptor agonist activity as well as serotonin and norepinephrine reuptake inhibition and alpha-2 receptor

agonism. Little parent drug activity at opioid receptors and limited active metabolite formation mean this drug has limited efficacy for acute pain in dogs [44–46]. Cats, however, readily produce the active metabolite responsible for opioid effect, O-desmethyltramadol, and therefore have demonstrated analgesic effects in acute pain models [47,48]. Use of tramadol for inflammatory or neuropathic pain states in dogs produces very modest analgesic effects and best utilization of this drug is as an adjunct to other analgesics [49]. Tramadol administered orally is generally well tolerated in dogs but can cause profuse salivation in cats, presumably due to a bitter taste.

Caution is advised when prescribing monodrug therapy or multimodal therapy using drugs that inhibit reuptake of serotonin or have serotonergic effects (tramadol, amitriptyline, trazadone), particularly if animals are on other therapies that have serotonergic effects as the development of serotonin syndrome is possible [50].

Amantadine

Amantadine, an antiviral, is the primary oral N-methyl-D-aspartate (NMDA) antagonist currently used in small animal veterinary medicine. The NMDA receptor is activated with prolonged or significant afferent C-fiber stimulation, which occurs in tissue and/or nerve injury, causing depolarization of second-order neurons in the dorsal horn of the spinal cord. Preventing activation of the NMDA receptor or treating temporally summated C-fiber activity-induced sensitization (wind-up) with an NMDA receptor antagonist will reduce hypersensitivity and may also demonstrate an analgesic-sparing effect. While data for the opioid-sparing effect are conflicting in cats, this may be due to limitations in the model (acute nociception) as opposed to lack of effect that has been demonstrated in a hypersensitivity model [51,52]. In a canine population with osteoarthritis, amantadine was demonstrated to have a NSAID-sparing effect [53] and a single case report demonstrating efficacy with a neuropathic pain condition [54].

Gabapentin

Gabapentin, an antiepileptic medication, has been used in the management of neuropathic pain in humans. While its exact mechanism of action is unknown, gabapentin is known to bind the alpha-2 delta-1 subunit of voltage-gated calcium channels that are present in the superficial laminae of the spinal cord dorsal horn and in the dorsal root ganglia. Data on efficacy of gabapentin in neuropathic pain syndromes are limited. Data in dogs are conflicting but dosing might be insufficient in some studies [55–58].

Cat data are limited to case reports, including trauma cases, and appear more positive although a control population was not available due to the nature of the information (case reports) [59–62]. Sedation and ataxia are common side-effects that can be minimized by adjusting the dosing schedule (reducing the dose or increasing dosing interval).

Tricyclic Antidepressants

Tricyclic antidepressants such as amitriptyline inhibit reuptake of serotonin and norepinephrine, thereby enhancing neurotransmitter activity in central nerve terminals and producing analgesic effects in neuropathic pain syndromes. Analgesia is also produced by augmentation of bulbospinal tone. Little information is available on analgesic efficacy or dosing in dogs and cats [63,64].

Lidocaine Patches

The transdermal lidocaine patch (Lidoderm) allows administration of lidocaine at local tissue concentrations high enough to produce clinically effective local analgesia without inducing complete sensory block, while producing systemic plasma concentrations far below those capable of producing local anesthetic toxicity [65,66]. Lidocaine patches may be used to provide local analgesia

for skin abrasions, lacerations, and severe local skin irritation and itching (hot spots).

The patches are supplied as a 10×14 cm adhesive patch that, unlike fentanyl patches, may be cut into strips or smaller sizes with a scissors prior to removing the protective liner to adapt to various anatomic uses. Clipping the hair where the patch will be applied is recommended but further skin preparation (application of a depilatory or alcohol) is not recommended as this will alter the pharmacokinetics. While original guidelines recommended not covering incisions or open wounds, recent data suggest that while plasma concentrations are higher when placed over mucosal surfaces, they are still well below toxic levels and local skin irritation was not appreciated [67]. The lidocaine patch can be covered with a dressing or bandage and changes in temperature (e.g. heating pad, forced warm air blanket) are tolerated without affecting drug deposition [68]. Generally, one to two patches trimmed into strips to line an incision is sufficient for most dogs. A single patch trimmed to line an incision is usually sufficient in cats. Patches can be left in place for up to 3 days without causing skin irritation while providing a local anesthetic effect. The patch should be disposed of in a way that prevents unintended human or animal exposure.

References

1 Wiese AJ. Assessing pain: pain behaviors. In: *Handbook of Veterinary Pain Management*, 3rd edn (eds Gaynor JS, Muir WW). Elsevier, St Louis, 2015, pp. 67–97.

2 Wiese AJ, Muir WW, Wittum TE. Characteristics of pain and response to analgesic treatment in dogs and cats examined at a veterinary teaching hospital emergency service. *J Am Vet Med Assoc* 2005;226:2004–2009.

3 Hansen B, Hardie E. Prescription and use of analgesics in dogs and cats in a veterinary teaching hospital: 258 cases (1983–1989). *J Am Vet Med Assoc* 1993;202:1485–1494.

4 Reid J, Scot EM, Calvo G, et al. Definitive Glasgow acute pain scale for cats: validation and intervention level. *Vet Rec* 2017;180;449.

5 Epstein ME, Rodanm I, Griffenhagen G, et al. 2015 AAHA/AAFP pain management guidelines for dogs and cats. *J Feline Med Surg* 2015;17:251–272.

6 Benito J, Depuy V, Hardie E, et al. Reliability and discriminatory testing of a client-based metrology instrument, feline musculoskeletal pain index (FMPI) for the evaluation of degenerative joint disease-associated pain in cats. *Vet J* 2013;196:368–373.

7 Gruen ME, Griffith E, Thomson A, et al. Detection of clinically relevant pain relief in cats with degenerative joint disease associated pain. *J Vet Intern Med* 2014;28:346–350.

8 Brown DC, Boston RC, Coyne JC, et al. Ability of the Canine Brief Pain Inventory to detect response to treatment in dogs with osteoarthritis. *J Am Vet Med Assoc* 2008;233:1278–1283.

9 Brown DC, Bell M, Rhodes L. Power of treatment success definitions when the Canine Brief Pain Inventory is used to evaluate carprofen treatment for the control of pain and inflammation in dogs with osteoarthritis. *Am J Vet Res* 2013;74: 1467–1473.

10 Hielm-Björkman AK, Rita H, Tulamo RM. Psychometric testing of the Helsinki chronic pain index by completion of a questionnaire in Finnish by owners of dogs with chronic signs of pain caused by osteoarthritis. *Am J Vet Res* 2009;70:727–734.

11 Walter S, Gruss S, Limbrecht-Ecklundt K, et al. Automatic pain quantification using autonomic parameters. *Psychol Neurosci* 2014;7:363–380.

12 Keel M, Trentz O. Pathophysiology of polytrauma. *Injury* 2005;36:691–709.

13 Wise AJ, Yaksh TL. Nociception and pain mechanisms. In: *Handbook of Veterinary Pain Management*, 3rd edn (eds Gaynor JS, Muir WW). Elsevier, St Louis, 2015, pp. 10–41.

14 Svensson CI, Yaksh TL. The spinal phospholipase-cyclooxygenase-prostanoid cascade in nociceptive processing. *Annu Rev Pharmacol Toxicol* 2002;42: 553–583.

15 Malchow RJ, Black IH. The evolution of pain management in the critically ill trauma patient: Emerging concepts from the global war on terrorism. *Crit Care Med* 2008;36:S346–357.

16 Benitez ME, Roush JK, McMurphy R, et al. Clinical efficacy of hydrocodone-acetaminophen and tramadol for control of postoperative pain in dogs following tibial plateau leveling osteotomy. *Am J Vet Res* 2015;76:755–762.

17 KuKanich B. Pharmacokinetics of acetaminophen, codeine, and the codeine metabolites morphine and codeine-6-glucuronide in healthy Greyhound dogs. *J Vet Pharmacol Ther* 2010;33:15–21.

18 Martins TL, Kahvegian MA, Noel-Morgan J, et al. Comparison of the effects of tramadol, codeine, and ketoprofen alone or in combination on postoperative pain and on concentrations of blood glucose, serum cortisol, and serum interleukin-6 in dogs undergoing maxillectomy or mandibulectomy. *Am J Vet Res* 2010;71:1019–1026.

19 Egger CM, Duke T, Archer J, et al. Comparison of plasma fentanyl concentrations by using three transdermal fentanyl patch sizes in dogs. *Vet Surg* 1998;27:159–166.

20 Kyles AE, Papich M, Hardie EM. Disposition of transdermally administered fentanyl in dogs. *Am J Vet Res* 1996; 57: 715–719.

21 Lee DD, Papich MG, Hardie EM. Comparison of pharmacokinetics of fentanyl after intravenous and transdermal administration in cats. *Am J Vet Res* 2000;61:672–667.

22 NADA. Simbadol Freedom of Information Summary. NADA, Rockville, 2014.

23 Giordano T, Steagall PV, Ferreira TH, et al. Postoperative analgesic effects of intravenous, intramuscular, subcutaneous or oral transmucosal buprenorphine administered to cats undergoing ovariohysterectomy. *Vet Anaesth Analg* 2010;37: 357–366.

24 Jones CJ, Budsberg SC. Physiologic characteristics and clinical importance of the cyclooxygenase isoforms in dogs and cats. *J Am Vet Med Assoc* 2000;217:721–729.

25 Luna SPL, Bastilio AC, Steagall PVM, et al. Evaluation of adverse effects of long-term oral administration of carprofen, etodolac, flunixin meglumine, ketoprofen and meloxicam in dogs. *Am J Vet Res* 2007;68:258–264.

26 Hanson PD, Brooks KC, Case J, et al. Efficacy and safety of firocoxib in the management of canine osteoarthritis under field conditions. *Vet Ther* 2006;7:127–140.

27 Pollmeier M, Toulemonde C, Fleishman C, et al. Clinical evaluation of firocoxib and carprofen for the treatment of dogs with osteoarthritis. *Vet Rec* 2006;159:547–551.

28 Doig PA, Purbrick KA, Hare JE, et al. Clinical efficacy and tolerance of meloxicam in dogs with chronic osteoarthritis. *Can Vet J* 2000;41:296–300.

29 Raekallio MR, Hielm-Bjorkman AK, Kejonen J, et al. Evaluation of adverse effects of long-term orally administered carprofen in dogs. *J Am Vet Med Assoc* 2006;15:876–880.

30 Wallace JL. NSAID gastropathy and enteropathy: distinct pathogenesis likely necessitates distinct prevention strategies. *Br J Pharm* 2012;165:67–74.

31 Surdyk KK, Sloan DL, Brown SA. Renal effects of carprofen and etodolac in euvolemic and volume-depleted dogs. *Am J Vet Res* 2012;73:1485–1490.

32 Mathews KA. Nonsteroidal anti-inflammatory analgesics: indications and contraindications for pain management in dogs and cats. *Vet Clin North Am Small Anim Pract* 2000;30:783-804.

33 Mathews KA. Pain management for the pregnant, lactating, and neonatal to pediatric cat and dog. *Vet Clin North Am Small Anim Pract* 2008;38:1291–1308.

34 Bennett WM, Henrich WL, Stoff JS. The renal effects of nonsteroidal anti-inflammatory drugs: summary and recommendations. *Am J Kidney Dis* 1996;28(Suppl 1):S56–62.

35 Schmid VB, Seewald W, Lees P, et al. In vitro and ex vivo inhibition of COX isoforms by robenacoxib in the cat: a comparative study. *J Vet Pharmacol Ther* 2010;33:444–452.

36 Sano T, King JN, Seewald W, et al. Comparison of oral robenacoxib and ketoprofen for the treatment of acute pain and inflammation associated with musculoskeletal disorders in cats: a randomised clinical trial. *Vet J* 2012;193:397–403.

37 Kamata M, King JN, Seewald W, et al. Comparison of injectable robenacoxib versus meloxicam for peri-operative use in cats: results of a randomised clinical trial. *Vet J* 2012;193:114–118.

38 King JN, King S, Budsberg SC, et al. Clinical safety of robenacoxib in feline osteoarthritis: results of a randomized, blinded, placebo-controlled clinical trial. *J Feline Med Surg* 2016;18:632–642.

39 Speranza C, Schmid V, Giraudel JM, et al. Robenacoxib versus meloxicam for the control of peri-operative pain and inflammation associated with orthopaedic surgery in cats: a randomised clinical trial. *BMC Vet Res* 2015;11:79.

40 Lebkowska-Wieruszewska B, De Vito V, Owen H et al. Pharmacokinetics of grapiprant, a selective EP4 prostaglanding PGE2 receptor antagonist, after 2 mg/kg oral and i.v. administration in cats, *J Vet Pharmacol Ther* 2017; 40:e11–e15.

41 Lin CR, Amaya F, Barret L, et al. Prostaglandin E2 receptor EP4 contributes to inflammatory pain hypersensitivity. *J Pharmacol Exp Ther* 2006;319: 1096–1103.

42 Sugimoto Y, Narumiva S, Prostaglanding E receptors. *J Biol Chem* 2007;282:11613–11617.

43 Rausch-Derra L, Huebner M, Wofford J, et al. A prospective, randomized masked, placebo-controlled multisite clinical study of grapiprant, an EP4 prostaglanding receptor antagonist (PRA), in dogs with osteoarthritis. *J Vet Intern Med* 2016;30:756–763.

44 KuKanich B, Papich MG. Pharmacokinetics and antinociceptive effects of oral tramadol hydrochloride

administration in greyhounds. *Am J Vet Res* 2011;72:256–262.

45 Kögel B1, Terlinden R, Schneider J. Characterization of tramadol, morphine and tapentadol in an acute pain model in Beagle dogs. *Vet Anaesth Analg* 2014;41: 297–304.

46 Benitez ME, Roush JK, KuKanich B, et al. Pharmacokinetics of hydrocodone and tramadol administered for control of postoperative pain in dogs following tibial plateau leveling osteotomy. *Am J Vet Res* 2015;76:763–770.

47 Pypendop BH, Ilkiw JE. Pharmacokinetics of tramadol, and its metabolite O-desmethyl tramadol, in cats. *J Vet Pharmacol Ther* 2008;31:52–59.

48 Pypendop BH, Siao KT, Ilkiw JE. Effects of tramadol hydrochloride on the thermal threshold in cats. *Am J Vet Res* 2009;70:1465–1470.

49 Malek S, Sample SJ, Schwartz Z, et al. Effect of analgesic therapy on clinical outcome measures in a randomized controlled trial using client-owned dogs with hip osteoarthritis. *BMC Vet Res* 2012;8:185.

50 Indrawirawan Y, McAlees T. Tramadol toxicity in a cat: case report and literature review of serotonin syndrome. *J Feline Med Surg* 2014;16:572–578.

51 Siao KT, Pypendop BH, Escobar A, et al. Effect of amantadine on oxymorphone-induced thermal antinociception in cats. *J Vet Pharmacol Ther* 2012;35:169–174.

52 Snijdelaar DG, van Rijn CM, Vinken P, et al. Effects of pre-treatment with amantadine on morphine induced antinociception during second phase formalin responses in rats. *Pain* 2005;119:159–167.

53 Lascelles BD1, Gaynor JS, Smith ES, et al. Amantadine in a multimodal analgesic regimen for alleviation of refractory osteoarthritis pain in dogs. *J Vet Intern Med* 2008;22:53–59.

54 Madden M, Gurney M, Bright S. Amantadine, an N-Methyl-d-aspartate antagonist, for treatment of chronic neuropathic pain in a dog. *Vet Anaesth Analg* 2014;41:440–441.

55 Aghighi SA, Tipold A, Piechotta M, et al. Assessment of the effects of adjunctive gabapentin on postoperative pain after intervertebral disc surgery in dogs. *Vet Anaesth Analg* 2012;39:636–646.

56 Wagner AE, Mich PM, Uhrig SR, et al. Clinical evaluation of perioperative administration of gabapentin as an adjunct for postoperative analgesia in dogs undergoing amputation of a forelimb. *J Am Vet Med Assoc* 2010;236:751–675.

57 KuKanich B, Cohen RL. Pharmacokinetics of oral gabapentin in greyhound dogs. *Vet J* 2011;187:133–135.

58 Crociolli GC, Cassu RN, Barbero RC, et al. Gabapentin as an adjuvant for postoperative pain management in dogs undergoing mastectomy. *J Vet Med Sci* 2015;77:1011–1015.

59 Lorenz ND, Comerford EJ, Iff I. Long-term use of gabapentin for musculoskeletal disease and trauma in three cats. *J Feline Med Surg* 2013;15:507–512.

60 Vettorato E, Corletto F. Gabapentin as part of multi-modal analgesia in two cats suffering multiple injuries. *Vet Anaesth Analg* 2011;38:518–520.

61 Steagall PV, Monteiro-Steagall BP. Multimodal analgesia for perioperative pain in three cats. *J Feline Med Surg* 2013;15:737–743.

62 Steagall PV, Benito J, Monteiro-Steagall BP. Analgesic effects of gabapentin and buprenorphine in cats undergoing ovariohysterectomy using two pain-scoring systems: a randomized clinical trial. *J Feline Med Surg* 2017 Sep 1 [Epub ahead of print].

63 Cashmore RG, Harcourt-Brown TR, Freeman PM, et al. Clinical diagnosis and treatment of suspected neuropathic pain in three dogs. *Aust Vet J* 2009;87: 45–50.

64 Norkus C, Rankin D, KuKanich B. Pharmacokinetics of intravenous and oral amitriptyline and its active metabolite nortriptyline in Greyhound dogs. *Vet Anaesth Analg* 2015;42:580–589.

65 Ko J, Weil A, Maxwell L, et al. Plasma concentrations of lidocaine in dogs following lidocaine patch application. *J Am Anim Hosp Assoc* 2007;43:280–283.

66 Ko JC, Maxwell LK, Abbo LA, et al. Pharmacokinetics of lidocaine following the application of 5% lidocaine patches to cats. *J Vet Pharmacol Ther* 2008;31: 359–367.

67 Joudrey SD, Robinson DA, Kearney MT, et al. Plasma concentrations of lidocaine in dogs following lidocaine patch application over an incision compared to intact skin. *J Vet Pharmacol Ther* 2015;38:575–580.

68 Weil AB, Ko J, Inoue T. The use of lidocaine patches. *Compend Contin Educ Vet* 2007;29:208–210, 212, 214–216.

199

Approach to the Aggressive or Fearful Emergency Room Patient

Selena L. Lane, DVM, DACVECC and Benjamin M. Brainard, VMD, DACVAA, DACVECC

College of Veterinary Medicine, University of Georgia, Athens, GA, USA

Introduction

Dogs and cats are presented to the emergency room (ER) for a wide range of reasons, from traumatic injury and critical illness to lacerations or gastrointestinal upset. The veterinary patient arriving to the ER may be agitated, which can compound fear, anxiety, and pain associated with injury or illness. The combination of these and other patient factors can result in aggression directed towards veterinary clinicians, staff, and even the client. Aggressive behavior in the veterinary patient can be frustrating, dangerous for personnel, and time-consuming, and may ultimately result in delayed therapy for severe or life-threatening illness. Recognizing, anticipating, and mitigating this behavior in the ER patient will reduce stress and the chance of injury to both staff and patient. The utilization of proper restraint techniques can improve the experience for the client, patient, and veterinary personnel.

Patient Fear and Aggression

Dogs and cats can exhibit fearful or aggressive behavior during ER evaluation, regardless of their typical demeanor outside the hospital setting. Patient aggression may be influenced by arousal, excessive stimulation, pain, anxiety, and fear. Fear is an emotional response that spurs an animal to avoid potentially dangerous or harmful situations [1]. Fear is common in veterinary patients, particularly cats, and can be aggravated with forceful restraint (such as scruffing the skin of the neck). The unfamiliar sights and smells of the ER, rapid movements by staff and other animals, and loud noises can compound this fear [2]. Aggression

associated with fear can result in unpredictable behaviors, and may also occur due to pain and discomfort. Additionally, if a pet has previously had negative experiences at veterinary clinics, or has an acute exacerbation of a chronic disease, they can become anxious, anticipating a negative outcome, resulting in fearful or aggressive behavior [3]. Other aspects of the ER visit, such as bright ambient lighting and visual contact with other patients, may contribute to fear [4]. If feasible, the cage or carrier of a fearful animal should be covered to decrease visual stimulation (e.g. using a towel over the opening) and help to calm the animal [4].

Recognizing Fear and Aggression in Dogs and Cats

All veterinary staff should be comfortable with the recognition of fear- or aggression-specific behaviors. From a distance, the animal's posture, eyes, ear, lip, and tail position should be evaluated. Fearful or aggressive behaviors in dogs and cats include cowering in the corner of the room or carrier, trembling, low head carriage with eyes averted, eyes that dart between areas of focus or stare, a tucked tail, or hiding under exam room furniture [3,5,6]. Dogs and cats may pant, or stand or sit with one paw raised [6]. A cat that lashes its tail, or just the tip of the tail, from side to side indicates agitation, annoyance, or arousal [5]. Ears flattened against the head, particularly in the cat, indicate a defensive behavior, which may progress to aggression [2]. In more aggressive and assertive animals, the ears may be positioned forward. Pupil size can correlate to the degree of intensity of the situation, becoming mydriatic with fear. Oblong pupils in the cat can signal aggression [5]. Pain and medications (e.g. opioids) can also affect pupil size. Aggressive dogs may display threatening behaviors, such as lip lifting, growling, barking, lunging, and biting. Aggressive cats may display hissing, growling, swatting, and biting [7]. However, displacement behavior such as yawning, smacking and licking of the lips in the dog or grooming in the cat can also signal a fear or anxiety-inducing situation [2,7].

If these behaviors are noted, care should be taken to avoid escalation to more aggressive, defensive behavior [7]. Animals that are extremely distressed may void urine, feces, or anal gland secretions, and may frantically try to escape from the situation, while others may freeze and not interact at all [4].

Techniques for Patient Handling and Physical Restraint

The veterinary staff should be comfortable utilizing tools for restraint and handling of aggressive patients. The use of pharmacological restraint techniques may also help to alleviate distress in patients, and if the animal is anticipated to react or does react poorly to physical restraint techniques, pharmacological restraint may be indicated (see below).

Client Communication

If the owner knows that a particular patient may be aggressive at the facility, the owner may be able to safely place a muzzle on the pet immediately prior to presenting for triage examination. If a pet displays severe aggressive behavior, clear communication with the client is necessary to ensure that the pet owner understands the need for manual or pharmacological restraint, as well as the veterinary personnel's genuine concern for the well-being of the pet.

Approaching the Patient

If the animal is in a travel carrier on presentation, opening the door, standing to the side of the open door, and talking softly to the dog or cat may encourage it to walk out of the carrier on its own. Emergency stabilization, however, may necessitate rapid manual removal of the pet from the carrier. Removal of the detachable top of pet carriers can improve access to the pet, and the fearful patient may be more amenable to handling by this route. This approach may also be safer for ER personnel. Any animal that requires assistance to be removed from a car should be muzzled prior to removal; this protects the lifters if the animal is unpredictably painful and bites, but also because the pet

may feel threatened as a stranger enters into a familiar place. If the patient walks into the ER on a leash, avoid confrontation by approaching the pet from the side, without direct eye contact. Avoid backing the pet into a corner or reaching over the head to grab the leash or collar [7]. Slip leashes should be used to control dogs, as the dog's own collar may slip off the neck if the dog resists handling. Talking to the pet in a comforting and soft tone throughout the examination can help reduce stress, fear, and anxiety. Avoid exposing the patient to excessive stimuli or noises (e.g. large numbers of people surrounding the treatment table, clippers, or monitor alarms) during triage evaluation.

Cats are often co-operative enough to be restrained on a table by using one hand or arm to restrain the body and the other hand to restrain the head. Many people will scruff the neck skin to restrain a fractious cat but this can increase fear and spark aggressive behavior [2]. If the cat requires restraint of the head, use the three middle fingers to massage the top of the head (between the ears), and the thumb and pinkie fingers to control the cat's head by firmly gripping it just below the ramus of the mandible [2]. This can allow full restraint of the cat's head while avoiding the stress and arousal associated with scruffing.

Towels are extremely helpful for restraint of fearful or aggressive cats and small dogs. Cats can be restrained by wrapping the body and limbs in a heavy towel in a burrito-like fashion. Once wrapped, limbs may be carefully withdrawn as needed, for procedures such as intravenous catheter placement or blood pressure measurement. A towel rolled length-wise can also be used to aid in restraint of small to medium-sized dogs, as it can be placed around the neck at arm's length and crossed over itself behind the head to facilitate placement of a muzzle. Care should be taken that the towel is not held too tightly around the patient's neck. Towels placed over the head or eyes of fearful animals may also help to calm them, especially in the context of manual restraint [4]. For anxious or fearful animals that are hospitalized, a tight-fitting body wrap or shirt (e.g. Thundershirt, ThunderWorks, Durham, NC) can provide a comforting and calming sensation. In postoperative patients, these wraps also protect surgical wounds.

Muzzles

Muzzles should be available for use in fearful or aggressive patients. They come in a variety of shapes, sizes, and are made of nylon, plastic, or leather. Most muzzles fit snugly over the pet's muzzle and latch or buckle behind the ears. Makeshift muzzles made from gauze or tape can be configured in the hospital to aid in restraint of the aggressive animal, especially those who might not allow placement of a regular muzzle. Snug-fitting muzzles should not be left on the patient any longer than necessary, as the muzzle closes the mouth and prevents panting, commonly seen in the anxious or fearful patient and necessary for temperature regulation [7]. Muzzles can also interfere with emesis and predispose to aspiration of vomitus. Basket-type muzzles allow the patient to pant effectively and are sometimes easier to place, because they are formed into shape, allowing rapid placement over the face [7]. Muzzles that restrict breathing should be avoided in the emergency patient with respiratory difficulty or in brachycephalic dogs. Cat muzzles cover both the mouth and eyes to aid in handling of the fractious cat. These cone-shaped muzzles may also be used for brachycephalic breeds, as they generally do not obstruct respiration and can also protect the eyes, depending on the size of the dog.

Other Manual Restraint Tools

Nets may assist in handling very aggressive or feral cats. There are also commercially- available nets on a metal clamshell frame (e.g. EZ-Nabber, Campbell Pet Company, Brush Prairie, WA). Once in the net, pharmacological restraint can be administered through the mesh to facilitate further examination. Leather gloves that cover the hands and forearm are available for holding smaller fractious patients and provide protection from bites and scratches; however, they are bulky and limit the dexterity of the handler.

Control poles, or "rabies poles," are used only with extremely dangerous and aggressive dogs. Restraint of the head with the control pole allows safe administration of intramuscular drugs for sedation. The dog should never be dragged, yanked, pulled, or lifted with the control pole, as this may cause injury. The control pole should be used only when other more humane or less threatening options are not feasible [7].

Pharmacologic Restraint of the Aggressive or Fearful Patient

Delivery of Pharmacological Agents for Restraint

If physical restraint is unsuccessful or dangerous for the veterinary staff or patient, pharmacological restraint may aid with patient handling. If the patient allows placement of an intravenous catheter, IV administration of sedatives results in rapid onset of action.

Intramuscular injection may be more feasible, and can be administered while the animal is muzzled, still inside the travel carrier, or even when distracted while exiting the exam room. For smaller dogs and cats, commercially available squeeze cages can stabilize the animal to allow rapid, accurate IM injections. For larger dogs, an exam room door or large chain-link cage door can make a modified squeeze cage. The dog is walked into a corner where the door meets the wall and the end of the leash is fed through the hinge of the door. The leash is held tight by an assistant on the other side of the door, and the door is swung against the dog, creating a "squeeze cage" between the door and wall. An IM injection can then be given.

Although it is ideal to verify that an IM injection is not accidently administered IV, this may not be possible in the aggressive animal. Rather, the syringe can be held with the plunger in the palm of the hand so that the needle and medications can be introduced in one firm movement. The authors prefer the epaxial muscles for this type of injection, as there is less danger of accidental injection in the nerves of the hindlimb.

If the handler cannot safely approach the animal to give an injection, commercially available pole syringes can be used to safely administer medications. Anesthetic gas induction chambers can be considered for sedation of aggressive small dogs, cats, non-domestic species and wildlife; however, this methodology results in exposure of personnel to high concentrations of inhalant gas, and the patient cannot be closely monitored during induction [8].

Pharmacological Agents for Use in Aggressive Animals

Various medications can be administered to the fearful or aggressive animal to allow for handling and treatment in the emergency situation (Table 199.1). A neuroleptanalgesic combination of a tranquilizer and an opioid is the safest combination for sedation in patients with unknown cardiovascular status, but may only provide light sedation, rather than heavy sedation or anesthesia. It may be necessary to subsequently place a muzzle and restrain the patient for IV catheter placement. With IV access, additional sedative or anesthetic drugs can be administered to deepen sedation or induce anesthesia. Additional drugs may also be given by the IM route. Opioids given alone may result in emesis, and the practitioner must remain vigilant and rapidly remove tight-fitting muzzles if nausea becomes apparent (i.e. ptyalism).

Anesthetic protocols involving dissociative anesthetics (e.g. ketamine or tiletamine) are preferred by the authors for aggressive patients, as the dissociative agent

Table 199.1 Suggested doses of sedative drugs for the fearful or aggressive veterinary patient and special considerations for their use.

Drug	Dose	Effects	Special considerations
Opioids: should be combined with tranquilizer (e.g. benzodiazepine, phenothiazine, alpha-2 agonist) for optimal sedation	Butorphanol 0.2–0.5 mg/kg IV, IM [9]	Good sedative, minimal analgesia	Minimal cardiovascular depression; respiratory depression at higher doses (applies to all opioids)
			Can partially reverse sedation secondary to administration of pure mu-opioids
	Morphine 0.5–2 mg/kg IM [11]	Very good sedative and analgesia	Can cause histamine release, nausea
	Hydromorphone 0.1–0.2 mg/kg IV, IM, SC [9]	Moderate sedative, good analgesic effects	May cause panting, nausea, and vomiting
	Methadone 0.05–0.6 mg/kg IV; 0.5–1 mg/kg IM [10,11]	Good sedative and analgesic effects	Lower incidence of nausea and vomiting relative to other opioids [11]
			May cause mild peripheral and pulmonary vasoconstriction [10]
Benzodiazepines: must be combined with opioid or dissociative agent for sedation of aggressive patients	Midazolam 0.1–0.5 mg/kg IV, IM [9]	Centrally acting muscle relaxant, anxiolytic, mild tranquilizer	Minimal cardiovascular and respiratory depression [12]
	Diazepam 0.1–0.5 mg/kg, IV [9]	Some amnesic effects	Can see paradoxical excitement and agitation after administration [9]
			May see more aggressive behavior after administration due to disinhibition of fear response [13]
			Do not use alone in aggressive animals
Phenothiazines: must be combined with opioid or dissociative agent for sedation of aggressive patients	Acepromazine 0.005–0.05 mg/kg IV, IM [9] Can give up to 0.1 mg/kg in single dose (not to exceed 3 mg total in dogs) [9]	Good tranquilizer and sedative	May take up to 40 min for full effect
			May cause hypotension, particularly in hypovolemic patients [9]
			Good for sedation in patients with respiratory distress; minimal respiratory depression
Alpha-2 agonists	Dexmedetomidine 0.5–20 μg/kg (0.0005–0.0020 mg/kg) IV, IM, PO [11]	Good sedation, muscle relaxation, and analgesia	Need higher doses of dexmedetomidine in highly agitated animals; response may be variable or animal may appear refractory to effects of the drug
	Medetomidine 1.0–20 μg/kg (0.001–0.0020 mg/kg) IV, IM, PO		Do not use as sole agent in aggressive animals
	Xylazine 0.5–1 mg/kg IV; 2.2 mg/kg IM [9]		Significant cardiovascular depression: decreases cardiac output, bradycardia, peripheral vasoconstriction
			May cause vomiting in cats
Dissociative anesthetics	Ketamine 5–10 mg/kg IV, IM [9,11]	Excellent tranquilization and sedation	Recommended to use ketamine in combination with a tranquilizer (e.g. benzodiazepine, alpha-2 agonist) to provide good muscle relaxation
	Tiletamine/zolazepam 5–15 mg/kg IM [11]	Useful adjunct to analgesia	Ketamine alone or combined with an alpha-2 agonist may be sprayed directly into an aggressive cat's mouth [11]
			May note erratic behavior during recovery and muscle twitching, leading to increased body temperature
			Use lower doses (0.5–2 mg/kg) in patients with suspected heart disease or cardiovascular dysfunction
			Increases intracranial and intraocular pressure
			Dose-dependent respiratory depression

(Continued)

Table 199.1 *(Continued)*

Drug	Dose	Effects	Special considerations
General anesthetic	Alfaxalone 5 mg/kg IV, IM (cats) and 5–10 mg/kg IV, IM (dogs) [14,15]	Excellent sedation and muscle relaxation Minimal cardiorespiratory depression	May cause dysphoria or ataxia in cats [14] May cause transient muscular tremors and staggering gait in dogs Dose-dependent hypoxemia and hypoventilation at higher doses [15] Can cause hypotension May cause apnea if administered rapidly IV

IM, intramuscular; IV, intravenous; PO, by mouth (*per os*); SC, subcutaneous.

impairs the animal's ability to act on aggressive influences. Dissociative anesthetics have minimal effect on cardiorespiratory function.

Alpha-2 agonist drugs should not be used alone for sedation of aggressive patients. They are associated with unpredictable sedation and unanticipated arousal. They also result in significant alterations in vascular tone and heart rate, which may not be tolerated in patients with known or unknown cardiovascular disease. Alpha-2 agonists increase urine output, and should not be used in patients who are unable to void urine. In patients where alpha-2 agonists are anticipated to be safe, their combination with opioid or dissociative anesthetics will result in a safer and more reliable immobilization. In patients that present an open mouth (e.g. a hissing cat), the combination of dexmedetomidine and ketamine may be squirted into the mouth for excellent sedation by transmucosal absorption.

Benzodiazepines should never be given alone to aggressive animals, as disinhibition may worsen the animal's aggressive tendencies. Combined with opioid or dissociative drugs, however, benzodiazepines result in synergy that provides good sedation and muscle relaxation (neuroleptanalgesia).

Opioids, benzodiazepines, and alpha-2 agonist drugs also have specific reversal agents, so the effects of sedation can be fully or partially removed following the ER exam or if adverse effects are seen (Table 199.2).

Every patient's physical and pharmacological restraint protocol should take into account their overall demeanor and suspected underlying disease process (Table 199.3). In most cases, the judicious use of sedatives, tranquilizers, and anxiolytics in combination with safe, careful physical restraint will result in a successful and less stressful ER experience for the patient, veterinary staff, and client.

Table 199.2 Suggested doses of reversal agents for sedated, aggressive veterinary patients.

Drug	Reversal class	Dose	Special considerations
Naloxone	Opioid antagonist	0.02–0.04 mg/kg IV, IM [11]	Duration of effect 30 min to 1 h May need to redose if inadequate reversal seen
Flumazenil	Benzodiazepine antagonist	0.01 mg/kg IV, IM [11]	May need to repeat due to short half-life (1 h)
Atipamezole	Alpha-2 adrenergic antagonist	Give IM at equal volume of alpha-2 agonist sedative administered or at 5 times the dose of medetomidine/dexmedetomidine [11] Can be given IV if needed in emergency	May reverse effects rapidly; caution in aggressive patients

IM, intramuscular; IV, intravenous.

Table 199.3 Suggested drug combinations for use in aggressive veterinary patients; all sedation doses given IV or IM, except where noted.

Commonly encountered patients	Drug combinations	Dose	Special considerations
Fearful or difficult, minimally aggressive dogs or cats	Butorphanol	0.2 mg/kg	Useful for short or non-painful procedures, such as radiographs or IV catheter placement
	Midazolam	0.2 mg/kg	
	+/− Dexmedetomidine	2–4 mg/kg	
Dogs or cats requiring moderate sedation	Butorphanol	0.2 mg/kg	Consider hydromorphone, morphine, or oxymorphone instead of butorphanol if procedure may be painful
	Midazolam	0.2 mg/kg	
	Dexmedetomidine or ketamine or telazol	3–5 mg/kg (dexmed) or 2–5 mg/kg (ketamine) or 2–5 mg/kg (telazol)	
Heavy sedation for aggressive dogs or cats	Butorphanol	0.2 mg/kg	Cats may require higher dexmedetomidine doses
	Midazolam	0.2 mg/kg	Consider other opioids for painful procedures
	Ketamine	5–10 mg/kg	Caution with use of dexmedetomidine in animals with severe aggressive behavior or with possible cardiac disease
	or		
	Dexmedetomidine	5–20 µg/kg	Dose reduce alfaxalone when used in combination with dexmedetomidine
	or	1–5 mg/kg	
	Alfaxalone	5–20 µg/kg	
	Dexmedetomidine		
Fearful or difficult, aggressive dogs or cats	Dexmedetomidine	2–10 mg/kg TM	Useful for initial restraint and IV catheter placement
	Ketamine	5–10 mg/kg TM	

IM, intramuscular; IV, intravenous; SC, subcutaneous, TM, transmucosal.

References

1 Overall KL. Fears, anxieties and stereotypes. In: *Clinical Behavioral Medicine for Small Animals.* Mosby, St Louis, 1997, p. 213.

2 Rodan I. Understanding feline behavior and application for appropriate handling and management. *Top Compani Anim Med* 2010;25:178–188.

3 Döring D, Roscher A, Scheipl F, et al. Fear-related behavior of dogs in veterinary practice. *Vet J* 2009;182:38–43.

4 Herron ME, Shreyer T. The pet-friendly veterinary practice: a guide for practitioners. *Vet Clin Small Anim* 2014;44:451–481.

5 Overall KL. *Normal feline behavior. In: Clinical Behavioral Medicine for Small Animals.* Mosby, St Louis, 1997, pp. 45–76.

6 Yin S. Simple handling techniques for dogs. *Compend Contin Educ Vet* 2007;29:352–358.

7 Moffat K. Addressing canine and feline aggression in the veterinary clinic. *Vet Clin Small Anim* 2008;38:983–1003.

8 Bednarski RM. Dogs and cats. In: *Lumb and Jones' Veterinary Anesthesia and Analgesia*, 4th edn (eds Tranquilli WJ, Thurmon JC, Grimm KA). Blackwell Publishing, Oxford, 2007, p. 712.

9 Papich MG. *Saunders Handbook of Veterinary Drugs: Small and Large Animal.* Elsevier Saunders, St Louis, 2011.

10 Murrell J. Clinical use of methadone in cats and dogs. *Companion Anim* 2011;16:56–61.

11 Plumb DC. *Plumb's Veterinary Drug Handbook.* Wiley-Blackwell, Oxford, 2015.

12 Jones DJ, Stehling LC, Zauder HL. Cardiovascular responses to diazepam and midazolam maleate in the dog. *Anesthesiology* 1979;51:430–434.

13 Overall KL. Behavioral pharmacology. In: *Clinical Behavioral Medicine for Small Animals.* Mosby, St Louis, 1997, p. 307.

14 Rodrigo-Mocholi D, Belda E, Bosmans T, et al. Clinical efficacy and cardiorespiratory effects of intramuscular administration of alfaxalone alone or in combination with dexmedetomidine in cats. *Vet Anaesth Analgesia* 2016;43:291–300.

15 Tamura J, Ishizuka T, Fukui S, et al. The pharmacological effects of the anesthetic alfaxalone after intramuscular administration to dogs. *J Vet Med Sci* 2015;77:289–296.

Section 8

Unique Emergency Medicine Topics

200

Antimicrobial Therapy in the Emergency Patient

Steven Epstein, DVM, DACVECC

School of Veterinary Medicine, University of California, Davis, CA, USA

Introduction

The frequency and distribution of emergency room visits amongst dogs and cats per year are unknown, although dogs are reported to present 2–3 times more frequently than cats [1,2]. In the United States 3% of emergency department visits were reported to have a primary diagnosis of infectious and parasitic diseases in 2011 [3], while it is estimated that 500 000 adults and nearly 100 000 children are treated annually for severe sepsis in US emergency departments [4,5].

The criteria for defining the systemic inflammatory response syndrome (SIRS) have been variably reported in dogs and cats (see Chapter 159). Sepsis is clinically diagnosed by the presence of SIRS and a documented or suspected infection. Sepsis has most recently been defined in human medicine as a life-threatening organ dysfunction caused by a dysregulated host response to infection while septic shock is a subset of sepsis in which underlying circulatory and cellular/metabolic abnormalities are profound enough to substantially increase mortality [6].

When considering antimicrobial needs in the veterinary emergency patient with an infectious disease, the patient may fall into one of three categories: a stable patient who will be treated on an outpatient basis, a patient with sepsis that requires hospitalization, or a critically ill patient with severe sepsis or septic shock. The level of illness affects the choice and route of administration of antimicrobials as dogs and cats with severe sepsis and subsequent organ dysfunction have increased mortality rates [7,8]. Therefore, identification of a patient in the emergency room with sepsis is of paramount importance to help guide antimicrobial administration.

General Considerations for Antimicrobial Selection

When choosing an antimicrobial, elements that should be considered include the following; patient-related factors, micro-organism-related factors, and antimicrobial-related factors, and asking the question, does this patient truly need an antimicrobial? Comprehensive coverage of appropriate antimicrobial choice for the wide variety of diseases for stable outpatient conditions is beyond the scope of this chapter, and consultation with a textbook for individual scenarios is recommended. However, the principles presented here should still be used to guide selection.

Major host factors to consider include the presence of renal or hepatic dysfunction, signalment, a documented allergy or intolerance to an antimicrobial, and prior antimicrobial use. The adverse effects of the antimicrobial may preclude the choice based on these host factors (e.g. aminoglycosides with pre-existing renal disease, clindamycin with liver failure, trimethoprim-sulfamethoxazole in Dobermans, etc.)

Important micro-organism factors that influence antimicrobial choice include the predicted bacteria at the site of infection, any intrinsic resistance to antimicrobials those bacteria may possess (e.g. *Pseudomonas aeruginosa* are resistance to amoxicillin and most cephalosporins), and local resistance data. Differing antimicrobial resistance patterns have been reported regionally in veterinary medicine [9] and human medicine [10]. Creation of a summary of antimicrobial susceptibilities of bacterial isolates submitted over a time period at one institution (an antibiogram) may increase antimicrobial stewardship in the emergency room and improve empiric decision making (Figure 200.1) [11].

UC Davis William R. Pritchard Veterinary Medical Teaching Hospital Canine and Feline 2014-2015 Antibiogram

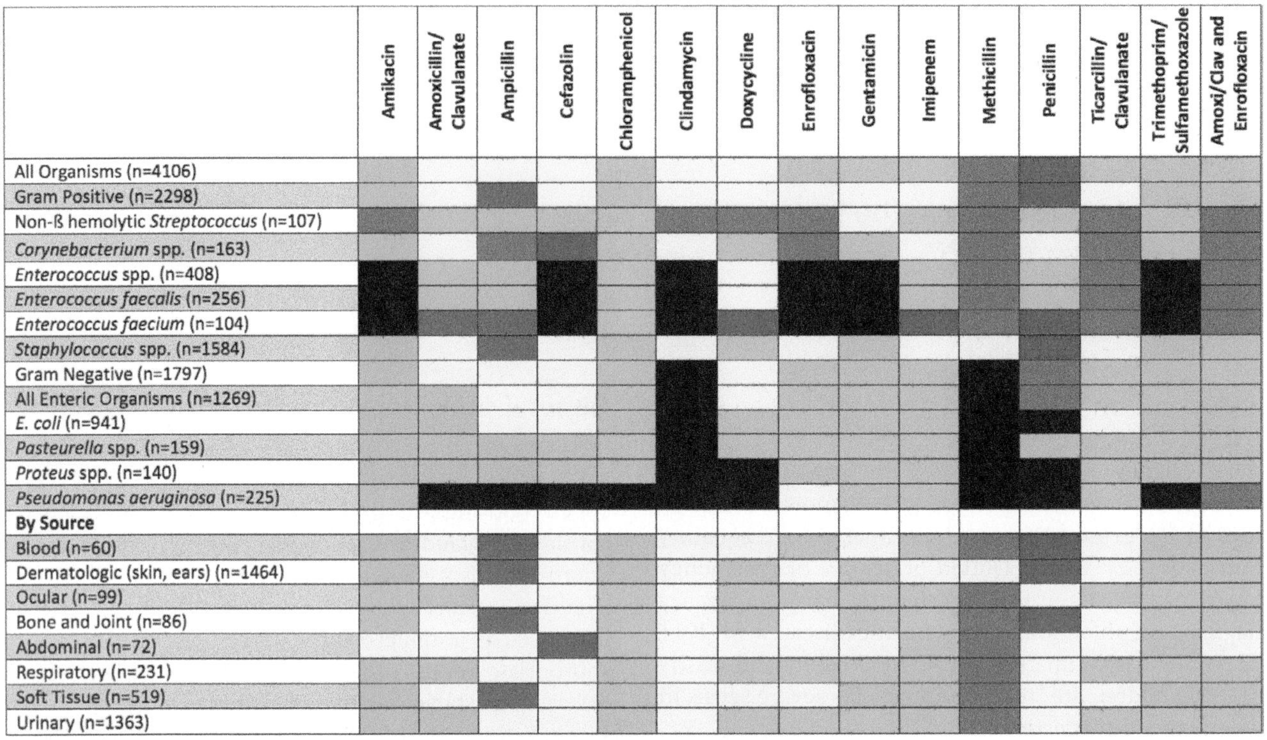

	Amikacin	Amoxicillin/ Clavulanate	Ampicillin	Cefazolin	Chloramphenicol	Clindamycin	Doxycycline	Enrofloxacin	Gentamicin	Imipenem	Methicillin	Penicillin	Ticarcillin/ Clavulanate	Trimethoprim/ Sulfamethoxazole	Amoxi/Clav and Enrofloxacin
All Organisms (n=4106)															
Gram Positive (n=2298)															
Non-ß hemolytic *Streptococcus* (n=107)															
Corynebacterium spp. (n=163)															
Enterococcus spp. (n=408)															
Enterococcus faecalis (n=256)															
Enterococcus faecium (n=104)															
Staphylococcus spp. (n=1584)															
Gram Negative (n=1797)															
All Enteric Organisms (n=1269)															
E. coli (n=941)															
Pasteurella spp. (n=159)															
Proteus spp. (n=140)															
Pseudomonas aeruginosa (n=225)															
By Source															
Blood (n=60)															
Dermatologic (skin, ears) (n=1464)															
Ocular (n=99)															
Bone and Joint (n=86)															
Abdominal (n=72)															
Respiratory (n=231)															
Soft Tissue (n=519)															
Urinary (n=1363)															

The information needs to be considered in light of selection of the most appropriate drug for the bacteria cultured, and in light of the anatomic site (i.e., drug penetration) and patient factors.
This should not be used as a substitute for culture and susceptibility testing.
Green>70% susceptibility, Yellow 40-70%, Red <40%, Blue= insufficient/not applicable data, and Black=intrinsic resistance

Figure 200.1 Example of an antibiogram for use in the emergency room to help guide empiric antimicrobial selection in dogs and cats. It is important to note that an antibiogram is specific to an institution and the information provided cannot be applied at other facilities.

Antimicrobial-specific factors that may affect selection are various. Whether the antimicrobial is bacteriostatic versus bactericidal should play a role in critically ill patients, but probably not in outpatient therapy, with more ill patients receiving a bactericidal choice. Other factors to consider include whether the antimicrobial can penetrate to the site of infection, the potential toxicity/adverse effects of the antimicrobial, and any potential drug–drug interactions.

Antimicrobial utilization increased 36% globally from 2000 to 2010 in human medicine [12] and an estimated 142 000 visits to the emergency department per year secondary to adverse events associated with antimicrobial therapy occurred in the US [3]. Unnecessary prescriptions of antimicrobials in the stable emergency room outpatient are common and represent an area for improved antimicrobial stewardship in both human [13] and veterinary medicine. Examples of areas for improved stewardship in the veterinary emergency room outpatients may include cats with lower urinary tract or upper respiratory tract signs not due to bacterial causes, patients with

fevers with no documented infections, and patients with asymptomatic bacteriuria without high risk of ascending infection [14].

Approach to Antimicrobial Selection for Patients with Sepsis

Obtaining a Culture

Patients that present to the emergency room and are diagnosed with sepsis should have a sample taken for bacterial culture and antimicrobial susceptibility testing. This will allow for confirmation of an infectious organism and the appropriateness of the antimicrobial choice.

The ideal source to culture would be the one suspected to harbor the infection. If that source is not easily obtainable (e.g. pneumonia, central nervous system infection, etc.) then blood cultures can be obtained. Ideally, the culture would be obtained prior to commencing antimicrobial therapy. In patients with severe sepsis or septic shock, if the culture can be obtained without creating a > 45-minute delay, then antimicrobial therapy should be delayed until the culture is obtained. However, in this subset of patients, if there would be an anticipated delay in obtaining the culture of > 45 minutes, then antimicrobials should be commenced as soon as possible [15].

There are no guidelines for patients that present with clinical signs of sepsis, but not severe sepsis or septic shock on how long a delay is considered acceptable. However, given the usual lack of information at presentation for these patients, it is the author's recommendation to treat any sick patient suspected of having sepsis as having severe sepsis until proven otherwise.

Timing of Antimicrobial Administration

The Surviving Sepsis guidelines recommend the administration of effective intravenous antimicrobials within the first hour of recognition of septic shock (grade 1B) and severe sepsis without septic shock (grade 1C) [15]. A major impetus for these recommendation was the study by Kumar et al. which demonstrated that each hour delay in initiating therapy following hypotension increased mortality by 7.6% [16], as well as many other studies in ICUs demonstrating a relationship between timing of antimicrobial administration and mortality [17–19].

Recently, there has been a focus on the impact of timing on antimicrobial administration for patients presenting to the emergency department. In both human and veterinary medicine, it has been documented that having protocols in place for emergency patients can be effective in reducing the time from presentation to antimicrobial administration [20,21]. For humans presenting to the emergency department with sepsis, numerous studies have failed to show an association with the timing of antimicrobial administration and mortality [22–27] while one study documented a survival benefit in patients receiving appropriate antimicrobials within 1 hour of triage or qualification for early goal-directed therapy [28]. It should be noted that one of these prospective studies in patients with septic shock documented a survival benefit to receiving antimicrobials prior to recognition of shock, although hourly delays did not change the mortality rate [27]. Additionally, two of these studies suggest that in a subgroup of more critically ill patients, there is a mortality benefit to early antimicrobial use in the emergency room [22,24]. Aside from mortality, the longer duration to antimicrobial initiation in severe sepsis and septic shock has been associated with increased rates of acute kidney injury, organ dysfunction, and length of hospital stay [19,29,30].

Given these conflicting findings on mortality, the lack of standardization for appropriateness of the antimicrobials, and the potential benefit of decreased organ dysfunction, it is still recommended to attempt to initiate antimicrobial therapy in the first hour if severe sepsis or septic shock is suspected for veterinary patients in the emergency room.

Empiric Antimicrobial Selection (Escalation Versus De-Escalation Therapy)

Escalation therapy involves selecting an antimicrobial with a narrow spectrum of activity that will likely cover the pathogen causing the suspected infection. After 24–72 hours when culture and susceptibility results are received, the antimicrobial choice may be validated or switched if resistance is documented. This is the standard approach to any outpatient or stable patient requiring hospitalization with sepsis. De-escalation therapy consists of the empiric administration of broad-spectrum antimicrobials aimed to cover all pathogens most frequently related to the infection, including multidrug-resistant (MDR) pathogens. When culture and susceptibility results are available, the spectrum of activity of the antimicrobials is then narrowed if possible or, rarely, it may need to be broadened. A de-escalation approach may be considered appropriate for patients with severe sepsis or septic shock.

This approach is justified, as it is associated with lower mortality in humans and may prevent development of MDR pathogens. The American Thoracic Society recommends it for patients with pneumonia at risk for MDR bacteria [31], as does the Surviving Sepsis Campaign [15]. De-escalation therapy has been shown to be feasible and beneficial in human ICUs [32,33] and has not been shown to increase the level of MDR carriage [34].

Identification of cats and dogs with an increased risk of carrying a MDR pathogen is important as it allows the clinician to alter their antimicrobial choice to one with a broader spectrum, or potentially to choose a tier two (e.g. third-generation cephalosporin) or three (e.g. carbapenem, vancomycin) antimicrobial empirically. In veterinary medicine, prior antimicrobial use within the last 30–90 days has been the factor most frequently associated with the presence of an MDR pathogen [35–41]. Additionally, duration of hospitalization [37–39,42], duration of ICU hospitalization or a surgical procedure [40], and need for mechanical ventilation [43] have been associated with increased MDR pathogen identification. While the veterinarian can justify an empiric tier three antimicrobial for a patient with severe sepsis or septic shock based on documentation of the above risk factors as long as there is a pending culture and susceptibility, there are the ethical considerations of using these antimicrobials and the potential spread of MDR pathogens [44,45]. A list of empiric antimicrobial choices for various situations in which an animal presents with severe sepsis or septic shock is presented in Table 200.1.

Table 200.1 Suggested empiric antimicrobial drug choices for intravenous use in dogs and cats with severe sepsis or septic shock pending the results of culture and susceptibility (which should be followed by reduction in spectrum when possible).

Situation	Antimicrobial drug	Intravenous dosage	Spectrum of activity
Scenario 1			
Patients with no recent antimicrobial history (30 days) and community-acquired infection	Ampicillin/sulbactam OR Clindamycin AND Amikacin	50 mg/kg q6h 12 mg/kg q8h 15 mg/kg q24h	Gram-negative bacteria, streptococci, susceptible staphylococci and enterococci, most anaerobes
Scenario 2			
Patients in scenario 1 with acute kidney injury or chronic kidney disease*	Ampicillin/sulbactam OR Clindamycin AND Enrofloxacin	50 mg/kg q8h 12 mg/kg q8h Dogs: 15 mg/kg first dose then 10 mg/kg q24h	Most gram-negative bacteria, anaerobes, streptococci, and susceptible staphylococci and enterococci. Not effective for MDR gram-negative bacteria
Scenario 3			
Patients with recent antimicrobial use or hospital-acquired infection	Third-generation cephalosporin with anti-*Pseudomonas* activity Cefotaxime Ceftazidime	30 mg/kg q8h 30 mg/kg q8h	Gram-negative rods including *Pseudomonas* and streptococci. Not active against methicillin-resistant staphylococci and enterococci[†]
Scenario 4			
Patients that developed new-onset or worsening severe sepsis/septic shock while on a third-generation cephalosporin	Meropenem	12 mg/kg q8h	MDR aerobic gram-negative bacteria, streptococci, and anaerobes
AND/OR	AND/OR		
have risk factors for methicillin-resistant *Staphylococcus* or MDR *Enterococcus*	Vancomycin	15 mg/kg q8h	Methicillin-resistant staphylococci and MDR enterococci

Dosages are for intravenous administration in animals with normal hepatic and renal function (except scenario 2).
*Further dosage reduction may be indicated based on assessment of renal function by serum creatinine.
[†]If an anaerobic bacterium is suspected, metronidazole can be added, or can be combined with vancomycin if methicillin-resistant staphylococci or MDR enterococci are considered likely.
MDR, multidrug resistant.

Pharmacokinetic and Pharmacodynamic Considerations

In the emergency room, there are a variety of pharmacokinetic/pharmacodynamic (PK/PD) parameters that can be important for patients with sepsis. Antimicrobials that require significantly higher concentrations to kill bacteria than are required to prevent replication are considered bacteriostatic. A bactericidal antimicrobial is one where the concentration required to kill is similar to that for preventing growth. When dealing with patients in the emergency room with any form of sepsis, a bactericidal antimicrobial that can be given intravenously would be the ideal.

In a dog or cat with severe sepsis or septic shock, there is often an increase in capillary permeability. This causes a fluid shift from the intravascular to the interstitial space. This can result in increasing the volume of distribution for many of the hydrophilic antimicrobials (beta-lactams and aminoglycosides) and thereby lowering the concentration of these antimicrobials in the interstitial fluid [46]. Lipophilic antimicrobials such as enrofloxacin are largely unaffected by this process. As most infections occur in the interstitial fluid of tissues, this lower concentration of hydrophilic antimicrobials has the potential to decrease their efficacy. As a result, the initial dose of these antimicrobials should be increased in patients with severe sepsis or septic shock to achieve the same desired interstitial concentrations as in a non-septic patient [10].

Another important PK/PD parameter to consider is the effect of hypoalbuminemia on distribution of antimicrobials. As albumin is the major circulating protein, when it is decreased in septic patients, this can result in an increased unbound fraction of antimicrobial for drugs that have high protein binding (e.g. doxycycline). This higher unbound fraction will result in a greater concentration of antimicrobial, but this is usually offset during fluid resuscitation as the volume of distribution is increased, resulting in lower plasma concentrations [46]. As a result, a larger or more frequent dose may be needed in these patients to achieve effective antimicrobial concentrations.

Additionally, due to diminished microvascular perfusion associated with severe sepsis and septic shock, there can be decreased antimicrobial delivery to sites of infection such as the soft tissues. In multiple studies, this effect has translated to a significant decrease in antimicrobial concentration in interstitial fluid compared to plasma levels [47,48]. The clinician must also take into account whether there is hepatic dysfunction or AKI present which can lead to decreased clearance of hepatically metabolized or renally cleared antimicrobials.

With all of these important PK/PD changes that can occur in patients with severe sepsis or septic shock, a general guiding principle for antimicrobial use is to give the maximum dose that will not create a risk for toxicity in that particular patient.

Duration of Antimicrobial Administration

The ideal duration of antimicrobial use in veterinary medicine has been minimally evaluated. Two studies evaluating short-term (3 day) versus long-term (10 or 14 days) antimicrobial use in dogs with uncomplicated urinary tract infections showed no difference in clinical cures [49,50]. Recent evidence from human medicine suggests a shorter duration of therapy (7 days) may be effective in certain situations [51,52]. The Surviving Sep-

sis guidelines suggest that the duration of therapy should typically be 7–10 days if clinically indicated, although acknowledging that there is a group of patients in which longer courses may be appropriate [15]. Antimicrobial duration driven by biomarkers such as procalcitonin has shown promise in human medicine, but until this biomarker can be reliably measured and validated in veterinary species, it cannot be recommended.

At this time, no definitive recommendation can be made as to the optimal duration of antimicrobial use. However, short duration should be considered in patients where the source of the infection has been drained or removed, and which are considered immunocompetent.

Source Control

As important as antimicrobials are in the treatment of infectious disease in the emergency patient, the clinician should not undervalue the concept of source control. If the infected tissue is amenable to drainage or removal, this should occur as soon as possible after resuscitation efforts are completed [15]. Failure to achieve adequate source control as well as inappropriate antibiotic choice can be the cause for mortality [53].

Conclusion

There are multiple factors to consider when choosing antimicrobial therapy for the emergency room patient. The recommendations made here should be considered as guidelines and not absolutes as the individual patient may need modifications based on a variety of factors. For difficult-to-manage infections, consultation with an infectious disease specialist may be beneficial for optimal patient outcome.

References

1 Wells RJ, Gionfriddo JR, Hackett TB, Radecki SV. Canine and feline emergency room visits and the lunar cycle: 11,940 cases (1992–2002). *J Am Vet Med Assoc* 2007;231(2):251–253.

2 Drobatz KJ, Syring R, Reineke E, Meadows C. Association of holidays, full moon, Friday the 13th, day of week, time of day, day of week, and time of year on case distribution in an urban referral small animal emergency clinic. *J Vet Emerg Crit Care* 2009;19(5):479–483.

3 Centers for Disease Control and Prevention. National Hospital Ambulatory Medical Care Survey: 2015 Emergency Department Summary Tables. https://www.cdc.gov/nchs/data/nhamcs/web_

tables/2015_ed_web_tables.pdf. Accessed 12 May, 2018.

4 Wang HE, Shapiro NI, Angus DC, Yealy DM. National estimates of severe sepsis in United States emergency departments. *Crit Care Med* 2007;35(8):1928–1936.

5 Singhal S, Allen MW, McAnnally JR, Smith KS, Donnelly JP, Wang HE. National estimates of emergency department visits for pediatric severe sepsis in the United States. *PeerJ* 2013;1:e79.

6 Singer M, Deutschman CS, Seymour CW, et al. The Third International Consensus Definitions for Sepsis and Septic Shock (Sepsis-3). *JAMA* 2016;315(8):801–810.

7 Brady CA, Otto CM, van Winkle TJ, King LG. Severe sepsis in cats: 29 cases (1986–1998). *J Am Vet Med Assoc* 2000;217(4):531–535.

8 Kenney EM, Rozanski EA, Rush JE, et al. Association between outcome and organ system dysfunction in dogs with sepsis: 114 cases (2003–2007). *J Am Vet Med Assoc* 2010;236(1):83–87.

9 Shaheen BW, Boothe DM, Oyarzabal OA, Smaha T. Antimicrobial resistance profiles and clonal relatedness of canine and feline Escherichia coli pathogens expressing multidrug resistance in the United States. *J Vet Intern Med* 2010;24(2):323–330.

10 Green RS, Gorman SK. Emergency department antimicrobial considerations in severe sepsis. *Emerg Med Clin North Am* 2014;32(4):835–849.

11 May L, Cosgrove S, L'Archeveque M, et al. A call to action for antimicrobial stewardship in the emergency department: approaches and strategies. *Ann Emerg Med* 2013;62(1):69–77.

12 Van Boeckel TP, Gandra S, Ashok A, et al. Global antibiotic consumption 2000 to 2010: an analysis of national pharmaceutical sales data. *Lancet Infect Dis* 2014;14(8):742–750.

13 Trinh TD, Klinker KP. Antimicrobial stewardship in the emergency department. *Infect Dis Ther* 2015;4(Suppl 1):39–50.

14 Weese JS, Blondeau JM, Boothe D, et al. Antimicrobial use guidelines for treatment of urinary tract disease in dogs and cats: Antimicrobial Guidelines Working Group of the International Society for Companion Animal Infectious Diseases. *Vet Med Int* 2011;2011:263768.

15 Dellinger RP, Levy MM, Rhodes A, et al. Surviving Sepsis Campaign: international guidelines for management of severe sepsis and septic shock, 2012. *Intensive Care Med* 2013;39(2):165–228.

16 Kumar A, Haery C, Paladugu B, et al. The duration of hypotension before the initiation of antibiotic treatment is a critical determinant of survival in a murine model of Escherichia coli septic shock: association with serum lactate and inflammatory cytokine levels. *J Infect Dis* 2006;193(2):251–258.

17 Kumar A, Ellis P, Arabi Y, et al. Initiation of inappropriate antimicrobial therapy results in a fivefold reduction of survival in human septic shock. *Chest* 2009;136(5):1237–1248.

18 Ferrer R, Martin-Loeches I, Phillips G, et al. Empiric antibiotic treatment reduces mortality in severe sepsis and septic shock from the first hour: results from a guideline-based performance improvement program. *Crit Care Med* 2014;42(8):1749–1755.

19 Weiss SL, Fitzgerald JC, Balamuth F, et al. Delayed antimicrobial therapy increases mortality and organ dysfunction duration in pediatric sepsis. *Crit Care Med* 2014;42(11):2409–2417.

20 Roman CP, Poole SG, Dooley MJ, Smit V, Mitra B. Implementation of hospital-wide reform at improving access and flow: impact on time to antibiotics in the emergency department. *Emerg Med Australas* 2016;28:133–137.

21 Abelson AL, Buckley GJ, Rozanski EA. Positive impact of an emergency department protocol on time to antimicrobial administration in dogs with septic peritonitis. *J Vet Emerg Crit Care* 2013;23(5):551–556.

22 Wisdom A, Eaton V, Gordon D, Daniel S, Woodman R, Phillips C. INITIAT-E.D.: Impact of timing of INITIation of Antibiotic Therapy on mortality of patients presenting to an Emergency Department with sepsis. *Emerg Med Australas* 2015;27(3):196–201.

23 Ryoo SM, Kim WY, Sohn CH, et al. Prognostic value of timing of antibiotic administration in patients with septic shock treated with early quantitative resuscitation. *Am J Med Sci* 2015;349(4):328–333.

24 Jalili M, Barzegari H, Pourtatabaei N, et al. Effect of door-to-antibiotic time on mortality of patients with sepsis in emergency department: a prospective cohort study. *Acta Med Iran* 2013;51(7):454–460.

25 Sterling SA, Miller WR, Pryor J, Puskarich MA, Jones AE. The impact of timing of antibiotics on outcomes in severe sepsis and septic shock: a systematic review and meta-analysis. *Crit Care Med* 2015;43(9):1907–1915.

26 Vilella AL, Seifert CF. Timing and appropriateness of initial antibiotic therapy in newly presenting septic patients. *Am J Emerg Med* 2014;32(1):7–13.

27 Puskarich MA, Trzeciak S, Shapiro NI, et al. Association between timing of antibiotic administration and mortality from septic shock in patients treated with a quantitative resuscitation protocol. *Crit Care Med* 2011;39(9):2066–2071.

28 Gaieski DF, Mikkelsen ME, Band RA, et al. Impact of time to antibiotics on survival in patients with severe sepsis or septic shock in whom early goal-directed therapy was initiated in the emergency department. *Crit Care Med* 2010;38(4):1045–1053.

29 Bagshaw SM, Lapinsky S, Dial S, et al. Acute kidney injury in septic shock: clinical outcomes and impact of duration of hypotension prior to initiation of antimicrobial therapy. *Intensive Care Med* 2009;35(5):871–881.

30 Zhang D, Micek ST, Kollef MH. Time to appropriate antibiotic therapy is an independent determinant of postinfection ICU and hospital lengths of stay in patients with sepsis. *Crit Care Med* 2015;43(10):2133–2140.

31 American Thoracic Society. Guidelines for the management of adults with hospital-acquired, ventilator-associated, and healthcare-associated pneumonia. *Am J Respir Crit Care Med* 2005;171(4):388–416.

32 Lee CC, Lee NY, Chen PL, et al. Impact of antimicrobial strategies on clinical outcomes of adults with septic shock and community-onset Enterobacteriaceae bacteremia: de-escalation is beneficial. *Diagn Microbiol Infect Dis* 2015;82(2):158–164.

33 Joung MK, Lee JA, Moon SY, et al. Impact of de-escalation therapy on clinical outcomes for

intensive care unit-acquired pneumonia. *Crit Care* 2011;15(2):R79.

34 Gonzalez L, Cravoisy A, Barraud D, et al. Factors influencing the implementation of antibiotic de-escalation and impact of this strategy in critically ill patients. *Crit Care* 2013;17(4):R140.

35 Proulx A, Hume DZ, Drobatz KJ, Reineke EL. In vitro bacterial isolate susceptibility to empirically selected antimicrobials in 111 dogs with bacterial pneumonia. *J Vet Emerg Crit Care* 2014;24(2):194–200.

36 Dickinson AE, Summers JF, Wignal J, Boag AK, Keir I. Impact of appropriate empirical antimicrobial therapy on outcome of dogs with septic peritonitis. *J Vet Emerg Crit Care* 2015;25(1):152–159.

37 Gibson JS, Morton JM, Cobbold RN, Filippich LJ, Trott DJ. Risk factors for multidrug-resistant Escherichia coli rectal colonization of dogs on admission to a veterinary hospital. *Epidemiol Infect* 2011;139(2):197–205.

38 Gibson JS, Morton JM, Cobbold RN, Filippich LJ, Trott DJ. Risk factors for dogs becoming rectal carriers of multidrug-resistant Escherichia coli during hospitalization. *Epidemiol Infect* 2011;139(10): 1511–1521.

39 Gibson JS, Morton JM, Cobbold RN, Sidjabat HE, Filippich LJ, Trott DJ. Multidrug-resistant E. coli and enterobacter extraintestinal infection in 37 dogs. *J Vet Intern Med* 2008;22(4):844–850.

40 Ogeer-Gyles J, Mathews KA, Sears W, Prescott JF, Weese JS, Boerlin P. Development of antimicrobial drug resistance in rectal Escherichia coli isolates from dogs hospitalized in an intensive care unit. *J Am Vet Med Assoc* 2006;229(5):694–699.

41 Leite-Martins L, Mahu MI, Costa AL, et al. Prevalence of antimicrobial resistance in faecal enterococci from vet-visiting pets and assessment of risk factors. *Vet Rec* 2015;176(26):674.

42 Hamilton E, Kruger JM, Schall W, Beal M, Manning SD, Kaneene JB. Acquisition and persistence of antimicrobial-resistant bacteria isolated from dogs and cats admitted to a veterinary teaching hospital. *J Am Vet Med Assoc* 2013;243(7):990–1000.

43 Epstein SE, Mellema MS, Hopper K. Airway microbial culture and susceptibility patterns in dogs and cats with respiratory disease of varying severity. *J Vet Emerg Crit Care* 2010;20(6):587–594.

44 Morley PS, Apley MD, Besser TE, et al. Antimicrobial drug use in veterinary medicine. *J Vet Intern Med* 2005;19(4):617–629.

45 Weese JS, Giguere S, Guardabassi L, et al. ACVIM consensus statement on therapeutic antimicrobial use in animals and antimicrobial resistance. *J Vet Intern Med* 2015;29(2):487–498.

46 Varghese JM, Roberts JA, Lipman J. Antimicrobial pharmacokinetic and pharmacodynamic issues in the critically ill with severe sepsis and septic shock. *Crit Care Clin* 2011;27(1):19–34.

47 Roberts JA, Roberts MS, Robertson TA, Dalley AJ, Lipman J. Piperacillin penetration into tissue of critically ill patients with sepsis – bolus versus continuous administration? *Crit Care Med* 2009;37(3):926–933.

48 Joukhadar C, Frossard M, Mayer BX, et al. Impaired target site penetration of beta-lactams may account for therapeutic failure in patients with septic shock. *Crit Care Med* 2001;29(2):385–391.

49 Westropp JL, Sykes JE, Irom S, et al. Evaluation of the efficacy and safety of high dose short duration enrofloxacin treatment regimen for uncomplicated urinary tract infections in dogs. *J Vet Intern Med* 2012;26(3):506–512.

50 Clare S, Hartmann FA, Jooss M, et al. Short- and long-term cure rates of short-duration trimethoprim-sulfamethoxazole treatment in female dogs with uncomplicated bacterial cystitis. *J Vet Intern Med* 2014;28(3):818–826.

51 Pugh R, Grant C, Cooke RP, Dempsey G. Short-course versus prolonged-course antibiotic therapy for hospital-acquired pneumonia in critically ill adults. *Cochrane Database Syst Rev* 2015;8: CD007577.

52 Barrett J, Edgeworth J, Wyncoll D. Shortening the course of antibiotic treatment in the intensive care unit. *Expert Rev Anti-Infect Ther* 2015;13(4): 463–471.

53 Tellor B, Skrupky LP, Symons W, High E, Micek ST, Mazuski JE. Inadequate source control and inappropriate antibiotics are key determinants of mortality in patients with intra-abdominal sepsis and associated bacteremia. *Surg Infect* 2015;16(6): 785–793.

201

Disaster Medicine

Lee Palmer, DVM, MS, DACVECC, NREMT-T, WEMT, CCRP

K9 Tactical Emergency Casualty Care Working Group, Auburn, AL, USA

What is a Disaster?

By definition, a *disaster* is a catastrophic event involving widespread loss of human life, economic and logistical hardship, and environmental damages to the point that it overwhelms the affected community's existing resources to recover on its own [1,2]. Many use the terms *disaster* and *emergency* synonymously, but an emergency is better defined as a natural or man-made incident in which a community has the resources to recover without the need for outside help an [2], ongoing emergency may quickly deplete a community's resources and become a true disaster at any moment.

Each disaster is unique. It may occur at any time; result from a natural phenomenon (e.g. earthquake, hurricane, tornado, flood, etc.) or man-made incident (e.g. terrorist attack, structural fire/collapse, chemical spill, etc.); involve only a few to a large number of casualties; last only a few days or endure over several weeks; and involve a few to many different species of animals. It is therefore impossible to predict exactly what one may encounter prior to arriving at the disaster site.

During Hurricane Katrina, it was reported that along with the traditional household pet (e.g. dogs and cats), other species of large animals (e.g. horses and cattle) as well as wildlife and exotics (e.g. foxes, raccoons, deer, etc.) were also in need of rescue and medical aid [3]. Considering how specialized veterinary medicine has become, it is prudent for veterinary personnel to briefly review the main points of veterinary medicine applicable to species they may encounter during a disaster, but that they do not routinely care for. For example, a small animal practitioner in a response team should consider reviewing basic equine medicine principles in order to support the medical needs of search-and-rescue horses.

The Human–Animal Bond During a Disaster

When a disaster strikes, companion animals experience the same risk for injuries and mortality as people. Today, society expects that injured and stranded animals will be given appropriate and timely veterinary care during disaster recovery efforts. From a small animal standpoint, experience from previous disaster events has shown that the loss and/or suffering of companion animals may greatly affect the community's overall psychological well-being [4–6].

It is estimated that over 50% of US households have pets, and six out of 10 pet owners consider their pets to be family members [7]. Interestingly, some data has shown pet ownership to be a major risk factor for evacuation failure during natural disasters [5,6]. Although several risk factors for pet-related evacuation failures have been identified [5,6], one reason was due to the fact that in the past, the priority for evacuation was saving human life; as such, people were forced to leave their pets behind [3–5]. Particularly during Hurricane Katrina, complications from this arose when people would choose not to evacuate and leave their pets behind or, if evacuated, they would re-enter an unstable disaster site to retrieve their animals [3–5]. People who failed to evacuate not only placed themselves at risk for serious injury or death, but they also put first responders in danger as they entered the unsafe environment to rescue these people.

Although it is hard to determine an exact number, it was estimated that 40 000–50 000 animals were lost during Hurricane Katrina [4]. The animal-related issues that occurred during Hurricane Katrina left thousands of animals stranded to die or become severely ill. Coupled with the poor sanitary conditions in the wake of massive flooding, multiple infectious diseases as well as a public health risk developed in the area. With vigilant media coverage bringing the events of Katrina to national attention, a large public outcry and demand for action were generated [4,6].

After seeing the impact of the human–animal bond during Hurricane Katrina, the American Veterinary Medical Association (AVMA) published *Placing the Human–Animal Bond in Context in the Face of Disasters* which stated: "When disaster strikes, saving animals means saving people – human and animal health and welfare are inextricably intertwined" [6]. In the wake of Hurricane Katrina and in order to ensure that animal-related issues did not repeat themselves in the future, Congress enacted the Pet Evacuation and Transportation Standards (PETS) Act in 2006 [4,8]. The PETS Act was enacted so that individuals no longer have to leave their pets behind during an evacuation or rescue operation. It requires state and local government entities to incorporate the needs of individuals with household pets and service animals into their disaster preparedness and recovery plans. In addition, the PETS Act granted the Federal Emergency Management Agency (FEMA) the authority to assist these agencies with developing and approving the standards of their plans.

Post Hurricane Katrina, two additional alliances were also created to help mitigate the animal-related issues encountered during Katrina for future incidents: the National Animal Rescue and Sheltering Coalition (NARSC) (http://thenarsc.org/) and the National Alliance for State Animal and Agricultural Emergency Programs (NASAAEP) (www.nasaaep.org). The NARSC is a coalition of national organizations in the areas of animal welfare, care, rescue, and control. Its mission is to "identify, prioritize and find collaborative solutions to major human-animal emergency issues." The NASAAEP's primary goal is to foster a network between all emergency management stakeholders to facilitate effective communications, information sharing, and planning at all levels of government and response. In addition, the NASAAEP has developed "Best Practices" guidelines to address key animal issues that may be encountered during an emergency or disaster (http://nasaaep.org/best-practices/) to include: animal decontamination; animal evacuation and transportation; animal search and technical rescue; community preparedness and outreach; disaster veterinary care; emergency animal sheltering; planning and resource management; zoo disaster preparedness.

Organizational Structure

Disaster medicine is multidisciplinary. It consists of multiple levels of organizational involvement consisting of local, state, and federal governments, tribal and territorial governments, and private sector entities that have a

functional need and vested interest in the community (e.g. local businesses, voluntary and non-profit organizations, academic institutions, individuals, and families) [9]. This multifaceted disaster management team is what the FEMA defines as the "whole community" [10], reinforcing that effective disaster management and preparedness is a shared responsibility of everyone involved, not just governmental entities.

Each of the three levels of government (e.g. local, state, federal) has an increasing span of responsibility. The intention is that each level maintains responsibility for managing emergencies in its jurisdiction until no longer feasible, at which point it may request assistance from the next higher level of government [9]. Most local municipalities have an emergency management representative or a designated Office of Emergency Management (OEM). County OEMs are primarily responsible for emergency preparedness and response planning as well as continued risk assessment for the communities within their locale. State OEMs provide assistance to all local municipalities within their state. Subsequent to a disaster or emergency, the governor may allocate resources (to include National Guard resources) to communities that lack the resources to recover from a disaster on their own. If a state's resources become depleted or overwhelmed, the governor may request aid from the federal government.

At the federal level, FEMA acting under the Department of Homeland Security has the most direct, primary role for overseeing and co-ordinating the nation's disaster management program [9]. Besides evaluating its own capability in responding to a large-scale, nationwide disaster, the federal government also assists and provides guidance to each state in developing and implementing state disaster management plans as well as allocating resources and assistance to support recovery efforts for communities in which the state's resources are depleted or insufficient. The National Incident Management System (NIMS) is an essential foundation of FEMA's National Preparedness System [9,11]. The NIMS provides all levels of government, non-governmental, and private sector organizations with a standardized template and systematic approach for collaboratively managing disaster events across the full spectrum of potential threats and hazards regardless of size or complexity [11].

Within the NIMS is the Incident Command System (ICS) which is a fundamental element for organizing and managing on-scene emergency or disaster response operations [9,12,13]. The ICS provides a unified command and control framework and establishes a common organizational chain of command for co-ordinating the activities of all agencies (federal, state, local, tribal, private sector, and non-governmental) involved in the response. Implementation of an ICS lessens the chances for miscommunication and ensures appropriate resources and personnel are directed and utilized where they are most needed; therefore, an effective ICS ensures that the disaster is resolved as quickly and efficiently as possible. The ICS is applicable to a wide array of disaster events to include different disciplines and complexities, small- and large-scale operations, near- and long-term operations, as well as natural, man-made, and terrorist events. Any personnel that may become part of a disaster response team or may have involvement with disaster or emergency management should receive training in NIMS and ICS (www.fema.gov/incident-command-system-resources) [14,15].

Veterinary Disaster Response Programs

The federal National Veterinary Response Team (NVRT) and the AVMA Veterinary Medical Assistance Team (VMAT) are two complementary animal response programs [16,17]. They facilitate veterinary emergency preparedness plans as well as animal rescue and recovery operations during an actual disaster event. As part of the Health and Human Services (HHS) National Disaster Medicine System (NDMS), the NVRT is a federal program that operates under the ICS [17], as the primary federal resource for the treatment of animals affected during a disaster. Members of the NVRTs are private citizens (veterinarians, public health safety officers, veterinary technicians, epidemiologists, logisticians, communications specialists, and other support personnel) who, once activated to respond to a disaster, are then compensated as federal employees.

From 1993 to 2007, the AVMA VMATs worked in partnership with the HHS and, when activated, the VMAT deployed as a federal entity [16]. Following Hurricane Katrina, restructuring of the government led to the AVMA relaunching the VMAT program as a private non-governmental organization. VMAT members are now volunteers and only receive reimbursement for travel, housing, and *per diem* expenses.

The main functions of the AVMA VMATS are to provide:

- early assessment teams to assess veterinary conditions, infrastructure, and resources
- basic veterinary treatment teams to augment local veterinary resources in providing primary field care
- training on emergency-related topics (e.g. animal emergency preparedness and response) to animal health authorities, veterinary medical associations, emergency first responders, and other relevant emergency management organizations.

Phases of Disaster Management

Disaster and emergency management involves more than just those actions taken to respond and rebuild a community after a disaster strikes. It involves a lifecycle of events that the FEMA has categorized into four strategic phases: *mitigation* of hazards, *preparedness* for and *response* to an emergency or disaster, and then *recovery* from the effects of the disaster [9,13,18].

Mitigation

Mitigation strategies are "preventive" in nature, are typically implemented prior to a disaster event and are intended to prevent the occurrence of and/or lessen the damaging effects of an emergency or disaster [9,13,18]. Examples include buying flood and fire insurance or building your home away from high-risk floodplains or high seismic activity zones. For coastal communities located in a "hurricane belt," state and local governments establish building codes and zoning requirements and construct barriers such as levees to help mitigate the severity and degree of structural damage. These actions not only reduce the need for reconstruction after a hurricane but also help diminish the loss of life and property.

In regard to companion animals, small animal practitioners should take an active role in educating their clients on mitigating strategies that may help safeguard their pets. For example, ensuring their animals remain up-to-date on preventive healthcare and that they have a method for positively identifying their pets (e.g. microchip, photos, etc.) in case they are separated from them during a disaster or relief operation. Veterinary clinics, humane societies, and other animal shelters should develop emergency procedures and evacuation plans for the animals in their care. These facilities should provide copies of their plans to the state emergency management agency. In addition to developing plans, it is advocated that veterinary clinics and animal facilities procure suitable containers to transport their animals during evacuations [18].

Preparedness

Preparedness planning enhances the whole community's ability to respond to a disaster [9,13,18]. FEMA developed a National Preparedness Goal to outline what is meant for the nation, and particularly a community, to be prepared for a disaster. The goal states, "A secure and resilient nation with the capabilities required across the whole community to prevent, protect against, mitigate, respond to, and recover from the threats and hazards that pose the greatest risk" [19]. General examples of preparedness planning include identifying potential disaster risk areas (e.g. floodplains), locating and mapping out viable evacuation routes, installing public alert and warning systems (e.g. tornado sirens), and identifying back-up community services and utility needs (e.g. power generators, fresh water supply, sewage disposal methods, etc.) [9,18,20].

Veterinarians should identify their local OEMS and become aware of the resources that may be available to them during a disaster. Veterinary personnel may decide to join a regional disaster response team. They may utilize their expertise to help develop and implement predisaster preparedness plans, establish relationships with community relief organizations (e.g. American Red Cross), provide animal handling and first aid training to emergency responders, and participate in conducting disaster response drills. Preplanning may include mapping out viable animal shelters and veterinary clinics for injured and displaced animals, identifying resources for transporting animals out of the disaster zone, establishing alternative sources of power for heating and lighting for veterinary clinics and shelters (e.g. electrical power generators), identifying viable evacuation routes for animals housed in animal and veterinary facilities located within a disaster zone, identifying communication equipment, and establishing caches of veterinary supplies and resources in key areas for immediate availability. Plans for humane euthanasia of critically ill or injured animals as well as disposal for animals that are euthanized or may have died during the disaster should also be taken into account. In planning for potential prolonged recovery operations, preventive health programs should be developed for sheltered animals to prevent the development and spread of disease.

Small animal practitioners may work with, educate, and train various groups and organizations within their community. They may work with local animal shelters, humane societies, and animal control agencies to guide them on appropriate animal care principles, first aid, and decontamination procedures. Together, they should develop a plan for fostering/adopting animals that are not reclaimed by their owners during or after the disaster incident. Search and rescue units may need guidance on animal care, handling, and restraint, techniques for sheltering in place with injured or critically ill animals; and techniques for extraction of injured and or trapped animals. It is also important that rescue teams have a method for properly identifying animals and then reuniting the animals with their owners.

The general public should be made aware of available public resources, actions for emergency sheltering of animals, available community warning systems, and contact information for key agencies or organizations in case a disaster does arise. As part of their general health and wellness discussion, the practitioner and/or staff

should consider educating animal owners about making arrangements for their pets in case of evacuation (e.g. identify designated safe havens and caregivers), keeping emergency supplies (e.g. food, water, flashlights, batteries, etc.) on hand in case they need to shelter in place, and maintaining emergency first aid and evacuation kits. Pet owners may be directed to organizations such as the Humane Society of the United States, the AVMA, the American Red Cross, and other organizations that provide online resources to help pet owners prepare for a disaster.

Veterinary clinics should also prepare for disaster scenarios, particularly considering they may need to shelter animals in place for days to weeks. The AVMA has developed a brochure which defines the essential elements that a veterinary practice's disaster plan should include [20].

- Emergency relocation of animals
- Medical record back-up
- Continuity of operations
- Security
- General emergency planning
- Fire prevention
- Insurance and legal issues

The brochure is available for download at: https://ebusiness.avma.org/ProductCatalog/product.aspx?ID=139.

Preparedness planning is only effective if everyone involved is aware of their roles and responsibilities, is properly trained in disaster management principles, and the disaster plan is actually practiced and rehearsed on a routine basis. After each rehearsal, a formal debriefing should be conducted to identify deficiencies as well as aspects of the plan that worked well. All personnel that may be involved in a disaster should also receive some formal training in disaster and emergency management. FEMA's Emergency Management Institute offers several free online courses and its Center for Domestic Preparedness also offers high-quality comprehensive preparedness training programs for emergency responders [21]. Other organizations such as the Humane Society, AVMA, and various academic institutions offer varying degrees of emergency management training [22–24].

Response

Response actions take place during and after the incident and include actions taken to prevent further loss of life and property during a disaster [9,18]. During a disaster, veterinary personnel play a key role as animal advocates by ensuring the welfare and needs of animals are covered during the response. Although providing medical aid to injured and sick animals is part of a veterinary disaster response, it often makes up only a small portion of the disaster veterinarian's duties. Other common responsibilities a veterinarian may have during a response include working with the humane society and local animal shelter to retrieve and shelter animals that have been abandoned, displaced or escaped from their owners during evacuation; assisting with the humane euthanasia and proper disposal of dead animals; arranging for the provision of food, water, and shelter for displaced animals; triaging and establishing a casualty collection point; counseling pet owners who have been separated from their animals; and serving as a liaison to maintain communications between key relief agencies, governmental organizations, and the incident command structure.

An important duty of a disaster veterinarian is providing support and aid for the operational working canines or OpK9s (search and rescue and law enforcement canines) that are involved in the recovery efforts. Many disaster responses employ OpK9s to assist with human recovery. As an advocate for OpK9s, it is the on-site veterinarian's responsibility to ensure not only that these dogs are given timely medical care when they suffer an injury or illness, but also that preventive measures are implemented to prevent injury and illness from occurring (e.g. dehydration, exhaustion, etc.). Lessons learned from past disaster events (e.g. Oklahoma City, World Trade Center on 9/11, Haiti, Oso, Washington, etc.) demonstrated that the overall number of OpK9 injuries was actually quite small [25–28]. Most were footpad injuries and cuts/abrasions on the limbs, mainly subsequent to OpK9s having to traverse over sharp surfaces and structural damage. Other common problems included fatigue, gastrointestinal problems, dehydration, and ocular irritations. Awareness of past lessons learned will help increase the chance of future successes.

Recovery

Recovery activities typically start after the event, but may occur concurrently with response efforts after immediate

basic life-sustaining needs of the community have been addressed. The focus of recovery efforts is directed towards actions needed to return a community and its infrastructure to near-normal conditions. Depending upon the complexity and severity of damage inflicted by the disaster, recovery efforts may last a few weeks to a few years. A key task during the recovery period is evaluating the incident to identify lessons learned. Communities may then use this information to develop measures to mitigate the effects of future incidents. A debriefing with all agencies and organizations involved in the event should take place to identify what worked and what didn't. An after action report is generated and distributed to all organizations and personnel involved in order to help them prepare for the next disaster.

Considerations the veterinarian may need to take into account are dealing with animal owners who lost their pets and filing insurance claims for injuries animals may have suffered during the disaster. Also, health issues in pets may continue to manifest for weeks to months after the incident, particularly if an animal was exposed to any type of hazardous material and/or smoke inhalation [29,30]. Psychological issues may develop in the pet owner while behavioral issues develop in the pet, both of which the veterinarian may find themselves dealing with in the healing process [4,9].

Conclusion

Animals suffer the same risks for injury and death during a disaster as people do. Experience from previous disaster events has demonstrated that the well-being of household pets and service animals during the disaster response and recovery efforts may have a large impact on the psychological healing of a community. As such, it is vital that veterinarians become involved in their community's disaster preparedness activities and become aware of the main concepts and structures of disaster medicine.

References

1 World Health Organization website. Available at: http://www.who.int/hac/about/definitions/en/ (accessed 20 February 2018).
2 Oliver C. The definition and history of disasters. In: *Catastrophic Disaster Planning and Response*. Taylor and Francis, Boca Raton, 2010, pp. 7–9.
3 Lanman LL, Wingfield WE. Disaster Response Overview. Proceedings of the International Veterinary Emergency and Critical Care Symposium, 2006. Available at: www.vin.com/members/cms/project/

defaultadv1.aspx?id=3857223&pid=11222&catid =&&n=22&sx=11381595 (accessed 20 February 2018).
4 Hunt MG, Bogue K, Rohrbaugh N. Pet ownership and evacuation prior to Hurricane Irene. *Animals* 2012;28;2(4):529–539.
5 Heath SE, Voeks SK, Glickman LT. Epidemiologic features of pet evacuation failure in a rapid-onset disaster. *J Am Vet Med Assoc* 2001;218:1898–1904.
6 American Veterinary Medical Association (AVMA). Human–Animal Bond – Disaster Preparedness.

Available at: www.avma.org/kb/resources/reference/human-animal-bond/pages/human-animal-bond-disaster-preparedness.aspx (accessed 20 February 2018).

7   American Veterinary Medical Association (AVMA). US Pet Ownership and Demographics Sourcebook (2012). Available at: www.avma.org/KB/Resources/Statistics/Pages/Market-research-statistics-US-Pet-Ownership-Demographics-Sourcebook.aspx (accessed 20 February 2018).

8   Pets Evacuation and Transportation Standards Act of 2006 Public Law 109–308. Available at: www.gpo.gov/fdsys/pkg/PLAW-109publ308/pdf/PLAW-109publ308.pdf (accessed 20 February 2018).

9   Engelke HT. Emergency management during disasters for small animal practitioners. *Vet Clin North Am Small Anim Pract* 2009;39(2):347–358.

10 Federal Emergency Management Agency. Whole Community. Available at: www.fema.gov/whole-community (accessed 20 February 2018).

11 Federal Emergency Management Agency. National Incident Management System (NIMS). Available at: www.fema.gov/national-incident-management-system (accessed 20 December 2015)

12 Federal Emergency Management Agency. Incident Command System (ICS) Resources. Available at: www.fema.gov/incident-command-system-resources (accessed 20 February 2018).

13 Madigan J, Dacre I. Preparing for veterinary emergencies: disaster management and the Incident Command System. *Rev Sci Tech* 2009;28(2):627–633.

14 Federal Emergency Management Agency, Emergency Management Institute. Independent study program courses. Available at: http://training.fema.gov/IS/crslist.asp (accessed 20 February 2018).

15 Federal Emergency Management Agency, Emergency Management Institute. Available at: https://training.fema.gov/emi.aspx (accessed 20 February 2018).

16 American Veterinary Medical Association (AVMA). Veterinary Medical Assistance Teams (VMAT). Available at: www.avma.org/vmat (accessed 20 February 2018).

17 United States Department of Health and Human Services. National Veterinary Response Team (NVRT). Available at: https://www.phe.gov/Preparedness/responders/ndms/ndms-teams/Pages/nvrt.aspx (accessed 20 February 2018).

18 American Veterinary Medical Association (AVMA). Emergency Preparedness and Response Guide. Available at: https://ebusiness.avma.org/files/productdownloads/emerg_prep_resp_guide.pdf (accessed 20 February 2018).

19 Federal Emergency Management Agency. National Preparedness Goal. Available at: http://www.fema.gov/national-preparedness-goal (accessed 20 February 2018).

20 American Veterinary Medical Association (AVMA). Disaster Preparedness for Veterinary Practices. Available at: https://ebusiness.avma.org/files/productdownloads/vet_practices_brochure.pdf (accessed 20 February 2018).

21 Center for Domestic Preparedness. Available at: https://cdp.dhs.gov/about/ (accessed 20 February 2018).

22 American Red Cross. Plan & Prepare. Available at: www.redcross.org//prepare (accessed 20 February 2018).

23 Humane Society of the United States. Disaster Preparedness. Available at: www.humanesociety.org/about/departments/disaster_preparedness.html?credit=web_id281031178 (accessed 20 February 2018).

24 American Veterinary Medical Association (AVMA). Disaster Preparedness for Veterinarians. Available at: www.avma.org/kb/resources/reference/disaster/pages/default.aspx?utm_source=prettyurl&utm_medium=web&utm_campaign=redirect&utm_term=disaster (accessed 20 February 2018).

25 Otto CM, Downend AB, Serpell JA, Ziemer LS, Saunders HM. Medical and behavioral surveillance of dogs deployed to the World Trade Center and the Pentagon from October 2001 to June 2002. *J Am Vet Med Assoc* 2004;225:861–867.

26 Slensky KA, Drobatz KJ, Downend AB, Otto CM. Deployment morbidity among search-and-rescue dogs used after the September 11, 2001, terrorist attacks. *J Am Vet Med Assoc* 2004;225(6):868–873.

27 Gordon LE. Injuries and illnesses among urban search-and-rescue dogs deployed to Haiti following the January 12, 2010, earthquake. *J Am Vet Med Assoc* 2012; 240(4):396–403.

28 Gordon LE. Injuries and illnesses among Federal Emergency Management Agency-certified search-and-recovery and search-and-rescue dogs deployed to Oso, Washington, following the March 22, 2014, State Route 530 landslide. *J Am Vet Med Assoc* 2015;247(8):901–908.

29 Levy JK, Edinboro CH, Glotfelty CS, et al. Seroprevalence of Dirofilaria immitis, feline leukemia virus, and feline immunodeficiency virus infection among dogs and cats exported from the 2005 Gulf Coast hurricane disaster area. *J Am Vet Med Assoc* 2007;231:218–225.

30 Levy JK, Lappin MR, Glaser AL, Birkenheuer AJ, Anderson TC, Edinboro CH. Prevalence of infectious diseases in cats and dogs rescued following Hurricane Katrina. *J Am Vet Med Assoc* 2011;238(3):311–317.

202

Working Dogs in the Emergency Room

Cynthia M. Otto, DVM, PhD, DACVECC, DACVSMR, CCRT

Penn Vet Working Dog Center, University of Pennsylvania, Philadelphia, PA, USA

Occupations

Working dogs represent a unique group of patients that require veterinary care. The dogs are generally highly trained and typically work very closely with an individual handler. Professional working dogs can be broken down into three major categories: police/patrol/military, detection, and service. Many of the risks and special considerations for working dogs will also apply to sport and performance dogs.

Police/Patrol/Military

These dogs generally are partnered with a police or military handler. The dog is trained to protect the handler above all else. Most of these dogs are not "attack dogs" but rather they are trained to bite and hold a suspect. Well-trained police dogs should be able to guard a suspect without contact. After release of a bite, the suspect should be able to even pet the dog. If the dog perceives a threat to the handler, however, he will initiate action (bite) without a command. In addition to criminal apprehension, these dogs are typically also trained to identify an odor, whether it is explosives, narcotics or human remains. As a rule, the handler should be with the police dog whenever possible for examination. Most handlers will muzzle the dog for an examination. Using a calm approach in an examination, paying close attention to the dog's body language and avoiding threatening positions (e.g. hovering over the head and direct eye contact) will often make an exam more manageable; however, some police dogs will not be able to be examined without sedation. In some situations, the dog will be hospitalized and away from the handler. In this case, it is important to know the common commands used for the dog (and in what language!).

Odor Detection

There are numerous canine detection careers. Search and rescue (SAR) dogs are commonly owned by private citizens who volunteer their time and efforts in searches. Although some dogs may be owned by an organization, they still work and are certified with a designated handler. These dogs may work in urban/disaster or wilderness (wide area) environments and may search for live humans or human remains. Other examples of detection dog careers include explosive detection, drug detection, bed bug detection, and several fields of conservation work, to name a few. All of these dogs typically work with a specific handler/owner. These dogs range from high energy to relatively calm. Depending on their job, they may or may not be friendly with people or other dogs. Search and rescue dogs must not display any aggression toward humans or other dogs. Despite their extensive training, these dogs, especially the high-energy dogs, are often not comfortable during veterinary visits. Due to the relationship with the handler, these handlers should remain with their dogs during examinations whenever possible.

Assistance/Service

According to the federal government through the Americans with Disabilities Act (ADA) [1], a service dog is defined as one that has been trained to perform tasks directly related to the disability of that dog's handler. Although guide and hearing dogs have a long history, the field of service dogs has expanded exponentially in recent years. Now dogs are trained to provide services for a variety of different disabilities. Autism dogs are particularly useful with children, as they help to keep the child from bolting and help with social adaptation. Dogs for veterans and other individuals with posttraumatic stress disorder (PTSD) provide the security to allow the individuals to interact within society. These dogs, while trained for the individual needs of the handler, will often provide a physical barrier ('block") between the handler and other individuals. They can provide a "look out" so the handler is not taken by surprise and they often wake up individuals experiencing night terrors. Many service

Textbook of Small Animal Emergency Medicine, First Edition. Edited by Kenneth J. Drobatz, Kate Hopper, Elizabeth Rozanski and Deborah C. Silverstein.
© 2019 John Wiley & Sons, Inc. Published 2019 by John Wiley & Sons, Inc.
Companion Website: www.wiley.com/go/drobatz/textbook

dogs are also trained to provide stability or retrieve objects for their handlers with physical disabilities.

Medical detection dogs are a fairly recent addition to the service dog field. Dogs are trained to alert diabetic individuals to drops or sudden increases in blood sugar. Epilepsy alert dogs anticipate the onset of a seizure and can help facilitate the safety of their handler. Emotional support and therapy dogs do not fall under the definition of a service dog (although some state or local laws may include these dogs). According to the ADA guidelines, if it is not obvious that the dog is a service animal, only two specific questions may be asked: (1) is the dog a service animal required because of a disability? and (2) what work or task has the dog been trained to perform? People are not allowed to request any documentation for the dog, require that the dog demonstrate its task, or inquire about the nature of the person's disability [1].

Service dogs should be examined with the handler present whenever possible. Clear explanations of all the procedures should accommodate the person's disability. For example, a blind person will need a clear narration of each step of an exam or procedure, whereas a deaf person will need written or signed information.

Occupational Hazards

Common Conditions

Working dogs have occupational risks based on their exposure, their trained tasks, and their breed (Table 202.1). Emergency care of traumatic injuries is expected to be common in working dogs. The risk of specific trauma will depend on the job and the environment.

Blast injury is likely highest in military working dogs (MWD), although explosive detection dogs and urban search and rescue dogs could be at risk. Gunshot wounds can be a hazard for most working dogs. For MWD in a battlefield setting, catastrophic injury is common, with frequent thoracic and extremity injuries [2]. In police dogs, gunshot wounds are a recognized risk, but there is no information about gunshot injuries specific to police dogs [3]. Wilderness

Table 202.1 Occupational hazards associated with various canine working disciplines.

Occupational hazards	Police/patrol/ military	Detection urban/disaster	Detection wilderness	Service/ assistance
Cause of injury/illness				
Trauma –bite wounds (i.e. dogs, other animals)	+	+	+	+
Trauma – blast	+ +	+	+/-	-
Trauma – blunt (i.e. falls, vehicles)	+ +	+ +	+	+
Trauma – gunshot	+ +	+	+	-
Trauma – impalement	+	+	+	-
Cold injury	+/-	+/-	+/-	-
Heat injury (i.e. exercise, confinement)	+ +	+ +	+ +	-
Infectious	+	+	+ +	+/-
Neoplasia	+ +	+ +	+ +	+ +
Toxin exposure	+	+	+	+
Body system				
Respiratory	-	-	-	-
Cardiac	-	-	-	-
Neurological (spinal cord, central)	+	+/-	+/-	+/-
Urogenital	+ +	+	+/-	+/-
Musculoskeletal (e.g. pad cuts, lacerations, lameness)	+ + +	+ + +	+ + +	+
Gastrointestinal (e.g. vomiting, diarrhea, GDV)	+ + +	+ +	+ +	+ +
Dermatological (e.g. dermatitis, otitis, atopy)	+ +	+ +	+ +	+ +
Dental	+ +	+/-	+/-	+/-
Ophthalmological	+	+	+	+

+ + +, very high risk; + +, high risk; +, moderate risk; +/-, low risk; -, negligible risk compared to pet dogs; GDV, gastric dilation-volvulus.

detection dogs may be at higher risk of being shot by hunters, whereas urban detection dogs may be at risk of being shot by criminals or police. In one study, the type of firearm did not influence outcome in gunshot wounds in pet animals [4]. Impalement injury can occur in any of the police or detection environments. Although no published reports describe impalement injuries in working dogs, anecdotal reports of injuries in both urban and rural settings exist.

Service dogs are unlikely to have a high risk of ballistic trauma or impalement, but guide dogs may be at risk of dog bites due to the inability of the handler to anticipate an attack. Police and other detection dogs are at risk of bite wounds when working off leash in environments where there are stray or wild animals. In addition, in training situations when the dogs are highly stimulated, fights could break out. Blunt trauma is a risk for working dogs, but it is unknown if the risk is higher than for pet dogs.

In general, working dogs will be under better control than pet dogs, but when they are on task (in pursuit or following an odor), they may not be environmentally aware, thus increasing the risk of being hit by a vehicle or falling from a height. Police dogs traveling in a vehicle involved in a high-speed chase are also at risk of injury if the vehicle crashes. Service dogs are expected to be at lower risk of vehicular trauma but may be at risk of being hit by a falling object if the handler is unable to anticipate or protect the dog from the incident.

One of the greatest concerns for police and detection dogs that work in adverse environments is heat stroke; in fact, it is one of the most common preventable causes of early retirement in MWD [4] (see Chapter147) Several news reports cite heat stroke deaths in police dogs in patrol cars where cooling systems failed. One case report detailed the prehospital resuscitation and successful outcome in such a case [5]. Heat stroke in working dogs cannot be defined by rectal temperature alone since many dogs will work with core body temperatures in excess of 106 °F (personal observation). Even if dogs do not succumb to heat injury, work in the heat can lead to dehydration and other complications as observed with search and rescue dogs [6–8]. Service dogs are expected to be at low risk of heat injury. Cold injury is uncommon in adult working dogs unless the dog is immobilized from injury and exposed to cold environments (e.g. open helicopter transport of MWD) (see Chapter 148). Swimming in cold water or cold exposure, however, can be associated with an acutely limp tail [9]. This condition, often called limber tail or swimmer's tail, can be acutely painful, requiring pain control.

Inhaled, ingested or topical toxin exposure is a risk for all working dogs (see Chapter 127). Drug and explosives detection dogs are at risk of exposure through inhaling or ingesting their training aids or the source they are seeking [10–14]. Current street narcotics may contain the potent opioids fentanyl or carfentanyl. If a dog inhales sufficient quantities of these drugs, they will show signs of intoxication which should be treated with naloxone. The dog will likely have the opioid on its fur and serve as a fomite. Handlers and individuals working with the exposed canine must be aware of the risk of opioid exposure to themselves from contact with the dog. Service dogs travel everywhere with their handlers and could ingest unrecognized toxins or medications that have fallen to the ground.

Infectious disease risk depends on the environment in which the dog is working. For wilderness (wide area) detection dogs, diseases spread by ticks or wild animals are a concern. For large-scale missions, congregating dogs can spread infectious disease such as kennel cough complex. If dogs travel, they can be exposed to endemic disease (e.g. heartworm or fungal disease in response to Hurricane Katrina).

The breeds that are commonly used as working and service dogs have a high incidence of cancer and may present acutely with the consequences, such as hemoabdomen or pericardial effusion (see Chapters 54 and 84). There is no evidence that environmental exposure during the 9/11 response increased the risk of cancer in search dogs [15]. Cancer is the cause of death in approximately 30% of service dogs and 40% of search and rescue dogs [15].

Common Systems Affected

There are no reports of cardiopulmonary risks associated with working occupations. Even dogs responding to 9/11 did not develop respiratory complications from their exposure [15].

In a study of police dogs in an urban emergency room, the most common reason for presentation was gastrointestinal disorders. Vomiting and diarrhea were more common than gastric dilation-volvulus (GDV), and more frequent in police dogs than in pet GSDs (Table 202.2) [16] (see Chapters 13 and 82) The second most frequent reason for emergency care was musculoskeletal injuries; again, lameness was more common in police dogs than in pet GSDs. Arthritis and orthopedic conditions are common in service dogs and may lead to their retirement. Non-combat injuries and illness in MWD were similar to those reported in police dogs, but more dermatological disease and soft tissue trauma, which included footpad injuries, were seen [17]. In SAR dogs, cuts and scrapes are frequent occurrences, and although most are minor, some may require emergency management (see Chapter 166) [6–8]. Many of the breeds used for working/service careers are at risk for allergies and skin disease. An acute ear infection in a working dog can impair their ability to work and will often require urgent care.

Spinal cord disease is the most common cause of retirement in MWD older than 5 years of age (see Chapters 24–26) [4]. Although some of these conditions can be chronic in nature (i.e. lumbosacral disease, degenerative myelopathy), acute disk rupture or fibrocartilaginous

Table 202.2 Primary problems of German Shepherd emergency hospital visits comparing police GSDs and pet (control) GSDs 7/2008–7/2010. Reproduced with permission of John Wiley & Sons, Ltd.

	Police GSD ES visits*		Pet (control) GSD ES visits*		P-values	Total ES visits[†]	
Cardiovascular	0	0.%	12	8.%	0.001	12	4.%
Dental	2	1.%	0	0.%	0.478	2	0.%
Dermatology	14	10.%	8	5.%	0.266	22	8.%
Gastrointestinal	39	28.3%	31	22.5%	0.333	70	25.4%
Vomiting/diarrhea	33	23.9%	17	12.3%	0.019	50	18.1%
GDV/bloat	2	1.4%	7	5.1%	0.175	9	3.3%
Other	4	2.9%	7	5.1%	0.538	11	4.0%
Neoplastic condition	5	3.6%	17	12.3%	0.014	22	8.0%
Nervous system	1	0.7%	12	8.7%	0.004	13	4.7%
Ophthalmology	2	1.4%	4	2.9%	0.680	6	2.2%
Orthopedic	35	25.4%	17	12.3%	0.009	52	18.8%
Appendicular	27	19.6%	5	3.6%	<0.001	32	11.6%
Axial	8	5.8%	12	8.7%	0.486	20	7.2%
Other	5	3.6%	4	2.9%	–	9	3.3%
Postoperative complications	2	1.4%	3	2.2%	–	5	1.8%
Respiratory	5	3.6%	6	4.3%	–	11	4.0%
Toxin exposure/ingestion	3	2.2%	6	4.3%	0.498	9	3.3%
Trauma/wound	21	15.2%	12	8.7%	0.138	33	12.0%
Urogenital	4	2.9%	6	4.3%	0.747	10	3.6%

*Total visits 138.
[†]Total visits 276.
GDV, gastric dilation-volvulus; GSD, German Shepherd; ES, emergency service.

infarcts will typically present as an acute emergency. Pet GSDs were seen for back conditions at an equal frequency as police GSDs [16] so these conditions may not be occupational hazards as much as breed risk.

Reproductive emergencies are uncommon in working dogs. Most police and MWD are sexually intact males, whereas most service dogs and SAR dogs have been spayed or castrated. Urinary tract problems were reported at an incidence rate of 1.3/1000 dog search hours during the 9/11 response [6]. Some of the urinary tract signs may have been complicated by dehydration.

Tooth fractures, especially those involving the canine teeth, in police/patrol warrant emergency care to attempt to preserve the integrity of the tooth. One study documented that 88% of teeth remained vital if treated within 48 hours of pulp exposure although this study did not specify if working dogs had a different outcome from pet dogs [18]. Other working dogs that are rewarded by tugging or have a tendency to chew on tennis balls or bones can suffer tooth damage that could predispose them to tooth fractures.

Eye injuries were not commonly reported in the SAR dogs that responded to the 9/11 terrorist attacks [6] or the earthquake in Haiti [7] (see Chapter 12). This is in contrast to reports of ocular infection and an eye injury in SAR dogs and an explosive detection dog respectively, during the response to the Oklahoma City bombing [19]. Routine saline flushing of the eyes is a common practice since the Oklahoma City experience and may be responsible for a decrease in ocular infections/irritations. Any eye injury in a working dog must be treated aggressively due to the potential career-ending impact of vision loss. Genetic eye disease is common in working dog breeds and can lead to progressive blindness.

Client Education

Educating handlers on the impact that any procedures or medications may have on the dogs' working performance is an important part of client communication. Another important aspect of handler education is providing them with the skills for basic first aid assessment of their dog. Emergency clinicians are uniquely positioned to help educate working dog handlers.

References

1 US Department of Justice. Americans with Disabilities Act. Frequently Asked Questions about Service Animals and the ADA. Available at: www.ada.gov/regs2010/service_animal_qa.html (accessed 20 February 2018).

2 Baker JL, Havas KA, Miller LA, Lacy WA, Schlanser J. Gunshot wounds in military working dogs in Operation Enduring Freedom and Operation Iraqi Freedom: 29 cases (2003–2009). *J Vet Emerg Crit Care* 2013;23(1):47–52.

3 Olsen LE, Streeter EM, DeCook RR. Review of gunshot injuries in cats and dogs and utility of a triage scoring system to predict short-term outcome: 37 cases (2003–2008). *J Am Vet Med Assoc* 2014;245(8):923–929.

4 Evans RI, Herbold JR, Bradshaw BS, Moore GE. Causes for discharge of military working dogs from service: 268 cases (2000–2004). *J Am Vet Med Assoc* 2007;231(8):1215–1220.

5 Le Clair T. Hot dogs: not just backyard fun: a K-9 heat injury case study. *J Spec Ops Med* 2011;11(3):66–68.

6 Slensky K, Drobatz K, Downend A, Otto C. Deployment morbidity among search and rescue dogs from 9/11. *J Am Vet Med Assoc* 2004;225(6):868–873.

7 Gordon LE. Injuries and illnesses among urban search-and-rescue dogs deployed to Haiti following the January 12, 2010, earthquake. *J Am Vet Med Assoc* 2012;240(4):396–403.

8 Gordon LE. Injuries and illnesses among Federal Emergency Management Agency-certified search-and-recovery and search-and-rescue dogs deployed to Oso, Washington, following the March 22, 2014, State Route 530 landslide. *J Am Vet Med Assoc* 2015;247(8):901–908.

9 Steiss J, Braund K, Wright J, et al. Coccygeal muscle injury in English Pointers (limber tail). *J Vet Intern Med* 1999;13(6):540–548.

10 Gwaltney-Brant SM, Murphy LA, Wismer TA, Albretsen JC. General toxicologic hazards and risks for search-and-rescue dogs responding to urban disasters. *J Am Vet Med Assoc* 2003;222(3):292–295.

11 Wismer TA, Murphy LA, Gwaltney-Brant SM, Albretsen JC. Management and prevention of toxicoses in search-and-rescue dogs responding to urban disasters. *J Am Vet Med Assoc* 2003;222(3):305–310.

12 Murphy LA, Gwaltney-Brant SM, Albretsen JC, Wismer TA. Toxicologic agents of concern for search-and-rescue dogs responding to urban disasters. *J Am Vet Med Assoc* 2003;222(3):296–304.

13 Llera RM, Volmer P.A. Toxicologic hazards for police dogs involved in drug detection. *J Am Vet Med Assoc* 2006;228(7):1028–1032.

14 Fishkin RA, Stanley SW, Langston CE. Toxic effects of cyclonite (C-4) plastic explosive ingestion in a dog. *J Vet Emerg Crit Care* 2008;18(5):537–540.

15 Otto C, Downend A, Moore G, et al. Medical surveillance of search dogs deployed to the World Trade Center and Pentagon: 2001–2006. *J Environ Health* 2010;73(2):12–21.

16 Parr JR, Otto CM. Emergency visits and occupational hazards in German shepherd police dogs (2008–2010). *J Vet Emerg Crit Care* 2013;23(6):591–597.

17 Takara MS, Harrell K. Noncombat-related injuries or illnesses incurred by military working dogs in a combat zone. *J Am Vet Med Assoc* 2014;245(10):1124–1128.

18 Clarke DE. Vital pulp therapy for complicated crown fracture of permanent canine teeth in dogs: a three-year retrospective study. *J Vet Dent* 2001;18(3):117–121.

19 Duhaime RA, Norden D, Corso B, Mallonee S, Salman MD. Injuries and illnesses in working dogs used during the disaster response after the bombing in Oklahoma City. *J Am Vet Med Assoc* 1998;212(8):1202–1207.

203

Approach to Unowned and Shelter/Rescue Animals in the Emergency Room
April Paul, DVM, DACVECC

Tufts VETS, Walpole, MA, USA

Introduction

Animals may be presented to the ER by non-owners/agents under various circumstances. Each ER should develop its own policy for each case, based upon local laws and hospital administration. Policies may vary depending upon location as well as prior agreements, local resources, and goals of the hospital management. It is exceedingly useful to have developed a relationship with local shelters and animal law enforcement. Find out if they have veterinarians on staff as this will help to guide your treatment plan. If they have veterinarians, they can possibly provide continued care after emergency stabilization and may be able to provide future surgical intervention, follow-up, and medications. If they don't have a veterinarian on staff, they probably use a veterinary clinic(s) that can help to care for the animals; these hospitals can be a resource as well.

Boarding kennels or pet sitters may present animals without knowledge of the owners' wishes or a method to contact the true owner. In these cases, it can be challenging to know the appropriate step; for minor illness or injuries, treatment is typically provided, and when the owner is reached, arrangements can be made for follow-up or payment. Some boarding kennels and pet sitters will arrange for payment as well. Professional kennels are more likely to have a contact for the owner, but in some cases the contact also does not know the owner's wishes, particularly if a catastrophic illness (e.g. GDV, IVDD, hemoabdomen) has developed. There is generally no easy answer in these cases; if the family veterinarian is reachable, then they often have knowledge of the individual's general approach to pet care. In other cases, while ongoing efforts to reach the owners should be made, it may be that the emergency clinician, in consultation with hospital administration and any potential agents, may need to make decisions, if life-saving treatment is required.

Animal control officers (ACO) may present animals that they have recently found or, less likely, that have been in custody either during a hold period or while waiting for a criminal trial. Most towns have a small amount of resources in their budget to support the care of unowned injured animals or those animals in their custody. However, it is essential that a clear understanding of the goals and expense of treatment is reached before proceeding with more severe injuries. Recently, in Connecticut, a Great Dane on "death row" for killing another dog, which had been in custody for almost a year, developed and was surgically treated for a colonic torsion while awaiting a final verdict for euthanasia at the expense of the town [1]. ACOs represent useful resources for the emergency clinician and good relationships should be fostered.

Animals may be presented for urgent care after potential cruelty cases; in these cases, in addition to providing care for the patient, it is essential to determine what type of forensic information will be required if the case is ultimately prosecuted. Cruelty cases brought in by ACOs generally require full work-ups for legality purposes. Remember to gather evidence – the presenting officer may have done this, but make sure evidence is obtained prior to changing the appearance of animal (such as shaving matted fur, bathing, etc.). Photographs and video may be needed to document the way an animal looks – remember that the animal should be considered as evidence. Also, you may need to collect evidence such as the fur and anything on the animals to save for use later. Every detail that you find on physical examination should be recorded in the medical record. Remember that the medical record could end up in court, so everything said should be straightforward without personal opinions.

Things that are especially important to keep in mind for your exam include the animal's demeanor, body condition score, and pain score. Make sure you obtain a weight and a TPR. Note any external parasites,

Textbook of Small Animal Emergency Medicine, First Edition. Edited by Kenneth J. Drobatz, Kate Hopper, Elizabeth Rozanski and Deborah C. Silverstein.
© 2019 John Wiley & Sons, Inc. Published 2019 by John Wiley & Sons, Inc.
Companion Website: www.wiley.com/go/drobatz/textbook

scars, wounds or injuries which should be described in detail. Give as much information as you can in the objective section of your record. Write reports in plain language without medical terminology so that records in court are understandable by the judge and jury. Starting with the subjective section, keep this as short as possible since this may be contested in court. Make sure the objective section is thorough and everything is well documented. The assessment section should include every problem and also every possible differential without any personal bias to the situation. In potential starvation cases, it is important to note the animal's reaction to food. An animal that is sick and not starved may not want to eat. An animal that is starved typically is ravenous. This should be noted in your exam notes.

Tests for cruelty cases will be tailored towards what the cruelty charge is about. Animals suspected to have been abused or used in dog fighting likely will need radiographs to document new or old fractures. Animals suspected to be starved will likely need laboratory testing, fecals, and imaging to rule out other underlying causes of malnutrition. Animals that are brought in for cruelty should be treated like any other animal and their response to treatment should be well documented. These animals will likely be kept in custody, potentially for long periods of time. In cases of starvation, it is very important to remember about refeeding syndrome. Refeed them very slowly and monitor their electrolytes. It is difficult for most people to work with these animals and not feed them, but it could be detrimental, so sticking to a strict feeding regimen should be encouraged. Resources are available to veterinarians to help address these cases [2]. In some states (e.g. Massachusetts), veterinarians are considered mandatory reporters of possible abuse cases, and the policy of hospitals should support this.

Animals may also be presented by Good Samaritans, who have found a stray or injured animal. Uninjured animals may be directed to a local shelter, but injured animals should be cared for, with consultation with local ACOs and in support of hospital policies. A microchip scanner should be available and used in any unowned animals to attempt to locate owners. Animals with unclear vaccine history should be vaccinated against rabies and species-specific infectious disease on admit.

Breed-specific or general rescue groups may present animals for care. These cases are usually more straightforward as most groups have an individual in charge of payment and deciding about treatment. These groups are also a vital resource for unowned animals matching specific descriptions (e.g. boxer rescue) or for helping owners of pets belonging to specific breeds. In some cases, rescue groups may require counseling as to the predicted outcome and benefit for specific treatments, and each dollar spent is then a dollar that is subsequently unavailable for another patient. Common presenting conditions in rescue include infectious diseases, neglect, and trauma. It is wise to recall that nationwide efforts to rehome dogs and to a lesser extent cats have results in the potential appearance of dogs with infectious but non-endemic or common local disease (e.g. histoplasmosis in a puppy from Louisiana that was rehomed in Maine).

Common infectious diseases in felines include panleukopenia, upper respiratory disease, and retroviral infections. Common infectious diseases in canines include parvovirus, kennel cough or canine infectious respiratory disease, and distemper. Ringworm is another common infectious disease found in shelter animals and should be on your differential list for skin lesions. It is important to remember that animals with suspected infectious diseases should be treated in isolation to prevent further disease spread to other patients and also to protect them from other diseases to which they may be more susceptible. Proper disinfection protocols should be performed to prevent disease spread in the ER. Specific infectious disease management is covered elsewhere in this text.

Spay/neuter complications may present in shelter animals or in animals that were spayed/neutered at high-volume clinics. It is best to not always assume the worst case scenario, as spay-neuter clinics have exceedingly low rates of significant complications. Many times, the complications will be simple, like seromas. Keep in mind that not every animal that comes in with a swelling associated with their surgery site needs an ultrasound. Often, palpating the linea will allow better assessment of the swelling. Usually, once a linea dehiscence occurs, the whole suture line does, so it should be easy to tell if there is a defect. If you are unsure, it is easy enough to aspirate the swelling to determine if it is a seroma. Most spay/neuter complications can be dealt with by the initial veterinarian unless there is obvious dehiscence. Antibiotics and an e-collar are a quick and easy fix until follow-up can occur. It is useful, as with all veterinary hospitals that refer to your emergency service, to have contact numbers of owners/administrators in case of a dramatic out-of-hours complication.

Remember to think of shelters as your clients. Involve them in your decision-making process. Try to think of what is most humane for the animal. A shelter may not want to fix or treat an animal that is aggressive and has little chance of being adopted. It is helpful for you to provide information on behavior to the shelter so that can help in their decision on how to proceed with treatment. You would not want to put an animal through unnecessary tests, treatment, surgery, etc. if it is only going to go to the shelter and be euthanized. Sometimes it is also important for shelters to euthanize very sick animals for the greater good, to help save other animals if they can get a diagnosis from necropsy. This also pertains to finances, as spending thousands of dollars on one animal leaves less money for others.

References

1 http://bristolobserver.com/2016/12/28/dog-lingering-on-citys-animal-death-row-getting-surgery-on-citys-dime/ (accessed 20 February 2018).

2 www.vetinvestigator.com/ (accessed 20 February 2018).

204

Euthanasia Considerations
Katherine J. Goldberg, DVM, LMSW

Whole Animal Veterinary Geriatrics & Hospice Services, Ithaca, NY, USA

Introduction

Emergency medicine encompasses much hope and promise, but also stress and disappointment for both clients and clinicians. Their focus on serious illness and injury means that emergency veterinarians will deal with a significant amount of death – occurring from progression of disease or injury, as well as euthanasia. Precise mortality and euthanasia rates in veterinary emergency facilities are unknown, but it has been estimated that veterinarians experience death five times more than human physicians [1]. Assuming overall higher rates of death per shift in emergency compared with general practice, the emergency veterinarian is involved in some of the highest rates of death in veterinary medicine.

The impact of euthanasia on veterinarians is considerable [2–7]. While frequent euthanasia and end-of-life discussions can be some of the most challenging aspects of emergency medicine, multiple opportunities exist to minimize emotional distress, maximize goal-concordant care, and ensure sufficient thoughtfulness in euthanasia considerations. This chapter aims to help clinicians understand and navigate several unique aspects of euthanasia in the veterinary emergency setting, expose clinicians to some newer concepts related to veterinary end-of-life care, and improve clinician comfort and competency in these important areas.

Emotional Aspects of Euthanasia in the Emergency Setting

Rapport

Euthanasia in the emergency setting may be particularly stressful since veterinarians typically do not have long-term relationships with their patients and clients. Developing rapport with clients quickly is an essential skill of the emergency clinician. This becomes especially important for end-of-life discussions. Asking the client to share non-medical information about the pet can be a means of establishing rapport quickly. For example, "*Can you tell me what Molly's favorite thing to do was when she was healthy?*" This often helps clients relax by recalling positive memories, and also assures them that you care about their pet as an individual. Simple statements such as "*I know this is hard/painful/scary/unexpected. I am here to support you through it*" are extremely effective in achieving partnership with clients and setting the stage for shared decision making.

Goals of Care Discussions in the Emergency Setting

Research in human medicine regarding end-of-life preferences consistently demonstrates positive outcomes from early goals of care (GOC) discussions [8–11]. This is an area for further exploration within veterinary medicine. The Serious Illness Conversation Guide [10] has recently been modified for veterinary use [12] (Figure 204.1). A full discussion of GOC conversations is beyond the scope of this chapter but the guide provides a basic framework that may be used in the emergency setting to facilitate serious illness and end-of-life conversations for veterinary patients. Understanding the nuances of client beliefs and preferences enables clinicians to provide goal-concordant care.

Beliefs Regarding Aid in Dying

It is essential that emergency clinicians understand their clients' beliefs regarding euthanasia. It is often assumed by veterinary professionals that euthanasia is acceptable to clients but this is not universally the case. Acceptance or opposition is also rarely absolute. Stated opposition to euthanasia generally falls into three categories:

- a fundamental philosophic or religious opposition
- an emotional tie that requires exploration, i.e. fear from previous experience, misunderstanding regarding

Textbook of Small Animal Emergency Medicine, First Edition. Edited by Kenneth J. Drobatz, Kate Hopper, Elizabeth Rozanski and Deborah C. Silverstein.
© 2019 John Wiley & Sons, Inc. Published 2019 by John Wiley & Sons, Inc.
Companion Website: www.wiley.com/go/drobatz/textbook

Serious Veterinary Illness Conversation Guide

CLINICIAN STEPS

☐ **Set up**
- Thinking in advance
- Is this okay?
- Hope for best, prepare for worst
- Benefit for patient/family
- No decisions necessary today

☐ **Guide** (right column)

☐ **Act**
- Affirm commitment
- Make recommendations about next steps
  - Acknowledge medical realities
  - Summarize key goals/priorities
  - Describe treatment options that reflect both
- Document conversation

Katherine Goldberg, DVM
Whole Animal Veterinary Geriatrics & Hospice Services

© 2015 Ariadne Labs: A Joint Center for Health Systems Innovation (www.ariadnelabs.org) and Dana-Farber Cancer Institute

CONVERSATION GUIDE

Understanding

What is your understanding now of where _____ is with his/her illness?
What questions do you have about information your family veterinarian has already shared with you?

Information Preferences

How much information about _____'s illness would you like from me? How much additional information do you feel you need to help make decisions?

FOR EXAMPLE:
Some families like to have lots of information about what to expect, others do not. Some people are very comforted by lots of diagnostic information and some people find this stressful.

Prognosis

Share prognosis as a range, tailored to information preferences. Understand that euthanasia as end point for most patients has tremendous impact on "prognosis". What is acceptable for one family may not be for another.

Goals

If _____'s situation worsens, what are your most important goals?

Fears / Worries

What are your biggest fears and worries about _____'s health?

Function

What abilities or activities are so critical to _____'s life that you can't imagine him/her living without them?

Trade-offs

If _____ becomes sicker, how much are you willing to go through for the possibility of gaining more time together?

Aid in Dying

What are your beliefs surrounding euthanasia?

Figure 204.1 Serious Veterinary Illness Care Conversation Guide. Reproduced with permission of Ariadne Labs (https://portal.ariadnelabs.org).

procedure, particular connection to the pet that makes purposeful ending of life feel unacceptable

- a *preference* for unaided death but euthanasia may be acceptable under certain circumstances. It is important for the clinician to determine what those circumstances are.

Some of the most common end-of-life communication challenges can be avoided by *asking* clients what their feelings are regarding euthanasia. This is ideally done by the veterinarian, but may also be done by nursing staff or even incorporated into emergency room (ER) paperwork just like code status for CPR orders. Wording on paperwork such as *"Difficult Discussions: Understanding Your Preferences"* can help frame this solicitation of information positively, reiterating that the ER team values shared decision making.

Palliative sedation is a topic of much discussion within human medicine and is deserving of attention within the veterinary profession [13–18]. Palliative sedation can be very useful in situations where clients are resistant to euthanasia, yet the patient cannot be kept comfortable while still conscious. Most emergency veterinarians are quite competent in anesthesia and analgesia for their patients; drawing upon this knowledge with the goal of alleviating suffering via continuous sedation can be a useful tool in some of the most challenging end-of-life situations.

Technical Aspects of Euthanasia in the Emergency Setting

Procedural Considerations: Pharmacology and Technique

Most emergency patients will already have established venous access via intravenous catheter(s). Therefore, the technical aspects of euthanasia in the emergency setting are usually straightforward. Whether or not to administer pre-euthanasia sedation or injectable anesthesia (i.e. propofol) must be determined on a case-by-case basis. Level of stress and alertness of the patient, and any particular emotional needs of the client should be considered. Benefits of pre-euthanasia medication include achieving stage 3 of anesthesia prior to administration of euthanasia solution, which can be helpful for client-witnessed euthanasia. Clients may have close physical contact with sedated or anesthetized patients, which can be meaningful for some families, especially if they have not been able to touch their pet since the onset of illness or injury. Sedation also provides relief from suffering such as air hunger, pain, and seizure activity while clients cope with the imminent loss of their pet and say goodbye.

It is essential that clients are not rushed into euthanasia to relieve clinical signs; euthanasia is an irreversible solution to patient suffering. Adequate analgesia and symptom management must be provided while euthanasia decision making is taking place. In the most severe cases, intubation and injectable anesthesia may be provided when patients require immediate relief but clients are not yet ready to euthanize. This may be considered a brief form of palliative sedation, and can be a useful tool for all involved.

In situations where intravenous access has not been established, or cannot be established due to peripheral edema, seizure activity, limited personnel, or other challenges, several options remain. Clinicians should be familiar with alternative routes to intravenous euthanasia, and corresponding drug dosage adjustments (Table 204.1). In particular, intrarenal euthanasia is a useful technique in anesthetized cats and has been shown to be similar in effect to intravenous euthanasia [19].

Procedural Considerations: Treatment Area and Patient Preparation

While treatment and intensive care areas are familiar to veterinarians and their teams, clients may be significantly affected by the experience of being in these surroundings with a sick or injured pet. Remembering that the various sights, smells, sounds, and general atmosphere can be traumatic to clients is important for providing compassionate care. A growing body of research in human medicine describes the mental health impact of intensive care on patients' family members [20–23]. It is likely that families of veterinary patients are at similar risk, and this is an area for future investigation in veterinary critical care. A keen awareness of treatment area conditions while clients are present is essential; this includes the physical cleanliness of the area, condition of patients, as well as professional behavior and language of veterinarians and staff. Many veterinary hospitals have systems in place to inform staff that clients are present, such as flags or blinking lights.

Ideally, euthanasia would occur in a designated location, away from a busy treatment area or intensive care unit (ICU); however, this is not always possible. When euthanasia must occur in a treatment area or ICU, several simple steps may be taken to improve the client (and staff) experience. Remove all equipment with noisy or visible displays; they are not necessary during euthanasia, can be distracting to clients, and intensify the "medical" nature of the dying experience. Intubated patients would ideally be extubated immediately prior to euthanasia, after discussion with the clients

Table 204.1 Euthanasia methods: injectable euthanasia solutions

Route	Pros	Cons	Dose
Intravenous (IV)	Rapid death, 30 sec Reliable	Locating vein Quality of vein Extravasation Seizuring pet	1 mL/10 lb
Intracardiac (IC)	Seizuring pet No venous access	Requires anesthesia, injectable or inhalant Technical skill Client response	1 ml/10 lb + 2–5 mL
Intraperitoneal (IP)	Easy No sedation required for pure barbiturate solution Slower death may be preferred by clients	Prolonged time to death, 15–25 min possible (but usually 8–10) Verify death closely	3 mL/10 lb
Intrahepatic	Easy Improved uptake over IP Respiratory arrest rapid Rapid death, 2 min	Requires anesthesia, injectable or inhalant Death may be prolonged if extrahepatic injection	2 mL/10 lb
Intrarenal	Easier than IV in volume-depleted cats Rapid death, 30–60 sec	Requires anesthesia, injectable or inhalant Technical skill	3–6 mL/cat
Oral	Aggressive animals Safe, limited human contact	Unreliable Unpalatable Verify death closely	3 mL/10 lb PO (solution) 1 tsp/40 lb PO (powder)

Adapted from Cooney et al. [53] and Cooney [54].
PO, by mouth (*per os*).

regarding what will happen next. For example, "*We are going to get Molly ready for you and then we'll bring you back in to say goodbye.*" Preparation of the patient for euthanasia can often occur while consent forms and aftercare paperwork are being taken care of, depending on the practice's particular procedures. Extubation will require continued sedation if the patient is oxygen dependent, to prevent air hunger. However, most clients would prefer to have the last image of their pet without a tube. Removing any barriers to physical contact is especially important around the head and face of the patient, where clients are likely to be gathering for euthanasia. Clients may appreciate being able to hold smaller patients during euthanasia. Informing clients of the possibility of involuntary eliminations, and draping blankets with waterproof backing on the client's lap is a good idea in this situation in case they occur, although many clients who wish to hold their pets do not mind getting soiled.

Patient preparation for client-witnessed euthanasia includes cleaning up any major visible wounds, body fluids, or soiled linens whether the patient has been hospitalized for weeks or hours. Disconnecting the patient from all machines, capping the intravenous catheter, rewrapping it with clean materials if necessary, and draping a large clean blanket (in good condition, no holes or stains) over the body, leaving the head and neck exposed, is a respectful demonstration of care and compassion for the patient and will positively affect the client experience.

During the euthanasia procedure, the team can facilitate focus on the patient and minimize surrounding distractions by bringing the family to the patient's head and making sure they can sit down if they want to. Providing tissues and a clean trash bin is important. Asking if clients have been present for euthanasia before, explaining the procedure and physiological responses to death, and answering any questions that the clients may have are essential. This step may have been completed prior to gathering around the patient. If so, it is important to reiterate the key steps of the procedure and obtain clear verbal consent indicating that the clients are ready to proceed prior to administering drugs.

It is also important to confirm death after listening to the patient with a stethoscope, using clear language that cannot be misinterpreted. Although in the vast majority of cases, saying *"S/he's gone"* is sufficient, there have been situations where clients do not understand that their pet is dead. Discretion as to whether to reiterate *"S/he has died"* may be left up to the individual veterinarian; however, it may be necessary, especially with very distraught clients.

Procedural Considerations: Client Visiting with Deceased Patients

Clients will often visit with deceased patients, even if they do not choose to be present for euthanasia. Families with small children may elect to have only adults present for euthanasia, but wish to have children view the deceased pet so that they know s/he has died. Clients may also come into the hospital after they have been notified via phone that their pet has died. These visits should be prepared for with care, as if they are a client-witnessed euthanasia. Most often, deceased patients can be moved out of the treatment area for visiting; this is strongly recommended even if clients are only visiting briefly. No matter where the visit takes place, it is important that no evidence of aftercare preparation is in view, such as garbage bags, cremation paperwork, body tags. While some of these things may appear to be of minimal significance, it is important to remember that the manner in which veterinarians handle patient death has the potential to alleviate or aggravate client grief. Research shows that veterinarians have significant influence on client coping with pet loss [4,24–26].

Current Concepts in Veterinary End-of-Life Care

Veterinary–Social Work Partnerships

Veterinary social work is an emerging field with innumerable benefits for patients, clients, and veterinary professionals [27–30]. The human needs that arise in relationships with animals, particularly in end-of-life situations, are tremendous. Veterinary hospitals are encouraged to partner with social workers who are experienced in grief and bereavement, and who embrace a strengths-based approach to human–animal interactions. Emergency practices in particular stand to benefit from social work support, given their highly stressful and emotionally charged environments.

Veterinary Hospice and Palliative Care

In parallel with a rising interest in end-of-life care for people, increased attention is currently being given to death and dying within veterinary medicine [31–33]. Interest in hospice and palliative care (HPC) for companion animals is on the rise [34–48], and emergency veterinarians in particular are likely to benefit from referral relationships with HPC providers. These relationships enable smooth transitions to home care, expanding the available options for emergency and critical care cases. Building networks of these providers is invaluable for cases that may require support beyond what is typical for a particular veterinary hospital.

Client Request for Home Death

Much attention has been given to preferred place of death (PPD) in human medicine [49–52]. While similar research in veterinary medicine is lacking, it is possible that client preferences regarding place of death may carry over into preferences for their companion animals. Emergency veterinarians should be aware that clients might not want their pets to die in the hospital, even if death is imminent. Clients may wish to spend final hours or days with their pet in a familiar setting where they can receive the support of friends and family, and express their grief more openly. Referral relationships with mobile practitioners are useful in cases where home is the PPD. Incorporating place of death preferences into end-of-life conversations is good standard practice for emergency veterinarians. Euthanasia is rarely an emergency procedure; relief of suffering is what must be done urgently. Clients should be able to choose the time, manner, and place of their pet's death.

Conclusion

Life and death decisions are frequently made in the ER. Severe presenting signs, uncertain outcomes, emotional and financial stress, and legal availability of euthanasia for animals all contribute to the reality of euthanasia as a procedure commonly performed by emergency veterinarians. Fortunately, several steps can be taken to minimize the negative impact that euthanasia may have on clients and the entire veterinary team. Engaging in goals of care conversations, prioritizing emotional support for clients, self-care for veterinarians, and relief of suffering for patients are important practices that will enable euthanasia to be performed well, and placed in an appropriate context within emergency medicine.

References

1 Hart LA, Hart BL. Grief and stress from so many animal deaths. *Compan Anim Pract* 1987;1:20–21.

2 Schneider BJ. Euthanasia and the veterinarian. *Can Vet J* 1996;37(4):217–218.

3 Rollin BE. Euthanasia, moral stress, and chronic illness in veterinary medicine. *Vet Clin North Am Small Anim Pract* 2011;41(3):651–659.

4 Morris P. Managing pet owners' guilt and grief in veterinary euthanasia encounters. *J Contemp Ethnogr* 2012;41(3):337–365.

5 Hart LA, Hart BL, Mader B. Humane euthanasia and companion animal death: caring for the animal, the client, and the veterinarian. *J Am Vet Med Assoc* 1990;197(10):1292–1299.

6 Fogle B, Abrahamson D. Pet loss: a survey of the attitudes and feelings of practicing veterinarians. *Anthrozoos* 1990;3(3):143–150.

7 Tran L, Crane MF, Phillips JK. The distinct role of performing euthanasia on depression and suicide in veterinarians. *J Occup Health Psychol* 2014;19(2): 123–132.

8 Bernacki RE, Block SD, American College of Physicians High Value Care Task Force. Communication about serious illness care goals: a review and synthesis of best practices. *JAMA Intern Med.* 2014;174(12):1994–2003.

9 You JJ, Downar J, Fowler RA, et al. Barriers to goals of care discussions with seriously ill hospitalized patients and their families. *JAMA Intern Med* 2015;175(4):549.

10 Bernacki RE, Block SD. Serious illness communications checklist. *Virtual Mentor* 2013;15(12):1045–1049.

11 Bernacki RE, Block SD. Communication about serious illness care goals. *JAMA Intern Med.* 2014;174(12):1994.

12 Goldberg K. Serious Veterinary Illness Conversation Guide. Adapted from Serious Illness Conversation Guide, Ariadne Labs, Dana-Farber Cancer Institute, 2015.

13 Quill TE, Lo B, Brock DW, Meisel A. Last-resort options for palliative sedation. *Ann Intern Med* 2009;151(6):421–424.

14 Claessens P, Menten J, Schotsmans P, Broeckaert B. Palliative sedation: a review of the research literature. *J Pain Symptom Manage* 2008;36(3):310–333.

15 Maltoni M, Scarpi E, Nanni O. Palliative sedation for intolerable suffering. *Curr Opin Oncol* 2014;26(4): 389–394.

16 Alonso-Babarro A, Varela-Cerdeira M, Torres-Vigil I, Rodríguez-Barrientos R, Bruera E. At-home palliative sedation for end-of-life cancer patients. *Palliat Med* 2010;24(5):486–492.

17 Materstvedt LJ, Bosshard G. Deep and continuous palliative sedation (terminal sedation): clinical-ethical and philosophical aspects. *Lancet Oncol* 2009;10(6):622–627.

18 Sinclair CT, Stephenson RC. Palliative sedation: assessment, management, and ethics. *Hosp Physician* 2006;42(3):33–38.

19 Cooney K, Coates J, Leach L, Hrenchir K. Intrarenal injection of pentobarbital sodium for euthanasia in cats: 131 cases (2010–2011). Presented at the AVMA Humane Endings Symposium, 2014.

20 Jones C, Skirrow P, Griffiths RD, et al. Post-traumatic stress disorder-related symptoms in relatives of patients following intensive care. *Intensive Care Med* 2004;30(3):456–460.

21 Azoulay E, Pochard F, Kentish-Barnes N, et al. Risk of post-traumatic stress symptoms in family members of intensive care unit patients. *Am J Respir Crit Care Med* 2005;171(9):987–994.

22 Lautrette A, Darmon M, Megarbane B, et al. A communication strategy and brochure for relatives of patients dying in the ICU. *N Engl J Med* 2007;356(5):469–478.

23 Kross EK, Engelberg R, Gries C. ICU care associated with symptoms of depression and posttraumatic stress disorder among family members of patients who die in the ICU. *Chest* 2011;139(4):795.

24 Fernandez-Mehler P, Gloor P, Sager E, Lewis FI, Glaus TM. Veterinarians' role for pet owners facing pet loss. *Vet Rec* 2013;172(21):555.

25 Adams CL, Bonnett BN, Meek AH. Predictors of owner response to companion animal death in 177 clients from 14 practices in Ontario. *J Am Vet Med Assoc* 2000;217(9):1303–1309.

26 Adams CL, Bonnett BN, Meek AH. Owner response to companion animal death: development of a theory and practical implications. *Can Vet J* 1999;40(1):33–39.

27 Cohen SP. The role of social work in a veterinary hospital setting. *Vet Clin North Am Small Anim Pract* 1985;15(2):355–363.

28 Larkin M. For human needs, some veterinary clinics are turning to a professional. *J Am Vet Med Assoc* 2015;248(1):8–12.

29 Moger S. Speaking of Loss: perspectives on hospice and professional grief counseling. *Am Anim Hosp Assoc Trends* 2015;November:28–33.

30 Strand E. Veterinary Social Work Program. University of Tennessee, Knoxville. Available at: http://www.vetsocialwork.utk.edu/ (accessed 20 February 2018).

31 Dickinson GE, Roof PD, Roof KW. A survey of veterinarians in the US: euthanasia and other end-of-life issues. *Anthrozoos* 2011;24(2):167–174.

32 Dickinson GE, Roof PD, Roof KW. End of life issues in United States veterinary medicine schools. *Soc Anim* 2010;18:152–162.

33 Dickinson GE, Paul ES. UK veterinary schools: emphasis on end-of-life issues. *Vet Rec* 2014;174.

34 Bishop GA, Long CC, Carlsten KS, Kennedy KC, Shaw JR. The Colorado State University Pet Hospice Program: end-of-life care for pets and their families. *J Vet Med Educ* 2008;35(4):525–531.

35 Richtel M. All dogs may go to heaven. These days, some go to hospice. New York Times, 2013. Available at: http://www.nytimes.com/2013/12/01/business/

all-dogs-may-go-to-heaven-these-days-some-go-to-hospice.html (accessed 20 February 2018).

36 Jarolim E. AAHA Trends: spreading the word on hospice care. *Am Anim Hosp Assoc Trends* 2014;May:39–42.

37 Shearer TS. Preface: the role of the veterinarian in hospice and palliative care. *Vet Clin North Am Small Anim Pract* 2011;41(3):3–5.

38 Jessup DA, Scott CA. Hospice in a zoologic medicine setting. *J Zoo Wildl Med* 2011;42(2):197–204.

39 Monti DJ. JAVMA News: Pawspice, an option for pets facing the end. *J Am Vet Med Assoc* 2000;217(7):969.

40 Rezendes A. JAVMA News: More veterinarians offering hospice. *J Am Vet Med Assoc* 2006;229(4):484–485.

41 Nolen RS. JAVMA News: Protecting pet hospice. *J Am Vet Med Assoc* 2007;231(12);1793–1794.

42 Bittel E. Hospice Care Symposium 2008: reflections. *J Am Holist Vet Med Assoc* 2008;28(2):25–28.

43 Osborne M. JAVMA News: Pet hospice gaining momentum. *J Am Vet Med Assoc* 2009;234(8):998–999.

44 Feldmann B. Letter to the editor: Comments on 'elements of, and factors important in, veterinary hospice'. *J Am Vet Med Assoc* 2011;238(5):563.

45 Johnson CL, Patterson-Kane E, Lamison A, Noyes HL. JAVMA Commentary: elements of, and factors important in, veterinary hospice. *J Am Vet Med Assoc* 2011;238(2):148–150.

46 Cooney K. Offering hospice care for pets. *Vet Rec* 2015;177(11):i–ii.

47 Goldberg K. Letter to the editor: In-home euthanasia versus hospice. *J Am Vet Med Assoc* 2015;246(4):401–402.

48 Kahler SC. JAVMA News: The end-all practice: home euthanasia. *J Am Vet Med Assoc* 2015;246(1):14–16.

49 Fields A, Finucane AM, Oxenham D. Discussing preferred place of death with patients: staff experiences in a UK specialist palliative care setting. *Int J Palliat Nurs* 2013;19(11):558–565.

50 Tolle SW. Oregon's low in-hospital death rates: what determines where people die and satisfaction with decisions on place of death? *Ann Intern Med* 1999;130(8):681.

51 Thomas C, Morris S, Clark D. Place of death: preferences among cancer patients and their carers. *Soc Sci Med* 2004;58(12):2431–2444.

52 Meeussen K, van den Block L, Bossuyt N, et al. GPs' awareness of patients' preference for place of death. *Br J Gen Pract* 2009;59(566):665–670.

53 Cooney KA, Chappell JR, Callan RJ, Connally BA. Veterinary Euthanasia Techniques: A Practical Guide. John Wiley and Sons, Chichester, 2012.

54 Cooney KA. In-home Pet Euthanasia Techniques: The Veterinarian's Guide to Helping Families and Their Pets Say Goodbye in the Comfort of Home. Kathleen Cooney, 2011. Available from Amazon.

205

Emergency Room Design and Staffing Models

Jan P. Kovacic, DVM, DACVECC

Horizon Veterinary Services, Appleton, WI, USA

Introduction

In human healthcare, "emergency care" is often defined as the diagnosis and treatment of acute injury and/or illness that pose an immediate risk to life or long-term health. Similarly, but at a lower severity of illness, "urgent care" is defined as the diagnosis and treatment of medical conditions that are serious or acute but pose no immediate threat to life and health but that require medical attention within 24 hours.

In veterinary medicine, the term "emergency" applies to both urgent and emergent conditions – those that a pet caretaker and a doctor agree require immediate attention no matter what the problem. This may involve medical, surgical, reproductive, or even non-medical issues. There is a general rule in veterinary emergency practice that if a client believes that their pet's problem is an emergency, it is until proven otherwise.

Designing a facility for emergency care extends to all phases of hospital planning – location, accessibility, hours of operation, facility, equipment, drugs, supplies, medical staff, and management. All veterinarians are confronted with an emergency at one time or another, independent of their workplace or type of practice – teaching hospital, referral center, emergency clinic, general practice, vaccine clinic, spay/neuter clinic, or even a mobile house-call practice. In addition, an emergency can occur anywhere at any time. Every space is a potential emergency room, including a client's car, a parking lot, or an outdoor exercise area. A practical design for providing excellent emergency care is a challenge that extends to all aspects of hospital design.

General Design Concepts

Goals

Emergency response depends on readiness. Doctors must be educated and current. Staff must be trained, capable of caring for multiple patients simultaneously, and able to shift into "high gear" when under pressure. The hospital's armamentarium of equipment, drugs, and supplies must be adequate to the task. The hospital design should reflect the organization and efficiency needed to respond rapidly and effectively in an emergency.

Ideally, an emergency hospital should be central to the population it serves. It should be very accessible (no more than one turn off a major highway) and easy to find. Signage should be highly visible, particularly at night. Emergency parking should be available close to an entrance that permits rapid transfer of a patient to an emergency room (ER) or response area. This area should be organized and maintained ready for an emergency at any time. Staff should be immediately available to respond to an emergency, including receptionists to process information and care co-ordinators who are ready to support anxious or grieving clients. Because emergencies also occur with in-hospital patients, this level of readiness should be established in multiple areas of the hospital. This includes, in addition to the primary ER, the ICU, surgery, procedures, radiology, or any room where anesthesia is performed or unstable patients are treated or housed.

Limitations

There is another general rule in emergency practice that you can't always have what you want, or even what you need. You can only have what you can afford. We must often compromise on our goal to provide the highest level of readiness due to limitations on our resources. There are communities too small to support a 24/7 emergency center, and general practitioners must fill that role in a general practice setting, often on call at night. There are always financial constraints that affect hospital design, equipment purchases, and staffing levels. There are shortages in the supply of quality emergency doctors and technicians as the work is stressful and most emergency hours

Textbook of Small Animal Emergency Medicine, First Edition. Edited by Kenneth J. Drobatz, Kate Hopper, Elizabeth Rozanski and Deborah C. Silverstein.
© 2019 John Wiley & Sons, Inc. Published 2019 by John Wiley & Sons, Inc.
Companion Website: www.wiley.com/go/drobatz/textbook

are nights and weekends. For practical reasons, staffing levels are based on an average anticipated caseload so it is not uncommon for a very busy shift to overwhelm the resources of even the most prepared practice. The cost of quality care is already high and steadily increasing faster than the overall inflation rate. Pet owners are already stressed to meet these costs. The "ideal" design must yield to practical and affordable considerations.

Practical Design

Quality care is still possible within the constraints of the imposed limitations. Facilities can be built on cheaper commercial or even industrial land. Construction costs can be controlled with intelligent choices of structural and design elements; still expensive at up to $500 + (2016) per square foot, but still half the cost of a comparable human hospital. The hospital design focuses on making effective use of space, minimizing hallways, and designing rooms that can support multiple functions.

In smaller clinics, equipment is shared among several areas, which is an acceptable compromise since the spaces are small and time is not wasted moving resources from one area to another. The primary treatment room serves as the ER with space dedicated to immediate response. Staff are cross-trained, with receptionists and technicians often serving as care co-ordinators in addition to their primary functions. There is a premium on technician training as they can be called upon to play a role often performed by a veterinarian in a larger, multidoctor facility.

In large hospitals, each major service should be ready for emergency response. This usually includes ER, ICU, medical procedures, and surgery departments but can extend to oncology, imaging, and other areas. With the possibility of an emergency occurring anywhere, the design must still be flexible, permitting the patient to quickly and safely get to an emergency response area, or the personnel, equipment, and medical supplies to quickly get to the patient. The cost of independently equipping multiple areas in the hospital can be considerable. A practical design can be accomplished using mobile cart systems, lightweight mobile equipment, an alert staff, and an excellent system of in-hospital communication so that the range of effective ER response can be extended from a few rooms to all areas of the hospital.

Entrance

Current building codes that establish access requirements for handicapped persons also benefit the emergency patient. Lighting for vehicle ingress and egress must meet minimum standards. Handicapped parking must be generous and a similar design should be used for emergency parking near the entrance. Parking lot slope cannot be excessive, access to the entrance must be without obstacles, curbs must be cut to permit wheelchair use, entry doors must be large enough with hold-open function or automatic openers. These design elements all permit medical staff and gurneys to reach a patient that cannot be carried in by an owner.

Ideally, hospital design provides for a separate emergency entrance or entrances to permit rapid access to an ER. If only the main entrance is available, there should be a straight path from waiting room to ER, through the exam room area, that is as short as possible. A gurney should be stationed near emergency entrances to shorten response time.

Reception

Reception areas should have sight lines to the parking lot and emergency parking area. The front desk should be designed so that a receptionist does not have to leave this area to do their job while observing waiting patients at the same time. The phone, intercom, and/or paging system should be robust and able to rapidly call for assistance when needed at the front of the hospital. Each phone should be paired with a laminated list of emergency conditions – those client complaints that a receptionist can easily recognize, either on the phone or in the waiting room, that these are problems that should be addressed immediately.

Waiting Room

Client waiting areas should be partitioned so that families and pets can find some personal space. If possible, cats should be separated from dogs, and fractious dogs (and boisterous children) should be separated from others by the design of the waiting room. The challenge is to provide these areas of separation while keeping clients and pets visible to hospital staff. Children should have their own area with games, toys, and television. Adults should have access to television to help endure longer waiting times. Current hospital design tends toward smaller waiting rooms in favor of adding more exam rooms. The exam rooms double as personal waiting areas for individual families and pets and help to ease the stress of a waiting room full of clients and patients.

Exam Rooms

A well-designed exam room can serve as a receiving room, a waiting room, a consultation room, a grieving

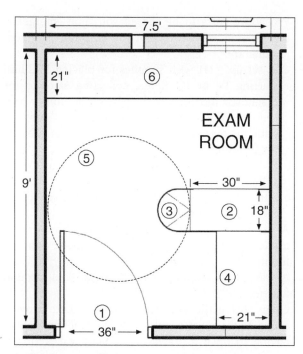

1. Single entry door
2. Fixed exam table, 30" above floor level (AFL)
3. Folding 12" exam table extension
4. Doctor's work space, 42" AFL
5. ADA-compliant wheelchair access
6. Full room width client bench seating, 18" AFL

Figure 205.1 Compact exam room design.

room, a room for patient history and examination, a client education room, and a discharge room. It is unusual for an exam room to be used for emergency procedures or treatments, except in the context of minor, outpatient urgent care.

Current hospital design plans for a smaller waiting room and more exam rooms. In addition, exam rooms can be designed smaller than the traditional 8' × 10' space thought to be the minimum size. With careful design, 10 exam rooms can be built in the space normally filled by eight (Figure 205.1).

Historically, exam rooms were designed with a hallway on each side with a separate entry door for clients on one side and doctors on the opposite side. Considerable space can be saved by creating a pod of exam rooms, each room with a single door with rooms aligned on each side of a semi-private hallway that is accessed from the waiting area at one end and the private, secure, staff-only area toward the back of the hospital. Client seating is in the back of the room with the doctor's workspace near the door. The doctor and staff can enter and leave the room at will without disrupting the client or patient.

Veterinarians may have strong opinions about having sinks in exam rooms, but with the high cost of plumbing and the trend toward all procedures being performed away from the client, a single sink can serve all exam rooms in a pod.

Visitation, Consulting, and Grieving Rooms

If the facility and the budget are large enough, there may be benefit to planning client rooms that are not as stark as the typical exam room. Space dedicated for client privacy and comfort can be a good investment, and may be used for consultation, grieving, or visiting a hospitalized pet that is well enough to be moved from its cage or run. These rooms can be designed with more subdued lighting, more comfortable furniture, and rugs on the floor. If this space is to be used for patient visits, an oxygen outlet should be provided. This type of room can also be fitted with a folding exam table to be used when extra examination space is needed.

Emergency Room

Ideally, whatever space is designed for a practice's primary emergency response would be dedicated to that response so that an incoming emergency patient had immediate access to the workspace, supplies, and equipment needed for their urgent care. These resources would be reserved strictly for emergency use and considered to be so vital to that purpose that they would never be taken for use elsewhere in the hospital. However, for most practices, the cost to duplicate the space, equipment, drugs, and supplies is simply too high, so they are used in support of the non-emergency caseload as well.

Most small and medium-sized hospitals (3000–12 000 square feet) integrate their emergency patient care into their central treatment area. During the day, it shares functionality with the non-emergency caseload of the hospital. If the facility is open nights, weekends, and holidays, this area becomes the ER. This room is usually at the center of the hospital where staff tend to converge and where, because the hospital is small, the room is in reasonably close proximity to everything needed for patient care.

To serve as an efficient ER, the treatment room must be organized, equipped, and supplied for the task. Both wet and dry treatment tables should be available, organized along a wall as peninsula projections or in the center of the room in treatment islands. Oxygen, suction, waste gas, plumbing, and electrical lines to any island should arise from the floor below the island and *not* be installed in columns that extend to the ceiling. Contractors may resist this design element since installation is considerably more difficult, but patients and hospital staff benefit from having unobstructed lines of sight around the room.

High-intensity surgical lighting should be installed in the ceiling centered on each treatment table within easy reach. IV tubing and med gas lines should not interfere with the overhead exam lights or with access to the patient, so IV hangers should be installed on medical carts or on the exam light columns overhead. Medical gas connections for oxygen, suction, and waste gas should be at the end of each treatment table along with a bracket to hang a suction canister. These items should be recessed below the end of the table, along with electrical outlets and a switch for a small shop vacuum installed inside the cabinet for vacuuming clipped hair.

Emergency room practitioners have different opinions on whether "readiness" means that all emergency drugs and supplies should be out in the open or whether well-labeled drawers and cabinets provide an adequate level of accessibility without the clutter. This author prefers multiple levels of organization, all in close proximity to the treatment tables.

1. A "crash" cart reserved for cardiopulmonary resuscitation. On or in the cart should be:
   o a bag of balanced electrolyte solution with an attached administration set, pressure infuser, and infusion pump
   o a biphasic defibrillator with connected external paddles
   o a multiparameter patient monitor capable of displaying ECG, NIBP, SaO_2, temperature, and $ETCO_2$
   o endotracheal tubes and laryngoscope
   o Ambu bag and oxygen masks
   o supplies for intravenous and intraosseous catheterization
   o supplies for obtaining diagnostic samples
   o bandage material
   o examination and surgical gloves
   o a surgical pack and supplies
   o chest and abdominal retractors
   o tourniquets.
2. An oxygen flowmeter plugged into the oxygen fixture at the treatment table attached to a patient line. An E-series oxygen tank attached to the crash cart is acceptable if the hospital does not have piped medical gas lines.
3. A surgical suction regulator plugged into the suction fixture at the treatment table attached to a suction canister, suction tubing and a Yankauer or Poole suction catheter. A Gomco or similar suction pump on the crash cart is acceptable if the hospital does not have central suction.

4. Procedure carts to be shared with non-emergency patients for use throughout the hospital. The most popular are:
   o a "set-up" cart with supplies for placing IV lines, starting IV or IO fluids, collecting samples for diagnostic testing, and for performing minor procedures. This is used with almost all hospitalized patients, permitting the crash cart to be reserved for CPR only
   o a bandage cart containing bandage, casts, and splint materials
   o a treatment cart to organize and deliver scheduled medication for hospitalized patients.
5. A gas anesthesia machine, preferably with an anesthetic ventilator and a multiparameter patient monitor.
6. A cart with a small, highly mobile ultrasound machine.
7. Open bins at the treatment table islands to provide access to the most commonly used supplies without having to open a drawer or cabinet, e.g. syringes, tape, bandage material, gauze, etc.
8. Cabinets and drawers throughout the treatment room containing those items that are used for both emergency and non-emergency patients.

The ER room should be designed to array all of these elements around central treatment tables. Islands arranged in an "H" pattern allow for four patient tables in close proximity – two wet tables, one fixed dry table, and one docking station for a mobile lift gurney. With one or more such islands in the center of the room, the periphery of the room can be used for storage cabinets, rolling stock (crash cart, procedure carts, anesthetic machine, ultrasound machine), cages, and for doors leading to surrounding rooms.

A room designated exclusively for use as an ER is probably practical only in very large hospitals with a large daytime emergency caseload and the space available for this single use. Design and organization are similar to that described above, with a minimum of two patient tables. This space has the advantage that it does not interfere with more routine non-emergency care, does not add to the stress of the quieter pace in the treatment room, and can be located to permit client access without entrance into the main treatment area.

Other Hospital Space

Hospital space surrounding the primary treatment room or ER is considered to be "prime real estate," reserved for important patient support functions. Unfortunately, as larger and larger hospitals are constructed, everything cannot be close to the ER. A list of hospital space assigned by proximity to the ER and designed to optimize patient support might be as follows.

Nurses' Workstation

This is an area for medical staff to complete records and other administrative tasks while maintaining close observation of emergency patients. It may be part of the main treatment/ER room or in a room in close proximity with large windows for observation.

Doctors' Workstation

This is compact desk space where doctors can complete records, make phone calls, access the hospital library, or consult with colleagues. This should be an enclosed area with a large window wall that permits monitoring of all activity in the treatment/ER room.

Intensive Care

In a 2016 study bt VECCS and Horizon Veterinary Services, nearly 90% of emergency care providers reported that they had primary ICU patient responsibility while working emergency shifts. Even though the quiet, contemplative environment of the ICU seems only remotely related to the hectic pace of a busy ER, this joint responsibility means that these hospital areas need to be closely associated. Only in very large hospitals in which these services can be manned separately can they be separated in the facility.

Radiology

Digital technology permits safer and more rapid radiological assessment of the emergency patient. Radiology rooms should be easily accessed from the departments that need rapid access to this technology – ER and surgery.

Laboratory

The dramatic advances in point-of-care testing will eventually mean that hand-held analyzers can be used in the ER and the main hospital laboratory can be located farther away. At this time, rapid laboratory access and rapid turnaround times are still a high priority for the ER, the ICU, and the surgery department.

Care Co-ordinator Workstation

These are the people who bond the client to the medical staff. They maintain client communication while the medical staff are busy with patient care. Care co-ordinators must have easy access to both clients and medical personnel so this bond is not broken.

Surgery

A number of surgical procedures are carried out in the ER, including open chest CPR, emergency tracheotomy, laparotomy or thoracotomy for massive hemorrhage control, and minor wound repair. Usually, patients that require less urgent or more extensive surgery are stabilized in the ER so that they can be moved safely to a more remote surgery department. That said, many emergency rooms in large practices are designed with a dedicated surgical suite nearby.

Isolation

There are differing opinions on the best strategy for the design and location of isolation rooms. Many patients that should be isolated present through the emergency service. Once identified, they should be housed and treated in an area away from other patients at risk. Placing this area close to the ER seems appropriate, but also invites contamination between these areas. An isolation room more remote in the hospital with a vestibule for storing supplies and for decontamination after contact with patients is also an acceptable solution. The space should include a wet table and everything necessary to care for the patient. The room should have audio and video monitoring displayed in the nurses' and doctors' workstations. It should also have an outside entrance and isolated exercise yard.

Advanced Imaging (CT and MRI)

Magnetic resonance imaging studies are unlikely to be performed on emergency patients until they are stable enough to undergo a fairly long anesthetic procedure. On the other hand, multi-slice CT scanners are becoming more affordable, making for more rapid studies that can be performed with minimal, if any, sedation. CT is becoming a more useful tool for the assessment of the emergency patient and future hospital design should consider placing this imaging modality closer to the ER.

Other Design Considerations for the Emergency Room

Flooring

Flooring is the Achilles heel of a veterinary facility. It should be impervious but ideally soft underfoot. It should be stain resistant and bacteriostatic or even bactericidal.

The flooring material should be seamless and coved onto walls and cabinet bases to eliminate open seams where fluids and debris can collect, unable to be cleaned. The surface should be smooth to allow easy movement of carts and gurneys but not so smooth as to be slippery when wet. There is no perfect flooring system and many poor ones. Most reasonable solutions are sheet goods with heat-sealed seams, or epoxy or epoxy/acrylic troweled-on materials that harden in place and create a seamless floor cover. Newer acrylic combination products show promise and have the advantage that repairs can be made seamlessly.

Lighting

The trend in lighting design to save energy is to provide less overhead general lighting and to rely on more focused task lighting. Many building codes now make this a requirement and limit the amount of general lighting that can be installed. Hospitals can benefit from this approach, but should still recognize areas that should be brighter than a normal office building would be. Extra general overhead lighting should ideally be provided in the parking lot, waiting rooms, exam rooms, ER, ICU, and isolation. Dimmable lighting should be provided in imaging rooms, ICU, anesthesia recovery, wards, and visitation rooms.

Plumbing

Stainless steel is an obvious choice for handwashing stations, patient wet tables, dog runs, or anywhere there is a drain. Exam room sinks can be replaced with one sink in the hallway of each exam pod. Wet tables should be equipped with sprayers and a garbage disposal if local building code allows. Fixtures should be single spout with a single lever mixer to permit one-handed operation. The area around the entrance, the run wards, and outdoor exercise areas should have hose bibs. Building codes will often require a drinking fountain in public areas or near public bathrooms.

Heating, Ventilation, and Cooling

Multiple, independent heating and cooling ventilation systems are required to separate public, interface, private, and animal housing areas. Systems are often overdesigned when the designer tries to meet the air exchange standards of an animal housing facility such as a boarding kennel. In a hospital, most odors result from contamination with feces, urine, vomitus, or body fluids that are more serious threats to patients and staff than just the odor. An inexpensive solution for odor control is to install high-capacity switched exhaust fans, able to dump the entire air volume in a room within minutes.

Surgery rooms should have Hepa filters or at least laminar flow supply and return vents installed at the periphery of the room. Isolation should have its own HVAC (usually a mini-split system) with negative pressure in the room so all air flow around the door is inward. All return air should be exhausted to the outside when the room is occupied. Ceiling fans can be used help to circulate air downward into runs.

Electrical System

The electrical system must be robust and even smaller clinics will require at least 400 amp service. If possible, circuits to computers and lab equipment should be conditioned or the equipment should have surge protection. Back-up power should be provided, either with battery power or a generator. Multiple outlets or high-density plug strips will be needed in the laboratory and in any area where patient care involves multiple pumps, monitors, warmers, clippers, and other electrical devices.

Security

The front entrance or vestibule should be locked during off-hours and controlled from the reception desk. Access to the clinical areas of the hospital should be limited and controlled with electronic locks that can be armed when security is needed between public and private areas. Narcotics cabinets must be double-locked and monitored. Video monitoring is recommended throughout the exterior and interior of the hospital, with focus on important areas that include the entrance, reception desk, isolation, narcotics storage, and outdoor exercise areas. Video monitoring can also be used to monitor cages and runs where emergency or ICU patients are housed. Some hospitals monitor and record video and audio feeds from exam rooms to minimize risk to hospital personnel, to use in the event of any dispute or legal action, or even for staff training purposes.

Cart Systems

To prevent duplication of expensive equipment and supplies, cart systems are becoming more popular. Carts have the advantage of organizing supplies and equipment for a targeted task (e.g. initial patient set-up, scheduled treatment for patients in wards, bandaging, anesthesia monitoring, computer record keeping) and can be stationed anywhere near the patient when needed, but stored along a wall or in a ready room when not in use. They have the added advantage that they can be rolled to central supply when they need to be restocked.

Medical Gases

Emergency rooms and ICUs use a large quantity of oxygen. This can be supplied by an appropriately sized oxygen generator, liquid oxygen tanks, or a manifold of large H tanks. Oxygen should be piped to outlets in walls where anesthesia is performed, above cages and runs to provide supplemental oxygen, and in the face of treatment stations for both purposes. Overhead oxygen lines should be avoided if possible, or at least strategically placed to not interfere with patient lighting or patient access. Oxygen alarms must be audible throughout the hospital.

A hospital-grade compressor to provide both surgical suction and waste anesthetic gas scavenging should be part of the medical gas system. Smaller clinics can realize savings with low-tech scavenging systems and point-of-care portable suction pumps. Nitrogen may be needed in surgical suites for power tools, although surgeons are more commonly opting for electrical devices.

Cages and Runs

Stainless steel is the best choice for animal housing. Laminate cages have an advantage in cost and can be installed with an in-floor heating system, but they are not as cleanable or as durable. Any electrical heating system should be closely monitored so patients are not burned. Heating patients with warmed air or water blankets is preferred, but these systems are much more cumbersome to use on awake patients.

Cages should be banked in two tiers. Modules of three cages, one 36" high × 48" wide below and two 30" high × 24" wide above, can be arranged in line to provide efficient accommodation anywhere patients are housed. Above each module is a shallow cabinet that contains fluid pumps, hanging fluid bags, and patient monitors that support the patients housed below.

Run doors and walls should be stainless steel with an impervious floor of epoxy or acrylic blend sloping to a drain. The floors can be heated at reasonable cost. The drain should be selected to minimize the likelihood of a dog's nail or digit being trapped. If glass is used in the run door to improve patient monitoring, the lower one-third of the door should be stainless steel wire to permit hanging pumps and monitors and to permit air circulation in the run. Overhead ceiling fans can improve this circulation. Runs should be equipped with multiple places to hang pumps and monitors, preferably outside the cage or on the cage door. In ER and ICU areas, oversize runs are required to permit access to a recumbent patient from at least three sides.

Design Summary

All the elements of a practical hospital design capable of providing excellent care for emergency patients anywhere in the hospital can be seen in Figure 205.2.

Staffing the Emergency Room

Staffing the ER is an administrative challenge. Emergency care has become increasingly more sophisticated, requiring greater levels of expertise from both doctors and medical staff. Emergency patient care demands constant vigilance and meticulous attention to detail with little room for error. The caseload is unpredictable – a staff schedule can be created to cover an average shift, but it can easily be overwhelmed on any given shift. Emergency work is highly stressful due to the volatility of clients and caseload. It is also not conducive to a "normal" lifestyle in which people typically do not work nights, weekends, and holidays.

The cost of staffing an ER can exceed 60% of the budget and is rising due to a shortage of applicants for emergency positions. The cost of medical care in general increases at a rate 2–3 times faster than the increase in the average cost of living. Staffing challenges will only increase in the foreseeable future.

How emergency services are coping with these challenges can be summarized in the results of a 2016 survey performed by Horizon Veterinary Services and the Veterinary Emergency and Critical Care Society. The results are listed below.

- Over 1000 responses were obtained from emergency service personnel from all regions of the United States.
- 77% of responders were female, with 83% younger than 50 years old.
- Emergency services are either provided during routine general practice office hours (8am–6pm Monday through Saturday), emergency clinic hours (5 or 6pm–8 or 9am Monday through Friday and all day weekends and holidays), or central hospital hours 24/7.
- 47% of respondents have at least one board-certified ACVECC diplomate on staff.
- 24% use other specialists to provide emergency services.
- 21% employ ACVECC residents, 10% other residents, 19% E/CC interns, and 32% rotating interns.
- 87% employ regular emergency doctors.
- 21% employ part-time and relief doctors.
- 88% of reporting hospitals use certified technicians, 81% non-certified technical assistants.

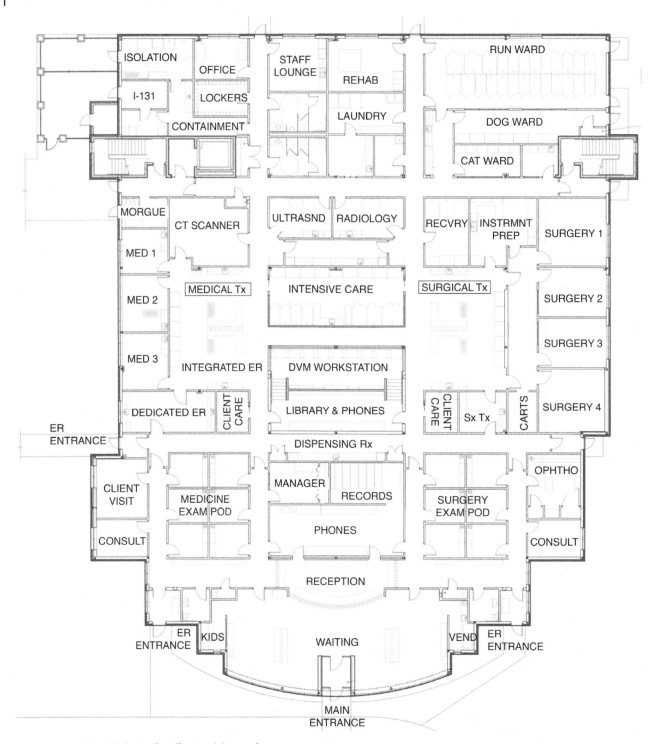

Figure 205.2 Hospital design for effective delivery of emergency services.

- 80% are staffed with a separate team of receptionists, 23% with care co-ordinators, 35% with dedicated kennel staff, and 45% with managers on duty at least part of the emergency shifts.
- 69% are structured as a single business, 31% are an association of multiple businesses.
- 21% of responding hospitals are owned by large corporations that own more than 50 practices, 11% by medium-sized companies that own 11–50 practices, and 20% by groups that own 2–10 practices.
- Ownership interest is held by all types of hospital personnel: 70% are doctors, 7% medical staff, and 6% managers.
- Caseload ranges from less than 1000 patient visits per year to over 20 000 per year. Dividing hospitals into four groups based on number of patient visits, the lower quartile sees 1000–3500/year, the second quartile 3500–6000/year, the third quartile 6000–12 000/year, and the upper quartile 12 000–20 000/year. Seven percent of hospitals have over 20 000 patient visits each year.
- 60% of the caseload is canine, 37% feline, and 3% avian and exotic.
- Staffing levels are highly variable and dependent on caseload. For each doctor on duty, there are typically 2–2.5 technicians, 0.3–0.5 receptionists (i.e. shared among 2–3 doctors), 0.5–1 assistant, and 0–0.5 care co-ordinators. The use of care co-ordinators and separate kennel staff increases with higher caseloads.
- An emergency doctor will typically see 5–10 cases on a weekday shift, 5–20 cases on a weeknight shift, 5–15 cases on a weekend day shift, 5–25 cases on a weekend night shift, and 5–30 cases on a holiday shift.
- 88% of emergency doctors have primary ICU patient responsibility when working an emergency shift.
- 83% of emergency doctors have surgical responsibility, with the majority performing procedures, wound repair, laparotomies, and management of penetrating wounds of the abdomen and thorax. Only 19% perform thoracotomies.
- Emergency doctors work full or part time; 70% are scheduled for 12–16 shifts per month.
- The vast majority of responding doctors have worked less than 25 years in emergency practice. Only 4% have been in emergency practice for over 25 years.
- 44% of doctors are paid by salary, 17% by the greater of salary or production, 24% by base salary plus production, 6% by production only, and 9% hourly.
- Over 70% of doctors receive benefits that include health insurance, dues and license fees, continuing education, paid personal days, and retirement plans. 10% participate in a formal profit sharing plan. 32% receive unscheduled bonuses.
- Emergency doctor income (from all sources) ranges from less than $10 000 per year to over $1 000 000 per year.
- Earnings from the practice of emergency medicine range from less than $10 000 to over $500 000 per year.
- 70–88% of doctors receive no additional income from general practice, teaching, training, administrative duties, or veterinary practice ownership.
- 78% of doctors have some level of ownership interest in their practice or their owner corporation.
- The majority of emergency practitioners average from $300–600 per transaction, with a range from $200–3000.
- Doctors give a passing grade for quality to themselves, their colleagues, their support staff, their equipment, the level of collaboration, and their practice overall.
- Doctors give <70% approval to their building, their owners, and their managers.
- Most emergency doctors plan to retire before the age of 60.

206

Conflict in the Emergency Room

Jim Wohl, DVM, MPA, DACVIM, ACVECC

University of Connecticut, Storrs, CT, USA

Introduction

Conflict can be defined as a form of competition for perceived or actual incompatible needs, goals, desires, ideas, or resources [1]. When managed constructively in the ER, conflict can harness intellectual growth, foster innovation, promote change, and even enhance relationships. Left unattended, conflict can be a destructive influence on patient care, profitability, and quality of life for ER personnel. The negative organizational consequences of a high-conflict work environment include internal competition, visible disputes, sabotage, inefficiency, low productivity, low morale, and withholding knowledge [2]. Consequences can be equally destructive to individuals. Resignation, absenteeism, going slow, complaints, legal suits, gossip, anonymous attacks, fear of loss of privacy, loss of dignity, and fear of retaliation and labelling are typical results affecting individuals. These individual concerns can be more acute for women, minorities, and non-traditionals who experience a greater risk of being stigmatized as troublemakers rather than as self-confident professionals [3].

The ER has many features that contribute to a high-conflict environment. Time-sensitive high-stake decision making on patient care, a high expectation for spontaneity, demanding clients, scarce resources, informal and formal hierarchy, shared responsibilities associated with shift transition, team-managed care, and high levels of uncertainty about the effect of medical interventions are just a sampling of contributory environmental characteristics of emergency medicine. Working long hours within this compassion fatigue-inducing milieu are highly trained and driven clinicians, administrators, technicians, and professional staff, many of whom are competitive by nature and may be drawn to veterinary medicine for deeply personal reasons involving their core values. In such an environment, embracing the inevitability of conflict permits caretakers of the workplace culture to focus on diverting destructive conflict toward constructive ends.

Leaders in the ER with management and policy-making authority have special responsibility in transforming conflict. At the same time, nearly every individual, regardless of their positional authority, can influence the way conflict is managed although undoubtedly, some individuals will be more predisposed to collegiality than others. An understanding of the environmental factors of the ER, the nature of interpersonal conflict, and the role management can play in influencing a culture of conflict competence can be the tools for transforming destructive conflict in the ER.

Interpersonal Conflict

The interpersonal dimension of conflict within the ER setting is composed of the characteristics of the individual members of the emergency service. Each member's personal history, style of approaching conflictual situations, communication preferences, and values will affect the ways in which disputes manifest in the ER. When two or more people in the ER are involved in a conflict, the goals of the parties can be analyzed as content, relationship, identity, or process oriented [4].

Content goals refer to the substance of the disagreement or the topic of what is being disputed. For example, during a dispute between two clinicians over patient management decisions, the parties typically describe the problem in terms of content (the conflict is over the best treatment for the patient). Generally, conflicts that solely involve content goals are resolvable or, even when left unresolved, are handled professionally and are rarely destructive to the organizational culture or co-workers (e.g. agreeing to disagree). Indeed, when a conflict is destructive, it is likely that other goals, in addition to the content, are present for those involved even though the parties themselves would describe the conflict as having to do solely with the content.

In such cases, some combination of *relationship*, *identity*, and/or *process* goals is almost always present. Relationship goals are emotionally based and center on hierarchy, power, or social roles between the parties in conflict. Often, a sense of injustice, offense, and victimization is an unspoken driver of the conflict (that, again, is usually described in terms of content only). A relationship-based conflict driver for a clinician in a dispute over a treatment plan may be the perception that the counterpart clinician's decision to change the treatment only occurred because of another unrelated problem in their relationship (e.g. rivalries, prior offensive interaction, differences in philosophical approaches).

Identity goals involve a party's self-esteem, face, or social identity and can be quite powerful drivers of conflict and are typically unarticulated. Identity goals imply a psychological and emotional basis where the importance of the conflict is connected to how one sees oneself. For the clinician driven by identity goals, the change in treatment plan represents a judgment of the quality of their expertise, or even their value as a human being.

Process goals as drivers of destructive conflict involve how decisions are made or how conflicts get resolved. In an organizational setting like an ER, process goals may involve perceived inconsistency in following policy, differing opinion on best practices, and lines of authority. In the preceding example over treatment plans, a process-oriented driver of the conflict may be disagreement as to whether treatment plans should be guided by evidence-based best practice or the autonomy of a clinician's judgment.

In particular, relationship and identity goals, when projected onto the content of a dispute, can explain the severity or rigidity of a party's response.

Further complicating the analysis of interpersonal conflict is the fact that each party to a dispute is driven by their own personal combination of goals (Figure 206.1). Despite the variability of the combination of goals, some

people can seemingly specialize in one or another type of goal. Analysis in the conflict literature describes threats to "core concerns" such as appreciation, personal autonomy, feelings of affiliation to colleagues, personal status, and professional role as drivers of interpersonal conflict [5].

In a given conflict, an individual's conflict style can be understood as a balance between (a) how concerned the person is about achieving their preferred outcome in the dispute, and (b) how concerned he or she is for their counterpart's ability to achieve their preferences [6]. For example, a team member who is highly focused on achieving their own outcome but negligibly interested in their counterpart's interests is said to have a *competitive* conflict style (Figure 206.2). Conversely, one who is mostly concerned with their counterpart's satisfaction at the expense of their own concerns would demonstrate an *accommodating* style. An *avoiding* style suggests that the person is most interested in averting a conflict to the degree that they will ignore their own potential beneficial outcomes as well as those of their counterparts.

Compromising and *collaborative* styles reflect approaches that share some combination of pursuing one's own and the counterpart's goals with an important difference. An individual with a collaborative style seeks to optimize the outcomes for themselves and their counterpart and this approach necessitates more time and effort in discussing the range of outcomes sought by each party. A compromise mode instead seeks an equal or fair outcome in which the attainment of goals for each (or, often, the lack of attainment for each) approximates one another.

It is helpful in understanding this aspect of conflict theory to know that although individuals tend to gravitate to one particular conflict style as a regular response, all people are generally capable of demonstrating each of the five conflict styles depending on the situation. Broadening the exposure of conflicts outside the workplace, it's easy to imagine various circumstances when one might

Figure 206.1 Often, conflicts are presented about a specific topic or issue – a content issue. However, there are almost always underlying relational and identity goals and often these categories of issues overlap. C, content; I, identity; P, process; R, relationship,

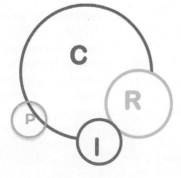

Party A's Goals/Issues

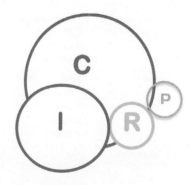

Party B's Goals/Issues

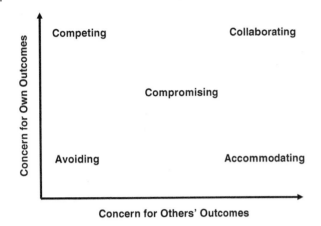

Figure 206.2 The conflict style demonstrated by a party in conflict reflects a balance between two competing goals: concern about one's own outcomes and concern about the counterpart's outcomes.

choose any of the styles (Table 206.1). Exploring the style options one has in responding to conflict or examining the appropriateness of the styles exhibited in a past situation can be a very helpful tool towards transforming workplace conflicts. Intuitively, most people can imagine

Table 206.1 Features of various conflict styles that might be adopted by a party to a conflict and characteristics of the conflict that are appropriate for each style. Evaluating conflict styles can elucidate perceptions of the conflict and the relationships involved or whether the adopted style is appropriate for the conflict situation.

Conflict style	Features	When appropriate
Avoiding	Quick, no effort, leaves possible solutions unachieved	Unimportant issues Ongoing relationship unimportant No time unavailable for engagement
Competitive	Quick, minimal to moderate effort, leaves counterpart goals unmet	Important issues Ongoing relationship unimportant Little time available for engagement
Accommodating	Quick, minimal to moderate effort, leaves own goals unmet	Unimportant issues Ongoing relationship important Little time available for engagement
Compromising	Quick, minimal to moderate effort, goals partially met for both	Important issues Ongoing relationship important Some time available for engagement
Collaborative	Takes time, maximal effort, goals optimized for both	Creative solutions needed for important issues Ample time available for engagement

what different actions they may have adopted, how the communication would have changed, and in what ways the trajectory of the conflict would have changed if one of the parties had chosen an alternative style in approaching a past conflict.

Other perspectives from the conflict theory and communication literature can illuminate the nature of interpersonal conflict in the ER. Incompatibility of communication styles contribute as much to conflict as the intersection of conflict styles. Communication styles have been described as action oriented, process oriented, people oriented, and idea oriented [7,8]. When discussing a work-related plan in the ER (e.g. case rounds, therapeutic planning, new facilities, training of staff), a person's communication style and language reflect the aspects of the topic that is most important to them (Table 206.2). Differences in communication priorities during such interactions can be fertile ground for conflicts. Differential power between interlocutors due to seniority, position, expertise, or decision-making responsibility can amplify this stylistic miscommunication. Indeed, initial assessment of new employees' competence or ability to "hit the ground running" is often more a reflection of their communication compatibility with supervisors than their task-related capabilities. Contrasting communication styles can obviously exacerbate attempts at dialogue during interpersonal conflicts.

Enhancing Constructive Conflict

Leadership's role in fostering a culture of conflict competence focuses on controlling the environmental stressors that foment conflict where possible, establishing good management practices, and empowering ER team members with the skills and abilities to respond to conflicts constructively. Practice considerations regarding workflows, proper staffing, and clear lines of authority can mitigate the time stress, chaos, and uncertainty that breed conflict. In-depth awareness of and a prophylactic approach towards veterinary regulations and employment law are obvious ways to limit destructive conflict. Adhering to clear and consistent practices regarding decision making, rather than an *ad hoc* style of change management, can also be a key stress reliever for staff. Understanding what types of decisions will be made by what type of process (e.g. group decisions, decision by a single leader after soliciting input, feedback system for revisiting decisions) is often more important to the environment than the actual decisions themselves.

Attention to identifying patterns where conflicts commonly arise can reveal to leaders in the ER where policy or practices require change or clarity. For example, the potential for conflict between people exists whenever

Table 206.2 Typical characteristics of people and the language used in four communication styles. Differences in communication styles can be a source of conflict itself as well as explaining how attempts to resolve conflicts through dialogue can escalate conflict.

Orientation	They talk about...	They are...
Action	Results, responsibility, objectives, feedback, performance, experience, productivity, challenge, efficiency, achievements, moving ahead, change, decisions	Pragmatic, direct, impatient, decisive, quick (jumping from one thing to another), energetic, challenging of others
Process	Facts, trying out procedures, analysis, planning, observations, organizing, proof, controlling, details, testing	Systematic, logical, factual, verbose, unemotional, cautious, patient
People	People, self-development, needs, sensitivity, motivations, awareness, teamwork, co-operation, communications, beliefs, feelings, values, team spirit, expectations, understanding, relations	Spontaneous, empathetic, warm, subjective, emotional, perceptive, sensitive
Idea	Concepts, what's new in the field, innovation, creativity, interdependence, opportunities, new ways, possibilities, new methods, grand designs, improving issues, problems, potential alternatives	Imaginative, charismatic, difficult to understand, ego-centered, unrealistic, creative, full of ideas, provocative

opposition is expressed towards an individual or group. The focus of opposition may be ideas, behaviors, or decisions. Opposition is expressed across the dimensions of clarity (direct or indirect opposition) and intensity (high or low intensity) [9]. Highly conflict-competent work environments typically utilize direct and low-intensity communication when expressing opposition rather than other combinations of expression (direct-high intensity, indirect-low intensity, indirect-high intensity).

Voluminous resources on effective management practices and leadership skills can assist leaders in aligning management's role with the mission of the ER [10–12]. The salutary effects of coherent management style and workplace policies can be supplemented with specific approaches that empower all team members.

1. Provide negotiations skills training (or mediation training) to all team members with supervisory responsibility and non-supervisory staff who express an interest. Negotiation and/or mediation trainings can be completed in short frequent sessions, are fun, and instill effective communications skills that focus on surfacing people's interests when conflicts arise. Transitioning the dialogue from one of blame and demands for some desired outcome (positions) toward dialogue based on what people want and why (their interests) can be the most effective method to pivot conflict toward a constructive experience [13].

2. Develop and then articulate to team members specific methods by which leadership will respond to episodes of unprofessional behavior [14]. Disciplinary responses have three components: the swiftness with which they are delivered, the certainty that they will be delivered, and the severity of the response. It has been argued that when swiftness and certainty are constantly present, severity becomes the least important component [15].

Equally important is empowering non-supervisory staff to confront episodes of unprofessional behavior informally themselves. Excellent trainings, videos, and short articles are available for staff [16]. A cornerstone to empowering both management and non-supervisory staff to confront unprofessional behavior in the workplace involves distinguishing whether the behavior is an isolated episode, a pattern of behavior, or focused on the relationship between the people involved in the unwanted behaviors [17].

3. Incorporate communication, practice management, conflict management, and leadership articles or topics into the in-house continuing education framework. When done sporadically, such sessions can be a welcome diversion from the medical or hospital policy-oriented topics and help reinforce commitment to conflict competence.

4. Reward team members who contribute to civility and respect in the work environment. Identifying this contribution as a specific domain in annual performance evaluations (rather than a component of a more vague categorical dimension such as "works well in a team") signals that handling conflict constructively is a priority and provides acknowledgment to those who are enhancing conflict competence in the ER.

5. Communication protocols, consensus statements, and Circles can be effective tools for smaller units within the ER setting to break through long-standing negative behaviors affecting morale. Communication protocols are a form of consensus-building exercise that focuses on answering three or so process-oriented questions on how to respond when someone in the unit is causing a problem for another [18]. The goal is for the unit to arrive at a consensus agreement to follow the process they develop in the

protocol. A Circle is a central element of restorative practices and formalizes a way to discuss a problem or address harm that has occurred to a team member [19]. It is essential that participation in these practices is voluntary. They are likely to do more harm than good if the people involved do not buy in or the practice is imposed on perceived problem units. When embraced voluntarily, they can be transformative to units plagued with destructive conflict.

Conclusion

Managing conflict in the ER requires attention to the environmental setting inherent to emergency practice, the people working in the ER setting, and the ways in which management and leaders can influence the workplace culture. Despite the challenges in high-conflict ERs, remaining mindful of two realities provides some degree of optimism. First is that the goal is not to eliminate conflict but rather to capitalize on its occurrence and harness conflicts toward constructive ends. The second is the fallacy that "everyone needs to be on board" for effective culture change to occur. Results of research in conflict studies and game theory suggest that if just 25% of people in a given work environment are committed to co-operation, significant culture change can ensue over time [20,21]. Leaders in the ER can therefore provide their greatest service in allowing those 25% (or hopefully more) to thrive.

References

1 Consortium on Negotiation and Conflict Resolution. *Basic Mediation Manual*. Summer Institute on Conflict in Higher Education, Jekyll Island, Atlanta, GA, 2005.
2 Constantino CA, Merchant CS. *Designing Conflict Management Systems*. Jossey-Bass, San Francisco, 1996.
3 Rowe M. Dispute resolution in the nonunion environment: an evolution toward integrated systems for conflict management. In: *Workplace Dispute Resolution* (ed. Gleason SE). Michigan State University Press, East Lansing, 1976.
4 Wilmot WW, Hocker JL. *Interpersonal Conflict*, 2nd edn. McGraw-Hill, Boston, 2007.
5 Fisher R, Shapiro D. *Beyond Reason: Using Emotions as You Negotiate*. Viking, New York, 2005.
6 Thomas K, Kilmann RH. *Thomas–Kilmann Conflict Mode Instrument*. Xicom Inc., Sterling, 1974.
7 Casse P. *Training for the Cross-Cultural Mind*. SIETAR International, Washington DC, 1979, pp. 125–132.
8 Youker R. Communication Style Instrument: a team building tool. Proceedings of the PMI Seminars and Symposium, October 17–20, 1979, Atlanta, GA, pp. 796–799.
9 Weingart LE, Behfar KJ, Bendersky C, Todorova G, Jehn KA. The directness and oppositional intensity of conflict expression. *Acad Manage Rev* 2015;40(2):235–262.
10 Collins JC. *Good to Great: Why Some Companies Make the Leap … And Others Don't*. HarperBusiness, New York 2001.
11 Lencioni P. *Death by Meeting: A Leadership Fable … About Solving the Most Painful Problem in Business*. Jossey-Bass, San Francisco, 2004.
12 Hersey P, Blanchard KH, Johnson DE. *Management of Organizational Behavior: Leading Human Resources*, 8th edn. Prentice Hall, Upper Saddle River, 2001.
13 Fisher R, Ury W. *Getting to Yes: Negotiating Agreement Without Giving In*, 2nd edn. Penguin Books, New York, 1991.
14 Hickson GB, Pichert JW, Webb LE, Gabble SG. A complementary approach to promoting professionalism: identifying, measuring, and addressing unprofessional behaviors. *Acad Med* 2007;82(11):1040–1048.
15 Kleiman MAR. Smart on crime. *Democracy J* 2013;28:51–63.
16 Vital Smarts. Position Papers. Available at: www.vitalsmarts.com/resource-center/?fwp_resource_type=position-paper (accessed 20 February 2018).
17 Patterson K, Grenny J, McMillan R, Switzler A, Maxwell D. *Crucial Accountability: Tools for Resolving Violated Expectations, Broken Commitments, and Bad Behavior*, 2nd edn. McGraw-Hill, Boston, 2013.
18 Hoover L. Developing Departmental Communication Protocols. Available at: www.campus-adr.org/cmher/print/hoover4_1.pdf (accessed 20 February 2018).
19 Zehr H. *The Little Book of Restorative Justice*. Good Books, New York, 2014.
20 Mayer B. *The Conflict Paradox: Seven Dilemmas at the Core of Disputes*. Jossey-Bass, San Francisco, 2015.
21 Axelrod R, Hamilton W. *The Evolution of Cooperation*. Basic Books, New York, 1984.

207

Maximizing Communication

Laura D. Garrett, DVM, DACVIM

College of Veterinary Medicine, University of Illinois Urbana-Champaign, Urbana, IL, USA

Core Communication Skills

Too often, the ability to communicate with clients effectively is considered an inherent skill – you either have it or you don't. However, a multitude of studies in the field of human medicine, from all over the world, have shown that the skills involved in communication can be defined and, indeed, learned [1–6]. Several constructs exist by which to outline and describe techniques for communication. This chapter will focus on the four core communication skills: open-ended questions, reflective listening, empathy, and non-verbals, and how they can be used in an ER setting. Applying the skills requires intent; in interacting with the client, one must attend not only to *what* is being said but *how* it is being said. Studies in human medicine, including in the emergency setting, confirm that patient satisfaction and clinical outcome are associated with the doctor's communication skills [7–15].

Open-Ended Questions

Open-ended questions start with "what" or "how" and they invite the client to tell the history in their own words. Open-ended questions are not only important in obtaining an accurate history, they also greatly increase the client–veterinarian bond by allowing a client to tell their story, a key part of feeling understood and valued as a person. This "story telling" does not need to be very long; using other core skills such as reflective listening and empathy, a veterinarian can guide the answers in situations where they may be lengthy. Very often, open-ended questions save time in an interview, as they allow the veterinarian to understand the true nature of the client's concerns without misleading answers that the use of only closed questions may provide. Closed questions may be necessary when the case presents in crisis; these questions can be softened by a quick empathy statement and then signposting, or informing of what will be

happening. "I can't imagine how scary this is for you. I'm going to need to ask you a series of quick questions so we can get started taking care of Bertie. I'll send a technician to get a more complete history and give you an update as soon as possible; that may be 30–45 minutes."

Open-ended questions are not just for history taking; they play a vital role in discussions of treatment options and prognosis and can help prevent misunderstanding in difficult conversations. For example, rather than asking "Are you thinking about euthanasia?" and having an owner get upset because they were not, ask "What are your thoughts about options from here?" Also, "ask rather than tell" is a great rule of thumb. When a new diagnosis has been made, asking a client what they know about the disease, rather than jumping into a description of the problem, can save time and avoid unnecessary client education. This asking not only allows the clinician to begin the discussion at an appropriate level, but also importantly shows the client that their knowledge is valued; this leads to a better client–veterinarian bond as the client feels treated as a unique and important individual.

Reflective Listening

Reflective listening involves paraphrasing what the client said or how they appear (which relates to empathy). The classic stem, or starter, for a reflective statement is "What I hear you saying is…". Other stems may feel more natural and include "So, you are saying…," "It sounds like…," "You are…" A complete statement could be something like: "It sounds like you are worried that Turner is having a hard time breathing right now." The client can then correct if that is not their main concern, or if correct, can feel a sense of relief or gratitude that the clinician listened to and understands them. Reflective listening allows for improved information accuracy between the client and the clinician and also improved connection between them.

Textbook of Small Animal Emergency Medicine, First Edition. Edited by Kenneth J. Drobatz, Kate Hopper, Elizabeth Rozanski and Deborah C. Silverstein.
© 2019 John Wiley & Sons, Inc. Published 2019 by John Wiley & Sons, Inc.
Companion Website: www.wiley.com/go/drobatz/textbook

Empathy

Empathy is the skill of imagining standing in the other person's shoes and showing that imagining back to the person. Empathy does not mean one feels what the client feels, but rather that one can try to imagine what the client has or is experiencing. Showing empathy is a key part in building rapport with a client. Just feeling empathy is not enough; the client will not know the clinician has it if they do not show it. Empathy can be shown in both verbal and non-verbal ways. Reflective statements can be used to show empathy verbally. Expression of empathy by the veterinarian has been shown to correlate with improved client satisfaction [16]. When thinking about how to show empathy, consider the three key points of having a client know that they are seen, heard, and accepted.

"Being seen" means not only physically seen, but seen as an individual person and not just a client. Ways to reflect back to the client that they are seen are to comment on a unique aspect of that individual unrelated to their pet's medical concerns, such as their clothing (for example, if they are wearing a sport team's logo), their pet's collar, etc. It is also important that the client knows they are seen as a person when it comes to the medical issues, and that their emotions about these issues are noticed. A good way to show this is by verbally stating what is seen: "You seem worried," "You look very scared." While this may seem awkward or obvious at first, clients appreciate having their concerns noted and bond more with the clinician who shows it.

Strong client emotions are daunting. A common fear is that the client's emotion, once acknowledged, will escalate. In actuality, validating the client's emotions often allows them to focus back on the situation at hand and move on in the discussion about their pet. A statement as simple as "It must be so hard to hear that your beloved pet has a life-threatening condition" can be grounding for a client and allow them to refocus on the medical conversation. Other non-verbal means to show a client they are seen is to use an appropriate speaking tone and rate, such as quiet, slower speaking in times of sadness. Handing a box of tissues to a crying client is an effective and helpful means of showing empathy.

"Being heard" is similar to being seen; the veterinarian not only needs to listen to the client but needs to show them that they are heard, and ideally understood. Saying something like "It sounds like a terrible night" is both quick and effective at showing empathy.

"Being accepted" is an inherent desire in everyone, and this acceptance will help an owner to be open and honest with the clinician and also to voice concerns or questions that they may be embarrassed to mention otherwise. It also helps clients to work through difficult problems and

see the veterinarian as supportive as opposed to adversarial. There are several categories of statements that can be made to help a client feel accepted, and intentionally using these will take conscious effort but can be of great benefit in improving the client–clinician bond. These types of statements include:

- non-judgmental comment: "You were in a very difficult situation."
- normalizing comment: "We see many dogs that escape from their yard and get injured."
- self-disclosing comment: "My cat gets into fights too."

Intentionally expressing empathy becomes even more critical with clients for whom it is difficult to naturally feel empathy; verbally showing acceptance via the above phrases can help the client–veterinarian bond even for clients with whom it is very hard to bond.

Non-Verbal Aspects

Non-verbal cues of both the veterinarian and client play a role in all discussions. The stress of working in the ER may be portrayed to clients non-verbally, and unintentionally, by the clinician and can heighten the challenges in these communications. Self-awareness and control of body position, speaking tone and volume, eye contact, etc. are crucial to help create a feeling of safety and comfort for the client. Shaping these non-verbal attributes adds no additional time to the visit, and the improved atmosphere will help clients to develop trust and make decisions more quickly. Monitoring the client's tone of voice, rate of speaking, and physical stance, such as clutching the animal to their body, is an excellent way to assess the client's level of comfort with and comprehension of what they are being told. If a disconnect is noted between the client's words and their non-verbal cues, the non-verbal message is more accurate and needs to be addressed. If the response to "How does that sound?" is a hesitant "Fine" with eyes looking at the floor, the client clearly is not fine with things. Paying attention to that fact and opening discussion about concerns at that time will often save misunderstanding and upset in the future.

Breaking the News/Presenting the Diagnosis

Clients need time to adjust to the idea that their pet has a serious illness or injury, yet in an ER setting such time may not be available. Small "sound bites" work best, especially for people who are feeling overwhelmed. For example, prepare the client for the most likely diagnosis before test results are back. "One of the most likely causes of such a big belly like this is a twisted stomach.

We would like to take x-rays; I'll let you know what we find as soon as I can." Explaining things in layperson's terms is always important in communication with a pet owner, but it is even more critical in the highly charged discussions surrounding emergency situations. Clients can easily become overwhelmed by the crisis, and may be too distraught or embarrassed to ask for explanations about what they don't understand.

Offering Options

Once the diagnosis is made, it is still important to keep the information provided on a basic level. Even with prior warning that the diagnosis could be serious, some clients may be shocked and not be able to take in all they are being told. Providing information about treatment and prognosis should be done verbally and, ideally, in writing to make sure that the facts are clear. While clients may seem to understand, because much of the information may be new or frightening, they may not remember what they are told. Be prepared to repeat and use reflective listening and empathy during this difficult time for the clients.

In discussing treatment options, it is important to present a range of options, and also to balance presenting options with not overwhelming an owner with too many choices. Once some information has been provided, use open-ended questions to ascertain a client's thoughts or more specifically goals or limitations. This question can be phrased with an opening empathy statement: "I've covered a lot of information at what must be a very difficult time for you. What are your thoughts about the options I presented?" "What are your goals for treatment?"

Specific Pointers

When asking a client if they have questions, an open-ended "What questions do you have for me?" is much more welcoming and likely to elicit an embarrassing or reluctant concern than the close-ended "Do you have any questions?" While this open invitation may seem a recipe for disaster in the ER, and would not be recommended when a critical case is ongoing, many clients state that they do not have questions, and the appreciation generated by the openness will be an asset in future interactions.

Lastly, just say no to "but"! Be conscious of the use of the word "but", especially after an empathy statement, and replace it with "and" or separation of the sentence into two sentences. "But" negates the empathy – think of it as saying "but I don't care." "I can see how hard it is for you to leave Fiona overnight, but it's what's best for her" versus "I can see how hard it is for you to leave Fiona, and it's what's best for her." Both of these statements are true, no "but" is needed. "However" is just a "but" in a tuxedo; in other words, "however" also argues against the empathy.

Conclusion

Applying core communication skills in an emergency setting can help provide comfort to a pet owner, allow the clinician to get accurate information, guide diagnostic and treatment decisions, and overall allow the patient to be diagnosed and treated in a timely manner. These skills will also increase the bond clients have with the ER clinician and thus increase client satisfaction in a difficult time.

References

1 Fallowfield L, Jenkins V, Farewell V, Solis-Trapala I. Enduring impact of communication skills training: results of a 12-month follow-up. *Br J Cancer* 2003;89(8):1445–1449.
2 Gordon GH. Care not cure: dialogues at the transition. *Patient Educ Couns* 2003;50(1):95–98.
3 Lukman H, Beevi Z, Yeap R. Training future doctors to be patient-centred: efficacy of a communication skills training (CST) programme in a Malaysian medical institution. *Med J Malaysia* 2009;64(1):51–55.
4 Nikendei C, Bosse HM, Hoffmann K, et al. Outcome of parent-physician communication skills training for pediatric residents. *Patient Educ Couns* 2010;82(1):94–99.
5 Shama ME, Meky FA, Abou El Enein NY, Mahdy MY. The effect of a training program in communication skills on primary health care physicians' knowledge, attitudes and self-efficacy. *J Egypt Public Health Assoc* 2009;84(3-4):261–283.
6 Stiefel F, Barth J, Bensing J, et al. Communication skills training in oncology: a position paper based on a consensus meeting among European experts in 2009. *Ann Oncol* 2010;21(2):204–207.
7 Sandhu H, Dale J, Stallard N, Crouch R, Glucksman E. Emergency nurse practitioners and doctors consulting with patients in an emergency department: a comparison of communication skills and satisfaction. *Emerg Med J* 2009;26(6):400–404.
8 Shilling V, Jenkins V, Fallowfield L. Factors affecting patient and clinician satisfaction with the clinical consultation: can communication skills training

for clinicians improve satisfaction? *Psychooncology* 2003;12(6):599–611.

9 Stewart M, Brown JB, Donner A, et al. The impact of patient-centered care on outcomes. *J Fam Pract* 2000;49(9):796–804.

10 Wanzer MB, Booth-Butterfield M, Gruber K. Perceptions of health care providers' communication: relationships between patient-centered communication and satisfaction. *Health Commun* 2004;16(3):363–383.

11 Fitzpatrick N, Breen DT, Taylor J, et al. Parental satisfaction with paediatric care, triage and waiting times. *Emerg Med Australas* 2014;26(2):177–182.

12 Menendez ME, Chen NC, Mudgal CS, Jupiter JB, Ring D. Physician empathy as a driver of hand surgery patient satisfaction. *J Hand Surg* 2015;40(9):1860–1865 e2.

13 Locke R, Stefano M, Koster A, Taylor B, Greenspan J. Optimizing patient/caregiver satisfaction through quality of communication in the pediatric emergency department. *Pediatr Emerg Care* 2011;27(11):1016–1021.

14 Rutherford KA, Pitetti RD, Zuckerbraun NS, Smola S, Gold MA. Adolescents' perceptions of interpersonal communication, respect, and concern for privacy in an urban tertiary-care pediatric emergency department. *Pediatr Emerg Care* 2010;26(4):257–273.

15 Clark NM, Cabana MD, Nan B, et al. The clinician-patient partnership paradigm: outcomes associated with physician communication behavior. *Clin Pediatr* 2008;47(1):49–57.

16 McArthur ML, Fitzgerald JR. Companion animal veterinarians' use of clinical communication skills. *Aust Vet J* 2013;91(9):374–380.

208

Basics of Clinical Study Design

Kenneth J. Drobatz, DVM, MSCE, DACVIM, DACVECC

University of Pennsylvania, Philadelphia, PA, USA

Introduction

The anatomy of designing clinical research usually includes six major areas: the research question, choosing the appropriate subjects, planning the measurement, choosing the type of study to answer the question, analyzing the data, and writing the final manuscript for publication.

The Research Question

The clinical research question should pass the test of "Is the answer to this question useful to the care of our patients? Will the answer lead to better care of our patients or will it provide insight into the pathophysiology of disease?" The question doesn't have to appeal to everyone but it should be a question that will at least provide useful information, however you define "useful." Your clinical question should be succinct and straightforward. It should ask a very pointed question and should not be vague. For example, "Does radiographically determined vertebral heart size predict the presence of heart disease in cats with respiratory distress?" or "Does intravenous normal saline lower potassium faster than intravenous Normosol-R in cats with urethral obstruction?" Try to avoid vague terms and be as specific as possible. Starting with a clear and answerable question makes the research project that much easier to perform and the results easier to interpret.

Not all research projects involve specific questions. Some of the most common studies in veterinary clinical medicine are purely descriptive reports of disease conditions. Although this type of study is relatively low in the hierarchy of evidence-based medicine, clinical veterinary medicine has not fully characterized even the most common diseases. These types of clinical reports form the basis for the generation of hypotheses regarding etiology, diagnosis, prognosis,

and therapy which can be tested with analytic studies (see below).

While developing the research question, you should review the electronic library databases to see if this question has been answered in the clinical literature. There is no sense in reinventing the wheel but corroboration of previous evidence does have value. Unfortunately, journal editors and reviewers are not always open to corroboration of previous studies and you may end up performing a study that is rejected "because it has been done before." If an appropriately performed literature search does not come up with a study that has answered your clinical question, then clinical research to answer that question appears warranted.

Choosing the Appropriate Subjects

One of the major goals of clinical research is to infer the findings from the animals in the study to the general population of animals that have that condition. This is called "external validity" or "generalizability." No one necessarily cares what happens to one set of animals if it only happens to that specific group. What clinicians care about is whether the study findings can be applied to their clinic patients with that condition. Therefore, selection of the animals to be studied should keep this generalizability in mind. For example, a study of diabetics referred to a teaching hospital may not be a good group to generalize to diabetics seen in general practice. You must keep in mind the target population you are trying to generalize to and make sure that the inclusion and exclusion criteria help meet that goal.

To clearly specify the group of animals to study, you must thoroughly define the parameters that must be included – whether they need to be male or female, neutered or intact or both, age range, breeds, condition (how that condition is determined). For example, in a study performed by Clifford et al. entitled "Magnetic

Textbook of Small Animal Emergency Medicine, First Edition. Edited by Kenneth J. Drobatz, Kate Hopper, Elizabeth Rozanski and Deborah C. Silverstein.
© 2019 John Wiley & Sons, Inc. Published 2019 by John Wiley & Sons, Inc.
Companion Website: www.wiley.com/go/drobatz/textbook

resonance imaging (MRI) of canine focal splenic and hepatic lesions" the patient population was clearly specified as follows:

> Twenty-five cases were prospectively enrolled for MR imaging at the Matthew J. Ryan Veterinary Hospital of the University of Pennsylvania (VHUP). Criteria for case recruitment included an abdominal ultrasound, owner consent for MR imaging, and either lesion biopsy or fine-needle aspiration. Case selection was also based upon the availability of MR imaging and patient's health status, specifically, critical patients requiring immediate surgery were not selected due to timing constraints of MR imaging accessibility.

The last statement, though not specifically stated as such, is an exclusion criterion. There were animals that filled all the inclusion criteria but had to be excluded because of how critically ill they were. You can see from these specifications that you would have to put in the discussion how this study could apply to critically ill patients, because these patients were not part of the study group. You can see, based on the principles of MRI, that justification for this generalization can easily be made, but again, it was not proven by this study.

Once the inclusion and exclusion criteria have been specified, then you must identify the accessible population. Is it all animals that present with the condition to your clinic or would it be too difficult to get all animals? Perhaps you only need a representative sample. It is important that if you are not taking every case that fits the inclusion and exclusion criteria, you must be careful that you truly have a random sample of your accessible population; otherwise you could end up with a biased sample that is not representative of the population to which you want to generalize your findings.

Planning and Recording the Measurements

When planning your study, it is important to determine which variables will be assessed; these will depend upon your research question and study population. In general, when in doubt about whether you should record something, record it! You can always eliminate it later, but you can't add data that you didn't record (particularly in a prospective study).

The types of variables most commonly used in clinical veterinary research are categorical variables and continuous variables. Categorical variables are unordered categories such as sex, blood type, breed, dead, alive, etc. These variables are statistically described using counts, proportions, percentages etc. The most common statistics assessing categorical variables are relative risk, odds

ratios, chi-square, regression, and Fisher's exact test. Ordinal variables are categorical variables but there is an inherent order to the categories. Examples include degree of pain, body condition score or anesthetic risk category. Descriptive statistics for this type of variable include what was mentioned for categorical variables but also can be described by median and minimum and maximum values. These can be analyzed using statistics mentioned for categorical variables as well as the Mann–Whitney (Wilcoxon rank sum test) test and rank correlation.

Continuous variables have an infinite number of values (e.g. weight, rectal temperature). Discrete variables have a finite scale (e.g. heart rate, number of times vomiting per day – you can't have half of a heart beat or one-third of a vomiting episode). Discrete variables that are ordered and have a large number of possible values can be statistically treated similar to continuous variables. Depending upon whether the data are normally distributed or not, continuous and ordered discrete variables can be described by mean and standard deviation, median and quartiles or range, and statistically analyzed using t-test, Mann–Whitney test, Kruskal–Wallis test, analysis of variance, correlation. and regression.

In general, a continuous or ordered discrete variable should be recorded as such and not dichotomized. Dichotomizing loses information. Dichotomization can always be performed later even if the data are recorded as continuous or ordered discrete, but one cannot convert data recorded as dichotomous or categorical into continuous or ordered discrete.

For most statistical programs, data recording on an Excel spreadsheet works well. If you are working with a statistician, consult with him or her regarding how the data should be recorded on the spreadsheet prior to entering the data.

Choosing the Study Design

There are a variety of different clinical study designs that fall into two general types: analytic studies and descriptive studies. Analytic studies include the experimental study, prospective cohort study, retrospective cohort study, and case control study. Descriptive studies include analyses of secular trends, case series, and case reports. Each of these studies provides different types of information and levels of evidence.

Case Report

A case report is a clinical description of a single patient. Its primary use is for hypothesis generation and it has limited generalizability (or how much or how reasonable it is to apply the findings in this one case to the overall population of animals with that condition). Case reports in the veterinary literature tend to describe unusual conditions or techniques.

Case Series

A case series is a clinical description of a number of animals with a disease. This type of study is primarily used to characterize an illness or a technique. Its main limitation is that there is no control group and therefore you cannot determine which factors in the description are unique to the condition. Case series are relatively common in the veterinary literature.

Analysis of Secular Trends

Analysis of secular trends is a study comparing geographic and/or time trends of a condition to trends in risk factors for that condition. Its primary use is for rapid and easy support for or against hypotheses, but the primary limitation is that you cannot differentiate among those hypotheses consistent with the data. This is not a commonly used study design in small animal veterinary medicine.

Case Control Study

The case control study is one of the more commonly used analytic study designs in clinical small animal medicine. It compares diseased patients (cases) to non-diseased patients (controls), looking for differences in risk factors. It is primarily used for the study of any number of risk factors or etiologies for a single disease. It is particularly useful for studying rare diseases. One of the biggest limitations is trying to avoid specific biases. In addition, selecting proper controls can be very challenging.

Cohort Study

This type of study is not commonly used in veterinary medicine. It compares animals with a risk factor or exposure to other animals without that risk factor or exposure, looking at differences in outcome. This study design is used when evaluating any number of outcomes from a single risk factor or exposure. Depending upon the length of time between exposure and outcome, this type of study, when done on a prospective basis, can be very prolonged.

Experimental Study or Randomized Control Trial

In an experimental study, the investigator controls the risk factor/exposure of interest and randomization is generally used. This study provides the most convincing evidence of causality. An excellent example of this type of study is the randomized control trial, the gold standard of clinical study designs, in which a group of animals are randomly allocated by the investigator to two or more treatment groups and the outcomes evaluated. Theoretically, if performed properly and with a large enough sample size, the groups will only differ with respect to the treatment they have been assigned and nothing else. The major disadvantage to this type of study is cost, depending on what you are studying.

Retrospective Versus Prospective Studies

Studies can also be categorized by the timing of data collection. In a prospective study, data are collected by looking forward and obtaining new data after the start of the study. Retrospective studies look "backward" at data that have already been collected for other reasons. The advantage of prospectively collected data is that the nature of the data, the definition of inclusion and exclusion criteria, the definitions of signs/symptoms and other factors can be determined ahead of time and are consistent throughout the study. The variability in retrospective studies tends to be much greater because the data were collected for reasons other than for the purpose of the study at hand. This variability can decrease the power (the ability to detect a difference between two groups) of the study. It addition, it is more difficult with retrospective studies to determine the directionality of events or what occurred first and what happened later.

Many of the different study designs described above can be performed on a retrospective or prospective basis, except for randomized clinical trials which must be performed in a prospective manner.

Analysis

To gain the most from the data of a study, you should be fairly familiar with statistics. Most statistical evaluations of veterinary clinical studies are relatively straightforward, but inappropriate application of statistics can result in erroneous conclusions from the data. In addition, you should plan in advance what should be analyzed and things that are analyzed should make biological sense. Analyzing anything and everything without any rationale enhances the probability of a type I error (finding something significant when it truly is not). Planning in advance what should be analyzed and limiting it to what makes sense will minimize errors.

If you decide to analyze variables that are a *post hoc* decision, correction to a more rigorous P-value for those extra multiple comparisons may minimize type I error.

There are different thoughts on multiple comparisons but the author's philosophy is that if you had a prior hypothesis about certain variables, then P-value comparison adjustments for those comparisons should not be necessary. Opinions differ regarding this point.

Presenting the Results

Once you have performed your study, collected the data and analyzed it, you must report your findings. You should choose a journal that is appropriate for your topic and will capture the readers who would benefit most from your findings. Once you have decided which journal, you should read their "Instructions to Authors" so that you can format your manuscript to their specifications. It is much easier to do this before beginning writing because journals vary in their format style and how data should be reported.

The *title* of your manuscript should accurately represent your study. The *abstract* should be a short and concise synopsis of the paper. It should be to the point, yet adequately describe the study design, what was studied, the results, and pertinent conclusions. The *introduction* should bring the reader rapidly up to date with what is known about the topic of the manuscript. It is not meant to be a review of all the literature on the topic. The goal of the introduction is to "build a case" for why the study was performed. It should be concise and the information should be directly relevant to the objective of the study. The final culmination of the introduction should be a statement of the purpose or objectives of the study.

The *materials and methods* should be thorough and clearly stated. The goal of materials and methods is to give the reader the ability to repeat the study exactly as it was performed. Materials and methods generally include explicitly stated inclusion and exclusion criteria for the animals in the study and how the animals were initially identified. A clear description of the study design and all parameters that were evaluated is also an integral component of this section. Explicit description of analytic methods used in the measurement of certain parameters should also be provided or referenced appropriately to the original study that developed the assay. Statistical methods are also described in the materials and methods section and should include all tests performed.

Results should have a logical presentation to them and are most easily presented in "chunks" of related data. The best papers are ones that are focused on their objective and collect data relevant to their objective or hypothesis. Interpretative statements do not belong in the results section and are more appropriate to the discussion section.

The first paragraph of the *discussion* should summarize the findings and significance of the study. There should be organization to the discussion and it should follow a logical order and not jump from point to point. Many authors follow the order of how the results were presented. The discussion points should be focused on the findings of the study and their significance. Conclusions should be limited to the facts provided by the study and anything beyond that should be explicitly stated as conjecture or speculation by the authors. It is allowed and often helpful for the authors to provide speculation about the findings, as they are often the experts in the area of study. Any discussion about no difference or statistically non-significant findings in the study should include information about the power of the study. Without a discussion on power, any discussion of no difference between groups should be viewed with caution. Finally, many discussions will introduce possible future studies of interest based on their results and conclusions.

Further Reading

Hennekens CH, Buring JE. *Epidemiology in Medicine.* Little, Brown, Boston/Toronto, 1987.

Hulley SB, Cummings SR. *Designing Clinical Research.* Williams and Wilkins, Baltimore, 1988.

209

Designing and Participating in Clinical Trials

Dorothy Cimino Brown, MS, DVM, DACVS

Elanco Animal Health, Greenfield, IN, USA

Clinical Trial Design

Because of the potential to minimize biases, randomized controlled clinical trials (RCTs) are the "gold standard" study design methodology by which practitioners make decisions about the efficacy of interventions, such as drugs, devices or procedures studied for diagnostic, therapeutic or prophylactic value. Therefore, the RCT, more than any other study design methodology, can have a powerful and immediate impact on patient care. Whether the results of a clinical trial are truly unbiased, however, depends on the many features of how the trial was designed and implemented.

Controlled Clinical Trial Design

Defining the Study Population

Ideally, study subjects in a trial are representative of patients routinely seen in practice. Narrow inclusion and exclusion criteria confine enrollment to a subset of patients with the disease. This makes analysis of results more straightforward (internal validity) but may impose limitations on how useful the results are to a practitioner (generalizability).

Balancing internal validity with generalizability occurs early in trial protocol development. Internal validity is always the primary concern, because generalizing results of an invalid study, one with biases in design or uncontrolled confounding factors, is not useful. Figure 209.1 describes the progression of defining the study population from the reference population to the actual study participants, with cats with urinary obstruction as an example. Describing the inclusion and exclusion criteria for the study and documenting the number of qualified subjects whose owners opt not to include their animal in the study, along with their reason for choosing not

to participate, allows the reader of the study to decide whether the results are generalizable to the population of animals that they regularly treat.

Defining the Control Group

Placebo-treated controls are often ideal, as they can be used to obtain an unbiased estimate of the effects of an intervention by subtracting the effects in the control group from the effects in the treated group. The control group may receive placebo only or may receive standard of care intervention in addition to placebo. How the control group is defined is determined by the question the study is intended to answer, how the intervention is intended to be used in practice, and the characteristics of the study population which may make a placebo-only control group impossible or unethical.

Assignment to Intervention Versus Control Groups

Randomization minimizes bias in the assignment of animals to intervention or control groups by ensuring that each study subject has the same chance of being placed in either group. Then, with an adequate sample size, the study groups tend to be comparable with respect to all variables except for the intervention being studied. Selection bias occurs when study subjects with one or more influencing factors appear more frequently in one study group than in another. For example, if younger age is associated with better outcome in dogs with gastric dilation-volvulus (GDV) and the proportion of younger study subjects is greater in the intervention group than in the control group, there could be an observed benefit of the intervention that did not really exist. Randomization ensures that dogs of every age are evenly distributed amongst the study groups.

The ultimate power of randomization is that even factors that are not known to be important at the time the trial is initiated end up being evenly distributed amongst

Textbook of Small Animal Emergency Medicine, First Edition. Edited by Kenneth J. Drobatz, Kate Hopper, Elizabeth Rozanski and Deborah C. Silverstein.
© 2019 John Wiley & Sons, Inc. Published 2019 by John Wiley & Sons, Inc.
Companion Website: www.wiley.com/go/drobatz/textbook

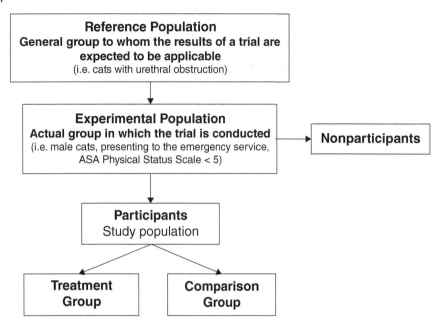

Figure 209.1 The progression of defining the study population from the reference population to the actual study participants, with cats with urinary obstruction as an example. Describing the inclusion and exclusion criteria for the study and documenting the number of screened subjects not enrolled, along with the reason for non-enrollment, allows the reader of the study to decide whether the results are generalizable to the population of animals that they regularly treat.

groups. For example, if it were discovered after the GDV trial was reported that thin dogs do better than obese dogs, the results of the trial would still be valid because randomization would have roughly equally allocated obese and thin dogs between the study groups, thus negating the potential for body condition to bias the results. To effectively eliminate selection bias, randomization must include two important processes [1].

Generation of a Random Sequence

The first step of randomization involves generation of an unpredictable allocation sequence based on a random procedure. The most common method of generating a random sequence is via computer, but random number tables and flipping a coin to generate a sequence are also appropriate. Other methods of generating an allocation scheme, such as alternating assignments between intervention and control groups or assigning animals to groups according to day of the week or hospital number, are systematic methods of allocation but are not appropriate for randomization because the sequence cannot be concealed.

Allocation Concealment

The second step of randomization is concealment of the randomization sequence (allocation concealment), preventing those admitting subjects to the trial from knowing the upcoming assignments. This is distinctly different from blinding, discussed later in this chapter, which pertains to being unaware of the animals' treatment group as data are collected on the outcome of interest *after* the

animal is enrolled in the study. Randomization concealment ensures that those screening candidates for inclusion and exclusion criteria have no way of knowing to which group the animal will be allocated *prior* to it being randomized. While certain studies cannot be blinded, it is *always* possible to conceal the randomization scheme.

Traditionally, biomedical researchers focus on only the sequence generation process of randomization, but concealment is crucially important. When a system of assignment is known, there is potential for bias. For example, in a study in which dogs enrolled on Tuesdays receive intervention A and dogs enrolled on Thursdays receive intervention B, even if individuals screening animals do not know what interventions A and B are, if they believe that dogs enrolled on Thursdays are "doing better," they may consciously or subconsciously enroll dogs with different prognostic factors to different groups. Knowledge of the next assignment can also lead to exclusion of animals on the basis of prognosis because they would have been allocated to the perceived inappropriate group.

Without adequate allocation concealment, even random, unpredictable assignment sequences can be undermined, allowing individual preferences to influence the assignment of animals to groups such that important differences between groups result, affecting the study outcome.

Concealment can appear to be a challenge in studies involving emergency and critical care medicine because services, such as a pharmacy that would keep the concealed randomization scheme, may not be available

24 hours a day. A valid approach in these instances is to have the pharmacy generate the random sequence and then allocate that sequence to sequentially numbered opaque-sealed envelopes which are then housed in the emergency and critical care units. After an animal is screened for study inclusion, if it qualifies, the next envelope in the sequence is opened to reveal to which group that animal is allocated.

Blinding and Outcome Assessment

Observation bias occurs when knowledge of a study subject's group allocation influences identification of relevant events during the study. For example, if investigators know which animals received an active intervention, they may monitor that group more closely than the control group in a way that could seriously affect the trial outcome. If an owner knows their dog is receiving an active intervention, they are likely to overreport improvement, whereas those who know their dog is in the control group are likely to overreport no improvement (or perhaps deterioration). This leads to exaggerated estimates of intervention benefits. Blinding of investigators and owners to which group animals are allocated prevents these biases [2–4].

The potential for observation bias is related to the subjectivity of the outcomes under study. If an outcome for a trial is change in lactate levels, observation bias is unlikely because lactate measurement cannot be affected by knowledge of the animal's study group. In contrast, when the outcome of interest is subjective, such as owner or veterinarian assessment of pain, knowledge of the animal's group allocation could affect the pain score attributed to that animal. Blinding also mitigates the problem that owners administering a known active drug to their pet may be sensitized to its condition and may tend to ascribe every sign or unusual occurrence to the intervention, thus increasing the side-effect profile of that group. To obtain unbiased estimates of intervention effect, regardless of whether the outcome measured is subjective or objective, is to subtract the effect documented in the control group from the effect documented in the intervention group.

Placebo Effects

Placebo effects are improvements documented in a control group with no active intervention. Commonly, the assumption is that the animals are not really improved, but merely a bias of owners or investigators who want to believe that animals in the study are improving. However, animals in a control group can actually improve, even with no active intervention. This can be due to regression to the mean.

Many diseases, particularly chronic ones, have waxing and waning signs and symptoms. Owners may seek out enrollment in a trial when those signs and symptoms are at a peak. Over time, even without intervention, these animals will cycle back to their average level of symptom burden or disability. In these cases, animals in control groups can show improvement even with no intervention. The animals have indeed improved. One way to combat regression to the mean in the design of trials is, when possible, to screen animals for study inclusion when interested owners present them for consideration for inclusion, but delay baseline data collection until a follow-up visit occurs 7–10 days later.

Minimizing placebo effects in the design of the study provides the benefit of needing fewer animals enrolled to document a significant difference between groups.

Sample Size Considerations

A trial undertaken with an insufficient number of animals is of little scientific value and can be scientifically harmful if the results are misinterpreted as demonstrating that an intervention has no effect when, in fact, the sample size was not sufficient to draw that conclusion. Performing a sample size calculation requires data on the outcome of interest in the target population to be studied. This often comes from the literature. When data for a sample size calculation do not exist, a pilot study can be undertaken to collect data on a small group of animals which are then used to determine the sample size required for the larger controlled study. The target sample size for the study is increased above that suggested by the sample size calculation to maintain the ability to identify a significant difference between groups, even if some animals are lost to follow-up or do not follow the protocol as intended, because ideally, even animals that do not comply with the protocol are included in the analysis.

Statistical Analysis

A statistical testing plan is developed during study design and is necessary to perform the sample size calculation. Ideally, an intention-to-treat analysis is planned, which means that once animals are randomized to a study group, their outcomes data must be analyzed along with those of all others in that group, regardless of whether there is compliance with their assigned regimen in the protocol. In other words, "once randomized, always analyzed" [5,6]. While the goal is to study the effect of the intervention, randomization is done only on the basis of *offering* it. To preserve the power of randomization, the data must be analyzed on this basis. Only the entire groups allocated by randomization are truly comparable.

If analyses are performed on a subset of animals randomized to a group, it is impossible to achieve balance in the distribution of unknown factors that had originally been achieved through randomization and the results of the subgroup of compliers may be biased.

Clinical Trial Implementation

Recruitment

Even meticulously designed trials fail if an appropriate number of animals are not enrolled. The ability to recruit animals is dependent on the owner incentive to include their animal as well as the recruiting budget available to reach out to owners of potential study participants. Many times, access to care for their pet that is financially covered by the study sponsor is a major incentive, as well as access to interventions that may not be available outside a trial. While owners are informed that their animal may not directly benefit from inclusion in a trial, many are very invested in the concept that the information gained by choosing to include their animal will benefit other animals and potentially people in the future. Owners balance these incentives with potential risks and time commitment of the study. Studies that are very long or require many visits can be more difficult to achieve adequate recruitment.

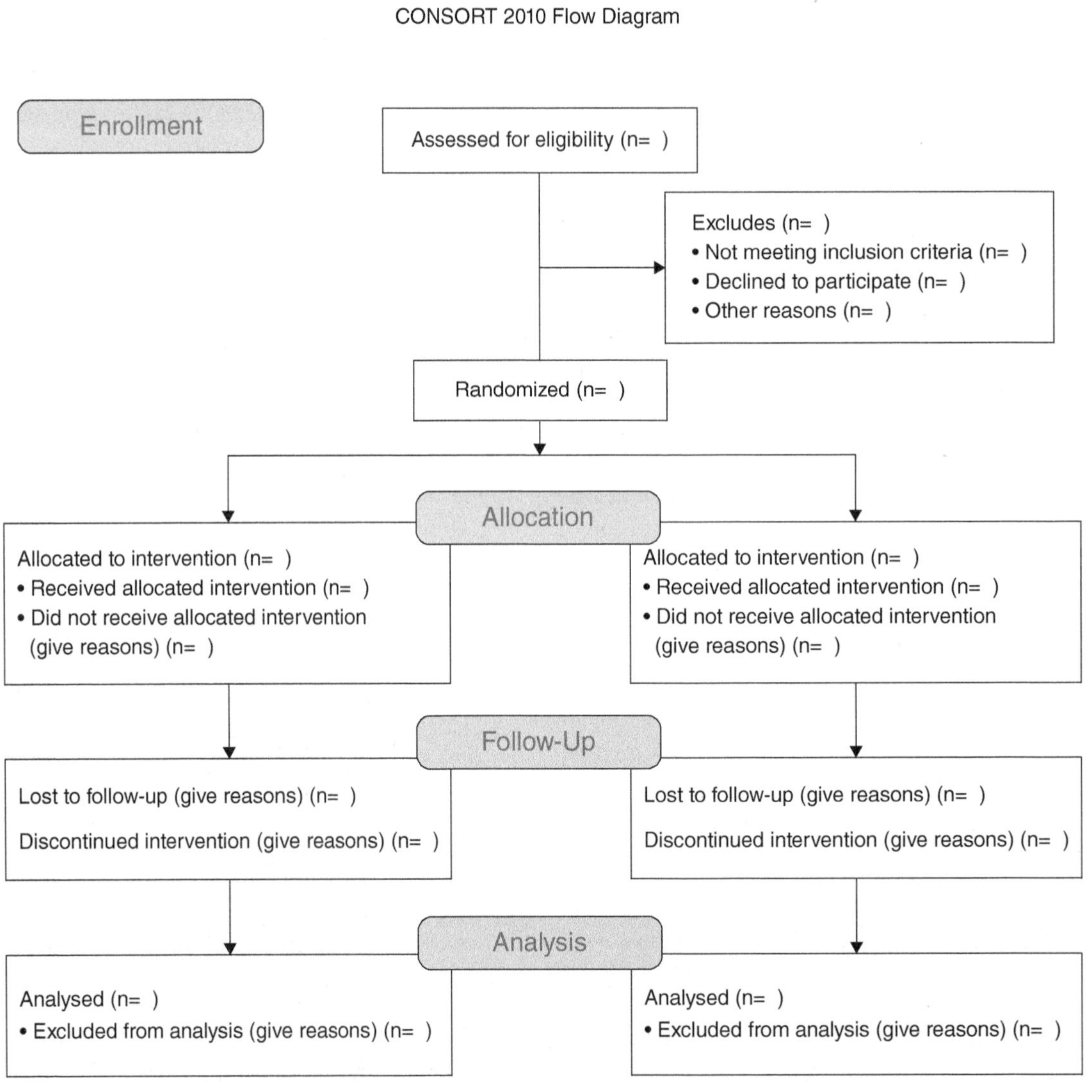

CONSORT 2010 Flow Diagram

Figure 209.2 The study participant flow chart recommended by the Consolidated Standards of Reporting Trials (CONSORT) Group [7]. The CONSORT guidelines are adopted by most biomedical journals for reporting RCTs, with this flow chart in particular required for publication of study results.

It is best to have a recruitment strategy based on how difficult it might be to enroll animals as well as how quickly the study needs to be completed. While recruiting from the hospital population may eventually allow one to achieve the appropriate sample size, active recruitment outside the hospital clientele is often needed to complete enrollment. Cost-effective methods of outside recruitment include social media campaigns and lawn signs in local dog parks. When a large number of animals need to be recruited in a short period of time, more extensive and expensive recruiting methods are often necessary, including print ads in local or regional papers, or local radio ads.

Data Collection

Data are collected using data capture forms (DCFs) designed for the study to ensure complete data collection. DCFs support both primary (real-time) data collection and secondarily recorded data originating elsewhere (e.g. the medical record). While electronic data capture systems are becoming more available, DCFs are most commonly paper based. The data are then transcribed into a database for analysis, but DCFs are saved for future reference.

Meticulous data collection is crucial to successful trial completion. This is true both for animals enrolled in the study and those that are screened but not enrolled. Figure 209.2 is the study participant flow chart that is recommended by the Consolidated Standards of Reporting Trials (CONSORT) Group [7]. The CONSORT guidelines are adopted by most biomedical journals for reporting RCTs, with this flow chart in particular required for publication of study results. The CONSORT statement also contains a 25-item checklist which focuses on reporting how the trial was designed, analyzed, and interpreted

Good Clinical Practice

Good Clinical Practice (GCP) is an international ethical and scientific quality standard for the design, performance, analysis, and reporting of clinical trials [8]. While compliance with GCP is required for trials registered with regulatory agencies such as the Food and Drug Administration (FDA) [9], all investigators interested in the design of high-quality clinical trials should be aware of these guidelines and use a minimum trial implementation standard that is in the "spirit" of GCP.

References

1 Brown DC. Control of selection bias in parallel-group controlled clinical trials in dogs and cats: 97 trials (2000–2005). *J Am Vet Med Assoc* 2006;229(6):990–993.

2 Giuffrida MA, Agnello KA, Brown DC. Blinding terminology used in reports of randomized controlled trials involving dogs and cats. *J Am Vet Med Assoc* 2012;241(9):1221–1226.

3 Halpern SD. Evaluating preference effects in partially unblinded, randomized clinical trials. *J Clin Epidemiol* 2003;56(2):109–115.

4 Hrobjartsson A, Thomsen AS, Emanuelsson F, et al. Observer bias in randomised clinical trials with binary outcomes: systematic review of trials with both blinded and non-blinded outcome assessors. *BMJ* 2012;344:e1119.

5 Brown DC. Sources and handling of losses to follow-up in parallel-group randomized clinical trials in dogs and cats: 63 trials (2000–2005). *Am J Vet Res* 2007;68(7):694–698.

6 Sargeant JM, Thompson A, Valcour J, et al. Quality of reporting of clinical trials of dogs and cats and associations with treatment effects. *J Vet Intern Med* 2010;24(1):44–50.

7 Begg C, Cho M, Eastwood S, et al. Improving the quality of reporting of randomized controlled trials. The CONSORT statement. *JAMA* 1996;276(8):637–639.

8 Vijayananthan A, Nawawi O. The importance of Good Clinical Practice guidelines and its role in clinical trials. *Biomed Imag Intervent J* 2008;4(1):e5.

9 US Department of Health and Human Services Food and Drug Administration Center for Veterinary Medicine. Guidance for Industry. Good Clinical Practice. VICH GL9. Final Guidance 2011. Available at: www.fda.gov/downloads/AnimalVeterinary/GuidanceComplianceEnforcement/GuidanceforIndustry/ucm052417.pdf (accessed 21 February 2018).

Index

Note: page numbers in *italics* refer to figures and those in **bold** to tables (figures and tables are only indicated when they are separated from their text references).